Mediterranean Diet Cookbook For Beginners 2021

15-Week Meal Plan to Burn Fat and Get Healthy | 1100+ Recipes Ready in 30 Minutes with Easily Accessible Ingredients Which are Light on Your Pocket

Bianca Carter

DISCLAIMER

Neither the publisher nor the author is engaged in rendering legal or any other professional service through this book. If expert assistance is required, the services of appropriate professionals should be sought. The publisher and the author shall have neither liability nor responsibility to any person or entity concerning any loss or damage caused directly or indirectly by the professional by using the information in this book.

Table of Contents

Introduction

The term "diet" for most of us spells out deprivation, extreme hunger, and bland and boring foods that we are forced to eat in order to lose weight. However, with the Mediterranean diet, none of those apply.

The Mediterranean diet is endowed with an unlimited assortment of fresh, healthy, natural, and wholesome foods from all food groups. Although there is a greater focus on certain components, no natural components are excluded.

Mediterranean diet devotees can enjoy their favorite dishes as they learn to appreciate how nourishing the freshest healthy and natural foods can be.

This diet is primarily based on the eating habits of the original inhabitants of the coasts of Greece, Italy, Spain, Morocco, and France. Because of their temperate climate and location, seasonal fruit, vegetables, and seafood from these regions' nutritional foundation.

The easiest way to understand the Mediterranean diet is to picture eating as though it's summer every day. It might also give you a déjà vu moment by reminding you of the foods you enjoyed most on a summer vacation or at the beach. In truth, there is never a dull moment with the Mediterranean diet!

All fun aside, the Mediterranean diet will help you find great pleasure in food, knowing that every bite you take will provide your body with the healthiest nutrition.

When your food tastes like you are on a perpetual vacation, its easy ad exciting to stay on the bandwagon!

3 Benefits Of The Mediterranean Diet

If we take an in-depth look at the Mediterranean diet, it's not a *diet* per se as a weight-loss tool—it's more of a lifestyle and a culinary tradition for the people of the Mediterranean region. Its primary focus is on whole grains, fruit and vegetables, seafood, nuts, olive oil, and a glass of wine now and then. This diet is part of a culture that appreciates the freshest components, is prepared in a simple but tasty way, and is shared with friends and family in a laid-back environment.

1. Most of us understand the vitality of eating a clean and well-balanced diet for improved health and better quality of life, but very few of us place this into practice. With most of us spending a greater percentage of our days at work, we tend to opt for fast and easy options for the food we eat. In fact, in many cases, fast food, frozen dinners from food stores, and processed foods are our first options.
   Over the years, people have stopped eating seasonal worldwide foods because we can now access all kinds of food all year round. What's more, cooking meals from scratch seems to be an unnecessary hassle, considering our overburdened schedules & the time it requires to make a good meal. As a result, we are eating foods that are made in a plant instead of food that grows like a plant. Our diets are characterized by over-processed foods, unhealthy fats, truckloads of sugar, and lots and lots of artificial ingredients, the names of which most of us can't even pronounce.
2. Perhaps one of the greatest attributes of the Mediterranean diet is the fact that it is very simple and direct. You have not to be an expert to make the meals, as you will learn in our recipes section. Eat less red meat and more fish—especially fatty fish rich in omega-3 fatty acids—cook with olive oil, and eat fruit, vegetables, whole grains, and nuts several times a day.
3. Unlike many popular diets, many of which are fads, the Mediterranean diet encourages healthy fats from olive oil, nuts, seeds, fish, and avocado. Sometimes, the occasional glass of red wine lowers your risk of heart disease.

15 Week Meal Plan

Week 1						
	Breakfast & Brunch Recipes	**Lunch Recipes**	**Dinner recipes**	**Side Dishes Recipes**	**Snacks & Appetizer Recipes**	**Dessert Recipes**
Day 1	Croque Madame -80	Beef & broccoli -61	Noodle Soup -104	Roasted Green Bean -93	Greek White Pizza With Roasted Tomatoes -144	Whole Wheat Mango Loaf -69
Day 2	Quiche, Crepes and Souffles -45	Roasted Fennel & Mushroom -93	Tortilla Soup -105	Thai-style Chicken Salad with Spicy Peanut -103	Greek Wedge Salad -126	Almond and Cherry Muffins -100
Day 3	Huevos Rancheros -81	Wilted Spinach Salad With Warm Bacon -86	Roasted Green Bean -93	Classic Tuna Salad -103	Greek Green Goddess Cobb Salad -127	Banana Mango Bread -69
Day 4	Breakfast Enchiladas -46	Roasted Green Bean -93	Buttered Cinnamon-sugar Croutons -114	Vietnamese-style Beef Noodle -106	Quinoa-Stuffed Squash Boats -144	Mango Soufflé -69
Day 5	Huevos Rancheros -81	Roasted Fennel & Mushroom -93	Roasted Green Bean -93	Classic Tuna Salad -103	Greek Wedge Salad -126	Red Wine Poached Pears -56
Day 6	Coconut Pomegranate Oatmeal -59	Beef & broccoli -61	Deli-style Colesla -96	Classic Chicken Noodle -104	Steak Bites -123	Lemon and Chia Biscotti -133
Day 7	Croque Madame -80	Deli-style Colesla -96	Sautéed Wild Mushroom -114	Shrimp Salad -103	Crispy Salmon With Lemony Asparagus -127	Pear Tart Tatin -56

Week 2

	Breakfast & Brunch Recipes	Lunch Recipes	Dinner recipes	Side Dishes Recipes	Snacks & Appetizer Recipes	Dessert Recipes
Day 1	Mushrooms Omelet -70	Pork Braised with Dried Fruits and Cipollini Onions 155	Tortilla Soup -105	Pad Thai -65	Greek Pesto Corkscrew -130	Mango Ice Cream -79
Day 2	Huevos Rancheros -81	Roasted Fennel & Mushroom -93	Buttered Cinnamon-sugar Croutons -114	Beef Noodle Soup -106	Roasted Fish -141	Almond and Cherry Muffins -100
Day 3	Zucchini Pancakes -33	Roasted Green Bean & Potato Salad With Radicchio 93	Deli-style Colesla -96	Pork chops -141	Italian Egg Bake -129	Banana Mango Bread-69
Day 4	Cacao & Raspberry Chia Pudding -101	Wilted Spinach Salad With Warm Bacon -86	Hearty Lentil Soup -115	X Pad Thai -65 shrimp	Greek Green Goddess Cobb Salad -127	Red Wine Poached Pears -56
Day 5	Breakfast Enchiladas -46	Deli-style Colesla -96	Hearty Lentil Soup -115	Pork chops -141	Shrimp & Seafood Couscous Paella -180 scallops	Apple Upside-Down Cake -189
Day 6	Watercress Smoothie -123	Roasted Green Bean -93	Buttered Cinnamon-sugar Croutons -114	Pad Thai -65	Butternut Squash Soup -114	Cherry Blondies -109
Day 7	Croque Madame -80	Roasted Green Bean -93	Tortilla Soup -105	Pork chops -141	Steak Bites -123	Almond and Cherry Muffins -100

Week 3						
	Breakfast & Brunch Recipes	**Lunch Recipes**	**Dinner recipes**	**Side Dishes Recipes**	**Snacks & Appetizer Recipes**	**Dessert Recipes**
Day 1	Huevos Rancheros -81	Roasted Fennel & Mushroom -93	Chicken enchilada/tortilla soup -105	Shrimp Salad -103	Greek Wedge Salad -126	Lemon and Chia Biscotti -133
Day 2	Cacao & Raspberry Chia Pudding -101	Pork Braised with Dried Fruits and Cipollini Onions -155	Deli-style Colesla -96	Classic Tuna Salad -103	Crispy Salmon With Lemony Asparagus -127	Pear Tart Tatin -56
Day 3	Huevos Rancheros -81	Wilted Spinach Salad With Warm Bacon -86	Buttered Cinnamon-sugar Croutons -114	Classic Tuna Salad -103	Greek Green Goddess Cobb Salad -127	Red Wine Poached Pears -56
Day 4	Coconut Pomegranate Oatmeal -59	Roasted Green Bean -93	Balsamic chicken -136	chicken salad -42	Roasted Fish -141	Banana Mango Bread-69
Day 5	Espinacase la Catalana -112	Balsamic chicken -136	Chicken enchilada/tortilla soup -105	Celery Root Salad With Apple & Parsley -102	Butternut Squash Soup -114	Almond and Cherry Muffins -100
Day 6	Mushrooms Omelet -70	Roasted Green Bean -93	Deli-style Colesla -96	Shrimp Salad -103	Mediterranean Orange-Glazed Pork -144	Cherry Blondies -109
Day 7	Cacao & Raspberry Chia Pudding -101	Balsamic chicken -136	Chicken enchilada/tortilla soup -105	chicken salad -42	Greek White Pizza With Roasted Tomatoes -144	Pineapple Popsicles -57

Week 4						
	Breakfast & Brunch Recipes	**Lunch Recipes**	**Dinner recipes**	**Side Dishes Recipes**	**Snacks & Appetizer Recipes**	**Dessert Recipes**
Day 1	Coconut Pomegranate Oatmeal -59	Pork Braised with Dried Fruits and Cipollini Onions -155	Hearty Lentil Soup -115	Thai-style Chicken Salad With Spicy Peanut -103	Steak Bites -123	Mango Ice Cream -79
Day 2	Eggplant and Yogurt -92	Roasted Fennel & Mushroom -93	Hearty Lentil Soup -115	Classic Tuna Salad -103	Chicken Marinade -128	Mango Ice Cream -79
Day 3	Huevos Rancheros -81	Balsamic chicken -136	Sautéed Wild Mushroom -114	BBQ chicken salad -42	Mediterranean-Style Greek Pasta -141	Red Wine Poached Pears -56
Day 4	Filled Crepes -45	Tabbouleh -94	French onion soup 106	Classic Tuna Salad -103	Greek Green Goddess Cobb Salad -127	Pear Clafoutis -55
Day 5	Cacao & Raspberry Chia Pudding -101	Roasted Green Bean & Radicchio -93	French onion soup 106	Shrimp Salad -103	Mediterranean Grilled Balsamic Chicken -136	Almond and Cherry Muffins -100
Day 6	Eggs in Purgatory -33	Herbed Baked Goat -85	Sautéed Wild Mushroom -114	Shrimp Salad -103	Seafood Couscous Paella -180	Cherry Blondies -109
Day 7	Mushrooms Omelet -70	Tabbouleh -94	Hearty Lentil Soup -115	Celery Root Salad With Apple & Parsley -102	Crispy Salmon With Lemony Asparagus -127	Banana Mango Bread-69

Week 5						
	Breakfast & Brunch Recipes	**Lunch Recipes**	**Dinner recipes**	**Side Dishes Recipes**	**Snacks & Appetizer Recipes**	**Dessert Recipes**
Day 1	Baba Ghanoush -122	lentils -58	Tortilla Soup -105	Classic Tuna Salad -103	Mediterranean-Style Greek Pasta -141	Pear Clafoutis -55
Day 2	Huevos Rancheros -81	Roasted Fennel & Mushroom -93	Buttered Cinnamon-sugar Croutons -114	Shrimp Salad -103	Steak Bites -123	Mango Ice Cream -79
Day 3	Breakfast Enchiladas -46	Pork Braised with Dried Fruits and Cipollini Onions -155	lentils -58	Celery Root Salad With Apple & Parsley -102	Greek Wedge Salad -126	Mango Ice Cream -79
Day 4	Huevos Rancheros -81	Lentils -65	Tortilla Soup -105	Classic Tuna Salad -103	Mediterranean-Style Greek Pasta -141	Banana Mango Bread-69
Day 5	Coconut Pomegranate Oatmeal -59	Wilted Spinach Salad With Warm Bacon -86	Vietnamese-style Beef Noodle Soup -106	Garlic Chips -113	Greek Pesto Corkscrew -130	Mango Ice Cream -79
Day 6	Coconut Pomegranate Oatmeal -59	Roasted Fennel & Mushroom -93	Deli-style Colesla -96	Garlic Chips -113	Greek Green Goddess Cobb Salad -127	Apple Upside-Down Cake -189
Day 7	Watercress Smoothie -123	Lentils -65	lentils -58	Shrimp Salad -103	Italian Egg Bake -129	Lemon and Chia Biscotti -133

Week 6						
	Breakfast & Brunch Recipes	**Lunch Recipes**	**Dinner recipes**	**Side Dishes Recipes**	**Snacks & Appetizer Recipes**	**Dessert Recipes**
Day 1	Huevos Rancheros -81	Pork Braised with Dried Fruits and Cipollini Onions -155	Tortilla Soup -105	Classic Tuna Salad -103	Mediterranean-Style Greek Pasta -141	Pear Clafoutis -55
Day 2	Cacao & Raspberry -59	Roasted Green Bean & Potato Salad With Radicchio -93	Chia Pudding Buttered Cinnamon-sugar Croutons -114	Garlic Chips -113	Quinoa-Stuffed Squash Boats -144	Pineapple Popsicles -57
Day 3	Zucchini Pancakes -33	Deli-style Colesla -96	Hearty Lentil Soup -115	Celery Root Salad With Apple & Parsley -102	Butternut Squash Soup -114	Mango Ice Cream -79
Day 4	Huevos Rancheros -81	Lentils -65	Tortilla Soup -105	Classic Tuna Salad -103	Mediterranean-Style Greek Pasta -141	Pear Clafoutis -55
Day 5	Eggplant and Yogurt -92	Roasted Green Bean & Potato Salad With Radicchio -93	Deli-style Colesla -96	Buttered Cinnamon-sugar Croutons -114	Roasted Fish -141	Banana Mango Bread-69
Day 6	Huevos Rancheros -81	Pork Braised with Dried Fruits and Cipollini Onions -155	Chia Pudding Buttered Cinnamon-sugar Croutons -114	Garlic Chips -113	Crispy Salmon With Lemony Asparagus -127	Pear Clafoutis -55
Day 7	Coconut Pomegranate Oatmeal -59	Deli-style Colesla -96	Hearty Lentil Soup -115	Classic Tuna Salad -103	Steak Bites -123	Pineapple Popsicles -57

Week 7						
	Breakfast & Brunch Recipes	**Lunch Recipes**	**Dinner recipes**	**Side Dishes Recipes**	**Snacks & Appetizer Recipes**	**Dessert Recipes**
Day 1	Baba Ghanoush -122	Pork Braised with Dried Fruits and Cipollini Onions -155	Tortilla Soup 105	Classic Tuna Salad -103	Greek Wedge Salad -126	Apple Upside-Down Cake -189
Day 2	Cacao & Raspberry Chia Pudding -101	Wilted Spinach Salad With Warm Bacon -86	Buttered Cinnamon-sugar Croutons -114	Garlic Chips -113	Greek Wedge Salad -126	Pear Tart Tatin -56
Day 3	Espinacase la Catalana -112	Lamb curry -50	Hearty Lentil Soup -115	Classic Chicken Noodle -104	Greek Wedge Salad -126	Red Wine Poached Pears -56
Day 4	Filled Crepes -45	Lamb curry -50	Tortilla Soup -105	Shrimp Salad -103	Seafood Couscous Paella -180	Pear Clafoutis -55
Day 5	Cacao & Raspberry 59	Fried baby Carrot with shrimps	Hearty Lentil Soup -115	Chia Pudding -101	Garlic Chips Greek Green Goddess Cobb Salad -127	Banana Mango Bread-69
Day 6	Coconut Pomegranate Oatmeal -59	Deli-style Colesla -96	Buttered Cinnamon-sugar Croutons -114	Creamy Green Pea Soup -113	Butternut Squash Soup -114	Pear Tart Tatin -56
Day 7	Watercress Smoothie -123	Wilted Spinach Salad With Warm Bacon -86	Lamb curry -50	Celery Root Salad With Apple & Parsley -102	Mediterranean Orange-Glazed Pork -144	Pineapple Popsicles -57

Week 8						
	Breakfast & Brunch Recipes	**Lunch Recipes**	**Dinner recipes**	**Side Dishes Recipes**	**Snacks & Appetizer Recipes**	**Dessert Recipes**
Day 1	Huevos Rancheros -81	Roasted Fennel & Mushroom -93	Buttered Cinnamon-sugar Croutons -114	Celery Root Salad With Apple & Parsley -102	Steak Bites -123	Pear Clafoutis -55
Day 2	Zucchini Pancakes -33	Wilted Spinach Salad With Warm Bacon -86	Pesto pasta -108	Stuffed Squash -144	Roasted Fish -141	Red Wine Poached Pears -56
Day 3	Baba Ghanoush -122	Pork Braised with Dried Fruits and Cipollini Onions -155	Pesto pasta -180	Shrimp Salad -103	Mediterranean Grilled Balsamic Chicken -136	Pineapple Popsicles -57
Day 4	Breakfast Enchiladas -46	Lamb curry -50	Beef Noodle Soup -106	Creamy Green Pea Soup -113	Quinoa-Stuffed Squash Boats -144	Pear Clafoutis -55
Day 5	Coconut Pomegranate Oatmeal -59	Roasted Fennel & Mushroom -93	Roasted Green Bean -93	Creamy Green Pea Soup -113	Quinoa-Stuffed Squash Boats -144	Pear Tart Tatin -56
Day 6	Cacao & Raspberry Chia Pudding -102	Pesto pasta -108	Beef Noodle Soup -106	Buttered Cinnamon-sugar Croutons -114	Mediterranean-Style Greek Pasta -141	Apple Upside-Down Cake -189
Day 7	Breakfast Enchiladas -46	Wilted Spinach Salad With Warm Bacon -86	Tortellini -75	Stuffed Squash -144	Greek Wedge Salad -126	Banana Mango Bread-69

Week 9						
	Breakfast & Brunch Recipes	**Lunch Recipes**	**Dinner recipes**	**Side Dishes Recipes**	**Snacks & Appetizer Recipes**	**Dessert Recipes**
Day 1	Huevos Rancheros -81	Deli-style Colesla -96	Buttered Cinnamon-sugar Croutons -114	Pesto pasta -108	Seafood Couscous Paella -180	Red Wine Poached Pears -56
Day 2	Eggplant and Yogurt -92	Roasted Fennel & Mushroom -93	Hearty Lentil Soup -115	Tortellini -75	Pizza With Roasted Tomatoes	Pear Clafoutis -55
Day 3	Baba Ghanoush -122	Pork Braised with Dried Fruits and Cipollini Onions -155	Deli-style Colesla -96	lentils -58	Mediterranean-Style Greek Pasta -141	Banana Mango Bread-69
Day 4	Filled Crepes -45	Roasted Fennel & Mushroom -93	Buttered Cinnamon-sugar Croutons -114	Pesto pasta -108	Greek Wedge Salad -126	Apple Upside-Down Cake -189
Day 5	Eggs in Purgatory -33	Roasted Green Bean & Potato Salad With Radicchio -93	Beef Noodle Soup -106	lentils -58	Crispy Salmon With Lemony Asparagus -127	Mango Ice Cream -79
Day 6	Breakfast Enchiladas -46	Pesto pasta -108	Vietnamese-style Beef Noodle Soup -106	Creamy Green Pea Soup -113	Greek Green Goddess Cobb Salad -127	Pear Tart Tatin -56
Day 7	Western Omelet -80	Beef Noodle Soup -106	Tortellini soup -75	Shrimp Salad -103	Butternut Squash Soup -114	Red Wine Poached Pears -56

Week 10						
	Breakfast & Brunch Recipes	**Lunch Recipes**	**Dinner recipes**	**Side Dishes Recipes**	**Snacks & Appetizer Recipes**	**Dessert Recipes**
Day 1	Asparagus Omelet -80	Burritos -46.	Pad Thai -65	Classic Tuna Salad -103	Greek Wedge Salad -126	Cherry Blondies -109
Day 2	Croque Madame -80	Wilted Spinach Salad With Warm Bacon -86	Burritos -46.	Celery Root Salad With Apple & Parsley -102	Roasted Fish -141	Mango Ice Cream -79
Day 3	Huevos Rancheros -81	Stir fry -134	Sautéed Wild Mushroom -114	Tortellini soup -75	Steak Bites -123	Pear Clafoutis -55
Day 4	Coconut Pomegranate Oatmeal -59	Deli-style Colesla -96	Buttered Cinnamon-sugar Croutons -114	Creamy Green Pea Soup -113	Greek Pesto Corkscrew -130	Mango Ice Cream -79
Day 5	Cacao & Raspberry Chia Pudding -101	Wilted Spinach Salad With Warm Bacon -86	Hearty Lentil Soup -115	Buttered Cinnamon-sugar Croutons -114	Italian Egg Bake -129	Pear Tart Tatin -56
Day 6	Zucchini Pancakes -33	Burritos -46.	Deli-style Colesla -96	Celery Root Salad With Apple & Parsley -102	Seafood Couscous Paella Herry -180	Chery Blondies -109
Day 7	Mushrooms Omelet -70	Deli-style Colesla -96	Sautéed Wild Mushroom -114	White chicken chili -36	Chicken Marinade -128	Red Wine Poached Pears -56

Week 11						
	Breakfast & Brunch Recipes	**Lunch Recipes**	**Dinner recipes**	**Side Dishes Recipes**	**Snacks & Appetizer Recipes**	**Dessert Recipes**
Day 1	Huevos Rancheros -81	Roasted Green Bean & Potato Salad With Radicchio -93	Roasted Fennel & Mushroom -93	Thai-style Chicken Salad With Spicy Peanut -103	Crispy Salmon With Lemony Asparagus -127	Banana Mango Bread-69
Day 2	Quiche, Crepes and Souffles -45	Stir fry -134	Deli-style Colesla -96	Creamy Green Pea Soup -113	Quinoa-Stuffed Squash Boats -144	Pineapple Popsicles -57
Day 3	Espinacase la Catalana -112	Roasted Fennel & Mushroom -93	Pad Thai -65	Clam chowder -35	Crispy Salmon With Lemony Asparagus -127	Lemon and Chia Biscotti -133
Day 4	Coconut Pomegranate Oatmeal -59	Deli-style Colesla -96	Hearty Lentil Soup -115	White chicken chili -36	Mediterranean-Style Greek Pasta -141	Lemon and Chia Biscotti -133
Day 5	Breakfast Enchiladas -46	Pork Braised with Dried Fruits and Cipollini Onions -155	Roasted Fennel & Mushroom -93	Buttered Cinnamon-sugar Croutons -114	Seafood Couscous Paella -180	Apple Upside-Down Cake -189
Day 6	Cacao & Raspberry Chia Pudding -101	Burritos -46.	Roasted Fennel & Mushroom -93	Classic Tuna Salad -103	Greek Wedge Salad -126	Red Wine Poached Pears -56
Day 7	Quiche, Crepes and Souffles -45	Stir fry -134	Sautéed Wild Mushroom -114	Creamy Green Pea Soup -113	Steak Bites -123	Pear Clafoutis -55

Week 12						
	Breakfast & Brunch Recipes	**Lunch Recipes**	**Dinner recipes**	**Side Dishes Recipes**	**Snacks & Appetizer Recipes**	**Dessert Recipes**
Day 1	Eggs in Purgatory -33	Roasted Green Bean & Potato Salad With Radicchio -93	Sautéed Wild Mushroom -114	tortilla soup -105	Chicken Marinade -128	Cherry Blondies -109
Day 2	Espinacase la Catalana -112	Pork Braised with Dried Fruits and Cipollini Onions -155	Deli-style Colesla -96	Thai-style Chicken Salad With Spicy Peanut -103	Greek Green Goddess Cobb Salad -127	Lemon and Chia Biscotti -133
Day 3	Huevos Rancheros -81	Wilted Spinach Salad With Warm Bacon -86	Burritos -46	Chicken enchilada/Tortila Soup -105	Greek Wedge Salad -126	Pear Tart Tatin -56
Day 4	Quiche, Crepes and Souffles -45	Burritos -46.	Buttered Cinnamon-sugar Croutons -114	Creamy Green Pea Soup -113	Greek Pesto Corkscrew -130	Pear Tart Tatin -56
Day 5	Breakfast Enchiladas -46	Deli-style Colesla -96	Burritos -46	Buttered Cinnamon-sugar Croutons -114	Greek Wedge Salad -126	Banana Mango Bread-69
Day 6	Breakfast Enchiladas -46	Burritos -46	Sautéed Wild Mushroom -114	Thai-style Chicken Salad With Spicy Peanut -103	Roasted Fish -141	Cherry Blondies -104
Day 7	Coconut Pomegranate Oatmeal -59	Roasted Fennel & Mushroom -93	Deli-style Colesla -96	Buttered Cinnamon-sugar Croutons -114	Seafood Couscous Paella -180	Red Wine Poached Pears -56

Week 13						
	Breakfast & Brunch Recipes	**Lunch Recipes**	**Dinner recipes**	**Side Dishes Recipes**	**Snacks & Appetizer Recipes**	**Dessert Recipes**
Day 1	Quiche, Crepes and Souffles -45	Chicken parmesan -181	Cumin Pork chops -141	Thai-style Chicken Salad With Spicy Peanut -103	Steak Bites -123	Lemon and Chia Biscotti -133
Day 2	Eggs in Purgatory -33	Roasted Green Bean & Potato Salad With Radicchio -93	Tortilla Soup 105	Creamy Green Pea Soup -113	Crispy Salmon With Lemony Asparagus -127	Almond and Cherry Muffins -100
Day 3	Eggplant and Yogurt -92	Pork Braised with Dried Fruits and Cipollini Onions -155	Pork chops -141	Celery Root Salad With Apple & Parsley -102	Seafood Couscous Paella -180	Lemon and Chia Biscotti -133
Day 4	Breakfast Enchiladas -46	Chicken parmesan -181	Hearty Lentil Soup -115	White chicken chili -36	Greek Green Goddess Cobb Salad -127	Mango Ice Cream -79
Day 5	Filled Crepes -45	Wilted Spinach Salad With Warm Bacon -86	Buttered Cinnamon-sugar Croutons -114	Classic Tuna Salad -103	Chicken wings -87	Pineapple Crumble -79
Day 6	Coconut Pomegranate Oatmeal -59	Stir fry -134	Stuffed Pork chops -141	Classic Tuna Salad -103	Roasted Fish -141	Red Wine Poached Pears -56
Day 7	Cacao & Raspberry Chia Pudding -101	Deli-style Colesla -96	Sautéed Wild Mushroom -114	White chicken chili -36	Greek Wedge Salad -126	Pineapple Crumble -79

Week 14						
	Breakfast & Brunch Recipes	**Lunch Recipes**	**Dinner recipes**	**Side Dishes Recipes**	**Snacks & Appetizer Recipes**	**Dessert Recipes**
Day 1	Breakfast Enchiladas -46	Pork Braised with Dried Fruits and Cipollini Onions -155	Meatloaf -142	Thai-style Chicken Salad With Spicy Peanut -103	Fried Leeks	Pineapple Crumble -79
Day 2	Croque Madame -80	Orange chicken -60	Sautéed Wild Mushroom -114	Classic Chicken Noodle -104	Greek Green Goddess Cobb Salad -127	Almond and Cherry Muffins -100
Day 3	Zucchini Pancakes -33	Beef & broccoli -61	Meatloaf -142	Buttered Cinnamon-sugar Croutons -114	Stuffed pork chops	Pineapple Popsicles -57
Day 4	Mushrooms Omelet -70	Chicken parmesan -181	Sautéed Wild Mushroom -114	Classic Tuna Salad -103	Mediterranean Orange-Glazed Pork -144	Lemon and Chia Biscotti -133
Day 5	Baba Ghanoush -122	Beef & broccoli -61	Meatloaf -142	Celery Root Salad With Apple & Parsley -102	Mediterranean-Style Greek Pasta -141	Red Wine Poached Pears -56
Day 6	Quiche, Crepes and Souffles -45	Roasted Green Bean & Potato Salad With Radicchio -93	Sautéed Wild Mushroom -114	Buttered Cinnamon-sugar Croutons -114	Quinoa-Stuffed Squash Boats -144	Pineapple Crumble -79
Day 7	Coconut Pomegranate Oatmeal -59	Roasted Fennel & Mushroom 93	Hearty Lentil Soup -115	Buttered Cinnamon-sugar Croutons -114	Steak Bites -123	Mango Ice Cream -79

Week 15						
	Breakfast & Brunch Recipes	**Lunch Recipes**	**Dinner recipes**	**Side Dishes Recipes**	**Snacks & Appetizer Recipes**	**Dessert Recipes**
Day 1	Cacao & Raspberry Chia Pudding -101	Pork Braised with Dried Fruits and Cipollini Onions -155	Sautéed Wild Mushroom -114	Classic Chicken Noodle -104	Quinoa-Stuffed Squash Boats -144	Pineapple Crumble -79
Day 2	Croque Madame -80	Deli-style Colesla -96	Buttered Cinnamon-sugar Croutons -114	Thai-style Chicken Salad With Spicy Peanut -103	Fried Leeks -113	Pineapple Crumble -79
Day 3	Breakfast Enchiladas -46	Beef & broccoli -61	Sautéed Wild Mushroom -114	Celery Root Salad With Apple & Parsley -102	Smoked Salmon -54	Almond and Cherry Muffins -100
Day 4	Eggs in Purgatory -33	Wilted Spinach Salad With Warm Bacon -86	Buttered Cinnamon-sugar Croutons -114	Classic Chicken Noodle -104	Mediterranean-Style Greek Pasta -141	Red Wine Poached Pears -56
Day 5	Quiche, Crepes and Souffles -45	Roasted Fennel & Mushroom 93	Deli-style Colesla -96	Classic Tuna Salad -103	Greek Wedge Salad -126	Pineapple Crumble -79
Day 6	Cacao & Raspberry Chia Pudding -101	Chicken parmesan -181	Wilted Spinach Salad With Warm Bacon -86	Classic Chicken Noodle -104	Greek Green Goddess Cobb Salad -127	Apple Pie -189
Day 7	Croque Madame -80	Beef & broccoli -61	Chicken parmesan -181	Celery Root Salad With Apple & Parsley -102	Steak Bites -123	Almond and Cherry Muffins -100

1125 Mediterranean Diet Recipes

Mediterranean Dash Diet

Breakfast & Brunch Recipes

1. Spinach Frittata

Prep Time: *1 Minutes* | *Cook Time:* *35 Minutes* | *Servings:* *6*

Ingredients:

- 6 servings
- 2 tbsp. olive oil or avocado oil 1 Zucchini sliced 1 cup torn fresh spinach
- 2 tbsp. sliced green onions
- 1 tsp. crushed garlic salt and pepper to taste 1/3 cup coconut milk
- 6 eggs

Directions:

1. Heat olive oil in a skillet over medium heat. Add zucchini and cook until tender. Mix in spinach, green onions and garlic. Season with salt and pepper. Continue cooking until spinach is wilted.
2. In a bowl, beat eggs and coconut milk together. Pour into the skillet over the vegetables. Reduce heat to low cover and cook until eggs are firm (5 to 7 minutes).

2. Superfoods Naan Pancakes Crepes

Prep Time:5 Minutes | *Cook Time:* *35 Minutes* | *Servings:* *2*

Ingredients:

- ½ cup almond flour ½ cup Tapioca Flour 1 cup Coconut Milk Salt
- coconut oil

Directions:

- *Mix all the ingredients together.*
- *After heating a pan over medium heat and pour the batter to desired thickness; once the batter looks firm, flip it over to cook the other side.*
- *If you want this to be a dessert crepe or pancake, then omit the salt. You can add minced garlic or ginger in the batter if you want or some spices.*

3. Frittata with Broccoli and Tomato

Prep Time: *15 Minutes* | *Cook Time:* *30 Minutes* | *Servings : 6*

Ingredients:

- 2 large eggs
- Salt Ground black pepper 1 tsp. Olive oil or cumin oil ½ cup broccoli
- ½ cup sliced tomatoes Crushed red pepper flakes and a 1 Tbsp. chopped chives (optional)

Directions:

1. 2 large eggs are whisking in a small bowl. Present with salt and ground black pepper and set aside. Heat 1 tsp.
2. Oil in a medium skillet over medium heat. Add broccoli and tomatoes and cook, tossing approx. 1 minute. Add eggs; cook, occasionally stirring until just set about 1 minute. Stir in cheese.
3. Sprinkle with crushed red pepper flakes and chives.

4. Frittata with Green and Red Peppers

Prep Time:2 *Minutes* | *Cook Time:* *10 Minutes* | *Servings:* *2*

Ingredients:

- 2 large eggs
- Salt Ground black pepper 1 tsp. olive oil or avocado oil ½ cup each chopped green and red peppers

Directions:

1. 2 large eggs are whisking in a small bowl. Present with salt and ground black pepper and set aside. Heat 1 tsp.
2. Olive oil in a medium skillet. Add peppers and cook, tossing approx. 1 minute.
3. Add eggs; cook, occasionally stirring until just set about 1 minute.

5. Eggs in Purgatory

Prep Time: *15 Minutes* | *Cook Time:* *10 Minutes* | *Servings:* *2*

Ingredients:

- 2 large eggs
- Salt 1 clove garlic chopped.
- 1 tsp. Olive oil or avocado oil 1 cup chopped tomatoes 1 Tbsp. Hot red pepper flakes and 1 Tbsp. cilantro

Directions:

1. Heat 1 tsp. Oil in a medium skillet over medium heat. Add garlic, chopped tomatoes and red pepper flakes and cook, tossing approx. 15 minutes.
2. Add eggs and cook until eggs are done. Sprinkle with salt and cilantro.

6. Frittata with Carrots Green Peas and Asparagus

Prep Time: *15 Minutes* | *Cook Time:* *10 Minutes* | *Servings: 4*

Ingredients:

- 2 large eggs
- Salt Ground black pepper 1 tsp. Olive oil or avocado oil ½ cup cooked green peas ½ cup chopped carrot ½ cup asparagus 1 tbsp. fresh dill

Directions:

1. 2 large eggs are whisking in a small bowl. Present with salt and ground black pepper and set aside. Heating 1 tsp.
2. Oil in a skillet over medium heat. Add carrots and asparagus and cook, tossing approx. 5 minutes. Add cooked and drained green peas. Add eggs; cook, occasionally stirring until just set about 1 minute. Sprinkle with dill.

7. Zucchini Scrambled Eggs

Prep Time: *6 Minutes* | *Cook Time:* *10 Minutes* | *Servings : 6*

Ingredients

- 1 tsp coconut oil 4 eggs
- 1 Tbs water
- 1 zucchini sliced
- ground black pepper to taste

Directions:

1. Whisk 4 large eggs in a small bowl. Present with salt and ground black pepper and set aside. Heat 1 tsp. Olive oil in a skillet. Add sliced zucchini and cook, tossing until wilted (approx. 3 minutes). Set aside.
2. Add eggs and cooked completely, stirring occasionally. Serve with zucchini on the aside.

8. Frittata with Asparagus and Tomato

Prep Time:8 *Minutes* | *Cook Time:* *10 Minutes* | *Servings: 2*

Ingredients:

- 2 large eggs
- Salt Ground black pepper 1 tsp. olive oil or avocado oil 1 cup asparagus
- ½ cup sliced tomatoes

Directions:

- Whisk 2 large eggs in a small bowl. Present with salt and ground black pepper and set aside. Heat 1 tsp. Oil in a medium skillet over medium heat. Add asparagus and cook, tossing approx. 4-5 minutes. Add tomatoes and eggs and cook, occasionally stirring until just set about 1 minute. Sprinkle with dill (optional).

9. Eggs with Zucchini Onions and Tomato

Prep Time: *15 Minutes* | *Cook Time:* *10 Minutes* | *Servings:* *2*

Ingredients:

- 2 large eggs
- Salt Ground black pepper 1 tsp. olive oil or avocado oil
- 1/3 cup sliced
- zucchini 1/3 cup chopped onions 1/3 cup sliced tomato Crushed red pepper flakes and a pinch of dill (optional)

Directions:

1. Mix 2 eggs in a small bowl. Present with salt and ground black pepper and set aside. Heat 1 tsp. Olive oil in a skillet. Add zucchini, onions and tomatoes and cook tossing until wilted (approx. 3-4 minutes). Add eggs and cook until just set.

10. Frittata with Tomatoes and Spinach

Prep Time: *15 Minutes* | *Cook Time:* *10 Minutes* | *Servings:* *2*

Ingredients:

- 2 large eggs
- Salt Ground black pepper 1 tsp. olive oil or avocado oil ½ cup sliced tomatoes 1/3 cup spinach

Directions:

1. Whisk 2 large eggs in a small bowl. Season with salt and ground black pepper and set aside. Heat 1 tsp. Olive oil in a medium skillet over medium heat. Add baby spinach and tomatoes and cook, tossing until wilted (approx. 1 minute). Add eggs; cook, occasionally stirring until just set about 1 minute.

11. Zucchini Pancakes

Prep Time: *15 Minutes* | *Cook Time:* *10 Minutes* | *Servings:* *4*

Ingredients:

- 2 medium zucchini
- 2 tbsp. chopped onion
- 3 beaten eggs 6 to 8 tbsp. Almond flour 1 tsp. Salt
- ½ tsp. ground black pepper
- coconut oil

Directions:

1. Heat the oven to 300 degrees F.
2. Grate the zucchini into a bowl and mix in the onion and eggs. Stir in 6 tbsp of the flour, salt and pepper.
3. Heat a large sauté pan over medium heat and add coconut oil to the pan. When the oil is hot lower the heat to medium-low and adds batter into the pan. Baked the pancakes for about 2 minutes on each side until browned. Place the pancakes in the oven.

12. Savoury Superfoods Pie Crust

Prep Time: *15 Minutes* *Cook Time:* *8 Minutes* *Servings: 6*

Ingredients:

- DF
- 11/4 cups blanched almond flour 1/3 cup tapioca flour
- ¾ tsp. Finely ground sea salt
- ¾ tsp. Paprika
- ½ tsp. ground cumin
- 1/8 tsp. ground white pepper
- ¼ cup coconut oil 1 large egg

Directions:

1. Place almond flour tapioca flour, sea salt, vanilla egg and coconut sugar (if you use coconut sugar) in the bowl of a food processor. Process 2-3 times to combine. Add oil and raw honey (if you use raw honey) and pulse with several one-second pulses and then let the food processor run until the mixture comes together. Move the dough onto a plastic wrap sheet. Wrap and then press the dough into a 9-inch disk. Refrigerate for 30 minutes.
2. Remove plastic wrap. Press dough onto the bottom and up the sides of a 9-inch buttered pie dish. Crimp a little bit the edges of the crust. Cool in the refrigerator for 20 minutes. Tp put the oven rack in the middle after heating the oven to 375F. Put in the oven and bake until golden brown.

13. Spinach Quiche

Prep Time: *15 Minutes* *Cook Time:* *8 Minutes* *Servings: 8*

Ingredients:

- 1 Precooked and cooled Savory Superfoods Pie Crust
- 8 ounces organic spinach cooked and drained
- 6 ounces cubed pork 2 medium shallots thinly sliced and sautéed
- 4 large eggs 1 cup coconut milk ¾ tsp. Salt ¼ tsp. freshly ground black pepper

Directions:

1. Brown the pork in coconut oil and then add the spinach and shallots. Set aside once done.
2. Preheat oven to 350F. In a large bowl, combine eggs, milk, salt and pepper. Whisk until foamy. Add in about ¾ of the drained filling mixture reserving the other ¼ to "top" the quiche. Pour egg mixture into crust and place remaining filling on top of the quiche.
3. Place quiche in the oven in the centre of the middle rack and bake undisturbed for 45 to 50 minutes.

14. Mushroom Quiche

Prep Time: *15 Minutes* *Cook Time:* *8 Minutes* *Servings: 2*

Ingredients:

- 1 Precooked and cooled Savory Superfoods Pie Crust
- 1 cup sliced mushrooms 6 ounces cubed pork 2 medium shallots thinly sliced and sautéed
- 4 large eggs 1 cup coconut milk ¾ tsp. Salt ¼ tsp. freshly ground black pepper

Directions:

1. Brown the pork in coconut oil and then add the mushrooms and shallots. Set aside once done.
2. Preheat oven to 350F. In a large bowl, combine eggs, milk, salt and pepper. Whisk until foamy. Add in about ¾ of the drained filling mixture reserving the other ¼ to "top" the quiche. Pour egg mixture into crust and place remaining filling on top of the quiche.
3. Place quiche in the oven in the centre of the middle rack and bake undisturbed for 45 to 50 minutes.

15. Tomato Quiche

Prep Time: *15 Minutes* *Cook Time:* *25 Minutes* *Servings:2*

Ingredients:

- 1 Precooked and cooled Savory Superfoods Pie Crust
- 1 cup sliced tomatoes 6 ounces cubed pork 2 medium shallots thinly sliced and sautéed
- 4 large eggs 1 cup coconut milk ¾ tsp. Salt ¼ cup. Arugula ¼ tsp. freshly ground black pepper

Directions:

1. Brown the pork and shallots in coconut oil. Set aside once done.
2. Preheat oven to 350F. In a large bowl, combine eggs, milk, salt and pepper. Whisk until foamy. Add in about ¾ of the drained filling mixture and tomatoes, reserving the other ¼ to "top" the quiche. Pour egg mixture into crust and place remaining filling on top of the quiche.
3. Place quiche in the oven in the centre of the middle rack and bake undisturbed for 45 to 50 minutes. Sprinkle with arugula.

16. WHITE BEAN SOUP WITH WINTER VEGETABLES

Prep Time: *5 Minutes* *Cook Time:* *25 Minutes* *Servings: 6*

INGREDIENTS:

- ounces Pancetta, cut into 1-inch cubes
- 12 cups water, plus extra as needed
- 1 lb dried cannellini beans (2 cups), picked over & rinsed
- 1 large onion, unpeeled & halved, and 1 small onion,
- chopped four garlic cloves, unpeeled, as well as 3 garlic cloves, minced
- 1 bay leaf
- Salt & pepper
- 1/4 cup of extra-virgin olive oil, and extra for serving 2 small carrots, diced medium
- 2 celery ribs, diced medium
- small leeks, white & light green parts only, halved lengthwise, sliced crosswise into 1/2-inch pieces, & rinsed thoroughly
- ounces kale stemmed & leaves cut into 1/2-inch strips
- ounces escarole stemmed & leaves cut into 1/2-inch strips
- 6 ounces red potatoes, diced medium
- 1 (14.5-ounce) can diced tomatoes, drained
- 1 sprig of fresh rosemary

DIRECTIONS:

1. Cook pancetta in the oven over medium heat till just golden, 8 to 10 mins.
2. Include water, beans, halved onion, unpeeled garlic cloves, bay leaf, & 1 Tsp. Salt & bring to boil over medium-high heat.
3. Cover pot partially reduces heat to low, & simmer, occasionally stirring, till beans are almost tender, 1 to 1 1/4 hrs.
4. Remove beans from heat, cover, & let stand till beans are tender, about 30 mins.
5. Drain beans, reserving cooking liquid. Discard pancetta, onion, unpeeled garlic cloves, & bay leaf. Sprinkle beans in an even layer on a rimmed baking sheet & let cool.
6. Beans are cooling; heat oil in a pot over medium heat till shimmering.
7. Include carrots, celery, leeks, & chopped onion & cook, occasionally stirring, till softened but not browned, about 7 mins.
8. Stir in minced garlic & cook till fragrant, about 30 seconds. Include enough water to reserved bean cooking liquid to equal 9 cups & Include to pot with kale & escarole.
9. Increase heat to medium-high & bring to boil, cover, reduce heat to low, & simmer 30 mins. Include potatoes & tomatoes, cover, & cook till potatoes are tender, about 20 mins.
10. Include cooled beans in the pot, increase heat to medium-high, & bring to simmer.
11. Submerge rosemary in liquid, cover, & let stand off the heat for 15 to 20 mins.
12. Discard rosemary & season with salt & pepper to taste. Ladle soup into containers, drizzle with olive oil, & serve.

17. QUICK TUSCAN WHITE BEAN SOUP

Prep Time: *5 Minutes* *Cook Time:* *15 Minutes* *Servings: 6*

INGREDIENTS:

- 6 ounces pancetta, cut into 1-inch cubes
- Tbsps. extra-virgin olive oil, plus extra for serving
- 1 small onion, chopped
- 3 garlic cloves, minced
- Salt & pepper
- 3 1/2 cups water
- (15-ounce) cans cannellini beans, rinsed
- 1 sprig of fresh rosemary Balsamic vinegar for serving

DIRECTIONS:

1. Cook pancetta in the oven over medium heat till just golden, 8 to 10 mins.
2. Discard pancetta & Include oil to pot with rendered pancetta fat.
3. Include onion & cook, occasionally stirring, till softened, 5 to 6 mins.
4. Stir in garlic & cook till fragrant, about 30 seconds.
5. Include beans, 1/2 Tsp. Salt, & 3 1/2 cups water. Increase heat to medium-high & bring to simmer.
6. Submerge rosemary in liquid; cover & let stand off heat 15 to 20 mins.
7. Discard rosemary & season with salt & pepper to taste.
8. Ladle soup into containers, drizzle with olive oil, & serve, passing balsamic vinegar separately.

18. BLACK BEAN SOUP

Prep Time: *5 Minutes* *Cook Time:* *35 Minutes* *Servings: 4*

INGREDIENTS:

- 5 cups water, plus extra as needed
- lb dried black beans (2 cups), picked over & rinsed
- 4 ounces ham steak, trimmed
- 2 bay leaves
- 1/8 Tsp. baking soda
- 1 Tsp. salt
- 3 Tbsps. olive oil
- large onions, chopped fine
- 1 large carrot, chopped fine
- 3 celery ribs, chopped fine
- 1/2 Tsp. salt
- 5-6 garlic cloves, minced
- 1/2 Tsp. red pepper flakes
- 1 1/2 Tbsps. ground cumin
- cups low-sodium chicken broth
- 2 Tbsps. cornstarch
- 2 Tbsps. water
- 2 Tbsps. lime juice
- GARNISHES:
- Lime wedges
- Minced fresh cilantro
- Red onion diced fine
- Avocado halved, pitted, & diced
- Sour cream

DIRECTIONS:

1. Place water, beans, ham, bay leaves, & baking soda in a large saucepan with a tight-fitting lid. Bring to boil over medium-high heat. Using a large spoon, skim foam from the surface as needed.
2. Stir continuously in salt, reduce heat to low, cover, & simmer briskly till beans are tender, 1 1/4 to 1 1/2 hrs (if after 1 1/2 hrs the beans are not tender include 1 cup more water & continue to simmer till tender); do not drain beans.
3. Discard bay leaves. Remove ham steak, cut into 1/4-inch cubes, & set aside.
4. Heat oil in a Dutch oven over medium-high heat till shimmering. Include onions, carrot, celery, & salt & cook, occasionally stirring, till vegetables are soft & lightly browned, 12 to 15 mins.

5. Reduce heat to medium-low; include garlic, pepper flakes, & cumin & cook, constantly stirring, till fragrant, about 3 mins.
6. Stir in beans, bean cooking liquid, & chicken broth. Increase heat to medium-high & bring to boil, then reduce heat to low & simmer, uncovered, occasionally stirring, until it completely blends flavours, about 30 mins.
7. Ladle 1¹/2 cups beans & 2 cups liquid into a food processor or blender, process till smooth, & return to pot.
8. Stir together cornstarch & water in a small container till combined, then gradually stir half of the cornstarch batter into soup.
9. Take it to boil over medium-high heat, occasionally stirring, to fully thicken. If soup is still thinner than desired once boiling, stir remaining cornstarch batter to recombine & gradually stir batter into soup; return to boil to fully thicken.
10. Off heat, stir in lime juice & reserved ham; ladle soup into containers & serve immediately, passing garnishes separately.(If necessary, thin it with additional chicken broth when reheating)

19. CLASSIC CORN CHOWDER

Prep Time: 5 Minutes | *Cook Time: 55 Minutes* | *Servings: 3*

INGREDIENTS:

- 10 ears corn, husks & silk removed
- ounces salt pork, rind removed, cut into two 1-inch cubes
- 1 Tbsp. unsalted butter
- 1 large onion, preferably Spanish, chopped fine
- 2 garlic cloves, minced
- Tbsps. all-purpose flour
- cups low-sodium chicken broth
- ounces red potatoes, cut into ¹/4-inch cubes
- 2 cups whole milk
- 1 Tsp. Minced fresh thyme or ¹/4 Tsp. dried 1 bay leaf
- 1 cup heavy cream
- 2 Tbsps. minced fresh parsley Salt & pepper

DIRECTIONS:

1. Using paring knife, cut kernels from 4 ears of corn (you should have about 3 cups).
2. Grate kernels from leftover 6 ears on large holes of a box grater into the container, and then firmly scrape each pulp remaining on cobs with the back of butter knife or vegetable peeler (you should have 2 generous cups grated kernels & pulp).
3. Sauté salt pork in a Dutch oven over medium-high heat, turning with tongs & pressing down on pieces to render fat, till cubes are crisp & golden brown, about 10 mins.
4. Reduce heat to low, stir in butter & onion, cover, & cook till onion is softened for about 12 mins.
5. Remove salt pork & reserve. Include garlic & sauté till fragrant, about 1 min. Whisk in flour & cook, constantly stirring, about 2 mins.
6. Whisking constantly, gradually Include broth. Include grated corn & pulp, potatoes, milk, thyme, bay leaf, & reserved salt pork & bring to boil.
7. Reduce heat to medium-low & simmer till potatoes are almost tender, 8 to 10 mins.
8. Include reserved corn kernels & heavy cream & return to simmer. Simmer till corn kernels are tender yet still slightly crunchy, about 5 mins. Discard bay leaf & salt pork. Stir in parsley, season with salt & pepper to taste, & serve immediately.

20. MODERN CORN CHOWDER

Prep Time: 5 Minutes | *Cook Time: 20 Minutes* | *Servings: 5*

INGREDIENTS:

- 3 Tbsps. unsalted butter
- 1 onion, chopped fine
- 4 slices of bacon, halved lengthwise, then cut crosswise into ¹/4-inch pieces 2 Tbsps. minced fresh thyme
- Salt & pepper
- ¹/4 cup all-purpose flour
- 5 cups water
- ounces red potatoes, cut into ¹/2-inch cubes
- 1 cup half-and-half Sugar
- 3 Tbsps. chopped fresh basil

DIRECTIONS:

1. Using paring knife, cut kernels from corn (you should have 5 to 6 cups).
2. Holding cobs over the second container, use the back of a butter knife or vegetable peeler to firmly scrape any pulp remaining on the cobs into the container (you should have 2 to 2¹/2 cups of pulp).
3. Shift pulp to the centre of the clean kitchen towel set in a medium container. Wrap towel tightly around pulp & squeeze tightly till dry.
4. Discard pulp in towel & set corn juice aside (you should have about ²/3 cup of juice).
5. Melt butter in the oven over medium heat. Include onion, bacon, thyme, 2 Tbps. salt, & 1 Tsp. pepper & cook, stirring frequently, till onion is softened & beginning to brown, 8 to 10 mins.
6. Stir continuously□ in flour & cook, constantly stirring, for 2 mins.
7. Whisking constantly, gradually Include water & then bring to boil. Include corn kernels & potatoes.
8. Return to simmer, reduce heat to medium-low, & cook till potatoes have softened 15 to 18 mins.
9. Shift 2 cups chowder to blender & process till smooth, 1 to 2 mins. Return puree to the pot, stir in half-and-half, & return to simmer.
10. Remove pot from heat & stir in reserved corn juice. Season with salt, pepper, & up to 1 Tbsp. Sugar to taste. Sprinkle with basil & serve.

21. NEW ENGLAND CLAM CHOWDER

Prep Time: 5 Minutes | *Cook Time: 20 Minutes* | *Servings: 2*

INGREDIENTS:

- 3 cups water
- lbs medium hard-shell clams, such as cherrystones, scrubbed
- 2 slices bacon, chopped fine
- 2 onions, chopped fine
- 2 celery ribs, chopped fine
- 1 Tsp. Minced fresh thyme leaves or ¹/4 Tsp. dried
- ¹/3 cup all-purpose flour
- 3 (8-ounce) bottles of clam juice
- 1¹/2 lbs Yukon of Gold potatoes, peeled and cut into ¹/2-inch pieces
- bay leaf
- cup heavy cream
- Tbsps. minced fresh parsley Salt & pepper

DIRECTIONS:

1. Bring water to boil in a Dutch oven. Include clams, cover, & cook for 5 mins.
2. Stir clams thoroughly, cover, & continue to cook till they just begin to open, 2 to 5 mins.
3. As clams open, Shift them to a large container & let cool slightly. Discard any unopened clams.
4. Measure out & reserve 2 cups clam steaming liquid, avoiding any gritty sediment that has settled on the bottom of the pot. Use a paring knife to remove clam meat from shells & chop coarsely.
5. In a clean Dutch oven, cook bacon over medium heat till crisp, 5 to 7 mins. Stir in onions & celery & cook till vegetables are softened, 5 to 7 mins.
6. Stir in thyme & cook till fragrant, about 30 seconds. Stir in flour & cook for 1 min.
7. Gradually whisk in bottled clam juice & reserved clam steaming liquid, scraping up any browned bits & smoothing out any lumps.
8. Stir in potatoes & bay leaf & bring to boil. Reduce to gentle simmer & cook till potatoes are tender, 20 to 25 mins.
9. Stir in cream & return to brief simmer.
10. Off heat, remove bay leaf, stir in parsley, & season with salt & pepper to taste. Stir in chopped clams, cover, & let stand till clams are warmed through, about 1 min. Serve.

22. RICH & VELVETY SHRIMP BISQUE

Prep Time: 5 Minutes | *Cook Time: 15 Minutes* | *Servings: 4*

INGREDIENTS:

- lbs extra-large shell-on shrimp (21 to 25 per lb)
- 3 Tbsps. olive oil
- ¹/3 cup brandy or cognac, warmed
- Tbsps. unsalted butter
- 1 small carrot, chopped fine
- 1 small celery rib, chopped fine
- 1 small onion, chopped fine
- 1 garlic clove, minced
- ¹/2 cup all-purpose flour
- (8-ounce) bottles clam juice 1¹/2 cups dry white wine
- 1 (14.5-ounce) can diced tomatoes, drained
- 1 cup heavy cream
- 1 Tbsp. lemon juice
- 1 sprig fresh tarragon Pinch cayenne pepper
- 2 Tbsps. dry sherry or Madeira Salt & pepper

DIRECTIONS:

1. Peel ¹/2 lb shrimp, reserving shells, & cut each peeled shrimp into thirds & set aside. Pat dry reserved shells & remaining unpeeled shrimp with paper towels.
2. Heat 12-inch pan over high heat till very hot, about 3 mins.
3. Include 1¹/2 Tbsps. Oil & swirl to coat the bottom of the pan. Include half of the shell on shrimp & half of the reserved shells & cook till shrimp are deep pink & outsides are lightly browned, about 2 mins.
4. Shift shrimp to medium container & repeat with remaining 1¹/2 Tbsps. Oil, shell-on shrimp, & shells.
5. Return the first batch of shrimp to the pan.
6. Off heat, pour brandy over shrimp & let warm through, about 5 seconds.
7. Wave lit match over cooking wok till brandy ignites, then shake cooking wok to distribute flames.
8. When flames subside, shift shrimp & shells to the food processor & process till batter resembles a fine meal, about 10 seconds.
9. Heat butter in the oven over medium heat. Include carrot, celery, onion, garlic, & ground shrimp & shells.
10. Cover & cook, frequently stirring, till vegetables are slightly softened & batter is fragrant about 5 mins.
11. Include flour & cook, constantly stirring, till thoroughly combined, about 1 min. Stir in clam juice, wine, & tomatoes, scraping cooking wok bottom with a wooden spoon to loosen any browned bits.
12. Cover, increase heat to medium-high, & bring to boil. Reduce heat to low & simmer, frequently stirring, till soup is thickened & flavours meld, about 20 mins.
13. Strain bisque through a fine-mesh strainer into a medium container, pressing on solids to extract as much liquid as possible.
14. Wash & dry Dutch oven, return strained bisque to the pot, & stir in cream, lemon juice, tarragon, & cayenne.
15. Bring to simmer over medium-high heat. Include reserved peeled & cut shrimp & simmer till shrimp are firm but tender about 1¹/2 mins.
16. Discard tarragon, stir in sherry, season with salt & pepper to taste, & serve.

23. CREOLE-STYLE SHRIMP & SAUSAGE GUMBO

Prep Time: 5 Minutes | *Cook Time: 55 Minutes* | *Servings: 6*

INGREDIENTS:

- 1¹/2 lbs small shrimp (51 to 60 per lb), peeled & deveined; shells reserved 3¹/2 cups ice water
- (8-ounce) bottle clam juice ¹/2 cup vegetable oil
- ¹/2 cup all-purpose flour 2 onions, chopped fine
- red bell pepper stemmed, seeded, & chopped fine
- celery rib, chopped fine
- garlic cloves, minced
- 1 Tsp. dried thyme Salt & pepper Cayenne pepper
- 2 bay leaves
- 1 lb of smoked sausage, such as andouille or kielbasa, sliced ¹/4 inch thick
- ¹/2 cup minced fresh parsley leaves
- 4 scallions, sliced thin

DIRECTIONS:

1. Bring reserved shrimp shells & 4¹/2 cups water to boil in a stockpot or large saucepan over medium-high heat. Reduce heat to medium-low & simmer for 20 mins.
2. Strain stock & Include ice water & clam juice (you should have about 8 cups of tepid stock, 100 to 110 degrees); discard shells. Set stock aside.
3. Heat oil in the oven or large saucepan over medium-high heat till it registers 200 degrees on an instant-read thermometer, 1¹/2 to 2 mins.
4. Reduce heat to medium & gradually stir in flour with a wooden spatula or spoon, making sure to work out any lumps that may form. Stirring constantly, reaching into corners of the pan, till batter has toasty aroma & is deep reddish-brown, about 20 mins.
5. Include onions, bell pepper, celery, garlic, thyme, 1 Tsp. Salt, & ¹/4 Tsp.
6. Cayenne to roux & cook, frequently stirring, till vegetables soften, 8 to 10 mins. Include 4 cups reserved stock in a slow, steady stream while stirring vigorously. Stir in remaining 4 cups stock. Increase heat to high & bring to boil.
7. Reduce heat to medium-low, skim foam from the surface with a wide spoon.
8. Include bay leaves, & simmer, uncovered, about 30 mins, skimming foam as it rises to surface. (Batter can be covered & set aside for several hrs or refrigerated for up to 2 days. Reheat when ready to proceed.)
9. Stir in sausage & continue simmering to blend flavours, about 30 mins. Stir in shrimp & simmer till cooked through, about 5 mins.

10. Off heat, stir in parsley & scallions & season with salt, pepper, & cayenne to taste. Discard bay leaves & serve immediately.

24. SIMPLE BEEF CHILI WITH KIDNEY BEANS

Prep Time: *Cook Time:* *Servings: 6*
5 Minutes *25 Minutes*

INGREDIENTS:

- Tbsps. vegetable oil
- onions chopped fine
- red bell pepper, stemmed, seeded, & cut into 1/2-inch pieces
- 6 garlic cloves, minced
- 1/4 cup chilli powder
- 1 Tbsp. ground cumin
- Tbsps. ground coriander
- 1 Tsp. red pepper flakes
- 1 Tsp. dried oregano
- 1/2 Tsp. cayenne pepper
- lbs 85 per cent lean ground beef
- (15-ounce) can red kidney beans, rinsed
- (28-ounce) can diced tomatoes, drained with juice reserved
- (28-ounce) can tomato puree Salt
- Lime wedges

DIRECTIONS:

1. Heat oil in the oven over medium heat till shimmering but not smoking.
2. Include onions, bell pepper, garlic, chilli powder, cumin, coriander, pepper flakes, oregano, & cayenne & cook, occasionally stirring, till vegetables are softened & beginning to brown, about 10 mins.
3. Increase heat to medium-high & Include half of the beef. Cook, breaking up.
4. Pieces with a spoon, till no longer pink & just beginning to brown, 3 to 4 mins. Include remaining beef & cook, breaking up pieces with spoon, till no longer pink, 3 to 4 mins.
5. Include beans, tomatoes, tomato puree, & 1/2 Tsp. Salt; turn it to boil, then reduce heat to low & simmer, covered, occasionally stirring, for 1 hr.
6. Remove cover & continue to simmer 1 hr longer, occasionally stirring (if chilli begins to stick to the bottom of the pot, stir in 1/2 cup water & continue to simmer), till beef is tender & chilli is dark, rich, & slightly thickened.
7. Season with salt to taste. Serve with lime wedges & condiments, if desired.

25. CHILI CON CARNE

Prep Time: *Cook Time:* *Servings: 4*
5 Minutes *55 Minutes*

INGREDIENTS:

- Tbsps. ancho chilli powder or 3 chiles (about 1/2 ounce), toasted & ground
- Tbsps. new Mexican chilli powder or 3 medium chiles (about 3/4 ounce), toasted & ground
- Tbsps. cumin seeds, toasted
- Tbsps. dried oregano, preferably Mexican 7 1/2 cups plus 2/3 cup water
- 1 (4-lb) chuck-eye roast, trimmed & cut into 1-inch pieces salt & pepper
- slices bacon, cut into 1/4-inch pieces
- 1 onion, chopped fine
- 5 garlic cloves, minced
- 4–5 small jalapeño chiles, stemmed, seeded, & minced
- cup canned crushed tomatoes or plain tomato sauce
- 2 Tbsps. lime juice
- 5 Tbsps. Masa or 3 Tbsps. cornstarch

DIRECTIONS:

1. Combine chilli powders, cumin, & oregano in the small container & stir in 1/2 cup water to form a thick paste; set aside.
2. Season beef with 2 Tbsps. Salt; set aside.
3. Cook bacon in the oven over medium-low heat till crisp, about 10 mins.
4. Using a slotted spoon, Shift bacon to the paper towel-lined plate. Pour all but 2 Tbsps. Fat into a small container; set aside.
5. Increase heat to medium-high & sauté the meat in 4 batches till well browned on all sides, about 5 mins per batch, including an additional 2 Tbsps.
6. Bacon fat to pot as necessary. Reduce heat to medium & Include 3 Tbsps. Bacon fat to now-empty pan.
7. Include onion & cook till softened, 5 to 7 mins. Include garlic & jalapeños & cook till fragrant, about 1 min. Include chile paste & cook till fragrant, 2 to 3 mins.
8. Include reserved bacon & browned beef, crushed tomatoes, lime juice, & 7 cups water & bring to simmer.
9. Continue to simmer till meat is tender & juices are dark, rich, & starting to thicken, about 2 hrs.
10. Mix masa with remaining 2/3 cup water (or cornstarch with 3 Tbsps. water) in a small container to form a smooth paste.
11. Increase heat to medium, stir in pasta, & simmer till thickened, 5 to 10 mins.
12. Season with salt & pepper to taste & serve.

26. ULTIMATE BEEF CHILI

Prep Time: *Cook Time:* *Servings: 2*
5 Minutes *15 Minutes*

INGREDIENTS:

- Salt
- 8 ounces (1 1/4 cups) dried pinto beans, picked over & rinsed
- dried ancho chiles, stemmed, seeded, & torn into 1-inch pieces 2–4 dried de árbol chiles, stemmed, seeded, & split into 2 pieces
- 3 Tbsps. cornmeal
- 2 Tbsps. dried oregano
- 2 Tbsps. ground cumin
- 2 Tbsps. cocoa
- 2 1/2 cups low-sodium chicken broth 2 onions, cut into 3/4-inch pieces
- 3 small jalapeño chiles, stemmed, seeded, & cut into 1/2-inch pieces 3 Tbsps. vegetable oil
- 4 garlic cloves, minced
- 1 (14.5-ounce) can diced tomatoes
- 2 Tbsps. molasses
- 3 1/2 lbs blade steak, 3/4 inch thick, trimmed & cut into 3/4-inch pieces 1 (12-ounce) bottle mild lager, such as Budweiser

DIRECTIONS:

1. Combine 3 Tbsps. Salt, 4 quarts water, & beans in a Dutch oven & bring to boil over high heat. Remove pot from heat, cover, & let stand 1 hr. Drain & rinse well.
2. Set oven rack to lower-middle setting & heat oven to 300 degrees.
3. Place ancho chiles in the 12-inch pan set over medium-high heat; toast, frequently stirring, till the flesh is fragrant, 4 to 6 mins, reducing heat if chiles begin to smoke.
4. Shift to food processor & cool. Do not wash out the pan.
5. Include de árbol chiles, cornmeal, oregano, cumin, cocoa, & 1/2Tsp. Salt to food processor with toasted ancho chiles; process till finely ground, about 2 mins.
6. With processor running, slowly Include 1/2 cup broth till smooth paste forms, about 45 seconds, scraping downsides of the container as necessary.
7. Shift paste to a small container. Place onions in now-empty processor & pulse till roughly chopped, about 4 pulses. Include jalapeños & pulse till the consistency of chunky salsa, about 4 pulses, scraping down container as necessary.
8. Heat 1 Tbsp. Oil in a Dutch oven overheats medium to high flame.
9. Include onion batter & cook, occasionally stirring, till the moisture has evaporated & vegetables are softened, 7 to 9 mins.
10. Include garlic & cook till fragrant, about 1 min. Include chile paste, tomatoes, & molasses; stir till chile paste is thoroughly combined.
11. Include remaining 2 cups broth & drained beans; bring to boil, then reduce heat to simmer.
12. Meanwhile, heat 1 Tbsp. Oil in 12-inch pan over medium-high heat till shimmering. Pat beef dry with paper towels & sprinkle with 1 Tsp. Salt.
13. Include half of beef & cook till browned on all sides, about 10 mins. Shift meat to a Dutch oven.
14. Include half of the beer to the pan, scraping up browned bits from the bottom of the pan, & bring to simmer. Shift beer to Dutch oven.
15. Repeat with remaining 1 Tbsp. oil, remaining steak, & remaining beer. Stir to combine & return batter to simmer.
16. Cover pot & Shift to oven. Cook till meat & beans are fully tender, 1 1/2 to 2 hrs.
17. Let chilli stand, uncovered, for 10 mins. Stir well, season with salt to taste, & serve. (Chili can be refrigerated for up to 3 days.)

27. WHITE CHICKEN CHILI

Prep Time: *Cook Time:* *Servings: 2*
5 Minutes *35 Minutes*

INGREDIENTS:

- lbs bone-in split chicken breasts or thighs, trimmed salt & pepper
- Tbsp. vegetable oil, plus extra as needed
- 3 jalapeño chiles
- 3 poblano chiles, stemmed, seeded, & cut into large pieces
- 3 New Mexican chile peppers, stemmed, seeded, & cut into large chunks 2 onions, cut into large pieces
- 6 garlic cloves, minced
- Tbsp. ground cumin
- 1 1/2 Tbsps. ground coriander
- (15-ounce) cans cannellini beans, rinsed
- 3 cups low-sodium chicken broth
- 3 Tbsps. lime juice (2 limes)
- 1/4 cup minced fresh cilantro
- scallions, sliced thin

DIRECTIONS:

1. Season chicken with 1 Tsp. Salt & 1/4 Tsp. Pepper.
2. Heat oil in a Dutch oven after setting medium-high heat till just smoking. Include chicken, skin side down, & cook without moving till the skin is golden brown, about 4 mins.
3. Using tongs, flip chicken & lightly brown on another side, about 2 mins. Shift chicken to plate; remove & discard skin.
4. While chicken is browning, remove & discard ribs & seeds from 2 jalapeños, then mince jalapeños & set aside. Process half of poblano Chiles, New Mexican chiles, & onions in the food processor till the consistency of chunky salsa, 10 to 12 pulses, scraping down sides of container halfway through.
5. Shift batter to the medium container. Repeat with remaining poblano chiles, New Mexican chiles, & onions; combine with the first batch (do not wash food processor).
6. Pour off all but 1 Tbsp. Fat from Dutch oven (including additional vegetable oil if necessary) & reduce heat to medium. Include minced jalapeños, chile batter, garlic, cumin, coriander, & 1/4 Tsp. Salt.
7. Cover & cook, occasionally stirring, till vegetables have softened, about 10 mins. Remove pot from heat.
8. Shift 1 cup cooked vegetable batter to the now-empty food processor.
9. Include 1 cup beans & 1 cup broth & process till smooth, about 20 seconds.
10. Include vegetable-bean batter, remaining 2 cups broth, & chicken breasts to Dutch oven & bring to boil over medium-high heat.
11. Reduce heat to medium-low & simmer, covered, occasionally stirring, till chicken registers 160 degrees (175 degrees if using thighs), 15 to 20 mins (40 mins if using thighs).
12. Shift chicken to a large plate. Stir in remaining beans & continue to simmer, uncovered, till beans are heated through & chilli has thickened slightly about 10 mins.
13. Mince remaining jalapeño, reserving & mincing ribs & seeds, & set aside. After cooling enough to handle, shred chicken into bite-size pieces, discarding bones.
14. Stir shredded chicken, lime juice, cilantro, scallions, & remaining minced jalapeño (with seeds if desired) into chilli & return to simmer.
15. Season with salt & pepper to taste & serve.

28. LIGHTER CHICKEN & DUMPLINGS

Prep Time:□*5* *Cook Time:*□*20* *Servings: 4*
Minutes *Minutes*

INGREDIENTS:

- 2 1/2 lbs bone-in chicken thighs, trimmed
- Salt & pepper
- Tbsps. vegetable oil
- small onions, chopped fine
- carrots, peeled & cut into 3/4-inch pieces
- 1 celery rib, chopped fine
- 1/4 cup dry sherry
- cups low-sodium chicken broth
- 1 Tsp. minced fresh thyme
- 1 lb chicken wings
- 1/4 cup chopped fresh parsley
- cups (10 ounces) all-purpose flour
- 1 Tsp. sugar
- 1 Tsp. salt
- 1/2 Tsp. baking soda
- 3/4 cup buttermilk, chilled
- 4 Tbsps. unsalted butter, melted & hot
- 1 large egg white

DIRECTIONS:

1. Pat chicken thighs for drying with paper towels & season with 1 Tsp. Salt & 1/4 Tsp. Pepper. Heat oil in a Dutch oven after setting medium-high heat till shimmering.
2. Include chicken thighs, skin side down, & cook till the skin is crisp & well browned, 5 to 7 mins. Using tongs, flip chicken pieces & brown on the second side, 5 to 7 mins longer; Shift to a large plate. Discard all but 1 Tsp. Fat from the pot.

3. Include onions, carrots, & celery to now-empty pot; cook, occasionally stirring, till caramelized, 7 to 9 mins.
4. Mix the sherry and remove the brown spots from the bottom of the pool. Mix the broth and thyme. Put the juicy chicken thighs back into the pan and add the chicken wings.
5. Simmer for 45-55 minutes, cover and cook until the thigh meat can't stand being stabbed and sticking to the bones.
6. Remove pot from heat & Shift chicken to cutting board. Allow broth to settle for 5 mins, then skim fat from the surface.
7. When cool enough to handle, remove & discard chicken skin. With the fingers or a fork, pick up the meat from the chicken thighs (and wings, if desired) & cut it into 1-inch pieces.
8. Return the beef to the pan. (At the end, the stew cooled to room temperature, then refrigerated for up to 2 days. Bring to a boil over medium-low heat before continuing.)
9. Whisk flour, sugar, salt, & baking soda in a large container. Combine buttermilk & melted butter in a medium container, stirring till butter forms small clumps; whisk in egg white.
10. Include buttermilk batter to dry ingredients & stir with a rubber spatula till just incorporated & batter pulls away from sides of the container.
11. Return stew to simmer, stir in parsley, & season with salt and Pepper to taste. Using greased Tbsp. Measure each scoop level amount of batter & drop over the top of the stew, spacing about 1/4 inch apart.
12. Wrap lid of Dutch oven with a clean kitchen towel (keeping towel away from heat source) & cover pot.
13. Simmer gently till dumplings have doubled in size & toothpick inserted into the centre comes out clean, 13 to 16 mins. Serve immediately.

29. QUICK CHICKEN FRICASSEE

Prep Time: 5 Minutes *Cook Time: 20 Minutes* *Servings: 4*

INGREDIENTS:

- lbs boneless, skinless chicken breasts and/or thighs, trimmed salt & pepper
- Tbsp. unsalted butter
- Tbsp. olive oil
- lb cremini mushrooms, trimmed & sliced 1/4 inch thick
- onion, chopped fine
- 1/4 cup dry white wine
- Tbsp. all-purpose flour
- garlic clove, minced
- 1 1/2 cups low-sodium chicken broth
- 1/3 cup sour cream
- 1 large egg yolk
- 1/2 Tsp. freshly grated nutmeg
- Tbsps. lemon juice
- Tbsps. minced fresh tarragon

IDIRECTIONS:

1. Chicken pat after drying with paper towels & season with 1 Tsp. Salt & 1/2 Tsp. Pepper. Heat butter & oil in the 12-inch pan over medium-high heat till butter is melted.
2. Place chicken in the pan & cook till browned, about 4 mins. Using tongs, flip chicken & cook till browned on the second side, about 4 mins longer. Shift chicken to a large plate.
3. Include mushrooms, onion, & wine to the now-empty pan & cook, occasionally stirring, till the liquid has evaporated & mushrooms are browned, 8 to 10 mins.
4. Include flour & garlic; cook, constantly stirring, 1 min. Include broth & bring the batter to boil, scraping up browned bits the bottom of the pan includes chicken & any accumulated juices into the pan.
5. Reduce heat to medium-low, cover, & simmer till breasts register 160 degrees & thighs register 175 degrees, 5 to 10 mins.
6. Shift chicken to clean platter & tent loosely with aluminium foil.
7. Whisk sour cream & egg yolk together in a medium container. Whisking constantly, slowly stir 1/2 cup hot sauce into the sour cream batter to temper.
8. Stirring constantly, slowly pour sour cream batter into the simmering sauce. Stir in nutmeg, lemon juice, & tarragon; return to simmer.
9. Present with salt & pepper for taste, pour sauce over chicken, & serve.

Dinner Recipes

30. COQ AU VIN

Prep Time: 5 Minutes *Cook Time: 15 Minutes* *Servings: 6*

INGREDIENTS:

- chicken leg quarters (about 3 lbs), trimmed, thighs & drumsticks separated salt & pepper
- (750-ml) bottle medium-bodied red wine 2 1/2 cups low-sodium chicken broth
- Tsp. Dried thyme
- parsley stems plus 2 Tbsps. minced fresh parsley
- 1 bay leaf
- 5 slices thick-cut bacon, cut into 1/4-inch pieces
- 6-7 Tbsps. unsalted butter, room temperature
- large carrot, chopped coarse,
- large onion, chopped coarsely
- 2 shallots, peeled & quartered
- 2 garlic cloves, skin on & smashed
- 1 1/2 Tbsps. tomato paste
- 3/4 cup frozen pearl onions, thawed

DIRECTIONS:

1. Ounces white mushrooms, trimmed & halved if medium or quartered if large 2-3 Tbsps. All-purpose flour chicken pat dry with paper towels & season with salt & pepper; set aside.
2. Bring red wine & chicken broth to boil in a large saucepan; reduce heat to medium-high & simmer till reduced to about 4 cups, about 20 mins.
3. Assemble thyme, parsley, & bay leaf together in a double layer of cheesecloth & tie securely with kitchen twine to form bouquet garni.
4. Therefore, cook bacon in a Dutch oven over medium heat till the fat has rendered & bacon is crisp, 5 to 7 mins. Remove bacon with slotted spoon to the paper towel-lined plate; set aside.
5. Heat 1 Tbsp. Butter with rendered bacon fat; Include carrot, onion, shallots, & garlic & sauté till lightly browned 10 to 15 mins. Press vegetables against side of cooking wok with a slotted spoon to squeeze out as much fat as possible; Shift vegetables to cooking wok with reduced wine batter (off heat) & discard all but 1 Tbsp. Fat from Dutch oven.
6. Include 1 Tbsp. Butter to Dutch oven & heat over medium-high heat. Include chicken (in batches if necessary to avoid overcrowding) & cook till well browned, 12 to 16 mins.
7. Shift chicken to plate; set aside. Pour off fat from Dutch oven; return to heat & Include wine-vegetable batter. To bring to boil, browned bits from the bottom of the pan .
8. Include browned chicken, bouquet garni, & tomato paste, bring to simmer, then reduce to low & simmer gently, partially covered, till chicken is tender, flipping once, 45 to 60 mins.
9. While chicken & sauce are cooking, heat 2 Tbsps. The butter melted in a medium pan over medium-low heat.
10. Include pearl onions & cook, occasionally stirring, till lightly browned & almost cooked through, 5 to 8 mins. Include mushrooms, season with salt, cover, increase heat to medium, & cook till mushrooms release their liquid, about 5 mins.
11. Uncover, increase heat to high, & boil till liquid evaporates & onions & mushrooms are golden browns, 2 to 3 mins longer. Shift onions & mushrooms to plate with bacon; set aside.
12. Shift chicken to platter & tent loosely with aluminium foil. Strain sauce through a fine-mesh strainer into the large measuring cup, pressing on solids to release as much liquid as possible.
13. Return sauce to cooking wok & skim the fat off the surface. For each cup of sauce, mash 1 Tbsp. each butter & flour in a small container or plate to make beurre manié (you should have 2 to 3 Tbsps. each of butter and flour).
14. Bring sauce to boil & whisk in beurre manié till smooth. Include reserved chicken, bacon, onions & mushrooms; season with salt & pepper to taste, reduce heat to medium-low, & simmer gently to warm through & blend flavours, about 5 mins.
15. Present with salt & pepper to taste & stir in minced parsley. Shift chicken to a serving platter, pour sauce over chicken, & serve immediately.

31. CHICKEN BOUILLABAISSE

Prep Time: 5 Minutes *Cook Time: 35 Minutes* *Servings: 2*

INGREDIENTS:

- lbs bone-in chicken pieces (breasts, thighs, & drumsticks, with breasts cut in half), trimmed
- 2 Tbsps. olive oil
- large leek, white & light green parts only, halved lengthwise, sliced thin, & washed thoroughly
- small fennel bulb, stalks discarded, halved, cored, & sliced thin
- 4 garlic cloves, minced
- Tbsp. tomato paste
- Tbsp. All-purpose flour 1/4 Tsp. Saffron threads 1/4 Tsp. cayenne pepper
- 3 cups low-sodium chicken broth
- (14.5-ounce) can diced to
- small garlic cloves, minced 1/4 Tsp. cayenne pepper 1/2 cup vegetable oil
- 1/2 cup plus 2 Tbsps. extra-virgin olive oil Salt & pepper
- matoes, drained
- ounces Yukon Gold potatoes, cut into 3/4-inch pieces 1/2 cup dry white wine
- 1/4 cup pastis or Pernod
- 1 (3-inch) strip orange zest
- 1 Tbsp. chopped fresh tarragon or parsley
- 3 Tbsps. water
- 1/4 Tsp. saffron threads
- 1 (12-inch) baguette
- Tbsps. lemon juice
- 1 large egg yolk
- Tbsps. Dijon mustard

DIRECTIONS:

1. Set oven racks to middle & lower settings & heat oven to 375 degrees. Chicken after drying with paper towels & season with salt & pepper. Heat oil in a Dutch oven after setting medium-high heat till just smoking.
2. Include chicken pieces, skin side down, & cook without moving till well browned 5 to 8 mins. Using tongs, flip chicken & brown another side, about 3 mins. Shift chicken to a large plate.
3. Include leek & fennel & cook, often stirring, till vegetables begin to soften & turn translucent about 4 mins. Include garlic, tomato paste, flour, saffron, & cayenne & cook till fragrant, about 30 seconds. Include broth, tomatoes, potatoes, wine, pastis, & orange zest; bring to simmer.
4. Reduce heat to medium-low & simmer for 10 mins.
5. Nestle chicken thighs & drumsticks into the simmering liquid with the skin above the surface of the liquid; cook, uncovered, 5 mins.
6. Nestle breast pieces into the simmering liquid, Setting pieces as necessary to ensure skin stays above the surface of the liquid. Bake on the middle rack, uncovered, till breasts register 145 degrees & thighs/drumsticks register 160 degrees 10 to 20 mins.
7. While chicken cooks, microwave water & saffron in a medium microwave-safe container till water is steaming, 10 to 20 seconds. Let sit for 5 mins.
8. Cut a 3-inch piece off the baguette; remove & discard crust. Tear crustless bread into 1-inch chunks (you should have about 1 cup).
9. Stir bread pieces & lemon juice into saffron-infused water; soak 5 mins. By using a whisk, mash soaked bread batter till uniform paste forms, 1 to 2 mins.
10. Whisk in egg yolk, mustard, garlic, & cayenne till smooth for 15 seconds. Mixing constantly, drizzle in vegetable oil in a steady stream till smooth mayonnaise-like consistency is reached, scraping down container as necessary. Slowly whisk in 1/2 cup olive oil in a steady stream till smooth. Season with salt & pepper to taste.
11. Cut remaining baguette into 3/4-inch-thick slices. To keep slices in a single layer on a rimmed baking sheet. Drizzle with remaining 2 Tbsps. Olive oil & season with salt & pepper to taste.
12. Bake on lower rack till light golden brown (can be toasted while bouillabaisse is in the oven), 10 to 15 mins.
13. Remove bouillabaisse & croutons from oven. Setting oven rack 6 inches from broiler element & heat broiler.
14. Return bouillabaisse to oven & cook till chicken skin is crisp & breast registers 160 degrees & drumsticks/thighs register 175 degrees, 5 to 10 mins (smaller pieces may cook faster than larger pieces; remove individual pieces as they reach correct temperature).
15. Shift chicken pieces to a large plate. Skim excess fat from broth. Stir tarragon into broth & season with salt & pepper to taste. Shift broth & potatoes to a large shallow serving container & top with chicken pieces.
16. Drizzle 1 Tbsp. Rouille over each portion & spread 1 Tsp. rouille on each crouton. Serve, floating 2 croutons in each container & passing remaining croutons & rouille separately.

32. CHICKEN CACCIATORE WITH PORTOBELLO MUSHROOMS & SAGE

Prep Time: 5 Minutes *Cook Time: 25 Minutes* *Servings: 4*

INGREDIENTS:

- (5-to 7-ounce) bone-in chicken thighs, trimmed salt & pepper
- Tsp. olive oil
- onion, chopped
- medium portobello mushroom caps, cut into 3/4-inch cubes
- 4 garlic cloves, minced
- 1 1/2 Tbsps. all-purpose flour
- 1 1/2 cups dry red wine
- 1/2 cup low-sodium chicken broth
- (14.5-ounce) can diced tomatoes, drained
- 2 Tbsps. minced fresh thyme
- Parmesan cheese rind (optional)
- Tbsps. minced fresh sage

DIRECTIONS:

1. Season chicken with salt & pepper.
2. Heat oil in a Dutch oven after setting medium-high heat till shimmering, about 2 mins.
3. Include 4 chicken thighs, skin side down, & cook without moving till the skin is crisp & well browned, about 5 mins. Using tongs, flip chicken & brown on the second side, about 5 mins longer. Shift chicken to large plate; brown remaining 4 chicken thighs, Shift to the plate, & set aside.
4. Drain off all but 1 Tbsp. Fat from the pot. Include onion, mushrooms, & 1/2 Tsp. salt & cook over medium-high heat, stirring occasionally, till vegetables are beginning to brown, 6 to 8 mins. After cooling enough to handle, remove & discard skin.
5. Include garlic in the pot & cook till fragrant, about 30 seconds. Stir in flour & cook, constantly stirring, about 1 min. Include wine, scraping browned bits from the bottom of the pot. Stir in broth, tomatoes, thyme, cheese rind if using 1/2 Tsp. Salt (omit salt if using cheese rind) & pepper to taste.
6. Submerge chicken pieces in liquid & bring to boil; cover, reduce heat to low, & simmer till chicken is tender & cooked through, about 45 mins, turning chicken pieces halfway through cooking.
7. Discard cheese rind, stir in sage, season with salt & pepper to taste, & serve.

33. CHICKEN CHASSEUR

Prep Time: *5 Minutes* | *Cook Time:* *55 Minutes* | *Servings: 2*

INGREDIENTS:

- (10-to 12-ounce) bone-in split chicken breasts, trimmed salt & pepper
- 2 Tbsps. vegetable oil
- ounces white mushrooms, trimmed & sliced 1/8 inch thick
- 1 shallot, minced
- 3 Tbsps. brandy or cognac
- 1/2 cup dry white wine
- 3 1/2 cups low-sodium chicken broth
- 1/3 cup canned diced tomatoes, drained
- Tbsps. unsalted butter, cut into 4 pieces & chilled
- 1 Tbsp. minced fresh parsley
- 1 Tbsp. minced fresh tarragon

DIRECTIONS:

1. Set oven rack to middle setting; heat oven to 400 degrees. Season chicken with salt & pepper. Heat oil in the 12-inch pan over medium-high heat till almost smoking.
2. Include chicken, skin side down, & cook without moving till the skin is crisp & well browned, 5 to 8 mins. Using tongs, flip chicken & brown on the second side, about 5 mins longer. Place browned chicken, skin side up, on baking sheet & set aside.
3. Pour off all but 2 Tbsps. Fat from pan. Include mushrooms & cook over medium-high heat till mushrooms start to brown, 6 to 8 Mins. Reduce heat to medium & Include shallot; cook till softened, about 1 min longer.
4. Off heat, Include brandy & let warm through, about 5 seconds.
5. Wave lit match over the pan to ignite, then shake cooking wok to distribute flames.
6. When flames subside, return pan to medium-high heat, Include wine, & scrape browned bits from the bottom of the pan. Simmer till reduced to glaze, about 3 mins.
7. Include broth & tomatoes & simmer till liquid, mushrooms, & tomatoes measure 1 1/2 cups, about 25 mins.
8. While sauce simmers, place chicken in the oven. Cook till chicken registers 160 degrees, 15 to 20 mins. Shift chicken pieces to serving platter & tent loosely with aluminium foil.
9. When the sauce is properly reduced, whisk in butter, 1 piece at a time, till melted & incorporated.
10. Include parsley & tarragon & season with salt & pepper to taste. Spoon sauce over chicken & serve immediately.

34. CHICKEN PROVENÇAL

Prep Time: *5 Minutes* | *Cook Time:* *25 Minutes* | *Servings: 2*

INGREDIENTS:

- (5-to 7-ounce) bone-in chicken thighs, trimmed salt
- Tbsp. extra-virgin olive oil
- small onion, chopped fine
- 6 garlic cloves, minced
- anchovy fillet, rinsed & minced 1/8 Tsp. cayenne pepper
- cup dry white wine
- (14.5-ounce) can diced tomatoes, drained
- cup low-sodium chicken broth
- 2 1/2 Tbsps. tomato paste
- 1 1/2 Tbsps. chopped fresh thyme
- Tsp. chopped fresh oregano
- Tsp. herbes de Provence (optional)
- bay leaf
- 1 1/2 Tbsps. grated lemon zest
- 1/2 cup niçoise olives pitted
- Tbsp. chopped fresh parsley

DIRECTIONS:

1. Set oven rack to lower-middle setting; heat oven to 300 degrees.
2. Present both sides of the chicken with salt. Heat 1 Tsp. Oil Heat oil in a Dutch oven after setting medium-high heat till shimmering.
3. Include 4 chicken thighs, skin side down, & cook without moving till the skin is crisp & well browned, about 5 mins. Using tongs, flip chicken & brown on the second side, about 5 mins longer; Shift to a large plate.
4. Repeat with remaining 4 chicken thighs & Shift to plate; set aside. Discard all but 1 Tbsp. Fat from the pot.
5. Include onion to fat in Dutch oven & cook, occasionally stirring, over medium heat till browned, about 4 mins.
6. Include garlic, anchovy, & cayenne; cook, constantly stirring, till fragrant, about 1 min. Cover the wine and scrape the brown pieces off the bottom of the pan.
7. Stir in the tomatoes, chicken stock, tomato paste, thyme, oregano, Provencal herbs (if used) and bay leaves.
8. Remove & discard skin from chicken thighs, then submerge the chicken in liquid & Include accumulated chicken juices in the pot.
9. The heat increased from low to high, bring to simmer, cover, & Shift pot to oven; cook till chicken offers no resistance about 1 1/4 hrs.
10. Using a slotted spoon, Shift chicken to serving platter & tent with aluminium foil. Dutch oven set over high heat, stir in 1 Tsp. Lemon zest, bring to boil, & cook, occasionally stirring, till slightly thickened & reduced to 2 cups, about 5 mins. Stir in olives & cook till heated through about 1 min.
11. Meanwhile, mix remaining 1/2 Tsp. Parsley. The spoon sauce over chicken, drizzle chicken with remaining 2 Tbsps. Olive oil, sprinkle with parsley batter, & serve.

35. CHICKEN PAPRIKASH

Prep Time: *5 Minutes* | *Cook Time:* *20 Minutes* | *Servings: 6*

INGREDIENTS:

- (5-to 7-ounce) bone-in chicken thighs, trimmed salt & pepper
- Tsp. Vegetable oil
- large onion, halved & sliced thin
- large red bell pepper, stemmed, seeded, halved widthwise, & cut into 1/4-inch strips
- large green bell pepper, stemmed, seeded, halved widthwise, & cut into 1/4-inch strips 3 1/2 Tbsps. paprika
- Tbsp. all-purpose flour
- 1/4 Tsp. dried marjoram
- 1/2 cup dry white wine
- (14.5-ounce) can diced tomatoes, drained 1/3 cup sour cream
- 2 Tbsps. chopped fresh parsley

DIRECTIONS:

1. Set oven rack to lower-middle setting; heat oven to 300 degrees.
2. Present both sides of chicken with salt & pepper. Heat oil in a Dutch oven after setting medium-high heat till shimmering.
3. Include 4 chicken thighs, skin side down, & cook without moving till the skin is crisp & well browned, about 5 mins. Using tongs, flip chicken & brown on the second side, about 5 mins longer; Shift to a large plate. Repeat with remaining 4 chicken thighs & Shift to plate; set aside.
4. After the chicken is cooling, remove & discard skin. Discard all but 1 Tbsp. Fat from pan.
5. Include onion to fat left in Dutch oven & cook, occasionally stirring, over medium heat till softened, 5 to 7 mins. Include bell peppers & cook, occasionally stirring, till onions are browned & peppers are softened, about 3 mins.
6. Stir in 3 Tbsps. Paprika, flour, & marjoram & cook, constantly stirring, till fragrant, about 1 min.
7. Include wine, scraping up browned bits from the bottom of the pot; stir in tomatoes & 1 Tsp. Salt. Include chicken & any accumulated juices, submerging them in vegetables; bring to a simmer, then cover & place the pot in the oven.
8. After cooking till chicken is no longer pink when cut into with paring knife, about 30 mins. Remove pot from oven.
9. Combine sour cream & remaining 1/2 Tbsp. Paprika in a small container.
10. Place chicken on individual plates. Stir a few Tbsps. Of sauce into sour cream to temper, then stir batter back into the sauce in the pot.
11. Spoon sauce & peppers over chicken, sprinkle with parsley, & serve immediately

36. CHICKEN CANZANESE

Prep Time: *5 Minutes* | *Cook Time:* *15 Minutes* | *Servings: 4*

INGREDIENTS:

- 1 Tbsp. olive oil
- ounces prosciutto (1/4 inch thick), cut into 1/4-inch pieces
- 4 garlic cloves, sliced thin
- 8 (5-to 7-ounce) bone-in chicken thighs, trimmed salt & pepper
- Tbsps. all-purpose flour
- cups dry white wine
- cup low-sodium chicken broth
- 12 whole fresh sage leaves
- sprig fresh rosemary leaves removed & minced fine, stem reserved
- 4 whole cloves
- 2 bay leaves
- 1/4–1/2 Tsp. red pepper flakes
- Tbsps. unsalted butter
- 1 Tbsp. lemon juice

DIRECTIONS:

1. Set oven rack to lower-middle setting & heat oven to 325 degrees.
2. Heat 1 Tsp. Oil in 12-inch oven-safe pan over medium heat till shimmering. Include prosciutto & cook, frequently stirring, till just starting to brown, about 3 mins.
3. Include garlic slices & cook, frequently stirring, till garlic is golden brown, about 1 1/2 mins. Using a slotted spoon, Shift garlic & prosciutto to a small container & set it aside. Do not rinse the pan.
4. Increase heat to medium-high; include remaining 2 Tbsps. Oil & heat till just smoking. Chicken pat after drying with paper towels & season with pepper.
5. Include chicken, skin side down, & cook without moving till well browned 5 to 8 mins. Using tongs, flip chicken & brown on the second side, about 5 mins longer. Shift chicken to a large plate.
6. Remove all but 2 Tbsps. fat from pan. Sprinkle flour over fat & cook, constantly stirring, for 1 min.
7. Slowly Include wine & broth; bring to simmer, scraping up browned bits from the bottom of the pan. Cook till liquid is slightly reduced, 3 mins.
8. Stir in sage leaves, rosemary stem, cloves, bay leaves, pepper flakes, & reserved prosciutto & garlic.
9. Nestle chicken into liquid, skin side up (skin should be above the surface of the liquid), & bake, uncovered, till fork slips easily in & out meat, but meat is not falling off bones, about 1 1/4 hrs. (Check the chicken after 15 mins; broth should be barely bubbling.
10. Shift chicken to serving platter & tent with aluminium foil. Remove & discard sage leaves, rosemary stem, cloves, & bay leaves.
11. Place pan over high heat & bring sauce to boil. Cook till sauce is reduced to 1 1/4 cups, 2 to 5 mins. Off heat, stir in minced rosemary, butter, & lemon juice.
12. Season with salt & pepper to taste. Pour sauce around chicken & serve.

37. MOROCCAN CHICKEN WITH OLIVES & LEMON

Prep Time: *5 Minutes* | *Cook Time:* *20 Minutes* | *Servings: 4*

INGREDIENTS:

- 1 1/4 Tbsps. paprika
- 1/2 Tsp. ground cumin
- 1/2 Tsp. ground ginger
- 1/4 Tsp. cayenne pepper
- 1/4 Tsp. ground coriander
- 1/4 Tsp. ground cinnamon
- (2-inch) strips lemon zest
- 5 garlic cloves, minced
- 1 (3 1/2- to 4-lb) whole chicken, cut into 8 pieces (4 breast pieces, 2 thighs, 2 drumsticks), trimmed, wings discarded
- Salt & pepper
- Tbsp. olive oil

- large onion, halved & sliced 1/4 inch thick 1 3/4 cups low-sodium chicken broth
- Tbsp. honey
- carrots, peeled & cut crosswise into 1/2-inch-thick rounds, very large pieces cut into half-moons
- cup cracked green olives, pitted & halved
- 3 Tbsps. lemon juice
- 2 Tbsps. chopped fresh cilantro

DIRECTIONS:

1. Combine paprika, cumin, ginger, cayenne, coriander, & cinnamon in the small container & set aside. Mince 1 strip lemon zest & combine with 1 Tsp. Minced garlic & mince together till reduced to a fine paste; set aside.
2. Present both sides of chicken pieces with salt & pepper. Heat oil in a Dutch oven after setting medium-high heat till beginning to smoke.
3. Include chicken pieces, skin side down, & cook without moving till the skin is deep golden, about 5 mins. Using tongs, flip chicken pieces & brown on the second side, about 4 mins longer.
4. Shift chicken to large plate; when cool enough to handle, remove & discard skin. Pour off & discard all but 1 Tbsp. Fat from the pot.
5. Include onion & 2 remaining lemon zest strips to pot & cook, occasionally stirring, till onion slices have browned but still retain their shape, 5 to 7 mins (Include 1 Tbsp. water if cooking wok gets too dark).
6. Include remaining 4 Tbsps. Garlic & cook, stirring, till fragrant. Include spices & cook, constantly stirring, till darkened & very fragrant, 45 seconds to 1 min.
7. Stir in broth & honey, scraping up browned bits from the bottom of the pot. Include thighs & drumsticks, reduce heat to medium, & simmer for 5 mins.
8. Include carrots & breast pieces with any accumulated juices to the pot, arranging breast pieces in a single layer on top of carrots. Cover, reduce heat to medium-low, & simmer till breast pieces register 160 degrees, 10 to 15 mins.
9. Shift chicken to plate & tent with aluminium foil. Include olives to pot; increase heat to medium-high & simmer till the liquid has thickened slightly & carrots are tender, 4 to 6 mins.
10. Return chicken to pot & stir in garlic butter, lemon juice, & cilantro; season with salt & pepper to taste. Serve immediately.

38. BOUILLABAISSE-STYLE FISH STEW

Prep Time:	*Cook Time:*	*Servings: 4*
5 Minutes	*35 Minutes*	

INGREDIENTS:

- 1 1/2 lbs skinless fish fillets, cut into 1-to 1 1/2-inch cubes
- ounces medium shrimp (41 to 50 per lb) peeled & deveined, shells reserved
- ounces large sea scallops, tendons removed & scallops halved
- 1/3 cup shredded fresh basil
- 1/4 cup olive oil
- Tbsps. Pernod
- garlic cloves, minced
- 2 Tbsps. salt
- 1/2 Tsp. saffron threads
- 1/4 Tsp. red pepper flakes
- 2 onions, chopped
- fennel bulb stalks discarded, halved, cored, & chopped
- large carrot, chopped
- 1/4 cup olive oil
- garlic heads, outer papery skin removed, heads intact
- 1 (750-ml) bottle dry white wine
- 2 (28-ounce) can diced tomatoes, drained with juice reserved
- 3 lbs fish frames, cleaned & cut into 6-inch pieces 4 cups water
- large leeks, white & light green parts only, halved lengthwise, chopped, & washed thoroughly
- bunch fresh parsley stems only
- 5 sprigs of fresh thyme
- 2 bay leaves
- 2 Tbsps. whole black peppercorns
- 2 Tbsps. salt
- 8 (2-inch) strips orange zest (2 oranges)
- 1/2 Tsp. saffron threads
- lbs mussels, scrubbed & debearded GARLIC TOASTS

DIRECTIONS:

1. Combine all the ingredients.
2. Bring to simmer on the medium-high heat, pressing down on fish bones occasionally with a spoon to submerge till stock is rich & flavorful, about 1 hr.

39. RED PEPPER ROUILLE

Prep Time:	*Cook Time:*	*Servings: 6*
5 Minutes	*25 Minutes*	

INGREDIENTS:

- Red pepper
- oil
- salt

DIRECTIONS:

1. Combine all ingredients (except shrimp shells) in a large container. Toss well, cover flush with plastic wrap, & refrigerate for 4 hrs.
2. Meanwhile, stir onions, fennel, carrot, & oil together in a large stockpot or Dutch oven.
3. Cover pot & set over medium-low heat; cook, frequently stirring, till vegetables are fragrant, about 15 mins.
4. Place garlic in a large heavy-duty zipper-lock bag & seal. Smash garlic with a rolling pin or meat labour till flattened.
5. Include smashed garlic to vegetables & continue to cook, frequently stirring, till vegetables are dry & just beginning to stick, about 15 mins longer.
6. Include wine & stir to scrape the pot bottom, then Include tomatoes with their juice, fish frames, shrimp shells, water, leeks, parsley stems, thyme, bay leaves, peppercorns, & salt.
7. Bring to simmer on the medium-high heat, pressing down on fish bones occasionally with a spoon to submerge till stock is rich & flavorful, about 1 hr.
8. Strain stock through a large fine-mesh strainer into a large container or container (you should have about 9 cups); rinse & wipe out stockpot & return strained stock to the pot.
9. Bring stock to boil over high heat & simmer till reduced to 8 cups, about 10 mins. Off heat, Include orange zest & saffron & let stand for 10 mins to infuse flavours. Strain stock through fine-mesh strainer; set aside.
10. Return fish broth to clean stockpot & bring to boil over high heat.
11. Stir in marinated fish & shellfish & mussels, cover pot, & return to simmer; cook for 7 mins, stirring occasionally. Off heat, cover & let stand till fish is cooked through & mussels have opened about 2 mins.
12. Garnish and serve with salt & pepper to taste, ladle into containers, & float 1 garlic toast topped with a dollop of rouille in each container. Serve immediately.

40. GARLIC TOASTS

Prep Time:	*Cook Time:*	*Servings: 2*
5 Minutes	*20 Minutes*	

INGREDIENTS:

- lb country-style French bread, cut into ten 1/2-inch-thick slices (remainder reserved for rouille if using for bouillabaisse)
- garlic cloves, peeled & halved
- 3 Tbsps. olive oil

DIRECTIONS:

1. Setting oven rack 6 inches from broiler element & heat broiler.
2. Arrange bread slices in a single layer on a baking sheet; broil till lightly toasted, about 1 1/2 mins.
3. Flip slices & rub the second side of each slice with raw garlic, then brush with oil.
4. Broil till light golden brown, about 1 1/2 mins longer.

41. HEARTY TUSCAN BEAN STEW

Prep Time:	*Cook Time:*	*Servings: 2*
5 Minutes	*55 Minutes*	

INGREDIENTS:

- Salt & pepper
- lb dried cannellini beans (2 cups), picked over & rinsed
- Tbsp. extra-virgin olive oil, plus extra for drizzling
- ounces pancetta, cut into 1/4-inch pieces
- 1 large onion, chopped
- 2 carrots, peeled & cut into half-inch pieces 2 celery ribs, cut into 1/2-inch pieces
- 8 garlic cloves, peeled & crushed
- 4 cups low-sodium chicken broth
- 3 cups water
- 2 bay leaves
- 1 lb kale or collard greens, stemmed & leaves chopped into 1-inch pieces 1 (14.5-ounce) can diced tomatoes, drained
- 1 sprig of fresh rosemary slices country white bread, and 1 1/4 inch thick, broiled till golden brown on both sides & rubbed with the garlic clove (optional)

DIRECTIONS:

1. Dissolve 3 Tbsps. Salt in 4 quarts of cold water large container or container. Include beans & soak at room temperature for at least 8 hrs or up to 24 hrs. Drain & rinse well.
2. Set oven rack to lower-middle setting & heat oven to 250 degrees. Heat oil & pancetta in a Dutch oven over medium heat.
3. Cook, occasionally stirring, till pancetta is lightly browned & fat has rendered, 6 to 10 mins.
4. Include onion, carrots, & celery & cook, occasionally stirring, till vegetables are softened & lightly browned, 10 to 16 mins. Stir in garlic & cook till fragrant, about 1 min. Stir in broth, water, bay leaves, & soaked beans.
5. Increase heat to high & bring to simmer. Cover pot, Shift to the oven, & cook till beans are almost tender (very centre of beans will still be firm), 45 mins to 1 hr.
6. Remove pot from oven & stir in kale & tomatoes. Return pot to oven & continue to cook till beans & greens are fully tender, 30 to 40 mins longer.
7. Remove pot from oven & submerge rosemary in the stew. Cover & let stand 15 mins.
8. Discard bay leaves & rosemary & season stew with salt & pepper to taste.
9. If desired, use the back of the spoon to press some beans against the side of the pot to thicken the stew.
10. Serve over toasted bread, if desired, & drizzle with olive oil.

42. FRENCH PORK & WHITE BEAN CASSEROLE (CASSOULET)

Prep Time:	*Cook Time:*	*Servings: 4*
5 Minutes	*35 Minutes*	

INGREDIENTS:

- Salt & pepper
- lb dried cannellini beans (2 cups), picked over & rinsed
- 2 celery ribs
- bay leaf
- 4 sprigs of fresh thyme
- 1 1/2 lbs fresh French garlic sausage
- ounces salt pork rinsed 1/4 cup vegetable oil
- 1 (1 1/2-lb) pork shoulder, cut into 1-inch chunks 1 large onion, chopped fine
- 2 carrots, peeled & cut into 1/4-inch pieces
- garlic cloves, minced
- Tbsp. tomato paste 1/2 cup dry white wine
- (14.5-ounce) can diced tomatoes
- 4 cups low-sodium chicken broth
- 4 slices hearty white sandwich bread
- 1/2 cup chopped fresh parsley

DIRECTIONS:

1. Dissolve 2 Tbsps. Salt in 4 quarts of cold water container or container. Include beans & soak at room temperature for at least 8 hrs or up to 24 hrs. Drain & rinse well.
2. Set oven rack to lower-middle setting & heat oven to 300 degrees. Using kitchen twine, tie together celery, bay leaf, & thyme.
3. Place sausage & salt pork in a medium saucepan & Include cold water to cover by 1 inch; bring to boil over high heat. Reduce heat to simmer & cook 5 mins.
4. Shift sausage to the cutting board, allow to cool slightly, then cut into 1-inch pieces. Remove salt pork from water; set aside.
5. Heat 2 Tbsps. Oil in a Dutch oven after setting medium-high heat till beginning to smoke. Include sausage pieces & brown on all sides, 8 to 12 mins total. Shift to the medium container.
6. Include pork shoulder & brown on all sides, 8 to 12 mins total.
7. Include onion & carrots; cook, constantly stirring, till onion is translucent, about 2 mins. Include garlic & tomato paste & cook, constantly stirring, till fragrant, 30 seconds.
8. Return sausage to Dutch oven; Include white wine, scraping browned bits from the bottom of the pan. Cook till slightly reduced, about 30 seconds. Stir in tomatoes, celery bundle, & reserved salt pork.
9. Stir in broth & beans, pressing beans into an even layer, including up to 1 cup water so beans are at least partially submerged (beans may still break the surface of the liquid).
10. Increase heat to high & bring to simmer. Cover pot, Shift to the oven, & cook till beans are tender, about 1 1/2 hrs.
11. Remove celery bundle & salt pork & discard. (Alternatively, dice salt pork & return to the casserole.) Using a large spoon, skim fat from the surface & discard.
12. Season with salt & pepper to taste. Increase oven temperature to 350 degrees & bake, uncovered, 20 mins.

13. Meanwhile, pulse bread & the remaining 2 Tbsps. Oil in the food processor till crumbs are no larger than 1/8 inch, 8 to 10 pulses.
14. Shift to the medium container, Include parsley, & toss to combine. Season with salt & pepper to taste.
15. Sprinkle 1/2 cup bread-crumb batter evenly over casserole; bake, covered, 15 mins. Remove lid & bake 15 mins longer.
16. Sprinkle remaining bread-crumb batter over top of casserole & bake till topping is golden brown, about 30 mins. Let rest 15 mins before serving.

43. OLD-FASHIONED BEEF STEW

Prep Time: *5 Minutes* *Cook Time:* *35 Minutes* *Servings: 3*

INGREDIENTS:

- (3-lb) boneless beef, & cut into 11/2-inch pieces
- Salt & pepper
- Tbsps. vegetable oil
- 2 onions, chopped coarsely
- garlic cloves, minced
- Tbsps. all-purpose flour
- 1 cup full-bodied red wine
- 2 cups low-sodium chicken broth
- 2 bay leaves
- 1 Tsp. dried thyme
- 1 lb small red potatoes, peeled & halved 4 large carrots, peeled & sliced 1/4 inch thick 1 cup frozen peas, thawed
- 1/4 cup minced fresh parsley

DIRECTIONS:

1. Heat oven to 300 degrees. Season beef with 11/2 Tbsps. salt & 1 Tsp. pepper; toss to coat.
2. Heat 2 Tbsps. Oil over medium-high heat. After heating, the meat turns into brown colour on all sides in 2 batches, about 5 mins per batch, including the remaining 1 Tbsp. Oil if necessary.
3. Remove meat & set aside. Include onions to now-empty pot & cook till almost softened 4 to 5 mins.
4. Reduce heat to medium & Include garlic; cook till fragrant, about 30 seconds.
5. Stir in flour; cook till lightly coloured, 1 to 2 mins. Include wine, scraping up browned bits on the bottom of the pot.
6. Include broth, bay leaves, & thyme & bring to simmer. Include meat & return to simmer. Cover & place in oven & simmer 1 hr.
7. Remove pot from oven, Include potatoes & carrots, cover, & return to oven.
8. Simmer till meat is just tender, about 1 hr. Remove stew from the oven. 3. Stir in peas & let stand 5 mins.
9. Stir in parsley, season with salt & pepper to taste, & serve.

44. MODERN BEEF STEW

Prep Time: *5 Minutes* *Cook Time:* *55 Minutes* *Servings:8*

INGREDIENTS:

- 2 garlic cloves, minced
- anchovy fillets, rinsed & minced
- 1 Tbsp. tomato paste
- (4-lb) & cut into 11/2-inch pieces
- 2 Tbsps. vegetable oil
- large onion halved & sliced 1/8 inch thick
- 4 carrots, peeled & cut into 1-inch pieces
- 1/4 cup all-purpose flour
- cups red wine
- cups low-sodium chicken broth
- 4 ounces salt pork, rinsed
- bay leaves
- 4 sprigs of fresh thyme
- lb Yukon Gold potatoes, cut into 1-inch pieces 11/2 cups frozen pearl onions, thawed
- 2 Tbsps. unflavored gelatin 1/2 cup water
- cup frozen peas, thawed salt & pepper

DIRECTIONS:

1. Set oven rack to lower-middle setting & heat oven to 300 Degrees. Combine garlic & anchovies in a small container; press with the back of a fork to form a paste. Stir in tomato paste & set aside.
2. Pat meat dry with paper towels. Do not season. Heat 1 Tbsp. Oil in a Dutch oven until just starting to smoke.
3. Include half of beef & cook till well browned on all sides, about 8 mins. Shift beef to a large plate.
4. Repeat with remaining beef & remaining 1 Tbsp. Oil, leaving the second batch of meat in the pot after browning.
5. Reduce heat to medium & return the first batch of beef to pot. Stir in onion & carrots & cook, scraping the bottom of cooking wok to loosen browned bits, till onion is softened, 1 to 2 mins.
6. Include garlic batter & cook, constantly stirring, till fragrant, about 30 seconds. Include flour & cook, constantly stirring, till no dry flour remains, about 30 seconds.
7. Slowly include wine, scraping the bottom of the cooking wok to loosen browned bits. Increase heat to high & simmer till wine is thickened & slightly reduced, about 2 mins.
8. Stir in broth, pork, bay leaves, & thyme. Bring to simmer, cover, Shift to the oven, & cook for 11/2 hrs.
9. Remove pot from oven; remove & discard bay leaves & salt pork.
10. Stir in potatoes, cover, return to oven, & cook till potatoes are almost tender, about 45 mins.
11. Using a large spoon, skim excess fat from the surface of the stew.
12. Stir in pearl onions; cook over medium heat till potatoes & onions are cooked through & fork slips easily in & out of beef (meat should not be falling apart), about 15 mins.
13. Meanwhile, sprinkle gelatin over water in the small container & allow it to soften for 5 mins.
14. Increase heat to high, stir in softened gelatin batter & peas; simmer till the gelatin is fully dissolved & stew is thickened, about 3 mins.
15. Season with salt & pepper to taste; serve. (Stew can be refrigerated for up to 2 days.)

Side Dishes Recipes

45. BACON & SUN-DRIED TOMATO PHYLLO TARTS

Prep Time: *15 Minutes* *Cook Time:* *30 Minutes* *Servings: 5*

INGREDIENTS:

- 2 tsp olive oil
- ¾ cup chopped onion (about 1 medium)
- ¾ cup chopped green pepper (about 1 small)
- ¾ cup of chopped sweet red pepper (about 1 small)
- 1 garlic clove, minced
- Dash dried oregano
- 3 packages (1.9 ounces each) frozen miniature phyllo tart shells
- 1 package (8 ounces) cream cheese, softened
- 1 ½ tsp lemon juice
- 1/8 tsp salt
- 1 egg, lightly beaten
- ½ cup oil-packed sun-dried tomatoes, chopped and patted dry
- 2 bacon strips, cooked and crumbled
- 1 tbsp of minced fresh basil or 1 tsp of dried basil
- ½ cup crushed butter-flavoured crackers
- ½ cup shredded cheddar cheese

Directions:

1. Preheat oven to 350°. In a big skillet, heat oil over medium-high heat. Add onion and peppers; cook and stir 6-8 minutes or until tender. Add garlic and oregano; cook 1 minute longer. Cool completely.
2. Place tart shells on ungreased baking sheets. In a big bowl, beat cream cheese, lemon juice and salt until smooth.
3. Add egg; beat on reduce speed just until blended. Stir in tomatoes, bacon, basil and onion mixture.
4. Spoon 2 tsp filling into each tart shell. Top each with ½ tsp crushed crackers and ½ tsp cheddar cheese.
5. Bake 10-12 minutes or until set. Present warm.
6. FREEZE OPTION Freeze cooled baked pastries in freezer containers. To use, reheat pastries on a baking sheet in a preheated 350° oven for 15-18 minutes or until heated through.

46. CRAWFISH BEIGNETS WITH CAJUN DIPPING SAUCE

Prep Time: *15 Minutes* *Cook Time:* *35 Minutes* *Servings: 3*

INGREDIENTS:

- 1 egg, beaten
- 1 pound chopped cooked crawfish tail meat or shrimp
- 4 green onions, chopped
- 1 ½ tsp butter, melted ½ tsp salt
- ½ tsp cayenne pepper 1/3 cup bread flour Oil for deep-fat frying
- ¾ cup mayonnaise
- ½ cup ketchup
- ¼ tsp prepared horseradish, optional ¼ tsp hot pepper sauce 1.
- In a big bowl, add the egg, crawfish, onions, butter, salt and cayenne.
- Stir in flour until blended.

Directions:

1. An electric skillet or deep fryer is heating oil to 375°. Drop tbsps of batter, a few at a time, into the hot oil.
2. Fry until golden brown on both sides. Drain on paper towels.
3. In a small size bowl, add the mayonnaise, ketchup, horseradish if desired and pepper sauce. Present with beignets.

47. SPANAKOPITA PINWHEELS

Prep Time: *15 Minutes* *Cook Time:* *20 Minutes* *Servings: 4*

INGREDIENTS:

- 1 medium onion, finely chopped
- 2 tbsps olive oil
- 1 tsp of dried oregano
- 1 clove of garlic, minced
- 2 packs (10 oz each) frozen minced spinach, thawed and pressed dry
- 1 package (17.3 oz) Frozen Puff Pastries, Thaw 1.

Directions:

1. Heat oil in a skillet and then sauté onions until tender. Add oregano and garlic. Boil for 1 more minute.
2. Add spinach. Cook for at least 3 minutes or until the liquid evaporates. Transfer the spinach mixture to a large bowl. Cold.
3. Add feta cheese and eggs to the spinach mixture. Mix well. Open the puff pastry. Spread each sheet with half of the spinach mixture within an inch of the edge. Roll jelly-roll style.
4. Cut into 12 inches each. Some part. Place cut side down on a greased baking sheet.
5. Bake at 400° for 18-22 minutes or until golden brown.

48. MIXED OLIVE CROSTINI

Prep Time: *15 Minutes* *Cook Time:* *25 Minutes* *Servings:4*

INGREDIENTS:

- 1 can (4 ¼ ounces) chopped ripe olives ½ cup pimiento-stuffed olives, finely chopped ½ cup grated Parmesan cheese ¼ cup butter, softened
- 1 tbsp olive oil
- 2 garlic cloves, minced
- ¾ cup shredded part-skim mozzarella cheese ¼ cup minced fresh parsley

Directions:

1. 1 French bread baguette (10 ½ ounces) 1. In a small size bowl, add the first six ingredients; stir in mozzarella cheese and parsley.

2. Cut baguette into 24 slices; place on an ungreased baking sheet. Spread with olive mixture.
3. Broil 3-4 in. from the heat for 2-3 minutes or until edges are lightly browned, and cheese is melted.

49. CHAMPION CHICKEN PUFFS

Prep Time: *15 Minutes* | *Cook Time:* *25 Minutes* | *Servings: 3*

INGREDIENTS:

- 4 ounces cream cheese, softened
- ½ tsp garlic powder
- ½ cup of shredded cooked chicken
- 2 tubes (8 ounces each) of refrigerated crescent rolls

Directions:

1. Whisk cream cheese and garlic powder in a small bowl until smooth. Stir the chicken.
2. Roll out the crescent dough. Divide it into 16 triangles. Cut each triangle in half lengthwise to make two triangles. add 1 teaspoon
3. The chicken mixture is in the middle of each. Fold the short side over the filling. Close and roll up by pressing the sides.
4. Put the 1 inch apart on a greased baking sheet. Bake at 375° for 12-14 minutes or until golden brown. come warm

50. MINIATURE SHEPHERD'S PIES

Prep Time: *15 Minutes* | *Cook Time:* *25 Minutes* | *Servings: 4*

INGREDIENTS:

- ½ pound ground beef
- 1/3 cup finely chopped onion ¼ cup finely chopped celery 3 tbsp finely chopped carrot
- 1 ½ tsp all-purpose flour 1 tsp dried thyme
- ¼ tsp salt
- 1/8 tsp ground nutmeg
- 1/8 tsp of pepper
- 2/3 cup of beef broth
- 1/3 cup of frozen petite peas 2 packages (17.3 ounces each) frozen puff pastry, thawed
- 3 cups mashed potatoes

Directions:

1. Preheat oven to 400°. In a large skillet, cook the beef, onions, celery and carrots over medium heat until the beef is no longer pink. Thin.
2. Stir in the flour, thyme, salt, nutmeg and pepper until smooth. Add broth gradually. Take to a boil; cook and stir continuously for 2 minutes or until sauce thickens. Stir the peas. Heat passing. Separately.
3. Open the puff pastry. Use 2 inches of flour. The circular cutter cut 12 circles from each sheet (keep the rest for other use). Slide the puff pastry circles on the bottom and top of the non-greasy side of a mini muffin cup.
4. Fill each with 1 teaspoon of beef mixture. Top or pipe with 1 tbsp mashed potatoes. Bake 13-16 minutes or until heated and potatoes are slightly browned. come warm

51. BRIE-APPLE PASTRY BITES

Prep Time: *15 Minutes* | *Cook Time:* *20 Minutes* | *Servings: 4*

INGREDIENTS:

- 1 package (17.3 ounces) of frozen puff pastry, thawed
- 1 round (8 ounces) of Brie cheese, cut into ½-inch cubes 1 medium apple, chopped
- 2/3 cup sliced almonds ½ cup chopped walnuts ¼ cup dried cranberries Ground nutmeg

Directions:

1. Open puff pastry; cut each sheet into 24 squares. Gently press the square into the bottom of the greased 48 mini muffin cups.
2. Add cheese, apples, nuts and cranberries. Spoon in the cup. Bake at 375° for 12-15 minutes or until cheese is melted. Sprinkle with nutmeg.

52. SWEDISH MEATBALLS

Prep Time: *15 Minutes* | *Cook Time:* *25 Minutes* | *Servings: 6*

INGREDIENTS:

- 2/3 cup evaporated milk
- 2/3 cup chopped onion
- ¼ cup fine dry bread crumbs
- ½ tsp salt
- ½ tsp allspice
- Dash pepper
- 1 pound lean ground beef (90% lean)
- 2 tsp butter
- 2 tsp beef bouillon granules
- 1 cup hot water
- ½ cup cold water
- 2 tbsps all-purpose flour
- 1 cup evaporated milk
- 1 tbsp lemon juice

Directions:

1. Add 2/3 cup evaporated milk, onion, crumbs, salt, allspice and pepper. Add meat; mix well, chill. Shape meat mixture into 1-in. balls.
2. In a big skillet, brown meatballs in butter. Dissolve bouillon in hot water; pour over meatballs and bring to boil over medium heat. Cover; simmer for 15 minutes.
3. Meanwhile, blend together cold water and flour. Remove meatballs from skillet, skim fat from pan juices and rePresent juices.
4. Stir 1 cup evaporated milk and flour/water mixture into pan juices in skillet; cook, uncovered, over reduce heat, stirring until sauce thickens.
5. Return meatballs to skillet. Stir in lemon juice. Present with cooked noodles that have been tossed with poppy seeds and butter.

53. SWEET SAUSAGE ROLLS

Prep Time: *15 Minutes* | *Cook Time:* *30 Minutes* | *Servings: 5*

INGREDIENTS:

- 1 tube (8 ounces) refrigerated crescent rolls
- 24 miniature smoked sausage links
- ½ cup butter, melted
- ½ cup chopped nuts
- 3 tbsps honey
- 3 tbsps brown sugar

Directions:

1. Unroll crescent dough and separate into triangles; cut each lengthwise into three triangles. Place sausages on the wide end of triangles; roll up tightly.
2. Add the remaining ingredients in an 11x7-in. Baking dish. Arrange sausage rolls, seam side down, in butter mixture. Bake, uncovered, at 400° for 15-20 minutes or until golden brown.

54. PEANUT SHRIMP KABOBS

Prep Time: *15 Minutes* | *Cook Time:* *35 Minutes* | *Servings: 3*

INGREDIENTS:

- ¼ cup sugar
- ¼ cup reduced-sodium soy sauce
- ¼ cup reduced-fat creamy peanut butter
- 1 tbsp water
- 1 tbsp canola oil
- 3 garlic cloves, minced
- 1 ½ pound of uncooked medium shrimp, peeled and deveined

Directions:

1. In a small saucepan, add the first six ingredients until smooth. Cook and stir over medium-reduce heat until blended and sugar is dissolved. Set aside 6 tbsps sauce.
2. On eight metal or soaked wooden skewers, thread the shrimp. Brush with remaining peanut sauce. By Using long-handled tongs, moisten a paper towel with cooking oil and coat the grill rack.
3. Grill kabobs, covered, overheat or broil 4 in. from the heat for 4-6 minutes or until shrimp turn pink, turning once.
4. Brush with reserved sauce before serving.

55. CRAB RANGOON

Prep Time: *15 Minutes* | *Cook Time:* *43 Minutes* | *Servings: 2*

INGREDIENTS:

- 3 ounces reduced-fat cream cheese
- 1/8 tsp garlic salt
- 1/8 tsp Worcestershire sauce
- ½ cup lump crabmeat, drained
- 1 green onion, chopped
- 14 wonton wrappers

Directions:

1. In a small size bowl, add the cream cheese, garlic salt and Worcestershire sauce until smooth. Stir in crab and onion. Place 2 cupfuls in the centre of each wonton wrapper. Moisten edges with water; bring corners to centre over filling and press edges together to seal.
2. Place on a baking sheet coated with cooking spray. Lightly spray wontons with cooking spray. Bake at 425° for 8-10 minutes or until golden brown. Present warm.

56. CORN FRITTERS WITH CARAMELIZED ONION JAM

Prep Time: *15 Minutes* | *Cook Time:* *23 Minutes* | *Servings: 2*

INGREDIENTS:

- 1 big sweet onion, halved and thinly sliced
- 1 tbsp olive oil
- 2 tsp balsamic vinegar
- 1/3 cup apple jelly
- 1/3 cup canned diced tomatoes
- 1 tbsp tomato paste
- 1/8 tsp curry powder
- 1/8 tsp of ground cinnamon
- Dash salt and pepper
- FRITTERS
- 2 cups of biscuit/baking mix
- 1 can (11 ounces) gold and white corn, drained
- 2 eggs, lightly beaten
- ½ cup 2% milk
- ½ cup sour cream
- ½ tsp salt
- Oil for frying

Directions:

1. Fry the onions in oil In a small frying pan until golden brown. Add vinegar. Cook and stir for 2-3 minutes. Separately.
2. In a small saucepan, combine the jelly, tomatoes, tomato paste, curry powder, cinnamon, salt and pepper. Cook over medium heat for 5-7 minutes or until done. Add the onion mixture. Cook for 3 minutes and stir. Set aside and keep warm.
3. In a small bowl, add cake mix, corn, eggs, milk, sour cream and salt until added.
4. Heat the oil to 375° in a fryer or electric skillet. In the hot oil, drop the dough, stacking a little at a time a tablespoon. Fry on each side or until golden brown, 1 minute. Drain the water on a paper towel. Serve warm with jam.

57. GREEK PIZZAS

Prep Time: *15 Minutes* | *Cook Time:* *45 Minutes* | *Servings: 6*

INGREDIENTS:

- 4 pita bread (6 inches)
- 1 cup reduced-fat ricotta cheese
- ½ tsp garlic powder
- (10 ounces) one pkg of frozen chopped spinach, thawed and then squeezed dry
- 3 medium tomatoes, sliced
- ¾ cup crumbled feta cheese
- ¾ tsp dried basil

Directions:

1. Place pita bread on a baking sheet. Add ricotta cheese and garlic powder; spread over pitas. Top with spinach, tomatoes, feta cheese and basil.
2. Bake it at least at 400° for 12-15 minutes or until bread is lightly browned.

58. BACON & FONTINA STUFFED MUSHROOMS

Prep Time: *Cook Time:* *Servings: 3*
15 Minutes *23 Minutes*

INGREDIENTS:

- 4 ounces cream cheese, softened
- 1 cup (4 ounces) of shredded fontina cheese 8 bacon strips, cooked and crumbled
- 4 green onions, chopped
- ¼ cup chopped oil-packed sun-dried tomatoes 3 tbsps minced fresh parsley
- 24 big fresh mushrooms (about 1 ¼ pound), stems removed 1 tbsp olive oil

Directions:

1. Preheat oven to 425°. In a small size bowl, mix the first six ingredients until blended. Arrange mushroom caps in a greased 15x10x1-in. Baking pan, stem side up. Spoon about 1 tbsp filling into each.
2. Spread tops with olive oil. Bake it, uncovered, 9-11 minutes or until it turn golden brown and mushrooms are tender.

59. ALMOND CHEDDAR APPETIZERS

- 1 cup mayonnaise
- 2 tsp Worcestershire sauce
- 1 cup (4 ounces) shredded sharp cheddar cheese 1 medium onion, chopped
- ¾ cup of slivered almonds chopped 6 bacon strips, cooked and crumbled
- 1 loaf (1 pound) French bread

1. In a bowl, add the mayonnaise and Worcestershire sauce; stir in cheese, onion, almonds and bacon.
2. Cut bread into ½-in. slices; sprinkle with cheese mixture. Divide slices in half; place on a greased baking sheet. 8- in 400 degree oven minutes or until foamy.
3. FROZEN OPTION Lay raw appetizers in one layer on a baking sheet. Freeze it for 1 hour.
4. Put off from pan and store in an airtight container for up to 2 months. When ready to use, place the thawed appetizer on a greased baking sheet. Bake at 400° for 10 minutes or until warm and frothy.

60. MINI TERIYAKI TURKEY SANDWICHES

Prep Time: *Cook Time:* *Servings: 4*
15 Minutes *25 Minutes*

INGREDIENTS:

- (2 pounds each) 2 boneless skinless turkey breast halves
- 2/3 cup of packed brown sugar
- 2/3 cup of reduced-sodium soy sauce
- ¼ cup cider vinegar
- 3 garlic cloves, minced
- 1 tbsp minced fresh ginger root
- ½ tsp pepper
- 2 tbsps cornstarch
- 2 tbsps cold water
- 20 Hawaiian sweet rolls
- 2 tbsps butter, melted

Directions:

1. Place turkey in a 5-or 6-qt. Reduce cooker. In a small size bowl, add brown sugar, soy sauce, vinegar, garlic, ginger and pepper; pour over turkey. Cook, covered, on reducing 5-6 hours or until the meat is tender.
2. Remove turkey from reducing cooker. In a small size bowl, combine cornstarch and cold water until smooth; gradually stir into cooking liquid.
3. When cool enough, shred meat with two forks and return meat to reduce cooker. Cook, covered, on high 30- minutes or until sauce is thickened.
4. Preheat oven to 325°. Split rolls and brush cut sides with butter; place on an ungreased baking sheet, cut side up.
5. Bake 8-10 minutes or until toasted and golden brown. Spoon 1/3 cup turkey mixture on roll bottoms. Replace tops.
6.

61. SUMMER TEA SANDWICHES

Prep Time: *Cook Time:* *Servings: 2*
15 Minutes *35 Minutes*

INGREDIENTS:

- ½ tsp dried tarragon ½ tsp salt, divided ¼ tsp pepper 1 pound boneless skinless chicken breasts
- ½ cup reduced-fat mayonnaise 1 tbsp finely chopped red onion
- 1 tsp dill weed
- ½ tsp lemon juice 24 slices soft multigrain bread, crusts removed
- 1 medium cucumber, thinly sliced
- ¼ medium cantaloupe, cut into 12 thin slices 1. Add the tarragon,
- ¼ tsp salt and pepper; rub over chicken. Place it on a baking sheet that is coated with cooking spray.

Directions:

1. Bake it at least 350° for 20-25 minutes or until a thermometer reads 170°. Cool to room temperature; thinly slice.

Snacks And Appetizer Recipes

62. SEAFOOD SALAD MINI CROISSANTS

Prep Time: ***Cook Time:78*** ***Servings: 5***
15 Minutes ***Minutes***

INGREDIENTS:

- ½ cup mayonnaise
- 1 tbsp snipped fresh dill
- 1 tbsp minced chives
- 1 tbsp lemon juice
- ½ tsp salt
- ¼ tsp pepper
- ½ pound imitation lobster ½ pound cooked small shrimp, peeled and deveined and coarsely chopped 10 miniature croissants, split

Directions:

1. In a big bowl, add the mayonnaise, dill, chives, lemon juice, salt and pepper. Stir in lobster and shrimp. Cover and refrigerate until serving. Present on croissants.
2. In a small size bowl, add the mayonnaise, onion, dill, lemon juice and remaining salt; spread over 12 bread slices. Top with cucumber, chicken, cantaloupe and remaining bread. Cut sandwiches in half diagonally. Present immediately.

63. CHIPOTLE SLIDERS

Prep Time: *Cook Time:* *Servings: 4*
15 Minutes *20 Minutes*

INGREDIENTS:

- 1 package (12 ounces) Hawaiian sweet rolls, divided
- 1 tsp salt
- ½ tsp of pepper
- 8 tsp of minced chipotle peppers in adobo sauce, divided
- 1 ½ pounds ground beef
- 10 slices pepper Jack cheese
- ½ cup mayonnaise

Directions:

1. Add 2 rolls to the food processor. The process of demolition. Make it into a large bowl. Now add salt, pepper and 6 tsp chopped chives. Mix the beef into the dough and mix well. Make 10 columns.
2. Cook the covered burgers on medium heat for 3-4 minutes on both sides or until the thermometer reads 160° and the water is clear. Top with cheese. Bake for 1 minute or until cheese is melted.
3. Remove the rest of the rolls, turn them over and heat over medium heat for 30-60 seconds or until fully cooked.
4. Add mayonnaise and remaining chipotle peppers; spread over roll bottoms. Top each with a burger. Replace roll tops.

64. CHICKEN SALAD PARTY SANDWICHES

Prep Time: *Cook Time:* *Servings: 3*
5 Minutes *15 Minutes*

Ingredients:

- 4 cups cubed cooked chicken breast
- 1 ½ cups dried cranberries
- 2 celery ribs, finely chopped
- 2 green onions, thinly sliced
- ¼ cup chopped sweet pickles
- 1 cup fat-free mayonnaise
- ½ tsp curry powder
- ¼ tsp coarsely ground pepper
- ½ cup chopped pecans, toasted
- 15 whole wheat dinner rolls
- Torn leaf lettuce

Directions:

1. In a bowl, now add the first five ingredients. In a small size bowl, add the mayonnaise, curry and pepper. Add to chicken mixture; toss to coat. Chill until serving.
2. Stir pecans into chicken salad. Present on rolls lined with lettuce

65. STATE FAIR SUBS

Prep Time: *Cook Time:* *Servings: 6*
15 Minutes *20 Minutes*

Ingredients:

- 1 loaf (1 pound unsliced) French bread
- 2 eggs
- ¼ cup milk
- ½ tsp pepper
- ¼ tsp salt
- 1 pound bulk Italian sausage
- 1 ½ cups chopped onion
- 2 cups (8 ounces) of shredded part-skim mozzarella cheese

Directions:

1. Cut the bread in half lengthwise. Drill holes carefully in the top and bottom of the loaf, leaving about an inch.
2. Husks. Diced bread. In a large bowl, shake together the eggs, milk, pepper and salt. Add slices of bread and stir to coat. Separately.
3. In a frying pan over high heat, cook the sausages and onions until the meat is no longer pink. Thin.
4. Add to bread dough. Spoon for filling in breadcrumbs; Sprinkle with cheese. Wrap each in foil. Bake it at least 400° for 20-25 minutes or until cheese is melted. Cut French bread into 1-serving-sized pieces

66. PARTY PITAS

Prep Time: *Cook Time:* *Servings: 4*
15 Minutes *22 Minutes*

INGREDIENTS:

- 4 whole-wheat pita pocket halves
- 1/3 cup Greek vinaigrette ½ pound thinly sliced deli turkey 1 jar (7 ½ ounces) roasted sweet red peppers, drained and patted dry 2 cups fresh baby spinach
- 24 pitted Greek olives
- 24 frilled toothpicks

Directions:

1. Brush insides of pita pockets with vinaigrette; fill with turkey, peppers and spinach. Cut each pita into six wedges.
2. Thread olives onto toothpicks; use to secure wedges.

67. BAJA CHICKEN & SLAW SLIDERS

Prep Time: *15 Minutes* | *Cook Time:* *25 Minutes* | *Servings: 6*

INGREDIENTS:

- ¼ cup reduced-fat sour cream ½ tsp grated lime peel ¼ tsp lime juice SLAW
- 1 cup broccoli coleslaw mix
- 2 tbsps finely chopped sweet red pepper
- 2 tbsps finely chopped sweet onion
- 2 tbsps of minced fresh cilantro
- 2 tsp of chopped seeded jalapeno pepper 2 tsp of lime juice
- 1 tsp of sugar
- SLIDERS
- (4 ounces each) 4 boneless skinless chicken breast halves ½ tsp of ground cumin
- ½ tsp of chilli powder
- ¼ tsp of salt
- ¼ tsp of coarsely ground pepper 8 Hawaiian sweet rolls, split
- 8 small lettuce leaves
- 8 slices tomato

Directions:

1. In a small size bowl, add sour cream, lime peel and lime juice. In another small size bowl, add slaw ingredients. Refrigerate sauce and slaw until serving.
2. Cut each chicken breast in half wide; flatten to -in. Thickness. Sprinkle with spices.
3. Wet a paper towel with cooking oil; using long-handled tongs, rub on grill rack to lightly coat.
4. Grill chicken, covered, over medium heat or roast 4 inches from heat 4 to 7 minutes on each side or until no longer pink.
5. Toast bread, cut side down, 30-60 seconds or until toasted. Serve grilled chicken on a roll with lettuce, tomatoes, sauce, and slaw.

68. ONION BEEF AU JU

Prep Time: *15 Minutes* | *Cook Time:* *25 Minutes* | *Servings: 4*

INGREDIENTS:

- 1 beef rump roast (4 pounds) 2 tbsps canola oil
- 2 big sweet onions, cut into ¼-inch slices 6 tbsp butter, softened, divided
- 5 cups water
- ½ cup of reduced-sodium soy sauce 1 envelope onion soup mix
- 1 garlic clove, minced
- 1 tsp browning sauce, optional
- 1 loaf (1 pound) French bread
- 1 cup (4 ounces) shredded Swiss cheese

Directions:

1. Bake chocolate on all sides in oil in a Dutch oven over medium heat. Thin. In a large frying pan, add 2 tablespoons of butter and saute the onions until soft. Add water, soy sauce, soup mix, garlic, and browning sauce if desired. Pour over roast.
2. Wrap and cook at 325° for 2 hours or until meat is tender. Leave the meat for about 10 minutes, then slice thinly.
3. Put the meat back into the juice pan. Separate the bread lengthwise. Cut into 3 inches. Part. Brush with the remaining butter. Place it on the pan.
4. Bake 4-6 inches of bread over heat for 2-3 minutes or until golden brown. Sprinkle with beef and onions.
5. Sprinkle with cheese. Bake for 1-2 minutes or until cheese is melted. Serve bread with pan juice.

69. HAWAIIAN BEEF SLIDERS

Prep Time: *15 Minutes* | *Cook Time:* *45 Minutes* | *Servings: 4*

INGREDIENTS:

- 1 can (20 ounces) unsweetened crushed pineapple
- 1 tsp pepper
- ¼ tsp salt
- 1 ½ pounds lean ground beef (90% lean)
- ¼ cup reduced-sodium soy sauce
- 2 tbsp ketchup
- 1 tbsp white vinegar
- 2 garlic cloves, minced
- ¼ tsp crushed red pepper flakes
- 18 miniature whole wheat buns
- Baby spinach leaves
- 3 centre-cut bacon strips, cooked and crumbled
- Sliced jalapeno peppers, optional

Directions:

1. Drain pineapple, reserving juice and 1 ½ cups pineapple (save remaining pineapple for another use). In a big bowl, add ¾ cup reserved crushed pineapple, pepper and salt.
2. Crumble beef over mixture and mix well. Shape into 18 patties; place in two 11x7-in. Dishes.
3. In a small size bowl, add soy sauce, ketchup, vinegar, garlic, pepper flakes and reserved pineapple juice. Pour half of the marinade into each dish; cover and refrigerate for 1 hour, turning once.
4. Drain and discard marinade. Moisten a paper towel with cooking oil by using long-handled tongs, coat the grill rack lightly.
5. Grill patties, covered, over medium heat or broil 4 in. from heat 4-5 minutes on each side or until a thermometer reads 160° and juices run clear.
6. Grill buns, uncovered, 1-2 minutes or until toasted. Present burgers on buns with spinach, remaining pineapple, bacon and jalapeno peppers if desired.

70. TUNA TEA SANDWICHES

Prep Time: *15 Minutes* | *Cook Time:* *21 Minutes* | *Servings: 4*

INGREDIENTS:

- 1 can (6 ounces) light water-packed tuna, drained and flaked 1 to 2 tbsps mayonnaise
- ¼ tsp lemon-pepper seasoning 4 tbsps crumbled goat cheese
- 4 slices multigrain bread, crusts removed 4 big fresh basil leaves

Directions:

1. In a small size bowl, add the tuna, mayonnaise and lemon pepper. Spread 1 tbsp of goat cheese on each slice of bread.
2. Spread two slices with tuna mixture; top with basil leaves and remaining bread. Cut in half or into desired shapes.

71. MINI MUFFULETTA

Prep Time: *15 Minutes* | *Cook Time:* *40 Minutes* | *Servings: 4*

INGREDIENTS:

- 1 jar (10 ounces) of pimiento-stuffed olives, drained and chopped
- 2 cans (4 ¼ ounces each) chopped ripe olives
- 2 tbsps balsamic vinegar
- 1 tbsp red wine vinegar
- 1 tbsp olive oil
- 3 garlic cloves, minced
- 1 tsp dried basil
- 1 tsp dried oregano
- 6 French rolls, split
- ½ pound thinly sliced hard salami
- ¼ pound sliced provolone cheese
- ½ pound thinly sliced Cotto salami
- ¼ pound sliced part-skim mozzarella cheese

Directions:

1. In a big bowl, add the first eight ingredients; set aside. Holreduce out tops and bottoms of rolls, leaving ¾-in. Clams (discard the discarded bread or save it for other uses).
2. Apply the olive mixture above and below the roll. Coat the bottom of the roll with hard salami, provolone cheese, Coto salami and mozzarella cheese. Change the top.
3. Wrap tightly with plastic wrap. Cool overnight. Cut each into six pieces. Secure it with a toothpick.

72. ANTIPASTO-STUFFED BAGUETTES

Prep Time: *15 Minutes* | *Cook Time:* *29 Minutes* | *Servings: 6*

INGREDIENTS:

- 1 can (2 ¼ ounces) sliced ripe olives, drained
- 2 tbsps olive oil
- 1 tsp lemon juice
- 1 garlic clove, minced
- 1/8 tsp each dried basil, thyme, marjoram and rosemary, crushed
- 2 French bread baguettes (10 ½ ounces each)
- 1 package (4 ounces) crumbled feta cheese
- ½ pound thinly sliced Genoa salami
- 1 cup fresh baby spinach
- 1 jar (7 ¼ ounces) of roasted red peppers, drained and chopped
- 1 can (14 ounces) of water-packed artichoke hearts, rinsed, drained and quartered

Directions:

1. Put the olives, oil, lemon juice, garlic and spices in a blender. Cover and process until olives are cut. Set aside 1/3 cup of the olive mixture (refrigerate the remaining mixture for other uses).
2. Cut the top 1/3 of each baguette. Carefully drill a hole in the bottom, leaving a -in. Peel (discard the discarded bread or save it for another use).
3. Apply the olive mixture to the bottom of each bread. Sprinkle with feta cheese. Fold the salami slices in half and put them on top of the cheese. Sprinkle with spinach, red pepper and artichoke need. Replace the top of the bread. Wrap the bread tightly in foil.
4. Refrigerate for at least 3 hours or overnight. Preheat oven to 350° to serve cold or warm.
5. Place the bread wrapped in foil on a baking sheet. Bake for 20-25 minutes or until heated. Cut into pieces. Secure it with a toothpick.

73. DELI SANDWICH PARTY PLATTER

Prep Time: *15 Minutes* | *Cook Time:* *45 Minutes* | *Servings: 6*

INGREDIENTS:

- 1 bunch of green leaf lettuce
- 2 pounds sliced of deli turkey
- 2 pounds sliced of deli roast beef
- 1 pound sliced of deli ham
- 1 pound thinly sliced hard salami
- 2 cartons (7 ounces each) of roasted red pepper hummus 2 cartons (6 ½ ounces each) garden vegetable cheese spread Assorted bread and mini bagels

Directions:

1. set lettuce leaves on a serving platter; top with deli meats, rolled up if desired. Present with hummus, cheese spread, bread and bagels.'

74. HAM 'N' CHEESE BISCUIT STACKS

Prep Time: *15 Minutes* | *Cook Time:* *30 Minutes* | *Servings: 8*

INGREDIENTS:

- 2 tubes (12 ounces each) refrigerated buttermilk biscuits
- ¾ cup stone-ground mustard, divided
- ½ cup butter softened
- ¼ cup chopped green onions
- ¼ cup mayonnaise
- ¼ cup honey
- 10 thick slices of deli ham
- 10 slices Swiss cheese
- 2 ½ cups of shredded romaine
- 40 frilled toothpicks
- 20 pitted ripe olives and drained and patted dry
- 20 pimiento-stuffed olives, drained and patted dry

Directions:

1. 2 inches apart on a greased baking sheet. Sprinkle each spoonful of mustard. Bake for 8-10 minutes or until golden brown. Remove from pan with wire rack to cool.

2. Put the butter and onion in a small bowl. In another bowl, add mayonnaise, honey and remaining mustard. Cut each piece of ham into rectangles. Cut each piece of cheese into four triangles.
3. Divide each biscuit in half. Grease the floor with the butter mixture. Layer 1 ham slice, 1 cheese slice, and 1 tablespoon romaine on each bottom of the biscuit.
4. Spread mustard mixture over biscuit tops; place over romaine. Thread toothpicks through olives; insert into stacks. Refrigerate leftovers.

75. CITRUS SPICED OLIVES

Prep Time: *15 Minutes* *Cook Time:* *55 Minutes* *Servings: 3*

INGREDIENTS:

- ½ cup white wine ¼ cup canola oil 3 tbsps salt-free seasoning blend
- 4 garlic cloves, minced
- ½ tsp crushed red pepper flakes 2 tsp each grated orange, lemon and lime peels 3 tbsps each orange, lemon and lime juices 4 cups mixed pitted olives

Directions:

1. Whisk until blended. Add olives and toss to coat. Refrigerate, wrapped, at least 4 hours before serving.
2.

Dessert Recipes

76. Lemon Glazed Raspberry Cake

Prep Time: *15 Minutes* *Cook Time:* *60 Minutes* *Servings: 8*

Ingredients:

- 1 cup whole wheat flour
- 1 cup all-purpose flour
- 2 tsp baking powder
- 1 pinch of salt
- 2/3 cup sugar
- 2 eggs
- ½ cup low-fat milk
- 1 tsp lemon zest
- 1 cup fresh raspberries
- Glaze:
- juice from ½ lemon
- 1 ½ cups powdered sugar

Directions:

1. In a bowl, stir the flours with the baking powder and a pinch of salt, then set aside.
2. In another bowl, stir the butter with the sugar until creamy and fluffy, then add the eggs, one by one. Start incorporating the flour stir, alternating it with milk. Carefully fold in the raspberries, then convert the batter into a 9-inch round cake pan.
3. Bake in the before heating oven at 350F for 30-40 minutes or until golden brown and fragrant.
4. To make the glaze: Stir the juice with powdered sugar until it reaches the desired consistency. It should be thick but still runny. Add the glaze over the chilled cake and let it rest for 1 hour in the refrigerator.

77. Chocolate Pear Cake

Prep Time: *15 Minutes* *Cook Time:* *45 Minutes* *Servings: 8*

Ingredients:

- 3 oz chocolate, chopped
- 3 oz butter
- 3 egg yolks
- 3 egg whites
- 3 oz sugar
- 3 oz chopped walnuts
- 4 ripe pears, peeled, halved and cored, then sliced
- 1 pinch of salt
- 1 tablespoon dark rum

Directions:

1. Place the chocolate as well as butter in a heavy pan and heat it on low flame until melted.
2. Add the rum and remove from heat. Let it cool to room temperature.
3. In a bowl, stir the egg yolks with the sugar until creamy, fluffy and pale in colour. Carefully stir in the chocolate, then fold in the chopped hazelnuts. In another bowl, whip the egg whites with a pinch of salt, then gently fold them into the chocolate base.
4. Grease and flour a 9-inch round cake pan with butter and flour it slightly. Spoon the batter into the pan, arrange the pears on top and bake in the before heating oven at 250F for 30-40 minutes. The cake will rise then deflate, but that is how it should look like.
5. Serve when completely chilled with a dollop of fresh cream if you want.

78. Pear Frangipane Tart

Prep Time: *15 Minutes* *Cook Time:* *60 Minutes* *Servings: 4*

Ingredients:

- Crust:
- 2 cups low-fat chocolate biscuits
- 3 oz butter, melted
- Pears:
- 4 small pears
- 2 cups red wine
- 1 cinnamon stick
- 1-star anise
- ½ cup brown sugar
- Frangipane filling:
- ½ cup sugar
- 3 oz butter
- 2 eggs
- ¼ cup cocoa powder
- 3 oz almond meal
- 1 tsp rum
- ¼ tsp almond extract

Directions:

1. To make the crust: Simply stir the biscuits in a food processor until ground, then pour in the melted butter. To convert the structure into a 10-inch tart pan and press it on the bottom and sides of the pan until all even.
2. To prepare the pears: Pour the wine in a saucepan and add the sugar, cinnamon stick and star anise. Bring to a boil, then add the pears, peeled, cored and halved.
3. Cook on minimum heat for about 15 minutes, then remove from heat and let them cool in the syrup. To convert them in a sieve to drain, but keep the syrup and put it back on the heat. Cook it until reduced by half.
4. To make the frangipane filling: Stir the butter with the sugar until creamy and fluffy, and then now add the eggs, one by one, followed by the cocoa powder and almond meal.
5. Add the rum and almond extract as well. Spread this stir in the pan, over the crust and top with pear halves.
6. Bake in the before heating oven at 350F for 30-40 minutes.

79. Pear and Applesauce Muffins

Prep Time: *15 Minutes* *Cook Time:* *5 Minutes* *Servings: 8*

Ingredients:

- 1 cup applesauce
- ½ cup brown sugar
- 1 cup all-purpose flour
- 2/3 cup whole wheat flour
- 1 tsp baking powder
- 1 tsp baking soda
- 1 tsp cinnamon
- 1 pinch nutmeg
- 1/8 tsp ground cloves
- 3 oz butter, softened
- 2 eggs
- 2 pears, peeled, cored and sliced
- 1 pinch of salt

Directions:

1. In a bowl, stir the butter continuously with the sugar until creamy and fluffy. Add the eggs, one after another, then the cinnamon, nutmeg and applesauce. Sift the flours with the baking powder, baking soda and a pinch of salt and incorporate this stir into the batter.
2. Line a muffin tin with special papers and spoon the batter evenly between the muffin cups. Top with a few pear slices and bake in the before heating oven at 350F for 20-25 minutes or until golden brown and fragrant.

80. Pear and Raisin Cobbler

Prep Time: *15 Minutes* *Cook Time:* *8 Minutes* *Servings: 4*

Ingredients:

- Pears:
- 2 pounds pears, peeled, cored and cubed
- ½ cup brown sugar
- 1 tablespoon cornstarch
- ¼ cup raisins
- Batter:
- 4 oz butter
- 1 cup whole wheat flour
- ½ tsp baking powder
- 1 pinch of salt
- 2 tbsp sugar
- ¾ cup low-fat milk
- 1 pinch nutmeg
- 1/8 tsp cinnamon

Directions:

1. In a bowl, stir the pear cubes with brown sugar, cornstarch and raisins.
2. 3To convert the stir into a deep dish baking pan (9x13-inches). Set aside.To make the batter: Stir the flour with the butter until sandy. Add the sugar, nutmeg and cinnamon, then pour in the milk, stirring well. Spread the butter over the pears and bake in the before heating oven at 350F for 30-40 minutes. Serve warm topped with a scoop of caramel ice cream.

Breakfast & Brunch Recipes

81. Buttermilk Pancakes

Prep Time: *15 Minutes* *Cook Time:* *6 Minutes* *Servings: 2*

Ingredients:

- 2 cups all-purpose flour
- 3 tbsp cane sugar
- 3 tsp baking powder
- 1 tsp baking soda
- 1 tsp salt
- 2 cups buttermilk
- 6 tbsp butter
- 1 tsp vanilla
- eggs Maple Syrup Confectioners' sugar

Directions:

1. Combine all together with the flour, sugar, baking soda, as well as baking powder, and salt.
2. Use another bowl to combine the buttermilk, butter, eggs, and vanilla.
3. Slowly add the buttermilk mixture to the flour mix. Mix to blend. Set the batter on the counter for 5 minutes
4. Heat a griddle or skillet. It needs to be hot, but not overly hot. When the griddle is at the right temperature, add a tablespoon of butter.
5. Use half a cup of batter per pancake. Place the batter on the grill. Flip it when the top starts to bubble.
6. Use up the entire batter. Place pancakes on a platter. Top with syrup or confectioners' sugar.

82. Johnnycakes

Prep Time: *15 Minutes* *Cook Time:* *22 Minutes* *Servings: 6*

Ingredients:

- 1 cup ground cornmeal ½ tsp salt 1/3 cup water 1 cup milk

Directions:

1. Mix the cornmeal and the salt.
2. Warm up the milk and water. Pour into cornmeal mix.
3. Butter a skillet and a tablespoon to drop the batter.
4. Fry the johnnycakes until browned on both sides.
5. Serve with applesauce or butter.

83. Apple Pancakes

Prep Time: *15 Minutes* *Cook Time:* *12 Minutes* *Servings: 8*

Ingredients:

- 2 Granny Smith apples, peeled and cut into small, thin slices ¼ cup cane sugar
- 3 tsp cinnamon
- 3 beaten eggs
- tsp salt ½ cup flour ½ cup milk ½ tsp vanilla
- ½ cup sweet butter

Directions:

1. Preheat oven to 425 degrees.
2. Mix together the cinnamon and sugar.
3. In another bowl, whip the eggs, flour, milk, salt, and vanilla until the mixture is smooth.
4. Melt the butter in a skillet. Add the apples and the cinnamon sugar. Stir and cook for 5 minutes.
5. Place the batter in a baking dish. Pour the apples on top of the batter.
6. Bake for 20 minutes.
7. Flip the pancake upside down on a plate. Once the pancake deflates (it will), cut and serve.

84. Almond Pancakes

Prep Time: *15 Minutes* *Cook Time:* *115 Minutes* *Servings: 6*

Ingredients:

- 1 ¾ cups cake flour
- ¼ cup almond flour
- ¼ cup instant-cooking oats
- 2 tsp baking soda
- 1 tsp salt
- 2 eggs
- ½ cup sliced almonds

Directions:

1. Mix together the flours, oats, baking soda and salt.
2. Use a second bowl to stir together the eggs and buttermilk.
3. Mix the egg/milk mixture into the flour and stir until all ingredients are well-blended.
4. Grease a skillet and add a quarter cup of batter. Top the batter with some almonds.
5. Cook the pancake until browned on one side, then flip.
6. Repeat with the rest of the batter.

85. Belgian Waffles

Prep Time: *15 Minutes* *Cook Time:* *16 Minutes* *Servings: 4*

Ingredients:

- 2 cups cake flour
- 2 tsp baking powder
- ½ tsp salt
- 4 large eggs, cut into whites and yolks
- 2 tbsp cane sugar
- ½ tsp vanilla
- 4 tbsp sweet butter
- 2 cups milk
- Vegetable cooking spray

Directions:

1. Preheat the waffle iron.
2. Transfer the flour, baking powder and salt into a bowl.
3. In another bowl, beat the yolks and sugar until well-blended.
4. Mix in the vanilla, butter, and milk and use a whisk to mix.
5. Plus the egg mix to the flour mix. Blend well.
6. Whip the egg whites with a hand mixer. Fold the egg whites into the batter.
7. Spray the waffle iron with vegetable spray.
8. Transfer some of the batters to the waffle iron.
9. Cook until waffles are nice and brown.

86. Chocolate Waffle

Prep Time: *15 Minutes* *Cook Time:* *20 Minutes* *Servings: 4*

Ingredients:

- 1 ½ cups all-purpose flour
- 4 tbsp sugar
- ½ cocoa powder
- 1 ½ tsp baking powder
- 1 tsp salt
- 3 large eggs
- 2 tbsp sweet butter
- 1 tsp vanilla
- 1/3 cup buttermilk
- cup chocolate chips Vegetable spray

Directions:

1. Preheat waffle iron.
2. Mix together the flour, cocoa, baking powder, and salt.
3. Use another bowl to beat the eggs, vanilla, and butter. Add the buttermilk and mix.
4. Mix in the chocolate chips and combine.
5. Let batter sit for 10 minutes.
6. Spray the waffle iron with vegetable spray.
7. Transfer batter to the waffle iron.
8. Cook until waffles are golden brown on each side.
9. Repeat with all of the batters. Keep the waffles warm.

87. Quiche, Crepes and Souffles

Prep Time: *15 Minutes* *Cook Time:* *25 Minutes* *Servings: 4*

Ingredients:

- 1 9-inch store-bought piecrust
- Salt and pepper to taste
- 1 cup diced ham
- 4 eggs
- cup half-and-half 1/8 tsp nutmeg
- 8 oz. diced Swiss cheese

Directions:

1. Preheat oven to 375 degrees.
2. Mix together the eggs, ham, half-and-half, nutmeg, and cheese.
3. Season to taste.
4. Transfer the eggs to the pre-made crust.
5. Bake for 35 minutes.

88. Filled Crepes

Prep Time: *15 Minutes* *Cook Time:* *23 Minutes* *Servings: 4*

Ingredients:

- 1 cup flour
- 1 cup milk
- cup heavy cream
- ½ tsp baking powder ¼ cup sweet butter
- ½ cup sliced mushrooms 1 chopped onion
- 1 tablespoon flour
- 1 cup cream
- 1 cup diced ham
- Salt and pepper to taste

Directions:

1. Mix together the milk, flour, baking powder and chill overnight.
2. Melt half of the butter in a crepe pan. Add ¼ cup of the batter.
3. Turn and rotate the crepe pan. Cook until one side is golden brown, then flip and cook the other side.
4. Repeat until batter is used up.
5. Melt the remaining butter and saute the mushrooms and the onions. Mix in the ham, and add the flour and the milk to thicken the filling.
6. Divide the filling between the crepes. Roll the crepe closed.

89. Cheese Souffle

Prep Time: *15 Minutes* *Cook Time:* *22 Minutes* *Servings: 2*

Ingredients:

- ¼ cup grated Parmesan cheese 5 tbsp sweet butter
- 2 tbsp all-purpose flour
- 2 tbsp pastry flour
- 1 cup heavy cream
- ¾ cup water

- `2 cups of shredded cheddar cheese Salt and pepper to taste
- 6 eggs, divided into whites and yolks.

Directions:

1. Preheat oven to 350 degrees.
2. Butter a 2-qrt souffle dish. Dust the bottom of the dish with the Parmesan cheese.
3. Use a saucepan to melt the butter. Add both flours. Mix vigorously.
4. While continuing to whisk, add the cream and water. Add the remaining Parmesan, cheddar, and salt and pepper.
5. Stir until mixture boils.
6. Take the saucepan off the stove and add the yolks. Whisk until integrated.
7. Pour the mixture into a bowl and let sit.
8. Beat the egg whites with a hand mixer for 5 minutes.
9. Add the egg whites into the egg mixture.
10. Transfer the soufflé into the soufflé dish.
11. Bake for 40 minutes.

90. Ham and Cheese Soufflé

Prep Time: 15 Minutes *Cook Time: 17 Minutes* *Servings: 8*

Ingredients:

- 3 tbsp sweet butter 1 chopped shallot 2 tbsp. Cake flour 1 1/2 cups whole milk 4 oz. Grated mild cheddar 1/2 tsp.
- Mustard powder 6 eggs, divided into whites and yolks Salt and pepper to taste 4 oz.
- Chopped ham 1 1/2 tbsp. chopped chives

Directions:

1. Melt 2 tablespoons butter in a saucepan. Mix in the shallots and stir for 2 minutes.
2. Stir in the flour.
3. Add the milk. Keep whisking until smooth.
4. Let the mixture simmer for 5 minutes. It should be thick by then.
5. Add the cheddar, salt and pepper, and egg yolks.
6. Keep stirring for 4 minutes.
7. Pour the mixture into a bowl and stir in the chives and ham.
8. After completely cover with plastic and refrigerate it for half an hour.
9. Preheat the oven to 375 degrees.
10. Butter a soufflé dish.
11. Beat the eggs whites with a hand mixer until they are stiff.
12. Fold the whites into the cheese mix.
13. Pour the batter into the soufflé dish.
14. Bake for 40 minutes.

91. Breakfast Enchiladas

Prep Time: 15 Minutes *Cook Time: 12 Minutes* *Servings: 4*

Ingredients:

- 1/3 cup butter
- 1/3 cup all-purpose flour
- 3 cups whole milk
- 8 oz. shredded Cheddar cheese
- 4 tbsp chopped chilis
- ½ tsp salt

Directions:

1. Melt the butter, then add the flour.
2. Stir until the mixture is smooth.
3. Put the milk, keep whisking until the mixture is thickened.
4. Place pan on the counter and stir in all of the other ingredients.

92. Sausage Twist

Prep Time: 15 Minutes *Cook Time: 18 Minutes* *Servings: 2*

Ingredients:

- 1 frozen pizza dough
- 1 pkg. breakfast sausage
- ½ cup chopped olives
- 4 oz. shredded Mozzarella cheese
- cup feta cheese 1 large egg

Directions:

1. Preheat oven to 400 degrees.
2. Flatten out the dough on a baking sheet.
3. Top the dough with sausage, olives and cheeses.
4. Fold the dough over the filling and make diagonal cuts on top.
5. Beat the egg and brush over the dough.
6. Bake for 20 minutes.
7. The dough should be a light brown.
8. Slice the dough into six portions.

93. Breakfast Burritos

Prep Time: 15 Minutes *Cook Time: 19 Minutes* *Servings: 4*

Ingredients:

- 1 package hot breakfast sausage
- 1 cup chopped green pepper
- 1 chopped jalapeno peppers
- 8 large eggs
- 2 tbsp whole milk
- 4 oz. cream cheese
- 8 flour tortillas
- Use whatever toppings you like:
- Shredded cheese
- Black Beans
- Chopped avocado
- Salsa

Directions:

1. The sausage, pepper and jalapeno pepper are frying for 10 minutes.
2. Drain the fat, but leave sausages in the skillet.
3. Mix the eggs and the milk. Add the mixture to the skillet.
4. Cook until the eggs are just are completely cooked. Mix the cream cheese and continue cooking until the cream cheese is blended. Keep the mixture warm.
5. Warm the tortillas in a skillet.
6. Divide the sausage mixture onto each tortilla. Roll up the tortilla and fold to close.
7. Repeat with all of the tortillas.
8. Place the toppings in a separate bowl.

94. Stuffed French Toast

Prep Time: 15 Minutes *Cook Time: 10 Minutes* *Servings: 5*

Ingredients:

- 3 cups of cubed bread
- 8 large eggs
- 8 oz. cream cheese
- cup honey 1 ¼ cups milk

Directions:

1. Blend the eggs, milk, and honey in a bowl.
2. After putting half of the bread on the bottom of a 9 x 13-inch baking dish.
3. Top with the cream cheese and the remaining bread.
4. Top the bread with the egg mixture, making sure to coat all, and chill overnight.
5. Bake at 350 degrees for 35 minutes.
6. Top with butter or syrup.

95. Breakfast Frittata

Prep Time: 15 Minutes *Cook Time: 10 Minutes* *Servings: 3*

Ingredients:

- 6 slices of chopped bacon
- 1 cup diced green peppe2
- Salt and pepper to taste
- 1 cup diced cooked potatoes
- 10 beaten eggs
- 2 oz. feta cheese

Directions:

1. Fry the bacon in a skillet. When bacon is crispy, mix in the green pepper.
2. Stir for approximately 3 minutes.
3. To put out the skillet from the stove and drain any excess fat. Add the salt and pepper.
4. Place the skillet back on the stove and mix in the diced potatoes. Stir for approximately 2 minutes. Add the eggs. Stir for 5 minutes. Eggs should still be soft.
5. Top frittata with the feta cheese.
6. Preheat the broiler.
7. Broil frittatas for 5 minutes.

96. Breakfast Enchiladas

Prep Time: 15 Minutes *Cook Time: 15 Minutes* *Servings: 2*

Ingredients:

- 1 lb. mild ground pork sausage
- 3 tbsp sweet butter
- 4 sliced scallions
- 3 tbsp chopped cilantro
- 14 large eggs
- Salt and pepper to taste
- 8 flour tortillas
- 4 oz. shredded Monterey Jack cheese

Directions:

1. Crumble and fry the sausage in a skillet. Drain on a paper towel.
2. Use another skillet to melt the butter.
3. Add the scallions, eggs, salt and pepper and cook for 5 minutes.
4. Place the mixture in a bowl and mix in the sausage and 1 cup of cheese sauce (see recipe below).
5. Divide the mix onto each tortilla.
6. Roll up the tortilla and transfer them to a buttered 9 x 13 baking dish.
7. Top with the rest of the cheese sauce and the Monterey Jack.
8. Bake for half an hour at 350 degrees.

Lunch Recipes

97. DAUBE PROVENÇAL

Prep Time: 14 Minutes *Cook Time: 15 Minutes* *Servings: 6*

INGREDIENTS:

- 3/4 ounce dried porcini mushrooms, rinsed
- 2 cups water
- (3 1/2-lb) boneless beef trimmed & cut into 2-inch pieces
- Tsp. salt
- Tsp. pepper
- 4 Tbsps. olive oil
- 5 ounces salt pork, rind removed
- carrots, peeled & cut into 1-inch rounds
- 2 onions, halved & sliced 1/8 inch thick
- garlic cloves, sliced thin
- Tbsps. tomato paste 1/3 cup all-purpose flour
- 1 (750-ml) bottle red wine
- 1 cup low-sodium chicken broth
- 4 (2-inch) strips orange zest, cut lengthwise into thin strips 1 cup niçoise olives, pitted
- 3 anchovy fillets, rinsed & minced
- sprigs fresh thyme, tied together with kitchen twine
- 2 bay leaves
- 1 (14.5-ounce) whole tomatoes, drained & cut into 1/2-inch pieces 2 Tbsps. minced fresh parsley

DIRECTIONS:

1. Microwave 1 cup water & mushrooms in a covered container till steaming, about 1 min. Lift mushrooms from liquid with fork & chop into 1/2-inch pieces (you should have about 1/4 cup).
2. Strain liquid through a paper towel-lined fine-mesh strainer into a medium container. Set mushrooms & liquid aside.
3. Set oven rack to lower-middle setting; heat oven to 325 degrees. Pat beef dry & season with salt & pepper. Heat 2 Tbsps. Oil in a Dutch oven after setting medium-high heat till shimmering.
4. Include half of beef & cook without moving till well browned, about 2 mins per side. Shift meat to the medium container. Repeat with remaining oil & remaining meat.
5. Reduce heat to medium & Include salt pork, carrots, onions, garlic, & tomato paste to now-empty pot; cook, occasionally stirring, till lightly brown, about 2 mins.
6. Stir in flour & cook, constantly stirring, about 1 min. Slowly Include wine, scraping the bottom of the cooking wok to loosen browned bits.
7. Include broth, remaining 1 cup water, & beef with any accumulated juices. Increase heat to medium-high & bring to simmer.
8. Stir in mushrooms & their liquid, orange zest, 1/2 cup olives, anchovies, thyme, & bay leaves, arranging beef.
9. After completely covered by a liquid, partially cover pot & place in oven. Cook till fork slips easily in & out of beef (meat should not be falling apart), 2 1/2 to 3 hrs.
10. Discard salt pork, thyme, & bay leaves. Include tomatoes & remaining 1/2 cup olives & cook over medium-high heat till heated for about 1 min.
11. Cover pot & let the stew sit for about 5 mins. Using a large spoon, skim the fat from the surface of the stew.
12. Stir in parsley & serve.

98. HUNGARIAN BEEF STEW

Prep Time: 5 Minutes | *Cook Time: 15 Minutes* | *Servings: 4*

INGREDIENTS:

- (3 1/2- to 4-lb) boneless beef, trimmed, & cut into 1 1/2-inch pieces
- Salt & pepper
- 1/3 cup paprika
- cup jarred roasted red peppers, rinsed & patted dry
- 2 Tbsps. tomato paste
- Tbsp. white vinegar
- Tbsps. vegetable oil
- 4 large onions, chopped fine
- 4 large carrots, peeled & cut into 1-inch-thick rounds 1 bay leaf
- 1 cup beef broth, warmed
- 1/4 cup sour cream (optional)

DIRECTIONS:

1. Set oven rack to lower-middle setting & heat oven to 325 degrees. Season meat evenly with 1 Tsp. Salt & let stand 15 mins.
2. Process paprika, roasted peppers, tomato paste, & 2 Tbsps. Vinegar in the food processor till smooth, 1 to 2 mins, scraping down sides as needed.
3. Combine oil, onions, & 1 Tsp. salt in Dutch oven; cover andset over medium heat.
4. Cook, occasionally stirring, till onions soften but have not yet begun to brown, 8 to 10 mins.
5. Stir in paprika butter; cook, occasionally stirring, till onions stick to the bottom of the pan, about 2 mins.
6. Include beef, carrots, & bay leaf; stir till beef is well coated. Using a rubber spatula, press the sides of the pot. Cover pot & Shift to oven.
7. Cook till meat is almost tender & the surface of the liquid is 1/2 inch below the top of the meat, 2 to 2 1/2 hrs, stirring every 30 mins.
8. Remove pot from oven & Include enough beef broth so that surface of the liquid is 1/4 inch from the top of the meat (beef should not be fully submerged).
9. Return covered pot to oven & continue to cook till fork slips easily in & out of beef, about 30 mins longer.
10. Using a large spoon, skim fat from the surface of stew; stir in remaining Tsp. Vinegar & sour cream, if using.
11. Remove bay leaf, season with salt & pepper to taste, & serve. (Stir sour cream into the reheated stew just before serving.)

99. CARBONNADE À LA FLAMANDE (BELGIAN BEEF, BEER, & ONION STEW)

Prep Time: 15 Minutes | *Cook Time: 45 Minutes* | *Servings: 4*

INGREDIENTS:

- 3 1/2 lbs blade steaks, 1 inch thick, trimmed & cut into 1-inch pieces salt & pepper
- 3 Tbsps. vegetable oil
- lbs onions, halved & sliced 1/4 inch thick
- 1 Tbsp. tomato paste
- garlic cloves, minced
- Tbsps. all-purpose flour 3/4 cup low-sodium chicken broth 3/4 cup beef broth
- 1 1/2 cups beer
- sprigs fresh thyme, tied with kitchen twine
- Two bay leaves
- 1 Tbsp. cider vinegar

DIRECTIONS:

1. Set oven rack to lower-middle setting; heat oven to 300 degrees. Beef pat drying with paper towels & season with salt & pepper. Heat 2 Tbsps. After setting over medium-high heat till beginning to smoke; Include about one-third of beef in the pot. Cook without moving till well browned, 2 to 3 mins; using tongs, turn each piece & continue cooking till the second side is well browned about 5 mins.
2. Longer. Shift browned beef to the medium container. Repeat with 2 Tbsps. oil & half of the remaining meat. (If drippings in the bottom of the pot are very dark, Include about 1/2 cup of chicken or beef broth & scrape cooking wok bottom with a wooden spoon to loosen browned bits; pour liquid into a container with browned beef, then proceed.) Repeat once more with 2 Tbsps. Oil & remaining beef.
3. Include remaining 1 Tbsp. Oil to empty Dutch oven reduces heat to medium-low. Include onions, 1/2 Tsp. Salt & tomato paste; cook, scraping the bottom of the pot to loosen browned bits, till onions have released some moisture, about 5 mins. Increase heat to medium & continue to cook, occasionally stirring, till onions are lightly browned, 12 to 14 mins. Stir in garlic & cook till fragrant, about 30 seconds. Include flour & stir till onions are evenly coated & flour is lightly browned for about 2 mins. Stir in chicken & beef broths, scraping cooking wok bottom to loosen browned bits. Mixing in beer, thyme, bay leaves, vinegar, browned beef with any accumulated juices, & salt & pepper to taste. Increase heat to medium-high & bring to simmer, stirring occasionally; cover partially, then place the pot in the oven. Cook till fork slips easily in & out of beef, about 2 hrs.
4. Discard thyme & bay leaves. Season with salt & pepper to taste & serve.

100. BEEF BURGUNDY

Prep Time: 20 Minutes | *Cook Time: 18 Minutes* | *Servings: 8*

INGREDIENTS:

- ounces salt pork, rind removed & reserved, salt pork cut into 1 by 1/4 by 1/4-inch pieces
- 2 onions, chopped coarsely
- 2 carrots, chopped coarsely
- 1 head garlic, cloves separated & crushed but unpeeled
- 1/2 ounce dried porcini mushrooms, rinsed (optional)
- sprigs fresh parsley, torn into pieces
- 6 sprigs of fresh thyme
- 2 bay leaves, crumbled
- 1/2 Tsp. whole black peppercorns
- (4-to 4 1/4-lb) boneless beef chuck-eye roast pulled apart at seams, trimmed, & cut into 1 1/2- to 2-inch chunks
- Salt & pepper
- 2 1/2 cups water
- Tbsps. unsalted butter, cut into 4 pieces 1/3 cup all-purpose flour
- 1 3/4 cups low-sodium chicken broth
- (750-ml) bottle red wine
- Tsp. tomato paste
- cup frozen pearl onions, thawed
- Tbsp. unsalted butter
- Tbsp. sugar
- Salt & pepper
- 3/4 cup water
- ounces white mushrooms, trimmed, whole if small, halved if medium, quartered if large
- 2 Tbsps. brandy
- 3 Tbsps. minced fresh parsley

DIRECTIONS:

1. Bring salt pork, reserved salt pork rind, & 3 cups water to boil in a medium saucepan over high heat. Boil 2 mins, then drain well.
2. Cut two 22-inch lengths of cheesecloth & place them on top of each other. Wrap onions, carrots, garlic, porcini mushrooms, parsley, thyme, bay leaves, peppercorns, & blanched salt pork rind in cheesecloth & set in Dutch oven. Set oven rack to lower-middle setting & heat oven to 300 degrees.
3. Heat salt pork in a large pan over medium heat & cook till lightly browned & crisp, about 12 mins. Using a slotted spoon, Shift to pot; pour off all but 2 Tbsps. Fat & reserve. Season beef with salt & pepper. Increase heat to high & brown half of beef in a single layer, turning once or twice, till deep brown, about 7 mins; Shift browned beef to pot. Pour 1/2 cup water into pan & scrape cooking wok to loosen browned bits; Include liquid to the pot.
4. Return pan to high heat & Include 2 Tbsps. Reserved pork fat; swirl to coat cooking wok bottom. When fat begins to smoke, remaining brown beef in a single layer, turning once or twice, till deep brown, about 7 mins; Shift browned beef to pot. Pour 1/2 cup water into pan & scrape cooking wok to loosen browned bits; Include liquid to the pot.
5. Melt butter in a now-empty pan over medium heat. Whisk in flour till evenly moistened & cook, constantly whisking, till batter has toasty aroma & resembles light-coloured peanut butter, about 5 mins.
6. Gradually whisk in chicken broth & remaining 1 1/2 cups water; increase heat to medium-high & bring to simmer, frequently stirring, till thickened. Pour batter into pot. Include 3 cups wine, tomato paste, & salt & pepper to taste to pot & stir to combine. Set pot over high heat & bring to boil. Cover & Shift to oven; cook till meat is tender, 2 1/2 to hrs.
7. After removing the pot carefully from the oven and using tongs, Shift vegetable & herb bouquet to a strainer set over the pot. Press out the liquid into the pot & discard the bouquet. With a slotted spoon, remove beef to medium container; set aside. Allow braising liquid to settle for 15 mins; with a large spoon, skim fat from surface & discard.
8. Bring liquid in the pot to boil over medium-high heat. Simmer briskly, occasionally stirring to ensure that bottom is not burning, till sauce is reduced to about 3 cups & thickened to the consistency of heavy cream, 15 to 25 mins.
9. While reducing the sauce, bring pearl onions, butter, sugar, 1/4 Tsp. Salt, & 1/2 cup water to boil in a medium pan over high heat; cover & reduce heat to medium-low & simmer, shaking cooking wok occasionally, till onions are tender about 5 mins. Uncover, increase heat to high, & simmer till all liquid evaporates, about 3 mins. Include mushrooms & 1/4 Tsp. Salt; cook, occasionally stirring, till liquid released by mushrooms evaporates & vegetables are browned & glazed about 5 mins. Shift vegetables to a large plate & set them aside. Include remaining 1/4 cup water to pan & stir to loosen browned bits. When cooking wok bottom & sides are clean, Include liquid to reducing the sauce.
10. When the sauce has been less to about 3 cups & thickened the heavy cream, low heat to medium-low; stir in beef, mushrooms & onions (and any accumulated juices), remaining wine from the bottle, & brandy into the pot. Cover pot & cook till just heated through, 5 to 8 mins. Season with salt & pepper to taste & serve, sprinkling individual servings with minced parsley.

101. CLASSIC POT ROAST

Prep Time: 20 Minutes | *Cook Time: 18 Minutes* | *Servings: 2*

INGREDIENTS:

- (3 1/2- to 4-lb) boneless beef chuck-eye roast pulled apart at seams & trimmed Kosher salt & pepper
- Tbsps. unsalted butter
- onions, halved & sliced thin
- large carrot, peeled & chopped
- celery rib, chopped
- garlic cloves, minced 2–3 cups beef broth
- 3/4 cup dry red wine
- 1 Tbsp. tomato paste
- 1 bay leaf
- 1 sprig fresh thyme plus 1/4 Tsp. chopped
- 1 Tbsp. balsamic vinegar
- Season pieces of meat with 1 Tbsp. Salt, in rimmed baking sheet, & let stand at room temperature for 1 hr.

DIRECTIONS:

1. Set oven rack to lower-middle setting & heat oven to 300 degrees. Butter melting in a Dutch oven set over medium heat. Include onions & cook, occasionally stirring, till softened & beginning to brown, 8 to 10 mins. Include carrot & celery; continue to cook, occasionally stirring, for about 5 mins. Include garlic & cook till fragrant, about 30 seconds. Stir in 1 cup broth, 1/2 cup wine, tomato paste, bay leaf, & thyme sprig; bring to simmer. Beef pat drying with the paper towels & season with pepper mixed 3 pieces of kitchen twine around each piece of meat into an even shape.

2. aluminium foil & cover with lid; Shift pot to oven. Cook beef till fully tender & fork slips easily in & out of meat, 3¹/2 to 4 hrs, turning meat halfway through cooking.
3. Shift roasts to carving board & tent loosely with foil. Strain liquid through a fine-mesh strainer into the 4-cup liquid measuring cup. Discard bay leaf & thyme sprig. Shift vegetables to a blender. Let liquid settle for 5 mins, then skim fat; Include beef broth to bring the liquid amount to 3 cups. Include liquid to blender & blend till smooth, about 2 mins. Shift sauce to medium saucepan & bring to simmer over medium heat.
4. Meanwhile, remove twine from roasts & slice against the grain into ¹/2-inch-thick slices. Shift meat to a serving platter. Stir remaining ¹/4 cup wine, chopped thyme, & vinegar into gravy & season with salt & pepper to taste. Spoon half of the gravy over meat; pass the remaining gravy separately.

102. FRENCH-STYLE POT ROAST

Prep Time: 19 Minutes *Cook Time: 17 Minutes* *Servings: 3*

INGREDIENTS:

- (4-to 5-lb) boneless beef chuck-eye roast pulled apart at seams & trimmed Kosher salt & pepper
- (750-ml) bottle red wine
- sprigs fresh parsley plus 2 Tbsps. minced
- 2 sprigs of fresh thyme
- 2 bay leaves
- 3 slices thick-cut bacon, cut into ¹/4-inch pieces 1 onion, chopped fine
- 3 garlic cloves, minced
- 1 Tbsp. all-purpose flour
- 2 cups beef broth
- 4 carrots, peeled & cut on the bias into 1¹/2-inch pieces 2 cups frozen pearl onions, thawed
- 3 Tbsps. unsalted butter
- 2 Tbsps. sugar
- ³/4 cup water
- ounces white mushrooms, trimmed, halved if small & quartered if large
- 1 Tbsp. unflavored gelatin

DIRECTIONS:

1. Season pieces of meat with 2 Tbsps. Salt, in rimmed baking sheet, & let rest at room temperature for 1 hr.
2. Meanwhile, bring wine to simmer in a large saucepan over medium-high heat. Cook till reduced to 2 cups, about 15 mins. Using kitchen twine, tie parsley sprigs, thyme sprigs, & bay leaves into a bundle.
3. Beef pat drying with paper towels & season generously with pepper. Mixed with 3 pieces of kitchen twine around each piece of meat to keep it from falling apart.
4. Set oven rack to lower-middle setting & heat oven to 300 degrees. Cook bacon in an oven of a Dutch after setting medium-high heat, occasionally stirring, till crisp, 6 to 8 mins. Using a slotted spoon, Shift bacon to the paper towel-lined plate & reserve. Pour off all but 2 Tbsps. Fat. Return Dutch oven to medium-high heat & heat till fat begins to smoke. Include beef to pot & brown on all sides, 8 to 10 mins total. Shift beef to a large plate & set aside.
5. Reduce heat to medium; Include onion & cook, occasionally stirring, till beginning to soften, 2 to 4 mins. Include garlic, flour, & reserved bacon; cook, constantly stirring, till fragrant, about 30 seconds. Include reduced wine, broth, & herb bundle, scraping the bottom of the pot to loosen browned bits. Return roast & any accumulated juices to pot; increase heat to high & bring the liquid to simmer, then place a large sheet of aluminium foil over pot & cover tightly with lid. Set pot in oven & cook, using tongs to turn beef every hr, till fork slips easily in & out of meat, 2¹/2 to 3 hrs, including carrots to pot after 2 hrs. After meat cooks, bring pearl onions, butter, sugar, & ¹/2 cup water to boil in a large pan over medium-high heat. Reduce heat to medium, cover, & cook till onions are tender, 5 to 8 mins. Uncover, increase heat to medium-high, & cook till all liquid evaporates, 3 to 4 mins. Include mushrooms & ¹/4 Tsp. Salt; cook, occasionally stirring, till vegetables are browned & glazed, 8 to 12 mins. Remove from heat & set aside. Place remaining ¹/4 cup cold water in the small container & sprinkle gelatin on top.
6. Shift beef to carving board; tent with foil to keep warm. Let
7. Braising liquid settle, about 5 mins; using a large spoon, skim fat from surface. Remove herb bundle & stir in the onion-mushroom batter. Bring liquid to simmer over medium-high heat & cook till batter is slightly thickened & reduced to 3¹/4 cups, 20 to 30 mins. Season sauce with salt & pepper to taste. Include softened gelatin & stir till completely dissolved.
8. Remove twine from roasts & discard. Slice meat against the grain into ¹/2-inch-thick slices. Divide meat among warmed containers or Shift to platter; arrange vegetables around meat, pour sauce over the top, & sprinkle with minced parsley. Serve immediately.

103. BEEF BRAISED IN BAROLO

Prep Time: 22 Minutes *Cook Time: 20 Minutes* *Servings: 4*

INGREDIENTS:

- (3¹/2-lb) boneless beef chuck-eye roast pulled apart at seams & trimmed
- 4 ounces pancetta, cut into ¹/4-inch cubes 2 onions, chopped
- 2 carrots, chopped
- 2 celery ribs, chopped
- Tbsp. tomato paste
- 3 garlic cloves, minced
- Tbsp. All-purpose flour ¹/2 Tsp. sugar
- (750-ml) bottle Barolo wine
- (14.5-ounce) can diced tomatoes, drained
- 10 sprigs fresh parsley
- sprig fresh rosemary
- sprig fresh thyme, plus 1 Tsp. minced

DIRECTIONS:

1. 2Set oven rack to middle setting; heat oven to 300 degrees. Beef pat drying with paper towels, season with salt & pepper & tie both pieces together with kitchen twine. Place pancetta in 8-quart Dutch oven; cook over medium heat, occasionally stirring, till browned & crisp, about 8 mins. Using a slotted spoon, Shift the pancetta to the paper towel-lined plate & set it aside. Pour off all but 2 Tbsps. Fat; set Dutch oven over medium-high heat & heat till beginning to smoke. Include beef to pot & cook till well browned on all sides, about 8 mins. Shift beef to a large plate & set aside.
2. Reduce heat to medium; include onions, carrots, celery, & tomato paste to pot & cook, occasionally stirring, till vegetables begin to soften & brown, about 6 mins. Include garlic, flour, sugar, & reserved pancetta; cook, constantly stirring, till fragrant, about 30 seconds. Include wine & tomatoes, scraping the bottom of the cooking wok to loosen browned bits; Include parsley, rosemary, & thyme sprigs. Return roast & any accumulated juices to pot; increase heat to high & bring the liquid to boil, then place a large sheet of aluminium foil over pot & cover tightly with lid. Set pot in oven & cook, using tongs to turn beef every 45 mins, till fork slips easily in & out of meat, about 3 hrs.
3. 4Shift beef to carving board; tent with foil to keep warm. Let braising liquid settle, about 5 mins; using a large spoon, skim fat from the surface. Include minced thyme, bring the liquid to boil over high heat, & cook, whisking vigorously to help vegetables break down, till batter is thickened & reduced to about 3¹/2 cups, about 18 mins. Strain liquid through a large fine-mesh strainer, pressing on solids to extract as much liquid as possible; you should have 1¹/2 cups strained sauce (if necessary, return the strained sauce to Dutch oven & reduce to 1¹/2 cups). Discard solids in strainer. Season sauce with salt & pepper to taste.
4. Remove twine from roasts & discard. Slice meat against the grain into ¹/2-inch-thick slices. Divide meat among warmed containers or plates; pour about ¹/4 cup sauce over the top & serve immediately.

104. BEEF STROGANOFF

Prep Time: 35 Minutes *Cook Time: 12 Minutes* *Servings: 8*

INGREDIENTS:

- 1¹/4 lbs sirloin steak tips, trimmed & cut lengthwise with grain into 4 equal pieces 2 Tbsps. soy sauce
- lb white mushrooms, trimmed & quartered
- Tbsp. dry mustard
- Tbsps. hot water
- 1 Tsp. sugar Salt & pepper
- 1 Tbsp. vegetable oil
- 1 onion, chopped fine
- 4 Tbsps. all-purpose flour
- Tbsps. tomato paste 1¹/2 cups beef broth
- ¹/3 cup plus 1 Tbsp. white wine or dry vermouth ¹/2 cup sour cream
- 1 Tbsp. chopped fresh parsley or dill

DIRECTIONS:

1. Poke using a fork or finger each piece of steak 10 to 12 times. Place in baking dish; rub both sides evenly with soy sauce. Covered with plastic wrap & let it cool into refrigerate for at least 15 mins or up to 1 hr.
2. While meat marinates, place mushrooms in a medium container, cover, & microwave till mushrooms have decreased in volume by half, 4 to 5 mins (there should be as much as ¹/4 cup liquid in a container). Drain mushrooms & set aside; discard liquid. Combine mustard, water, sugar, & ¹/2 Tsp. Pepper in a small container till smooth paste forms; set aside.
3. Pat steak pieces dry with paper towels & season with pepper. Heat oil in the 12-inch pan over medium-high heat till just smoking. Place steak pieces in the pan & cook till browned on all sides & meat registers 125 to 130 degrees, 6 to 9 mins. Shift meat to a large plate & set it aside while cooking sauce.
4. 5Include mushrooms, onion, & ¹/2 Tsp. Salt to pan & cook till vegetables begin to brown & dark bits form on the bottom of the pan, 6 to 8 mins. Include flour & tomato paste & cook, constantly stirring, till onions & mushrooms are coated, about 1 min. Stir in beef broth, ¹/3
5. 6cup wine, & mustard paste & bring to simmer, scraping the bottom of the cooking wok to loosen browned bits. Reduce heat to medium & cook till sauce has reduced slightly & begun to thicken, 4 to 6 mins.
6. While sauce is reducing, cut steak pieces across grain into ¹/4-inch-thick slices. Stir meat & any accumulated juices into the thickened sauce & cook till beef has warmed through, 1 to 2 mins. Remove cooking wok from heat & let any bubbles subside. Stir in sour cream & remaining Tbsp. Wine; season with salt & pepper to taste. Sprinkle with parsley & serve.

105. POT-AU-FEU

Prep Time: 15 Minutes *Cook Time: 35 Minutes* *Servings: 2*

INGREDIENTS:

- onions, chopped
- carrots, chopped
- 1 celery rib, chopped
- Tbsps. vegetable oil
- 1 (3-lb) beef chuck-eye roast, trimmed & tied
- lbs beef short ribs (about 5 large ribs), trimmed & tied
- 2 lbs beef shanks, 1¹/2 inches thick, trimmed & tied
- cups water
- 3 bay leaves
- 1 Tsp. whole black peppercorns
- 5 whole cloves
- 1 large head garlic, outer papery skins removed & top third of head cut off & discarded
- sprigs fresh parsley
- 8 sprigs of fresh thyme
- 1 Tbsp. salt
- lbs small red potatoes, halved if larger than 1¹/2 inches
- Tbsps. salt
- 1¹/2 lbs carrots, peeled, halved crosswise, thicker half quartered lengthwise, thinner half halved lengthwise
- 1¹/2 lbs parsnips, peeled, halved crosswise, thicker half quartered lengthwise, thinner half halved lengthwise
- 1 lb green beans, trimmed
- ¹/4 cup chopped fresh parsley
- baguette, sliced thick
- Dijon mustard or whole grain mustard Sea salt
- Cornichons Prepared horseradish

DIRECTIONS:

1. Combine onions, carrots, celery, & oil in a large stockpot; cook, covered, over low heat, frequently stirring, till vegetables are softened but not browned, 8 to 10 mins. (If vegetables begin to brown before softening, Include 1 Tbsp. water & continue to cook.) Include roast, ribs, shanks, water, bay leaves, peppercorns, & cloves; increase heat to medium-high & bring to boil, using a large spoon to skim any fat. Reduce heat to low & simmer, uncovered, for 2¹/2 hrs, the skimming surface of fat every 30 mins.
2. Include garlic, parsley stems, thyme, & salt. Simmer till the tip of the paring knife inserted into meats meets little resistance, 1 to 1¹/2 hrs.
3. Using tongs, Shift roast, ribs, shanks, & garlic to a large carving board & tent with aluminium foil after straining the broth through a mesh strainer lined with double layer cheesecloth into a large container. Let broth settle for at least 5 mins; using a large spoon, skim fat from the surface.
4. While broth settles, rinse out stockpot & Include potatoes, salt, & 16 cups water; bring to boil over high heat & cook for 7 mins. Include carrots & parsnips & cook for 3 mins. Include green beans & cook for 4 mins. Using a slotted spoon, Shift
5. Vegetables to large serving platter & tent with foil.

6. Using tongs, squeeze garlic cloves out of skins & into a small serving container. Remove twine from roast & separate roast at its seams; cut roast across the grain into 1/2-inch-thick slices & Shift to platter with vegetables. Remove twine from shanks & ribs & arrange on a platter. Ladle about 1 cup broth over meat & vegetables & sprinkle with parsley. Serve, ladling broth over individual servings & passing garlic, baguette, & condiments separately.

106. BRAISED BONELESS BEEF SHORTRIBS

Prep Time: 18 Minutes *Cook Time: 16 Minutes* *Servings: 8*

INGREDIENTS:

- 3 1/2 lbs boneless beef short ribs, trimmed
- Kosher salt & pepper
- Tbsps. vegetable oil
- large onions, sliced thin
- 1 Tbsp. tomato paste
- 6 garlic cloves, peeled
- cups red wine
- 1 cup beef broth
- large carrots, peeled & cut into 2-inch pieces
- sprigs fresh thyme
- 1 bay leaf
- 1/4 cup cold water
- 1/2 Tsp. unflavored gelatin

DIRECTIONS:

1. Set oven rack to lower-middle setting & heat oven to 300 degrees. Beef pat drying with paper towels & season with 2 Tbsps. salt & 1 Tsp. pepper. Heat 1 Tbsp. Oil in over medium-high heat of oven till smoking. Include half of beef & cook, without moving, till well browned, 4 to 6 mins. Turn beef & continue to cook on the second side till well browned, 4 to 6 mins longer, low heat if fat begins to smoke. Shift beef to the medium container. Repeat with remaining 1 Tbsp. Oil & meat.
2. Reduce heat to medium, Include onions, & cook, occasionally stirring, till softened & beginning to brown, 12 to 15 mins. (If onions begin to darken too quickly, Include 1 to 2 Tbsps. water to the pan.) Include tomato paste & cook, constantly stirring, till it browns on sides & bottom of the pan, about 2 mins. Include garlic & cook till fragrant, about 30 seconds. Increase heat to medium-high, Include wine & simmer, scraping the bottom of cooking wok to loosen browned bits, till reduced by half, 8 to 10 mins. Include broth, carrots, thyme, & bay leaf. Include beef & any accumulated juices to pot; cover & bring to simmer. Shift pot to oven & cook, turning meat twice during cooking, till fork slips easily in & out of meat, 2 to 2 1/2 hrs.
3. Place water in the small container & sprinkle gelatin on top; let stand at least 5 mins. Using tongs, Shift meat & carrots to serving platter & tent with aluminium foil. Straining liquid through a fine-mesh strainer into a fat separator or container, compression on solids to remove liquid as possible; discard solids. Let liquid settle for 5 mins & strain off fat. Return cooking liquid to pot & cook over medium heat till reduced to 1 cup, 5 to 10 mins. Remove from heat & stir in gelatin batter; season with salt & pepper to taste. Pour sauce over meat & serve.

107. SHORT RIBS BRAISED IN RED WINE WITH BACON, PARSNIPS, & PEARL ONIONS

Prep Time: 25 Minutes *Cook Time: 23 Minutes* *Servings: 6*

INGREDIENTS:

- lbs bone-in English-style beef short ribs, trimmed, or bone-in flanken-style beef short ribs, trimmed
- cups dry red wine
- large onions, chopped
- 2 carrots, chopped
- 1 large celery rib, chopped
- 9 garlic cloves, chopped
- 1/4 cup all-purpose flour
- 4 cups low-sodium chicken broth
- (14.5-ounce) can diced tomatoes, drained 1 1/2 Tbsps. minced fresh rosemary
- Tbsp. minced fresh thyme
- 3 bay leaves
- 1 Tsp. tomato paste
- 6 slices bacon, cut into 1/4-inch pieces
- ounces parsnips, peeled & cut diagonally into 3/4-inch pieces
- 1 cup frozen pearl onions, thawed
- 1/4 Tsp. granulated sugar
- 1/4 Tsp. salt
- Tbsps. chopped fresh parsley

DIRECTIONS:

1. 2Set oven rack to lower-middle setting & heat oven to 450 degrees. Arrange short ribs bone side down in single layer in large roasting pan; season with salt & pepper. Roast till meat begins to brown, about 45 mins; drain off all liquid. Return cooking wok to oven & continue to cook till meat is well browned, 15 to 20 mins longer. (For flanken-style short ribs, continue to cook till browned, about 8 mins; using tongs, flip each piece & cook till the second side is browned, about 8 mins longer.) Shift ribs to a large plate; set aside. Drain off & reserve fat. Reduce oven temperature to 300 degrees. Heat roasting cooking wok on 2 stovetop burners over medium heat; Include wine & bring to simmer, scraping up browned bits. Set cooking wok with wine aside.
2. Heat 2 Tbsps. Reserved fat in a Dutch oven over medium-high heat; Include onions, carrots, & celery & cook, occasionally stirring, till vegetables soften, about 12 mins. Include garlic & cook till fragrant, about 30 seconds. Stir in flour till combined, about 45 seconds. Stir in wine from roasting pan, broth, tomatoes, rosemary, thyme, bay leaves, tomato paste, & salt & pepper to taste. Bring to boil & Include ribs, completely submerging meat in liquid; return to boil, cover, Shift to the oven, & simmer till ribs are tender, 2 to 2 1/2 hrs. Shift pot to wire rack & cool, partially covered, till warm, about 2 hrs.
3. Shift ribs to large plate & discard loose bones. Strain braising liquid into the medium container, pressing out liquid from solids; discard solids. Cover ribs & liquid separately & refrigerate overnight. (Ribs & liquid can be refrigerated for up to 3 days.)
4. In a Dutch oven, cook bacon over medium heat till just crisp, 8 to 10 mins; using a slotted spoon, Shift to a paper towel-lined plate. Include parsnips, pearl onions, sugar, & salt to pot & cook over high heat, occasionally stirring, till browned, about 5 mins. Spoon off & discard solidified fat from the reserved braising liquid. Include defatted liquid & bring to simmer, stirring occasionally; season with salt & pepper to taste. Submerge ribs in liquid, return to simmer. Reduce heat to medium & cook, partially covered, till ribs are heated through & vegetables are tender, about 5 mins longer; gently stir in bacon. Divide ribs & sauce among individual containers sprinkle each with 1 Tbsp. Parsley, & serve.

108. ONION-BRAISED BEEF BRISKET

Prep Time: 25 Minutes *Cook Time: 23 Minutes* *Servings: 6*

INGREDIENTS:

- (4-to 5-lb) beef brisket, flat cut preferred, trimmed salt & pepper
- Vegetable oil
- 2 1/2 lbs onions, halved & sliced 1/2 inch thick
- Tbsp. brown sugar
- 3 garlic cloves, minced
- Tbsp. tomato paste
- Tbsp. paprika
- 1/8 Tsp. cayenne pepper
- Tbsps. all-purpose flour
- 1 cup low-sodium chicken broth
- 1 cup dry red wine
- 3 bay leaves
- 3 sprigs fresh thyme
- Tbsps. cider vinegar

DIRECTIONS:

1. Set oven rack to lower-middle setting & heat oven to 300 degrees. Line 13 by a 9-inch baking dish with two 24-inch-long sheets of 18-inch-wide heavy-duty foil, setting sheets perpendicular to each Other & allowing excess foil to extend beyond edges of the pan. Pat the brisket dry with a paper towel. Place the brisket with the fat side on a cutting board. Using a dinner fork, pierce the meat through the fat layer about 1 inch. Present both sides of the brisket with salt and pepper.
2. Heat 1 Tsp. Oil in a 12-inch pan over medium-high heat till oil just begins to smoke. Place brisket, fat side up, in a pan (brisket may climb up sides of the pan); weight brisket with a heavy Dutch oven or cast-iron pan & cook till well browned about 7 mins. Remove Dutch oven; using tongs, flip brisket & cook on the second side without weight till well browned, about 7 mins longer. Shift brisket to a platter.
3. Pour off all but 1 Tbsp. Fat from cooking wok (or, if brisket was lean, Include enough oil to fat in the pan to equal 1 Tbsp.); stir in onions, sugar, & 1/4 Tsp. Salt & cook over medium-high heat, occasionally stirring, till onions are softened, 10 to 12 mins. Include garlic & cook, frequently stirring, till fragrant, about 1 min; Include tomato paste & cook, stirring to combine, till paste darkens, about 2 mins. Include paprika & cayenne & cook, constantly stirring, till fragrant, about 1 min. Include flour & cook, constantly stirring, till well combined, about 2 mins. Include broth, wine, bay leaves, & thyme, stirring to scrape up browned bits from pan; bring to simmer & simmer for 5 mins to fully thicken.
4. 4Pour sauce & onions into a foil-lined baking dish. Nestle brisket, fat side up, in sauce & onions. Fold foil extensions over & seal (do not tightly crimp foil because foil must later be opened to test for doneness). Place in oven & cook till fork slips easily in & out of meat, 3 1/2 to 4 hrs (when testing for doneness, open foil with caution as contents will be steaming). Carefully open foil & let brisket cool at room temperature, 20 to 30 mins.
5. 1Shift brisket to large container; set fine-mesh strainer over container & strain sauce over brisket. Discard bay leaves & thyme from onions & Shift onions to a small container. Cover both containers with plastic wrap, cut vents in plastic, & refrigerate overnight.
6. About 45 mins before serving, Set oven rack to lower-middle setting; heat oven to 350 degrees. While oven heats, Shift cold brisket to a carving board. Scrape off & discard any fat from the surface of the sauce, then heat sauce in a medium saucepan over medium heat till warm, skimming any fat on the surface with a wide shallow spoon. Slice brisket against grain into 1/4-inch-thick slices & place slices in 13 by 9-inch baking dish. Stir reserved onions & vinegar into warmed sauce & season with salt & pepper to taste. To put the sauce over brisket slices, cover the baking dish with foil, & bake till heated through 25 to 30 mins. Serve immediately.

109. NEW ENGLAND–STYLE CORNED BEEF & CABBAGE

Prep Time: 15 Minutes *Cook Time: 45 Minutes* *Servings: 6*

INGREDIENTS:

- 1/2 cup kosher salt
- Tbsp. black peppercorns, cracked
- Tbsp. dried thyme
- 2 1/4 Tbsps. ground allspice
- 1 1/2 Tbsps. paprika
- 2 bay leaves, crumbled
- (4-to 6-lb) beef brisket, preferably point cut, trimmed, rinsed, & patted dry 7–8 lbs vegetables, chosen from categories below
- Carrots, peeled & halved crosswise, thin end halved lengthwise, thick end quartered lengthwise.
- Rutabagas (small), peeled & halved crosswise; each half cut into 6 chunks Turnips, peeled & quartered.
- Red potatoes (small), scrubbed & left whole
- Boiling onions (small), peeled & left whole
- Green cabbage (1 small head), uncored & cut into 6 to 8 wedges
- Parsnips, peeled & halved crosswise, thin end halved lengthwise, thick end quartered lengthwise
- Brussels sprouts, trimmed

DIRECTIONS:

1. Combine salt, peppercorns, thyme, allspice, paprika, & bay leaves in a small container. Poke brisket about 30 times on each side with a fork or metal skewer. Rub each side evenly with salt batter; place in the 2-gallon zipper- Lock bag, forcing out as much air as possible. Place in cooking wok large enough to hold it, cover with second, similar-size pan, & weight with 2 bricks or heavy cans. Refrigerate 5 to 7 days for storing, turning once a day.
2. Rinse brisket & pat it dry. Place brisket in a large stockpot, Include water to cover, & bring to boil, skimming the surface. Cover & simmer till the skewer inserted in the thickest part of brisket slides out easily, 2 to 3 hrs.
3. Heat oven to 200 degrees. Shift meat to a large platter & ladle about 1 cup cooking liquid over the top to keep it moist. Cover with aluminium foil & set in the oven.
4. Include vegetables from category 1 to pot & bring to boil; cover & simmer till vegetables begin to soften, about 10 mins. Include vegetables from category 2 & bring to boil; cover & simmer till all vegetables are tender, 10 to 15 mins longer.
5. Meanwhile, remove meat out of the oven & slice across the grain into 1/4-inch slices. Shift vegetables to a platter, drizzle with broth, & serve.

110. BRAISED LAMB SHOULDER CHOPS WITH TOMATOES & RED WINE

Prep Time: 10 Minutes *Cook Time: 8 Minutes* *Servings: 4*

INGREDIENTS:

- lamb shoulder chops, about 3/4 inch thick, trimmed salt & pepper
- 2 Tbsps. olive oil
- small onion, chopped fine
- 2 small garlic cloves, minced
- 1/3 cup dry red wine
- cup canned whole peeled tomatoes, chopped
- 2 Tbsps. minced fresh parsley

DIRECTIONS:

1. 2Season chops with salt & pepper. Heat 1 Tbsp. Oil in a 12-inch pan over medium-high heat. Brown chops, in batches, if necessary, on both sides, 4 to 5 mins. Set aside.
2. 3Pour off fat from the pan. Include remaining 1 Tbsp. Oil & heat over medium heat. Include onion & cook till softened, about 4 mins. Include garlic & cook till fragrant, about 30 seconds longer. Include wine & simmer till reduced by half, scraping to loosen browned bits from the bottom of the pan, 2 to 3 mins. Stir in tomatoes, then return chops to pan. Reduce heat to low & cover & simmer till chops are cooked through & tender, 15 to 20 mins.
3. Shift chops to individual plates. Stir parsley into the sauce & simmer till sauce thickens 2 to 3 mins. Present with salt & pepper to taste, spoon sauce over each chop, & serve.

111. LAMB SHANKS BRAISED IN RED WINE WITH HERBES DE PROVENCE

Prep Time: 35 Minutes *Cook Time: 11 Minutes* *Servings: 6*

INGREDIENTS:

- (12-to 16-ounce) lamb shanks, trimmed salt & pepper
- 2 Tbsps. vegetable oil
- carrots, peeled & cut into 2-inch pieces
- 2 onions, sliced thick
- 2 celery ribs, cut into 2-inch pieces
- 4 garlic cloves, minced
- 2 Tbsps. tomato paste
- 1 Tbsp. herbes de Provence
- 2 cups dry red wine
- cups low-sodium chicken broth

DIRECTIONS:

1. Set oven rack to middle setting & heat oven to 350 degrees. Pat lamb shanks dry & season with salt. After heating oil in a Dutch oven over medium-high heat till just smoking. Brown half of shanks on all sides, 7 to 10 mins. Shift shanks to large plate & repeat with remaining Tbsp. Oil & remaining lamb shanks.
2. Drain all but 2 Tbsps. Fat off the pan. Include carrots, onions, celery, garlic, tomato paste, herbes de Provence, & pinch salt & cook till vegetables are just starting to soften, 3 to 4 mins. Mixing in wine, then broth, scraping up browned bits on the bottom of the pan.
3. Bring to simmer, cover the pot, Shift to the oven, & cook for 1 1/2 hrs.
4. 5Uncover & continue to cook till tops of shanks are browned, about 30 mins. Flip shanks & continue to cook till remaining sides are browned & fork slips easily in & out of shanks, 15 to 30 mins longer.
5. Remove pot from oven & let rest for 15 mins. Using tongs, Shift shanks & vegetables to a large plate & tent with aluminium foil. Skim fat from braising liquid & season with salt & pepper to taste. To change the shanks to braising liquid to warm through before serving.

DINNER

112. RAS AL HANOUT

Prep Time: 10 Minutes *Cook Time: 8 Minutes* *Servings: 4*

INGREDIENTS:

- allspice berries
- cardamom pods
- whole black peppercorns
- 1 (1/2-inch) cinnamon stick
- 1 Tbsp. ground ginger
- 1 Tsp. fennel seeds
- 1 Tsp. coriander seeds
- 1 Tsp. ground nutmeg
- 1/2 Tsp. anise seeds
- 1/2 Tsp. cumin seeds
- 1/8 Tsp. red pepper flakes
- 1/8 Tsp. mace

DIRECTIONS:

1. Combine all ingredients and, using a spice grinder, grind to a fine powder.
2. Shift to a small container.

113. CHICKEN TIKKA MASALA

Prep Time: 20 Minutes *Cook Time: 18 Minutes* *Servings: 2*

INGREDIENTS:

- 1 Tsp. salt
- 1/2 Tsp. ground cumin
- 1/2 Tsp. ground coriander
- 1/4 Tsp. cayenne pepper
- lbs boneless, skinless chicken breasts, trimmed
- 1 cup plain whole-milk yoghurt
- Tbsps. vegetable oil
- Tbsp. grated fresh ginger
- Two garlic cloves, minced
- Tbsps. vegetable oil
- One onion, chopped fine
- 2 garlic cloves, minced
- 2 Tbsps. grated fresh ginger
- 1 fresh serrano chile, ribs & seeds removed, flesh minced 1 Tbsp. tomato paste
- 1 Tbsp. garam masala
- 1 (28-ounce) can crushed tomatoes
- 2 Tbsps. sugar
- Salt
- 2/3 cup heavy cream
- 1/4 cup chopped fresh cilantro1

DIRECTIONS:

1. Combine salt, cumin, coriander, & cayenne in a small container. Sprinkle both sides of the chicken with spice batter, pressing gently so the batter adheres. Place chicken on a plate, cover with plastic wrap, & refrigerate for 30 to 60 mins. Meanwhile, whisk yoghurt, oil, ginger, & garlic together in the large container & set aside.
2. Heating oil a over medium heat till shimmering. Include onion & cook, frequently stirring, till lightly golden, 8 to 10 mins. Include garlic, ginger, serrano, tomato paste, & garam masala & cook, frequently stirring, till fragrant, about 3 mins. Include crushed tomatoes, sugar, & 1/2 Tsp. Salt & bring to boil. Reduce heat to medium-low, cover, & simmer for 15 mins, stirring occasionally. Stir in cream & return to simmer. Remove cooking wok from heat & cover to keep warm.
3. While sauce simmers, setting oven rack 6 inches from heating element & heat broiler. Using tongs, dip chicken into yoghurt batter (chicken should be coated with a thick layer of yoghurt) & arrange on a wire rack set in an aluminium foil-lined rimmed baking sheet or broiler pan. Discard excess yoghurt batter. Broil chicken till thickest part registers 160 degrees & exterior is lightly charred in spots, 10 to 18 mins, flipping chicken halfway through cooking.
4. Let chicken rest 5 mins, cut into 1-inch chunks & stir into warm sauce (do not simmer chicken in sauce). Mixed in cilantro, and present with salt to taste, & serve.

114. INDIAN LAMB CURRY WITH WHOLE SPICES

Prep Time: 20 Minutes *Cook Time: 18 Minutes* *Servings: 2*

INGREDIENTS:

- 1 1/2 (3-inch-long) cinnamon sticks
- whole cloves
- green cardamom pods
- 8 black peppercorns
- 1 bay leaf
- 1/4 cup vegetable oil
- 1 onion, sliced thin
- 1 1/2 lbs boneless leg meat
- cut into 3/4-inch cubes 2/3 cup crushed tomatoes
- 4 large garlic cloves, minced
- Tbsp. grated fresh ginger
- 2 Tbsps. ground cumin
- 2 Tbsps. ground coriander
- Tsp. ground turmeric
- 2 cups water
- jalapeño chile, cut in half lengthwise, stemmed & seeded
- 4 medium boiling potatoes, peeled & cut into 3/4-inch cubes 4
- Tbsps. chopped fresh cilantro

DIRECTIONS:

1. Combine ingredients in a small container.
2. 3And heat oil in a large Dutch oven after setting over medium-high heat till shimmering. Include spice blend & cook, stirring with a wooden spoon till cinnamon stick unfurls & cloves pop for about 5 seconds. Include onions & cook till softened, 3 to 4 mins.
3. Stir in lamb, tomatoes, garlic, ginger, cumin, coriander, turmeric, & 1/2 Tsp. Salt & cook, frequently stirring, till liquid evaporates, oil separates & turns orange, & spices begin to fry, 5 to 7 mins. Continue to cook, constantly stirring, till spices are very fragrant, about 30 seconds longer.
4. Include water & jalapeño. Bring to simmer, then reduce heat, cover, & simmer till meat is tender, 30 to 40 mins.
5. Include potatoes & cook till tender, about 15 mins. Stir in cilantro, simmer 3 mins, season with salt to taste, & serve.

115. INDIAN CURRY WITH POTATOES, CAULIFLOWER, PEAS, & CHICKPEAS

Prep Time: 15 Minutes *Cook Time: 35 Minutes* *Servings: 4*

INGREDIENTS:

- Tbsps. Sweet or mild curry powder 1 1/2 Tbsps. garam masala
- 1 (14.5-ounce) can diced tomatoes 1/4 cup vegetable oil
- onions, chopped fine
- ounces red potatoes, cut into 1/2-inch pieces)
- 3 garlic cloves, minced
- 1 Tbsp. grated fresh ginger
- 1–1 1/2 serrano chiles, minced
- 1 Tbsp. tomato paste
- 1/2 head cauliflower (1 lb), cored & cut into 1-inch florets
- (15-ounce) can chickpeas, rinsed 1 1/4 cups water
- Salt
- 1 1/2 cups frozen peas
- 1/4 cup heavy cream or coconut milk
- CONDIMENTS
- ONION RELISH (recipe follows)
- CILANTRO-MINT CHUTNEY (recipe follows)

DIRECTIONS:

1. Toast curry powder & garam masala in a small pan over medium-high heat, constantly stirring, till spices darken slightly & become fragrant, about 1 min. Shift to a small container & set it aside. Pulse tomatoes in the food processor till roughly chopped, 3 to 4 pulses.
2. Heat 3 Tbsps. Oil in a large over medium-high heat till shimmering. Include onions & potatoes & cook, occasionally stirring, till onions are caramelized & potatoes are golden brown on edges, about 10 mins. (Low heat to medium if onions darken too quickly.)
3. Reduce heat to medium. Clear centre of pot & Include remaining 1 Tbsp. Oil, garlic, ginger, serrano, & tomato paste & cook, constantly stirring, till fragrant, about 30 seconds. Include reserved toasted spices & cook, continually going about 1 min.

Include cauliflower & cook, constantly stirring, till spices coat florets, about 2 mins longer.

4. Include tomatoes, chickpeas, water, & 1 Tsp. Salt. Increase heat to medium-high & bring the batter to boil, scraping the bottom of the pot with a wooden spoon to loosen browned bits. Cover & reduce heat to medium. Simmer briskly, occasionally stirring, till vegetables are tender, 10 to 15 mins.
5. Stir in peas & cream & continue to cook till heated for about 2 mins. Present with salt to taste & serve immediately, passing condiments separately.

116. ONION RELISH

Prep Time: *8 Minutes* | *Cook Time:* *6 Minutes* | *Servings: 4*

INGREDIENTS:

- Tbsp. lime juice
- 1/2 Tsp. sugar
- 1/8 Tsp. salt
- Pinch cayenne pepper

DIRECTIONS:

1. Combine all ingredients in a medium container.

117. CILANTRO-MINT CHUTNEY

Prep Time: *6 Minutes* | *Cook Time:* *5 Minutes* | *Servings: 6*

INGREDIENTS:

- cups fresh cilantro leaves
- 1 cup fresh mint leaves
- 1/3 cup plain whole-milk yoghurt
- 1/4 cup finely chopped onion
- Tbsp. Lime juice 1 1/2 Tbsps. sugar
- 1/2 Tsp. Ground cumin 1/4 Tsp. salt

DIRECTIONS:

1. Grinding all ingredients in the food processor till smooth, about 20 seconds, scraping down sides of container halfway through.

118. STIR-FRIED SICHUAN GREEN BEANS

Prep Time: ***15 Minutes*** | ***Cook Time:*** ***40 Minutes*** | ***Servings: 8***

INGREDIENTS:

- Tbsps. soy sauce
- Tbsps. water
- Tbsp. dry sherry
- Tsp. sugar
- 1/2 Tsp. cornstarch
- 1/4 Tsp. ground white pepper
- 1/4 Tsp. red pepper flakes
- 1/4 Tsp. dry mustard
- 2 Tbsps. vegetable oil
- lb green beans, trimmed & cut into 2-inch pieces 1/4 lb ground pork
- 3 garlic cloves, minced
- Tbsp. grated fresh ginger
- scallions, white & light green parts only, sliced thin
- 1 Tsp. toasted sesame oil

DIRECTIONS:

1. Stir together soy sauce, water, sherry, sugar, cornstarch, white pepper, pepper flakes, & dry mustard in a small container till sugar dissolves.
2. Heat oil in 12-inch nonstick pan over high heat till just smoking. Include beans & cook, frequently stirring, till crisp-tender & skins are shrivelled & blackened in spots, 5 to 8 mins (reduce heat to medium-high if beans darken too quickly). Shift beans to a large plate.
3. Reduce heat to medium-high & Include pork in the pan. Cook, breaking pork into small pieces, till no pink remains, about 2 mins. Include garlic & ginger & cook, mashing batter into pan, till fragrant, 15 to 20 seconds. Stir sauce to recombine & return beans to the pan with sauce. Toss & cook till sauce is thickened, 5 to 10 seconds. Remove from heat & stir in scallions & sesame oil. Serve immediately.

119. STIR-FRIED EGGPLANT WITH GARLIC & BASIL SAUCE

Prep Time: *15 Minutes* | *Cook Time:* *44 Minutes* | *Servings: 6*

INGREDIENTS:

- 3 Tbsps. fish sauce
- Tsp. grated lime zest plus 1 Tbsp. juice
- Tbsp. light brown sugar
- 1/8 Tsp. red pepper flakes
- Tbsp. Plus 1 Tsp. vegetable oil
- eggplant, cut into 3/4-inch cubes
- 6 garlic cloves, minced
- Tbsp. grated fresh ginger
- 2 scallions, sliced thin
- 1/2 cup fresh basil leaves
- 1/2-inch pieces

DIRECTIONS:

1. Mixed together all ingredients in a small container till sugar is dissolved.
2. Heat 1 Tbsp. Oil in 12-inch nonstick pan over high heat till shimmering, 2 to 3 mins. Include eggplant & cook, stirring every 10 to 15 seconds, till browned & tender, 4 to 5 mins.
3. Clear centre of pan; Include remaining 1 Tsp. Oil, garlic, & ginger & cook, mashing batter into pan, till fragrant, 15 to 20 seconds. Stir batter into the eggplant. Include sauce & cook till thickened, 5 to 10 seconds. Off heat, stir in scallions & basil & serve immediately.

120. STIR-FRIED BROCCOLI & RED PEPPERS WITH PEANUT SAUCE

Prep Time: *14 Minutes* | *Cook Time:* *12 Minutes* | *Servings: 2*

INGREDIENTS:

- 3/4 cup coconut milk
- 1/4 cup water
- Tbsps. smooth peanut butter
- Tbsps. fish sauce
- Tsp. grated lime zest plus 1 Tbsp. juice
- Tbsp. light brown sugar
- 1/8 Tsp. red pepper flakes
- Tbsp. Plus 1 Tsp. Vegetable oil
- large red bell pepper, stemmed, seeded, & cut into 1/2-inch strips 10 ounces broccoli florets.
- Tsp. grated fresh ginger

DIRECTIONS:

1. 2Whisk all ingredients together in a small container till smooth.
2. Heat 1 Tbsp. Oil in 12-inch nonstick pan over high heat till shimmering, 2 to 3 mins. Include red pepper & broccoli & cook, stirring every 10 to 15 seconds, till just barely tender, about 2 mins. Clear centre of pan; Include remaining 1 Tsp. Oil, garlic, & ginger & cook, mashing batter into pan, till fragrant, 15 to 20 seconds. Stir batter into vegetables. Reduce heat to medium-low & stir in sauce batter. Simmer to heat through & blend flavours, about 1 min. Serve immediately.

121. STIR-FRIED CAULIFLOWER WITH THAI RED CURRY SAUCE

Prep Time: *15 Minutes* | *Cook Time:* *4 Minutes* | *Servings: 2*

INGREDIENTS:

- 1 cup coconut milk
- 3 Tbsps. fish sauce
- Tsp. grated lime zest plus 1 Tbsp. juice
- Tbsp. light brown sugar
- Tbsps. Red curry paste 1/8 Tsp. red pepper flakes
- Tbsp. Plus 1 Tsp. vegetable oil
- large head cauliflower (3 lbs), cored & cut into 3/4-inch florets
- 2 garlic cloves, minced
- Tsp. grated fresh ginger
- ounces snow peas, strings removed
- 2 Tbsps. minced fresh basil

DIRECTIONS:

1. 2Whisk all ingredients together in a small container till smooth.
2. Heat 1 Tbsp. Oil in 12-inch nonstick pan over high heat till shimmering, 2 to 3 mins. Include cauliflower & cook, occasionally stirring, till just barely tender, about 3 mins. Clear centre of pan; Include remaining 1 Tsp. Oil, garlic, & ginger & cook, mashing batter into pan, till fragrant, 15 to 20 seconds. Stir batter into the cauliflower. Reduce heat to medium-high & stir in sauce batter. Simmer, occasionally stirring, till cauliflower is just tender, about 2 mins. Include snow peas & continue to simmer till cauliflower is fully tender, about 3 mins longer. Sprinkle with basil.
3. Serve immediately.

122. STIR-FRIED BROCCOLI WITH CHILI-GARLIC SAUCE

Prep Time: *10 Minutes* | *Cook Time:* *8 Minutes* | *Servings: 6*

INGREDIENTS:

- 1/4 cup low-sodium chicken broth
- Tbsp. dry sherry
- 2 Tips. soy sauce
- 2 Tbsps. Asian chilli-garlic sauce
- Tsp. toasted sesame oil
- Tsp. cornstarch
- 2 garlic cloves, minced
- 1/8 Tsp. red pepper flakes
- 1 Tsp. Plus 1 Tbsp. vegetable oil
- 1 1/2 lbs broccoli, florets cut into 3/4-inch pieces, stalks peeled & cut on the bias into 1/4-inch-thick slices
- 1/4 Tsp. sugar

DIRECTIONS:

1. Whisk broth, sherry, soy sauce, chilli-garlic sauce, sesame oil, & cornstarch together in a small container. Combine garlic, pepper flakes, & 1 Tsp. Vegetable oil in a second small container.
2. Heat remaining 1 Tbsp. Vegetable oil in 12-inch nonstick pan over medium-high heat till just beginning to smoke. Include broccoli & sprinkle with sugar. Cook, frequently stirring, till broccoli is well browned, 8 to 10 mins.
3. Clear centre of the pan, Include oil-garlic batter & cook, mashing batter into pan, till fragrant, 15 to 20 seconds. Stir batter into broccoli. Include chicken broth batter & cook, constantly stirring, till florets are cooked through, stalks are crisp-tender, & sauce is thickened, 30 to 45 seconds. Serve.

123. STIR-FRIED SNOW PEAS WITH LEMON & PARSLEY

Prep Time: *10 Minutes* | *Cook Time:* *9 Minutes* | *Servings: 8*

INGREDIENTS:

- small shallot, minced
- Tbsp. vegetable oil
- Tsp. grated lemon zest plus 1 Tsp. juice Salt & pepper
- 1/8 Tsp. sugar
- ounces snow peas, strings removed
- 1 Tbsp. minced fresh parsley

DIRECTIONS:

1. Combine shallot, 1 Tsp. Oil & lemon zest in a small container. Combine 1/4 Tsp. Salt, 1/8 Tsp. Pepper & sugar in a second small container.
2. Heat remaining 2 Tbsps. Oil in 12-inch nonstick pan over high heat till just smoking. Include snow peas, sprinkle with salt batter, & cook, without stirring, for 30 seconds. Stir & continue to cook, without stirring, 30 seconds longer. Continue to cook, constantly stirring, till peas are crisp-tender, 1 to 2 mins longer.
3. Clear centre of the pan, Include shallot batter, & cook, mashing batter into pan, till fragrant, about 20 seconds. Stir batter into vegetables. Shift peas to container & stir in lemon juice & parsley. Season with salt & pepper to taste & serve.

124. STIR-FRIED PORTOBELLOS WITH GINGER-OYSTER SAUCE

Prep Time: 15 Minutes *Cook Time: 42 Minutes* *Servings: 4*

INGREDIENTS:

- 1/4 cup low-sodium broth of chicken or vegetable broth
- Tbsps. soy sauce
- Tbsps. sugar
- cup low-sodium chicken broth or vegetable broth
- 3 Tbsps. oyster sauce
- Tbsp. soy sauce
- Tbsp. cornstarch
- 2 Tbsps. toasted sesame oil
- Tbsps. grated fresh ginger
- 2 garlic cloves, minced
- 1/4 cup vegetable oil
- 1 1/2 lbs portobello mushroom caps, gills removed, cut into 2-inch wedges 3 carrots, peeled & sliced 1/4 inch thick on the bias
- 1/2 cup low-sodium chicken broth or vegetable broth 2 ounces snow peas, strings removed
- lb bok choy or napa cabbage, stalks or cores cut on the bias into 1/4-inch pieces & greens cut into 3/4-inch strips
- Tbsp. sesame seeds, toasted (optional)

DIRECTIONS:

1. Whisk all ingredients together in a small container.
2. Whisk all ingredients together in a second small container.
3. Combine ginger, garlic, & 1 Tsp.
4. Oil in the third small container & set aside. Heat 3 Tbsps. Vegetable oil in 12-inch nonstick pan over medium-high heat till shimmering. Include mushrooms & cook, without stirring, till browned on one side, 2 to 3 mins. (Pan will be crowded at first; arrange mushrooms in a single layer as they shrink.) Flip mushrooms over, reduce heat to medium, & cook till the second side is browned & mushrooms are tender about 5 mins. Increase heat to medium-high, Include glaze batter, & cook, constantly stirring, till glaze is thickened & mushrooms are coated, 1 to 2 mins. Shift mushrooms to plate. Rinse pan clean & dry with paper towels.
5. Heat 1 Tsp. Oil in pan over medium-high heat till just smoking. Include carrots & cook, occasionally stirring, till beginning to brown, 1 to 2 mins. Include 1 broth, cover, & cook till carrots are just tender, 2 to 3 mins. Uncover & cook till liquid evaporates, about 30 seconds. Shift carrots to plate with mushrooms.
6. Heat remaining 1 Tsp. Vegetable oil in the pan set over medium-high heat till just smoking. Include snow peas & bok choy stalks & cook, occasionally stirring, till beginning to brown & soften 1 to 2 mins. Include greens & cook, frequently stirring, till wilted, about 1 min.
7. Clear centre of the pan, Include ginger batter, & cook, mashing batter into pan, till fragrant, 15 to 20 seconds. Stir batter into greens.
8. Return vegetables to the pan, Include sauce, & cook, constantly stirring, till sauce is thickened & vegetables are coated, 2 to 3 mins. Shift to the platter, top with sesame seeds if using, & serve immediately.

125. HONEY-NUT ENDIVE APPETIZERS

Prep Time: 15 Minutes *Cook Time: 20 Minutes* *Servings: 3*

INGREDIENTS:

- 1/3 cup crumbled goat cheese 1/3 cup crumbled Gorgonzola cheese 1/3 cup pine nuts
- 1/3 cup chopped walnuts
- 1/3 cup golden raisins
- 4 bacon strips, cooked and crumbled
- 2 heads Belgian endive, separated into leaves
- 1/3 cup honey

Directions:

1. In a small size bowl, add the first six ingredients. Spoon into endive leaves. Spread honey over cheese mixture. Present immediately.

126. CARAMEL APPLE AND BRIE SKEWERS

Prep Time: 15 Minutes *Cook Time: 20 Minutes* *Servings: 2*

INGREDIENTS:

- 2 medium apples, cubed
- 1 log (6 ounces) Brie cheese, cubed
- ½ cup hot caramel ice cream topping
- ½ cup finely chopped macadamia nuts
- 2 tbsp dried cranberries

Directions:

1. On each of six wooden appetizer skewers, alternately thread apple and cheese cubes; place on a serving tray. Spread with caramel topping; sprinkle with macadamia nuts and cranberries.

127. THYME-SEA SALT CRACKERS

Prep Time: 15 Minutes *Cook Time: 20 Minutes* *Servings: 8*

INGREDIENTS:

- 2 ½ cups all-purpose flour
- ½ cup white whole wheat flour
- 1 tsp salt
- ¾ cup water ¼ cup plus 1 tbsp olive oil, divided 1 to 2 tbsps minced fresh thyme
- ¾ tsp sea or kosher salt 1.

Directions:

- Preheat oven to 375°. In a big bow whisk flours and salt. Gradually add water and ¼ cup oil, tossing with a fork until dough holds together when pressed. Divide dough into three portions.
- Roll each part of the dough 1/8 inch on a lightly floured surface. Thickness. Cut into 1½ inches of flour.
- Round cookies cutter. Place 1-in. Separately on a non-oiled baking sheet. Poke each cracker with a fork. Lightly comb with the remaining oil. Add thyme and sea salt and sprinkle over crackers.
- Baked it for 9-11 minutes or until the bottom is slightly browned.

128. SEAFOOD SALAD STUFFED SHELLS

Prep Time: 15 Minutes *Cook Time: 20 Minutes* *Servings: 2*

INGREDIENTS:

- 1 package (12 ounces) jumbo pasta shells
- 2 packages (8 ounces each) cream cheese, softened
- 1/3 cup mayonnaise 2 tsp sugar
- 1 ½ tsp lemon juice 1/8 tsp salt 1/8 tsp coarsely ground pepper 1/8 tsp cayenne pepper 3 cans (6 ounces each) lump crabmeat, drained
- ½ pound frozen cooked salad shrimp, thawed 12 green onions, finely chopped

Directions:

1. Cook pasta according to directions and drain and rinse in cold water. Cool to room temperature.
2. In a big bowl, add the cream cheese, mayonnaise, sugar, lemon juice, salt, pepper and cayenne. Gently stir in the crab, shrimp and onions. Stuff shells, about 2 tbsps in each. Cover and refrigerate for at least 1 hour.

129. BLUE CHEESE-STUFFED STRAWBERRIES

Prep Time: 15 Minutes *Cook Time: 20 Minutes* *Servings: 8*

INGREDIENTS:

- ½ cup balsamic vinegar
- 3 ounces fat-free cream cheese
- ½ cup crumbled blue cheese
- 16 big fresh strawberries
- 3 tbsp finely chopped pecans, toasted

Directions:

1. Place vinegar in a small saucepan. Let it boil cook until liquid is reduced by half. Cool to room temperature.
2. Meanwhile, in a small size bowl, beat cream cheese until smooth. Beat in blue cheese. Remove stems and scoop out centres from strawberries; fill each with about 2 tsp cheese mixture.
3. Sprinkle pecans over filling, pressing lightly. Chill until serving.
4. Spread with balsamic vinegar.

130. CUCUMBER-STUFFED CHERRY TOMATOES

Prep Time: 15 Minutes *Cook Time: 20 Minutes* *Servings: 2*

INGREDIENTS:

- 24 cherry tomatoes
- 1 package cream cheese, softened 2 tbsps mayonnaise
- ¼ cup finely chopped peeled cucumber 1 tbsp finely chopped green onion 2 tsp minced fresh dill

Directions:

1. Cut a thin slice off the top of each tomato. Scoop out and discard pulp; invert tomatoes onto paper towels to drain.
2. In a small size bowl, add cream cheese and mayonnaise until smooth; stir in the cucumber, onion and dill. Spoon into tomatoes. Refrigerate until serving.

131. STIR-FRIED PORTOBELLOS WITH SOY-MAPLE SAUCE

Prep Time: 25 Minutes *Cook Time: 23 Minutes* *Servings: 5*

INGREDIENTS:

- Tbsps. maple syrup
- 2 Tbsps. soy sauce
- 2 Tbsps. mirin
- 3/4 cup low-sodium chicken
- Tbsps. soy sauce
- 2 Tbsps. mirin
- 1 Tbsp. rice vinegar
- 1 Tbsp. cornstarch
- 2 Tbsps. toasted sesame oil
- garlic cloves, minced
- Tbsps. Grated fresh ginger 1/4 Tsp. red pepper flakes 1/4 cup vegetable oil
- 1 1/2 lbs portobello mushroom caps, gills removed, cut into 2-inch wedges 8 ounces green beans, trimmed
- 1/2 cup low-sodium chicken broth or vegetable broth
- red bell pepper stemmed, seeded, & cut into 3/4-inch pieces
- lb bok choy or napa cabbage, stalks or cores cut into 1/4-inch pieces on bias & greens cut into 3/4-inch strips
- 1/4 cup roasted cashews (optional)

DIRECTIONS:

1. FOR THE GLAZE:
   Mixing all ingredients together in a small container.
2. FOR THE SAUCE:
3. Mixing all ingredients together in a second small Container.
4. Combine garlic, ginger, pepper flakes, & 1 Tsp. Oil in the third small container & set aside. Heat 3 Tbsps. Vegetable oil in 12-inch nonstick pan over medium-high heat till shimmering. Include mushrooms & cook, without stirring, till browned on one side, 2 to 3 mins. (Pan will be crowded at first; arrange mushrooms in a single layer as they shrink). Flip mushrooms over, reduce heat to medium, & cook till the second side is browned & mushrooms are tender about 5 mins. Increase heat to medium-high, Include glaze batter, & cook, stirring, till glaze is thickened & mushrooms are coated, 1 to 2 mins. Shift mushrooms to plate. Rinse pan clean & dry with paper towels.

5. Heat 1 Tsp. Oil over medium-high heat till just smoking. Include green beans & cook, occasionally stirring, till beginning to brown, 1 to 2 mins. Include broth, cover, & cook till beans are just tender, 2 to 3 mins. Uncover & cook till liquid evaporates, about 30 seconds. Shift beans to plate with mushrooms.
6. Heat remaining 1 Tsp. Oil over medium-high heat till just smoking. Include bell pepper & bok choy stems & cook, occasionally stirring, till beginning to brown & soften 1 to 2 mins. Include greens & cook, frequently stirring, till wilted, about 1 min.
7. Clear centre of the pan, Include garlic batter, & cook, mashing batter into pan, till fragrant, 15 to 20 seconds. Stir batter into greens.
8. Return vegetables to the pan, Include sauce, & cook, stirring, till sauce is thickened & vegetables are coated about 1 min. Shift to a platter, top with cashews, if using, & serve immediately.

132. STIR-FRIED EGGPLANT WITH SWEET CHILI-GARLIC SAUCE

Prep Time: 20 Minutes *Cook Time: 18 Minutes* *Servings: 3*

INGREDIENTS:

- 1/4 cup low-sodium broth of chicken or vegetable broth
- Tbsps. soy sauce
- Tbsps. honey
- 3/4 cup low-sodium broth of chicken or vegetable broth
- Tbsps. soy sauce
- 2 Tbsps. honey
- 1 Tbsp. rice vinegar
- 1 Tbsp. cornstarch
- 1 Tsp. Asian chilli-garlic sauce
- 4 garlic cloves, minced
- 2 Tbsps. grated fresh ginger
- 1/4 cup plus 1 Tbsp. Vegetable oil
- large egg, lightly beaten 1/2 Tsp. salt
- 1 1/2 lbs eggplant, peeled & cut crosswise into 1 1/4-inch-thick rounds, each round cut into pie-shaped wedges
- 1/3 cup cornstarch
- 5 1/2 ounces broccoli florets
- 3/4 cup low-sodium broth of chicken or vegetable broth 1
- red bell pepper stemmed, seeded, & cut into 1/4-inch pieces
- lb bok choy or napa cabbage, stalks or cores cut into 1/4-inch pieces on bias & greens cut into 3/4-inch strips
- Tbsps. pine nuts, toasted & roughly chopped (optional)

DIRECTIONS:

1. Whisk all ingredients together in a small container.
2. Whisk all ingredients together in a second small container.
3. Combine garlic, ginger, & 1 Tsp. Oil in the third small container & set aside.
4. Whisk egg & salt together in a large container. Include eggplant, toss to coat, then Shift to clean container, allowing any excess egg to drip off. Sprinkle cornstarch over eggplant and, using a rubber spatula, toss to coat. Heat 1/4 cup oil in 12-inch nonstick pan over medium-high heat till shimmering. Include eggplant in single layer & cook, without moving, till golden brown on one side, 2 to 3 mins. Reduce heat to medium, flip the eggplant over gently, & continue to cook, shaking pan occasionally, till pieces are golden brown & softened for about 10 mins. (Some pieces may take longer than others; see note.) Increase heat to medium-high, Include glaze batter, & cook, stirring, till glaze is thickened & eggplant is coated, 1 to 2 mins. Shift eggplant to a large plate. Rinse pan clean & dry with paper towels.
5. Heat 1 Tsp. Oil over medium-high heat till just smoking. Include broccoli & cook, occasionally stirring, till beginning to brown, 1 to 2 mins. Include broth, cover, & cook till broccoli is just tender, 2 to 3 mins. Uncover & cook till liquid evaporates, about 30 seconds. Shift broccoli to plate with eggplant.
6. Heat 1 Tsp. Oil over medium-high heat till just smoking. Add Bell pepper & bok choy stems & cook, occasionally stirring, till beginning to brown & soften, 1 to 2 mins. Include greens & cook, frequently stirring, till wilted, about 1 min. Clear centre of the pan, Include garlic batter, & cook, mashing batter into pan, till fragrant, 15 to 20 seconds. Stir batter into greens.
7. Return vegetables to the pan, Include sauce, & cook, stirring, till sauce is thickened & vegetables are coated about 1 min. Shift to a platter, top with pine nuts, if using, & serve immediately.

Snacks And Appetizer Recipes

133. CHERRY-BRANDY BAKED BRIE

Prep Time: 15 Minutes *Cook Time: 20 Minutes* *Servings: 8*

INGREDIENTS:

- 1 round (8 ounces) Brie cheese
- ½ mug dried cherries
- ½ mug chopped walnuts
- ¼ mugs packed brown sugar
- ¼ mug brandy or unsweetened apple juice French bread baguette, sliced and toasted or assorted crackers

DIRECTIONS:

1. Preheat oven to 350°. Place cheese in a 9-in. pie plate. Mix cherries, walnuts, as well as brown sugar and brandy; spoon over cheese.
2. Bake 15-20 minutes or until cheese is softened.
3. Serve it with a baguette.

134. BUFFALO WING CHEESE MOLD

Prep Time: 15 Minutes *Cook Time: 20 Minutes* *Servings: 6*

INGREDIENTS:

- 2 packages cream cheese of 8 ounces each
- softened 2 celery ribs, finely chopped
- 2 mugs (8 ounces) crumbled blue cheese
- 1 cup shredded Monterey Jack cheese
- 1 ½ cup finely chopped cooked chicken breasts
- 3 tbsp buffalo wing sauce
- 1 French bread baguette (16 ounces)
- ¼ mug olive oil
- ½ cup shredded carrots, optional

DIRECTIONS:

1. In a bowl, mix the cream cheese, celery, blue and Monterey Jack cheeses. In a small bowl, combine chicken and
2. wing sauce.
3. Line a 1-qt. Bowl with plastic cover, overlapping the sides of the bowl. Spread 1 ½ mug of cream cheese mixture over the bottom and up the sides in a prepared bowl. Layer with the chicken mixture as well as the remaining cream cheese mixture. Bring plastic cover over cheese; press down smoothly. Now let it cool for about 4 hours or until firm.
4. Just before serving, cut the baguette into ¼-in. slices. To keep on an ungreased baking sheet, brush with oil. Bake at 375° for 10-12 minutes or until lightly browned.
5. Extract mould from the refrigerator and invert onto a serving plate. Extract bowl and plastic cover. Garnish with carrots if desired. Serve with toasted baguette slices.

135. CHUNKY MANGO GUACAMOLE

Prep Time: 15 Minutes *Cook Time: 21 Minutes* *Servings: 7*

INGREDIENTS:

- 3 medium ripe avocados, peeled and chopped 1 large mango, peeled and chopped 1 large tomato, chopped
- 1 small red onion, chopped
- ¼ mug chopped fresh cilantro 3 tbsp lime juice
- 1 tsp salt

DIRECTIONS:

1. Assorted fresh vegetables and tortilla chips In a large bowl, mix the first five ingredients; stir in lime juice and salt. Serve with vegetables and chips.

136. APPETIZER BLUE CHEESE LOGS

Prep Time: 15 Minutes *Cook Time: 24 Minutes* *Servings: 2*

INGREDIENTS:

- 1 package (8 ounces) cream cheese, softened
- 1 mug (4 ounces) shredded sharp cheddar cheese
- ½ mug crumbled blue cheese
- 1 ½ tsp curry powder
- 1 tbsp butter
- ½ mug finely chopped pecans
- 2 tbsps minced fresh parsley
- Assorted crackers

DIRECTIONS:

2. In a bowl, beat the cream cheese. Fold in cheddar cheese and blue cheese. Cover and let cool for at least 2 hours.
3. In a small frying pan, fry the buttered curry powder for 1-2 minutes. Add now the pecans and cook for 1 minute, stirring. Mix the parsley. Now Cooldown a bit. Roll the cheese mixture into two sticks about 5 inches long. Roll out the hazelnut mixture. Cover and cook until served. Serve with crackers.

137. CREAMY BLACK BEAN SALSA

Prep Time: 15 Minutes *Cook Time: 26 Minutes* *Servings: 5*

INGREDIENTS:

- 1 can (15 ounces) black beans,
- 1 ½ mug frozen corn, thawed
- 1 mug finely chopped sweet red pepper
- ¾ mug finely chopped green pepper ½ mug finely chopped red onion
- 1 tbsp minced fresh parsley
- ½ mug sour cream ¼ mug mayonnaise 2 tbsps red wine vinegar
- 1 tsp ground cumin
- 1 tsp chili powder
- ½ tsp salt
- ¼ tsp garlic powder
- 1/8 tsp pepper Tortilla chips

DIRECTIONS:

1. In a bowl, combine together the beans, corn, peppers, onion and parsley. Mix the sour cream, mayonnaise, vinegar and seasonings; spread over corn mixture and toss smoothly to coat.
2. Serve with tortilla chips. Let it cool leftovers.

138. CELEBRATION CHEESE BALL

Prep Time: 15 Minutes *Cook Time: 44 Minutes* *Servings: 12*

INGREDIENTS:

- 2 pkg (8 ounces each) of cream cheese, softened 1 mug grated Parmesan cheese
- 2 garlic cloves, minced

DIRECTIONS:

Let it cool for up to two weeks. Serve with crackers.
In a bowl, beat together the cream cheese, Parmesan cheese and garlic until blended. Cut into three portions.

139. PINE NUT-PESTO CHEESE BALL

Prep Time: 15 Minutes *Cook Time: 55 Minutes* *Servings: 12*

INGREDIENTS:

- 2 tbsp prepared pesto
- 2 tbsps minced fresh basil
- 2 tbsps plus ½ mug pine nuts, toasted, divided HORSERADISH-BACON

DIRECTIONS:

1. In a bowl, beat one portion of the cream cheese mixture and pesto altogether until blended. Stir in basil. Chop 2 tbsps pine nuts; stir into
2. Cheese mixture. Shape into a ball; roll in remaining pine nuts. Cover in plastic cover; chill until firm.

140. CHEESE BALL

Prep Time: *15 Minutes* *Cook Time:* *56 Minutes* *Servings: 6*

INGREDIENTS:

- 2 tbsp prepared horseradish
- ½ mug crumbled cooked bacon 1 green onion, finely chopped

DIRECTIONS:

1. In a bowl, beat one portion of the cream cheese mixture and horseradish altogether until blended. Stir in bacon and onion. Shape into a ball. Cover in plastic cover; chill until firm.

141. SALSA CHEESE BALL

Prep Time: *15 Minutes* *Cook Time:* *36 Minutes* *Servings: 8*

INGREDIENTS:

- 2 tbsps tomato paste
- 1/8 tsp salt 2 tbsps minced fresh cilantro
- 1 tbsp finely chopped onion
- 1 tbsp minced seeded jalapeno pepper Assorted crackers

DIRECTIONS:

1. In a small bowl, beat altogether one portion of cream cheese mixture, tomato paste and salt until blended. Stir in the cilantro, onion and jalapeno. Shape into a ball. Cover in plastic cover; chill until firm.

142. LOADED BAKED POTATO DIP

Prep Time: *15 Minutes* *Cook Time:* *5 Minutes* *Servings: 12*

INGREDIENTS:

- 2 mugs (16 ounces) sour cream
- 2 mugs (8 ounces) shredded cheddar cheese
- 8 centre-cut bacon or turkey bacon strips, chopped and cooked 1/3 mug minced fresh chives 2 tsp Louisiana-style hot sauce
- Hot cooked waffle-cut fries

DIRECTIONS:

1. In a bowl, comb the first five ingredients until blended; Let it cool until serving. Serve with waffle fries.

143. SMOKED SALMON CHEESE SPREAD

Prep Time: *15 Minutes* *Cook Time:* *32 Minutes* *Servings: 12*

INGREDIENTS:

- 2 pkg (8 ounces each) of cream cheese, softened 1 package (4 ounces) smoked salmon or lox
- 3 tbsp horseradish sauce
- 1 tbsp lemon juice
- 1 tbsp Worcestershire sauce
- ¼ tsp Creole seasoning ¼ tsp coarsely ground pepper Chopped walnuts and snipped fresh dill
- Assorted crackers

DIRECTIONS:

1. Place the first seven ingredients all together in a food processor; process until blended. Transfer to a serving dish; sprinkle with walnuts and dill. Refrigerate, covered, until serving. Serve with crackers.

Note *You can substitute 1 teaspoon of Creole seasoning with the following spices: tsp each of salt, garlic powder as well as paprika; And a pinch each of dried thyme, ground cumin, and cayenne pepper.*

144. PEACHY FRUIT DIP

Prep Time: *15 Minutes* *Cook Time:* *50 Minutes* *Servings: 12*

INGREDIENTS:

- 1 can (15 ¼ ounces) sliced or halved peaches, drained ½ mug marshmallow creme 1 package (3 ounces) cream cheese, cubed
- 1/8 tsp ground nutmeg Assorted fresh fruit

DIRECTIONS:

1. In a blender, combine together the first four ingredients; cover and blend until smooth. Serve with fruit.

145. ENLIGHTENED SPICY AVOCADO DIP

Prep Time: *15 Minutes* *Cook Time:* *5 Minutes* *Servings: 2*

INGREDIENTS:

- 2 medium ripe avocados, peeled and pitted
- ¼ mug fresh cilantro leaves ¼ mug reduced-fat sour cream ¼ mug lime juice 2 tbsp olive oil
- 1 garlic cloves, minced
- ¼ to ½ tsp prepared wasabi Assorted fresh vegetables

DIRECTIONS:

1. Put the first seven ingredients all together in a food processor; cover and process until smooth. Chill until serving. Serve with vegetables.

146. HOT COLLARDS AND ARTICHOKE DIP

Prep Time: *15 Minutes* *Cook Time:* *Minutes* *Servings: 8*

INGREDIENTS:

- 12 ounces of frozen chopped collard greens, thawed and squeezed dry
- 2 jars (7 ½ ounces each) marinated quartered artichoke hearts, drained and chopped
- 1 mug (8 ounces) sour cream
- 1 package (6 ½ ounces) garlic-herb spreadable cheese
- 1 mug grated Parmesan cheese
- 10 thick sliced of peppered bacon strips, cooked and crumbled
- ¾ mug mayonnaise
- 1 ½ mug (6 ounces) shredded part-skim mozzarella cheese, divided Garlic naan flatbreads, warmed and cut into wedges

DIRECTIONS:

1. In a bowl, combine together the first seven ingredients and 1 mug of mozzarella cheese altogether until blended. Transfer to a greased 11x7-in. Baking dish. Sprinkle with remaining mozzarella cheese.
2. Bake it unwrapped, at 350° for 20-25 minutes or until heated through and cheese is melted. Serve with naan.

147. CREAMY ARTICHOKE DIP

Prep Time: *15 Minutes* *Cook Time:* *20 Minutes* *Servings: 12*

INGREDIENTS:

- 2 cans (14 ounces each) of water-packed artichoke hearts, rinsed, drained and coarsely chopped 2 mugs of shredded part-skim mozzarella cheese 1 pkg of cream cheese, cubed 1 mug shredded Parmesan cheese
- ½ mug mayonnaise ½ mug shredded Swiss cheese 2 tbsp lemon juice
- 2 tbsps plain yoghurt
- 1 tbsp seasoned salt
- 1 tbsp chopped seeded jalapeno pepper 1 tsp garlic powder
- Tortilla chips

DIRECTIONS:

1. In a 3-qt slow cooker, combine together the first 11 ingredients. Wrap and cook on low for 1 hour or until heated through. Serve it with tortilla chips.

148. STRAWBERRY SALSA

Prep Time: *15 Minutes* *Cook Time:* *35 Minutes* *Servings: 2*

INGREDIENTS:

- 1 ½ mug sliced fresh strawberries 1 ½ mug chopped sweet red pepper
- 1 mug chopped green pepper
- 1 mug seeded chopped tomato
- ¼ mug chopped Anaheim pepper 2 tbsps minced fresh cilantro
- ½ tsp salt ½ tsp crushed red pepper flakes ¼ tsp pepper 2 tbsps plus 2 tsp honey
- 2 tbsps lemon juice

DIRECTIONS:

1. In a bowl, combine together the first nine ingredients. In a bowl, combine together honey and lemon juice; smoothly stir into the strawberry mixture. Cover and let it cool for at least 4 hours. Stir just before serving. Serve the salsa with a slotted spoon.

Dessert Recipes

149. Lemon Glazed Raspberry Cake

Prep Time: *15 Minutes* *Cook Time:* *35 Minutes* *Servings: 6*

Ingredients:

- 1 cup whole wheat flour
- 1 cup all-purpose flour
- 2 tsp baking powder
- 1 pinch of salt
- 2/3 cup sugar
- 2 eggs
- ½ cup low-fat milk
- 1 tsp lemon zest
- 1 cup fresh raspberries
- Glaze:
- juice from ½ lemon
- 1 ½ cups powdered sugar

Directions:

1. In a bowl, stir the flours with the baking powder and a pinch of salt, then set aside.
2. In another bowl, stir the butter with the sugar until creamy and fluffy, then add the eggs, one by one. Start incorporating the flour stir, alternating it with milk. Carefully fold in the raspberries, then convert the batter into a 9-inch round cake pan.
3. Bake in the before heating oven at 350F for 30-40 minutes or until golden brown and fragrant.
4. To make the glaze: Stir the juice with powdered sugar until it reaches the desired consistency. It should be thick but still runny. Add the glaze over the chilled cake and let it rest for 1 hour in the refrigerator.

150. Chocolate Pear Cake

Prep Time: *15 Minutes* *Cook Time:* *70 Minutes* *Servings: 8*

Ingredients:

- 3 oz chocolate, chopped
- 3 oz butter
- 3 egg yolks
- 3 egg whites
- 3 oz sugar
- 3 oz chopped walnuts
- 4 ripe pears, peeled, halved and cored, then sliced
- 1 pinch of salt
- 1 tablespoon dark rum

Directions:

1. Place the chocolate as well as butter in a heavy pan and heat it on low flame until melted.
2. Add the rum and remove from heat. Let it cool to room temperature.
3. In a bowl, stir the egg yolks with the sugar until creamy, fluffy and pale in colour. Carefully stir in the chocolate, then fold in the chopped hazelnuts. In another bowl,

whip the egg whites with a pinch of salt, then gently fold them into the chocolate base.

4. Grease and flour a 9-inch round cake pan with butter and flour it slightly. Spoon the batter into the pan, arrange the pears on top and bake in the before heating oven at 250F for 30-40 minutes. The cake will rise then deflate, but that is how it should look like.
5. Serve when completely chilled with a dollop of fresh cream if you want.

151. Pear Frangipane Tart

Prep Time: *15 Minutes* | *Cook Time:* *60 Minutes* | *Servings: 4*

Ingredients:

- Crust:
- 2 cups low-fat chocolate biscuits
- 3 oz butter, melted
- Pears:
- 4 small pears
- 2 cups red wine
- 1 cinnamon stick
- 1-star anise
- ½ cup brown sugar
- Frangipane filling:
- ½ cup sugar
- 3 oz butter
- 2 eggs
- ¼ cup cocoa powder
- 3 oz almond meal
- 1 tsp rum
- ¼ tsp almond extract

Directions:

1. To make the crust: Simply stir the biscuits in a food processor until ground, then pour in the melted butter. To convert the structure into a 10-inch tart pan and press it on the bottom and sides of the pan until all even.
2. To prepare the pears: Pour the wine in a saucepan and add the sugar, cinnamon stick and star anise. Bring to a boil, then add the pears, peeled, cored and halved.
3. Cook on minimum heat for about 15 minutes, then remove from heat and let them cool in the syrup. To convert them in a sieve to drain, but keep the syrup and put it back on the heat. Cook it until reduced by half.
4. To make the frangipane filling: Stir the butter with the sugar until creamy and fluffy, and then now add the eggs, one by one, followed by the cocoa powder and almond meal.
5. Add the rum and almond extract as well. Spread this stir in the pan, over the crust and top with pear halves.
6. Bake in the before heating oven at 350F for 30-40 minutes.

152. Pear and Applesauce Muffins

Prep Time: *15 Minutes* | *Cook Time:* *30 Minutes* | *Servings: 4*

Ingredients:

- 1 cup applesauce
- ½ cup brown sugar
- 1 cup all-purpose flour
- 2/3 cup whole wheat flour
- 1 tsp baking powder
- 1 tsp baking soda
- 1 tsp cinnamon
- 1 pinch nutmeg
- 1/8 tsp ground cloves
- 3 oz butter, softened
- 2 eggs
- 2 pears, peeled, cored and sliced
- 1 pinch of salt

Directions:

1. In a bowl, stir the butter continuously with the sugar until creamy and fluffy. Add the eggs, one after another, then the cinnamon, nutmeg and applesauce. Sift the flours with the baking powder, baking soda and a pinch of salt and incorporate this stir into the batter.
2. Line a muffin tin with special papers and spoon the batter evenly between the muffin cups. Top with a few pear slices and bake in the before heating oven at 350F for 20-25 minutes or until golden brown and fragrant.

153. Pear and Raisin Cobbler

Prep Time: *15 Minutes* | *Cook Time:* *45 Minutes* | *Servings: 6*

Ingredients:

- Pears:
- 2 pounds pears, peeled, cored and cubed
- ½ cup brown sugar
- 1 tablespoon cornstarch
- ¼ cup raisins
- Batter:
- 4 oz butter
- 1 cup whole wheat flour
- ½ tsp baking powder
- 1 pinch of salt
- 2 tbsp sugar
- ¾ cup low-fat milk
- 1 pinch nutmeg
- 1/8 tsp cinnamon

Directions:

1. In a bowl, stir the pear cubes with brown sugar, cornstarch and raisins.
2. 3To convert the stir into a deep dish baking pan (9x13-inches). Set aside.
3. To make the batter: Stir the flour with the butter until sandy. Add the sugar, nutmeg and cinnamon, then pour in the milk, stirring well. Spread the butter over the pears and bake in the before heating oven at 350F for 30-40 minutes. Serve warm topped with a scoop of caramel ice cream.

154. Pear and Honey Bread

Prep Time: *15 Minutes* | *Cook Time:* *35 Minutes* | *Servings: 6*

Ingredients:

- ½ cup brown sugar
- ½ cup honey
- ½ cup olive oil
- ½ cup applesauce
- 3 eggs
- 2 ¼ cups whole wheat flour
- 2/3 cup all-purpose flour
- 2 tsp baking powder
- 1 tsp all spices
- ½ tsp cinnamon
- 1 pinch of salt
- 1 tsp vanilla extract
- 2 tbsp chia seeds
- 5 pears, peeled and diced

Directions:

1. In a bowl, stir the oil with the brown sugar, honey and applesauce. Once well combined, add the eggs, vanilla extract, all spices and cinnamon.
2. Stir in the flours sifted with the baking powder. Fold in the diced pear, then evenly spread the batter between 2 small loaf pans.
3. Bake in the before heating oven at 350F for 40-50 minutes. The best way to check if it's done is to insert a skewer in the middle of the cake. If it comes out clean of any crumbs, it is done.
4. Let it cool in the pan before To converting on a serving plate.

155. Pear Clafoutis

Prep Time: *15 Minutes* | *Cook Time:* *35 Minutes* | *Servings: 2*

Ingredients:

- 4 small pears, peeled, cored and sliced
- 1/3 cup almond meal
- 1/3 cup whole wheat flour
- 1 cup milk
- 3 eggs
- 2 tbsp sugar
- 1 tsp vanilla extract
- 1 cup low-fat yoghurt
- 1 pinch of salt

Directions:

1. Grease with the use of butter a 9-inch round cake pan, then arrange the pear slices on the bottom of the pan. To make the batter, stir the almond meal with flour, sugar, and a pinch of salt, then stir in the milk, eggs, yoghurt and vanilla.
2. Give it a good stir until there are no lumps, then pour the batter into the pan, cover the pears. Bake in the before heating oven at 350F for 30-35 minutes or until set and fragrant. It is best to let it cool in the pan before To converting it to a serving plate.

156. Pear Galette

Prep Time: *15 Minutes* | *Cook Time:* *23 Minutes* | *Servings: 2*

Ingredients:

- Crust:
- 1 cup all-purpose flour
- 1 cup whole wheat flour
- 1 pinch salt
- 1 pinch baking powder
- 6 oz butter, cold, but into cubes
- 4-6 tbsp cold water
- Filling:
- 6 pears, peeled, cored and sliced
- 4 tbsp brown sugar
- ½ tsp cinnamon

Directions:

1. To make the crust: In a bowl, stir the flours with a pinch of salt and baking powder, then rub in the cold butter until the stricture looks sandy. Gradually add the water and stir until it comes together. Do not knead it as it will lose its flakiness. Give the Shape to the dough into a disc and then refrigerate for 30 minutes.
2. When done, convert on the back of a baking tray lined with baking paper and roll it out in a thin sheet (about 12-inch diameter).
3. Arrange the pear slices in the middle, top with sugar and cinnamon, then gather the edges of the galette to the middle, wrapping them over the pears.
4. Since you rolled it on the back of a tray, simply place it in the oven and bake at 350F for 30-40 minutes or until crisp and golden brown.

157. Pear and Ginger Crumble

Prep Time: ***15 Minutes*** | ***Cook Time:*** ***33 Minutes*** | ***Servings: 4***

Ingredients:

- 6 oz butter, cold and cubed
- 1 cup whole wheat flour
- 1 cup rolled oats, ground
- ½ cup brown sugar
- 2 oz hazelnuts, ground
- 1 egg
- 3 ripe pears, peeled, cored and sliced
- ½ tsp cinnamon
- 1 tsp ground ginger
- 1 pinch of salt

Directions:

1. In a bowl, stir the flour continuously with the ground rolled oats, sugar and hazelnuts. Pour a pinch of salt, then rub in the cold butter until sandy.
2. Stir in the egg and stir until it comes together. Divide the dough into 2 equal portions. Wrap one of them in plastic wrap and freeze it for 30 minutes.

3. The other half of the dough is placed on the bottom of a 9-inch square pan. by using your fingertips to press it until it's evenly distributed.
4. Top with pear slices stirred with cinnamon and ginger. Put off the other half of the dough from the freezer and grate it over the pear slices.
5. Bake in the before heating oven at 350F for 30-40 minutes or until golden brown and crisp.

158. Pear Tart Tatin

Prep Time: *15 Minutes* | *Cook Time:* *43 Minutes* | *Servings: 2*

Ingredients:

- 4 phyllo dough sheets
- ½ cup brown sugar
- ¼ tsp cinnamon
- 4 pears, peeled, cored and sliced
- butter to grease the skillet

Directions:

1. Grease 1 9-inch heavy skillet or pan with butter (make sure the skillet or pan does not have parts that can melt in the oven).
2. Sprinkle in the sugar and cinnamon, then arrange the pear slices. Cut the phyllo sheets in half and stack them together.
3. Top the apples with them and bake in the before heating oven at 400F for 5 minutes, then lower the heat to 350F and cook 20 more minutes.
4. When complete, remove it from the oven and quickly turn it upside down on a plate. Carefully lift the skillet to reveal the tart. Serve warm with vanilla ice cream or cold with a dollop of fresh cream.

159. Red Wine Poached Pears

Prep Time: *15 Minutes* | *Cook Time:* *43 Minutes* | *Servings: 4*

Ingredients:

- 4 large, ripe but firm pears
- juice from ½ lemon
- 3 cups red wine (choose a sweeter type of wine)
- ½ cup sugar
- 1-star anise
- 1 cinnamon stick
- 2 cardamom pods, crushed

Directions:

1. Add the wine into a large saucepan and stir in the sugar (add more if you are using a dry red wine). Stir in the cinnamon stick, star anise and cardamom pods. Bring to a boil.
2. In the meantime, peel the pears, but them in half, and remove the core with a spoon. Place them in cold water stirred with lemon juice to prevent them from oxidizing.
3. When the wine is boiling, carefully place the pears in the hot liquid, lower the heat and cook them for 20-30 minutes until tender.
4. Turn the heat off and let them cool in the red wine. When chilled, convert them on a plate, then put the pan and the wine back on the heat. Cook until reduced by half.
5. Serve the pears drizzled with the reduced wine syrup.

160. Mango Coconut Bread

Prep Time: *15 Minutes* | *Cook Time:* *53 Minutes* | *Servings: 2*

Ingredients:

- 1 cup all-purpose flour
- 2/3 cup whole wheat flour
- 1 tsp baking powder
- 1 tsp baking soda
- 1 ripe mango, pureed
- 1 ripe mango, diced
- 1 cup sugar
- 1 pinch of salt
- ½ tsp cinnamon
- ½ tsp ground ginger
- 3 eggs
- 3 oz butter, melted
- ½ cup desiccated coconut

Directions:

1. In a bowl, stir the flours with a pinch of salt and baking powder, as well as baking soda and spices. In another bowl, combine the pureed mango with the eggs and melted butter.
2. Pour this stricture into the flour and stir well. Fold in the mango pieces, then convert the batter into a loaf pan lined with baking paper.
3. Bake in the before heating oven at 350F for 30-40 minutes or until fragrant and golden brown.

161. Superfoods Oatmeal Breakfast

Prep Time: *Cook Time:* *Servings: 4*
15 Minutes *53 Minutes*

Ingredients:

- 1 cup cooked oatmeal
- 1 tsp. Of ground flax seeds 1 tsp. of sunflower seeds
- A dash of cinnamon
- Half of the tsp. of cocoa

Directions:

1. Cook oatmeal with hot water, and after that, mix all ingredients. Sweeten if you have to with few drops of raw honey. Optional: You can replace sunflower seeds with pumpkin seed or chia seed. You can add a handful of blueberries or any berries instead of cocoa.

162. Oatmeal Yogurt Breakfast

Prep Time: *Cook Time:* *Servings: 6*
15 Minutes *15 Minutes*

Ingredients:

- ½ cup dry oatmeal
- A handful of blueberries (optional)
- 1 cup of low-fat yoghurt

Directio:

1. Mix all ingredients and wait 20 minutes or leave overnight in the fridge if using steel cut oats.

163. Cocoa Oatmeal

Prep Time: *Cook Time:* *Servings: 2*
15 Minutes *5 Minutes*

Ingredients

- ½ cup oats
- 2 cups water
- A pinch tsp. Salt
- ½ tsp. Ground vanilla bean 2 tbsp. cocoa powder
- 1 tbsp. raw honey
- 2 tbsp. ground flax seeds meal a dash of cinnamon
- 2 egg whites

Directions:

1. In a saucepan over high heat, place the oats and salt. Cover with 3 cups water. Bring to a boil and cook for 3-5 minutes, stirring occasionally. Keep adding ½ cup water if necessary as the mixture thickens.
2. In a separate bowl, whisk 4 tbsp. Water into the 4 tbsp. Cocoa powder to form a smooth sauce. Add the vanilla to the pan and stir.
3. Turn the heat down to low. Add the egg whites and whisk immediately. Add the flax meal and cinnamon. Stir to combine. Remove from heat, add raw honey and serve immediately.

164. Pineapple Turnovers

Prep Time: *Cook Time:* *Servings: 3*
15 Minutes *3 Minutes*

Ingredients:

- 1 ½ cups whole wheat flour
- ½ cup all-purpose flour
- 6 oz cold butter, cubed
- 2 tablespoons sugar
- 1 pinch salt
- ½ teaspoon baking powder
- 1 egg
- 2-4 tablespoons cold water
- 1 large pineapple, peeled, cored and diced ½ teaspoon cinnamon
- 1 tablespoon brown sugar
- 1 tablespoon cornstarch

Directions:

1. In a bowl, mix the pineapple with sugar, cornstarch and cinnamon. Set aside. To make the dough, in a bowl, combine the flours with a pinch of salt and sugar. Rub in the butter until it looks sandy, then stir in the egg.
2. Add 1-2 tablespoons of water or more until the dough comes together and looks easy to work with. Transfer on a well-floured working surface and roll it out into a thin sheet. Cut the sheet into small squares.
3. Drop spoonfuls of pineapple filling in the middle of each square, then fold them over to form a triangle. Press the edges of the triangle slightly with your fingertips or a fork and transfer all the turnovers on a baking tray lined with baking paper.
4. Bake in after heating the oven at 400F for 5 minutes, then lower the heat at 350F and bake 10-15 more minutes until fluffed and golden brown.

165. Pineapple Cheesecake

Prep Time: *Cook Time:* *Servings: 8*
15 Minutes *35 Minutes*

Ingredients:

- Crust:
- 2 cups graham crackers
- 1 tablespoon powdered sugar
- 1 teaspoon vanilla extract
- 6 oz butter, melted
- Filling:
- 20 oz low-fat cream cheese
- 10 oz low-fat yoghurt
- 4 eggs
- 2 tablespoons cornstarch
- 1 teaspoon vanilla extract
- 1 teaspoon lemon zest
- ½ cup sugar
- Topping:
- 2 cups fresh pineapple cubes
- juice from 1 lemon
- 2 tablespoons brown sugar
- 1 tablespoon chopped mint leaves

Directions:

1. To make the crust, simply put all the ingredients in a food processor and pulse until well mixed and sandy. Transfer on a 9-inch round cake pan lined with baking paper and press it down on the bottom and sides of the pan either with your fingertips or the back of a spoon. It should be really packed. Set aside.
2. To make the filling: Add the cream cheese with the sugar and yoghurt, then add the eggs, vanilla and lemon zest, as well as the cornstarch. Pour this filling in the crust and bake in the preheated oven at 350F for 40-50 minutes or until it looks wobbly in the middle but slightly set. Remove it and let it cool in the pan.
3. To make the topping: Mix the pineapple cubes with sugar, lemon juice and chopped mint. Let it cool for at least one hour, then top the cheesecake with the pineapple cubes.

166. White Chocolate Pineapple Mousse

Prep Time: *Cook Time:* *Servings: 4*
15 Minutes *10 Minutes*

Ingredients:

- 5 oz white chocolate
- 1 oz butter
- 2 cups heavy cream
- 2 cups canned crushed pineapple, drained
- 1 teaspoon vanilla extract
- 4 oz ginger biscuits, crushed

Directions:

1. In a saucepan, bring half of the heavy cream to the boiling point, then remove from heat and stir in the chocolate. Mix until melted, then add the butter.
2. Keep it cool at room temperature, then fold in the remaining cream, whipped. Add the vanilla, then spoon the mousse into small serving glasses.
3. Top with crushed biscuits, then crushed pineapple and refrigerate at least 1 hour before serving.

167. Pineapple Popsicles

Prep Time: *Cook Time 0* *Servings: 2*
15 Minutes *Minutes*

Ingredients:

- 2 cups fresh chopped pineapple
- 1 ½ cup coconut milk
- ½ cup low-fat cream cheese
- 1 teaspoon vanilla extract
- 1 tablespoon mint leaves
- juice and zest from 1 lime
- ¼ cup brown sugar

Directions:

1. Mix the pineapple with the cream cheese, lime juice and zest and mint leaves into a blender and pulse until well pureed and smooth. Add the coconut milk and cream cheese, then the sugar.Pour the mixture into your popsicle moulds and freeze for at least 4 hours. To remove them from their moulds, sink them in hot water for 5 seconds

168. SPLIT PEA & HAM SOUP

Prep Time: *Cook Time:* *Servings: 6*
12 Minutes *04 Minutes*

INGREDIENTS:

- Tbsps. unsalted butter
- 1 large onion, chopped fine salt & pepper
- garlic cloves, minced
- 7 cups water
- ham steak (about 1 lb), skin removed, cut into quarters
- 3 slices thick-cut bacon
- lb green split peas (2 cups), picked over & rinsed
- sprigs fresh thyme
- bay leaves
- carrots, peeled
- 1 celery rib, divide into 1/2-inch pieces 1 recipe BUTTER CROUTONS

TECHNIQUE:

1. Heat butter in a Dutch oven over high heat. Include onion & 1/2 Tsp. Salt & cook, frequently stirring, till onion is softened, about 3 to 4 mins. Include garlic & cook till fragrant, about 30 seconds. Include water, ham steak, bacon, peas, thyme, & bay leaves. Increase heat to high & bring to simmer, frequently stirring to keep peas from sticking to the bottom. Reduce heat to low, cover, & simmer till peas are tender but Not falling apart, about 45 mins.
2. Remove ham steak, cover with aluminium foil or plastic wrap to prevent drying out, & set aside. Stir in carrots & celery & continue to simmer, covered, till vegetables are tender & peas have almost completely broken down, about 30 mins longer.
3. When cool enough, shred ham into small bite-size pieces. Remove & discard thyme, bay leaves, & bacon slices. Stir ham back into soup & return to simmer. Season with salt & pepper to taste & serve.

169. LENTILS

Prep Time: *Cook Time:* *Servings: 2*
10 Minutes *8 Minutes*

INGREDIENTS:

- slices bacon, cut into 1/4-inch pieces
- 1 large onion, chopped fine
- 2 carrots, peeled & chopped
- garlic cloves, minced
- (14.5-ounce) can diced tomatoes, drained
- bay leaf
- Tsp. minced fresh thyme
- ounces lentils (1 cup), picked over & rinsed
- 1 Tsp. salt Pepper
- 1/2 cup dry white wine
- 4 1/2 cups low-sodium chicken broth
- 1 1/2 cups water
- 1 1/2 Tsps. balsamic vinegar
- Tbsps. minced fresh parsley

TECHNIQUE:

1. Cook bacon in an oven over medium-high heat, occasionally stirring, till bacon is crisp, about 5 mins. Include onion & carrots & cook, occasionally stirring, till vegetables begin to soften about 2 mins. Include garlic & cook till fragrant, about 30 seconds. Stir in tomatoes, bay leaf, & thyme & cook till fragrant, about 30 seconds.
2. Stir in lentils & salt & season with pepper to taste. Cover, reduce heat to medium-low, & cook till vegetables are softened & lentils have darkened 8 to 10 mins.
3. Uncover, increase heat to high, Include wine, & bring to simmer. Include chicken broth & water, bring to boil, cover partially, & reduce heat to low. Simmer till lentils are tender but still hold their shape, 30 to 35 mins.
4. Remove bay leaf from pot & discard. Puree 3 cups soup in the blender till smooth, then return to pot. Stir in vinegar & heat soup over medium-low heat till hot, about 5 mins. Stir in 2 Tbsps. Parsley & serve, garnishing each container with remaining parsley.

170. PASTA E FAGIOLI

Prep Time: *Cook Time:* *Servings: 5*
15 Minutes *35 Minutes*

INGREDIENTS:

- Tbsp. extra-virgin olive oil, plus extra for drizzling
- 3 ounces pancetta, chopped fine
- onion, chopped fine
- celery rib, chopped fine
- 4 garlic cloves, minced
- 1 Tsp. dried oregano
- 1/4 Tsp. red pepper flakes
- anchovy fillets, rinsed & minced
- 1 (28-ounce) can diced tomatoes
- 1 Parmesan cheese rind
- 2 (15-ounce) cans cannellini beans, rinsed
- 3 1/2 cups low-sodium chicken broth
- 2 1/2 cups water
- 1 cup orzo
- 1/4 cup chopped fresh parsley
- ounces Parmesan cheese, grated (1 cup)

TECHNIQUE:

1. Heat oil in an oven over medium-high heat till shimmering. Include pancetta & cook, occasionally stirring, till beginning to brown, 3 to 5 mins. Include onion & celery & cook, occasionally stirring, till vegetables are softened, 5 to 7 mins. Include garlic, oregano, pepper flakes, & anchovies & cook, constantly stirring, till fragrant, about 1 min. Stir continuously in tomatoes, scraping up any browned bits from the bottom of the pan. Include Parmesan rind & beans & bring to boil, then reduce heat to low & simmer to blend flavours, 10 mins.
2. Include chicken broth, water, & 1 Tsp. Salt to pot. Increase heat to high & bring to boil. Include pasta & cook till al dente, about 10 mins.
3. Remove & discard Parmesan rind. Off heat, stir in 3 Tbsps. Parsley & season with salt & pepper to taste. Ladle soup into containers, drizzle with olive oil & sprinkle with remaining parsley. Serve immediately, passing grated Parmesan separately.

171. CREAMY CHICKEN

Prep Time: *Cook Time:* *Servings: 4*
12 Minutes *10 Minutes*

INGREDIENTS:

(1 1/2-lb) whole bone-in chicken breasts
1 Tbsp. vegetable oil Salt
celery ribs, cut into small dice
scallions, minced
3/4–1 cup mayonnaise
1 1/2–2 Tbsps. lemon juice
Tbsps. minced fresh parsley

TECHNIQUE:

1. 2Set oven rack to middle setting & heat oven to 400 degrees. Set breasts on a small, aluminium foil-lined rimmed baking sheet. Brush with oil & sprinkle generously with salt. Roast till chicken registers 160 degrees, 35 to 40 mins. Let cool to room temperature, remove skin & bones, & shred meat into bite-size pieces (about 5 cups).
2. Using the lesser amounts of mayonnaise & lemon juice, mix all salad ingredients (including chicken) together in a large container. Set flavor & consistency with additional mayonnaise & lemon juice & salt & pepper to taste. Serve. (Chicken salad can be refrigerated overnight.)

172. CHICKEN WITH ASPARAGUS & TOMATO

Prep Time: *Cook Time:* *Servings: 2*
35 Minutes *11 Minutes*

INGREDIENTS:

- 1/2 cup extra-virgin olive oil plus 1 additional Tbsp. 1/4 cup red wine vinegar
- 1/2 cup oil-packed sun-dried tomatoes, rinsed & minced 1 small garlic clove, minced
- Salt & pepper
- 1/2 lb asparagus, trimmed & cut on the bias into 1-inch lengths
- cup chopped fresh basil

Prep Time:* *11 Minutes ***Cook Time:* *9 Minutes***

Servings: 2

- recipe CLASSIC ROAST CHICKEN, cooled, meat removed & shredded into 2-inch pieces
- ounces goat cheese, crumbled (3/4 cup) (optional) 1/2 cup pine nuts, toasted

TECHNIQUE:

1. Puree 1/2 cup oil, vinegar, sun-dried tomatoes, garlic, 1/4 Tsp. Salt, & 1/2 Tsp. Pepper in the blender till smooth. Shift to the large container. 2. Heat remaining Tbsp. Oil in 10-inch nonstick pan over high heat till beginning to smoke; Include asparagus, 1/4 Tsp. Salt, & 1/4 Tsp. Pepper; cook till asparagus is browned & almost tender, about 3 mins, stirring occasionally. Shift to plate & let cool.
2. Include cooled asparagus & basil to vinaigrette; stir to combine. Include chicken & toss gently to combine; let stand at room temperature 15 mins. Season with salt & pepper to taste & sprinkle with goat cheese, if using, & pine nuts. Serve immediately.

173. CHICKEN WITH SPICY PEANUT DRESSING

Prep Time: *Cook Time:* *Servings: 6*
11 Minutes *9 Minutes*

INGREDIENTS:

- 1/2 cup canola oil
- Tbsps. smooth peanut butter 1/2 cup lime juice (3 to 4 limes)
- 2 Tbsps. water Salt & pepper
- small garlic cloves, minced
- Tops. grated fresh ginger
- Tbsps. Light brown sugar 1 1/2 Tips. red pepper flakes
- 1/2 cucumber, peeled, halved lengthwise, seeded, & cut into 1-inch-long matchsticks 1 carrot, peeled & shredded
- 4 scallions, sliced thin
- 3 Tbsps. minced fresh cilantro
- recipe CLASSIC ROAST CHICKEN, cooled, meat removed & shredded into 2-inch pieces
- 1/2 cup unsalted peanuts, toasted & chopped

TECHNIQUE:

1. Puree oil, peanut butter, lime juice, water, 1/4 Tsp. Salt, garlic, ginger, brown sugar, & pepper flakes in the blender till combined. Shift to the large container. 2. Include cucumber, carrot, scallions, & cilantro to vinaigrette; toss to combine. Include chicken & toss gently to combine; let stand at room temperature 15 mins. Season with salt & pepper to taste & sprinkle with peanuts. Serve immediately.

174. CHICKEN With ROASTED RED PEPPER

INGREDIENTS:

- 1 1/3 cups chopped jarred roasted red peppers
- 1/2 cup extra-virgin olive oil
- Tbsps. sherry vinegar or balsamic vinegar
- 1 small garlic clove, minced salt & pepper
- 2 celery ribs, sliced very thin
- 1/2 cup chopped pitted green olives
- Tbsps. minced fresh parsley
- 1 small shallot, minced
- 1/2 cup sliced almonds, toasted

TECHNIQUE:

1. Puree 2/3 cup roasted red peppers, oil, vinegar, garlic, 1/4 Tsp. Salt, & 1/2 Tsp. Pepper in the blender till smooth. Shift to a container.

Include celery, olives, parsley, shallot, & remaining 2/3 cup red peppers to vinaigrette; stir to combine. Include chicken & toss gently to combine; let stand at room temperature 15 mins. Season with salt & pepper to taste & sprinkle with almonds. Serve immediately.

.

175. Flax and Blueberry Vanilla Overnight Oats

Prep Time: *Cook Time:* *Servings: 4*
15 Minutes *35 Minutes*

Ingredients:

½ cup oats
¼ cup water
¼ cup low-fat yoghurt
½ tsp. Ground vanilla bean 1 tbsp. flax seeds meal A pinch of salt
Blueberries walnuts blackberries raw honey for topping

Directions:

1. 2Add the ingredients (except for toppings) to the bowl in the evening.
2. Refrigerate overnight.
3. In the morning, stir up the mixture. It should be thick. Add the toppings of your choice.

176. Apple Oatmeal

Prep Time: *Cook Time:0* *Servings: 2*
15 Minutes *Minutes*

Ingredients:

- 1 grated apple
- ½ cup oats
- 1 cup water
- Dash of cinnamon
- 2 tsp. raw honey

Directions:

1. Cook the oats with the water for 3-5 minutes.
2. Add grated apple and cinnamon. Stir in the raw honey.

177. Almond Butter Banana Oats

Prep Time: *Cook Time:* *Servings: 2*
15 Minutes *0 Minutes*

Ingredients:

- ½ cup oats
- ¾ cup water
- 1 egg white
- 1 banana 1 tbs. Flax seeds meal 1 tsp raw honey
- pinch cinnamon
- ½ tbs. almond butter

Directions:

1. Combine oats and water in a bowl. Egg white beat, then whisk it in with the uncooked oats.
2. Boil on the stovetop after checking consistency and continue to heat as necessary until the oats are fluffy and thick.
3. Mash banana and add to oats. Heat for 1-minute stir in flax, raw honey and cinnamon. Top with almond butter!

178. Coconut Pomegranate Oatmeal

Prep Time: *15 Minutes* *Cook Time:* *0 Minutes* *Servings:3*

Ingredients:

- ½ cup oats
- 1/3 cup coconut milk
- 1 cup water
- 2 tbs. shredded unsweetened coconut
- 1-2 tbs. Flax seeds meal 1 tbs. raw honey
- 3 tbs. pomegranate seeds
- Cook oats with coconut milk, water and salt.

Directions:

1. Stir in the coconut raw honey and flaxseed meal. Sprinkle with extra coconut and pomegranate seeds.

179. Banana Almond Overnight Oats

Prep Time: *15 Minutes* *Cook Time:* *0 Minutes* *Servings: 8*

Ingredients:

- ½ cup oats
- ½ cup coconut milk
- 1 banana 1 tbs. flax seeds meal 1 tsp raw honey
- pinch cinnamon
- 1 tsp dried cranberries 2 Brazil nuts ½ tbs. almond butter

Directions:

1. Make a smoothie with banana coconut milk, almond butter, honey and cinnamon. Stir in flax and oatmeal and leave overnight. Top with 1 tsp. Dried cranberries, Brazil nuts.

180. Walnut Oatmeal with Fresh Blueberries

Prep Time: *15 Minutes* *Cook Time:* *0 Minutes* *Servings: 3*

Ingredients:

- ½ cup blueberries
- ½ cup oats
- 1 cup water
- ½ cup walnuts Dash of cinnamon
- 2 tsp. raw honey

Directions:

1. Cook the oats with the water for 3-5 minutes.
2. Add walnuts and cinnamon. Stir in the raw honey. Top with blueberries

181. Raspberry cereal

Prep Time: *15 Minutes* *Cook Time:* *0 Minutes* *Servings: 4*

Ingredients:

- ½ cup raspberries
- ½ cup oats
- 1 cup water
- ½ cup sesame seeds
- Dash of cinnamon
- 2 tsp. raw honey

Directions:

1. 2Cook the oats with the water for 3-5 minutes.
2. Add sesame seeds and cinnamon. Stir in the raw honey. Top with raspberries

182. Strawberry Oatmeal

Prep Time: *15 Minutes* *Cook Time:* *0 Minutes* *Servings: 2*

Ingredients:

- ½ cup strawberries
- ½ cup oats
- 1 cup water
- 2 Tbsp. sunflower seeds
- 1 Tbsp. Raisins 2 tsp. raw honey

Directions:

1. Cook the oats with the water for 3-5 minutes.
2. Add sesame seeds and cinnamon. Stir in the raw honey. Top with raspberries

183. Kiwi Oatmeal

Prep Time: *15 Minutes* *Cook Time:* *0 Minutes* *Servings: 4*

Ingredients:

- 1 sliced kiwi
- ½ cup oats
- 1 cup water
- 2 Tbsp. pumpkin seeds
- 1 Tbsp. Raisins 2 tsp. raw honey

Directions:

1. Cook the oats with the water for 3-5 minutes.
2. Add sesame seeds and cinnamon. Stir in the raw honey. Top with raspberries

184. Coconut Chia Puddin

Prep Time: *15 Minutes* *Cook Time:* *0 Minutes* *Servings: 6*

Ingredients

- ¼ cup Chia seeds
- 1 cup coconut milk ½ tbs Royall jelly 1 tsp.
- Ground Vanilla Bean a pinch of Nutmeg Top with Blueberries

Directions:

1. Mix all ingredients except blueberries and leave overnight in the fridge. Top with blueberries.

185. Coconut Pomegranate Chia Pudding

Prep Time: *15 Minutes* *Cook Time:* *0 Minutes* *Servings: 6*

Ingredients

- ¼ cup Chia seeds
- 1 cup Coconut milk
- ½ tablespoon Raw honey
- ½ tablespoon Coconut flakes
- Top with Pomegranate seeds

Directions:

1. Mix all ingredients except pomegranate and leave overnight in the fridge. Top with pomegranate.

186. Yogurt & Mango Pudding

Prep Time: *15 Minutes* *Cook Time:* *0 Minutes* *Servings: 2*

Ingredients

- ¼ cup Chia seeds 1 ½ cup yoghurt 1 tablespoon raw honey
- ½ cup chopped Mango

Directions:

1. 2Mix 1 cup of yoghurt honey and chia seeds and leave overnight in the fridge.
2. Divide into 2 glasses, top each with ¼ cup yoghurt and ¼ cup mango.

187. Cacao & Raspberry Pudding

Prep Time: *15 Minutes* *Cook Time:* *0 Minutes* *Servings: 2*

Ingredients

- ¼ cup Chia seeds
- 1 cup coconut milk
- 1 tablespoon raw honey
- 1 Tsp. cacao powder
- ½ cup yoghurt
- ½ cup raspberrie

Directions:

1. Mix coconut milk, honey cacao and chia seeds and leave them overnight in the fridge.
2. Divide into 2 glasses, top each with ¼ cup yoghurt and ¼ cup raspberries.

Lunch Recipes

188. SPICY STIR-FRIED SESAME CHICKEN WITH GREEN BEANS & SHIITAKE MUSHROOMS SAUCE

Prep Time: *23 Minutes* *Cook Time:* *21 Minutes* *Servings: 8*

INGREDIENTS:

- 1/2 cup low-sodium chicken broth
- Tbsps. soy sauce
- 2 Tbsps. dry sherry
- 1 Tbsp. Plus 1 Tsp. Asian chilli-garlic sauce 1 Tbsp. Plus 1 Tsp. sugar
- 2 Tbsps. sesame seeds, toasted
- 1 Tsp. toasted sesame oil
- 1 Tsp. cornstarch
- 1 garlic clove, minced
- CHICKEN STIR-FRY
- 2 garlic cloves, minced
- 1 Tsp. grated fresh ginger
- Tbsps. Plus 2 Tbsps. vegetable oil 1/4 cup soy sauce
- 1/4 cup dry sherry 1 cup water
- 1 lb boneless, skinless chicken breasts, trimmed & sliced thin

- Tbsps. Plus 1 Tsp. toasted sesame oil
- Tbsp. cornstarch
- Tbsp. all-purpose flour
- lb green beans, trimmed & cut on the bias into 1-inch pieces
- 8 ounces shiitake mushrooms, stemmed & sliced 1/8 inch thick
- Tsp. sesame seeds, toasted

DIRECTIONS:

1. FOR THE SAUCE:
Mixing all ingredients together in a small container.
2. FOR THE STIR-FRY: Combine garlic, ginger, & 1 Tsp. Vegetable oil in the small container & set aside. Combine soy sauce, sherry, & water in a medium container. Include chicken & stir to break up clumps after covering with plastic wrap & refrigerate for at least 20 mins or up to 1 hr. Pour off excess liquid from the chicken.
3. Mix 2 Tbsps. Sesame oil, cornstarch, & flour in a medium container till smooth. Toss chicken in cornstarch batter till evenly coated.
4. Heat 2 Tbsps. Vegetable oil in 12-inch nonstick pan over high heat till smoking. Include half of the chicken to pan in even layer & cook, without stirring, till golden brown on the first side, about 1 min. Flip chicken pieces over & cook till lightly browned on the second side, about 30 seconds. Shift chicken to clean container. Repeat with 2 Tbsps. Vegetable oil & remaining chicken.
5. Include 1 Tbsp. Vegetable oil to pan & heat till just smoking. Include green beans & cook, occasionally stirring, 1 min. Include mushrooms & cook till mushrooms are lightly browned about 3 mins. Clear centre of the pan, Include garlic batter, & cook, mashing batter into pan, till fragrant, 15 to 20 seconds. Stir batter into beans & mushrooms & continue to cook till beans are crisp-tender, about 30 seconds.
6. Return chicken to pan. Whisk sauce to recombine, Include to the pan, reduce heat to medium, & cook, constantly stirring, till sauce is thickened & chicken is cooked through about 30 seconds. Shift to the platter, drizzle with the remaining 1 Tsp. Sesame oil, & sprinkle with sesame seeds. Serve immediately.

189. SWEET, SOUR, and SPICY ORANGE CHICKEN and BROCCOLI WITH CASHEWS

Prep Time: 15 Minutes | *Cook Time: 25 Minutes* | *Servings: 6*

INGREDIENTS:

- SAUCE
- 1/4 cup low-sodium chicken broth
- 1/4 cup orange juice
- 1/4 cup white vinegar
- Tbsps. soy sauce
- Tbsps. hoisin sauce
- 1 Tsp. cornstarch
- 1 Tbsp. sugar
- 1/2 Tsp. red pepper flakes
- CHICKEN STIR-FRY
- Two garlic cloves, minced
- 1 Tsp. grated fresh ginger
- Tbsps. Plus 1 Tsp. vegetable oil 1 1/4 cups water
- 1/4 cup soy sauce 1/4 cup dry sherry
- 1 lb boneless, skinless chicken breasts, trimmed & sliced thin 2 Tbsps. toasted sesame oil
- 1 Tbsp. cornstarch
- 1 Tbsp. all-purpose flour
- 1 cup unsalted cashews, toasted
- 1 1/2 lbs broccoli, florets cut into 1-inch pieces, stalks peeled & sliced on bias 1/4 inch thick
- medium scallions, sliced 1/4-inch thick on the bias

DIRECTIONS:

1. FOR THE SAUCE: Whisk ingredients together in the small container & set aside.
2. FOR THE STIR-FRY: Combine garlic, ginger, & 1 Tbsp. Vegetable oil in the small container & set aside. Combine 1 cup water, soy sauce, & sherry in a medium container. Include chicken & stir to break up clumps. Cover with a wrap of plastic and refrigerate for at least 20 mins or up to 1 hr. Pour off excess liquid from the chicken.
3. Mix sesame oil, cornstarch, & flour in a medium container till smooth. Toss chicken in cornstarch batter till evenly coated.
4. Heat 2 Tbsps. Vegetable oil in 12-inch nonstick pan over high heat till smoking. Include half of the chicken in an even layer & cook, without stirring, till golden brown on the first side, about 1 min. Flip chicken pieces over & cook till lightly browned on the second side, about 30 seconds. Shift chicken to clean container. Repeat with 2 Tbsps. Vegetable oil & remaining chicken.
5. Include remaining 1 Tbsp. Vegetable oil to pan & heat till just smoking. Include broccoli & cook 30 seconds. Include remaining 1/4 cup water, cover, & lower heat to medium-low. Cook broccoli till crisp-tender, about 3 mins, then Shift to a paper towel-lined plate. Include garlic butter in the pan, increase heat to medium-high, & cook, mashing batter into pan, till fragrant & golden brown, 15 to 20 seconds.
6. Return chicken to pan & toss to combine. Whisk sauce to recombine, Include to the pan, & cook, constantly stirring, till sauce is thickened & evenly distributed, about 1 min. Off heat, Include broccoli & cashews & stir to combine. Shift to a platter, sprinkle with scallions, & serve.

190. STIR-FRIED CHICKEN WITH BOK CHOY & CRISPY NOODLE CAKE

Prep Time: 19 Minutes | *Cook Time: 17 Minutes* | *Servings: 8*

INGREDIENTS:

- SAUCE
- 1/4 cup low-sodium chicken broth
- Tbsps. soy sauce
- 1 Tbsp. dry sherry
- 1 Tbsp. oyster sauce
- 1 Tsp. sugar
- 1 Tsp. cornstarch
- 1/4 Tsp. red pepper flakes
- NOODLE CAKE
- (9-ounce) package fresh Chinese noodles
- Tsp. salt
- scallions, sliced thin 1/4 cup vegetable oil
- CHICKEN STIR-FRY
- lb boneless, skinless chicken breasts, trimmed & sliced thin
- Tbsp. soy sauce
- Tbsp. dry sherry
- Tbsps. toasted sesame oil
- 1 Tbsp. cornstarch
- 1 Tbsp. all-purpose flour
- Tbsps. Plus 2 Tbsps. vegetable oil
- 1 Tbsp. grated fresh ginger
- One medium garlic clove, minced
- lb bok choy stalks cut on the bias into 1/4-inch pieces & greens cut into 1/2-inch strips
- small red bell pepper stemmed, seeded, & cut into 1/4-inch strips

DIRECTIONS:

1. FOR THE SAUCE: all ingredients will combine in a small container.
2. FOR THE NOODLE CAKE: Bring 6 quarts of water to boil in a large pot. Include noodles & salt & cook, often stirring, till almost tender, 2 to 3 mins. Drain noodles, then toss with scallions.
3. Heat 2 Tbsps. Oil in 12-inch nonstick pan over medium heat till shimmering. Spread noodles evenly across the bottom of the pan & press with a spatula to flatten them into the cake. Cook till crisp & golden brown, 5 to 8 mins.
4. Slide noodle cake onto a large plate. Include remaining 2 Tbsps. Oil to pan & swirl to coat. Invert noodle cake onto the second plate & slide it, browned side up, back into the pan. Cook until turn golden brown on the second side, 5 to 8 mins.
5. Slide noodle cake onto cutting board & let sit for at least 5 mins before slicing into wedges & serving. (Noodle cake can be Shifted to a wire rack set over a baking sheet & kept warm in a 200-degree oven for up to 20 mins.) Wipe out the pan by use of a wad of paper towels.
6. FOR THE STIR-FRY: While the noodles boil, toss chicken with soy sauce & sherry in the medium container & let marinate for 10 mins or up to 1 hr. Whisk sesame oil, cornstarch, & flour together in a large container. Combine 1 Tsp. Vegetable oil, ginger, & garlic in a small container.
7. Stir marinated chicken into cornstarch batter. Heat 2 Tbsp. Vegetable oil in a pan over high heat till just smoking. Include half of the chicken, break up any clumps, & cook without stirring till meat is browned at edges, about 1 min. Stir chicken & continue to cook till
8. They are cooked through, about 1 min longer—shift chicken to clean container & cover with aluminium foil to keep warm. Repeat with 2 Tbsp: vegetable oil & remaining chicken.
9. Include remaining 1 Tbsp. Vegetable oil to pan & return to high heat till just smoking. Include bok choy stalks & bell pepper & cook till lightly browned 2 to 3 mins.
10. Clear centre of the pan, Include ginger batter, & cook, mashing batter into pan, till fragrant, 15 to 20 seconds. Stir ginger batter into vegetables, then stir in bok choy greens & cook till beginning to wilt, about 30 seconds.
11. Stir in chicken with any accumulated juices. Whisk sauce to recombine, then Includes to pan & cook, constantly tossing, till sauce is thickened, about 30 seconds. Shift to a platter & serve with noodle cake.

191. TERIYAKI STIR-FRIED BEEF WITH GREEN BEANS & SHIITAKES

Prep Time: 15 Minutes | *Cook Time: 55 Minutes* | *Servings: 4*

INGREDIENTS:

- 1/2 cup low-sodium chicken broth
- Tbsps. soy sauce
- Tbsps. sugar
- Tbsp. mirin
- Tsp. cornstarch
- 1/4 Tsp. red pepper flakes
- BEEF STIR-FRY
- Tbsps. soy sauce
- 1 Tsp. sugar
- 1 (12-ounce) flank steak, trimmed & sliced thin across the grain on slight bias three garlic cloves, minced
- 1 Tbsp. grated fresh ginger
- Tbsps. vegetable oil
- ounces shiitake mushrooms stemmed & cut into 1-inch pieces
- 12 ounces green beans, trimmed & halved 1/4 cup water
- Three scallions, cut into 1 1/2-inch pieces, white & light green pieces quartered lengthwise

DIRECTIONS:

1. 2FOR THE SAUCE: Whisk all combine ingredients together in the small container & set aside.
2. FOR THE STIR-FRY: Combine soy sauce & sugar in a medium container. Include beef, toss well, & marinate for at least 10 mins or up to 1 hr, stirring once. Meanwhile, combine garlic, ginger, & 1 Tsp. Oil in a small container.
3. Drain beef & discard liquid. Heat 1 Tsp. Oil in 12-inch nonstick pan over high heat till just smoking. Include half of the beef in a single layer, break up any clumps, & cook, without stirring for 1 min. Stir beef & continue to cook till browned, 1 to 2 mins—shift beef to clean container. Repeat with 1 Tsp. Oil & remaining beef. Rinse pan clean & dry with paper towels.
4. Include remaining 1 Tbsp. Oil to pan & heat till just smoking. Include mushrooms & cook till beginning to brown, about 2 mins. Include green beans & cook, frequently stirring, till spotty brown, 3 to 4 mins. Include water, cover, & continue to cook till green beans are crisp-tender, 2 to 3 mins longer. Uncover the clear centre of the pan, & Include garlic batter. Cook, mashing batter into pan, till fragrant, 15 to 20 seconds. Stir batter into vegetables. Return beef & any accumulated juices to the pan, Include scallions, & stir to combine. Whisk sauce to recombine, Include to the pan, & cook, constantly stirring, till thickened, about 30 seconds. Serve.

192. STIR-FRIED BEEF WITH SNAP PEAS & RED PEPPERS

Prep Time: 15 Minutes | *Cook Time: 36 Minutes* | *Servings: 6*

INGREDIENTS:

- SAUCE
- 1/2 cup low-sodium chicken broth
- 1/4 cup oyster sauce
- Tbsps. dry sherry
- 1 Tbsp. sugar
- 1 Tsp. cornstarch
- BEEF STIR-FRY
- Tbsps. soy sauce
- 1 Tsp. sugar
- 1 (12-ounce) flank steak, trimmed & sliced thin across the grain on slight bias three garlic cloves, minced
- 1 Tbsp. grated fresh ginger
- Tbsps. vegetable oil
- 12 ounces sugar snap peas, stems & strings removed
- red bell pepper, stemmed, seeded, & cut into 1/4-inch slices
- 2 Tbsps. Water

DIRECTIONS:

1. 2FOR THE SAUCE: Whisk all combine ingredients all together in the small container & set aside.
2. 3FOR THE STIR-FRY: Combine soy sauce & sugar in a medium container. Include beef, toss well, & marinate for at least 10 mins or up to 1 hr, stirring once. Meanwhile, combine garlic, ginger, & 1 Tsp. Oil in a small container.
3. Drain beef & discard liquid. Heat 1 Tsp. Oil in 12-inch nonstick pan over high heat till just smoking. Include half of the beef in single Layer, break up any clumps, & cook, without stirring, for 1 min. Stir beef & continue to cook till browned, 1 to 2 mins—shift beef to clean container. Repeat with 1 Tsp. Oil & remaining beef. Rinse pan clean & dry with paper towels.
4. Include remaining 1 Tbsp. Oil to pan & heat till just smoking. Include snap peas & bell pepper & cook, frequently stirring, till vegetables begin to brown, 3 to 5 mins. Include water & continue to cook till vegetables are crisp-tender, 1 to 2 mins longer. Clear centre of the pan, Include garlic-ginger batter & cook, mashing batter into pan, till fragrant, 15 to 20 seconds. Stir batter into vegetables. Return beef & any accumulated juices to pan & stir to combine. Whisk sauce to recombine, Include to the pan, & cook, constantly stirring, till thickened, about 30 seconds. Serve.

193. TANGERINE STIR-FRIED BEEF WITH ONIONS & SNOW PEAS

Prep Time: *14 Minutes* *Cook Time:* *12 Minutes* *Servings: 2*

INGREDIENTS:

- SAUCE
- 3/4 cup tangerine juice (3 to 4 tangerines)
- 2 Tbsps. soy sauce
- Tbsp. light brown sugar
- Tsp. toasted sesame oil
- Tsp. cornstarch
- BEEF STIR-FRY
- 2 Tbsps. soy sauce
- Tsp. light brown sugar
- (12-ounce) flank steak, trimmed and sliced thin across the grain on a slight bias
- Three garlic cloves, minced
- Tbsp. grated fresh ginger
- Tbsp. black bean sauce
- Tsp. grated tangerine zest
- 1/4–1/2 Tsp. red pepper flakes
- 2 Tbsps. vegetable oil
- large onion halved & cut into 1/2-inch wedges
- 10 ounces snow peas, stems & strings removed
- 2 Tbsps. Water

DIRECTIONS:

1. 2FOR THE SAUCE: Whisk all combine ingredients all together in the small container & set aside.
2. FOR THE STIR-FRY: Combine soy sauce & sugar in a medium container. Include beef, toss well, & marinate for at least 10 mins or up to 1 hr, stirring once. Meanwhile, combine garlic, ginger, black bean sauce, tangerine zest, pepper flakes, & 1 Tsp. Vegetable oil in a small container.
3. Drain beef & discard liquid. Heat 1 Tsp. Vegetable oil in 12-inch nonstick pan over high heat till just smoking. Include half of the beef in a single layer, break up any clumps, & cook, without stirring for 1 min. Stir beef & continue to cook till browned, 1 to 2 mins—shift beef to clean container. Repeat with 1 Tsp. Vegetable oil & remaining beef. Rinse pan clean & dry with paper towels.
4. Include remaining 1 Tbsp. Vegetable oil to pan & heat till just smoking. Include onion & cook, frequently stirring, till beginning to brown, 3 to 5 mins. Include snow peas & continue to cook till spotty brown, about 2 mins longer. Include water & cook till vegetables are crisp-tender, about 1 min. Clear centre of the pan, Include garlic batter, & cook, mashing batter into pan, till fragrant, 15 to 20 seconds. Stir batter into vegetables. Return beef & any accumulated juices to pan & stir to combine. Whisk sauce to recombine, Include to the pan, & cook, constantly stirring, till thickened, about 30 seconds. Serve.

194. KOREAN STIR-FRIED BEEF WITH KIMCHI

Prep Time: *15 Minutes* *Cook Time:* *23 Minutes* *Servings: 2*

INGREDIENTS:

- SAUCE
- 1/2 cup low-sodium chicken broth
- Tbsps. soy sauce
- 1 Tbsp. sugar
- 1 Tsp. toasted sesame oil
- 1 Tsp. cornstarch
- BEEF STIR-FRY
- Tbsps. soy sauce
- 1 Tsp. sugar
- 1 (12-ounce) flank steak, trimmed & sliced thin across the grain on slight bias three garlic cloves, minced
- 1 Tbsp. grated fresh ginger
- Tbsps. vegetable oil
- cup kimchi, chopped into 1-inch pieces
- 4 ounces bean sprouts (2 cups)
- Five scallions, cut into 1 1/2-inch pieces, white & light green pieces quartered lengthwise.

DIRECTIONS:

1. FOR THE SAUCE: Whisk all combine ingredients together in the small container & set aside.
2. FOR THE STIR-FRY: Combine soy sauce & sugar in a medium container. Include beef, toss well, & marinate for at least 10 mins or up to 1 Hr. I am stirring once. Meanwhile, combine garlic, ginger, & 1 Tsp. Vegetable oil in a small container.
3. Drain beef & discard liquid. Heat 1 Tsp. Vegetable oil in 12-inch nonstick pan over high heat till just smoking. Include half of the beef in a single layer, break up any clumps, & cook, without stirring for 1 min. Stir beef & continue to cook till browned, 1 to 2 mins—shift beef to clean container. Repeat with 1 Tsp. Vegetable oil & remaining beef. Rinse pan clean & dry with paper towels.
4. Include remaining 1 Tbsp. Oil to pan & heat till just smoking. Include kimchi & cook, frequently stirring, till aromatic, 1 to 2 mins. Include bean sprouts & stir to combine. Clear centre of the pan, Include garlic batter, & cook, mashing batter into pan, till fragrant, 15 to 20 seconds. Stir batter into vegetables. Return beef & any accumulated juices to the pan, Include scallions, & stir to combine. Whisk sauce to recombine, Include to the pan, & cook, constantly stirring, till thickened, about 30 seconds. Serve.

195. STIR-FRIED RED CURRY BEEF WITH EGGPLANT

Prep Time: *26 Minutes* *Cook Time:* *24 Minutes* *Servings: 4*

INGREDIENTS:

- SAUCE
- 1/2 cup low-sodium chicken broth
- 3 Tbsps. coconut milk
- Tbsps. light brown sugar
- 1 Tbsp. lime juice
- 1 Tbsp. fish sauce
- 1 Tsp. cornstarch
- BEEF STIR-FRY
- 2 Tbsps. soy sauce
- Tsp. light brown sugar
- (12-ounce) flank steak, trimmed and then sliced thin across the grain on a slight bias
- Three garlic cloves, minced
- 1 1/2 Tips. red curry paste
- 2 Tbsps. vegetable oil
- medium eggplant (about 1 lb), peeled & cut into 3/4-inch cubes
- 2 cups fresh basil leaves Lime wedges

DIRECTIONS:

1. FOR THE SAUCE: Whisk all combine ingredients all together in the small container & set aside.
2. FOR THE STIR-FRY: Combine soy sauce & sugar in a medium container. Include beef, toss well, & marinate for at least 10 mins or up to 1 hr, stirring once. Meanwhile, combine garlic, curry paste, & 1 Tsp. Oil in a small container.Drain beef & discard liquid. Heat 1 Tsp. oil in 12-inch
3. Nonstick pan over high heat till just smoking. Include half of the beef in a single layer, break up any clumps, & cook, without stirring for 1 min. Stir beef & continue to cook till browned, 1 to 2 mins—shift beef to clean container. Repeat with 1 Tsp. Oil & remaining beef. Rinse pan clean & dry with paper towels.
4. Include remaining 1 Tbsp. Oil to pan & heat till just smoking. Include eggplant & cook, frequently stirring, till browned & no longer spongy, 5 to 7 mins. Clear centre of the pan, Include garlic-curry batter, & cook, mashing batter into pan, till fragrant, 15 to 20 seconds. Stir batter into the eggplant. Return beef & any accumulated juices to pan & stir to combine. Whisk sauce to recombine, Include to the pan along with basil, & cook, constantly stirring, till thickened, about 30 seconds. Serve, passing lime wedges separately.

196. STIR-FRIED BEEF & BROCCOLI WITH OYSTER SAUCE

Prep Time: *20 Minutes* *Cook Time:* *18 Minutes* *Servings: 4*

INGREDIENTS:

- SAUCE
- 5 Tbsps. oyster sauce
- Tbsps. low-sodium chicken broth
- 1 Tbsp. dry sherry
- 1 Tbsp. light brown sugar
- 1 Tsp. toasted sesame oil
- 1 Tsp. cornstarch
- BEEF STIR-FRY
- (1-lb) flank steak, trimmed & sliced thin across the grain on the slight bias (See Illustrations)
- Tbsps. soy sauce
- Six garlic cloves, minced
- 1 Tbsp. grated fresh ginger
- Tbsps. vegetable oil
- 1 1/4 lbs broccoli, florets cut into bite-size pieces, stalks peeled & cut on the bias into 1/8-inch-thick slices
- 1/3 cup water
- small red bell pepper stemmed, seeded, & cut into 1/4-inch pieces
- Three medium scallions, sliced 1/2-inch thick on the bias

DIRECTIONS:

1. 2FOR THE SAUCE: Whisk all ingredients in the small container & set aside.
2. FOR THE STIR-FRY: Combine beef & soy sauce in a medium container, toss to coat, & let marinate for 10 mins or up to 1 hr, stirring once. Meanwhile, combine garlic, ginger, & 1 1/2 Tips. Vegetable oil in a small container.
3. Drain beef & discard liquid. Heat 1 1/2 Tips. Vegetable oil in 12-inch nonstick pan over high heat till just smoking. Include half of the beef in a single layer, break up clumps, & cook, without stirring for 1 min. Stir beef & continue to cook till beef is browned, about 30 seconds—shift beef to the medium container. Repeat with 1 1/2 Tips: vegetable oil & remaining beef.
4. Include 1 Tbsp. Vegetable oil to pan & heat till just smoking. Include broccoli & cook for 30 seconds. Include water to the pan, cover, & lower heat to medium. Steam broccoli till crisp-tender, about 2 mins, then Shift to a paper towel-lined plate. Include remaining 1 1/2 Tips. Vegetable oil to the pan, increase heat to high & heat till just smoking. Include bell pepper & cook, frequently stirring, till spotty brown, about 1 1/2 mins. Clear centre of the pan, Include garlic batter, & cook, mashing batter into pan, till fragrant, 15 to 20 seconds, then stir batter into peppers.
5. Return beef & broccoli to pan & toss to combine. Whisk sauce to recombine, then Includes to pan & cook, constantly stirring, till sauce is thickened & evenly distributed, about 30 seconds. Shift to a platter, sprinkle with scallions, & serve.

197. STIR-FRIED THAI-STYLE BEEF WITH CHILES & SHALLOTS BEEF STIR-FRY

Prep Time: *25 Minutes* *Cook Time:* *23 Minutes* *Servings: 8*

INGREDIENTS:

- Tbsp. fish sauce
- Tsp. Light brown sugar 3/4 Tsp. Ground coriander 1/8 Tsp. ground white pepper
- 2 lbs blade steak, trimmed (See Illustrations) & cut crosswise into 1/4-inch-thick strips
- SAUCE & GARNISH
- Tbsps. fish sauce
- Tbsps. rice vinegar
- Tbsps. water
- Tbsp. light brown sugar
- Tbsp. Asian chilli-garlic sauce
- Three garlic cloves, minced
- 3 Tbsps. vegetable oil
- Three serrano or jalapeño chiles, stemmed, seeded, & sliced thin three shallots, peeled, quartered, & layers separated
- 1/2 cup of fresh mint leaves, large leaves are torn into bite-size pieces 1/2 cup fresh cilantro leaves
- 1/3 cup dry-roasted peanuts, chopped
- Lime wedges

DIRECTIONS:

1. FOR THE STIR-FRY: Combine fish sauce, sugar, coriander, & white pepper in a large container. Include beef, toss well to combine; marinate 15 mins.
2. FOR THE SAUCE & GARNISH: Stir together fish sauce, vinegar, water, sugar, & chilli-garlic sauce in a small container till sugar dissolves & set aside. In a second small container, mix garlic & 1 Tsp. Oil & set aside.
3. To prepare stir-fry, heat 2 Tips. Oil in 12-inch nonstick pan over high heat till just smoking. Include one-third of beef to pan in an even layer. Cook, without stirring, till well browned, about 2 mins, then stir & continue cooking till beef is browned around edges & no longer pink in the centre, about 30 seconds. Shift beef to the medium container. Repeat with 2 Tips: oil more & remaining meat in 2 more batches.
4. Reduce heat to medium; include the remaining 2 Tbsps. Oil to pan & swirl to coat. Include chiles & shallots & cook, frequently stirring, till beginning to soften, 3 to 4 mins. Clear centre of the pan, Include garlic oil, & cook, mashing batter into pan, till fragrant, 15 to 20 seconds. Stir garlic into chile batter. Include fish sauce batter in the pan, increase heat to high, & cook till slightly reduced & thickened about 30 seconds.
5. Return beef & any accumulated juices to pan & toss well to combine & coat with sauce. Stir in half of mint & cilantro. Serve immediately, sprinkling each serving with peanuts & remaining herbs & passing lime wedges separately.

198. SPICY STIR-FRIED PORK, ASPARAGUS & ONIONS WITH LEMONGRASS

Prep Time: 25 Minutes *Cook Time: 23 Minutes* *Servings: 6*

INGREDIENTS:

- SAUCE
- 1/3 cup low-sodium chicken broth
- 2 Tbsps. fish sauce
- Tbsp. light brown sugar
- 2 Tips. lime juice
- Tsp. cornstarch
- PORK STIR-FRY
- (12-ounce) pork tenderloin, trimmed & cut into thin strips
- Tsp. fish sauce
- Tsp. soy sauce
- lemongrass stalks, trimmed to bottom 6 inches & minced
- garlic cloves, minced
- 3/4 Tsp. red pepper flakes
- 31/2 Tbsps. vegetable oil
- lb asparagus, trimmed & cut on the bias into 2-inch lengths
- large onion, cut into 1/4-inch wedges
- 1/4 cup chopped fresh basil

DIRECTIONS:

1. FOR THE SAUCE: Whisk all ingredients in the small container & set aside.
2. FOR THE STIR-FRY: Combine pork, fish sauce, & soy sauce in a small container. Cover with a wrap of plastic & refrigerate for at least 20 mins or up to 1 hr. Meanwhile, combine lemongrass, garlic, pepper flakes, & 1 Tbsp. Oil in a small container.
3. Heat 11/2 Tips. Oil in 12-inch nonstick pan over high heat till just smoking. Include half of the pork to pan, break up any clumps, & cook, occasionally stirring, till well browned, about 2 mins—shift pork to the medium container. Repeat with 11/2 Tips: oil & remaining pork.
4. Include 1 Tbsp. Oil to the pan, Include asparagus, & cook, stirring every 30 seconds, till browned & almost tender, 4 to 5 mins. Shift to a container with pork. Include remaining 11/2 Tips. Oil to the pan, Include onion, & cook, occasionally stirring, till beginning to brown & soften about 2 mins. Clear centre of the pan, Include lemon grass batter, & cook, mashing batter into pan, till fragrant, about 1 min. Stir batter into the onion.
5. Return pork & asparagus to pan & toss to combine. Stir sauce to recombine, Include to the pan, & cook, constantly stirring, till sauce is thickened & evenly distributed, about 30 seconds. Shift to a platter, sprinkle with basil, & serve.

199. STIR-FRIED PORK, GREEN BEANS, & RED BELL PEPPER WITH GINGERY OYSTER SAUCE

Prep Time: 15 Minutes *Cook Time: 43 Minutes* *Servings: 6*

INGREDIENTS:

- SAUCE
- 1/3 cup low-sodium chicken broth
- 21/2 Tbsps. oyster sauce
- 1 Tbsp. dry sherry
- Tips. toasted sesame oil
- 1 Tsp. rice vinegar
- 1 Tsp. cornstarch
- 1/4 Tsp. ground white pepper
- PORK STIR-FRY
- (12-ounce) pork tenderloin, trimmed & cut into thin strips
- 2 Tips. soy sauce
- 2 Tips. dry sherry
- 2 Tbsps. grated fresh ginger
- Two garlic cloves, minced
- 3 Tbsps. vegetable oil
- 12 ounces green beans, trimmed & cut on the bias into 2-inch lengths
- large red bell pepper, stemmed, seeded, & cut into 3/4-inch squares
- Three scallions, sliced thin on the bias

DIRECTIONS:

1. FOR THE SAUCE: Whisk all ingredients in the small container & set aside.
2. FOR THE STIR-FRY: Combine pork, soy sauce, & sherry in a small container. Cover with a wrap of plastic & refrigerate for at least 20 mins or up to 1 hr. Meanwhile, combine ginger, garlic, & 11/2 Tips—oil in a small container.
3. Heat 11/2 Tips. Vegetable oil in 12-inch nonstick pan over high heat till smoking. Include half of the pork, break up any clumps, & cook, occasionally stirring, till well-browned, about 2 mins—shift pork to the medium container. Repeat with 11/2 Tips—vegetable oil & remaining pork.
4. Include 1 Tbsp. Vegetable oil to pan. Include green beans & cook, occasionally stirring, till spotty brown & crisp-tender, about 5 mins. Shift to a container with pork. Include remaining 11/2 Tbsps. Oil to the pan, Include bell pepper, & cook, frequently stirring, till spotty brown, about 2 mins.
5. Clear centre of the pan, Include ginger batter, & cook, mashing batter into pan, till fragrant, 15 to 20 seconds. Stir batter into the pepper.
6. Return pork & green beans to pan & toss to combine. Whisk sauce to recombine, Include to the pan, & cook, constantly stirring, till sauce is thickened & evenly distributed, about 30 seconds. Shift to a platter, sprinkle with scallions, & serve.

200. STIR-FRIED PORK, EGGPLANT, & ONION WITH GARLIC & BLACK PEPPER

Prep Time: 15 Minutes *Cook Time: 34 Minutes* *Servings: 5*

INGREDIENTS:

- SAUCE
- 21/2 Tbsps. fish sauce
- Tbsps. Plus 11/2 Tips. Soy sauce 21/2 Tbsps. light brown sugar
- Tbsps. low-sodium chicken broth
- Tips. lime juice
- Tsp. cornstarch
- PORK STIR-FRY
- (12-ounce) pork tenderloin, trimmed & cut into thin strips
- Tsp. fish sauce
- Tsp. soy sauce
- garlic cloves, minced
- 2 Tips. pepper
- 31/2 Tbsps. vegetable oil
- medium eggplant (1 lb), cut into 3/4-inch cubes
- large onion, cut into 1/4- to 3/8-inch wedges
- 1/4 cup roughly chopped fresh cilantro

DIRECTIONS:

1. FOR THE SAUCE: Whisk all ingredients combine in the small container & set aside.
2. FOR THE STIR-FRY: Combine pork, fish sauce, & soy sauce in a small container. Cover with a wrap of plastic & refrigerate for at least 20 mins or up to 1 hr. Meanwhile, combine garlic, pepper, & 1 Tbsp. Oil in the second small container & set aside.
3. Heat 11/2 Tips. Oil in 12-inch nonstick pan over high heat till just smoking. Include half of the pork, break up any clumps, & cook, occasionally stirring, till well-browned, about 2 mins—shift pork to the medium container. Repeat with 11/2 Tips: oil & remaining pork.
4. Include 1 Tbsp. Oil to pan. Include eggplant & cook, stirring every 30 seconds, till browned & no longer spongy, about 5 mins. Shift to a container with pork. Include remaining 11/2 Tips. Oil to the pan, Include onion, & cook, occasionally stirring, till beginning to brown & soften about 2 mins.
5. Clear centre of the pan, Include garlic-pepper batter, & cook, mashing batter into pan, till fragrant & beginning to brown, about 11/2 mins. Stir batter into onions.
6. Return pork & eggplant to pan & toss to combine. Whisk sauce to recombine, Include to the pan, & cook, constantly stirring, till sauce is thickened & evenly distributed, about 30 seconds. Shift to a platter, sprinkle with cilantro, & serve.

201. THAI PORK LETTUCE WRAPS

Prep Time: 35 Minutes ***Cook Time: 11 Minutes*** ***Servings: 3***

INGREDIENTS:

- (1-lb) pork tenderloin, trimmed & cut into 1-inch chunks 21/2 Tbsps. fish sauce
- Tbsp. white rice
- 1/4 cup low-sodium chicken broth
- shallots, peeled & sliced into thin rings
- 3 Tbsps. lime juice (2 limes)
- 3 Tbsps. roughly chopped fresh mint
- 3 Tbsps. roughly chopped fresh cilantro
- Tips. sugar
- 1/4 Tsp. red pepper flakes
- head Bibb lettuce (8 ounces), leaves separated

DIRECTIONS:

1. 2Place pork on a large plate in a single layer. Freeze meat till firm & starting to harden around edges but still pliable, 15 to 20 mins.
2. Place half of the meat in the food processor & pulse till roughly chopped, 5 to 6 pulses. Shift ground meat to medium container & repeat with remaining chunks. Stir 1 Tbsp. Fish sauce into ground meat, cover with plastic wrap, & refrigerate for 15 mins.
3. Toast rice in a small pan over medium-high heat, stirring constantly, till deep golden brown, about 5 mins. Shift to a small container & cool for 5 mins. Grind rice by using a spice grinder, mini food processor, or mortar & pestle till it resembles a fine meal, 10 to 30 seconds.
4. Bring broth to simmer in a 12-inch nonstick pan over medium-high heat. Include pork & cook, frequently stirring, till about half of pork is no longer pink, about 2 mins. Sprinkle 1 Tsp. of rice powder over pork and continue to cook, constantly stirring, till remaining pork is no pinker, 1 to 11/2 mins longer. Shift pork to a large container & let cool for 10 mins.
5. Include remaining 11/2 Tbsps. Fish sauce, remaining 2 Tbsps. Of Rice powder, shallots, lime juice, mint, cilantro, sugar, & pepper flakes to pork & toss to combine. Serve with lettuce leaves, spooning meat into leaves at the table.

202. STIR-FRIED SHRIMP WITH SNOW PEAS & RED BELL PEPPER IN HOT & SOUR SAUCE

Prep Time: *15 Minutes* *Cook Time:* *35 Minutes* *Servings: 4*

INGREDIENTS:

- SAUCE
- Tbsps. sugar
- Tbsps. white vinegar
- Tbsp. Asian chilli-garlic sauce
- Tbsp. dry sherry or Chinese rice cooking wine
- Tbsp. ketchup
- Tips. toasted sesame oil
- Tips. cornstarch
- Tsp. soy sauce
- SHRIMP STIR-FRY
- lb extra-large shrimp (21 to 25 per lb), peeled, deveined, & tails removed
- 3 Tbsps. vegetable oil
- Tbsp. Grated fresh ginger
- garlic cloves, one minced, one sliced thin 1/2 Tsp. salt
- One large shallot, sliced thin
- eight ounces snow peas or sugar snap peas, stems & strings removed one red bell pepper, stemmed, seeded, & cut into 3/4-inch pieces

DIRECTIONS:

1. FOR THE SAUCE: shake all ingredients together in the small container & set them aside.
2. FOR THE STIR-FRY: Combine shrimp with 1 Tbsp. Vegetable oil, ginger, minced garlic, & salt in a medium container. Let the shrimp marinate at 25 degrees for 30 mins.
3. Combine sliced garlic with shallot in a small container—heat 1 Tbsp. Vegetable oil in 12-inch nonstick pan over high heat till just smoking. Include snow peas & bell pepper & cook, frequently stirring, till vegetables begin to brown, 1 1/2 to 2 mins—shift vegetables to the medium container.
4. Heat remaining 1 Tbsp. Vegetable oil over high heat till just smoking. Include shallot batter & cook, frequently stirring, till just beginning to brown, about 30 seconds. Include shrimp, reduce heat to medium-low, & cook, frequently stirring, till shrimp are light pink on both sides, 1 to 1 1/2 mins. Stir sauce to recombine & Include to pan; return to high heat & cook, constantly stirring, till sauce is thickened & shrimp are cooked through 1 to 2 mins. Return vegetables to the pan, toss to combine, & serve.

203. STIR-FRIED SICHUAN-STYLE SHRIMP WITH ZUCCHINI, RED BELL PEPPER, & PEANUTS

Prep Time: *19 Minutes* *Cook Time:* *17 Minutes* *Servings: 8*

INGREDIENTS:

- SAUCE
- Tbsps. dry sherry or Chinese rice cooking wine
- 1 Tbsp. broad bean chilli paste
- 1 Tbsp. Asian chilli-garlic sauce
- 1 Tbsp. white vinegar or Chinese black vinegar
- Tips. soy sauce
- Tips. chilli oil or toasted sesame oil
- Tsp. sugar
- Tsp. cornstarch
- 1/2 Tsp. Sichuan peppercorns, toasted & ground (optional)
- SHRIMP STIR-FRY
- lb extra-large shrimp (21 to 25 per lb), peeled, deveined, & tails removed
- 3 Tbsps. vegetable oil
- Two garlic cloves, one minced, one sliced thin
- 1/2 Tsp. salt
- 1/2 cup dry-roasted peanuts
- jalapeño chile, stemmed, halved, seeded, & sliced thin on small bias zucchini, cut into 3/4-inch dice
- red bell pepper stemmed, seeded, & cut into 3/4-inch dice 1/2 cup fresh cilantro leaves

DIRECTIONS:

1. FOR THE SAUCE: shake all ingredients together in the small container & set them aside.
2. FOR THE STIR-FRY: Combine shrimp with 1 Tbsp. Vegetable oil, minced garlic, & salt in a medium container. Let shrimp marinate at room temperature for 30 mins.
3. Combine sliced garlic, peanuts, & jalapeño in a small container. Heat 1 Tbsp. Oil in 12-inch nonstick pan over high heat till just smoking. Include zucchini & bell pepper & cook, frequently stirring, till zucchini is tender & well browned, 2 to 4 mins—shift vegetables to the medium container.
4. Include remaining 1 Tbsp. Oil to pan & heat till just smoking. Include peanut butter & cook, frequently stirring, till just beginning to brown, about 30 seconds. Include shrimp, reduce heat to medium-low, & cook, frequently stirring, till shrimp are light pink on both sides, 1 to 1 1/2 mins. Stir sauce to recombine & Include in the pan. Return to high heat & cook, constantly stirring, till sauce is thickened & shrimp are cooked through 1 to 2 mins. Return vegetables to the pan, Include cilantro, toss to combine, & serve.

Dinner Recipes

204. STIR-FRIED SHRIMP WITH GARLICKY EGGPLANT, SCALLIONS, & CASHEWS

Prep Time: *15 Minutes* *Cook Time:* *15 Minutes* *Servings: 5*

INGREDIENTS:

- SAUCE
- Tbsps. soy sauce
- Tbsps. oyster sauce
- Tbsps. dry sherry or Chinese rice cooking wine
- Tbsps. sugar
- Tbsp. toasted sesame oil
- Tbsp. white vinegar
- 2 Tips. cornstarch
- 1/8 Tsp. red pepper flakes
- SHRIMP STIR-FRY
- lb extra-large shrimp (21 to 25 per lb), peeled, deveined, & tails removed
- 3 Tbsps. vegetable oil
- Six garlic cloves, one minced, five sliced thin
- 1/2 Tsp. salt
- large scallions, whites sliced thin & greens cut into 1-inch pieces 1/2 cup cashews
- 12 ounces eggplant, cut into 3/4-inch pieces

DIRECTIONS:

1. FOR THE SAUCE: shake all ingredients together in the small container & set them aside.
2. FOR THE STIR-FRY: Combine shrimp with 1 Tbsp. Vegetable oil, minced garlic, & salt in a medium container. Let shrimp marinate at room temperature for 30 mins. Combine sliced garlic with scallion whites & cashews in a small container. Heat 1 Tbsp. oil in 12-inch nonstick pan over high heat till I was just smoking. Include eggplant & cook, frequently stirring, till lightly browned, 3 to 6 mins. Include scallion greens & continue to cook till scallion greens begin to brown & eggplant is fully tender, 1 to 2 mins longer—shift vegetables to the medium container.
3. Include remaining 1 Tbsp. Oil to pan & heat till just smoking. Include scallion whites batter & cook, frequently stirring, till just beginning to brown, about 30 seconds. Include shrimp, reduce heat to medium-low, & cook, frequently stirring, till shrimp are light pink on both sides, 1 to 1 1/2 mins. Stir sauce to recombine & Include in the pan. Return to high heat & cook, constantly stirring, till sauce is thickened & shrimp are cooked through 1 to 2 mins. Return vegetables to the pan, toss to combine, & serve.

205. KUNG PAO SHRIMP

Prep Time: *15 Minutes* *Cook Time:* *35 Minutes* *Servings: 6*

INGREDIENTS:

- SAUCE
- 3/4 cup low-sodium chicken broth
- Tbsp. oyster sauce
- Tbsp. hoisin sauce
- Tips. Chinese black vinegar or plain rice vinegar
- Tips. toasted sesame oil
- 1 1/2 Tips. cornstarch
- SHRIMP
- lb of extra-large shrimp (21 to 25 per lb), peeled and deveined
- Tbsp. dry sherry or Chinese rice cooking wine
- Tips. soy sauce
- Three garlic cloves, minced
- Tips. grated fresh ginger
- 3 Tbsps. vegetable oil
- 1/2 cup dry-roasted peanuts
- Six small whole dried red chiles (each about 2 inches long)
- red bell pepper stemmed, seeded, & cut into 1/2-inch pieces
- Three scallions, sliced thin

DIRECTIONS:

1. FOR THE SAUCE: shake all ingredients together in a small container and Set aside.
2. FOR THE SHRIMP: Toss shrimp with sherry & soy sauce in the medium container & let marinate for 10 mins. Meanwhile, mix garlic, ginger, & 1 Tbsp. Oil in a small container. Combine peanuts & chiles in the second small container & set aside.
3. Heat 1 Tbsp. Oil in 12-inch pan over high heat till just smoking. Include shrimp & cook, stirring about every 10 seconds, till barely opaque, 30 to 40 seconds. Include peanuts & chiles & continue to cook till shrimp are almost completely opaque & peanuts have darkened slightly, 30 to 40 seconds longer. Shift batter to a container & set aside.
4. Include remaining 1 Tbsp. Oil to pan & return to high heat till just smoking. Include bell pepper & cook, occasionally stirring, till slightly softened, about 45 seconds. Clear centre of the pan, Include garlic batter, & cook, mashing into the pan, till fragrant, 10 to 15 seconds. Stir batter into peppers till combined.
5. Stir sauce to recombine, then Include to pan along with reserved shrimp, peanuts, & chiles. Cook, stirring & scraping up any browned bits till sauce has thickened to a syrupy consistency, about 45 seconds. Stir in scallions & serve immediately.

206. KUNG PAO CHICKEN

Prep Time ***35 Minutes*** ***Cook Time:*** ***12 Minutes*** ***Servings: 4***

INGREDIENTS:

- SAUCE
- 3/4 cup low-sodium chicken broth
- Tbsp. oyster sauce
- Tbsp. hoisin sauce
- Tips. Chinese black vinegar or plain rice vinegar
- Tips. toasted sesame oil
- 1 1/2 Tips. cornstarch
- CHICKEN
- lb of boneless, skinless chicken thighs, and then trimmed and divided into 1-inch pieces
- Tbsp. dry sherry or Chinese rice cooking wine
- Tips. soy sauce
- Three garlic cloves, minced
- Tips. grated fresh ginger
- 3 Tbsps. vegetable oil
- 1/2 cup dry-roasted peanuts
- Six small whole dried red chiles (each about 2 inches long)
- red bell pepper stemmed, seeded, & cut into 1/2-inch pieces
- Three scallions, sliced thin

DIRECTIONS:

1. FOR THE SAUCE: shake all ingredients together in the small container & set them aside.
2. FOR THE CHICKEN: Toss chicken with sherry & soy sauce in the medium container & let marinate for 10 mins. Meanwhile, mix garlic, ginger, & 1 Tbsp. Oil in a small container; set aside. Combine peanuts & chiles in the second small container & set aside.
3. Heat 1 Tbsp. Oil in 12-inch pan over high heat till just smoking. Include chicken & cook, without stirring, for 2 mins, allowing the chicken to brown on the first side. Stir & cook till no longer pink, 1 1/2 to 2 mins. Stir peanuts & chiles into chicken &

continue cooking till peanuts have darkened slightly, 30 to 40 seconds longer. Shift batter to a container & set aside.

4. Include remaining 1 Tbsp. Oil to pan & return to high heat till just smoking. Include bell pepper & cook, occasionally stirring, till slightly softened, about 45 seconds. Clear centre of the pan, Include garlic batter, & cook, mashing batter into pan, till fragrant, 10 to 15 seconds. Stir batter into peppers till combined.
5. Stir sauce to recombine, then Include to pan along with reserved chicken, peanuts, & chiles. Cook, stirring & scraping up any browned bits till sauce has thickened to a syrupy consistency, about 45 seconds. Stir in scallions & serve immediately.

207. FRIED RICE WITH PEAS & BEAN SPROUTS

***Prep Time:* 10 Minutes**

***Cook Time:* 9 Minutes**

Servings: 2

INGREDIENTS:

- 1/4 cup oyster sauce
- 1 Tbsp. soy sauce
- Tbsps. peanut oil or vegetable oil
- Two large eggs, lightly beaten
- 1 cup frozen peas, thawed
- Two garlic cloves, minced
- 6 cups of cold cooked white rice, large clumps broke up with fingers, 2 ounces (1 cup) bean sprouts
- Five scallions, sliced thin

DIRECTIONS:

1. Combine oyster sauce & soy sauce in a small container & set aside.
2. Heat 1 1/2 Tips. Oil in 12-inch nonstick pan over medium heat till shimmering. Include eggs & cook, without stirring, till they just begin to set, about 20 seconds. Scramble & break into small pieces with a wooden spoon; continue to cook, constantly stirring, till eggs are cooked through but not browned, about 1 min longer. Shift eggs to a small container & set them aside.
3. Include remaining 2 1/2 Tbsps. Oil to pan & heat over medium heat till shimmering. Include peas & cook, constantly stirring for about 30 seconds. Stir in garlic & cook till fragrant, about 30 seconds. Include rice & oyster sauce batter & cook, constantly stirring & breaking up rice clumps, till batter is heated through, about 3 mins. Include eggs, bean sprouts, & scallions & cook, constantly stirring, till heated through, about 1 min. Serve immediately.

208. FRIED RICE WITH SHRIMP, HAM, & SHIITAKES

Prep Time: 5 Minutes *Cook Time:* 15 Minutes *Servings: 4*

INGREDIENTS:

- 1/2 ounce dried shiitake mushrooms
- 1/4 cup oyster sauce
- 1 Tbsp. soy sauce
- 3 1/2 Tbsps. peanut oil or vegetable oil
- 2 large eggs, lightly beaten
- ounces small shrimp (51 to 60 per lb), peeled & deveined
- 1 cup frozen peas, thawed
- ounces sliced smoked ham, cut into 1/2-inch pieces
- 2 garlic cloves, minced
- cups cold cooked white rice, large clumps are broken up with fingers
- scallions, sliced thin

DIRECTIONS:

1. Cover dried shiitakes with 1 cup hot tap water in a small container. Microwave mushrooms, covered, for 30 seconds. Let sit till softened, about 5 mins. Lift mushrooms from liquid with a fork; discard liquid. Trim stems, slice into 1/4-inch strips, & set aside.
2. Combine oyster sauce & soy sauce in a small container & set aside.
3. Heat 1 1/2 Tbsps. Oil in 12-inch nonstick pan over medium heat till shimmering. Include eggs & cook, without stirring, till they just begin to set, about 20 seconds. Scramble & break into small pieces with a wooden spoon; continue to cook, constantly stirring, till eggs are cooked through but not browned, about 1 min longer. Shift eggs to a small container & set them aside.
4. Include 1 1/2 Tbsps. Oil to pan & heat over medium heat till shimmering. Include shrimp & cook, constantly stirring, till opaque and
5. Just cooked through, about 30 seconds. Shift shrimp to the container with eggs & set aside.
6. Include remaining 2 1/2 Tbsps. Oil to pan & heat over medium heat till shimmering. Include mushrooms, peas, & ham & cook, constantly stirring, for 1 min. Stir in garlic & cook till fragrant, about 30 seconds. Include rice & oyster sauce batter & cook, constantly stirring & breaking up rice clumps, till batter is heated through, about 3 mins. Include eggs, shrimp, & scallions & cook, continually stirring, till heated through, about 1 min. Serve immediately.

209. THAI-STYLE CURRIED CHICKEN FRIED RICE

Prep Time: 18 Minutes *Cook Time:* 16 Minutes *Servings: 2*

INGREDIENTS:

- Tbsps. fish sauce
- 1 Tbsp. soy sauce
- 1 Tbsp. dark brown sugar
- 1 lb boneless, skinless chicken breasts, trimmed & cut into 1-inch pieces
- 3 1/2 Tbsps. peanut oil or vegetable oil
- 2 large eggs, lightly beaten
- Tbsp. Plus 1 Tsp. curry powder
- large onion, sliced thin
- Thai green chiles stemmed, seeded, & minced (about 2 Tbsps.)
- 2 garlic cloves, minced
- 6 cups cold cooked white rice, large clumps are broken up with fingers
- scallions, sliced thin
- Tbsps. minced fresh cilantro Lime wedges

DIRECTIONS:

1. Combine fish sauce, soy sauce, & sugar in the small container & stir to dissolve sugar. Set aside. Season chicken with 1/2 Tsp. Salt; set aside.
2. Heat 1 1/2 Tbsps. Oil in 12-inch nonstick pan over medium heat till shimmering. Include eggs & cook, without stirring, till they just begin to set, about 20 seconds. Scramble & break into small pieces with a wooden spoon; continue to cook, constantly stirring, till eggs are cooked through but not browned, about 1 min longer. Shift eggs to a small container & set them aside.
3. Include 1 1/2 Tbsps. oil to pan & heat over medium heat till Shimmering. Include 1 Tsp. Curry powder & cook till fragrant, about 30 seconds. Include chicken & cook, constantly stirring, till cooked through, about 2 mins. Shift to the container with eggs & set aside.
4. Include remaining 2 1/2 Tbsps. Oil to pan & heat over medium heat till shimmering. Include onion & the remaining 1 Tbsp. Curry powder & cook, constantly stirring, till onion is softened, about 3 mins. Stir in chiles & garlic & cook till fragrant, about 30 seconds. Include rice & fish sauce batter & cook, constantly stirring & breaking up rice clumps, till batter is heated through, about 3 mins. Include eggs, chicken, scallions, & cilantro & cook, constantly stirring, till heated through, about 1 min. Serve immediately with lime wedges.

210. INDONESIAN-STYLE FRIED RICE

Prep Time: 25 Minutes *Cook Time:* 23 Minutes *Servings: 6*

INGREDIENTS:

- Tbsps. plus 1/2 cup vegetable oil
- cups jasmine or long-grain white rice rinsed 2 2/3 cups water
- 5 green or red Thai chiles stemmed
- 7 large shallots, peeled
- 4 large garlic cloves, peeled
- Tbsps. dark brown sugar
- Tbsps. light or mild molasses
- Tbsps. soy sauce
- Tbsps. fish sauce
- 4 large eggs
- ounces extra-large shrimp (21 to 25 per lb), peeled, deveined, tails removed, & cut crosswise into thirds
- large scallions, sliced thin Lime wedges

DIRECTIONS:

1. Heat 2 Tbsps. Oil in a large saucepan over medium heat till shimmering. Include rice & stir to coat grains with oil, about 30 seconds. Include water, increase heat to high, & bring to boil. Reduce heat to low, cover, & simmer till all liquid is absorbed about 18 mins. Off heat, remove lid & place clean kitchen towel folded in half over saucepan; replace the lid. Let stand till rice is just tender, about 8 mins. Spread cooked rice onto the rimmed baking sheet, set on a wire rack, & cool for 10 Mins. Shift to refrigerator & chill for 20 mins.
2. While rice is chilling, pulse chiles, 4 shallots, & garlic in the food processor till the coarse paste is formed, about 15 pulses, scraping downsides of the container as necessary. Shift batter to a small container & set aside. In a second small container, stir together brown sugar, molasses, soy sauce, fish sauce, & 1 1/4 Tbsps. Salt. Whisk eggs & 1/4 Tsp. Salt together in a medium container.
3. Thinly slice the remaining 3 shallots (you should have about 1 cup sliced shallots) & place in 12-inch nonstick pan with the remaining 1/2 cup oil. Heat over medium heat, constantly stirring, till shallots are golden & crisp, 6 to 10 mins. Using a slotted spoon, Shift shallots to the paper towel-lined plate & season with salt to taste. Pour off oil & reserve. Wipeout pan with paper towels 4. Heat 1 Tsp. Reserved oil in a now-empty pan over medium heat till shimmering. Include half of the eggs to pan, gently tilting cooking wok to evenly coat the bottom. Cover & cook till the bottom of the omelette is spotty golden brown & top is just set, about 1 1/2 mins. Slide omelette onto cutting board & gently roll up into a tight log. Using a sharp knife, cut the record crosswise into 1-inch segments (leaving segments rolled). Repeat with 1 Tsp. Reserved oil & remaining eggs.
4. Remove rice from the refrigerator & break up any large clumps with fingers. Heat 3 Tbsps. Reserved oil in the now-empty pan over medium heat till just shimmering. Include chile batter & cook till the batter turns golden, 3 to 5 mins. Include shrimp, increase heat to medium-high, & cook, constantly stirring, till exterior of shrimp is just opaque, about 2 mins. Push shrimp to sides of pan to clear centre; stir molasses batter to recombine & pour into the centre of the pan. When molasses batter bubbles, Include rice & cook, stirring & folding
5. Constantly, till shrimp is cooked, rice is heated through, & batter is evenly coated about 3 mins. Stir in scallions, remove from heat, & Shift to a serving platter. Garnish with egg segments, fried shallots, & lime wedges; serve immediately.

211. SESAME NOODLES WITH SHREDDED CHICKEN

Prep Time: 20 Minutes *Cook Time:* 18 Minutes *Servings: 5*

INGREDIENTS:

- SAUCE
- 1/4 cup sesame seeds, toasted
- 1/4 cup chunky peanut butter
- Tbsps. soy sauce
- 2 Tbsps. rice vinegar
- 2 Tbsps. light brown sugar
- 1 Tbsp. grated fresh ginger
- 2 garlic cloves, minced
- 1 Tsp. hot sauce
- Tbsps. hot water
- CHICKEN & NOODLES
- 1 1/2 lbs boneless, chicken breasts
- lb fresh Chinese noodles or 12 ounces dried spaghetti
- Tbsp. salt
- Tbsps. toasted sesame oil
- 4 scallions, sliced thin on the bias
- 1 carrot, grated

DIRECTIONS:

1. FOR THE SAUCE: Puree 3 Tbsps. Sesame seeds, peanut butter, soy sauce, vinegar, sugar, ginger, garlic, & hot sauce in blender or food processor, about 30 seconds. With machine running, Include hot water, 1 Tbsp. At a time, till sauce has the consistency of heavy cream.
2. FOR THE CHICKEN & NOODLES: Bring 6 quarts of water to boil in a large pot. Setting oven rack 6 inches from broiler element & heat Broiler. Spray broiler cooking wok top with vegetable oil spray, place chicken breasts on top, & broil till lightly browned, 4 to 8 mins. Flip chicken over & continue to broil till meat registers 160 to 165 degrees, 6 to 8 mins. Shift to a cutting board & let rest 5 mins. Shred chicken into bite-size pieces & set aside.
3. Include noodles & salt to boiling water & cook, occasionally stirring, till tender, about 4 mins for fresh or 10 mins for dried. Drain, then rinse under cold water till cool. Drain again, Shift to an enormous container, Include sesame oil, & toss to coat.

Include shredded chicken, scallions, carrot, & sauce & toss to combine. Divide among containers sprinkles with remaining 1 Tbsp. Sesame seeds, & serve.

212. SPICY SICHUAN NOODLES

Prep Time: *15 Minutes* *Cook Time:* *23 Minutes* *Servings: 2*

INGREDIENTS:

- 8 ounces ground pork
- 3 Tbsps. soy sauce
- Tbsps. Chinese rice cooking
- Tbsps. oyster sauce
- 1/4 cup peanut butter
- 1 Tbsp. rice vinegar
- 1-1 1/4 cups low-sodium chicken broth
- Tbsp. vegetable oil
- 6 garlic cloves, minced
- Tbsp. Grated fresh ginger 3/4 Tsp. red pepper flakes
- Tbsp. toasted sesame oil
- ounces dried Asian noodles or 1 lb fresh Asian noodles (width between linguine & fettuccine) or 12 ounces linguine
- 3 medium scallions, sliced thin
- 4 ounces bean sprouts (2 cups) (optional)
- Tbsp. Sichuan peppercorns, toasted & ground (optional)

DIRECTIONS:

1. 2Combine pork, 1 Tbsp. Soy sauce, wine, & pinch white pepper in a small container. Stir well & set aside. Whisk together oyster sauce, remaining 2 Tbsps. Soy sauce, peanut butter, vinegar, & pinch white pepper in a medium container. Whisk in chicken broth & set aside.
2. Bring 4 quarts of water to boil pot over high heat. Meanwhile, heat a 12-inch pan over high heat; include vegetable oil & swirl to coat. Include pork & cook, breaking meat into small pieces, till well browned, about 5 mins. Stir in garlic, ginger, & pepper flakes & cook till fragrant, about 1 min. Include peanut butter batter & bring to boil, whisking to combine, then reduce heat to medium-low & simmer to blend flavours, occasionally stirring about 3 mins. Stir in sesame oil.
3. While sauce simmers, Include noodles in boiling water & cook till tender. Drain noodles & divide among containers. Ladle sauce over noodles sprinkles with scallions & bean sprouts & ground Sichuan peppercorns if using. Serve immediately.

213. PAD THAI

Prep Time: *20 Minutes* *Cook Time:* *78 Minutes* *Servings: 3*

INGREDIENTS:

- Tbsps. tamarind paste 3/4 cup boiling water
- 3 Tbsps. fish sauce
- 3 Tbsps. sugar
- 1 Tbsp. rice vinegar
- 3/4 Tsp. cayenne pepper 1/4 cup vegetable oil
- 8 ounces dried rice stick noodles, about 1/8 inch wide
- large eggs
- 1/4 Tsp. salt
- ounces medium shrimp (41 to 50 per lb), peeled & deveined
- 3 garlic cloves, minced
- 1 shallot, minced
- 2 Tbsps. dried shrimp, chopped fine (optional)
- 2 Tbsps. Thai salted preserved radish (optional)
- 6 Tbsps. dry-roasted peanuts, chopped
- 6 ounces bean sprouts (3 cups)
- scallions, green parts only, sliced thin on the bias
- 1/4 cup fresh cilantro leaves (optional)
- Lime wedges

DIRECTIONS:

1. 2Soak tamarind paste in boiling water for about 10 mins, then push it through a mesh strainer to remove seeds & fibres & extract as much pulp as possible. Stir fish sauce, sugar, rice vinegar, cayenne, & 2 Tbsps. Oil into tamarind liquid & set aside.
2. Cover rice sticks with hot tap water in a large container; soak till softened, pliable, & limp but not fully tender, about 10 mins. Drain noodles & set them aside. Beat eggs & 1/8 Tsp. Salt in a small container; set aside.
3. Heat 1 Tbsp. Oil in 12-inch nonstick pan over high heat till just smoking. Include shrimp, sprinkle with remaining 1/8 Tsp. Salt, & cook, occasionally tossing, till shrimp are opaque & browned around the edges, about 3 mins. Shift shrimp to plate & set aside.
4. 5Off heat, Include remaining 1 Tbsp. Oil & swirl to coat. Include garlic & shallot, return to medium heat, & cook, constantly stirring, till light golden brown, about 1 1/2 mins. Include eggs & stir till scrambled & barely moist, about 20 seconds.
5. Include noodles and dried shrimp & salted radish, if using, to pan & toss to combine. Pour fish sauce batter over noodles, increase heat to high, & cook, constantly tossing, till noodles are evenly coated.
6. Scatter 1/4 cup peanuts, bean sprouts, all but 1/4 cup scallions, & cooked shrimp over noodles. Continue to cook, constantly tossing, till noodles are tender, about 2 1/2 mins (if not yet tender, Include 2 Tbsps. water to pan & continue to cook till tender). Shift noodles to a serving platter, sprinkle with remaining scallions, remaining 2 Tbsps. Peanuts & cilantro. Serve immediately, passing lime wedges separately.

214. PASTA WITH SAUTÉED MUSHROOMS & THYME

Prep Time: *16 Minutes* *Cook Time:* *14 Minutes* *Servings: 8*

INGREDIENTS:

- Tbsps. unsalted butter
- Tbsps. extra-virgin olive oil
- 4 large shallots, chopped fine
- ounces shiitake mushrooms stemmed & sliced 1/4 inch thick
- ounces cremini mushrooms, trimmed & sliced 1/4 inch thick salt & pepper
- 5 Tbsps. minced fresh thyme
- 3 garlic cloves, minced
- 1 1/4 cups low-sodium chicken broth
- 1/2 cup heavy cream
- Tbsp. lemon juice
- lb farfalle or campanelle
- ounces Parmesan cheese, grated (1 cup)
- Tbsps. minced fresh parsley

DIRECTIONS:

1. Heat butter & oil in a 12-inch pan over medium-high heat till butter is melted. Include shallots & cook till softened, about 4 mins. Include shiitake mushrooms & cook for 2 mins. Include cremini mushrooms & 1/2 Tsp. Salt & continue to cook, occasionally stirring, till mushrooms are lightly browned, about 8 mins. Stir in thyme & garlic & cook till fragrant, about 30 seconds. Shift mushrooms to the container. Include broth to now-empty pan & bring to boil, scraping up any browned bits. Off heat, stir in cream & lemon juice & season with salt & pepper to taste.
2. Hence, bring 4 quarts of water to boil in a large pot. Include pasta & 1 Tbsp. salt & cook, often stirring, till al dente. Reserve 1/2 cup cooking water, then drain pasta & return it to pot.
3. Include mushrooms, broth batter, Parmesan, & parsley to pasta & cook over medium-low heat, tossing to combine, till pasta absorbs most of the liquid, about 2 mins. Include reserved cooking water as needed to Set consistency. Serve immediately.

215. ORECCHIETTE WITH ESCAROLE & WHITE BEANS

Prep Time: *15 Minutes* *Cook Time:* *56 Minutes* *Servings: 4*

INGREDIENTS:

- Tbsps. olive oil
- garlic cloves, minced
- 2 Tbsps. Minced fresh oregano or 1/2 Tsp. dried
- head escarole (1 lb), trimmed & sliced 1/2 inch thick 3/4 cup water
- (15-ounce) can cannellini beans, rinsed
- ounces orecchiette (2 1/4 cups)

DIRECTIONS:

1. Heat oil in the 12-inch pan over medium heat till shimmering. Include garlic & oregano & cook till fragrant, about 30 seconds. Include escarole, 1 handful at a time, & cook till completely wilted, 4 to 5 mins.
2. Stir in water & bring to a gentle simmer. Cover, reduce heat to medium-low, & simmer gently for 5 mins. Stir in beans, body, & continue to simmer gently till flavours meld, 3 to 4 mins longer. Season with salt & pepper to taste.
3. Hence, bring 4 quarts of water to boil in a large pot. Include pasta & 1 Tbsp. salt & cook, often stirring, till al dente.
4. Reserve 1/2 cup cooking water, then drain pasta & return it to pot. Include sauce to pasta & toss to combine. Include reserved cooking water as needed to Set consistency. Serve.

216. PASTA WITH ARUGULA, GOAT CHEESE, & SUN-DRIED TOMATO PESTO

Prep Time: *35 Minutes* *Cook Time:* *11 Minutes* *Servings: 6*

INGREDIENTS:

- cup oil-packed sun-dried tomatoes, rinsed, patted dry, & chopped coarsely
- ounce Parmesan cheese, grated (1/2 cup)
- Tbsps. extra-virgin olive oil 1/4 cup walnuts, toasted
- 1 small garlic clove, minced Salt
- 1/8 Tsp. pepper
- 10 ounces baby arugula (10 cups)
- 3 ounces goat cheese, crumbled (3/4 cup)

DIRECTIONS:

1. Process tomatoes, Parmesan, oil, walnuts, garlic, 1/2 Tsp. Salt & pepper in a food processor till smooth, about 1 min, scraping down container as needed.
2. Hence, bring 4 quarts of water to boil in a large pot. Include pasta & 1 Tbsp. salt & cook, often stirring, till al dente. Reserve 3/4 cup cooking water, then drain pasta & return it to pot; immediately stir in arugula, 1 handful at a time, till wilted. Include pesto & 1/2 cup reserved cooking water to pasta & toss to combine.
3. Include remaining cooking water as needed to Set consistency. Serve immediately, passing goat cheese separately.

217. PASTA WITH GREEN OLIVE-SUN-DRIED TOMATO SAUCE & BREAD CRUMBS

Prep Time: *3 Minutes* *Cook Time:* *15 Minutes* *Servings: 8*

INGREDIENTS:

- slices hearty white sandwich bread, crusts removed & bread torn into quarters
- Tbsps. Plus 1 Tsp. Extra-virgin olive oil
- garlic cloves, minced
- anchovy fillets, rinsed & minced 1/4 Tsp. red pepper flakes
- (14.5-ounce) can diced tomatoes, drained with 1/2 cup juice reserved, tomato pieces chopped fine
- 1 1/2 cups pitted green olives, chopped
- cup oil-packed sun-dried tomatoes, rinsed, patted dry, & chopped fine
- lb spaghetti
- Tbsp. salt
- Tbsp. chopped fresh parsley

DIRECTIONS:

1. Pulse bread in the food processor to coarse crumbs, about 10 pulses. Heat 1 Tsp. Oil in 12-inch nonstick over medium heat till shimmering. Include bread crumbs & cook, often stirring, till crisp & golden brown, about 6 mins; Shift to the container. Wipe pan clean with paper towels.
2. Heat remaining 2 Tbsps. Oil, garlic, anchovies, & pepper flakes in a now-empty pan over medium heat. Cook, often stirring, till garlic turns golden but not brown, about 3 mins. Stir in diced tomatoes & cook till thickened slightly & dry about 5 mins. Stir in olives, sun-dried tomatoes, & reserved tomato juice & cook till heated through, about 1 min.
3. Hence, bring 4 of water to boil in a pot. Include pasta & salt & cook, often stirring, till al dente. Reserve 1/2 cup cooking water, then drain pasta & return it to pot. Include sauce & parsley to pasta & toss to combine. Include reserved cooking water as needed to Set consistency. Serve immediately, passing bread crumbs separately

Appetizers Recipes

218. EMALEE PAYNE EAU CLAIRE, WI

INGREDIENTS:

START TO FINISH: 10 MIN. • MAKES: 6 MUGS

- 2 mugs (16 ounces) sour cream
- 2 mugs mayonnaise
- 2 pounds bacon slices, 6 cooked and mashed plum tomatoes, finely chopped
- 3 green onions, chopped
- Additional minced meat and minced green onions, assorted crackers or chips (optional)

DIRECTIONS:

1. In a bowl, combine sour cream, mayonnaise, bacon, tomatoes and onions altogether. Let cool until served. Garnish with bacon and onions, if desired. Serve with crackers or chips.

219. MAMMA'S CAPONATA

Prep Time: *1 Minutes* *Cook Time:* *10 Minutes* *Servings: 2*

INGREDIENTS:

- 1 large eggplant, peeled and chopped
- ¼ mug plus 2 tbsps olive oil, divided
- 2 medium onions, chopped
- 2 celery ribs, chopped
- 2 cans (14 ½ ounces each) of diced tomatoes, undrained
- 1/3 mug chopped ripe olives
- ¼ mug red wine vinegar
- 2 tbsp sugar
- 2 tbsp capers, drained
- ½ tsp salt
- ½ tsp pepper
- French bread baguettes, sliced and toasted

DIRECTIONS:

1. Fry eggplant in a cup of oil in a Dutch oven until tender. Remove from pan and set separately. Fry the onion In the same frying pan and celery in the remaining oil until they wilt. Stir in tomatoes and eggplant. Bring it to a boil. Reduce heat. Simmer without lid for 15 minutes.
2. Add olives, vinegar, sugar, capers, salt and pepper. Boil again. Reduce heat. Boil uncovered for 20 minutes or until thickened. Serve warm or at room temperature with baguettes.

220. WARM BACON CHEDDAR SPREAD

Prep Time: *2 Minutes* *Cook Time:* *10 Minutes* *Servings: 6*

INGREDIENTS:

- 1 package (8 ounces) cream cheese, softened
- ½ mug mayonnaise
  - ¼ tsp dried thyme
  - 1/8 tsp pepper
  - 1 mug (4 ounces) shredded sharp cheddar cheese
  - 3 green onions, chopped
  - 8 bacon strips, cooked and crumbled, divided
  - ½ mug crushed Ritz crackers
  - Assorted crackers

DIRECTIONS:

1. Preheat oven to 350°. In a bowl, combine together cream cheese, mayonnaise, thyme and pepper. Stir it continuously in cheese, green onions and half the bacon. Transfer to a greased 3-mug baking dish.
2. Bake, uncovered, 13-15 minutes or until bubbly. Top with crushed crackers and remaining bacon. Serve with assorted crackers.

221. CHIPOTLE HAM 'N' CHEESE DIP

Prep Time: *2 Minutes* *Cook Time:* *12 Minutes* *Servings: 2*

INGREDIENTS:

- 2 pkg(8 ounces each) of cream cheese, cubed 1 can (12 ounces) evaporated milk
- 2 mugs (8 ounces) shredded Gouda cheese
- 1 mug (4 ounces) shredded cheddar cheese
- 2 tbsps chopped chipotle pepper in adobo sauce 1 tsp ground cumin
- 2 mugs diced fully cooked ham
- Fresh vegetables or tortilla chips

DIRECTIONS:

1. In a 3-qt slow cooker, combine together the first six ingredients. Cover and cook on low for 40 minutes.
2. Stir continuously in ham, and cook 20 minutes longer or until heated through. Serve warm with vegetables or chips.

222. HAM SALAD SPREAD

Prep Time: *8 Minutes* *Cook Time:* *10 Minutes* *Servings: 2*

INGREDIENTS:

- 3 mugs ground fully cooked ham
- 1 hard-cooked egg, chopped
- 2 tbsps finely chopped celery
- 2 tsp finely chopped onion
- 2 tsp sweet pickle relish
- ¾ mug mayonnaise 1 tbsp prepared mustard Assorted crackers

DIRECTIONS:

1. In a bowl, combine together the first five ingredients. Mix mayonnaise and mustard; add to ham mixture and mix well. Let it cool until serving. Serve with crackers.

223. PEPPERONI PIZZA DIP

Prep Time: *2 Minutes* *Cook Time:* *10 Minutes* *Servings: 2*

INGREDIENTS:

- 4 mugs (16 ounces) shredded cheddar cheese
- 4 mugs (16 ounces) shredded part-skim mozzarella cheese 1 mug of mayonnaise
- 1 jar (6 ounces) sliced mushrooms, drained
- 2 cans (2 ¼ ounces each) sliced ripe olives, drained 1 package (3 ½ ounces) pepperoni slices, quartered 1 tbsp dried minced onion
- Assorted crackers

DIRECTIONS:

1. In a 3-qt slow cooker, mix the cheeses, mayonnaise, mushrooms, olives, pepperoni and onion.
2. Wrap and cook on low for 1 ½ hour; stir continuously. Wrap and cook it for about 1 hour longer or until heated through. Serve with crackers.

224. GERMAN BEER CHEESE SPREAD

Prep Time: *3 Minutes* *Cook Time:* *10 Minutes* *Servings: 6*

INGREDIENTS:

- 1 pound of sharp cheddar cheese, divided into ½-inch cubes 1 tbsp Worcestershire sauce
- 1 ½ tsp prepared mustard 1 small garlic clove, minced
- ¼ tsp salt
- 1/8 tsp pepper
- 2/3 cup German or non-alcoholic beer assorted biscuits

DIRECTIONS:

1. Put the cheese in the food processor. Pulse until chopped, about 1 minute. Add Worcestershire sauce, mustard, garlic, salt and pepper. Add beer little by little at a time, continuing to process until the mixture is smooth and spreadable, about a minute.
2. Transfer to a serving bowl or gift bottle. Cover and refrigerate for up to 1 week. Serve with crackers.

225. PASSION FRUIT HURRICANES

Prep Time: *9 Minutes* *Cook Time:* *10 Minutes* *Servings: 6*

INGREDIENTS:

- 2 mugs passion fruit juice
- 1 mug plus 2 tbsps sugar
- ¾ mug lime juice ¾ mug light rum ¾ mug dark rum
- 3 tbsp grenadine syrup
- 6 to 8 mugs ice cubes
- Orange slices, starfruit slices and maraschino cherries

DIRECTIONS:

1. In a pitcher, mix the fruit juice, sugar, lime juice, rum and grenadine; stir until sugar is dissolved.
2. Spread into a hurricane or highball glasses filled with ice. Serve with orange slices, starfruit slices and cherries.

226. SWEET TEA CONCENTRATE

Prep Time: *3 Minutes* *Cook Time:* *35 Minutes* *Servings: 4*

INGREDIENTS:

- 2 medium lemons
- 4 mugs sugar
- 4 mugs water
- 1 ½ mug English breakfast tea leaves or 20 black tea bags 1/3 mug lemon juice EACH SERVING
- 1 mug cold water
- Ice cubes
- Citrus slices, optional
- Mint sprigs, optional

DIRECTIONS:

1. Extract peels from lemons; set fruit aside for garnish or save for another use.
2. In a saucepan, combine together sugar and water. Bring to a boil over medium heat. Minimize heat; simmer, unwrapped, for 3-5 minutes or until sugar is dissolved, stirring occasionally. Extract from the heat; add tea leaves and lemon peels. Close and steep
3. minute. Strain the tea finally and discard the tea leaves and lemon peel. Mix lemon juice. Cool to room temperature.
4. Convert to a container with a tight lid. Store in the refrigerator for up to 2 weeks.
5. Tea preparation In a tall glass, mix water and concentrate. Add ice. Add orange slices and mint twigs if desired.

227. WHITE SANGRIA

Prep Time: *5 Minutes* *Cook Time:* *12 Minutes* *Servings: 2*

INGREDIENTS:

- ¼ mug sugar ¼ mug brandy 1 mug sliced peeled fresh peaches or frozen sliced peaches, thawed 1 mug sliced fresh strawberries or frozen sliced strawberries, thawed 1 medium lemon, sliced
- 1 medium lime, sliced

- 3 mugs dry white wine, chilled
- 1 can (12 ounces) lemon-lime soda, chilled Ice cubes

DIRECTIONS:

1. In a pitcher, mix sugar and brandy until sugar is dissolved. Add remaining ingredients; stir smoothly to mix. Serve over ice.

228. ALL-OCCASION PUNCH

Prep Time:5 Minutes *Cook Time: 0 Minutes* *Servings: 2*

INGREDIENTS:

- 8 mugs cold water
- 1 can (12 ounces) of frozen lemonade concentrate, thawed plus ¾ mug thawed lemonade concentrate 2 litres ginger ale, chilled
- 1-litre cherry lemon-lime soda, chilled Ice ring, optional

DIRECTIONS:

1. In a large punch bowl, mix water and lemonade concentrate. Stir in ginger ale and lemon-lime soda. Top with an ice ring if desired. Serve punch immediately.
2. Desired. Serve punch immediately.

229. SPARKLING PEACH BELLINIS

Prep Time: 2 Minutes *Cook Time: 0 Minutes* *Servings: 3*

INGREDIENTS:

- 3 medium peaches, halved
- 1 tbsp honey
- 1 can (11.3 ounces) of peach nectar, chilled
- 2 bottles (750 millilitres each) champagne or sparkling grape juice, chilled
- place a baking sheet with a large piece of heavy-duty foil (aboutx 12 in.).

DIRECTIONS:

1. Place the peach halves cut side up on the foil. Drizzle honey. Turn the foil over the peaches and seal.
2. Bake it at least 375° for 25-30 minutes or until soft. Cool completely. Extract and remove the skin. Process the peaches in a cooking processor until soft.
3. Transfer the peach puree to the pitcher. Add honey and 1 bottle of champagne. Stir until blended. 12 Spread in a champagne flute or wine glass. Finish with the remaining champagne. Serve immediately.

230. FROZEN STRAWBERRY DAIQUIRIS

Prep Time: 15 Minutes *Cook Time: 0 Minutes* *Servings: 4*

INGREDIENTS:

- ¾ mug rum
- ½ mug thawed limeade concentrate
- 1 package (10 ounces) frozen sweetened sliced strawberries
- 1 to 1 ½ mugs ice cubes
- GARNISH
- Fresh strawberries

DIRECTIONS:

1. In a blender, mix the rum, limeade concentrate, strawberries and ice. Cover and process until smooth and thickened (use more ice for thicker daiquiris). Spread into cocktail glasses.
2. To garnish each daiquiri, cut a ½-in. slit into the tip of a strawberry; position berry on the rim of the glass.

231. PUMPKIN PIE SHOTS

Prep Time: 4 Minutes ***Cook Time: 35 Minutes*** ***Servings: 2***

INGREDIENTS:

- 1 envelope unflavored gelatin
- 1 mug cold water
- 1/3 mug canned pumpkin ¼ mug sugar
- ½ tsp pumpkin pie spice 1/3 mug butterscotch schnapps liqueur ¼ mug vodka
- 1 ½ tsp heavy whipping cream Sweetened whipped cream

DIRECTIONS:

1. In a saucepan, spread gelatin over cold water; let it stand for 1 minute. Heat and stir it continuously over low heat until gelatin is completely dissolved. Stir in pumpkin, sugar and pie spice; cook and stir until sugar is dissolved. Extract from heat. Stir in liqueur, vodka and cream.
2. Spread mixture into twelve 2-oz. shot glasses; Let it cool until set. Top with sweetened whipped cream.

232. BANANA NOG

Prep Time: 1 Minutes ***Cook Time: 15 Minutes*** ***Servings: 4***

INGREDIENTS:

- 3 mugs milk, divided
- 3 mugs half-and-half cream, divided
- 3 egg yolks
- ¾ mug sugar
- 3 large ripe bananas
- ½ mug light rum
- 1/3 mug creme de cacao
- 1 ½ tsp vanilla extract
- Whipped cream and baking cocoa, optional
- In a large, heavy saucepan, mix 1 ½ mug milk,
- 1 ½ mugs cream, egg yolks and sugar.

DIRECTIONS:

1. Now Cook and stir continuously over medium-low heat until mixture reaches 160° and is thick to coat the back of a metal spoon.
2. Put bananas in a food processor; cover and process until blended. Spread milk mixture into a pitcher; stir in the banana puree, rum, creme de cacao, vanilla, and remaining milk and cream. Cover and let it cool for at least 3 hours before serving.
3. Spread into chilled glasses. Garnish with whipped cream and spread with cocoa if desired.
4. CHEAT IT! Substitute 6 mugs of eggnog from the dairy case for the milk mixture prepared in the recipe. Stir the banana puree, rum, creme de cacao and vanilla into the eggnog. Garnish as desired.

233. MEXICAN HOT CHOCOLATE

Prep Time: 1 Minutes ***Cook Time: 35 Minutes*** ***Servings: 4***

INGREDIENTS:

- 4 mugs fat-free milk
- 3 cinnamon sticks
- 5 ounces 53% of cacao dark baking chocolate, coarsely chopped
- 1 tsp vanilla extract
- Additional cinnamon sticks, optional 1

DIRECTIONS:

1. In a saucepan, heat milk and cinnamon sticks overheat until bubbles form around the sides of the pan. Discard cinnamon. Whisk in chocolate until smooth.
2. Extract from the heat; stir in vanilla. Serve it in mugs with additional cinnamon sticks if desired.

Side Dishes Recipes

234. CRAB

Prep Time: 15 Minutes ***Cook Time: 35 Minutes*** ***Servings: 2***

INGREDIENTS:

- ½ cup finely chopped onion 3 tbsps butter
- 3 tbsps all-purpose flour
- ½ tsp salt 1 ½ cups half-and-half cream 2 egg yolks, lightly beaten
- 3 cans (6 ounces each) crabmeat, drained, flaked, and cartilage removed 1 tbsp Dijon mustard
- 2 tsp Worcestershire sauce
- 1 tsp minced chives
- TOPPING
- 1 cup soft bread crumbs
- 1 tbsp butter, melted

Directions:

1. In a big skillet, saute onion in butter until tender. Stir in flour and salt until blended. Gradually stir in cream until smooth. Take it to a boil, and cook and stir for 2 minutes or until thickened and bubbly. Remove from the heat.
2. Stir a small amount of hot mixture into egg yolks. Return all to the pan, stirring constantly. Bring to a gentle boil; cook and stir 2 minutes longer. Remove from the heat. Stir in the crab, mustard, Worcestershire sauce and chives.
3. Spoon into six greased 6-oz. ramekins or custard cups. Place on a baking sheet. Add bread crumbs and melted butter;
4. sprinkle over tops. Bake it at least 375° for 20-25 minutes or until topping is golden brown.

235. ITALIAN CHEESE WONTONS

Prep Time: 11 Minutes *Cook Time: 12 Minutes* *Servings: 6*

INGREDIENTS:

- 2 cups shredded Italian cheese
- 1 carton (15 ounces) ricotta cheese
- 1 egg, beaten
- 1 tbsp minced fresh parsley
- 1 garlic clove, minced
- ¼ tsp salt
- 1/8 tsp pepper
- 40 wonton wrappers
- Oil for deep-fat frying
- Marinara or spaghetti sauce warmed.

Directions:

1. Put the first 7 ingredients in a bowl.
2. Place the dumpling wrapper at one point toward you. (Keep the rest of the wrap covered with a damp paper towel until ready to use.)
3. Place 1 tbsp of filling in the centre of the wrap. Fold the bottom corner over the filling.
4. After the sides folding towards the centre of the overcharge. Roll towards the remaining points. Wet the top edge with water. Press to seal. Repeat. Refrigerate for 30 minutes.
5. After heating, heat the oil to 375° in an electric frying pan. Fry the wontons a little at a time.
6. Fry for 1-2 minutes on each side or until golden brown. Drain the water on a paper towel. Served with marinara.
7. Prepare stuffed dumplings the day before TO RUN. Fill your party day wontons. Cover with wet tissue and wrap and store in the refrigerator.

236. SPICY CHEESE CRACKERS

Prep Time: 15 Minutes *Cook Time: 45 Minutes* *Servings: 2*

INGREDIENTS:

- 1 ½ cups (6 ounces) shredded extra-sharp cheddar cheese ¾ cup all-purpose flour
- ½ tsp kosher salt

- ¼ tsp crushed red pepper flakes ¼ cup cold butter, cubed
- 1 to 2 tbsps half-and-half cream

Directions:

1. Place the cheese, flour, salt and pepper flakes in a food processor; process until blended. Now mix butter; pulse until butter is the size of peas. During pulsing, add just enough cream to form moist crumbs.
2. On a lightly floured surface, roll dough to 1/8-in. Thickness. Cut with a floured 3-in. holiday-shaped cookie cutter. Place 2 in. apart on greased baking sheets. Reroll scraps and repeat. Set the oven at 350° and bake for 13-17 minutes or until it turns golden brown. Set aside from pans to wire racks to cool completely. Store in an airtight container.

237. LEMONY FENNEL OLIVES

Prep Time: ***15 Minutes*** ***Cook Time:*** ***34 Minutes*** ***Servings: 2***

INGREDIENTS:

- 1 small fennel bulb
- 2 cups pitted ripe olives
- 1 small lemon, cut into wedges
- ½ tsp whole peppercorns
- ½ cup olive oil
- ½ cup lemon juice

Directions:

1. Trim fennel bulb and cut into wedges. Snip feathery fronds from fennel bulb; rePresent 2 tsp. Boil the brine in a small saucepan. Add dill. Boil uncovered for 1 minute or until soft. Rinse and rinse with cold water.
2. In a large bowl, place the fennel, olives, lemon slices, pepper and fennel leaves. Whisk off the oil and lemon juice. Pour in the olive mixture. Throw it on the court. Cover and refrigerate overnight.
3. Remove from refrigerator 1 hour before serving. Transfer to a serving bowl. Serve with a slotted spoon.

238. COCONUT SHRIMP

Prep Time: *15 Minutes* *Cook Time:* *83 Minutes* *Servings: 6*

INGREDIENTS:

- 18 uncooked jumbo shrimp (about 1 pound) 1/3 cup cornstarch ¾ tsp salt ½ tsp cayenne pepper 3 egg whites
- 2 cups flaked coconut
- Oil for deep-fat frying
- APRICOT-PINEAPPLE SALSA
- 1 cup diced pineapple
- ½ cup finely chopped red onion ½ cup apricot presents ½ cup minced fresh cilantro 2 tbsp lime juice
- 1 jalapeno pepper, seeded and chopped
- Salt and pepper to taste

Directions:

1. Peel and devein shrimp, leaving tails intact. Make a slit down the inner curve of each shrimp, starting with the tail; press lightly to
2. flatten. Add cornstarch, salt and cayenne pepper to dishes that need to be reduced. Separately. Beat the egg whites in the bowl until they form stiff peaks. If you place the coconut on another plate, it will shrink. Coat the shrimp with cornstarch mixture. Dip in egg whites and then coat with coconut.
3. Heat the oil at 375° in an electric skillet or fryer. Fry the prawns a little at a time, 1 to 1 minute on each side, or until golden brown. Drain the water on a paper towel.
4. Place the salsa ingredients in a bowl. Comes with shrimp.
5. ***Note*** Wear disposable gloves when slicing peppers. Oil can burn your skin. Do not touch your face.

239. BLUE CHEESE-ONION STEAK BITE

Prep Time: *12 Minutes* *Cook Time:* *17 Minutes* *Servings: 2*

INGREDIENTS:

- 3 big onions, thinly sliced into rings
- 3 tbsps butter
- 12 garlic cloves, minced
- 4 beef tenderloin steaks (6 ounces each)
- ¼ tsp salt
- ¼ tsp pepper
- 1 French bread baguette (10 ½ ounces), cut into ¼-inch slices
- SPREAD
- 4 ounces cream cheese, softened
- 1 cup (4 ounces) crumbled blue cheese
- 1/8 tsp salt
- 1/8 tsp pepper

Directions:

1. In a big skillet, saute onions in butter until softened. Reduce heat to medium-reduce; cook, occasionally stirring, for 30 minutes or until onions are golden brown. Add garlic; cook 1 minute longer.
2. Meanwhile, sprinkle beef with salt and pepper. Using long-handled tongs, moisten a paper towel with cooking oil and coat the grill rack.
3. Grill the covered steak over medium heat or overheat 4 inches (4 inches) on each side for 5-7 minutes, or until the meat is at the desired cooking level (for medium-rare, thermometer 145°, medium, 160°, well finished, 170°) °). Cut into thin slices.
4. Place bread on ungreased baking sheets. After setting the temperature at 400°, bake for 4-6 minutes or until lightly browned.
5. Meanwhile, place the cream cheese, blue cheese, salt and pepper in a food processor; cover and process until blended. Spread each bread slice with 1 tsp cheese mixture; top with steak and onions.

240. ASPARAGUS, BRIE & PARMA HAM CROSTINI

Prep Time: *15 Minutes* *Cook Time:* *56 Minutes* *Servings: 6*

INGREDIENTS:

- 12 asparagus spears
- 2 tbsp olive oil, divided
- 1/8 tsp salt
- 1/8 tsp pepper
- 12 slices French bread baguette (1/2 inch thick)
- 3 thin slices prosciutto (Parma ham) or deli ham,
- cut into thin strips 6 ounces Brie cheese, cut into 12 slices 1.
- Cut asparagus tips into 2-in. lengths. (Discard stalks or save for another use.) Place asparagus tips in a 15x10x1-in.

Directions:

1. Baking pan lined with foil. Spread with 1 tsp oil and toss to coat. Sprinkle with salt and pepper. Bake at 425° for 10-15 minutes or until crisp-tender.
2. Brush baguette slices on both sides with remaining oil. Place on a baking sheet. Broil for 1-2 minutes on each side or until toasted.
3. Top each slice with asparagus, prosciutto and cheese. Boiling for 2-3 minutes or until cheese is melted.

241. CLAMS CASINO

Prep Time: ***15 Minutes*** ***Cook Time:*** ***33 Minutes*** ***Servings: 2***

INGREDIENTS:

- 1 pound kosher salt
- 1 dozen fresh cherrystone clams
- 1/3 cup soft bread crumbs
- 3 tbsps minced fresh parsley, divided
- 2 tbsps olive oil
- 1 garlic clove, minced
- 1/8 tsp cayenne pepper
- 1/8 tsp coarsely ground pepper

Directions:

1. After heating the oven to 450 °. Salt in an oven-ready or 15x10x1-inch metal dish. Pan. Remove the peel, leaving the bottom peel. Drain liquid (save for other use). Place the clams in a salted baking dish.
2. Add soft breadcrumbs, 2 tablespoons parsley, oil, garlic, cayenne pepper and black pepper. Spoon over clams.
3. Bake for 15-18 minutes or until the clams are firm and the breading mixture is crispy and golden brown. Sprinkle with the remaining parsley. Present immediately.

242. LIGHTENED-UP VEGGIE PIZZA SQUARES

Prep Time: *15 Minutes* *Cook Time:* *23 Minutes* *Servings: 2*

INGREDIENTS:

- 2 tubes refrigerated reduced-fat crescent rolls
- 1 package (8 ounces) reduced-fat cream cheese
- 1 package (8 ounces) fat-free cream cheese
- ½ cup plain yoghurt
- 1/3 cup reduced-fat mayonnaise
- ¼ cup fat-free milk
- 1 tbsp dill weed
- ½ tsp garlic salt
- 1 cup shredded carrots
- 1 cup fresh cauliflowers, chopped
- 1 cup fresh broccoli florets, chopped
- 1 cup julienned green pepper
- 1 cup sliced fresh mushrooms
- 2 cans (2 ¼ ounces each) sliced ripe olives, drained
- ¼ cup finely chopped onion

Directions:

1. Spread out two crescent dough tubes and pound them into 15x10x 1 inch ungreased. Pan; Suture sutures and perforations. Set the oven at 375° and baked for 10-12 minutes or until golden brown. Cool completely on wire rack.
2. In a bowl, beat the cream cheese, yoghurt, mayonnaise, milk, dill and garlic salt until smooth. Spread over the crust. Sprinkle with carrots, cauliflower, broccoli, bell peppers, mushrooms, olives and onions. Completely covered and refrigerate for at least 1 hour.
3. Cut into squares. Refrigerate leftovers.

243. ENSENADA SHRIMP COCKTAIL

Prep Time: *15 Minutes* *Cook Time:0 Minutes* *Servings: 2*

INGREDIENTS:

- 1 pound peeled and deveined cooked medium shrimp 2 plum tomatoes, seeded and chopped
- 3 jalapeno peppers, seeded and chopped 1 serrano pepper, seeded and chopped
- ¼ cup chopped red onion 2 green onions, chopped
- 2 tbsps minced fresh cilantro
- 2 tbsps olive oil
- 1 tbsp rice vinegar
- 1 tbsp key lime juice or lime juice 1 tsp adobo seasoning Lime wedges

Directions:

1. In a big bowl, add the shrimp, tomatoes, peppers, onions and cilantro. Add the oil, vinegar, lime juice and seasoning; spread over shrimp mixture and toss to coat.
2. Refrigerate it for at least 1 hour. Using a slotted spoon, put shrimp mixture in cocktail glasses, about ½ cup in each. Garnish with lime wedges.
3. **NOTE** Wear disposable gloves when dividing hot peppers; the oils can burn skin. Avoid touching your face.

244. APRICOT-RICOTTA STUFFED CELERY

Prep Time: *15 Minutes* *Cook Time:* *35 Minutes* *Servings: 4*

INGREDIENTS:

- 3 dried apricots
- ½ cup part-skim ricotta cheese 2 tsp brown sugar
- ¼ tsp grated orange peel 1/8 tsp salt 5 celery ribs, cut into 1 ½ inch pieces

Directions:

1. Place apricots in a food processor.
2. Cover and process until finely chopped. Add the ricotta cheese, brown sugar, orange peel and salt; cover and process until blended. Stuff or pipe into celery.
3. Chill until serving.

245. MOTHER LODE PRETZELS

Prep Time: *15 Minutes* *Cook Time:* *67 Minutes* *Servings: 2*

INGREDIENTS:

- 1 package (10 ounces) pretzel rods
- 1 package (14 ounces) caramels
- 1 tbsp evaporated milk
- 1 ¼ cups miniature semisweet chocolate chips
- 1 cup plus 2 tbsps butterscotch chips
- 2/3 cup milk chocolate toffee bits
- ¼ cup chopped walnuts

Directions:

1. After cutting pretzel rods in half with a sharp knife, set aside. In a big saucepan over reduce heat, melt caramels with milk. In a large bowl, reduce the dish, adding chips, chips and walnuts.
2. Pour caramel mixture into 2 cups. Add sliced pretzel pieces, each two-thirds of the mixture, to caramel mixture (reheat in the mixer if the mixture is too thick for application). Let the caramel pass, then turn the pretzels into a chip mixture. Place on a covered baking sheet until set.
3. Store in an airtight container.

246. VEGGIE HAM CRESCENT WREATH

Prep Time: *15 Minutes* *Cook Time:* *20 Minutes* *Servings: 2*

INGREDIENTS:

- 2 tubes refrigerated crescent rolls
- ½ cup spreadable pineapple cream cheese
- 1/3 cup diced fully cooked ham
- ¼ cup finely chopped sweet yellow pepper ¼ cup finely chopped green pepper
- ½ cup chopped broccoli florets
- 6 grape tomatoes, quartered
- 1 tbsp chopped red onion

Directions:

1. Remove (do not loosen) the crescent paste from the tube. Cut each roll into eight pieces. Align by 11 inches. Circle the 14 inches without oil. Pizza pan.
2. Set the temperature at 375° and baked for 15-20 minutes or until golden brown. Let it cool for 5 minutes before carefully removing it onto a serving platter. Cool completely.

Dessert Recipes

247. Whole Wheat Mango Loaf

Prep Time: *15 Minutes* *Cook Time:* *88 Minutes* *Servings: 8*

Ingredients:

- 2 cups whole wheat flour
- 1 tsp baking powder
- 1 pinch of salt
- 1 tsp cinnamon
- ¼ tsp ground ginger
- 1 cup mango puree
- ½ cup coconut milk
- ¼ cup olive oil
- ¼ cup low-fat yoghurt
- ¼ cup maple syrup or honey
- ¼ cup chopped mango

Directions:

1. In a bowl, stir the flour with baking powder, salt, cinnamon and ground ginger. In another bowl, combine the mango puree with coconut milk, olive oil, yoghurt and maple syrup.
2. Pour this stricture over the flour and give it a quick stir. Spoon the batter into a loaf pan previously lined with baking paper, then bake in the before heating oven at 350F for 30-35 minutes. The best way to check if the loaf is done is to insert a skewer or toothpick in the middle. If it comes out clean of any crumbs, it is ready.
3. If not, cook for 5 more minutes and repeat the check.

248. Mango and Coconut Tart

Prep Time: *15 Minutes* *Cook Time:* *70 Minutes* *Servings: 2*

Ingredients:

- Crust:
- 1 cup sweetened coconut
- 1 cup whole wheat flour
- ½ cup all-purpose flour
- 6 oz butter, chilled and cubed
- 4 tbsp powdered sugar
- 3 tbsp mango puree
- Filling:
- 8 oz low-fat cream cheese
- ¼ cup brown sugar
- 1 cup heavy cream
- 1 tsp lime zest
- 2 tbsp mango puree
- Topping:
- 3 ripe mangoes, finely sliced

Directions:

1. To make the crust: In a bowl, stir the flours with the coconut and sugar, then rub in the chilled butter until sandy.
2. Stir in the mango puree and stir until the dough comes together. To convert it on a well-floured surface and roll it into a thin sheet. Place the sheet on a 10-inch tart pan and press it on the bottom and sides of the pan with your fingertips.
3. Bake in the before heating oven at 375F for 10-15 minutes until slightly golden brown. Remove from the oven and convert on a serving plate.
4. To make the filling: Whip the heavy cream in a bowl. In another bowl, stir the cream cheese continuously with the sugar and lime zest, then fold in the whipped cream and mango puree. Spread the filling over the crust.
5. Top the tart with mango slices and refrigerate at least 1 hour before serving.

249. Banana Mango Bread

Prep Time: *15 Minutes* *Cook Time:* *40 Minutes* *Servings: 6*

Ingredients:

- 2 oz butter, room temperature
- 1 cup sugar
- 2 eggs
- 3 bananas, mashed
- 1 cup low-fat yoghurt
- 1 tsp cinnamon
- 1 pinch salt
- 1 cup all-purpose flour
- 1 ¼ cup whole wheat flour
- 1 tsp baking soda
- 1 tsp baking powder
- 1 cup fresh mango
- 1 tsp vanilla extract

Directions:

1. In a bowl, stir the butter continuously with the sugar, then add the eggs, one by one. Stir in the bananas, vanilla and yoghurt, then incorporate the flours sifted with baking soda, baking powder and a pinch of salt.
2. Fold in the mango cubes and convert the batter into a loaf pan lined with baking paper. Bake in the before heating oven at 350F for 30-35 minutes or until golden brown and fragrant.
3. Let this bread cool in the pan before slicing.

250. Mango Soufflé

Prep Time: *15 Minutes* *Cook Time:* *33 Minutes* *Servings: 8*

Ingredients:

- 1 medium-size mango
- ¼ cup sugar
- 1 tsp lemon juice
- 2 egg yolks
- 2 egg whites
- 2 tbsp powdered sugar
- 1 pinch of salt
- butter to grease the ramekins

Directions:

1. Butter your ramekins well and sprinkle them with white sugar. Shake to remove the excess and set them aside.
2. Place the mango, sugar and lemon juice in a blender. Pulse to blend well, then fold in the egg yolks.
3. In a bowl, whip the egg whites by use of a pinch of salt until stiff, then add the powdered sugar and stir until a stiff, glossy meringue forms. Gently fold the meringue into the mango stricture, then spoon the stir into your ramekins.
4. Bake in the before heating oven at 350F for 20-25 minutes. Do not open the oven's door in the first 10 minutes, or they will deflate. Serve them immediately before deflating.

251. Mango and Chocolate Marbled Cake

Prep Time: *15 Minutes* *Cook Time:* *53 Minutes* *Servings: 2*

Ingredients:

- 1 cup all-purpose flour
- 1 cup whole wheat flour
- 1 tsp baking powder
- 1 tsp baking soda
- 1 pinch of salt
- ¼ cup vegetable oil
- ½ cup brown sugar
- 1 cup mango puree
- ¼ cup low-fat yoghurt
- ¼ cup low-fat milk
- 3 tbsp cocoa powder stirred with 2 tbsp warm water

Directions:

1. In a bowl, stir the flours with the baking powder, baking soda and a pinch of salt. In another bowl, combine the brown sugar with the mango puree, yoghurt and milk. Pour this stricture over the flour and give it a good stir. Divide the batter into 2 equal portions.
2. Spread half of it in a loaf pan lined with baking paper. Stirrer the remaining butter with the cocoa paste, then spread it in the pan over the mango batter.
3. Bake in the before heating oven at 350F for 30-40 minutes or until golden brown on top.

2. Eggsadded to the hot skillet along with smoked salmon. Stirring continuously, cook eggs until soft and fluffy. Remove from heat.
3. Top with avocado black pepper and chives to serve.

Breakfast & Brunch Recipes

252. Blueberry Chia Pudding

Prep Time: *5 Minutes* *Cook Time:* *10 Minutes* *Servings: 1*

Ingredients

- ¼ cup Chia seeds
- 1 cup coconut milk
- 1 tablespoon raw honey

Directions:

1. ½ cup blueberry smoothie ¼ cup chopped almonds Mix coconut milk honey blueberry smoothie and chia seeds and leave overnight in the fridge. Divide into 2 glasses and top each almond.

253. Egg pizza crust

Prep Time: *5 Minutes* *Cook Time:* *70 Minutes* *Servings: 1*

Ingredients:

- 3 eggs
- ½ cup of coconut flour
- 1 cup of coconut milk
- 1 crushed garlic clove

Directions:

1. Mix and make an omelette.

254. Omelet with Superfoods veggies

Prep Time: *10 Minutes* *Cook Time:* *16 Minutes* *Servings: 1*

Ingredients:

- 2 large eggs
- Salt Ground black pepper
- 1 tsp. olive oil or avocado oil
- 1 cup spinach
- cherry tomatoes and 1 spoon of yoghurt cheese Crushed red pepper flakes and a pinch of dill (optional)

Directions:

1. 2 large eggs are whisking in a small bowl. Present with salt and ground black pepper and set aside. Heat 1 tsp.
2. Olive oil in a skillet and medium heat. Add baby spinach tomatoes and cook, tossing until wilted (approx. 1 minute). Set aside.
3. Add eggs and cook until set. Add veggies and cheese on top of eggs. Flip eggs over cheese and veggies. Sprinkle with crushed red pepper flakes and dill.

255. Egg Muffins

Prep Time: *5 Minutes* *Cook Time:* *23 Minutes* *Servings: 1*

Ingredients:

- 8 eggs
- 1 cup diced green bell pepper
- 1 cup diced onion
- 1 cup spinach
- ¼ tsp. salt
- 1/8 tsp. ground black pepper
- 2 tbsp. water

Directions:

1. The oven after heating to 350 degrees F. Oil 8 muffin cups. Beat eggs together.
2. Mix in bell pepper, spinach, onion, salt, black pepper and water. Pour the mixture into muffin cups
3. Bake in the oven until muffins are done in the middle.

256. Smoked Salmon Scrambled Eggs

Prep Time: *0 Minutes* *Cook Time:* *5 Minutes* *Servings: 1*

Ingredients:

- 1 tsp coconut oil
- 4 eggs
- 1 Tbs water
- 4 oz smoked salmon sliced
- ½ avocado
- ground black pepper to taste
- 4 chives minced

Directions:

1. Heat a skillet over medium heat. Coconut oil is added to the pan when hot. Meanwhile, scramble eggs

257. Steak and Eggs

Prep Time: *5 Minutes* *Cook Time:* *15 Minutes* *Servings: 1*

Ingredients:

- ½ lb boneless beef steak or pork tenderloin ¼ tsp ground black pepper
- ¼ tsp sea salt (optional)
- 2 tsp coconut oil
- ¼ onion diced
- 1 red bell pepper diced
- 1 handful spinach or arugula
- 2 eggs

Directions:

1. Season sliced steak or pork tenderloin with sea salt and black pepper. Heat a sauté pan over high heat. Add 1 tsp coconut oil onions and meat when the pan is hot and sauté until the steak is slightly cooked.
2. Add spinach and red bell pepper and cook until the steak is done to your liking. Meanwhile, heat a small frypan over medium heat.
3. Add remaining coconut oil and fry two eggs. Top each steak with a fried egg to serve.

258. Broccoli Frittata

Prep Time: *12 Minutes* *Cook Time:* *23 Minutes* *Servings: 1*

Ingredients:

- 2 large eggs

Directions:

1. Salt Ground black pepper 1 tsp. Olive oil or avocado oil 1 cup Broccoli. 2 large eggs whisking in a small bowl. Present with salt and ground black pepper and set aside. Heating 1 tsp. Olive oil in a skillet.
2. Add broccoli and cook, tossing approx. 4-5 minutes. Add eggs; cook, occasionally stirring until just set.

259. Mushrooms Omelet

Prep Time: *14 Minutes* *Cook Time:* *23 Minutes* *Servings: 1*

Ingredients:

- 2 large eggs
- Salt Ground black pepper
- 1 tsp. olive oil or avocado oil
- 1 cup mushrooms

Directions:

1. 2 large eggs whiskin in a small bowl. Present with salt and ground black pepper and set aside. Heat 1 tsp.
2. Olive oil in a medium skillet. Add mushrooms and cook, tossing until slightly wilted (Approx. 3 minutes). Set aside. Add eggs and cook until set.
3. Add mushrooms on top of the eggs. Flip eggs over mushrooms.

260. Spinach Egg Bake

Prep Time: *5 Minutes* *Cook Time:* *14 Minutes* *Servings: 1*

Ingredients:

- 2 cups chopped red peppers or spinach
- 1 cup zucchini
- 2 tbsp. coconut oil
- 1 cup sliced mushrooms
- ½ cup sliced green onions
- 8 eggs
- 1 cup coconut milk
- ½ cup almond flour 2 tbsp. Minced fresh parsley
- ½ tsp. Dried basil
- ½ tsp. Salt
- ¼ tsp. ground black pepper

Directions:

1. Preheat oven to 350 degrees F. Put coconut oil in a skillet. Heat it to medium heat. Add mushrooms, onions, zucchini, and red pepper (or spinach) until vegetables are tender for about 5 minutes. Drain veggies and spread them over the baking dish.
2. Beat eggs in a bowl with milk flour, parsley basil, salt and pepper. Pour egg mixture into baking dish.
3. Bake in preheated oven until the centre is set (approx. 35 to 40 minutes).

261. Spinach Frittata

Prep Time: *1 Minutes* *Cook Time:* *15 Minutes* *Servings: 1*

Ingredients:

- 6 servings
- 2 tbsp. olive oil or avocado oil 1 Zucchini sliced 1 cup torn fresh spinach
- 2 tbsp. sliced green onions
- 1 tsp. crushed garlic salt and pepper to taste 1/3 cup coconut milk
- 6 eggs

Directions:

1. Heat olive oil in a skillet over medium heat. Add zucchini and cook until tender. Mix in spinach, green onions and garlic. Season with salt and pepper. Continue cooking until spinach is wilted.
2. In a bowl, beat eggs and coconut milk together. Pour into the skillet over the vegetables. Reduce heat to low cover and cook until eggs are firm (5 to 7 minutes).

262. Superfoods Naan Pancakes Crepes

Prep Time: *2 Minutes* | *Cook Time:* *14 Minutes* | *Servings: 1*

Ingredients:

- ½ cup almond flour ½ cup Tapioca Flour 1 cup Coconut Milk Salt
- coconut oil

Directions:

1. Mix all the ingredients together.
2. After heating a pan over medium heat and pour the batter to desired thickness; once the batter looks firm, flip it over to cook the other side.
3. If you want this to be a dessert crepe or pancake, then omit the salt. You can add minced garlic or ginger in the batter if you want or some spices.

263. Frittata with Broccoli and Tomato

Prep Time: *15 Minutes* | *Cook Time:* *53 Minutes* | *Servings: 1*

Ingredients:

- 2 large eggs
- Salt Ground black pepper 1 tsp. Olive oil or cumin oil ½ cup broccoli
- ½ cup sliced tomatoes Crushed red pepper flakes and a 1 Tbsp. chopped chives (optional)

Directions:

1. 2 large eggs are whisking in a small bowl. Present with salt and ground black pepper and set aside. Heat 1 tsp.
2. Oil in a medium skillet over medium heat. Add broccoli and tomatoes and cook, tossing approx. 1 minute. Add eggs; cook, occasionally stirring until just set about 1 minute. Stir in cheese.
3. Sprinkle with crushed red pepper flakes and chives.

264. Frittata with Green and Red Peppers

Prep Time: *5 Minutes* | *Cook Time:* *14 Minutes* | *Servings: 1*

Ingredients:

- 2 large eggs
- Salt Ground black pepper 1 tsp. olive oil or avocado oil ½ cup each chopped green and red peppers

Directions:

1. 2 large eggs are whisking in a small bowl. Present with salt and ground black pepper and set aside. Heat 1 tsp.
2. Olive oil in a medium skillet. Add peppers and cook, tossing approx. 1 minute.
3. Add eggs; cook, occasionally stirring until just set about 1 minute.

265. Eggs in Purgatory

Prep Time: *35 Minutes* | *Cook Time:* *23 Minutes* | *Servings: 1*

Ingredients:

- 2 large eggs
- Salt 1 clove garlic chopped.
- 1 tsp. Olive oil or avocado oil 1 cup chopped tomatoes 1 Tbsp. Hot red pepper flakes and 1 Tbsp. cilantro

Directions:

1. Heat 1 tsp. Oil in a medium skillet over medium heat. Add garlic, chopped tomatoes and red pepper flakes and cook, tossing approx. 15 minutes.
2. Add eggs and cook until eggs are done. Sprinkle with salt and cilantro.

266. Frittata with Carrots Green Peas and Asparagus

Prep Time: *5 Minutes* | *Cook Time:* *15 Minutes* | *Servings: 1*

Ingredients:

- 2 large eggs
- Salt Ground black pepper 1 tsp. Olive oil or avocado oil ½ cup cooked green peas ½ cup chopped carrot ½ cup asparagus 1 tbsp. fresh dill

Directions:

1. 2 large eggs are whisking in a small bowl. Present with salt and ground black pepper and set aside. Heating 1 tsp.
2. Oil in a skillet over medium heat. Add carrots and asparagus and cook, tossing approx. 5 minutes. Add cooked and drained green peas. Add eggs; cook, occasionally stirring until just set about 1 minute. Sprinkle with dill.

Lunch Recipes

267. PASTA WITH SUN-DRIED TOMATOES, RICOTTA, & PEAS

Prep Time: *5 Minutes* | *Cook Time:* *45 Minutes* | *Servings: 1*

INGREDIENTS:

- Tbsps. olive oil
- garlic cloves, minced
- 1/4 Tsp. red pepper flakes
- 12 ounces whole-milk ricotta (1 1/2 cups)
- cup oil-packed sun-dried tomatoes, rinsed, patted dry, & chopped coarse 1/4 cup grated Parmesan cheese, plus extra for serving
- 2 Tbsps. minced fresh mint Salt
- 1/4 Tsp. pepper
- lb medium shells
- cup frozen peas

DIRECTIONS:

1. 2Heat oil, garlic, & pepper flakes in a 10-inch pan over medium heat. Cook, often stirring, till garlic turns golden but not brown, about 3 mins. Shift batter to an enormous container, cool slightly, then stir in ricotta, tomatoes, Parmesan, mint, 1/2 Tsp. Salt & pepper.
2. While bringing 4 quarts of water to boil in a pot. Include pasta & 1 Tbsp. salt & cook, often stirring, till al dente. Reserve 3/4 cup cooking water, then drain pasta & return it to pot. Include ricotta batter & 1/2 cup cooking water to pasta & toss to combine. Include remaining cooking water as needed to Set consistency. Serve immediately, passing Parmesan separately.

268. PASTA WITH SUN-DRIED TOMATOES, CAULIFLOWER, & THYME-INFUSED CREAM

Prep Time: *5 Minutes* | *Cook Time:* *33 Minutes* | *Servings: 1*

INGREDIENTS:

- lb tagliatelle Salt
- Tbsps. unsalted butter
- 1 Tbsp. vegetable oil
- 1 head cauliflower (2 lbs), cored & cut into 3/4-inch florets
- 1/8 Tsp. pepper
- small red onion chopped fine 3/4 cup dry white wine
- 2 cups heavy cream
- cup oil-packed sun-dried tomatoes, rinsed, patted dry, & cut into 1/4-inch-thick strips
- Tbsp. minced fresh thyme
- ounce Parmesan cheese, grated (1/2 cup), plus extra for serving
- 1/4 cup chopped fresh parsley
- 1 1/2 Tbsps. balsamic vinegar
- 1/4 cup pine nuts, toasted

DIRECTIONS:

1. 2Bring 4 quarts of water to boil in a pot. Include pasta & 1 Tbsp. salt & cook, often stirring, till al dente. Reserve 1/2 cup cooking water, then drain pasta & return it to pot.
2. Meanwhile, heat 1 Tbsp. Butter & oil in the 12-inch pan over high heat till butter is melted. Include cauliflower, 1/3 cup water, 1/4 Tsp. Salt, & pepper, cover, & cook till cauliflower is crisp-tender, about 3 mins. Uncover & continue to cook, often stirring, till the water has evaporated & cauliflower is golden, about 3 mins longer; Shift to Plate.
3. Melt remaining 1 Tbsp. Butter in a now-empty pan over medium heat. Include onion & cook till softened, about 5 mins. Stir in wine, increase heat to medium-high, & cook till reduced & batter measures 1/2 cup, about 4 mins. Stir in cream, tomatoes, & thyme & bring to simmer. Off heat, remove any foam from the surface with a large spoon, then stir in cauliflower & 1/2 Tsp. Salt.
4. Include cauliflower batter, Parmesan, parsley, & vinegar to pasta & toss to combine. Serve immediately, sprinkling individual portions with nuts & passing Parmesan separately.

269. WHOLE WHEAT SPAGHETTI WITH ITALIAN SAUSAGE & FENNEL

Prep Time: *12 Minutes* | *Cook Time:* *10 Minutes* | *Servings: 1*

INGREDIENTS:

- ounces sweet Italian sausage, casings removed 1/4 cup extra-virgin olive oil
- 6 garlic cloves, minced
- 1/2 Tsp. red pepper flakes Salt
- 1 fennel bulb, stalks discarded, halved, cored, & sliced thin 1/2 cup pine nuts, toasted & chopped
- 1/2 cup roughly chopped fresh basil 2 Tbsps. lemon juice
- 1 lb whole wheat spaghetti
- 1-ounce Pecorino Romano cheese, grated (1/2 cup)

DIRECTIONS:

1. Brown sausage well in 12-inch nonstick pan over medium-high heat, breaking up any large pieces with a wooden spoon, about 5 mins. Remove sausage with slotted spoon & Shift to the paper towel-lined plate.
2. Combine oil, garlic, pepper flakes, & 1/2 Tsp. Salt in the container. Include fennel & 1/4 Tsp. Salt to fat left in pan & cook over medium heat till softened, about 5 mins. Clear centre of the pan, Include oil batter, & cook till fragrant, about 30 seconds. Stir batter into fennel & cook for 1 min. Off heat, stir in browned sausage, nuts, basil, & lemon juice.
3. While bringing 4 quarts of water to boil in a pot. Include pasta & 1 Tbsp. salt & cook, often stirring, till al dente. Reserve 3/4 cup cooking water, then drain pasta & return it to pot. Include sausage batter
4. And reserved cooking water to pasta & toss to combine. Season with salt to taste. Serve, passing Pecorino separately.

270. WHOLE WHEAT PASTA WITH GREENS, BEANS, PANCETTA, & GARLIC BREAD CRUMBS

Prep Time: *16 Minutes* | *Cook Time:* *122 Minutes* | *Servings: 1*

INGREDIENTS:

- slices hearty white sandwich bread, torn into quarters
- 3 Tbsps. olive oil
- 6 garlic cloves, minced salt & pepper
- 3 ounces pancetta, cut into 1/2-inch pieces 1 onion, chopped fine
- 1/4 Tsp. red pepper flakes
- 11/2 lbs kale or collard greens stemmed & leaves cut into 1-inch pieces 11/2 cups low-sodium chicken broth
- (15-ounce) can cannellini beans, rinsed
- lb whole wheat spaghetti
- ounces fontina cheese, shredded (1 cup)

DIRECTIONS:

1. Pulse bread in the food processor to coarse crumbs, about 10 pulses. Heat 2 Tbsps. Oil in 12-inch straight-sided sauté cooking wok over medium heat till shimmering. Include bread crumbs & cook, often stirring, till beginning to brown, 4 to 6 mins. Stir in half of garlic & 1/4 Tsp. Salt & continue to cook, often going, till garlic is fragrant & bread crumbs are dark golden brown, 1 to 2 mins longer; Shift to the container. Wipe cooking work clean with paper towels.
2. Heat remaining 1 Tbsp. Oil in a now-empty cooking wok over medium heat till shimmering. Include pancetta & cook till crisp, 5 to 7 mins. Remove pancetta with slotted spoon & Shift to the paper towel-lined plate.
3. Include onion to fat left in cooking wok & cook over medium heat till
4. Softened & lightly browned, 5 to 7 mins. Stir in remaining garlic & pepper flakes & cook till fragrant, about 30 seconds. Include half of greens & cook, occasionally tossing, till starting to wilt, about 2 mins. Include remaining greens, broth, & 3/4 Tsp. Salt & bring to simmer. Reduce heat to medium, cover (pan will be very full), & cook, occasionally tossing, till greens are tender, about 15 mins (batter will be somewhat soupy). Stir in beans & crisp pancetta.
5. Mean, bring 4 quarts of water to boil in a pot. Include pasta & 1 Tbsp. salt & cook, often stirring, till just shy of al dente. Reserve 1/2 cup cooking water, then drain pasta & return it to pot. Include greens batter to pasta & cook over medium heat, tossing to combine, till pasta absorbs most of the liquid, about 2 mins.
6. Off heat, stir in fontina. Include reserved cooking water as needed to Set consistency. Season with salt & pepper to taste & serve immediately, passing bread crumbs separately.

271. WHOLE WHEAT PASTA WITH GREENS, BEANS, TOMATOES, & GARLIC CHIPS

Prep Time: *33 Minutes* | *Cook Time:* *112 Minutes* | *Servings: 1*

INGREDIENTS:

- 3 Tbsps. olive oil, plus extra for drizzling
- 8 garlic cloves, peeled, 5 cloves sliced thin lengthwise & 3 cloves minced salt & pepper
- 1 onion, chopped fine
- 1/2 Tsp. red pepper flakes
- 11/4 lbs curly-leaf spinach stemmed & leaves cut into 1-inch pieces 3/4 cup low-sodium chicken broth
- (14.5-ounce) can diced tomatoes, drained
- (15-ounce) can cannellini beans, rinsed
- 3/4 cup pitted kalamata olives, chopped coarsely
- 1 lb whole wheat spaghetti
- ounces Parmesan cheese, grated fine (1 cup), plus extra for serving

DIRECTIONS:

1. Heat oil & sliced garlic in a 12-inch straight-sided sauté cooking wok over medium heat. Cook, often stirring, till garlic turns golden but not brown, about 3 mins. Remove garlic with a slotted spoon & Shift to the paper towel-lined plate. Sprinkle garlic lightly with salt.
2. Include onion to oil left in cooking wok & cook over medium heat till softened & lightly browned, 5 to 7 mins. Stir in minced garlic & pepper flakes & cook till fragrant, about 30 seconds. Include half of spinach & cook, occasionally tossing, till starting to wilt, about 2 mins. Include remaining spinach, broth, tomatoes, & 3/4 Tsp. Salt & bring to simmer. Reduce heat to medium, cover (pan will be very full), & cook, occasionally tossing, till spinach is thoroughly wilted, about 10 mins (batter will be somewhat soupy). Stir in beans & olives.
3. Hence, bring 4 quarts of water to boil in a large pot. Include pasta & 1 Tbsp. salt & cook, often stirring, till just shy of al dente. Reserve 1/2 cup cooking water, then drain pasta & return it to pot. Include greens batter to pasta & cook over medium heat, tossing to combine, till pasta absorbs most of the liquid, about 2 mins.
4. Off heat, stir in Parmesan. Include reserved cooking water as needed to Set consistency. Season with salt & pepper to taste & serve immediately, drizzling individual portions with oil & passing garlic chips & Parmesan separately.

272. PASTA WITH SIMPLE ITALIAN-STYLE MEAT SAUCE

Prep Time: *25 Minutes* | *Cook Time:* *60 Minutes* | *Servings: 1*

INGREDIENTS:

- ounces white mushrooms, trimmed & halved if small or quartered if large
- 1 slice hearty white sandwich bread, torn into quarters
- 2 Tbsps. whole milk Salt & pepper
- 1 lb 85 per cent lean ground beef
- 1 Tbsp. olive oil
- 1 large onion, chopped fine
- 6 garlic cloves, minced
- 1/4 Tsp. red pepper flakes
- Tbsp. tomato paste
- (14.5-ounce) can diced tomatoes, drained with 1/4 cup juice reserved
- Tbsp. Minced fresh oregano or 1 Tsp. dried
- (28-ounce) can crushed tomatoes
- 1/4 cup grated Parmesan cheese, for serving
- lbs spaghetti or linguine

DIRECTIONS:

1. 2Pulse mushrooms in the food processor till finely chopped, about 8 pulses, scraping down sides as needed; Shift to the container. Include bread, milk, 1/2 Tsp. Salt, & 1/2 Tsp. Pepper to now-empty food processor & pulse till paste forms, about 8 pulses. Include ground beef & pulse till batter is well combined, about 6 pulses.
2. Heating the oil in a saucepan over medium-high heat till just smoking. Include onion & mushrooms & cook till vegetables are softened & well browned, 6 to 12 mins. Stir in garlic, pepper flakes, & tomato paste & cook till fragrant & tomato paste starts to brown, about 1 Min. Stir in reserved tomato juice & 2 Tbsps. Fresh oregano, scraping up any browned bits. Stir in meat batter & cook, breaking up any large pieces with a wooden spoon, till no longer pink, about 3 mins, making sure that meat does not brown.
3. Stir in diced tomatoes & crushed tomatoes, bring to a gentle simmer, & cook till sauce has thickened & flavours meld about 30 mins. Stir in Parmesan & remaining 1 Tsp. Fresh oregano & season with salt & pepper to taste.
4. Meanwhile, bring 8 quarts of water to boil in a 12-quart pot. Include pasta & 2 Tbsps. salt & cook, often stirring, till al dente. Reserve 1/2 cup cooking water, then drain pasta & return it to pot. Include 1 cup sauce & reserved cooking water to pasta & toss to combine. Serve, passing remaining sauce & Parmesan separately.

273. PASTA WITH HEARTY ITALIAN MEAT SAUCE (SUNDAY GRAVY)

Prep Time: *30 Minutes* | *Cook Time:* *28 Minutes* | *Servings: 1*

INGREDIENTS:

- SAUCE
- 2 Tbsps. olive oil
- 21/4 lbs baby back ribs, cut into 2-rib sections salt & pepper
- lb hot Italian sausage
- 2 onions, chopped fine
- 11/4 Tbsps. dried oregano
- Tbsps. tomato paste
- 4 garlic cloves, minced
- 2 (28-ounce) cans of crushed tomatoes
- 2/3 cup beef broth
- 1/4 cup chopped fresh basil
- MEATBALLS & PASTA
- slices hearty white sandwich bread, 1/2 cup buttermilk
- 1 lb meatloaf mix
- ounces thinly sliced prosciutto, chopped fine
- ounce Pecorino Romano cheese, grated (1/2 cup) 1/4 cup chopped fresh parsley
- 2 garlic cloves, minced
- large egg yolk Salt
- 1/4 Tsp. red pepper flakes
- 1/2 cup olive oil
- 11/2 lbs spaghetti or linguine
- Grated Parmesan cheese

DIRECTIONS:

1. FOR THE SAUCE: Set oven rack to lower-middle setting & heat oven to 325 degrees. Heating oil in a Dutch oven over medium-high heat till just smoking. Pat ribs dry with paper towels & season with salt & pepper. Brown half of ribs well on both sides, 5 to 7 mins. Shift ribs to large plate & repeat with remaining ribs. After Shifting the second batch of ribs to plate, brown sausage well on all sides, 5 to 7 mins; Shift to plate.
2. Include onions & oregano to fat left in the pot & cook over medium heat, occasionally stirring, till onions are softened & lightly browned, 5 to 7 mins. Include tomato paste & cook, constantly stirring, till very dark, about 3 mins. Stir in garlic & cook till fragrant, about 30 seconds. Stir in crushed tomatoes & broth, scraping up any browned bits. Nestle browned ribs & sausage into the pot. Bring to simmer, cover, & Shift to oven. Cook till ribs are tender, about 21/2 hrs.
3. FOR THE MEATBALLS: While sauce cooks, mash bread & buttermilk in a large container using a fork. Let stand 10 mins. Mix in meatloaf mix, prosciutto, Pecorino, parsley, garlic, egg yolk, 1/2 Tsp. Salt & pepper flakes using hands. Pinch off & roll batter into 12 meatballs. Shift meatballs to a plate, cover with plastic wrap, & refrigerate till ready to use.
4. When the sauce is 30 mins from being done, heat oil in a large nonstick pan over medium-high heat till shimmering. Brown meatballs well on all sides, 5 to 7 mins; Shift to the paper towel-lined plate. Remove sauce from oven & remove fat from surface using a large spoon. Gently nestle browned meatballs into sauce. Cover, return pot to oven, & continue to cook till meatballs are just cooked through, about. 2 Mins.
5. After, bringing 6 quarts of water to boil in a pot. Include pasta & 2 Tbsps. salt & cook, often stirring, till al dente. Reserve 1/2 cup cooking water, then drain pasta & return it to pot.
6. Using tongs, Shift meatballs, ribs, & sausage to a serving platter & cut each sausage in half. Stir basil into sauce & season with salt & pepper to taste. Include 1 cup sauce & reserved cooking water to pasta & toss to combine. Serve, remaining passing sauce, meat platter, & Parmesan separately. (Sauce & meatballs can be cooled & refrigerated for up to 2 days.)

274. PASTA WITH RUSTIC SLOW-SIMMERED MEAT SAUCE

Prep Time: *15 Minutes* | *Cook Time:* *130 Minutes* | *Servings: 1*

INGREDIENTS:

- 1 Tbsp. olive oil
- 11/2 lbs beef short ribs, pork spareribs, or country-style pork ribs, trimmed salt & pepper
- onion, chopped fine 1/2 cup dry red wine
- (28-ounce) can whole tomatoes, drained with juice reserved, tomatoes chopped fine
- lb penne, ziti, or other short, tubular pasta Grated Parmesan cheese

DIRECTIONS:

1. Heat oil in a 12-inch pan over medium-high heat till just smoking. Pat ribs dry by use of paper towels & season with salt & pepper. Turn Brown ribs well on all sides, 8 to 10 mins; Shift to plate. Pour off all but 1 Tsp. Fat from pan, Include onion, & cook over medium heat till softened, about 5 mins. Stir continuously in wine, scraping up any browned bits. Bring to simmer & cook till wine reduces to glaze about 2 mins.
2. Stir in tomatoes & reserved tomato juice. Nestle browned ribs into the sauce and any accumulated juices, & bring to a gentle simmer. Reduce heat to low, cover, & simmer gently, turning ribs occasionally, till meat is very tender & falling off bones, 11/2 hrs (for pork spareribs or country-style ribs) to 2 hrs (for beef short ribs).

3. Shift ribs to clean plate, cool slightly, then shred meat into bite-size pieces, discarding fat & bones. Return shredded meat to the sauce, bring to simmer, & cook till heated through & thickened slightly for about 5 mins. Season with salt & pepper to taste. Bring four parts of water to boil in a large pot. Include pasta & 1 Tbsp. salt & cook, often stirring, till al dente. Reserve 1/2 cup cooking water, then drain pasta & return it to pot. Include sauce to pasta & toss to combine. Include reserved cooking water as needed to Set consistency. Serve immediately, passing Parmesan separately.

275. PASTA WITH CLASSIC BOLOGNESE SAUCE

Prep Time: *5 Minutes* *Cook Time:* *32 Minutes* *Servings: 1*

INGREDIENTS:

- 5 Tbsps. unsalted butter
- Tbsps. finely chopped onion
- Tbsps. minced carrot
- Tbsps. minced celery
- ounces meatloaf mix Salt
- cup whole milk
- cup dry white wine
- (28-ounce) can whole tomatoes, drained with juice reserved, tomatoes chopped fine
- lb linguine or fettuccine Grated Parmesan cheese

DIRECTIONS:

1. Melt 3 Tbsps. Butter in an oven of Dutch over medium heat. Include onion, carrot, & celery & cook till softened, 5 to 7 mins. Stir in meatloaf mix & 1/2 Tsp. Salt & cook, breaking up any large pieces with a wooden spoon, till no longer pink, about 3 mins.
2. Stir in milk, bring to simmer, & cook till the milk evaporates & only rendered fat remains 10 to 15 mins. Stir in wine, bring to simmer and
3. Cook till wine evaporates, 10 to 15 mins. Stir in tomatoes & reserved tomato juice & bring to simmer. Minimize heat to low so that sauce continues to simmer just barely, with an occasional bubble or two at the surface, till the liquid has evaporated, about 3 hrs. Season with salt to taste. 3. bring 4 quarts of water to boil in a large pot. Include pasta & 1 Tbsp. salt & cook, often stirring, till al dente. Reserve 1/2 cup cooking water, then drain pasta & return it to pot. Include sauce & the remaining 2 Tbsps. Butter to pasta & toss to combine. Include reserved cooking water as needed to Set consistency. Serve, passing Parmesan separately.

276. BEEF BOLOGNESE SAUCE

Prep Time: *35 Minutes* *Cook Time:* *33 Minutes* *Servings: 1*

INGREDIENTS:

- Substitute 12 ounces of 85 per cent lean ground beef for meatloaf mix.
- TEST KITCHEN TIP NO. 42 BOILING WATER—WHAT'S THE RUSH?
- WEEKNIGHT PASTA BOLOGNESE
- 1/2 cup water
- 1/2 ounce dried porcini mushrooms, rinsed
- 1 1/4 cups sweet white wine
- small carrot, peeled & cut into 1/2-inch pieces 1/3 cup finely chopped onion
- 3 ounces pancetta, sliced 1 inch thick & cut into 1-inch pieces
- (28-ounce) can whole tomatoes
- Tbsps. unsalted butter
- 1 Tsp. sugar
- One small garlic clove, minced
- 1 1/4 lbs meatloaf mix
- 1 1/2 cups whole milk
- Tbsps. tomato paste Salt
- 1/8 Tsp. pepper
- lb spaghetti or linguine Grated Parmesan cheese

DIRECTIONS:

1. Microwave water & mushrooms in a covered container till steaming, about 1 min. Let stand till softened, about 5 mins. Drain Mushrooms through a mesh strainer lined with a coffee filter, reserving liquid.
2. Bring wine to simmer in a 10-inch nonstick pan & cook till reduced & measures 2 Tbsps., about 20 mins; set aside.
3. Meanwhile, pulse carrot in a food processor till broken down into rough 1/4-inch pieces, about ten pulses. Include onion & pulse till vegetables are broken down to 1/8-inch pieces, about ten pulses; Shift vegetables to a small container. Process softened porcini till the healthy ground, about 15 seconds, scraping down container as needed; Shift to a container with onion & carrot. Process pancetta till pieces are no larger than 1/4 inch, 30 to 35 seconds, scraping down container as needed; Shift to a separate container. Pulse tomatoes with their juice till finely chopped, 6 to 8 pulses.
4. Melt butter in a 12-inch pan over medium-high heat. Include pancetta & cook, often stirring, till well browned, about 2 mins. Stir in chopped vegetable batter & cook till vegetables are softened about 5 mins. Stir in sugar & garlic & cook till fragrant, about 30 seconds. Stir in meatloaf mix & cook, breaking meat into 1-inch pieces with a wooden spoon for 1 min. Stir in milk & bring to simmer, breaking meat into 1/2-inch pieces. Constantly do cooking, often stirring, to break up the meat into small pieces, till most of the liquid has evaporated & meat begins to sizzle, 18 to 20 mins longer.
5. Stir in tomato paste & cook till combined, about 1 min. Stir in chopped tomatoes, reserved porcini soaking liquid, 1/4 Tsp. Salt, & pepper, bring to simmer, & cook till sauce is thickened but still moist, 12 to 15 mins. Stir in reduced wine & simmer till flavours meld, about 5 mins. 5. bring four parts. Water to boil in a large pot.
6. Include pasta & 1 Tbsp. salt & cook, often stirring, till al dente. Reserve 1/4 cup of the cooking water, then drain pasta & return it to pot. Include 2 cups sauce & 2 Tbsps—pasta water to pasta & toss to combine. Include remaining cooking water as needed to Set consistency. Serve, passing remaining sauce & Parmesan separately.

277. OLD-FASHIONED SPAGHETTI & MEATBALLS

Prep Time: *30 Minutes* *Cook Time:* *28 Minutes* *Servings: 1*

INGREDIENTS:

- MEATBALLS
- slices hearty white sandwich bread, crusts removed, bread torn into small pieces 1/2 cup buttermilk
- 12 ounces 85 per cent lean ground beef
- 4 ounces ground pork
- 1/4 cup grated Parmesan cheese
- Tbsps. Minced fresh parsley
- large egg yolk
- garlic clove, minced 3/4 Tsp. salt
- 1/8 Tsp. pepper Vegetable oil
- TOMATO SAUCE
- Tbsps. extra-virgin olive oil
- One garlic clove, minced
- 1 (28-ounce) can crushed tomatoes
- 1 Tbsp. minced fresh basil Salt & pepper
- lb spaghetti
- Tbsp. salt
- Grated Parmesan cheese

DIRECTIONS:

1. FOR THE MEATBALLS: Mash bread & buttermilk in a large container using a fork. Let stand 10 mins. Mix in ground beef, ground pork, Parmesan, parsley, egg yolk, garlic, salt & pepper is using hands. Pinch off & roll batter into 1 1/2-inch meatballs (about 14 meatballs total).
2. Include oil in the 12-inch pan till it measures 1/4 inch deep. Heat oil over medium-high heat till shimmering. Carefully Include meatballs in a single layer & cook till well browned on all sides, about 10 mins. Remove meatballs with a slotted spoon & Shift to the paper towel-lined plate. Discard remaining oil.
3. FOR THE SAUCE: Heat oil & garlic in a now-empty pan over medium heat. Cook, stirring often & scraping up any browned bits, till garlic turns golden but not brown, about 3 mins. Stir in tomatoes, bring to simmer, & cook till sauce thickens about 10 mins. Stir in basil & season with salt & pepper to taste. Gently nestle meatballs into sauce, bring to simmer, & cook, turning meatballs occasionally, till heated through, about 5 mins. (Sauce & meatballs can be cooled & refrigerated for up to 2 days.) 4. bring four parts of water to boil in a large pot. Include pasta & salt & cook, often stirring, till al dente. Reserve 1/2 cup cooking water, then drain pasta & return it to pot.
4. Include 1 cup sauce (without meatballs) to pasta & toss to combine. Include reserved cooking water as needed to Set consistency. Serve, topping individual portions with more tomato sauce & several meatballs & passing Parmesan separately.

278. CLASSIC SPAGHETTI & MEATBALLS FOR A CROWD

Prep Time: *40 Minutes* *Cook Time:* *38 Minutes* *Servings: 1*

INGREDIENTS:

- MEATBALLS
- 2 1/4 cups panko bread crumbs
- 1 1/2 cups buttermilk
- 1 1/2 Tbsps. unflavored gelatin
- 3 Tbsps. water
- lbs 85 per cent lean ground beef
- 1 lb ground pork
- 6 ounces thinly sliced prosciutto, chopped fine
- Three large eggs
- 3 ounces Parmesan cheese, grated (1 1/2 cups)
- 6 Tbsps. minced fresh parsley
- Three garlic cloves, minced
- 1 1/2 Tbsps. salt
- 1/2 Tsp. pepper
- SAUCE
- Tbsps. extra-virgin olive oil
- One large onion, grated
- Six garlic cloves, minced
- 1 Tsp. dried oregano
- 1/2 Tsp. red pepper flakes
- (28-ounce) cans crushed tomatoes
- 6 cups tomato juice
- 6 Tbsps. dry white wine Salt & pepper
- 1/2 cup minced fresh basil
- Tbsps. minced fresh parsley Sugar
- lbs spaghetti
- Tbsps. salt
- Grated Parmesan cheese

DIRECTIONS:

1. FOR THE MEATBALLS: Set oven racks to lower-middle & upper-middle settings & heat oven to 450 degrees. Set wire racks in 2 aluminium foil-lined rimmed baking sheets & spray racks with vegetable oil spray.
2. Combine bread crumbs & buttermilk in the large container & let sit, occasionally mashing with a fork, till smooth paste forms, about 10 mins. Meanwhile, sprinkle gelatin over water in the small container & allow it to soften for 5 mins.
3. Mix ground beef, ground pork, prosciutto, eggs, Parmesan, parsley, garlic, salt, pepper, & gelatin batter into the bread-crumb batter using hands. Pinch off & roll the batter into 2-inch meatballs (about 40 meatballs total) & arrange on prepared baking sheets. Bake till well browned, about 30 mins, switching & rotating baking sheets halfway through baking.
4. FOR THE SAUCE: While meatballs bake, heat oil in a Dutch oven over medium heat till shimmering. Include onion & cook till softened & lightly browned, 5 to 7 mins. Stir in garlic, oregano, & pepper flakes & cook till fragrant, about 30 seconds. Stir in crushed tomatoes, tomato juice, wine, 1 1/2 Tbsps. Salt, & 1/4 Tsp. Pepper, bring to simmer, & cook till thickened slightly for about 15 mins.
5. Remove meatballs from oven & reduce oven temperature to 300 Degrees. Gently nestle meatballs into sauce. Cover, Shift to the oven, & cook till meatballs are firm & sauce has thickened, about 1 hr. (Sauce & meatballs can be cooled & refrigerated for up to 2 days. To reheat, drizzle 1/2 cup of water over sauce, without stirring, & reheat on the lower-middle rack of a 325-degree oven for 1 hr.) 6. bring 10 parts of water to boil in a 12-quart pot. Include pasta & salt & cook, often stirring, till al dente. Reserve 1/2 cup cooking water, then drain pasta & return it to pot.
6. Gently stir basil & parsley into sauce & season with sugar, salt, & pepper to taste. Include 2 cups sauce (without meatballs) to pasta & toss to combine. Include reserved cooking water as needed to Set consistency. Serve, topping individual portions with more tomato sauce & several meatballs & passing Parmesan separately.

279. PASTA WITH CHICKEN, BROCCOLI, & SUN-DRIED TOMATOES

Prep Time: *25 Minutes* *Cook Time:* *23 Minutes* *Servings: 1*

INGREDIENTS:

- 4 Tbsps. unsalted butter
- lb boneless, skinless chicken breasts, trimmed & sliced crosswise 1/4 inch thick
- small onion, chopped fine salt & pepper
- Six garlic cloves, minced
- Tbsps. minced fresh thyme
- Tbsps. all-purpose flour
- 1/4 Tsp. red pepper flakes
- cups low-sodium chicken broth
- 1 cup dry white wine
- ounces Asiago or Parmesan cheese, grated (1 cup), plus extra for serving
- One cup oil-packed sun-dried tomatoes patted dry & cut into 1/4-inch strips 1 Tbsp. minced fresh parsley
- 1 1/2 lbs broccoli, florets cut into 1-inch pieces, stalks discarded
- ounces penne, ziti, or campanelle (2 1/2 cups) Lemon wedges (optional)

DIRECTIONS:

1. Melt 1 Tbsp. Butter in 12-inch nonstick pan over high heat. Include chicken, break up any clumps, & cook, without stirring, till meat is browned at edges, about 1 min. Stir chicken & continue to cook till almost all of the pink colour has disappeared, about 2 mins longer. Shift chicken to container; set aside.
2. Melt 1 Tbsp. Butter in a now-empty pan over medium heat.
3. Include onion & 1/4 Tsp. Salt & cook till softened & lightly browned, 5 to 7 mins. Stir in garlic, thyme, flour, & pepper flakes & cook till fragrant, about 30 seconds. Slowly whisk in chicken broth & wine, bring to simmer, & cook, occasionally stirring, till sauce has thickened slightly & measures 1 1/4 cups, about 15 mins.
4. Stir in cooked chicken, Asiago, tomatoes, parsley, & the remaining 2 Tbsps. Butter & cook till chicken is hot & cooked through about 1 min. Season with pepper to taste.
5. Take 4 quarts of water to boil in a large pot. Include broccoli & 1 Tbsp. salt & cook till broccoli is crisp-tender, about 2 mins. Remove broccoli using a slotted spoon & Shift to the paper towel-lined plate. Return water to boil, then Include pasta & cook, often stirring, till al dente. Reserve 1/2 cup cooking water, then drain pasta & return it to pot.
6. Include sauce & broccoli to pasta & toss to combine. Include reserved cooking water as needed to Set consistency. Serve immediately, passing Asiago & lemon wedges, if using, separately.

280. GARLICKY SHRIMP PASTA

Prep Time: *15 Minutes* | *Cook Time:* *36 Minutes* | *Servings: 1*

INGREDIENTS:

- lb large shrimp (31 to 40 per lb), peeled, deveined, & each shrimp cut into 3 pieces
- 3 Tbsps. Olive oil
- garlic cloves, peeled, five cloves minced & 4 cloves smashed salt & pepper
- lb penne, ziti, or other short, tubular pasta 1/4–1/2 Tsp. red pepper flakes
- 2 Tips. all-purpose flour
- 1/2 cup of dry vermouth
- 1/2 cup chopped fresh parsley 3 Tbsps. unsalted butter
- Tsp. lemon juice plus lemon wedges

DIRECTIONS:

1. Combine shrimp, 1 Tbsp. oil, one-third of minced garlic, & 1/4 Tsp. Salt in the container. Let shrimp marinate at 25 degrees for 20 mins.
2. Heat smashed garlic & remaining 2 Tbsps. Oil in 12-inch pan over medium-low heat, often stirring, till garlic turns golden but not brown, 4 to 7 mins. Off heat, remove the garlic with a slotted spoon & discard. Set pan with oil aside.
3. Take 4 quarts of water to boil in a large pot. Include pasta & 1 Tbsp. salt & cook, often stirring, till al dente. Reserve 1/2 cup cooking water, then drain pasta & return it to pot.
4. While pasta cooks, return pan to medium heat. Include shrimp along With marinade, spread into even layer, & cook, without stirring, till oil starts to bubble gently, 1 to 2 mins. Stir shrimp & continue to cook till almost cooked through, about 1 min longer. Remove shrimp with slotted spoon & Shift to clean container. Include remaining minced garlic & pepper flakes to pan & cook over medium heat till fragrant, about 30 seconds. Include flour & cook, constantly stirring, for 1 min. Slowly whisk in vermouth & cook for 1 min. Stir in clam juice & parsley & cook till batter starts to thicken, 1 to 2 mins. Off heat, whisk in butter till melted, then stir in lemon juice.
5. Include shrimp & sauce to pasta & toss to combine. Include reserved cooking water as needed to Set consistency—season with pepper to taste. Serve immediately, passing lemon wedges separately.

281. PASTA WITH FRESH CLAM SAUCE

Prep Time: *15 Minutes* | *Cook Time:* *35 Minutes* | *Servings: 1*

INGREDIENTS:

- lbs littleneck or cherrystone clams, scrubbed 1/2 cup dry white wine
- Pinch cayenne pepper 1/4 cup extra-virgin olive oil 2 garlic cloves, minced
- Two plum tomatoes, peeled, seeded, & minced salt & pepper
- 1 lb spaghetti or linguine 3/4 cup chopped fresh parsley

DIRECTIONS:

1. Bring clams, wine, & cayenne to boil in 12-inch straight-sided sauté pan, cover, & cook, shaking cooking wok occasionally, for 5 mins. Stir clams thoroughly, cover, & continue to cook till they just begin to open, 2 to 5 mins longer. As clams open, remove them by using a slotted spoon & Shift them to the container. Discard any unopened clams.
2. Drain steaming liquid through a fine-mesh strainer lined with a coffee filter, avoiding any gritty sediment that has settled on the bottom of the pan. Measure out & reserve 1 cup of liquid; set aside. (If necessary, Include water to make 1 cup.) Wipe out the pan with paper towels.
3. Heat oil & garlic in a now-empty cooking wok over medium heat. Cook, often stirring, till garlic turns golden but not brown, about 3 mins. Stir in tomatoes, increase heat to medium-high, & cook till tomatoes soften about 2 mins. Stir in littlenecks, cover, & cook till
4. all clams are completely opened about 2 mins.
5. Take 4 quarts of water to boil in a large pot. Include pasta & 1 Tbsp. salt & cook, often stirring, till al dente. Drain pasta & return it to pot. Include sauce & reserved clam steaming liquid to pasta & cook over medium heat, tossing to combine, till flavours meld, about 30 seconds. Stir in parsley & season with salt & pepper to taste. Serve immediately.

282. PASTA WITH MUSSELS

Prep Time: *5 Minutes* | *Cook Time:* *33 Minutes* | *Servings: 1*

INGREDIENTS:

- Serve this dish with crusty bread to help soak up the flavorful sauce.
- lb mussels, scrubbed & debearded 1/2 cup dry white wine
- Tbsp. olive oil
- Two garlic cloves, minced
- 1/2 Tsp. red pepper flakes
- Tsp. grated lemon zest plus 2 Tbsps. juice
- lb spaghetti or linguine Salt
- Tbsps. minced fresh parsley

DIRECTIONS:

1. Bring mussels & wine to boil in 12-inch straight-sided sauté pan, cover, & cook, shaking cooking wok occasionally, till mussels open, about 5 mins. As mussels open, remove them by using a slotted spoon & Shift them to a container. Discard any unopened mussels. (If desired, remove mussels from shells.) Drain steaming liquid through a fine-mesh strainer lined with a coffee filter, avoiding any gritty sediment that has settled on the bottom of the pan. Reserve liquid & set aside. Wipe out the pan with paper towels.
2. Heat oil, garlic, & pepper flakes in a now-empty cooking wok over medium heat. Cook, often stirring, till garlic turns golden but not brown, about 3 mins. Stir in reserved mussel steaming liquid, lemon zest, & lemon juice, bring to simmer, & cook till flavours meld, 3 to 4 mins. Stir in mussels, cover, & cook till heated for about 2 mins.
3. Take 4 quarts of water to boil in a large pot. Include pasta & 1 Tbsp. salt & cook, often stirring, till al dente. Reserve 1/2 cup cooking water, then drain pasta & return it to pot. Include sauce to pasta

283. TOMATO SAUCE WITH TUNA & GREEN OLIVES

Prep Time: *4 Minutes* | *Cook Time:* *23 Minutes* | *Servings: 1*

INGREDIENTS:

- Tbsps. olive oil
- 2 garlic cloves, minced
- (28-ounce) can whole tomatoes, drained with 3/4 cup juice reserved, tomatoes chopped coarsely
- (6-ounce) can tuna in olive oil, drained & shredded
- 2/3 cup pitted green olives, chopped coarsely
- 2 Tbsps. minced fresh parsley
- lb farfalle or fusilli

DIRECTIONS:

1. Heat oil & garlic in a large saucepan over medium heat. Cook, often stirring, till garlic turns golden but not brown, about 3 mins. Stir in tomatoes & reserved tomato juice, bring to simmer, & cook till tomatoes soften & sauce thickens slightly, about 15 mins. Stir tuna & olives into the sauce & continue to simmer till flavours meld, about 5 mins longer. Stir in parsley & season with salt & pepper to taste.
2. Take 4 quarts of water to boil in a large pot. Include pasta & 1 Tbsp. salt & cook, often stirring, till al dente. Reserve 1/2 cup cooking water, then drain pasta & return it to pot. Include sauce to pasta & toss to combine. Include reserved cooking water as needed to Set consistency. Serve immediately.

284. PANTRY PASTA SAUCES WITH TUNA

Prep Time: *12 Minutes* | *Cook Time:* *90 Minutes* | *Servings: 1*

INGREDIENTS:

- Tbsps. olive oil
- Tbsps. capers, rinsed
- 6 garlic cloves, minced
- 1/2 Tsp. red pepper flakes
- 1/2 cup dry white wine
- 2 (6-ounce) cans solid white tuna in water, drained & shredded salt & pepper
- 1 lb penne or fusilli
- 1/4 cup chopped fresh parsley
- 1 Tsp. grated lemon zest
- Tbsps. unsalted butter, cut into 6 pieces

DIRECTIONS:

1. 2Heat oil, capers, half of the garlic, & pepper flakes in a 12-inch pan over medium heat. Cook, often stirring, till garlic turns golden but not brown, about 3 mins. Stir in wine, bring to simmer, & cook till alcohol aroma has cooked off about 1 min. Stir in tuna & 2 Tbsps. Salt & cook, often stirring, till tuna is heated through, about 1 min.
2. Take 4 quarts of water to boil in a large pot. Include pasta & 1 Tbsp. salt & cook, often stirring, till al dente. Reserve 1/4 cup cooking water, then drain pasta & return it to pot. Include sauce, parsley, lemon zest, butter, & remaining garlic to pasta & toss to combine. Include reserved cooking water as needed to Set consistency. Present with salt as well as pepper, and then serve immediately.

285. SHRIMP FRA DIAVOLO WITH LINGUINE

Prep Time: *16 Minutes* | *Cook Time:* *17 Minutes* | *Servings: 1*

INGREDIENTS:

- lb linguine or spaghetti Salt
- lb large shrimp (31 to 40 per lb), peeled & deveined
- 6 Tbsps. extra-virgin olive oil
- Tsp. red pepper flakes, or to taste
- 1/4 cup cognac or brandy
- 12 garlic cloves, minced
- (28-ounce) can diced tomatoes, drained
- cup dry white wine

- 1/2 Tsp. sugar
- 1/4 cup minced fresh parsley

DIRECTIONS:

1. take 4 quarts of water to boil in a large pot. Include pasta & 1 Tbsp. salt & cook, often stirring, till al dente. Reserve 1/2 cup cooking water, then drain pasta & return it to pot.
2. Meanwhile, toss shrimp with 2 Tbsps. Oil, 1/2 Tsp. Red pepper flakes, & 3/4 Tsp. Salt. Heat 12-inch pan over high heat. Include shrimp, spread into an even layer, & cook, without stirring, till bottoms of shrimp turn spotty brown, about 30 seconds. Off heat, flip shrimp, then Include cognac & let warm through, about 5 seconds. Wave lit match over cooking wok till cognac ignites, then shake cooking wok to distribute flames. When flames subside, Shift shrimp to a container & set aside. Cool pan slightly, about 3 mins.
3. Heat 3 Tbsps. Oil & three-quarters of garlic in a now-empty pan over low heat. Cook, constantly stirring, till garlic foams & is sticky & straw-coloured about 10 mins. Stir in tomatoes, wine, sugar, 3/4 Tsp. Salt, & remaining 1/2 Tsp. Pepper flakes, increase heat to medium-high, & simmer till thickened, about 8 mins.
4. Stir continuously shrimp along with any accumulated juices, parsley, & remaining garlic into the sauce. Simmer till shrimp have heated through, about 1 min. Off heat, stir in remaining 1 Tbsp. Oil. Include 1/2 cup sauce (without shrimp) to pasta & toss to combine. Include reserved cooking water as needed to Set consistency. Serve immediately, topping individual containers with shrimp & more sauce.

286. FRESH EGG PASTA

Prep Time: *11 Minutes* | *Cook Time:* *50 Minutes* | *Servings: 1*

INGREDIENTS:

- cups all-purpose flour, plus extra as needed
- 3 large eggs, beaten water

DIRECTIONS:

1. Pulse flour in the food processor to aerate. Include eggs & process till dough forms a rough ball, about 30 seconds. (If dough resembles small pebbles, Include water, 1/2 Tsp. At that time, if dough sticks to the side of the container, Include flour, 1 Tbsp. at a time, & process till dough forms a rough ball.) 2.
2. Turn out dough ball & any small bits onto counter & knead by hand till dough is smooth, 1 to 2 mins. Cover with plastic wrap & set aside to relax for at least 15 mins or up to 2 hrs.
3. separate the dough into 5 pieces and, using a manual pasta machine, roll out the dough into sheets. (Leave pasta in sheets for filled & hand-shaped kinds of pasta or cut into long strands to make fettuccine.)

287. MEAT & RICOTTA RAVIOLI OR TORTELLINI

Prep Time: *35 Minutes* | *Cook Time:* *33 Minutes* | *Servings: 1*

INGREDIENTS:

- GARDEN TOMATO SAUCE
- Tbsps. unsalted butter
- 1 small onion, chopped fine
- 1 carrot, peeled & minced
- 1 (28-ounce) can crushed tomatoes Salt & pepper
- MEAT & RICOTTA FILLING
- Tbsp. olive oil
- 2 garlic cloves, minced
- 8 ounces 85 per cent lean ground beef, ground pork, or ground veal 8 ounces (1 cup) whole-milk ricotta cheese
- 1/4 cup grated Parmesan cheese
- 1/4 cup minced fresh basil
- 1 large egg yolk
- 1/4 Tsp. pepper
- All-purpose flour for dusting
- recipe FRESH EGG PASTA
- Tbsp. salt
- Grated Parmesan cheese

DIRECTIONS:

1. FOR THE SAUCE: To melting butter in a saucepan over medium heat. Include onion & carrot & cook till vegetables are softened for about 5 mins. Stir in tomatoes & 1/2 Tsp. Salt, bring to simmer, & cook till sauce thickens, about 1 hr. Season with salt & pepper to taste. Cover & set aside to keep warm. Bring back to simmer before cooking ravioli.) 2. FOR THE FILLING: Heat oil & garlic in a 10-inch pan over medium heat. Cook, often stirring, till garlic turns golden but not brown, about 3 mins.
2. Stir in ground beef & cook, breaking up any large pieces with a wooden spoon, till the fat is rendered & the meat is browned about 5 mins. Remove browned meat with a slotted spoon, Shift to a large container, & let cool slightly. Stir in ricotta, Parmesan, basil, egg yolk, & pepper till well combined.
3. Cover & refrigerate batter till cool, about 30 mins. (Filling can be refrigerated for up to 2 days.)
4. 3A. TO FORM RAVIOLI: Dust 2 rimmed baking sheets & counter with flour. Working with 1 pasta sheet at a time, cut the pasta into long rectangles measuring 4 inches across with a pizza wheel or sharp knife. Place rounded 1-Tsp. dollops of filling 1 inch from the bottom edge of dough & spaced about 1 1/4 inches apart. (If edges of dough seem dry, dab with water.)
5. Fold the top of pasta overfilling & press layers of dough together securely around each mound of filling to seal. Using a fluted pastry wheel, cut ravioli apart & trim edges.
6. Shift finished ravioli to prepared sheets & cover with damp kitchen towels. Repeat with remaining pasta & filling. (Towel-covered sheets of ravioli can be wrapped with plastic wrap & refrigerated for up to 4 hrs, or frozen; when completely frozen, ravioli can be Shifted to a zipper-lock bag & stored in the freezer for up to 1 month. Do not thaw ravioli before boiling.)
7. 3B. TO FORM TORTELLINI: Dust 2 rimmed baking sheets & counter with flour. Working with 1 pasta sheet at a time, cut the pasta into 2 1/2-inch squares with a pizza wheel or sharp knife. Place 1/2-Tsp. dollops of filling in the centre of each square. (If edges of dough seem dry, dab with water.)
8. Fold 1 corner of square diagonally over filling, leaving a thin border of bottom dough layer exposed. Press layers of dough together securely around the filling to seal. Lift each filled triangle & wrap the back of the triangle around the top of the index finger. Squeeze the bottom corners of the triangle together.
9. Slide filled pasta off a finger, Shift to prepared sheets, & cover with damp kitchen towels. Repeat with remaining pasta & filling. (Towel-covered sheets of tortellini can be Wrapped with plastic wrap & refrigerated for up to 4 hrs, or frozen; when completely frozen, tortellini can be Shifted to zipper-lock bag & stored in a freezer for up to 1 month. Do not thaw tortellini before boiling.) 4. Bring 4 quarts of water to simmer in a large pot. Include half of pasta & 1 Tbsp. Salt & cook, often stirring, till pasta is tender, about 2 mins (3 to 4 mins if frozen), Setting heat as needed to maintain a simmer. Remove pasta with slotted spoon & Shift to warm serving container.
10. Include some warm sauce in pasta, toss gently to combine, & cover to keep warm. Repeat with remaining pasta & Shift to a serving container. Include remaining sauce to the pasta, toss gently to combine, & serve immediately, passing Parmesan separately.

Side Dishes Recipes

288. CREAMSICLE MIMOSAS

Prep Time: *12 Minutes* | *Cook Time:* *67 Minutes* | *Servings: 1*

INGREDIENTS:

- 2 ½ mugs orange juice
- 1 mug half-and-half cream
- ¾ mug superfine sugar
- 4 tsp grated orange peel
- 2 bottles (750 millilitres each) champagne or other sparkling wine Fresh strawberries

DIRECTIONS:

1. Place the orange juice, cream, sugar and orange peel in a blender; cover and process until sugar is dissolved. Transfer to an 8-in. square dish. Freeze for 6 hours or overnight.
2. For each serving, scoop ¼ mug mix into a champagne glass; top with champagne. Garnish with a strawberry and serve
3. immediately.

289. SPARKLING CRANBERRY KISS

Prep Time: *5 Minutes* | *Cook Time:* *20 Minutes* | *Servings: 1*

INGREDIENTS:

- 6 mugs cranberry juice
- 1 ½ mug orange juice 3 mugs ginger ale Ice cubes
- Orange slices, optional

DIRECTIONS:

1. In a pitcher, mix cranberry juice and orange juice. Before serving, stir continuously in ginger ale; serve it over ice. If desired, serve with orange slices.

290. GINGER-GRAPEFRUIT FIZZ

Prep Time: *0 Minutes* | *Cook Time:* *10 Minutes* | *Servings: 1*

INGREDIENTS:

- 1 mug sugar
- 1 mug water
- ½ mug sliced fresh ginger root
- ½ tsp whole peppercorns
- ¼ tsp vanilla extract
- 1/8 tsp salt
- ¼ mug coarse sugar
- 3 mugs fresh grapefruit juice, chilled
- Ice cubes
- 4 mugs sparkling water, chilled

DIRECTIONS:

1. In a saucepan, take the first six ingredients to a boil. Reduce heat; simmer for 10 minutes. Let it cool until cold. Strain syrup, discarding ginger and peppercorns.
2. Using water, moisten the rims of eight cocktail glasses. Spread coarse sugar on a plate; hold every glass upside down and dip rims into sugar. Discard remaining sugar on a plate.
3. In a pitcher, mix grapefruit juice and syrup. Spread ½ mug into prepared glasses over ice; top with ½ mug sparkling water.

291. GERMAN BEER CHEESE SPREAD

Prep Time: *5 Minutes* | *Cook Time:* *20 Minutes* | *Servings: 1*

INGREDIENTS:

- 1 pound of sharp cheddar cheese, divided into ½-inch cubes 1 tbsp Worcestershire sauce
- 1 ½ tsp prepared mustard 1 small garlic clove, minced
- ¼ tsp salt
- 1/8 tsp pepper
- 2/3 cup German or non-alcoholic beer assorted biscuits

DIRECTIONS:

1. Put the cheese in the food processor. Pulse until chopped, about 1 minute. Add Worcestershire sauce, mustard, garlic, salt and pepper. Add beer little by little at a time, continuing to process until the mixture is smooth and spreadable, about a minute.
2. Transfer to a serving bowl or gift bottle. Cover and refrigerate for up to 1 week. Serve with crackers.

292. COQUITO

Prep Time: *12 Minutes* | *Cook Time:* *30 Minutes* | *Servings: 1*

INGREDIENTS:

- 1 can (15 ounces) cream of coconut
- 1 can of sweetened condensed milk
- 1 can (12 ounces) evaporated milk
- ½ mug water 1 tsp vanilla extract
- ½ tsp ground cinnamon ¼ tsp ground cloves 1 mug rum

DIRECTIONS:

1. Put in a blender the first seven ingredients; cover and process until blended. Let it cool until chilled. Stir in rum before serving.

293. SLOW COOKER CIDER

Prep Time:
0 Minutes

Servings: 1

Cook Time:
23 Minutes

INGREDIENTS:

- 2 cinnamon sticks (3 inches)
- 1 tsp whole cloves
- 1 tsp whole allspice
- 2 quarts apple cider
- ½ mug packed brown sugar 1 orange, sliced

DIRECTIONS:

1. Put cinnamon, cloves as well as allspice in a double of cheesecloth; take bring up corners of cloth and tie by using a string to form a bag.
2. Put cider and brown sugar in a 3-qt. Slow cooker; stir continuously until sugar dissolves. Add spice bag. Put orange slices on top. Wrap and cook on low for 2-3 hours or until heated through. Discard spice bag.

294. CHAI TEA MIX

Prep Time: *0 Minutes* | *Cook Time:* *10 Minutes* | *Servings:1*

INGREDIENTS:

- 3 mugs nonfat dry milk powder
- 1 ½ mug sugar 1 mug unsweetened instant tea
- ¾ mug vanilla powdered non-dairy creamer 1 ½ tsp ground ginger 1 ½ tsp ground cinnamon ½ tsp ground cardamom ½ tsp ground cloves OPTIONAL GARNISH
- Whipped cream

DIRECTIONS:

1. In a food processor, combine together all dry ingredients; cover and process until powdery. Store in an airtight container in a cool, as well as dry place for up to 6 months.
2. TO PREPARE 1 SERVING Dissolve 3 tbsps of mix in ¾ mug boiling water; stir well. Dollop with whipped cream if desired.

295. CERVEZA MARGARITAS

Prep Time: *0 Minutes* | *Cook Time:* *10 Minutes* | *Servings: 1*

INGREDIENTS:

- Lime slices and kosher salt, optional
- 1 can (12 ounces) lemon-lime soda, chilled
- 1 bottle (12 ounces) beer
- 1 can (12 ounces) frozen limeade concentrate, thawed ¾ mug tequila Crushed ice

DIRECTIONS:

1. If desired, use lime slices to moisten the rims of five margarita or cocktail glasses. Sprinkle salt on a plate; dip rims in salt. Set glasses aside.
2. In a pitcher, mix the soda, beer, limeade concentrate and tequila. Serve in prepared glasses over crushed ice.

296. BOURBON SLUSH

Prep Time: *5 Minutes* | *Cook Time:* *15 Minutes* | *Servings: 1*

INGREDIENTS:

7 mugs water
1 ½ mugs sugar 1 can (12 ounces) frozen orange juice concentrate 1 can (12 ounces) frozen lemonade concentrate 2 mugs strongly brewed tea, cooled
2 mugs bourbon
3 litres lemon-lime soda, chilled

DIRECTIONS:

1. In a Dutch oven, mix water and sugar; bring to a boil, stirring to dissolve sugar. Extract from heat.
2. Stir in orange juice and lemonade concentrate, tea, and bourbon. Transfer to freezer containers; freeze 12 hours or overnight.
3. To serve, place about ½ mug bourbon mixture in each glass; top with ½ mug soda.

297. GERMAN BEER CHEESE SPREAD

Prep Time: *1 Minutes* | *Cook Time:* *20 Minutes* | *Servings: 1*

INGREDIENTS:

- 1 pound of sharp cheddar cheese, divided into ½-inch cubes 1 tbsp Worcestershire sauce
- 1 ½ tsp prepared mustard 1 small garlic clove, minced
- ¼ tsp salt
- 1/8 tsp pepper
- 2/3 cup German or non-alcoholic beer assorted biscuits

DIRECTIONS:

1. Put the cheese in the food processor. Pulse until chopped, about 1 minute. Add Worcestershire sauce, mustard, garlic, salt and pepper. Add beer little by little at a time, continuing to process until the mixture is smooth and spreadable, about a minute.
2. Transfer to a serving bowl or gift bottle. Cover and refrigerate for up to 1 week. Serve with crackers.

298. PASSION FRUIT HURRICANES

Prep Time: *15 Minutes* | *Cook Time:* *35 Minutes* | *Servings: 1*

INGREDIENTS:

- 2 mugs passion fruit juice
- 1 mug plus 2 tbsps sugar
- ¾ mug lime juice ¾ mug light rum ¾ mug dark rum
- 3 tbsp grenadine syrup
- 6 to 8 mugs ice cubes
- Orange slices, starfruit slices and maraschino cherries

DIRECTIONS:

1. In a pitcher, mix the fruit juice, sugar, lime juice, rum and grenadine; stir until sugar is dissolved.
2. Spread into a hurricane or highball glasses filled with ice. Serve with orange slices, starfruit slices and cherries.

299. SWEET TEA CONCENTRATE

Prep Time: *5 Minutes* | *Cook Time:* *23 Minutes* | *Servings: 1*

INGREDIENTS:

- 2 medium lemons
- 4 mugs sugar
- 4 mugs water
- 1 ½ mug English breakfast tea leaves or 20 black tea bags 1/3 mug lemon juice EACH SERVING
- 1 mug cold water
- Ice cubes
- Citrus slices, optional
- Mint sprigs, optional

DIRECTIONS:

1. Extract peels from lemons; set fruit aside for garnish or save for another use.
2. In a saucepan, combine together sugar and water. Bring to a boil over medium heat. Minimize heat; simmer, unwrapped, for 3-5 minutes or until sugar is dissolved, stirring occasionally. Extract from the heat; add tea leaves and lemon peels. Close and steep
3. minute. Strain the tea finally and discard the tea leaves and lemon peel. Mix lemon juice. Cool to room temperature.
4. Convert to a container with a tight lid. Store in the refrigerator for up to 2 weeks.
5. Tea preparation In a tall glass, mix water and concentrate. Add ice. Add orange slices and mint twigs if desired.

300. WHITE SANGRIA

Prep Time: *12 Minutes* | *Cook Time:* *16 Minutes* | *Servings: 1*

INGREDIENTS:

- ¼ mug sugar ¼ mug brandy 1 mug sliced peeled fresh peaches or frozen sliced peaches, thawed 1 mug sliced fresh strawberries or frozen sliced strawberries, thawed 1 medium lemon, sliced
- 1 medium lime, sliced
- 3 mugs dry white wine, chilled
- 1 can (12 ounces) lemon-lime soda, chilled Ice cubes

DIRECTIONS:

1. In a pitcher, mix sugar and brandy until sugar is dissolved. Add remaining ingredients; stir smoothly to mix. Serve over ice.

301. ALL-OCCASION PUNCH

Prep Time: *5 Minutes* | *Cook Time:* *33 Minutes* | *Servings: 1*

INGREDIENTS:

- 8 mugs cold water
- 1 can (12 ounces) of frozen lemonade concentrate, thawed plus ¾ mug thawed lemonade concentrate 2 litres ginger ale, chilled
- 1-litre cherry lemon-lime soda, chilled Ice ring, optional

DIRECTIONS:

1. In a large punch bowl, mix water and lemonade concentrate. Stir in ginger ale and lemon-lime soda. Top with an ice ring if desired. Serve punch immediately.
2. Desired. Serve punch immediately.

302. SPARKLING PEACH BELLINIS

Prep Time: *5 Minutes* | *Cook Time:* *23 Minutes* | *Servings: 1*

INGREDIENTS:

- 3 medium peaches, halved
- 1 tbsp honey
- 1 can (11.3 ounces) of peach nectar, chilled
- 2 bottles (750 millilitres each) champagne or sparkling grape juice, chilled
- place a baking sheet with a large piece of heavy-duty foil (aboutx 12 in.).

DIRECTIONS:

1. Place the peach halves cut side up on the foil. Drizzle honey. Turn the foil over the peaches and seal.
2. Bake it at least 375° for 25-30 minutes or until soft. Cool completely. Extract and remove the skin. Process the peaches in a cooking processor until soft.
3. Transfer the peach puree to the pitcher. Add honey and 1 bottle of champagne. Stir until blended. 12 Spread in a champagne flute or wine glass. Finish with the remaining champagne. Serve immediately.

303. FROZEN STRAWBERRY DAIQUIRIS

Prep Time: *5 Minutes* | *Cook Time:* *0 Minutes* | *Servings: 1*

INGREDIENTS:

- ¾ mug rum
- ½ mug thawed limeade concentrate
- 1 package (10 ounces) frozen sweetened sliced strawberries
- 1 to 1 ½ mugs ice cubes
- GARNISH
- Fresh strawberries

DIRECTIONS:

1. In a blender, mix the rum, limeade concentrate, strawberries and ice. Cover and process until smooth and thickened (use more ice for thicker daiquiris). Spread into cocktail glasses.
2. To garnish each daiquiri, cut a ½-in. slit into the tip of a strawberry; position berry on the rim of the glass.

304. PUMPKIN PIE SHOTS

Prep Time: *3 Minutes* | *Cook Time:* *32 Minutes* | *Servings: 1*

INGREDIENTS:

- 1 envelope unflavored gelatin
- 1 mug cold water
- 1/3 mug canned pumpkin ¼ mug sugar
- ½ tsp pumpkin pie spice 1/3 mug butterscotch schnapps liqueur ¼ mug vodka
- 1 ½ tsp heavy whipping cream Sweetened whipped cream

DIRECTIONS:

1. In a saucepan, spread gelatin over cold water; let it stand for 1 minute. Heat and stir it continuously over low heat until gelatin is completely dissolved. Stir in pumpkin, sugar and pie spice; cook and stir until sugar is dissolved. Extract from heat. Stir in liqueur, vodka and cream.
2. Spread mixture into twelve 2-oz. shot glasses; Let it cool until set. Top with sweetened whipped cream.

305. BANANA NOG

Prep Time: *35 Minutes* | *Cook Time:* *45 Minutes* | *Servings: 1*

INGREDIENTS:

- 3 mugs milk, divided
- 3 mugs half-and-half cream, divided
- 3 egg yolks
- ¾ mug sugar
- 3 large ripe bananas
- ½ mug light rum
- 1/3 mug creme de cacao
- 1 ½ tsp vanilla extract
- Whipped cream and baking cocoa, optional
- In a large, heavy saucepan, mix 1 ½ mug milk,
- 1 ½ mugs cream, egg yolks and sugar.

DIRECTIONS:

1. Now Cook and stir continuously over medium-low heat until mixture reaches 160° and is thick to coat the back of a metal spoon.
2. Put bananas in a food processor; cover and process until blended. Spread milk mixture into a pitcher; stir in the banana puree, rum, creme de cacao, vanilla, and remaining milk and cream. Cover and let it cool for at least 3 hours before serving.
3. Spread into chilled glasses. Garnish with whipped cream and spread with cocoa if desired.
4. CHEAT IT! Substitute 6 mugs of eggnog from the dairy case for the milk mixture prepared in the recipe. Stir the banana puree, rum, creme de cacao and vanilla into the eggnog. Garnish as desired.

306. MEXICAN HOT CHOCOLATE

Prep Time: *12 Minutes* | *Cook Time:* *34 Minutes* | *Servings: 1*

INGREDIENTS:

- 4 mugs fat-free milk
- 3 cinnamon sticks
- 5 ounces 53% of cacao dark baking chocolate, coarsely chopped
- 1 tsp vanilla extract
- Additional cinnamon sticks, optional 1

DIRECTIONS:

1. In a saucepan, heat milk and cinnamon sticks overheat until bubbles form around the sides of the pan. Discard cinnamon. Whisk in chocolate until smooth.
2. Extract from the heat; stir in vanilla. Serve it in mugs with additional cinnamon sticks if desired.

307. CREAMSICLE MIMOSAS

Prep Time: *11 Minutes* | *Cook Time:* *32 Minutes* | *Servings: 1*

INGREDIENTS:

- 2 ½ mugs orange juice
- 1 mug half-and-half cream
- ¾ mug superfine sugar
- 4 tsp grated orange peel
- 2 bottles (750 millilitres each) champagne or other sparkling wine Fresh strawberries

DIRECTIONS:

1. Place the orange juice, cream, sugar and orange peel in a blender; cover and process until sugar is dissolved. Transfer to an 8-in. square dish. Freeze for 6 hours or overnight.
2. For each serving, scoop ¼ mug mix into a champagne glass; top with champagne. Garnish with a strawberry and serve immediately.

308. SPARKLING CRANBERRY KISS

Prep Time: *15 Minutes* | *Cook Time:0* *Minutes* | *Servings: 1*

INGREDIENTS:

- 6 mugs cranberry juice
- 1 ½ mug orange juice 3 mugs ginger ale Ice cubes
- Orange slices, optional

DIRECTIONS:

1. In a pitcher, mix cranberry juice and orange juice. Before serving, stir continuously in ginger ale; serve it over ice. If desired, serve with orange slices.

309. TEXAS TEA

INGREDIENTS:

- 1 mug cola
- 1 mug sour mix
- ½ mug vodka
- ½ mug gin
- ½ mug Triple Sec ½ mug golden or light rum ½ mug tequila Lemon or lime slices

DIRECTIONS:

1. In a pitcher, mix the first seven ingredients; serve over ice.

Snacks And Appetizer Recipes

310. CRAB-STUFFED SNOW PEAS

Prep Time: *10 Minutes* | *Cook Time:* *25 Minutes* | *Servings: 1*

INGREDIENTS:

- 1 can crab meat, drained, flaked, and cartilage removed
- 2 tbsps mayonnaise
- 1 tbsp chilli sauce or seafood cocktail sauce
- 1/8 tsp salt
- 3 drops hot pepper sauce
- Dash pepper
- 16 fresh snow peas

Directions:

1. In a small-size bowl, add the crab, mayonnaise, chilli sauce, salt, hot sauce and pepper.
2. Put the snow peas in the steaming basket. Place in a small saucepan over 1 inch of water. Bring to a boil; cover and steam for 30 seconds until tender. Drain the snow peas and immediately drop them into ice water. Drain and dry.
3. Cut the peas along the curved edges with a sharp knife. Spoon each crab mixture 1 tbsp.

311. CUCUMBER RYE SNACKS

Prep Time: *15 Minutes* | *Cook Time:* *35 Minutes* | *Servings: 1*

INGREDIENTS:

- 1 package (8 ounces) cream cheese, softened
- 2 tbsps mayonnaise
- 2 tsp Italian salad dressing mix
- 30 slices snack rye bread
- 30 thin slices of cucumber
- Fresh dill sprigs and chive blossoms

Directions:

1. In a bowl, beat the cream cheese, mayonnaise and dressing mix until blended. Let stand for 30 minutes.
2. Spread mixture on rye bread. Top each with a slice of cucumber, dill sprig and chive blossom. Cover and refrigerate until serving.

312. ASIAN TUNA BITES WITH DIJON DIPPING SAUCE

Prep Time: *5 Minutes* | *Cook Time:* *23 Minutes* | *Servings: 1*

INGREDIENTS:

- 3 tbsps Dijon mustard
- 2 tbsps red wine vinegar
- 2 tbsp reduced-sodium soy sauce
- 1 tbsp sesame oil
- 1 tsp hot pepper sauce
- 1 pound tuna steaks, cut into thirty 1-inch cubes Cooking spray
- ¼ cup sesame seeds ½ tsp salt ¼ tsp pepper 2 green onions, finely chopped

Directions:

1. In a small size bowl, whisk the first five ingredients; set aside. Spritz tuna with cooking spray. Sprinkle with sesame seeds, salt and pepper. In a big nonstick skillet, brown tuna on all sides in batches until medium-rare or slightly pink in the centre; remove from the skillet.
2. On each of the 30 wooden appetizers, skewered, and thread one tuna cube. Arrange on a serving platter. Garnish with onions. Present with sauce.

313. MARINATED SAUSAGE KABOBS

Prep Time: *5 Minutes* | *Cook Time:* *35 Minutes* | *Servings: 1*

INGREDIENTS:

- ¼ cup olive oil
- 1 tbsp white vinegar
- ½ tsp minced garlic
- ½ tsp dried basil
- ½ tsp dried oregano
- 12 ounces cheddar cheese, cut into ¾-in. cubes 1 can (6 ounces) pitted ripe olives, drained
- 4 ounces hard salami, cut into ¾-in. cubes 1 medium sweet red pepper, cut into ¾-inch pieces 1 medium green pepper, cut into ¾-inch pieces 1.

Directions:

1. In a plastic bag, add the first five ingredients; add the remaining ingredients. Seal bag and turn to coat; refrigerate for at least 4 hours. Drain and discard marinade.
2. For each kabob, thread one piece each of cheese, olive, salami and pepper onto a toothpick.

314. SMOKED SALMON PINWHEELS

Prep Time: *15 Minutes* | *Cook Time:* *19 Minutes* | *Servings: 1*

INGREDIENTS:

- 1 package (8 ounces) cream cheese, softened
- 1 tbsp snipped fresh dill
- 1 tbsp capers, drained
- ½ tsp garlic powder
- ½ tsp lemon juice
- 4 spinach tortillas (8 inches), room temperature
- ½ pound smoked salmon fillets, flaked

Directions:

1. In a small size bowl, add the cream cheese, dill, capers, garlic powder and lemon juice. Spread over tortillas; top with salmon. Roll up tightly.
2. Cut into 1-in. pieces; secure with toothpicks. Chill until serving. Discard toothpicks before serving. Refrigerate leftovers.

315. CHEESE STRAWS

Prep Time: *12 Minutes* | *Cook Time:* *50 Minutes* | *Servings: 1*

INGREDIENTS:

- ½ cup butter softened
- 2 cups shredded sharp cheddar cheese
- 1 ¼ cups all-purpose flour
- ½ tsp salt
- ¼ tsp cayenne pepper

Directions:

1. Preheat oven to 350°. In a big bowl, beat butter until light and fluffy. Beat in cheese until blended.
2. Add flour, salt and cayenne; stir into cheese mixture until a dough forms. Roll into a 15x6-in rectangle. Cut into thirty 6-in. strips. Gently place strips 1 in. apart on ungreased baking sheets.
3. Bake 15-20 minutes or until lightly browned. Let it cool for 5 minutes before removing pans to wire racks to cool completely. Store straws in an airtight container.

316. HONEY CHAMPAGNE FONDUE

Prep Time: *5 Minutes* | *Cook Time:* *30 Minutes* | *Servings: 1*

INGREDIENTS:

- ¼ cup finely chopped shallot 1 tbsp butter
- 1 garlic clove, minced
- 1 ¼ cups champagne 4 tsp cornstarch
- 1 tsp ground mustard
- ¼ tsp white pepper 1/3 cup honey 4 cups (16 ounces) shredded Swiss cheese 2 tbsp lemon juice
- Pinch ground nutmeg

Directions:

1. French bread cubes, tart apple slices or pear slices 1. In a big saucepan, saute shallot in butter until tender. Add garlic; cook 1 minute longer. Add the Champagne, cornstarch, mustard and pepper until smooth; gradually stir into pan. Take it to a boil; cook and stir for 2 minutes or until thickened.
2. Stir in honey; heat through. Remove from the heat. Add cheese and lemon juice; gradually stir into champagne mixture until melted. Keep warm. Sprinkle with nutmeg. Present with bread cubes, apple or pear slices.

317. CHICKEN SALAD IN BASKETS

Prep Time: *10 Minutes* | *Cook Time:* *34 Minutes* | *Servings: 1*

INGREDIENTS:

- 1 cup diced cooked chicken
- 3 bacon strips, cooked and crumbled
- 1/3 cup chopped mushrooms 2 tbsp chopped pecans
- 2 tbsps diced peeled apple
- ¼ cup of mayonnaise
- 1/8 tsp salt Dash pepper
- 20 slices bread
- 6 tbsps butter, melted
- 2 tbsps minced fresh parsley

Directions:

1. In a small size bowl, add the first five ingredients. Add mayonnaise, salt as well as pepper. Now Add to chicken mixture and stir to coat. Wrap and refrigerate until serving.
2. Preheat oven to 350 degrees. Cut each piece of bread into 3-inches. Round cookie cutter; Grease both sides with butter. Pour into non-oiled mini muffin cups. Bake 11-35 Minutes or until it turns golden brown and crispy.
3. After cooling for about 3 minutes, transfer it from the pan to the wire mesh and let it cool completely, then put 1 tablespoon of chicken salad in the breadbasket. Wrap and refrigerate for up to 2 hours. Sprinkle with parsley right before serving.

318. TAPAS MEATBALLS WITH ORANGE GLAZE

Prep Time: *15 Minutes* | *Cook Time:* *45 Minutes* | *Servings: 1*

INGREDIENTS:

- 1 egg, lightly beaten
- ¼ cup ketchup 1 small onion, finely chopped
- ½ cup soft bread crumbs ¼ cup minced fresh parsley 3 tsp paprika
- 2 garlic cloves, minced
- ½ tsp salt ½ tsp pepper 1 pound lean ground beef (90% lean) 2 ½ ounces feta cheese, cut into sixteen ½-in. cubes GLAZE
- 1 jar (12 ounces) orange marmalade ¼ cup orange juice 3 green onions, chopped, divided
- 1 jalapeno pepper, seeded and chopped

Directions:

1. Place the first 9 ingredients in a large bowl. Mash the beef into the mixture and mix well. Divide into 16 parts. Levelling. Sprinkle with each cheese. Make meatballs with the beef mixture around the cheese.
2. Place on a greased rack on a baking sheet that needs to be reduced. Bake uncovered at 400° for 20-25 minutes or until no longer pink. In a saucepan, heat the marmalade, orange juice, halves of the green onion and jalapenos.
3. Place the meatballs on a serving plate. Pour the glaze over it and gently stir to coat it. Garnish with the rest of the green onions.

Note *Wear disposable gloves when slicing peppers. Oil can burn your skin. Do not touch your face*

319. BEEF WELLINGTON APPETIZERS

Prep Time: *12 Minutes* | *Cook Time:* *122 Minutes* | *Servings: 1*

INGREDIENTS:

- 2 beef tenderloin steaks, divide into ½-inch cubes
- 2 tbsps olive oil, divided
- 1 ¼ cups chopped fresh mushrooms
- 2 shallots, chopped
- 2 garlic cloves, minced
- 1/3 cup sherry or chicken broth
- 1/3 cup heavy whipping cream
- ½ tsp salt
- 1/8 tsp pepper
- 1 tbsp of minced fresh parsley
- 1 package (17.3 ounces) of frozen puff pastry, thawed
- 1 egg, beaten
- HORSERADISH CREAM
- 1 cup sour cream
- ½ cup mayonnaise
- 2 tbsp prepared horseradish
- 1 tbsp minced chives
- ¼ tsp pepper
- Additional minced chives, optional

Directions:

1. In a big skillet, add brown beef in 1 tbsp oil. Remove and keep warm.
2. In the frying pan, now fry the mushrooms and shallots in the remaining oil until tender. Add garlic. Boil for 1 more minute. Mix the sherry and stir to release the brown pieces from the pan. Mix cream, salt and pepper.
3. Bring to a boil; Cook for about 7 minutes until the liquid has almost evaporated. Mix the beef and parsley. Set aside and keep warm.
4. Preheat oven to 400 degrees. Open the puff pastry on a lightly dusted surface. Roll each sheet to 12 inches. Box. Cut each into 16 squares.
5. Place 2 tablespoons of beef mixture in the centre of half of the box. Top with the rest of the squares; Close by pressing the edge with a fork. Place on a parchment-lined baking sheet. Cut a slit at the top. Brush with eggs. Bake it at least for 14-16 minutes or until golden brown.

320. KIWI TIKI TORCHES

Prep Time: *11 Minutes* | *Cook Time:* *31 Minutes* | *Servings: 1*

INGREDIENTS:

- 1 fresh pineapple, peeled and cut into 1-inch chunks 4 medium kiwifruits, peeled and cut into ¾-inch pieces 2 cups fresh strawberries, halved
- WHITE CHOCOLATE DIPPING SAUCE
- 1 cup heavy whipping cream
- 6 white chocolate Toblerone candy bars (3.52 ounces each), broken into pieces ¼ cup finely chopped macadamia nuts 1 to 2 tsp rum extract
- 1/3 cup flaked coconut, toasted 1. Alternately thread the pineapple, kiwi and strawberries onto 12 metal or wooden skewers; set aside. In a saucepan over heat, bring cream just to a boil. Reduce

Directions:

1. Heat to reduce; stir in Toblerone until melted. Remove from the heat; stir in nuts, and extract.
2. Transfer to a fondue pot and keep warm.
3. Sprinkle with coconut. Present with fruit kabobs.

321. PUMPKIN CHEESE PUFFS

Prep Time: *15 Minutes* | *Cook Time:* *50 Minutes* | *Servings: 1*

INGREDIENTS:

- 2 tbsp cream cheese, softened
- ½ tsp balsamic vinegar ½ cup water
- ¼ cup butter, cubed ¼ tsp salt
- ½ cup of all-purpose flour 4 drops yellow paste food colouring
- 1 drop red paste food colouring
- ½ cup grated Romano cheese 2 eggs

- 20 sprigs fresh Italian parsley, stems removed

Directions:

1. In a small size bowl, add cream cheese and vinegar. Cover and refrigerate. In a big saucepan, bring the water, butter and salt to a boil.
2. Mix the flour at a time and mix until a smooth ball is formed. Remove from heat. Leave it on for 5 minutes.
3. Add the yellow and red food colouring to a small bowl. Stir in the Romano cheese and food colouring to the mixture. Add eggs one at a time and beat well after each addition. Continue to beat until the dough is soft and shiny.
4. Lower it to the level of 3 inches. Separate on a greased baking sheet. Bake at 400° for 15-20 minutes or until slightly browned. Remove with wire rack to cool.
5. Use the tip of the star to represent the cream cheese mixture, putting the stems into the puff. Add parsley eggplant. Refrigerate leftover food.

322. DEVILED CRAB

Prep Time: *Cook Time:* *Servings: 1*
12 Minutes *20 Minutes*

INGREDIENTS:

- ½ cup finely chopped onion 3 tbsps butter
- 3 tbsps all-purpose flour
- ½ tsp salt 1 ½ cups half-and-half cream 2 egg yolks, lightly beaten
- 3 cans (6 ounces each) crabmeat, drained, flaked, and cartilage removed 1 tbsp Dijon mustard
- 2 tsp Worcestershire sauce
- 1 tsp minced chives
- TOPPING
- 1 cup soft bread crumbs
- 1 tbsp butter, melted

Directions:

1. In a big skillet, saute onion in butter until tender. Stir in flour and salt until blended. Gradually stir in cream until smooth. Take it to a boil, and cook and stir for 2 minutes or until thickened and bubbly. Remove from the heat.
2. Stir a small amount of hot mixture into egg yolks. Return all to the pan, stirring constantly. Bring to a gentle boil; cook and stir 2 minutes longer. Remove from the heat. Stir in the crab, mustard, Worcestershire sauce and chives.
3. Spoon into six greased 6-oz. ramekins or custard cups. Place on a baking sheet. Add bread crumbs and melted butter;
4. sprinkle over tops. Bake it at least 375° for 20-25 minutes or until topping is golden brown.

323. ITALIAN CHEESE WONTONS

Prep Time: *Cook Time:* *Servings: 1*
35 Minutes *23 Minutes*

INGREDIENTS:

- 2 cups shredded Italian cheese
- 1 carton (15 ounces) ricotta cheese
- 1 egg, beaten
- 1 tbsp minced fresh parsley
- 1 garlic clove, minced
- ¼ tsp salt
- 1/8 tsp pepper
- 40 wonton wrappers
- Oil for deep-fat frying
- Marinara or spaghetti sauce warmed.

Directions:

8. Put the first 7 ingredients in a bowl.
9. Place the dumpling wrapper at one point toward you. (Keep the rest of the wrap covered with a damp paper towel until ready to use.)
10. Place 1 tbsp of filling in the centre of the wrap. Fold the bottom corner over the filling.
11. After the sides folding towards the centre of the overcharge. Roll towards the remaining points. Wet the top edge with water. Press to seal. Repeat. Refrigerate for 30 minutes.
12. After heating, heat the oil to 375° in an electric frying pan. Fry the wontons a little at a time.
13. Fry for 1-2 minutes on each side or until golden brown. Drain the water on a paper towel. Served with marinara.

Dessert Recipes

324. Mango Ice Cream

Prep Time: *Cook Time:* *Servings: 1*
5 Minutes *135 Minutes*

Ingredients:

- 2 cups heavy cream
- 2 ripe mangoes, pureed
- 1 cup cream cheese
- ½ cup sugar
- 1 tablespoon lemon juice
- 1 tsp lemon zest
- 1 tsp vanilla extract

Directions:

1. Put the mangoes, sugar, lemon juice and zest in a blender and pulse until well blended and smooth. To convert into a bowl and stir in the cream cheese, followed by the heavy cream, whipped, and vanilla.
2. To convert the structure into your ice cream maker and churn according to your machine's instructions.
3. If you don't plan to serve it immediately, store it in an airtight container in the freezer until needed.

325. Pineapple Raisin Bread

Prep Time: *Cook Time:* *Servings: 1*
10 Minutes *23 Minutes*

Ingredients:

- 6 oz butter, melted
- 2/3 cup brown sugar
- 2 eggs
- 1 ¼ cup fresh crushed pineapple
- 1 tsp vanilla extract
- 1 cup whole wheat flour
- 1 cup all-purpose flour
- 1 tsp baking soda
- 1 tsp baking powder
- 1 pinch of salt
- ½ tsp cinnamon
- ½ cup dark chocolate chips
- ½ cup raisins

Directions:

1. In a bowl, transfer the flours with the salt, baking powder, baking soda, salt and cinnamon. Set aside.
2. In another bowl, stir the melted butter with the eggs, pineapple and vanilla. Pour this stricture over the flour and stir well, then fold in the chocolate chips and raisins.
3. Into a loaf pan, Spoon the batter that is lined with baking paper. Bake in the before heating oven at 350F for 30-40 minutes or until a skewer inserted in the middle of the bread comes out clean.

326. Pineapple and Coconut Cake

Prep Time: *Cook Time:* *Servings: 1*
15 Minutes *45 Minutes*

Ingredients:

- 1 ½ cup sweetened coconut flakes
- 2 eggs
- 1 cup low-fat sour cream
- 1 cup whole wheat flour
- ¾ cup all-purpose flour
- 1 tsp vanilla extract
- ½ tsp coconut extract
- 1 tsp baking powder
- ½ tsp baking soda
- 1 pinch of salt
- 6 oz butter, room temperature
- ½ cup sugar
- 2 cups crushed pineapple

Directions:

1. In a bowl, stir the eggs with the low-fat sour cream, vanilla and coconut extract. In another bowl, sift the flours with the baking powder, baking soda, a pinch of salt and coconut flakes.
2. In a different bowl, stir the butter with the sugar until fluffy and creamy, then start incorporating the flour, alternating it with the egg structure. When done, fold in the crushed pineapple. Spoon the batter into the prepared 9-inch cake pan (lined with baking paper or greased) and bake in the before heating oven at 350F for 30-35 minutes or until golden brown. When done, remove from the oven.
3. To convert on a serving plate and cover with powdered sugar just before slicing.

327. Pineapple Crumble

Prep Time: *Cook Time:* *Servings: 1*
15 Minutes *56 Minutes*

Ingredients:

- 1 large fresh pineapple, cut into cubes
- 2 cups graham crackers
- 5 oz butter, melted
- ½ cup brown sugar
- 2 tbsp coconut flakes

Directions:

1. Place the coconut cubes into a 9-inc square deep dish baking pan and set aside.
2. In a bowl, stir the ground graham cracker with the sugar and coconut flakes, then stir in the melted butter. Stir well, then spoon the stirirture over the pineapple in the pan, then bake in the before heating oven at 375F for 20-25 minutes or until soft and turn golden brown.
3. Serve immediately warm with a scoop of vanilla ice cream.

328. Grilled Pineapple with Caramel Sauce

Prep Time: *Cook Time:* *Servings: 1*
11 Minutes *22 Minutes*

Ingredients:

- Pineapple:
- 1 fresh pineapple
- 2 tbsp honey
- 1 oz butter
- Caramel sauce:
- 1 cup sugar
- 1/ 2 cup heavy cream
- 1 oz butter

Directions:

1. To grill the pineapple, firstly peel it, cut it in half and remove its core. Cut it into cubes and place them all on wooden skewers. Drizzle them with honey, then heat a grill pan over medium flame.
2. Brush the pan with butter, then place the pineapple in the pan. Grill it on all sides for 2-3 minutes, then remove it from the pan and make the caramel sauce.
3. To make the sauce, melt the sugar in a heavy saucepan, then stir in the heavy cream. Keep on heat and stir until smooth, then remove from heat and add the butter.
4. Serve the pineapple skewers drizzled with caramel sauce. If you want a more fresh aroma, you can marinate the pineapple into a lemon and mint dressing before grilling.

Breakfast & Brunch Recipes

329. Western Omelet

Prep Time: *Cook Time:* *Servings: 2*
15 Minutes *35 Minutes*

Ingredients:

- 2 tbsp sweet butter
- 6 large eggs
- ¼ cup chopped green pepper
- 1/3 cup chopped scallions (use onion if scallions not available) ¾ cup milk
- ¾ cup chopped ham
- Salt and pepper to taste

Directions:

1. 2Melt the butter in a skillet.
2. Whisk together the eggs with all of the other ingredients.
3. Pour egg mixture into skillet.
4. Cook one side, flip, and cook the other.
5. Don't overcook the omelette.

330. Asparagus Omelet

Prep Time: *Cook Time:* *Servings: 2*
15 Minutes *11 Minutes*

Ingredients:

- 1 pound asparagus
- 1 cup shredded Swiss cheese
- 8 large eggs
- 5 tbsp milk
- 4 tsp butter
- Salt and pepper to taste

Directions:

1. Cook asparagus until they are tender.
2. Shake the eggs with salt, pepper, and milk.
3. For each omelette, butter a skillet and add half a cup of the egg mix.
4. Don't scramble; just lift the edges occasionally and move the mixture around in the skillet.
5. Add ¼ cup of cheese and 4 asparagus spears to one side of the omelette.
6. Flip the other half of the omelette over the asparagus.
7. Cook until done and season with salt and pepper.

331. Vegetable Omelet

Prep Time: *Cook Time:* *Servings: 2*
15 Minutes *32 Minutes*

Ingredients:

- 2 tbsp virgin olive oil
- 1 chopped onion
- 6 oz. chopped zucchini
- 1 chopped green pepper
- Salt and pepper to taste
- 2 chopped tomatoes
- 8 large eggs
- ½ cup whole milk
- 4 tsp sweet butter

Directions:

1. Heat the oil in a skillet. Add now the vegetables, salt and pepper and cook until done.
2. 3Add the tomatoes.
3. Blend the eggs and milk in a bowl.
4. Using another skillet, add the butter and pour in the eggs.
5. Cook until eggs are still soft but set. Add the vegetables and fold the omelette.

332. Eggs Benedict

Prep Time: *Cook Time:* *Servings: 2*
15 Minutes *35 Minutes*

Ingredients:

- ½ cup butter
- 2 large egg yolks
- 1 tsp lemon juice
- ¼ cup hot water
- Salt and pepper to taste
- 12 ham slices cut very thin
- 6 large eggs
- 6 toasted and buttered English muffins

Directions:

1. Use a double boiler for the Hollandaise sauce. Mix the egg yolks and lemon juice on the top. Add 3 tablespoons of butter. Mix vigorously.
2. Place the water in the bottom and bring to boil.
3. Add the rest of the butter and continue beating. Beat until sauce thickens.
4. Remove the double boiler from the stove. Add salt and pepper to the sauce.
5. Spread out the ham on a baking dish and bake for 8 minutes, until the edges brown.
6. Pour water into a pan and bring to boil. Crack the eggs and carefully slide them into the water.
7. Lower the heat and cook eggs for about 3 to 4 minutes.
8. Place the muffins on individual plates.
9. Place 2 ham slices and an egg on each half. Drizzle with the sauce.

333. Eggs Florentine

Prep Time: *Cook Time:* *Servings: 2*
15 Minutes *15 Minutes*

Ingredients:

- 4 tbsp butter
- 4 tbsp flour
- Salt and pepper to taste
- ½ cup whole milk
- 10 oz. chopped frozen spinach
- 12 large eggs
- ¼ cup parmesan cheese

Directions:

1. Preheat the oven to 350 degrees.
2. Use a skillet to melt the butter. Mix in the flour, salt and pepper and blend with a wooden spoon or whisk.
3. Lower the heat and mix in the milk. Stir continuously as the mixture gets thick.
4. 5Lightly butter a muffin pan. Add 2 teaspoons of water to each muffin cup.
5. Crack the eggs and slide one into each cup.
6. Bake the eggs for 15 minutes.
7. While eggs are baking, heat the spinach in a microwave and drain the liquid.
8. Butter a 9 x 13 baking dish. Transfer the spinach to the baking dish. Divide the eggs over the spinach. Spread the sauce and the parmesan cheese over the eggs.
9. Bake eggs for 5 minutes or until the cheese is bubbly and just turning brown.

334. Breakfast in a Skillet

Prep Time: *Cook Time:* *Servings: 2*
15 Minutes *15 Minutes*

Ingredients:

- 5 chopped bacon slices
- 3 tbsp chopped onions
- 3 small potatoes, cooked and cubed
- 6 large eggs
- Salt and pepper to taste
- 1/3 cup shredded Cheddar cheese

Directions:

1. Fry the bacon in a skillet and now drain.
2. Use the drippings in the skillet to cook the onion and potatoes for approximately 5 minutes.
3. Whisk the eggs in a bowl and add to the skillet. Stir until eggs are cooked.
4. Season with salt and pepper.
5. Top the eggs with the bacon pieces and the cheese. Let the cheese melt.

335. Egg Croquettes

Prep Time: *Cook Time:* *Servings: 2*
15 Minutes *10 Minutes*

Ingredients:

- 6 hard-boiled eggs, finely chopped
- 2 tbsp chopped parsley
- 3 tbsp sweet butter
- ½ cup chopped onions
- 3 tbsp white flour
- ½ cup whole milk
- 1/3 cup shredded Cheddar cheese Salt and pepper to taste 1 ½ cups bread crumbs
- 2 large eggs

Directions:

1. Mix the chopped boiled eggs with the parsley.
2. Use a skillet to heat the butter and sauté the onions until they are softened.
3. Add the flour and milk to the skillet. Keep stirring until the mixture thickens.4
4. Mix in the Cheddar cheese and salt and pepper. Add the chopped boiled eggs.
5. Refrigerate for 3 hours.
6. Use your hands to form eggs in cylindrical patties. Roll patties in the bread crumbs to coat.
7. Heat vegetable oil in a skillet and cook patties until they turn brown, around 2 minutes.

336. Mexican Eggs

Prep Time: *Cook Time:* *Servings: 2*
15 Minutes *23 Minutes*

Ingredients:

- 3 large eggs ¼ cup black beans - canned 1 oz. shredded cheddar cheese 2 tbsp tangy salsa

Directions:

1. Beat the eggs. Add the beans and cheese.
2. Scramble the eggs until done.
3. Top the eggs with the salsa.

337. Croque Madame

Prep Time: *Cook Time:* *Servings: 2*
15 Minutes *43 Minutes*

Ingredients:

- 8 slices sourdough bread
- ½ cup butter at room temperature 4 slices of cooked ham
- 4 pieces of Gruyere cheese
- 4 large eggs

Directions:

1. Use half of the butter to spread on each slice of bread.
2. Pile a slice of ham and cheese on top of the bread and create sandwiches using the remaining bread slices.
3. Fry the sandwiches in a skillet. The cheese should be melted, and the bread should be browned.
4. Prepare the eggs:
5. Put enough water in a pan to wrap the eggs and add a tsp of olive oil.
6. Boil the water, then lower the temperature to a simmer.
7. Crack the eggs and slide them carefully into the water.
8. Turn off the stove and let the eggs sit until poached – 3 to 4 minutes.
9. By using a spoon to remove the poached eggs from a plate.
10. Melt the remaining half of the butter and add the parsley.
11. Transfer one sandwich each to 4 serving plates. Top the
12. sandwich with one poached egg.
13. Lightly pour the butter mix over the sandwiches.
14. Serve while hot.

338. Eggs and Spinach

Prep Time: 15 Minutes *Cook Time: 53 Minutes* *Servings: 2*

Ingredients:

- 2 tbsp virgin olive oil
- 1 chopped garlic clove
- 1 large can tomatoes, diced and without the liquid salt and pepper to taste
- 1 lb. spinach
- 6 eggs whites
- 6 egg yolks.

Directions:

1. Preheat oven to 400 degrees.
2. Use a skillet to heat the oil and sauté the garlic.
3. Mix in the tomatoes, salt and pepper. Let tomatoes warm, about 4 minutes
4. Add spinach leaves and continue to cook for another minute.
5. Place mixture in a 9 x 13 baking dish.
6. Whip eggs whites until they are fluffy. Spread over spinach.
7. Use a spoon to transfer the egg yolks onto the spinach.
8. Bake for 20 minutes.

339. Huevos Rancheros

Prep Time: 15 Minutes *Cook Time: 24 Minutes* *Servings: 2*

Ingredients:

- 12 corn tortillas
- 2 tbsp sweet butter
- 12 large eggs
- ¼ cup milk
- ½ teaspoon salt

Directions:

1. Toast the tortillas by placing each one in a skillet on medium heat. Cook both sides for 30 seconds. The tortilla should be soft.
2. Place the tortillas on a platter.
3. Melt the butter in a skillet.
4. Beat the eggs, salt and milk in a bowl. Cook in the skillet.
5. Transfer two warm tortillas on each plate and divide the scrambled eggs between them.
6. Serve with the following:
7. Chopped scallions and/or tomatoes Finely grated cheese Chopped peppers. Salsa Guacamole

340. Texas Eggs

Prep Time: 15 Minutes *Cook Time: 10 Minutes* *Servings: 2*

Ingredients:

- 1 jar spicy salsa
- 4 eggs
- Salt and pepper to taste
- 1 diced avocado
- cup sour cream 5 tbsp cilantro
- 4 oz. tortilla chips

Directions:

1. Heat up the salsa in a skillet.
2. Crack the eggs on top of the salsa. Season to taste.
3. Transfer the salsa and eggs to individual dinner plates.
4. Serve with tortilla chips, sour cream, avocado, and cilantro.

341. Baked Eggs

Prep Time: 15 Minutes *Cook Time: 30 Minutes* *Servings: 2*

Ingredients:

- 2 tbsp chopped basil and thyme
- 1 minced garlic clove
- 2 tbsp melted unsalted butter
- 3 tbsp heavy cream
- 6 eggs
- 4 tbsp ricotta
- Salt and pepper to taste

Directions:

1. Preheat the oven to 450 degrees.
2. Mix all together with the herbs and garlic in a bowl.
3. Whip together the butter and cream in another bowl.
4. Prepare a baking sheet with 6 ramekins.
5. Add the butter mix to the ramekins.
6. Bake for 2 minutes.
7. Take the baking sheet with ramekins out of the oven.
8. Crack the eggs and carefully slide one into each ramekin.
9. Add the herbs and the ricotta on top of the eggs.
10. Season with salt and pepper.
11. Bake the eggs for 5 minutes.
12. Serve the baked eggs immediately.

342. Polenta and Eggs

Prep Time: 15 Minutes *Cook Time: 23 Minutes* *Servings: 2*

Ingredients:

- ½ cup dried tomatoes
- 2 ½ cups milk
- 1 can chicken broth
- 1 cup yellow cornmeal
- 1/3 cup grated Parmesan cheese 1 tbsp virgin olive oil 1 sliced onion
- 1 small lemon
- 8 large eggs

Directions:

1. Place the dried tomatoes in some boiling water and let soak.
2. Heat up the milk and broth in a saucepan. Add the cornmeal and keep whisking.
3. Have the heat on medium and stir several times for about 15 minutes.
4. Add the Parmesan and blend. Let sit over low heat.
5. Remove the dried tomatoes from the water and drain them.
6. Heat the oil in a skillet. Toss in dried tomatoes and onions.
7. Cook until onions are softened, then take off the stove.
8. Use a deep pan and fill it halfway with water. Squeeze in the juice of the lemon.
9. When water is simmering, crack the eggs and transfer them carefully into the pan. Let the eggs simmer for 4 minutes, then removed and drain on a paper towel.
10. Transfer the polenta into individual serving dishes. Top each dish with 2 eggs.

343. Buttermilk Pancakes

Prep Time: 15 Minutes *Cook Time: 29 Minutes* *Servings: 2*

Ingredients:

- 2 cups all-purpose flour
- 3 tbsp cane sugar
- 3 tsp baking powder
- 1 tsp baking soda
- 1 tsp salt
- 2 cups buttermilk
- 6 tbsp butter
- 1 tsp vanilla
- eggs Maple Syrup Confectioners' sugar

Directions:

1. Combine all together with the flour, sugar, baking soda, as well as baking powder, and salt.
2. Use another bowl to combine the buttermilk, butter, eggs, and vanilla.
3. Slowly add the buttermilk mixture to the flour mix. Mix to blend. Set the batter on the counter for 5 minutes
4. Heat a griddle or skillet. It needs to be hot, but not overly hot. When the griddle is at the right temperature, add a tablespoon of butter.
5. Use half a cup of batter per pancake. Place the batter on the grill. Flip it when the top starts to bubble.
6. Use up the entire batter. Place pancakes on a platter. Top with syrup or confectioners' sugar.

Lunch Recipes

344. ARUGULA SALAD WITH FIGS,PROSCIUTTO, WALNUTS, & PARMESAN

Prep Time: 15 Minutes *Cook Time: 20 Minutes* *Servings: 2*

INGREDIENTS:

- 1/4 cup extra-virgin olive oil
- ounces thinly sliced prosciutto, cut into 1/4-inch-wide ribbons
- 3 Tbsps. balsamic vinegar
- 1 Tbsp. raspberry jam
- 1/2 cup dried figs stemmed & chopped into 1/4-inch pieces 1 small shallot, minced
- 5 ounces (5 cups) baby arugula
- 1/2 cup walnuts, toasted & chopped
- ounces Parmesan cheese, shaved into thin strips with a vegetable peeler (1 cup)

TECHNIQUE:

1. Heat 1 Tbsp. Oil in 10-inch nonstick pan over medium heat; Include prosciutto & fry till crisp, frequently stirring, about 7 mins. Using a slotted spoon, Shift to a paper towel-lined plate & set it aside to let cool.
2. Whisk vinegar & jam in a medium microwave-safe container stir in figs. Then, cover with plastic wrap, and cut several steam vents in plastic, & microwave on high till figs are plump, 30 seconds to 1 min. Whisk in the remaining 3 Tbsps. Oil, shallot, 1/4 Tsp. Salt, & 1/8 Tsp. Pepper; toss to combine. Let cool to room temperature.
3. Toss arugula & vinaigrette in a large container; season with salt & pepper to taste. Divide salad into different plates. Then top each with a portion of prosciutto, walnuts, & Parmesan. Serve immediately.

345. ARUGULA SALAD WITH GRAPES, FENNEL, GORGONZOLA, & PECANS

Prep Time: *15 Minutes* *Cook Time:* *40 Minutes* *Servings: 2*

INGREDIENTS:

- Tbsps. white wine vinegar
- Tbsps. extra-virgin olive oil
- 1 small shallot, minced
- 4 Tips. apricot jam
- Salt & pepper
- 1/2 small fennel bulb, fronds chopped (1/4 cup), stalks discarded, bulb sliced very thin (1 cup) 5 ounces (5 cups) baby arugula
- ounces red seedless grapes, halved lengthwise (1 cup)
- 3 ounces Gorgonzola cheese, crumbled (3/4 cup)
- 1/2 cup pecans, toasted & chopped

TECHNIQUE:

1. Whisk vinegar, oil, shallot, jam, 1/4 Tsp. Salt, & 1/4 Tsp. Pepper in a large container. Toss fennel bulb with vinaigrette; let stand 15 mins. Include arugula, fennel fronds, & grapes; toss & season with salt & pepper to taste. Divide individual salad plates; top each with a portion of Gorgonzola & pecans. Serve immediately.

346. ARUGULA SALAD WITH ORANGES, FETA, & SUGARED PISTACHIOS

Prep Time: *15 Minutes* *Cook Time:* *43 Minutes* *Servings: 2*

INGREDIENTS:

- 1/2 cup shelled pistachios
- large egg white, lightly beaten 1/3 cup sugar
- 2 large oranges
- 3 Tbsps. extra-virgin olive oil
- Tbsps. Plus 2 Tips. lemon juice
- 5 Tips. orange marmalade
- 1 small shallot, minced
- 1 Tbsp. minced fresh mint Salt & pepper
- 5 ounces (5 cups) baby arugula
- 3 ounces feta cheese, crumbled (3/4 cup)

TECHNIQUE:

1. Line 8-inch square baking cooking wok with parchment paper. Set oven rack to middle setting & heat oven to 325 degrees. Toss pistachios with egg white in a small container. Using a slotted spoon, Shift nuts to the prepared baking pan; discard excess egg white. Include sugar & stir till nuts are completely coated. Bake, stirring batter every 5 to 10 mins, till coating turns a nutty brown, 25 to 30 mins. Shift nuts to plate in a single layer & let cool.
2. Peel oranges cut them into segments, then halve segments & drain to remove excess juice. Whisk oil, lemon juice, marmalade, shallot, mint, 1/4 Tsp. Salt, & 1/8 Tsp. Pepper in a large container. Include arugula & oranges; toss & season with salt & pepper to taste. Divide salad into individual plates; top each with a portion of feta & sugared pistachios. Serve immediately.

347. ARUGULA SALAD WITH PEAR, ALMONDS, GOAT CHEESE, & APRICOTS

Prep Time: *15 Minutes* *Cook Time:* *50 Minutes* *Servings: 2*

INGREDIENTS:

- Tbsps. white wine vinegar
- 1 Tbsp. apricot jam
- 1/2 cup dried apricots, chopped into 1/4-inch pieces
- Tbsps. extra-virgin olive oil
- 1 small shallot, minced
- 1/4 small red onion, sliced very thin
- Salt & pepper
- 5 ounces (5 cups) baby arugula
- pear halved, cored, & sliced into 1/4-inch-thick slices 1/3 cup sliced almonds, toasted
- 3 ounces goat cheese, crumbled (3/4 cup)

TECHNIQUE:

1. Whisk vinegar & jam in a medium microwave-safe container; stir in apricots. Cover with plastic wrap, cut several steam vents in plastic, & microwave on high till apricots are plump, 30 seconds to 1 min. Whisk in oil, shallot, onion, 1/4 Tsp. Salt, & 1/8 Tsp. Pepper; toss to combine. Let cool to room temperature.
2. Toss arugula, pear, & vinaigrette in a large container; season with salt & pepper to taste. Divide salad into different individual plates; top each with a portion of almonds & goat cheese. Serve immediately.

348. SALAD WITH APPLE, CELERY, HAZELNUTS, & ROQUEFORT

Prep Time: *15 Minutes* *Cook Time:* *53 Minutes* *Servings: 2*

INGREDIENTS:

- Tbsps. cider vinegar
- Tbsps. extra-virgin olive oil
- 1 Tbsp. honey Salt & pepper
- 1 Braeburn or Fuji apple, cored, halved, & sliced very thin 2 celery ribs, sliced very thin on the bias
- 1 head red or green leaf lettuce (12 ounces), torn into bite-size pieces
- 1/4 cup chopped parsley
- 1/2 cup hazelnuts, toasted, skinned, & chopped fine
- ounces Roquefort cheese, crumbled (1 1/2 cups)

TECHNIQUE:

1. Whisk vinegar, oil, honey, 1/4 Tsp. Salt, & 1/8 Tsp. Pepper in a small container till combined. In a medium container, toss apple & celery with 2 Tbsps. Vinaigrette; let stand 5 mins.
2. Toss lettuce, parsley, & remaining vinaigrette in a large container; season with salt & pepper to taste. Divide greens among individual plates; top each with a portion of apple batter, nuts, & Roquefort. Serve immediately.

349. SALAD WITH FENNEL, DRIED CHERRIES, WALNUTS, & ROQUEFORT

Prep Time: *17 Minutes* *Cook Time:* *45 Minutes* *Servings: 2*

INGREDIENTS:

- Tbsps. red wine vinegar
- 2 Tips. honey
- 1/2 cup dried sweet cherries or cranberries
- 3 Tbsps. extra-virgin olive oil
- small fennel bulb, fronds chopped (1/4 cup), stalks discarded, bulb sliced very thin (1 cup)
- small head red or green leaf lettuce (8 ounces), torn into bite-size pieces
- small head radicchio (6 ounces), quartered, cored, & cut crosswise into 1/8-inch-wide strips
- 1/2 cup walnuts, toasted & chopped
- ounces Roquefort cheese, crumbled (1 1/2 cups)

TECHNIQUE:

1. Whisk vinegar & honey in a medium microwave-safe container; stir in cherries. Cover with plastic wrap, cut several steam vents in plastic, & microwave on high till cherries are plump, about 1 min. Whisk in oil, 1/4 Tsp. Salt, & 1/8 Tsp. Pepper; while the batter is still warm, Include sliced fennel bulb & toss to combine. Let cool to room temperature.
2. Toss lettuce, radicchio, fennel fronds, & dried cherry batter in a large container; season to taste with salt & pepper. Divide salad into different individual plates and top each with a portion of nuts & Roquefort. Serve immediately.

350. SALAD WITH ROASTED BEETS, FRIED SHALLOTS, & ROQUEFORT

Prep Time: *16 Minutes* *Cook Time:* *14 Minutes* *Servings: 2*

INGREDIENTS:

- 12 ounces beets, trimmed
- shallots, sliced thin & separated into rings (1 cup)
- 2 Tbsps. all-purpose flour Salt & pepper
- 6 Tbsps. extra-virgin olive oil
- 2 Tbsps. sherry vinegar
- 2 Tips. honey
- 6 ounces (6 cups) baby arugula
- 1 head Boston or Bibb lettuce (8 ounces), torn into bite-size pieces 6 ounces Roquefort cheese, crumbled (1 1/2 cups)

TECHNIQUE:

1. Set oven rack to lower-middle setting; heat oven to 400 degrees. Wrap each beet in aluminium foil & roast till paring knife can be inserted & removed with little resistance, 50 to 60 mins. Unwrap beets. After cooling enough to handle, peel & cut beets into 1/4-inch-thick wedges & place in a medium container.
2. While beets are roasting, toss shallots with flour, 1/4 Tsp. Salt, & 1/8 Tsp. Pepper in a medium container. Heat 3 Tbsps. Oil in 12-inch nonstick pan over medium-high heat till just smoking; Include shallots & cook, frequently stirring, till golden & crisped, about 5 mins. Using a slotted spoon, Shift shallots to a paper towel-lined plate.
3. Whisk the remaining 3 Tbsps. Oil, vinegar, honey, 1/4 Tsp. salt, and 1/8 Tsp. Pepper in a small container till combined. Include 1 Tbsp. Vinaigrette to beets, season beets with salt & pepper to taste, & toss to combine.
4. Toss arugula, lettuce, & remaining vinaigrette in a large container; season with salt & pepper to taste. Divide greens among individual plates; top each with a portion of beets, fried shallots, & Roquefort. Serve immediately.

351. SALAD WITH AVOCADO, TOMATOES, BACON, & ROQUEFORT

Prep Time: *16 Minutes* *Cook Time:* *14 Minutes* *Servings: 2*

INGREDIENTS:

- slices bacon, cut into 1/2-inch pieces
- 3 Tbsps. red wine vinegar
- 3 Tbsps. extra-virgin olive oil Salt & pepper
- 6 ounces cherry tomatoes, halved
- One avocado, halved, pitted, & cut into 1/4-inch pieces 6 ounces (6 cups) baby arugula
- One head Boston or Bibb lettuce (8 ounces), torn into bite-size pieces three scallions, green parts only, sliced thin
- 6 ounces Roquefort cheese, crumbled (1 1/2 cups)

TECHNIQUE:

1. Cook bacon in a 10-inch pan over medium heat till browned & crisped 5 to 7 mins; Shift with a slotted spoon to paper towel-lined plate & set aside.
2. Whisk vinegar, oil, 1/4 Tsp. Salt, & 1/8 Tsp. Pepper in a small container till combined.
3. In a medium container, toss tomatoes & avocado with 1 Tbsp. Vinaigrette, let sit for 5 mins.
4. Toss arugula, lettuce, & remaining vinaigrette in a large container; season with salt & pepper to taste. Divide greens among individual plates; top each with a portion of tomato batter, then sprinkle with a portion of bacon, scallions, & Roquefort. Serve immediately.

352. CLASSIC CAESAR SALAD

Prep Time: *16 Minutes* *Cook Time:* *24 Minutes* *Servings: 2*

INGREDIENTS:

- 2 garlic cloves, peeled
- 5 Tbsps. extra-virgin olive oil
- 1/2-3/4 loaf ciabatta, cut into 3/4-inch cubes (about 5 cups)

- 1/4 cup water
- 1/4 Tsp. salt
- 2 Tbsps. finely grated Parmesan
- 2–3 Tbsps. lemon juice
- 2 large egg yolks
- anchovy fillets, rinsed, patted dry, minced, & mashed to paste with a fork (1 Tbsp.) 1/2 Tsp. Worcestershire sauce
- 5 Tbsps. canola oil
- 5 Tips. extra-virgin olive oil
- 1 1/2 ounces Parmesan, grated fine (3/4 cup)
- Pepper
- 2–3 romaine lettuce hearts (12 to 18 ounces), cut into 3/4-inch pieces, rinsed, & dried

TECHNIQUE:

1. Press garlic with a garlic pressor or grate very fine on a rasp-style grater. Measure out 1/2 Tsp. Garlic paste for croutons & 3/4 Tsp. Garlic paste for dressing (discard remaining garlic). Combine 1 Tbsp. Oil & 1/2 Tsp. Garlic paste in a small container; set aside. Place bread cubes in a large container. Sprinkle with water and Salt. Toss, squeezing gently, so the bread absorbs water. Place remaining 4 Tbsps. Oil & soaked bread cubes in 12-inch nonstick pan. Cook over medium-high heat, frequently stirring, till browned & crisp, 7 to mins.
2. Remove pan from heat, push croutons to sides of pan to clear centre; Include garlic batter to clearing & cook with the residual heat of pan, seconds. Sprinkle with Parmesan; toss till garlic & Parmesan are evenly distributed. Shift croutons to container; set aside.
3. Whisk 2 Tbsps. Lemon juice & reserved 3/4 Tsp. Garlic pastes together in a large container. Let stand 10 mins.
4. Whisk egg yolks, anchovies, & Worcestershire into garlic batter. While constantly whisking, drizzle canola oil & olive oil into the container in a slow, steady stream till fully emulsified. Include 1/2 cup Parmesan & pepper to taste; whisk till incorporated.
5. Include romaine to dressing & toss to coat. Include croutons & mix gently till evenly distributed. Taste & season with an additional 1 Tbsp. Lemon juice. Serve immediately, passing the remaining 1/4 cup Parmesan separately.

353. GRILLED THAI BEEF SALAD

Prep Time:	*Cook Time:*	*Servings: 2*
15 Minutes	*12 Minutes*	

INGREDIENTS:

- Tsp. paprika
- Tsp. cayenne pepper
- Tbsp. white rice
- Tbsps. lime juice (2 limes)
- 2 Tbsps. fish sauce
- 2 Tbsps. water
- 1/2 Tsp. sugar
- 1 (1 1/2-lb) flank steak, trimmed
- Salt & roughly ground white pepper
- 4 shallots, sliced thin
- 1 1/2 cups fresh mint leaves, torn
- 1 1/2 cups fresh cilantro leaves
- Thai chile stemmed, seeded, & sliced thin into rounds seedless English cucumber, sliced 1/4 inch thick on the bias

TECHNIQUE:

1. Heat paprika & cayenne in 8-inch pan over medium heat; cook, shaking the pan, till fragrant, about 1 min. Shift to a small container. Return pan to medium-high heat, Include rice & toast, constantly stirring, till deep golden brown, about 5 mins. Shift to a small container & let cool 5 mins after grinding the rice into a mini food processor, or mortar & pestle till it resembles a fine meal, 10 to 30 seconds.
2. Whisk lime juice, fish sauce, water, sugar, & 1/4 Tsp. toasted Paprika batters in the large container & set aside.
3. 3A. Fully open the bottom vent. Large, lightweight chimney starter filled with charcoal briquettes (6 litres). When the top charcoal is partially covered with ash, pour an even layer over half of the grill. Put the grill in place and close and fully open the vent cover. Heat the grill until it is hot, about 5 minutes.
4. 3B.: Turn all burners to high, cover, & heat grill till hot, about 15 mins. Leave primary burner on high & turn off another burner (s).
5. Clean & oil grate. Season steak with salt & pepper. Place steak on grate over hot part of grill & cook till beginning to char & beads of moisture appear on outer edges of meat, 5 to 6 mins. Flip steak, continue to cook on the second side until meat registers 125 degrees, about 5 minutes longer. Shift to carving board, tent loosely with aluminium foil, & rest for 10 mins (or allow to cool to room temperature, about 1 hr).
6. Line large platter with cucumber slices. Slice of meat, against the grain, on the bias, into 1/4-inch thick slices. Shift sliced steak to the container with fish sauce batter; include shallots, mint, cilantro, chile, & half of rice powder, & toss to combine. Arrange steak over a cucumber-lined platter. Serve, passing remaining rice powder & toasted paprika batter separately.

354. GREEK SALAD

Prep Time:	*Cook Time:*	*Servings: 2*
12 Minutes	*10 Minutes*	

INGREDIENTS:

- 6 Tbsps. olive oil
- 3 Tbsps. red wine vinegar
- Tips. Minced fresh oregano 1 1/2 Tips. lemon juice
- 1 garlic clove, minced 1/2 Tsp. salt
- 1/8 Tsp. pepper
- 1/2 red onion, sliced thin
- cucumber, peeled, halved lengthwise, seeded, & cut into 1/8-inch-thick slices
- 2 romaine lettuce hearts (12 ounces), torn into 1 1/2-inch pieces 2 large tomatoes, cored, seeded, & cut into 12 wedges
- 1/4 cup chopped fresh parsley
- 1/4 cup torn fresh cup of mint jarred roasted red peppers, rinsed, patted dry, & cut into 2 by 1/2-inch strips 1/2 cup large pitted kalamata olives, quartered lengthwise
- ounces feta cheese, crumbled (1 1/4 cup)

TECHNIQUE:

1. Whisk all ingredients in a large container till combined. Include onion & cucumber to vinaigrette & toss; let stand 20 mins.
2. Include romaine, tomatoes, parsley, mint, & peppers to the container with onions & cucumbers; toss to coat with dressing.
3. Shift salad to wide, shallow serving container or platter; sprinkle Olives & feta over salad. Serve immediately.

355. SALAD NIÇOISE

Prep Time:	*Cook Time:*	*Servings: 2*
11 Minutes	*9 Minutes*	

INGREDIENTS:

- 3/4 cup extra-virgin olive oil
- 1/2 cup of lemon juice
- 1 shallot, minced
- Tbsps. minced fresh basil
- 1 Tbsp. minced fresh thyme
- Tips. minced fresh oregano
- 1 Tsp. Dijon mustard Salt & pepper
- 1 1/4 lbs small new red potatoes, quartered
- Salt & pepper
- Tbsps. dry vermouth
- heads Boston lettuce or Bibb lettuce (1 lb), torn into bite-size pieces
- (6-ounce) cans olive oil-packed tuna, drained
- small tomatoes, cored & cut into eighths
- 1 small red onion, sliced very thin
- 8 ounces green beans, trimmed & halved crosswise
- 4 FOOLPROOF HARD-COOKED EGGS, peeled & quartered
- 1/4 cup niçoise olives pitted
- 10–12 anchovy fillets, rinsed (optional)
- 2 Tbsps. capers, rinsed (optional)

TECHNIQUE:

1. Whisk oil, lemon juice, shallot, basil, thyme, oregano, & mustard in the medium container; season with salt & pepper to taste & set aside.
2. Bring potatoes & 4 quarts of cold water to boil in a large Dutch oven or stockpot over high heat. Include 1 Tbsp. Salt & cook till potatoes are tender when poked with a paring knife, 5 to 8 mins. With a slotted spoon, gently Shift potatoes to the medium container (do not discard boiling water). Toss warm potatoes with vermouth & salt & pepper to taste; let stand 1 min. Toss in 1/4 cup vinaigrette; set aside.
3. While potatoes cook, toss lettuce with 1/4 cup vinaigrette in a large container till coated. Set a bed of lettuce on a large, flat serving platter. Place tuna in the now-empty container & break up with a fork. Include 1/2 cup vinaigrette & stir to combine; mound tuna in centre of lettuce. Toss tomatoes, onion, 3 Tbsps. Vinaigrette, & salt & pepper to taste in the now-empty container; arrange tomato-onion batter in the mound at edge of lettuce bed. Arrange reserved potatoes in a separate mound at the edge of the lettuce bed.
4. Return water to boil; Include 1 Tbsp. Salt & green beans. Cook till tender but crisp, 3 to 5 mins. Meanwhile, fill the medium container with 1-quart water & 1 tray of ice cubes. Drain beans, Shift to ice water, & let stand till just cool, about 30 seconds; dry beans well on a triple layer of paper towels. Toss beans, 3 Tbsps. Vinaigrette, & salt & pepper to taste in the now-empty container; arrange in a separate mound at edge of lettuce bed.
5. Arrange eggs, olives, & anchovies, if using, in separate mounds at the edge of the lettuce bed. Drizzle eggs with remaining 2 Tbsps. Sprinkle the whole salad with capers, if using, & serve immediately.

356. CHEF'S SALAD

Prep Time:	*Cook Time:*	*Servings: 2*
12 Minutes	*10 Minutes*	

INGREDIENTS:

- Tbsps. extra-virgin olive oil
- 3 Tbsps. red wine vinegar
- 2 Tips. minced shallot
- 1 garlic clove, minced
- 1 Tsp. minced fresh thyme
- 1/4 Tsp. salt
- 1/8 Tsp. pepper
- cucumber, peeled, halved lengthwise, seeded, & sliced crosswise 1/4 inch thick
- 2 heads leaf lettuce, washed, dried, & torn into bite-size pieces (about 3 quarts) 8 ounces (8 cups) baby arugula
- 6 ounces radishes, trimmed, halved, & sliced thin
- 12 ounces cherry tomatoes, quartered if large
- FOOLPROOF HARD-COOKED EGGS, peeled & quartered
- ounces deli ham, sliced 1/4 inch thick & cut into 2-inch-long matchsticks
- ounces deli turkey, sliced 1/4 inch thick & cut into 2-inch-long matchsticks
- ounces sharp cheddar cheese, sliced 1/4 inch thick & cut into 2-inch-long matchsticks 1 1/2 cups GARLIC CROUTONS

TECHNIQUE:

2. Whisk all ingredients in a medium container till combined. Include cucumber to vinaigrette & toss; let stand 20 mins.
3. Toss lettuce, arugula, & radishes in a large, wide serving container. Include cucumbers & all but 1 Tbsp. Dressing & toss to combine. Season with salt & pepper to taste.
4. Remaining dressing in the container; arrange tomatoes around the perimeter of greens. Arrange egg wedges in-ring inside tomatoes & drizzle with any dressing in the container. Arrange ham, turkey, & cheese over the centre of greens; sprinkle with croutons & serve immediately.

357. CHEF'S SALAD WITH FENNEL, ASIAGO, & SALAMI

Prep Time:	*Cook Time:*	*Servings: 2*
12 Minutes	*10 Minutes*	

INGREDIENTS:

- Tbsps. extra-virgin olive oil
- 3 Tbsps. balsamic vinegar
- 1 Tsp. minced garlic
- 1/4 Tsp. salt
- 1/8 Tsp. pepper
- heads romaine lettuce (1 1/2 lbs), torn into bite-size pieces
- 4 ounces (4 cups) watercress, torn into 2-inch pieces
- 1 small fennel bulb, stalks discarded, halved, cored, & sliced thin
- 1/2 cup chopped fresh parsley
- cup jarred roasted red peppers, rinsed, patted dry, & cut crosswise into 1/2-inch-wide strips

- (14-ounce) can artichoke hearts, drained & halved
- ounces hard salami sliced 1/4 inch thick & cut into 2-inch-long matchsticks
- ounces deli turkey sliced 1/4 inch thick & cut into 2-inch-long matchsticks
- ounces Asiago cheese, crumbled (2 cups)
- 1 1/2 cups GARLIC CROUTONS
- 1/2 cup pitted kalamata olives, chopped

TECHNIQUE:

1. Whisk all ingredients in a medium container till combined.
2. Toss romaine, watercress, fennel, & parsley in a large serving container. Include all but 1 Tbsp. dressing & toss to Combine. Season with salt & pepper to taste. Toss peppers & artichokes in the remaining dressing, then arrange around the perimeter of greens. Arrange salami, turkey, & cheese over the centre of greens; top with croutons & olives. Serve immediately.

358. CHEF'S SALAD WITH SPINACH, CHICKEN, & GOUDA

Prep Time: *12 Minutes* | *Cook Time:* *10 Minutes* | *Servings: 2*

INGREDIENTS:

- Tbsps. extra-virgin olive oil
- 3 Tbsps. sherry vinegar
- 2 Tips. Dijon mustard
- 1 garlic clove, minced
- 1/4 Tsp. salt
- 1/8 Tsp. pepper
- slices thick-cut bacon, cut into 1/4-inch pieces
- 14 ounces (14 cups) flat-leaf spinach
- 1 small head radicchio (6 ounces), leaves separated & cut into 1/2-inch strips
    - Belgian endive (4 ounces), halved, cored, & cut crosswise into 1/2-inch strips (about 1 cup)
- 1/2 cup of fresh basil leaves, divided into bite-size pieces 1/2 red onion, sliced very thin
    - avocados, halved, pitted, & cut into 1/2-inch pieces
- ounces deli chicken breast sliced 1/4 inch thick & cut into 2-inch-long matchsticks
- ounces Gouda cheese (regular or smoked), sliced 1/4 inch thick & cut into 2-inch-long matchsticks
- 1/2 cups GARLIC CROUTONS

TECHNIQUE:

1. Whisk all ingredients in a medium container till combined.
2. Cook bacon in a 10-inch pan over medium heat, occasionally stirring, till crisp, 5 to 7 mins. Shift to a paper towel-lined plate. Combine spinach, radicchio, endive, & basil in a large serving container. Include onion & all but 1 Tbsp. Dressing & toss to combine. Season with salt & pepper to taste. Toss avocados in the remaining dressing in the container; arrange avocados around the perimeter of greens. Arrange Chicken & cheese over centre of greens; sprinkle with bacon & croutons & serve immediately.
3.

Dinner Recipes

359. FENNEL & APPLE CHOPPED SALAD

Prep Time: *11 Minutes* | *Cook Time:* *9 Minutes* | *Servings: 2*

INGREDIENTS:

- cucumber, peeled, halved lengthwise, seeded, & cut into 1/2-inch dice Salt & pepper
- Tbsps. extra-virgin olive oil
- Tbsps. white wine vinegar
- fennel bulb stalks discarded, halved, cored, & cut into 1/4-inch dice
- 2 apples, cored & cut into 1/4-inch dice
- 1/2 small red onion, chopped fine
- 1/4 cup chopped fresh tarragon
- romaine lettuce heart (6 ounces), cut into 1/2-inch pieces 1/2 cup walnuts, toasted & chopped
- 4 ounces goat cheese, crumbled (1 cup)

TECHNIQUE:

1. Combine cucumber & 1/2 Tsp. Salt in a colander set over container & let stands 15 mins.
2. Whisk oil & vinegar together in a large container. Include drained cucumber, fennel, apples, onion, & tarragon; toss & let stand at room temperature to blend flavours, 5 mins.
3. Include romaine & walnuts; toss to combine. Season with salt & pepper to taste. Divide salad among plates; top each with some goat cheese & serve.

360. MEDITERRANEAN CHOPPED SALAD

Prep Time: *11 Minutes* | *Cook Time:* *9 Minutes* | *Servings: 2*

INGREDIENTS:

- cucumber, peeled, halved lengthwise, seeded, & cut into 1/2-inch dice
- 10 ounces grape tomatoes, quartered salt & pepper
- 3 Tbsps. extra-virgin olive oil
- 3 Tbsps. red wine vinegar
- garlic clove, minced
- (15-ounce) can chickpeas, rinsed
- 1/2 cup pitted kalamata olives, chopped
- 1/2 small red onion, chopped fine
- 1/2 cup chopped fresh parsley
- romaine lettuce heart (6 ounces), cut into 1/2-inch pieces
- 4 ounces feta cheese, crumbled (1 cup)

TECHNIQUE:

1. Combine cucumber, tomatoes, & 1 Tsp. Salt in a colander set over container & let stands 15 mins.
2. Whisk oil, vinegar, & garlic together in a large container. Include drained cucumber & tomatoes, chickpeas, olives, onion, & parsley; toss & let stand at room temperature to blend flavours, 5 mins.
3. Include romaine & feta; toss to combine. Season with salt & pepper to taste & serve.

361. PEAR & CRANBERRY CHOPPED SALAD

Prep Time: *12 Minutes* | *Cook Time:* *10 Minutes* | *Servings: 2*

INGREDIENTS:

- cucumber, peeled, halved lengthwise, seeded, & cut into 1/2-inch dice Salt & pepper
- Tbsps. extra-virgin olive oil
- Tbsps. sherry vinegar
- red bell pepper stemmed, seeded, & cut into 1/4-inch pieces
- ripe but firm pear cut into 1/4-inch pieces
- 1/2 small red onion, chopped fine
- 1/2 cup dried cranberries
- romaine lettuce heart (6 ounces), cut into 1/2-inch pieces
- 4 ounces blue cheese, crumbled (1 cup)
- 1/2 cup shelled pistachios, toasted & chopped

TECHNIQUE:

1. Combine cucumber & 1/2 Tsp. Salt in a colander set over container & let stands 15 mins.
2. Whisk oil & vinegar together in a large container. Include drained cucumber, bell pepper, pear, onion, & cranberries; toss & let stand at room temperature to blend flavours, 5 mins.
3. Include romaine, blue cheese, & pistachios; toss to combine. Season with salt & pepper to taste & serve.

362. RADISH & ORANGE CHOPPED SALAD

Prep Time: *11 Minutes* | *Cook Time:* *9 Minutes* | *Servings: 2*

INGREDIENTS:

- cucumber, peeled, halved lengthwise, seeded, & cut into 1/2-inch dice Salt & pepper
- Tbsps. extra-virgin olive oil
- Tbsps. lime juice (2 limes)
- 1 garlic clove, minced
- 2 oranges
- 10 radishes, halved & sliced thin
- avocado, halved, pitted, & cut into 1/2-inch pieces 1/2 small red onion, chopped fine
- 1/2 cup fresh cilantro, chopped
- romaine lettuce heart (6 ounces), cut into 1/2-inch pieces
- 3 ounces Manchego cheese, shredded (3/4 cup)

TECHNIQUE:

1. Combine cucumber & 1/2 Tsp. Salt in a colander set over container & let stands 15 mins. Whisk oil, lime juice, & garlic together in a large container.
2. Peel oranges, making sure to remove all pith, & cut into 1/2-inch pieces. Include oranges, drained cucumber, radishes, avocado, onion, & cilantro; toss & let stand at room temperature to blend flavours, 5 mins.
3. Include lettuce, cheese, & pepitas; toss to combine. Season with salt & pepper to taste & serve.

363. CLASSIC COBB SALAD

Prep Time: *11 Minutes* | *Cook Time:* *9 Minutes* | *Servings: 2*

INGREDIENTS:

- 1/2 cup extra-virgin olive oil
- Tbsps. red wine vinegar
- Tips. lemon juice
- Tsp. Worcestershire sauce
- Tsp. Dijon mustard
- garlic clove, minced
- 1/2 Tsp. salt
- 1/4 Tsp. sugar
- 1/8 Tsp. pepper
- 3 boneless, skinless chicken breasts, trimmed salt & pepper
- large head romaine lettuce (14 ounces), torn into bite-size pieces
- 4 ounces (4 ounces) watercress, torn into bite-size pieces
- 10 ounces grape tomatoes, halved
- FOOLPROOF HARD-COOKED EGGS, peeled & cut into 1/2-inch cubes
- 2 avocados, halved, pitted, & cut into 1/2-inch pieces
- slices bacon, cut into 1/4-inch pieces, cooked in a 10-inch pan over medium heat till crisp, 5 to 7 mins, & drained
- ounces blue cheese, crumbled (1/2 cup)
- 3 Tbsps. minced fresh chives

TECHNIQUE:

1. Whisk all ingredients in a medium container Till well combined; set aside.
2. Season chicken with salt & pepper. Set oven rack to 6 inches from the broiler element; heat broiler. Spray broiler-pan top with vegetable oil spray; place chicken breasts on top & broil chicken till lightly browned 4 to 8 mins. Using tongs, flip chicken over & continue to broil till thickest part is no longer pink when cut into & registers about 160 degrees, 6 to 8 mins. When cool enough, cut the chicken into 1/2-inch cubes & set aside.
3. Toss romaine & watercress with 5 Tbsps. Vinaigrette in a large container till coated; arrange on a very large, flat serving platter. Place chicken in the now-empty container, Include 1/4 cup vinaigrette & toss to coat; arrange in a row along one edge of greens. Place tomatoes in a now-empty container, Include 1 Tbsp. Vinaigrette & toss gently to combine; arrange on the opposite edge of greens. Arrange eggs & avocado in separate rows near the centre of greens & drizzle with the remaining vinaigrette. Sprinkle bacon, cheese, & chives evenly over salad & serve immediately.

364. HERBED BAKED GOAT CHEESE

Prep Time: *11 Minutes* | *Cook Time:* *9 Minutes* | *Servings: 2*

INGREDIENTS:

- ounces white Melba toasts (2 cups)
- 1 Tsp. pepper
- large eggs
- 2 Tbsps. Dijon mustard
- Tbsp. minced fresh thyme

- Tbsp. minced fresh chives
- 12 ounces goat cheese, firm Extra-virgin olive oil

TECHNIQUE:

1. In a food processor Process Melba toasts to fine even crumbs, about 1 1/2 mins; Shift crumbs to a medium container & stir in pepper. Whisk eggs & mustard in a medium container till combined. Combine thyme & chives in a small container.
2. Using dental floss or dental floss, cut the cheese into 12 equal pieces. Roll each piece into a ball. Roll the balls one by one over the seasoning and cover lightly. Put 6 eggs on top of the egg mixture and turn it over to coat evenly. Transfer to the melba breadcrumbs, flip each piece and slide the breadcrumbs into the cheese. Roll each and every ball into a disk about 1/2 inch wide and 1 inch thick and place it on a baking sheet. Repeat this process with the remaining 6 kinds of cheese. Freeze the cheese until it becomes firm, about 30 minutes. Set the oven rack to a high setting. Preheat oven to 475 degrees.
3. Remove cheese from freezer & brush tops & sides evenly with olive oil. Bake till crumbs are golden brown & cheese is slightly soft, 7 to 9 mins (or 9 to 12 mins if cheese is completely frozen). Using Thin metal spatula, Shift cheese to paper towel-lined plate & let cool 3 mins before serving on top of greens.

365. SALAD WITH HERBED BAKED GOAT CHEESE & VINAIGRETTE

Prep Time: *12 Minutes* | *Cook Time:* *10 Minutes* | *Servings: 2*

INGREDIENTS:

- Tbsps. red wine vinegar
- 1 Tbsp. Dijon mustard
- 1 Tsp. minced shallot
- 1/4 Tsp. salt
- Tbsps. extra-virgin olive oil Pepper
- ounces (14 cups) mixed hearty salad greens
- 1 recipe HERBED BAKED GOAT CHEESE

TECHNIQUE:

1. Combine vinegar, mustard, shallot, & salt in a small container. Whisking constantly, drizzle in oil; season with pepper to taste.
2. Place greens in a large container, drizzle vinaigrette over, & toss to coat. Divide greens among individual plates; place 2 rounds of warm goat cheese on each salad. Serve immediately.

366. SALAD WITH APPLES, WALNUTS, DRIED CHERRIES, & HERBED BAKED GOAT CHEESE

Prep Time: *12 Minutes* | *Cook Time:* *10 Minutes* | *Servings: 2*

INGREDIENTS:

- 1 cup dried cherries
- Tbsps. cider vinegar
- 1 Tbsp. Dijon mustard
- 1 Tsp. minced shallot
- 1/4 Tsp. salt
- 1/4 Tsp. sugar
- Tbsps. extra-virgin olive oil Pepper
- 14 ounces (14 cups) mixed hearty salad greens
- Granny Smith apples, cored, quartered, & cut into 1/8-inch-thick slices 1/2 cup walnuts, toasted & chopped
- 1 recipe HERBED BAKED GOAT CHEESE
- Plump cherries in 1/2 cup hot water in a small container, about 10 mins; drain.

TECHNIQUE:

1. Combine vinegar, mustard, shallot, salt, & sugar in a small container. Whisking constantly, drizzle in oil; season with pepper to taste. Place greens in a large container, drizzle vinaigrette over, & toss to coat. Divide greens among individual plates; divide cherries, apples, & walnuts among plates; & place 2 rounds of goat cheese on each salad. Serve immediately.

367. SALAD WITH GRAPES, PINE NUTS, PROSCIUTTO, & HERBED BAKED GOAT CHEESE

Prep Time: *14 Minutes* | *Cook Time:* *12 Minutes* | *Servings: 2*

INGREDIENTS:

- Tbsps. balsamic vinegar
- 1 Tbsp. Dijon mustard
- 1 Tsp. minced shallot
- 1/4 Tsp. salt
- Tbsps. extra-virgin olive oil Pepper
- ounces (14 cups) mixed hearty salad greens 1 1/4 cups red seedless grapes, halved
- 1/2 cup pine nuts, toasted
- 6 ounces thinly sliced prosciutto
- 1 recipe HERBED BAKED GOAT CHEESE

TECHNIQUE:

1. Combine vinegar, mustard, shallot, & salt in a small container. Whisking constantly, drizzle in oil; season with pepper to taste. Place greens in a large container, drizzle vinaigrette over, & toss to coat. Divide greens among individual plates; divide grapes & pine nuts among plates; & arrange 2 slices of prosciutto & 2 rounds of goat cheese on every salad. Serve immediately.

368. FRESH SPINACH SALAD WITH CARROT, ORANGE, & SESAME

Prep Time: *11 Minutes* | *Cook Time:* *9 Minutes* | *Servings: 2*

INGREDIENTS:

- 6 ounces (6 cups) baby spinach
- carrots, peeled & shaved with vegetable peeler lengthwise into ribbons
- oranges, 1/2 Tsp. finely grated zest from one, both peeled & segmented
- scallions, sliced thin
- Tips. rice vinegar
- 1 small shallot, minced
- 1 Tsp. Dijon mustard
- 3/4 Tsp. mayonnaise
- 1/4 Tsp. salt
- 3 Tbsps. vegetable oil
- 1 1/2 Tbsps. toasted sesame oil
- Tbsp. sesame seeds, toasted

TECHNIQUE:

1. Place spinach, carrots, orange segments, & scallions in large container.
2. Combine orange zest, vinegar, shallot, mustard, mayonnaise, & salt in a small container. Whisk till batter appears milky & no lumps remain. Place vegetable oil & sesame oil in a liquid measuring cup. Whisking constantly, very slowly drizzle oils into the batter. If pools of oil gather over the top, stop the addition of oils & whisk batter well to combine, then resume whisking in oils in a slow stream. The vinaigrette should be glossy & lightly thickened.
3. Pour dressing over spinach batter & toss to coat; sprinkle with sesame seeds & serve immediately.

369. FRESH SPINACH SALAD WITH FENNEL & APPLES

Prep Time: *12 Minutes* | *Cook Time:* *10 Minutes* | *Servings: 2*

INGREDIENTS:

- 6 ounces (6 cups) baby spinach
- fennel bulb, fronds minced & 1/4 cup reserved, stalks discarded, bulb halved, cored, & sliced thin
- Golden Delicious apples, cored & cut into 1-inch-long matchsticks 1 1/2 Tips. Finely grated lemon zest plus 7 Tips. juice
- 1 small shallot, minced
- 1 Tbsp. Whole grain mustard 3/4 Tsp. mayonnaise
- 1/4 Tsp. salt
- 4 1/2 Tbsps. extra-virgin olive oil

TECHNIQUE:

1. Place spinach, fennel, fennel fronds, & apples in a large container.
2. Combine lemon zest & juice, shallot, mustard, mayonnaise, & salt in a small container. Whisk till batter appears milky & no lumps remain. Place oil in the liquid measuring cup. Whisking constantly, and very slowly drizzle oil into the batter. When pools of oil gather on the surface, stop the addition of oil & whisk batter well to combine, then resume whisking in oil in a slow stream. The vinaigrette should be glossy & lightly thickened.
3. Pour dressing over spinach batter & toss to coat. Serve immediately.

370. FRESH SPINACH SALAD WITH FRISÉE & STRAWBERRIES

Prep Time: *12 Minutes* | *Cook Time:* *10 Minutes* | *Servings: 2*

INGREDIENTS:

- 6 ounces (6 cups) baby spinach
- 1 head frisée (6 ounces) torn into 2-inch pieces
- ounces strawberries, hulled & quartered (2 cups)
- 2 Tbsps. chopped fresh basil
- 7 Tips. balsamic vinegar
- 1 small shallot, minced
- 1 Tsp. Dijon mustard
- 3/4 Tsp. mayonnaise
- 1/4 Tsp. salt
- 1/2 Tsp. pepper
- 4 1/2 Tbsps. extra-virgin olive oil

TECHNIQUE:

1. 2Place spinach, frisée, strawberries, & basil in a large container.
2. Combine vinegar, shallot, mustard, mayonnaise, salt, & pepper in a small container. Whisk till batter appears milky & no lumps remain. Place oil in the liquid measuring cup. Whisking continuously, very slowly drizzle oil into the batter. If pools of oil gather on the surface, stop the addition of oil & whisk batter well to combine, then resume whisking in oil in a slow stream. The vinaigrette should be glossy & lightly thickened.
3. Pour dressing over spinach batter & toss to coat. Serve immediately.

371. FRESH SPINACH SALAD WITH RADICCHIO & MANGO

Prep Time: *15 Minutes* | *Cook Time:* *35 Minutes* | *Servings: 2*

INGREDIENTS:

- 6 ounces (6 cups) baby small spinach head radicchio (6 ounces), halved, cored, & sliced very thin
- mango, peeled & cut into 1/2-inch pieces
- 1/4 cup chopped fresh cilantro
- Tsp. Finely grated lime zest plus 7 Tips. juice
- Tbsp. honey
- small shallot, minced
- Tsp. Dijon mustard
- 3/4 Tsp. mayonnaise
- 1/4 Tsp. salt
- 4 1/2 Tbsps. extra-virgin olive oil

TECHNIQUE:

1. Place spinach, radicchio, mango, & cilantro in a large container.
2. Combine lime zest & juice, honey, shallot, mustard, mayonnaise, & salt in a small container. Whisk till batter appears milky & no lumps remain. Place oil in a liquid measuring cup, so it is easy to pour. Whisking constantly, very slowly drizzle oil into the batter. If pools of oil gather on the surface, stop the addition of oil & whisk batter well to combine, then resume whisking in oil in a slow stream. The vinaigrette should be glossy & lightly thickened.
3. Pour dressing over spinach batter & toss to coat. Serve immediately.

372. WILTED SPINACH SALAD WITH WARM BACON DRESSING

Prep Time: *11 Minutes* | *Cook Time:* *9 Minutes* | *Servings: 2*

INGREDIENTS:

- ounces (6 cups) baby spinach
- 3 Tbsps. cider vinegar
- 1/2 Tsp. sugar
- 1/4 Tsp. pepper
- slices thick-cut bacon, cut into 1/2-inch pieces
- 1/2 red onion, chopped medium
- 1 small garlic clove, minced
- 3 FOOLPROOF HARD-COOKED EGGS, peeled & quartered

TECHNIQUE:

1. Place spinach in a large container. Stir vinegar, sugar, pepper, & salt together in a small container till sugar dissolves; set aside.
2. Cook bacon in a 10-inch pan over medium-high heat, occasionally stirring, till crisp, about 5 mins. Using a slotted spoon, Shift bacon to a paper towel-lined plate. Add the fat into a heatproof container, then return 3 Tbsps. Fat to the pan. Include onion to pan & cook over medium heat, frequently stirring, till slightly softened, about 3 mins; stir in garlic till fragrant, about 15 seconds. Include vinegar batter, then remove the pan from heat; working quickly, scrape the bottom of the pan by using a wooden spoon to loosen browned bits. Pour hot dressing over spinach, Include bacon, & toss gently with tongs till spinach is slightly wilted. Divide among individual plates, arrange egg quarters over each, & serve.

373. CREAMY DILL CUCUMBER SALAD

Prep Time: *11 Minutes* | *Cook Time:* *9 Minutes* | *Servings: 2*

INGREDIENTS:

- cucumbers (2 lbs), peeled, halved lengthwise, seeded, & sliced 1/4 inch thick
- 1 small red onion, sliced very thin
- 1 Tbsp. salt
- 1 cup sour cream
- Tbsps. cider vinegar
- 1 Tsp. sugar
- 1/4 cup minced fresh dill

TECHNIQUE:

1. Toss cucumber & onion with salt in a colander set over a large container. Weight cucumbers with a gallon-size zipper-lock bag filled with water; drain for 1 to 3 hrs. Rinse & pat dry.
2. Whisk constantly the remaining ingredients together in a medium container. Include cucumbers & onion; toss to coat. Serve chilled.

Side Dishes Recipes

374. BAKED REUBEN

Prep Time: *15 Minutes* | *Cook Time:* *50 Minutes* | *Servings: 2*

INGREDIENTS:

- 1 jar (32 ounces) sauerkraut, rinsed and well-drained 10 ounces sliced deli corned beef, chopped
- 2 mugs (8 ounces) shredded sharp cheddar cheese 2 mugs (8 ounces) shredded Swiss cheese
- 1 mug mayonnaise
- ¼ mug Russian salad dressing 1 tsp caraway seeds, optional Rye crackers

DIRECTIONS:

1. In a bowl, combine together the first six ingredients all together; stir in caraway seeds, if desired. Transfer to a greased 13x9-in. Baking dish. Bake at 350°
2. if desired. Transfer to a greased 13x9-in. Baking dish. Bake it at least 350° for 25-30 minutes or until bubbly. Serve dip with rye crackers.

375. FUN-DO FONDUE

Prep Time: *15 Minutes* | *Cook Time:* *45 Minutes* | *Servings: 2*

INGREDIENTS:

- 2 mugs (8 ounces) shredded Jarlsberg cheese
- ½ mug shredded Swiss cheese
- ¼ mug all-purpose flour
- ½ tsp ground mustard
- ½ tsp freshly ground pepper
- 1 mug heavy whipping cream
- 1 mug reduced-sodium chicken broth
- 1 tbsp honey
- 1 tsp of lemon juice
- Cubed French bread, sliced pears as well as assorted fresh vegetables

DIRECTIONS:

1. In a bowl, combine together the first five ingredients all together; toss to mix. In a saucepan, mix cream, broth and honey; bring just to a boil, stirring occasionally. Reduce heat to medium-low. Add ½ mug cheese mixture; constantly stir until almost completely melted. Continue adding cheese, ½ mug at a time, allowing the cheese to almost melt completely between additions. Stirring continuously until thickened and smooth. Stir in lemon juice.
2. Convert mixture to a heated fondue pot; keep fondue bubbling smoothly. Serve it with bread, pears and vegetables for dipping. If fondue becomes too thick, stir it continuously in a little additional broth.

376. ROASTED RED PEPPER HUMMUS

Prep Time: *15 Minutes* | *Cook Time:* *20 Minutes* | *Servings: 2*

INGREDIENTS:

- 2 large sweet red peppers
- 2 cans of garbanzo beans, rinsed as well as drained 1/3 mug lemon juice 3 tbsps tahini
- 1 tbsp olive oil
- 2 garlic cloves, peeled
- 1 ¼ tsp salt 1 tsp curry powder
- ½ tsp ground coriander ½ tsp ground cumin ½ tsp pepper Pita bread, warmed and cut into wedges, and reduced-fat wheat snack crackers Additional garbanzo beans or chickpeas, optional 1.

DIRECTIONS:

1. Bake the red chillies for about 5 minutes to 4 inches of heat until the skin blisters. Turn the pepper 1/4 turn with tongs. baking
2. Rotate until all sides are blistered and black. Immediately put the peppers in a bowl. Cover and leave for 15-20 minutes.
3. Peel off the burnt skin and discard. Extract the stems and seeds. Put the peppers in the food processor. Add nuts, lemon juice, tahini, oil, garlic and seasoning. Cover and process until smooth.
4. Transfer to a serving bowl. Serve with pita bread and crackers. Garnish with additional nuts if desired.

377. TROPICAL DIP

Prep Time: *15 Minutes* | *Cook Time:* *25 Minutes* | *Servings: 2*

INGREDIENTS:

- 1 can (8 ounces) crushed pineapple, undrained
- 1 pkg (3.4 ounces) of instant vanilla pudding mix
- ¾ mug cold 2% milk ½ mug flaked coconut ½ mug sour cream Toasted coconut
- Assorted fresh fruit

DIRECTIONS:

1. In a blender, mix the pineapple, pudding mix, milk, coconut and sour cream; cover and process for 30 seconds.
2. Convert to a serving bowl, and cover and let it cool for 30 minutes. Garnish with toasted coconut. Serve with fruit.

378. TOMATILLO SALSA

Prep Time: *15 Minutes* | *Cook Time:* *40 Minutes* | *Servings: 2*

INGREDIENTS:

- 8 tomatillos, husks extracted
- 1 medium tomato, quartered
- 1 small onion, cut into chunks
- 1 jalapeno pepper, seeded
- 3 tbsps fresh cilantro leaves
- 3 garlic cloves, peeled
- 1 tbsp lime juice
- ½ tsp salt ¼ tsp ground cumin 1/8 tsp pepper Tortilla chips

DIRECTIONS:

1. In a large saucepan, bring 4 mugs of water to a boil. Add tomatillos. Reduce heat; simmer, uncovered, for 5 minutes. Drain.
2. Place the tomatillos, tomato, onion, jalapeno, cilantro, garlic, lime juice and seasonings in a food processor. Cover and process until blended. Serve with chips.

NOTE *Wear disposable gloves when dividing hot peppers; the oils can burn skin. Avoid touching your face.*

379. ALMOND "FETA" WITH HERB OIL

Prep Time: ***15 Minutes***

Servings: 2

Cook Time: ***55 Minutes***

INGREDIENTS:

- 1 mug of blanched almonds
- ½ mug water
- ¼ mug lemon juice
- 5 tbsps olive oil, divided
- 1 garlic clove
- 1 ¼ tsp salt
- 1 ½ tsp minced fresh thyme or ½ tsp dried thyme
- ½ tsp minced fresh rosemary or 1/8 tsp dried rosemary, crushed
- Assorted crackers

DIRECTIONS:

1. Almonds in cold water. Put it in a large bowl. Add water to cover 3 inches. Cover and leave overnight.
2. Rinse the almonds and discard the liquid. Transfer to the food processor. Add a cup of water, lemon juice, 3 tbsp oil, garlic and salt. Cover and cook it for about 5-6 minutes or until soft.
3. Place four layers of cotton cloth on a large sieve and place on a large bowl. Spread the almond mixture in the prepared colander. Lift the edges of the fabric and tie them with string to make a bag.
4. Let it cool overnight.
5. Squeeze out any liquid; extract cheesecloth and discard liquid from bowl. convert ball to a parchment paper-lined baking sheet;
6. flatten into a 6-in. circle.
7. Bake it at least 200° for 35-40 minutes or until firm. Cool. Let it cool until chilled.
8. In a skillet, heat the thyme, rosemary and remaining oil over medium heat for 2 minutes. Cool it at 25 degrees. Drizzle over almond mixture. Serve with crackers.

380. YUMMY CHOCOLATE DIP

Prep Time: *Cook Time:* *Servings: 2*
15 Minutes *35 Minutes*

INGREDIENTS:

- ¾ mug semisweet chocolate chips
- 1 carton (8 ounces) whipped topping, divided
- ½ tsp ground cinnamon
- ½ tsp rum extract or vanilla extract Assorted fresh fruit or graham cracker sticks

DIRECTIONS:

1. In a microwave, melt chocolate chips; stir until smooth. Stir in ½ mug whipped topping, cinnamon and extract; cool for 5 minutes.
2. Fold in the remaining whipped topping. Serve with fruit. Let it cool leftovers.

381. PINEAPPLE-PECAN CHEESE SPREAD

Prep Time: *Cook Time:* *Servings: 2*
15 Minutes *22 Minutes*

INGREDIENTS:

- 2 pkg (8 ounces each) of cream cheese, softened
- 1 ½ mug (6 ounces) shredded cheddar cheese 1 mug chopped pecans, toasted, divided
- ¾ mug crushed pineapple, drained 1 can (4 ounces) chopped green chillies, drained
- 2 tbsp chopped roasted sweet red pepper
- ½ tsp garlic powder Assorted fresh vegetables

DIRECTIONS:

1. In a bowl, beat continuously cream cheese until smooth. Add the cheddar cheese, ¾ mug pecans, pineapple, chillies, red pepper and garlic powder; beat until mixed. Transfer to a serving dish. Cover and let it cool until serving.
2. Sprinkle with remaining pecans just before serving. Serve with vegetables.

382. HOT SAUSAGE & BEAN DIP

Prep Time: *Cook Time:* *Servings: 2*
15 Minutes *43 Minutes*

INGREDIENTS:

- 1 pound bulk hot Italian sausage
- 1 medium onion, finely chopped
- 4 garlic cloves, minced
- ½ mug dry white wine or chicken broth ½ tsp dried oregano ¼ tsp salt ¼ tsp of dried thyme
- 1 pkg (8 ounces) of cream cheese, softened
- 1 package (6 ounces) fresh baby spinach, coarsely chopped 1 can (15 ounces) white kidney or cannellini beans, rinsed and drained 1 mug chopped seeded tomatoes
- 1 mug (4 ounces) shredded part-skim mozzarella cheese ½ mug shredded Parmesan cheese Assorted crackers or toasted French bread baguette slices

DIRECTIONS:

1. 1.Preheat oven to 375°. In a large skillet, cook the sausages, onions and garlic over medium heat until the sausages are no longer pink, crushing the sausages into crumbs. Thin. Stir in the wine, oregano, salt and thyme. Take it to a boil and cook until the liquid is almost evaporated.
2. Add cream cheese. Stir until melted. Stir in the spinach, beans and tomatoes. Cook and stir it continuously until the spinach is wilted. Go to a greased 8-inch square or 1 qt. Cake cooking. Sprinkle with cheese.
3. Bake 20-25 minutes or until bubbly. Serve with crackers.

383. AVOCADO SHRIMP SALSA

Prep Time: *Cook Time:* *Servings: 2*
15 Minutes *33 Minutes*

INGREDIENTS:

- 1 pound of peeled as well as deveined cooked shrimp, chopped 2 medium tomatoes, seeded and chopped
- 2 medium ripe avocados, peeled and chopped
- 1 mug minced fresh cilantro
- 1 medium sweet red pepper, chopped
- ¾ mug thinly sliced green onions ½ mug chopped seeded peeled cucumber 3 tbsps lime juice
- 1 jalapeno pepper, seeded and chopped
- 1 tsp salt
- ¼ tsp pepper Tortilla chips

DIRECTIONS:

1. In a bowl, combine together the first 11 ingredients altogether. Serve it with tortilla chips.
2. NOTE Wear disposable gloves when dividing hot peppers; the oils can burn skin. Avoid touching your face.

384. CREAMY WASABI SPREAD

Prep Time: *Cook Time:* *Servings: 2*
15 Minutes *23 Minutes*

INGREDIENTS:

- 1 package (8 ounces) cream cheese
- ¼ mug prepared wasabi 2 tbsps sesame seeds, toasted
- 2 tbsps soy sauce
- Rice crackers

DIRECTIONS:

1. Put cream cheese on a dividing board; split it into two layers. Spread wasabi over the bottom half; replace the top layer.
2. Press both sides into sesame seeds. Place on a shallow serving plate; spread soy sauce around cheese. Serve with crackers

385. PICNIC VEGGIE DIP

Prep Time: *Cook Time:* *Servings: 2*
15 Minutes *23 Minutes*

INGREDIENTS:

- 1 mug mayonnaise
- 1 mug (8 ounces) sour cream
- 1 pkg (1.7 ounces) of vegetable soup mix 1 pkg (10 ounces) of frozen chopped spinach, thawed as well as squeezed dry 1 can of water chestnuts, drained and chopped Assorted fresh vegetables

DIRECTIONS:

1. In a bowl, combine together the mayonnaise, sour cream and soup mix. Stir in spinach and water chestnuts. Cover and let it cool for at least 2 hours. Serve with vegetables.

386. MEDITERRANEAN DIP WITH PITA CHIPS

Prep Time: *Cook Time:* *Servings: 2*
15 Minutes *27 Minutes*

INGREDIENTS:

- 12 pita pocket halves
- Cooking spray
- 1 ¾ tsp garlic powder, divided
- 12 ounces cream cheese, softened
- 1 mug (8 ounces) plain yoghurt
- 1 tsp dried oregano
- ¾ tsp ground coriander
- ¼ tsp pepper
- 1 large tomato, seeded and chopped
- 5 pepperoncini, sliced
- ½ mug pitted Greek olives, sliced
- 1 medium cucumber, seeded and diced
- 1/3 mug crumbled feta cheese
- 2 tbsps minced fresh parsley

DIRECTIONS:

1. 2divide each pita half into three wedges; separate every wedge into two pieces. Place on a non-oiled baking sheet. Spray both sides of the piece with cooking spray. Sprinkle with 1 tsp garlic powder.
2. 3Bake for 5-6 minutes on each side or at 350° minimum until golden brown. Cool on a wire rack.
3. In a bowl, add cream cheese, yoghurt, oregano, coriander, black pepper, and remaining garlic powder and mix. fried food
4. It will be 9 inches. Cake plate. Sprinkle with tomatoes, pepperoncini, olives, cucumbers, feta cheese and parsley. Serve with pita chips.

Note *Look for pepperoncini (pickled peppers) in the pickles and olives section of your grocery store.*

387. SUN-DRIED TOMATO SPREAD

Prep Time: *Cook Time:* *Servings: 2*
15 Minutes *90 Minutes*

INGREDIENTS:

- 2 pkg (8 ounces each) of cream cheese, softened 2 mugs of mayonnaise
- ¼ mug chopped onion 4 garlic cloves, minced
- 1 jar (7 ounces)of oil-packed sun-dried tomatoes, drained and chopped 2/3 mug chopped roasted sweet red peppers 2 mugs (8 ounces) shredded part-skim mozzarella cheese 2 mugs (8 ounces) shredded Italian cheese blend 1 mug shredded Parmesan cheese, divided
- Assorted crackers

DIRECTIONS:

1. In a bowl, add the cream cheese, onion, garlic and mayonnaise, until blended. Stir it continuously in tomatoes as well as red peppers. Now Stir in the mozzarella cheese, Italian cheese blend and ¾ mug of Parmesan cheese.
2. Transfer to a greased 13x9-in. Baking dish. Sprinkle with the remaining Parmesan cheese. Bake, unwrapped, at 350° for 18-22 minutes or until edges are bubbly and lightly browned. Serve with crackers.

Snacks And Appetizer Recipes

388. SWEET GINGERED CHICKEN WINGS

Prep Time: *Cook Time:* *Servings: 2*
15 Minutes *53 Minutes*

INGREDIENTS:

- 1 cup all-purpose flour
- 2 tsp salt
- 2 tsp paprika
- ¼ tsp pepper
- 24 chicken wings (about 5 pounds)
- sauce
- ¼ cup honey
- ¼ cup thawed orange juice concentrate
- ½ tsp ground ginger Minced fresh parsley, optional

Directions:

1. In a big resealable plastic bag, add flour, salt, paprika and pepper. Add chicken wings, a few at a time; seal bag and toss to coat. Divide wings between prepared baking pans. Bake 30 minutes.
2. In a small bowl, add honey, orange juice concentrate and ginger; brush over chicken wings. After baking, 25-30 minutes or until juices run clear. Preheat broiler. Broil wings 4 in. from heat 1-2 minutes or until lightly browned. If desired, sprinkle with parsley.

389. MOTHER LODE PRETZELS

Prep Time: *Cook Time:* *Servings: 2*
15 Minutes *15 Minutes*

INGREDIENTS:

- 1 package (10 ounces) pretzel rods
- 1 package (14 ounces) caramels
- 1 tbsp evaporated milk
- 1 ¼ cups miniature semisweet chocolate chips
- 1 cup plus 2 tbsps butterscotch chips
- 2/3 cup milk chocolate toffee bits
- ¼ cup chopped walnuts

Directions:

1. After cutting pretzel rods in half with a sharp knife, set aside. In a big saucepan over reduce heat, melt caramels with milk. In a large bowl, reduce the dish, adding chips, chips and walnuts.
2. Pour caramel mixture into 2 cups. Add sliced pretzel pieces, each two-thirds of the mixture, to caramel mixture (reheat in the mixer if the mixture is too thick for application). Let the caramel pass, then turn the pretzels into a chip mixture. Place on a covered baking sheet until set.
3. Store in an airtight container.

390. VEGGIE HAM CRESCENT WREATH

Prep Time: 15 Minutes | *Cook Time: 20 Minutes* | *Servings: 2*

INGREDIENTS:

- 2 tubes refrigerated crescent rolls
- ½ cup spreadable pineapple cream cheese
- 1/3 cup diced fully cooked ham
- ¼ cup finely chopped sweet yellow pepper ¼ cup finely chopped green pepper
- ½ cup chopped broccoli florets
- 6 grape tomatoes, quartered
- 1 tbsp chopped red onion

Directions:

1. Remove (do not loosen) the crescent paste from the tube. Cut each roll into eight pieces. Align by 11 inches. Circle the 14 inches without oil. Pizza pan.
2. Set the temperature at 375° and baked for 15-20 minutes or until golden brown. Let it cool for 5 minutes before carefully removing it onto a serving platter. Cool completely.
3. Spread cream cheese over wreath; top with ham, peppers, broccoli, tomatoes and onion. Store in the refrigerator.

391. HONEY-NUT ENDIVE APPETIZERS

Prep Time: 15 Minutes | *Cook Time: 63 Minutes* | *Servings: 2*

INGREDIENTS:

- 1/3 cup crumbled goat cheese 1/3 cup crumbled Gorgonzola cheese 1/3 cup pine nuts
- 1/3 cup chopped walnuts
- 1/3 cup golden raisins
- 4 bacon strips, cooked and crumbled
- 2 heads Belgian endive, separated into leaves
- 1/3 cup honey

Directions:

1. In a small size bowl, add the first six ingredients. Spoon into endive leaves. Spread honey over cheese mixture. Present immediately.

392. CARAMEL APPLE AND BRIE SKEWERS

Prep Time: 15 Minutes | *Cook Time: 60 Minutes* | *Servings: 2*

INGREDIENTS:

- 2 medium apples, cubed
- 1 log (6 ounces) Brie cheese, cubed
- ½ cup hot caramel ice cream topping
- ½ cup finely chopped macadamia nuts
- 2 tbsp dried cranberries

Directions:

2. On each of six wooden appetizer skewers, alternately thread apple and cheese cubes; place on a serving tray. Spread with caramel topping; sprinkle with macadamia nuts and cranberries.

393. THYME-SEA SALT CRACKERS

Prep Time: 15 Minutes | *Cook Time: 40 Minutes* | *Servings: 2*

INGREDIENTS:

- 2 ½ cups all-purpose flour
- ½ cup white whole wheat flour
- 1 tsp salt
- ¾ cup water ¼ cup plus 1 tbsp olive oil, divided 1 to 2 tbsps minced fresh thyme
- ¾ tsp sea or kosher salt 1.

Directions:

1. Remove (do not loosen) the crescent paste from the tube. Cut each roll into eight pieces. Align by 11 inches. Circle the 14 inches without oil. Pizza pan.
2. Set the temperature at 375° and baked for 15-20 minutes or until golden brown. Let it cool for 5 minutes before carefully removing it onto a serving platter. Cool completely.
3. Spread cream cheese over wreath; top with ham, peppers, broccoli, tomatoes and onion. Store in the refrigerator.

394. SEAFOOD SALAD STUFFED SHELLS

Prep Time: 15 Minutes | *Cook Time: 22 Minutes* | *Servings: 2*

INGREDIENTS:

- 1 package (12 ounces) jumbo pasta shells
- 2 packages (8 ounces each) cream cheese, softened
- 1/3 cup mayonnaise 2 tsp sugar
- 1 ½ tsp lemon juice 1/8 tsp salt 1/8 tsp coarsely ground pepper 1/8 tsp cayenne pepper 3 cans (6 ounces each) lump crabmeat, drained
- ½ pound frozen cooked salad shrimp, thawed 12 green onions, finely chopped

Directions:

1. Cook pasta according to directions and drain and rinse in cold water. Cool to room temperature.
2. In a big bowl, add the cream cheese, mayonnaise, sugar, lemon juice, salt, pepper and cayenne. Gently stir in the crab, shrimp and onions. Stuff shells, about 2 tbsps in each. Cover and refrigerate for at least 1 hour.

395. BLUE CHEESE-STUFFED STRAWBERRIES

Prep Time: 15 Minutes | *Cook Time: 35 Minutes* | *Servings: 2*

INGREDIENTS:

- ½ cup balsamic vinegar
- 3 ounces fat-free cream cheese
- ½ cup crumbled blue cheese
- 16 big fresh strawberries
- 3 tbsp finely chopped pecans, toasted

Directions:

1. Place vinegar in a small saucepan. Let it boil cook until liquid is reduced by half. Cool to room temperature.
2. Meanwhile, in a small size bowl, beat cream cheese until smooth. Beat in blue cheese. Remove stems and scoop out centres from strawberries; fill each with about 2 tsp cheese mixture.
3. Sprinkle pecans over filling, pressing lightly. Chill until serving.
4. Spread with balsamic vinegar.

396. CUCUMBER-STUFFED CHERRY TOMATOES

Prep Time: 15 Minutes | *Cook Time: 16 Minutes* | *Servings: 2*

INGREDIENTS:

- 24 cherry tomatoes
- 1 package cream cheese, softened 2 tbsps mayonnaise
- ¼ cup finely chopped peeled cucumber 1 tbsp finely chopped green onion 2 tsp minced fresh dill

Directions:

1. Cut a thin slice off the top of each tomato. Scoop out and discard pulp; invert tomatoes onto paper towels to drain.
2. In a small size bowl, add cream cheese and mayonnaise until smooth; stir in the cucumber, onion and dill. Spoon into tomatoes. Refrigerate until serving.

397. TIERED CHEESE SLICES

Prep Time: 15 Minutes | *Cook Time: 23 Minutes* | *Servings: 2*

INGREDIENTS:

- 1 package (8 ounces) cream cheese, softened
- ½ tsp hot pepper sauce ¼ tsp salt
- ¼ cup chopped pecans
- ¼ cup dried cranberries 2 packages
- deli-style cheddar cheese slices
- Assorted crackers

Directions:

1. In a big bowl, add the cream cheese, hot pepper sauce and salt. Stir in pecans and cranberries.
2. On a 12-in. square of aluminium foil, place two slices of cheese side by side; spread with 2-3 tbsps cream cheese mixture. Repeat layers six times. Top with two cheese slices. Fold foil around cheese and seal tightly. Let it cool for 8 hours or overnight. Cut in half lengthwise and then widthwise into ¼-in. slices. Present with crackers.

398. CRAB-STUFFED SNOW PEAS

Prep Time: 15 Minutes | *Cook Time: 55 Minutes* | *Servings: 2*

INGREDIENTS:

- 1 can crab meat, drained, flaked, and cartilage removed
- 2 tbsps mayonnaise
- 1 tbsp chilli sauce or seafood cocktail sauce
- 1/8 tsp salt
- 3 drops hot pepper sauce
- Dash pepper
- 16 fresh snow peas

Directions:

1. In a small-size bowl, add the crab, mayonnaise, chilli sauce, salt, hot sauce and pepper.
2. Put the snow peas in the steaming basket. Place in a small saucepan over 1 inch of water. Bring to a boil; cover and steam for 30 seconds until tender. Drain the snow peas and immediately drop them into ice water. Drain and dry.
3. Cut the peas along the curved edges with a sharp knife. Spoon each crab mixture 1 tbsp.

399. CUCUMBER RYE SNACKS

Prep Time: 15 Minutes | *Cook Time: 56 Minutes* | *Servings: 2*

INGREDIENTS:

- 1 package (8 ounces) cream cheese, softened
- 2 tbsps mayonnaise
- 2 tsp Italian salad dressing mix
- 30 slices snack rye bread

- 30 thin slices of cucumber
- Fresh dill sprigs and chive blossoms

Directions:

1. In a bowl, beat the cream cheese, mayonnaise and dressing mix until blended. Let stand for 30 minutes.
2. Spread mixture on rye bread. Top each with a slice of cucumber, dill sprig and chive blossom. Cover and refrigerate until serving.

400. ASIAN TUNA BITES WITH DIJON DIPPING SAUCE

Prep Time:	*Cook Time:*	*Servings: 2*
15 Minutes	*89 Minutes*	

INGREDIENTS:

- 3 tbsps Dijon mustard
- 2 tbsps red wine vinegar
- 2 tbsp reduced-sodium soy sauce
- 1 tbsp sesame oil
- 1 tsp hot pepper sauce
- 1 pound tuna steaks, cut into thirty 1-inch cubes Cooking spray
- ¼ cup sesame seeds ½ tsp salt ¼ tsp pepper 2 green onions, finely chopped

Directions:

1. In a small size bowl, whisk the first five ingredients; set aside. Spritz tuna with cooking spray. Sprinkle with sesame seeds, salt and pepper. In a big nonstick skillet, brown tuna on all sides in batches until medium-rare or slightly pink in the centre; remove from the skillet.

On each of the 30 wooden appetizers, skewered, and thread one tuna cube. Arrange on a serving platter. Garnish with onions. Present with sauce.

Dessert Recipes

401. Pineapple and Cream Cheese Tart

Prep Time:	*Cook Time:*	*Servings: 2*
15 Minutes	*40 Minutes*	

Ingredients:

- Crust:
- 2 cups graham cracker
- 6 oz butter, melted
- 1 tablespoon powdered sugar
- 1 tsp vanilla extract
- Filling:
- 18 oz low-fat cream cheese
- 2 tbsp vanilla extract
- ½ cup sugar
- 2 cups crushed pineapple

Directions:

1. To make the crust: Place the graham crackers in a food processor and pulse until ground, then add the sugar, vanilla and melted butter. Pulse until well combined, then convert the structure into a 9-inch round pan. Press it on the bottom and sides of the pan very well, either with your fingertips or with the back of a spoon. Refrigerate the crust until you make the filling.
2. To make the filling: Stir the cream cheese with the sugar until fluffy, then add the vanilla. Spread the cream cheese in the pan, over the crust, then top with the crushed pineapple. Refrigerate at least 1 hour before serving.

402. Pineapple Pavlova

Prep Time:	*Cook Time:*	*Servings: 2*
15 Minutes	*23 Minutes*	

Ingredients:

- 5 egg whites
- 1 pinch cream of tartar
- 5 tbsp sugar
- 1 tsp vanilla extract
- 2 cups pineapple cubes
- 1 oz butter
- 4 tbsp brown sugar
- juice from 1 lime

Direction

1. whip the egg whites by the use of the cream of tartar In a bowl until stiff peaks form, then gradually stir in the sugar. Whip until a stiff, glossy meringue forms. Line a baking tray with baking paper, then trace a 9-inch round shape on the paper. Spread the meringue in the circle. Make it thick and rustic.
2. It doesn't have to look perfect. Also, make a small well in the centre. Bake in the before heating oven at 300F for 1 ½ hour or until crisp on the outside and chewy on the inside. When done, remove it from the oven and let it cool while you make the topping.
3. Melt the butter in a heavy skillet, then add the sugar and stir until melted. Stir in the pineapple cubes and lime juice and cook on a medium flame for 5 minutes or until well coated in caramel and a bit tender.
4. To finish the dessert, just before serving, top the meringue with the caramelized pineapple

403. Pineapple Turnovers

Prep Time:	*Cook Time:*	*Servings: 2*
15 Minutes	*33 Minutes*	

Ingredients:

- 1 ½ cups whole wheat flour
- ½ cup all-purpose flour
- 6 oz cold butter, cubed
- 2 tbsp sugar
- 1 pinch salt
- ½ tsp baking powder
- 1 egg
- 2-4 tbsp cold water
- 1 large pineapple, peeled, cored and diced ½ tsp cinnamon
- 1 tablespoon brown sugar
- 1 tablespoon cornstarch

Directions:

1. In a bowl, stir the pineapple with the sugar, cornstarch and cinnamon. Set aside. To make the dough, in a bowl, combine the flours with a pinch of salt and sugar.
2. Rub in the butter until it looks sandy, then stir in the egg. Add 1-2 tbsp of water or more until the dough comes together and looks easy to work with. To convert on a well-floured working surface and roll it out into a thin sheet. Cut the sheet into small squares.
3. Drop spoonfuls of pineapple filling in the middle of each square, then fold them over to form a triangle. Press the edges of the triangle slightly with your fingertips or a fork and convert all the turnovers on a baking tray lined with baking paper.
4. Bake in the before heating oven at 400F for 5 minutes, then lower the heat at 350F and bake 10-15 more minutes until fluffed and golden brown.

404. Pineapple Cheesecake

Prep Time:	*Cook Time:*	*Servings: 2*
15 Minutes	*30 Minutes*	

Ingredients:

- Crust:
- 2 cups graham crackers
- 1 tablespoon powdered sugar
- 1 tsp vanilla extract
- 6 oz butter, melted
- Filling:
- 20 oz low-fat cream cheese
- 10 oz low-fat yoghurt
- 4 eggs
- 2 tbsp cornstarch
- 1 tsp vanilla extract
- 1 tsp lemon zest
- ½ cup sugar
- Topping:
- 2 cups fresh pineapple cubes
- juice from 1 lemon
- 2 tbsp brown sugar
- 1 tablespoon chopped mint leaves

Directions:

1. To make the crust, simply put all the ingredients in a food processor and pulse until well stirred and sandy. To convert on a 9-inch round cake pan lined with baking paper and press it down on the bottom and sides of the pan either with your fingertips or the back of a spoon. It should be really packed. Set aside.
2. To make the filling: Stir the cream cheese with the sugar and yoghurt, then add the eggs, vanilla and lemon zest, as well as the cornstarch. Pour this filling in the crust and bake in the before heating oven at 350F for 40-50 minutes or until it looks wobbly in the middle but slightly set. Remove from the oven and let it cool in the pan.
3. To make the topping: In a bowl, stir the pineapple cubes with the sugar, lemon juice and chopped mint. Let it infuse for about one hour, then top the cheesecake with the pineapple cubes.

405. White Chocolate Pineapple Mousse

Prep Time:	*Cook Time:*	*Servings: 2*
15 Minutes	*29 Minutes*	

Ingredients:

- 5 oz white chocolate
- 1 oz butter
- 2 cups heavy cream
- 2 cups canned crushed pineapple, drained
- 1 tsp vanilla extract
- 4 oz ginger biscuits, crushed

Directions:

1. In a saucepan, bring half of the heavy cream to the boiling point, then remove from heat and stir in the chocolate. Stir until melted, then add the butter. Let it cool at 25 degrees, then fold in the remaining cream, whipped.
2. Add the vanilla, then spoon the mousse into small serving glasses. Top with crushed biscuits, then crushed pineapple and refrigerate at least 1 hour before serving.

406. KIWI TIKI TORCHES

Prep Time:	*Cook Time:*	*Servings: 2*
15 Minutes	*35 Minutes*	

INGREDIENTS:

- 1 fresh pineapple, peeled and cut into 1-inch chunks 4 medium kiwifruits, peeled and cut into ¾-inch pieces 2 cups fresh strawberries, halved
- WHITE CHOCOLATE DIPPING SAUCE
- 1 cup heavy whipping cream
- 6 white chocolate Toblerone candy bars (3.52 ounces each), broken into pieces ¼ cup finely chopped macadamia nuts 1 to 2 tsp rum extract
- 1/3 cup flaked coconut, toasted 1. Alternately thread the pineapple, kiwi and strawberries onto 12 metal or wooden skewers; set aside. In a saucepan over heat, bring cream just to a boil. Reduce

Directions:

1. Heat to reduce; stir in Toblerone until melted. Remove from the heat; stir in nuts, and extract.
2. Transfer to a fondue pot and keep warm.
3. Sprinkle with coconut. Present with fruit kabobs.

407. Pineapple Crumble

Prep Time:	*Cook Time:*	*Servings: 2*
15 Minutes	*63 Minutes*	

Ingredients:

- 1 large fresh pineapple, cut into cubes
- 2 cups graham crackers
- 5 oz butter, melted
- ½ cup brown sugar
- 2 tbsp coconut flakes

Directions:

1. Place the coconut cubes into a 9-inc square deep dish baking pan and set aside.
2. In a bowl, stir the ground graham cracker with the sugar and coconut flakes, then stir in the melted butter. Stir well, then spoon the stirirture over the pineapple in the pan, then bake in the before heating oven at 375F for 20-25 minutes or until soft and turn golden brown.
3. Serve immediately warm with a scoop of vanilla ice cream.

408. Grilled Pineapple with Caramel Sauce

Prep Time: 15 Minutes | *Cook Time: 19 Minutes* | *Servings: 2*

Ingredients:

- Pineapple:
- 1 fresh pineapple
- 2 tbsp honey
- 1 oz butter
- Caramel sauce:
- 1 cup sugar
- 1/ 2 cup heavy cream
- 1 oz butter

Directions:

1. To grill the pineapple, firstly peel it, cut it in half and remove its core. Cut it into cubes and place them all on wooden skewers. Drizzle them with honey, then heat a grill pan over medium flame.
2. Brush the pan with butter, then place the pineapple in the pan. Grill it on all sides for 2-3 minutes, then remove it from the pan and make the caramel sauce.
3. To make the sauce, melt the sugar in a heavy saucepan, then stir in the heavy cream. Keep on heat and stir until smooth, then remove from heat and add the butter.
4. Serve the pineapple skewers drizzled with caramel sauce. If you want a more fresh aroma, you can marinate the pineapple into a lemon and mint dressing before grilling.

Breakfast & Brunch Recipes

409. Frittata with Asparagus and Tomato

Prep Time: 15 Minutes | *Cook Time: 44 Minutes* | *Servings: 2*

Ingredients:

- 2 large eggs
- Salt Ground black pepper 1 tsp. olive oil or avocado oil 1 cup asparagus
- ½ cup sliced tomatoes

Directions:

1. Whisk 2 large eggs in a small bowl. Present with salt and ground black pepper and set aside.
2. Heat 1 tsp. Oil in a medium skillet over medium heat. Add asparagus and cook, tossing approx. 4-5 minutes.
3. Add tomatoes and eggs and cook, occasionally stirring until just set about 1 minute. Sprinkle with dill (optional).

410. Eggs with Zucchini Onions and Tomato

Prep Time: 15 Minutes | *Cook Time:30 Minutes* | *Servings: 4*

Ingredients:

- 2 large eggs
- Salt Ground black pepper 1 tsp. olive oil or avocado oil
- 1/3 cup sliced
- zucchini 1/3 cup chopped onions 1/3 cup sliced tomato Crushed red pepper flakes and a pinch of dill (optional)

Directions:

1. Mix 2 eggs in a small bowl. Present with salt and ground black pepper and set aside. Heat 1 tsp. Olive oil in a skillet. Add zucchini, onions and tomatoes and cook tossing until wilted (approx. 3-4 minutes). Add eggs and cook until just set.

411. Frittata with Tomatoes and Spinach

Prep Time: 15 Minutes | *Cook Time: 55 Minutes* | *Servings: 2*

Ingredients:

- 2 large eggs
- Salt Ground black pepper 1 tsp. olive oil or avocado oil ½ cup sliced tomatoes 1/3 cup spinach

Directions:

1. Whisk 2 large eggs in a small bowl. Season with salt and ground black pepper and set aside. Heat 1 tsp. Olive oil in a medium skillet over medium heat. Add baby spinach and tomatoes and cook, tossing until wilted (approx. 1 minute). Add eggs; cook, occasionally stirring until just set about 1 minute.

412. Zucchini Pancakes

Prep Time: 15 Minutes | *Cook Time: 14 Minutes* | *Servings: 2*

Ingredients:

- 2 medium zucchini
- 2 tbsp. chopped onion
- 3 beaten eggs 6 to 8 tbsp. Almond flour 1 tsp. Salt
- ½ tsp. ground black pepper
- coconut oil

Directions:

1. Heat the oven to 300 degrees F.
2. Grate the zucchini into a bowl and mix in the onion and eggs. Stir in 6 tbsp of the flour, salt and pepper.
3. Heat a large sauté pan over medium heat and add coconut oil to the pan. When the oil is hot lower the heat to medium-low and adds batter into the pan. Baked the pancakes for about 2 minutes on each side until browned. Place the pancakes in the oven.

413. Savoury Superfoods Pie Crust

Prep Time: 15 Minutes | *Cook Time: 14 Minutes* | *Servings: 8*

Ingredients:

- DF
- 11/4 cups blanched almond flour 1/3 cup tapioca flour
- ¾ tsp. Finely ground sea salt
- ¾ tsp. Paprika
- ½ tsp. ground cumin
- 1/8 tsp. ground white pepper
- ¼ cup coconut oil 1 large egg

Directions:

1. Place almond flour tapioca flour, sea salt, vanilla egg and coconut sugar (if you use coconut sugar) in the bowl of a food processor. Process 2-3 times to combine. Add oil and raw honey (if you use raw honey) and pulse with several one-second pulses and then let the food processor run until the mixture comes together. Move the dough onto a plastic wrap sheet. Wrap and then press the dough into a 9-inch disk. Refrigerate for 30 minutes.
2. Remove plastic wrap. Press dough onto the bottom and up the sides of a 9-inch buttered pie dish. Crimp a little bit the edges of the crust. Cool in the refrigerator for 20 minutes. Tp put the oven rack in the middle after heating the oven to 375F. Put in the oven and bake until golden brown.

414. Spinach Quiche

Prep Time: 15 Minutes | *Cook Time: 22 Minutes* | *Servings: 2*

Ingredients:

- 1 Precooked and cooled Savory Superfoods Pie Crust
- 8 ounces organic spinach cooked and drained
- 6 ounces cubed pork 2 medium shallots thinly sliced and sautéed
- 4 large eggs 1 cup coconut milk ¾ tsp. Salt ¼ tsp. freshly ground black pepper

Directions:

1. Brown the pork in coconut oil and then add the spinach and shallots. Set aside once done.
2. Preheat oven to 350F. In a large bowl, combine eggs, milk, salt and pepper. Whisk until foamy. Add in about ¾ of the drained filling mixture reserving the other ¼ to "top" the quiche. Pour egg mixture into crust and place remaining filling on top of the quiche.
3. Place quiche in the oven in the centre of the middle rack and bake undisturbed for 45 to 50 minutes.

415. Mushroom Quiche

Prep Time: 5 Minutes | *Cook Time: 15 Minutes* | *Servings: 2*

Ingredients:

- 1 Precooked and cooled Savory Superfoods Pie Crust
- 1 cup sliced mushrooms 6 ounces cubed pork 2 medium shallots thinly sliced and sautéed
- 4 large eggs 1 cup coconut milk ¾ tsp. Salt ¼ tsp. freshly ground black pepper

Directions:

1. Brown the pork in coconut oil and then add the mushrooms and shallots. Set aside once done.
2. Preheat oven to 350F. In a large bowl, combine eggs, milk, salt and pepper. Whisk until foamy. Add in about ¾ of the drained filling mixture reserving the other ¼ to "top" the quiche. Pour egg mixture into crust and place remaining filling on top of the quiche.
3. Place quiche in the oven in the centre of the middle rack and bake undisturbed for 45 to 50 minutes.

416. Tomato Quiche

Prep Time: 15 Minutes | *Cook Time: 30 Minutes* | *Servings: 6*

Ingredients:

- 1 Precooked and cooled Savory Superfoods Pie Crust
- 1 cup sliced tomatoes 6 ounces cubed pork 2 medium shallots thinly sliced and sautéed
- 4 large eggs 1 cup coconut milk ¾ tsp. Salt ¼ cup. Arugula ¼ tsp. freshly ground black pepper

Directions:

1. Brown the pork and shallots in coconut oil. Set aside once done.
2. Preheat oven to 350F. In a large bowl, combine eggs, milk, salt and pepper. Whisk until foamy. Add in about ¾ of the drained filling mixture and tomatoes, reserving the other ¼ to "top" the quiche. Pour egg mixture into crust and place remaining filling on top of the quiche.
3. Place quiche in the oven in the centre of the middle rack and bake undisturbed for 45 to 50 minutes. Sprinkle with arugula.

417. Vegetarian Tomato Quiche

Prep Time: 15 Minutes | *Cook Time: 43 Minutes* | *Servings: 2*

Ingredients:

- 1 Precooked and cooled Savory Superfoods Pie Crust
- 2 cups sliced tomatoes 4 large eggs 1 cup coconut milk ¾ tsp. Salt
- ¼ cup. Fresh basil ¼ tsp. freshly ground black pepper

Directions:

1. Preheat oven to 350F. In a large bowl, combine eggs, milk, salt and pepper. Whisk until foamy. Pour egg mixture into crust and place sliced tomatoes on top of the quiche.
2. Place quiche in the oven in the centre of the middle rack and bake undisturbed for 45 to 50 minutes. Sprinkle with basil

418. Cottage Cheese Sesame Balls

Prep Time: 15 Minutes | *Cook Time: 23 Minutes* | *Servings: 2*

Ingredients:

- EF
- 16-ounce farmers cheese or cottage cheese
- 1 cup finely chopped almonds
- 1and ½ cups oatmeal

Directions:

1. In a large bowl, combine blended cottage cheese almonds and oatmeal. Make balls and roll in sesame seeds mix.

419. Tapenade

Prep Time: *15 Minutes* | *Cook Time:* *53 Minutes* | *Servings: 2*

Ingredients:

- ½ pound pitted mixed olives
- 2 anchovy fillets rinsed
- 1 small clove garlic minced
- 2 tbsp. capers
- 2 to 3 fresh basil leaves
- 1 tbsp. freshly squeezed lemon juice
- 2 tbsp. extra-virgin olive oil or cumin oiL

Directions:

1. Rinse the olives in cool water. All ingredients transfer into the bowl of a food processor. The process is to combine until it becomes a coarse paste. Traner to a bowl and serve

420. Red Pepper Dip

Prep Time: *1 Minutes* | *Cook Time:* *10 Minutes* | *Servings: 2*

Ingredients:

- 1 pound red peppers
- 1 cup farmers' cheese
- ¼ cup virgin olive oil or avocado oil 1 tbsp minced garlic
- Lemon juice, salt basil, oregano red pepper flakes to taste.

Directions:

1. Roast the peppers. Cover them and cool for about 15 minutes. Peel the peppers and remove the seeds and stems. Chop the peppers.
2. Traner the peppers and garlic to a food processor and process until smooth. Add the farmers' cheese and garlic and process until smooth. With the machine running, add olive oil and lemon juice. Add the basil oregano, red pepper flakes and ¼ tsp. Salt and process until smooth. Adjust the seasoning to taste. Pour to a bowl and refrigerate.

421. Roasted Garlic

Prep Time: *1 Minutes* | *Cook Time:* *3 Minutes* | *Servings: 6*

Ingredients:

- Heat the oven to 350 F.

Directions:

1. Rub olive oil into the top of each garlic head and place it cut side down on a foil-lined baking sheet. Bake until the cloves turn golden. Remove from the oven and let cool. Squeeze each head of garlic to expel the cloves into a bowl. Mash into a paste.

422. Eggplant and Yogurt

Prep Time: *15 Minutes* | *Cook Time:* *16 Minutes* | *Servings: 2*

Ingredients:

- Mix 1 pound chopped eggplant
- 3 unpeeled shallots and 3 unpeeled garlic cloves with ¼ cup olive oil salt and pepper on a baking sheet.

Directions:

1. After roasting at 400 degrees for half an hour. Cool and squeeze the shallots and garlic from their skins and chop. Mix with the eggplant almond ½ cup plain yoghurt dill and salt and pepper.

423. Caponata

Prep Time: *15 Minutes* | *Cook Time:* *33 Minutes* | *Servings: 2*

Ingredients:

- Coconut oil 2 large eggplants cut into large chunks 1 tsp. dried oregano
- Sea salt and black pepper
- small onion peeled and finely chopped
- cloves garlic peeled and finely sliced
- bunch of parsley leaves of small size and stalks finely chopped 2 tbsp. Salted capers rinsed, soaked, and drained 1 handful of green olives stones removed 2-3 tbsp. lemon juice
- 5 large ripe tomatoes roughly chopped coconut oil
- tbsp. slivered almonds lightly toasted optional

Directions:

1. After heating the coconut oil in a pan and add eggplant oregano and salt. After cooking on high heat for around 4 or 5 minutes. Add the onion, garlic and parsley stalks and continue cooking for another few minutes. Add drained capers and the olives, and lemon juice. When all the juice has evaporated, add the tomatoes and simmer until tender.
2. Present with salt and olive oil to taste before serving. Sprinkle with almonds.

Lunch Recipes

424. YOGURT-MINT CUCUMBER SALAD

Prep Time: *12 Minutes* | *Cook Time:* *10 Minutes* | *Servings: 4*

INGREDIENTS:

- cucumbers (2 lbs), peeled, halved lengthwise, seeded, & sliced 1/4 inch thick
- 1 small red onion, sliced very thin salt & pepper
- 1 cup plain low-fat yoghurt
- 2 Tbsps. extra-virgin olive oil
- 1/4 cup minced fresh mint
- 1 garlic clove, minced
- 1/2 Tsp. ground cumin

TECHNIQUE:

1. set over a large container. Toss cucumber & onion with 1 Tbsp. Salt in a colander. Weight cucumbers with a gallon-size zipper-lock bag filled with water; drain for 1 to 3 hrs. Rinse & pat dry.
2. Whisk yoghurt, oil, mint, garlic, cumin, & salt & pepper to taste in a medium container. Include cucumbers & onion; toss to coat. Serve chilled.

425. SESAME LEMON CUCUMBER SALAD

Prep Time: *9 Minutes* | *Cook Time:* *7 Minutes* | *Servings: 4*

INGREDIENTS:

- cucumbers (2 lbs), peeled, halved lengthwise, seeded, & sliced 1/4 inch thick
- 1 Tbsp. salt
- 1/4 cup rice vinegar
- 1 Tbsp. lemon juice
- Tbsps. toasted sesame oil
- Tips. sugar
- 1/8 Tsp. red pepper flakes, plus more to taste
- Tbsp. sesame seeds, toasted

TECHNIQUE:

1. Toss cucumber with salt in colander set over a large container. Weight cucumbers with a gallon-size zipper-lock bag filled with water; drain for 1 to 3 hrs. Rinse & pat dry.
2. Whisk the remaining ingredients continuously together in a medium container. Include cucumbers; toss to coat. Serve chilled or at room temperature.

426. SWEET-AND-TART CUCUMBER SALAD

Prep Time: *6 Minutes* | *Cook Time:* *4 Minutes* | *Servings: 2*

INGREDIENTS:

- cucumbers (2 lbs), peeled, halved lengthwise, seeded, & sliced 1/4 inch thick 1/2 red onion, sliced very thin
- 1 Tbsp. salt 1/2 cup rice vinegar
- 2 1/2 Tbsps. sugar
- small jalapeño chiles, seeded & minced (or more, to taste)

TECHNIQUE:

1. Toss cucumber & onion with salt in a colander set over a large container. Weight cucumbers with a gallon-size zipper-lock bag filled with water; drain for 1 to 3 hrs. Rinse & pat dry.
2. 3Bring 2/3 cup water & vinegar to boil in a small nonreactive saucepan over medium heat. Stir in sugar to dissolve; reduce heat & simmer 15 mins. Let cool to room temperature.
3. Meanwhile, mix cucumbers, onion, & jalapeños in a medium container. Pour dressing over cucumber batter; toss to coat. Serve chilled.

427. GREEK CHERRY TOMATO SALAD

Prep Time: *12 Minutes* | *Cook Time:* *10 Minutes* | *Servings: 8*

INGREDIENTS:

- 1 1/2 lbs cherry tomatoes, quartered
- Salt & pepper
- 1/2 Tsp. sugar
- 2 garlic cloves, minced
- 1/2 Tsp. dried oregano
- shallot, minced
- Tbsp. red wine vinegar
- 2 Tbsps. extra-virgin olive oil
- small cucumber, peeled, halved lengthwise, seeded, & cut into 1/2-inch dice 1/2 cup chopped pitted kalamata olives
- 4 ounces feta cheese, crumbled (1 cup)
- 3 Tbsps. chopped fresh parsley

TECHNIQUE:

1. Toss tomatoes, 1/4 Tsp. Salt & sugar in a medium container; let stand for 30 mins. Shift tomatoes to salad spinner & spin till seeds & excess liquid have been removed, 45 to 60 seconds, stirring to redistribute tomatoes several times during spinning. Return tomatoes to a container & set them aside. Strain tomato liquid through a fine-mesh strainer into Liquid measuring cup, pressing on solids to extract as much liquid as possible.
2. Bring 1/2 cup tomato liquid (discard any extra), garlic, oregano, shallot, & vinegar to simmer in a small saucepan over medium heat. Simmer till reduced to 3 Tbsps., 6 to 8 mins. Shift batter to a small container & let cool to room temperature, about 5 mins. Whisk in oil & pepper to taste till combined. Taste & season with up to 1/8 Tsp. Salt.
3. Include cucumber, olives, feta, dressing, & parsley in a container with tomatoes; toss gently & serve.

428. PITA BREAD SALAD WITH CUCUMBERS, CHERRY TOMATOES, & FRESH HERBS

Prep Time: *35 Minutes* | *Cook Time:* *11 Minutes* | *Servings: 2*

INGREDIENTS:

- cucumber, peeled, halved lengthwise, seeded, & cut into 1/4-inch dice Salt & pepper
- (6-inch) pita bread, several days old, torn into 1/2-inch pieces
- 12 ounces cherry tomatoes, halved
- 6 scallions, whites & 2 inches of greens, sliced thin 1/4 cup minced fresh mint
- 1/4 cup of minced fresh cilantro or parsley 1/2 cup extra-virgin olive oil

- 6 Tbsps. lemon juice (2 lemons)

TECHNIQUE:

1. Heat oven to 375 degrees. Put the cucumber in colander; sprinkle with 1/4 Tsp. Salt. Weight cucumbers with a gallon-size zipper-lock bag filled with water; drain to release most of the liquid, about 30 mins. Rinse & pat dry.
2. Put bread pieces on baking sheet; bake till crisp but not browned, 5 to 7 mins. Shift to large container; Include cucumber, tomatoes, scallions, & herbs, & toss well. In a small container, combine oil & lemon juice & salt & pepper to taste. Include to the large container, toss again, & serve immediately.

429. ITALIAN BREAD SALAD (PANZANELLA)

Prep Time: 14 Minutes | *Cook Time: 12 Minutes* | *Servings: 2*

INGREDIENTS:

- (1-lb) loaf rustic Italian or French bread, cut into 1-inch pieces (about 6 cups) 1/2 cup extra-virgin olive oil
- 1 1/2 lbs tomatoes, cored, seeded, & cut into 1-inch pieces 3 Tbsps. red wine vinegar
- cucumber, peeled, halved lengthwise, seeded, & sliced thin
- shallot, sliced thin
- 1/4 cup chopped fresh basil

TECHNIQUE:

1. Set oven rack to middle setting & heat oven to 400 degrees. Toss bread pieces with 2 Tbsps. Oil & 1/4 Tsp. Salt; set bread in a single layer on a rimmed baking sheet. Toast bread pieces till just starting to turn light golden, 15 to 20 mins, stirring halfway through baking. Set aside & let cool to room temperature.
2. Gently toss tomatoes & 1/2 Tsp. Salt in a large container. Shift to a colander set over container; set aside to drain for 15 mins, tossing occasionally.
3. Whisk the remaining 6 Tbsps. Oil, vinegar, & 1/4 Tsp. Pepper into tomato juices. Include bread pieces, toss to coat, & let stand for 10 mins, tossing occasionally.
4. Include tomatoes, cucumber, shallot, & basil to the container with bread pieces & toss to coat. Season with salt & pepper to taste & serve Immediately.

430. ROASTED BEET & CARROT SALAD WITH WATERCRESS

Prep Time: 8 Minutes | *Cook Time: 6 Minutes* | *Servings: 2*

INGREDIENTS:

- lb beets, peeled & cut into 1/2-inch thick wedges, wedges cut in half crosswise if beets are large
- lb carrots, peeled & cut on the bias into 1/4-inch-thick slices
- Tbsps. extra-virgin olive oil Salt & pepper
- 1/4 Tsp. sugar
- Tbsps. white wine vinegar
- 1 Tsp. honey
- 1 shallot, minced
- 6 ounces (6 cups) watercress, torn into bite-size pieces

TECHNIQUE:

1. Set oven rack to the lowest setting, place large rimmed baking sheet on rack, & heat oven to 500 degrees. Toss beets & carrots with 2 Tbsps. Oil, 1/2 Tsp. Salt, 1/4 Tsp. Pepper & sugar in a large container. put off baking sheet from oven and, working quickly, carefully Shift beets & carrots to hot baking sheet & spread in even layer. (Do not wash container.) Roast till vegetables are tender & well browned on one side, 20 to 25 mins (do not stir during roasting).
2. Meanwhile, whisk remaining Tbsp. Oil, vinegar, honey, shallot, 1/4 Tsp. Salt, & 1/8 Tsp. Pepper in the now-empty container.
3. Toss hot vegetables with vinaigrette & let cool to room temperature, about 30 mins. Stir in watercress, Shift to a serving platter, & serve.

431. ROASTED FENNEL & MUSHROOM SALAD WITH RADISHES

Prep Time: 12 Minutes | *Cook Time: 10 Minutes* | *Servings: 8*

INGREDIENTS:

- fennel bulbs, fronds chopped & 1/3 cup reserved, stalks discarded, bulbs quartered, cored, & cut crosswise into 1/2-inch-thick slices
- 1 1/4 lbs cremini mushrooms, trimmed & quartered if large or halved if the medium
- Tbsps. extra-virgin olive oil Salt & pepper
- 1/4 Tsp. sugar
- Tbsps. lemon juice
- 1 Tsp. Dijon mustard
- 4-6 radishes, cut in half & sliced thin (3/4 cup)

TECHNIQUE:

1. Set oven rack to the lowest setting, place large rimmed baking sheet on rack, & heat oven to 500 degrees. Toss fennel & mushrooms with 2 Tbsps. Oil, 1/2 Tsp. Salt, 1/4 Tsp. Pepper & sugar in a large container. set aside baking sheet from oven and, working quickly, carefully Shift fennel & mushrooms to hot baking sheet & spread in even layer. (Do not wash container.) Roast till vegetables are tender & well-browned on one side, 20 to 25 mins (do not stir during roasting).
2. Meanwhile, whisk remaining Tbsp. oil, lemon juice, mustard, 1/4 Tsp. Salt, & 1/8 Tsp. Pepper in the now-empty container.
3. Toss hot vegetables with vinaigrette & let cool to room temperature, about 30 mins. Stir in radishes & reserved fennel fronds, Shift to a serving platter, & serve.

432. ROASTED GREEN BEAN & POTATO SALAD WITH RADICCHIO

Prep Time: 12 Minutes | *Cook Time: 10 Minutes* | *Servings: 2*

INGREDIENTS:

- lb green beans, trimmed & cut into 1 1/2-inch pieces
- lb red potatoes, cut into 1/2-inch pieces
- Tbsps. extra-virgin olive oil Salt & pepper
- 1/4 Tsp. sugar
- Tbsps. red wine vinegar
- 1 small garlic clove, minced
- 1 small head radicchio (6 ounces), washed & cut into 2-inch by 1/4-inch slices (4 cups)

TECHNIQUE:

1. Set oven rack to the lowest setting, place large rimmed baking sheet on rack, & heat oven to 500 degrees. Toss beans & potatoes with 2 Tbsps. Oil, 1/2 Tsp. Salt, 1/4 Tsp. Pepper & sugar in a large container. set aside baking sheet from oven and, working quickly, carefully Shift beans & potatoes to hot baking sheet & spread in even layer. (Do not wash container.) Roast till vegetables are tender & well-browned on one side, 20 to 25 mins (do not stir during roasting).
2. Meanwhile, whisk the remaining 1 Tbsp. oil, vinegar, garlic, 1/4 Tsp. Salt, & 1/8 Tsp. Pepper in the now-empty container.
3. Toss hot vegetables with vinaigrette & let cool to room temperature, about 30 mins. Stir in radicchio, Shift to a serving platter, & serve.

433. ASPARAGUS, RED PEPPER, SPINACH SALAD WITH SHERRY VINEGAR & GOAT CHEESE

Prep Time: 10 Minutes | *Cook Time: 8 Minutes* | *Servings: 6*

INGREDIENTS:

- 6 Tbsps. extra-virgin olive oil
- red bell pepper stemmed, seeded, & cut into 1-by 1/4-inch strips
- lb asparagus, trimmed & divide on the bias into 1-inch lengths salt & pepper
- shallot, sliced thin
- Tbsp. Plus 1 Tsp. sherry vinegar
- garlic clove, minced
- 6 ounces (6 cups) baby spinach
- ounces goat cheese, cut into small chunks

TECHNIQUE:

1. Heat 2 Tbsps. Oil in 12-inch nonstick pan over high heat till beginning to smoke; Include red pepper & cook till lightly browned, about 2 mins, stirring only once after 1 min. Include asparagus, 1/4 Tsp. Salt, & 1/8 Tsp. Pepper; cook till asparagus is browned & almost tender, about 2 mins, stirring only once after 1 min. Stir in shallot & cook till softened & asparagus is crisp-tender, about 1 min, stirring occasionally. Shift to large plate & let cool 5 mins.
2. Meanwhile, whisk the remaining 4 Tbsps. Oil, vinegar, garlic, 1/4 Tsp. Salt, & 1/8-Tsp. Pepper in a medium container till combined. In a large container, toss spinach with 2 Tbsps. Dressing & divide among salad plates. Toss asparagus batter with remaining dressing & place a portion over spinach; divide goat cheese among salads & serve.

434. ASPARAGUS & MESCLUN SALAD WITH CAPERS, CORNICHONS & HARD-COOKED EGGS

Prep Time: 35 Minutes | *Cook Time: 11 Minutes* | *Servings: 2*

INGREDIENTS:

- 5 Tbsps. extra-virgin olive oil
- 1lb asparagus, trimmed & cut on the bias into 1-inch lengths salt & pepper
- Tbsps. white wine vinegar
- 1 small shallot, minced
- Tbsps. minced cornichons
- 1 Tsp. chopped capers
- Tips. chopped fresh tarragon
- 6 ounces (6 cups) mesclun
- 3 FOOLPROOF HARD-COOKED EGGS, peeled & chopped medium

TECHNIQUE:

1. Heat 1 Tbsp. Oil in 12-inch nonstick pan over high heat till beginning to smoke. Include asparagus, 1/4 Tsp. Salt, & 1/4 Tsp. Pepper; cook till browned & crisp-tender, about 4 mins, stirring once every min. Shift to large plate & let cool 5 mins.
2. Meanwhile, whisk the remaining 4 Tbsps. Oil, vinegar, shallot, cornichons, capers, tarragon, & 1/4 Tsp. Pepper in a medium container till combined. In a large container, toss mesclun with 2 Tbsps. Dressing & divide among salad plates. Toss asparagus with remaining dressing & place a portion over mesclun; divide chopped eggs among salads & serve.

435. ASPARAGUS, WATERCRESS, & CARROT SALAD WITH THAI FLAVORS

Prep Time: 83 Minutes | *Cook Time: 11 Minutes* | *Servings: 2*

INGREDIENTS:

- Tbsps. lime juice
- Tbsps. fish sauce
- Tbsps. water
- Tips. sugar
- small garlic clove, minced
- small jalapeño chile, minced
- carrots, peeled & cut into 2-inch-long matchsticks
- 1 Tbsp. peanut oil or vegetable oil
- 1 lb asparagus, trimmed & cut on the bias into 1-inch lengths 6 ounces (6 cups) watercress
- 1/4 cup chopped fresh mint
- 1/3 cup chopped unsalted roasted peanuts

TECHNIQUE:

1. Whisk lime juice, fish sauce, water, sugar, garlic, & jalapeño in a medium container till sugar dissolves. Reserve 1 Tbsp. In a large container, toss carrots with remaining dressing & set aside.
2. Heat oil in 12-inch nonstick pan over high heat till beginning to smoke; Include asparagus & cook till browned & crisp-tender, about 4 mins, stirring once every min. Shift to large plate & place in freezer 5 mins.
3. Toss watercress with reserved 1 Tbsp. Dressing & divide among salad plates. Toss asparagus & mint with carrot batter & place a portion over watercress; sprinkle salads with peanuts & serve.

436. ASPARAGUS & ARUGULA SALAD WITH CANNELLINI BEANS & BALSAMIC VINEGAR

Prep Time: *11 Minutes* *Cook Time:* *9 Minutes* *Servings: 4*

INGREDIENTS:

- Tbsps. extra-virgin olive oil 1/2 red onion, sliced 1/8 inch thick
- 1 lb asparagus, trimmed & cut on the bias into 1-inch lengths Salt & pepper
- 1 (15-ounce) cannellini beans, rinsed
- 2 Tbsps. Plus 2 Tbsps. balsamic vinegar
- 6 ounces (6 cups) baby arugula

TECHNIQUE:

1. Heat 2 Tbsps. Oil in 12-inch nonstick pan over high heat till beginning to smoke; stir in onion & cook till beginning to brown, about 1 min. Include asparagus, 1/4 Tsp. Salt, & 1/4 Tsp. Pepper; cook till asparagus is browned & crisp-tender, about 4 mins, stirring once every min. Off heat, stir in beans; Shift to large plate & let cool 5 mins.
2. Meanwhile, whisk the remaining 3 Tbsps. Oil, vinegar, 1/4 Tsp. Salt, & 1/8 Tsp. Pepper in a medium container till combined. In a large container, toss arugula with 2 Tbsps. Dressing & divide among salad plates. Toss asparagus batter with remaining dressing, place a portion over arugula, & serve.

437. ORANGE & RADISH SALAD WITH ARUGULA

Prep Time: *35 Minutes* *Cook Time:* *11 Minutes* *Servings: 2*

INGREDIENTS:

- 3 oranges
- 5 Tbsps. lime juice
- 1/4 Tsp. Dijon mustard
- 1/2 Tsp. Ground coriander, toasted in a small dry pan till fragrant, about 30 seconds 1/8 Tsp. salt
- Pepper
- 3 Tbsps. vegetable oil
- 4 ounces (4 cups) baby arugula
- radishes, quartered lengthwise & cut crosswise into 1/8-inch-thick slices

TECHNIQUE:

1. Peel oranges, making sure to remove all pith, & cut into 1/4-inch pieces. Place orange pieces in a mesh strainer set over the container; let stand to drain excess juice. Meanwhile, whisk lime juice, mustard, coriander, Salt, & pepper to taste in a large container till combined. Whisking constantly, gradually Include oil.
2. Include oranges, arugula, & radishes in the container & toss gently to mix. Divide salad into individual plates & drizzle with any dressing in a container; serve immediately.

438. ORANGE, AVOCADO, & WATERCRESS SALAD WITH GINGER-LIME VINAIGRETTE

Prep Time: *11 Minutes* *Cook Time:* *9 Minutes* *Servings: 2*

INGREDIENTS:

- 3 oranges
- Tbsp. lime juice
- Tbsp. minced fresh mint
- Tsp. Grated fresh ginger 1/4 Tsp. Dijon mustard
- Pinch cayenne pepper Salt
- 3 Tbsps. vegetable oil
- 1/4 small red onion, sliced very thin
- avocado
- 2 1/2 ounces (2 1/2 cups) watercress, torn into 2-inch pieces

TECHNIQUE:

1. Peel oranges, making sure to remove all pith, & cut into 1/4-inch pieces. Place orange pieces in a mesh strainer set over the container; let stand to drain excess juice. Meanwhile, whisk lime juice, mint, ginger, mustard, cayenne, & 1/8 Tsp. Salt in a large container till combined. Whisking constantly, gradually Include oil. Toss onion in dressing & set aside.
2. 3Halve & pit avocado; cut each half lengthwise to form quarters. Using a paring knife, slice flesh of each quarter (do not cut through the skin) lengthwise into fifths. Using soupspoon, carefully scoop the flesh out of skin & fan slices from each quarter onto individual plates; season avocado lightly with Salt.
3. Include oranges in a container with onion; toss to coat. Include watercress & toss gently. Divide watercress among individual plates, mounding it in the centre; place portion of orange pieces & onion on top of watercress.
4. Drizzle any dressing in a container over salad; serve immediately.

439. ORANGE-JÍCAMA SALAD WITH SWEET & SPICY PEPPERS

Prep Time: *12 Minutes* *Cook Time:* *10 Minutes* *Servings: 8*

INGREDIENTS:

- oranges
- Tbsps. Lime juice (2 limes) 1/4 Tsp. Dijon mustard
- 1/2 Tsp. ground cumin, toasted in a small dry pan till fragrant, about 30 seconds Salt
- 1/4 cup vegetable oil
- 1 jícama (1 lb), peeled & cut into 2-inch-long matchsticks
- 1 red bell pepper, stemmed, seeded & divide into 1/8-inch-wide strips
- jalapeño chiles stemmed, seeded, quartered lengthwise, then cut crosswise into 1/8-inch-thick slices
- 1/2 cup fresh cilantro, chopped
- scallions, green parts only, sliced thin on the bias

TECHNIQUE:

1. Peel oranges, making sure to remove all pith, & cut into 1/4-inch pieces. Place orange pieces in a mesh strainer set over the container; let stand to drain excess juice. Meanwhile, whisk lime juice, mustard, cumin, & 1/4 Tsp. Salt in a large container till combined. Whisking constantly, gradually Include oil.
2. Toss jícama & red bell pepper with 1/8 Tsp. Salt in a medium container till combined. Include jícama batter, oranges, jalapeños, cilantro, & scallions to a container with dressing & toss well to combine. Divide among individual plates, drizzle with any dressing in a container, & serve immediately.

Dinner Recipes

440. PAN-ROASTED PEAR SALAD WITH WATERCRESS, PARMESAN, & PECANS

Prep Time: *12 Minutes* *Cook Time:* *10 Minutes* *Servings: 2*

INGREDIENTS:

- (8-ounce) pears, quartered & cored 2 1/2 Tbsps. sugar
- Salt & pepper
- 2 Tbsps. Plus 2 Tbsps. olive oil 1/4 cup balsamic vinegar
- 1 small shallot, minced
- 1/2 head green leaf lettuce (6 ounces), torn into 1-inch pieces 4 ounces (4 cups) watercress
- 4 ounces Parmesan cheese, shaved into strips with vegetable peeler 3/4 cup pecans, toasted & chopped

TECHNIQUE:

1. Toss pears, 2 Tbsps. Sugar, 1/4 Tsp. Salt, & 1/8 Tsp. Pepper in a medium container. Heat 2 Tbsps. Oil in 12-inch pan over medium-high heat till just smoking. Include pears cut side down in single layer & cook till golden brown, 2 to 4 mins. By Using a small spatula or fork, tip each pear onto the second cut side; continue to cook till the second side is light brown, 2 to 4 mins longer. Turn off heat, leave the pan on the burner, & Include 2 Tbsps. Vinegar; gently stir till vinegar becomes glazy & coats pears, about 30 seconds. Shift pears to large plate & let cool to room temperature, about 45 mins. Cut each pear quarter crosswise into 1/2-inch pieces.
2. Whisk remaining 2 Tbsps. Oil, remaining 2 Tbsps. Vinegar, remaining 1/2 Tsp. Sugar & shallot together in a large container; season with Salt & pepper to taste. Include lettuce, watercress, & cooled pears in a container; toss & season with Salt & pepper to taste. Divide salad into individual plates; top each with portions of cheese & nuts. Serve immediately.

441. CLASSIC THREE-BEAN SALAD

Prep Time: *2 Minutes* *Cook Time:* *11 Minutes* *Servings: 6*

INGREDIENTS:

- cup red wine vinegar 3/4 cup sugar
- 1/2 cup canola oil
- 2 garlic cloves, minced Salt & pepper
- 8 ounces green beans, trimmed & cut into 1-inch lengths
- 8 ounces yellow wax beans, trimmed & cut into 1-inch lengths
- (15-ounce) can red kidney beans, rinsed
- 1/2 red onion, chopped medium
- 1/4 cup minced fresh parsley

TECHNIQUE:

1. Heat vinegar, sugar, oil, garlic, 1 Tsp. Salt & pepper to taste in a small saucepan over medium heat, occasionally stirring, till sugar dissolves, about 5 mins. Shift to a large container & let cool to room temperature.
2. Bring 3 parts of water to boil in a large saucepan over high heat. Include 1 Tbsp. Salt & green & yellow beans; cook till crisp-tender, about 5 mins. Meanwhile, fill the medium container with ice water. When beans are done, drain & immediately plunge into ice water to stop the cooking process; let sit till chilled, about 2 mins. Drain well.
3. Include green & yellow beans, kidney beans, onion, & parsley to vinegar batter; toss well to coat. Cover & refrigerate overnight to let flavours meld. Left it at room temperature 30 mins before serving. (Salad can be refrigerated for up to 4 days.)

442. TABBOULEH

Prep Time: *11 Minutes* *Cook Time:* *9 Minutes* *Servings: 2*

INGREDIENTS:

- 1/2 cup of bulgur, fine or medium grain, rinsed under running water & drained 1/3 cup lemon juice (2 lemons)
- 1/3 cup olive oil
- Salt
- 1/8 Tsp. cayenne pepper (optional)
- cups minced fresh parsley
- tomatoes, cored, halved, seeded, & cut into very small dice
- 4 scallions, minced
- Tbsps. Minced fresh mint or 1 Tsp. dried

TECHNIQUE:

1. Mix bulgur with 1/4 cup of the lemon juice in a medium container; set aside till grains are tender & fluffy, 20 to 40 mins, depending on age & type of bulgur.
2. Mix continuously remaining lemon juice, olive oil, salt to taste & cayenne, if desired. Mix bulgur, parsley, tomatoes, scallions, & mint; Include dressing & toss to combine. Cover & refrigerate to let the flavours blend, 1 to 2 hrs. Serve.

443. PASTA SALAD WITH PESTO

Prep Time: *12 Minutes* *Cook Time:* *10 Minutes* *Servings: 2*

INGREDIENTS:

- 3/4 cup pine nuts
- 2 garlic cloves, unpeeled
- Salt
- 1 lb farfalle
- Tbsps. extra-virgin olive oil
- 3 cups fresh basil leaves
- 1 ounce (1 cup) baby spinach
- 1/2 Tsp. pepper
- 2 Tbsps. lemon juice
- 1 1/2 ounces Parmesan cheese, grated fine (3/4 cup), plus extra for serving 6 Tbsps.

- mayonnaise
- ounces cherry tomatoes, quartered, or grape tomatoes, halved (optional)

TECHNIQUE:

1. Bring 4 parts of water to boil in a large pot over high heat. Toast pine nuts in a small dry pan over medium heat, shaking cooking wok occasionally, till just golden & fragrant, 4 to 5 mins.
2. When water is boiling, Include garlic & let cook for 1 min. Remove garlic with a slotted spoon & rinse under cold water to stop cooking; set aside & let cool. Include 1 Tbsp. Salt & pasta to water, stir to separate, & cook till tender (just past al dente). Reserve 1/4 cupcooking water, drain pasta, toss with 1 Tbsp. Oil, spread in a single layer on a rimmed baking sheet, & let cool to room temperature, about 30 mins.
3. When garlic is cool, peel & mince or press through a garlic press.
4. Place 1/4 cup nuts, garlic, basil, spinach, pepper, lemon juice, remaining 1/4 cup oil, & 1 Tsp. Salt in a container of food processor & process till smooth, scraping sides of the container as necessary. Include cheese & mayonnaise & process till thoroughly combined. Shift batter to a large serving container. Cover & refrigerate till ready to assemble the salad.
5. When pasta is cool, toss with pesto, including reserved pasta water, 1 Tbsp. At a time, till pesto evenly coats pasta. Fold in remaining 1/2cup nuts & tomatoes, if using; serve with extra Parmesan.

444. PASTA SALAD WITH BROCCOLI & OLIVES

Prep Time: *11 Minutes* | *Cook Time:* *9 Minutes* | *Servings: 2*

INGREDIENTS:

- Lbs broccoli (2 medium bunches), florets cut into bite-size pieces (7 cups) 1/2 Tsp. grated lemon zest plus 1/4 cup juice (2 lemons)
- Salt
- 1 garlic clove, minced
- 1/2 Tsp. red pepper flakes 1/2 cup extra-virgin olive oil
- 1 lb bite-size pasta such as fusilli, farfalle, or orecchiette
- 1/2 cup kalamata olives or other brine-cured variety, pitted & chopped 1/2 cup chopped fresh basil

TECHNIQUE:

1. Bring 4 parts of water to boil in a large pot over high heat. In a separate pot, blanch broccoli in boiling salted water till crisp-tender, about 2 mins; drain & let cool to room temperature.
2. Meanwhile, whisk lemon juice & zest, 3/4 Tsp. Salt, garlic, & pepper flakes in a large container; whisk in oil in a slow, steady stream till smooth.
3. Include pasta & 1 Tbsp. salt to boiling water. Cook till pasta is al dente & drain. Whisk dressing again to blend; Include hot pasta, cooled broccoli, olives, & basil; toss to mix thoroughly. Let cool to room temperature, Set seasonings, & serve. (Pasta salad can be refrigerated for up to 1 day; return to room temperature before serving.)

445. PASTA SALAD WITH EGGPLANT, TOMATOES, & BASIL

Prep Time: *11 Minutes* | *Cook Time:* *9 Minutes* | *Servings: 4*

INGREDIENTS:

- lb eggplant, cut into 1/2-inch-thick rounds
- 1/2 cup of extra-virgin olive oil, and extra for brushing on eggplant Salt & pepper
- 1/2 Tsp. grated lemon zest plus 1/4 cup juice & (2 lemons)
  - garlic clove, minced
- 1/2 Tsp. red pepper flakes
- lb bite-size pasta, such as fusilli, farfalle, or orecchiette
  - large tomatoes, cored, seeded, & cut into 1/2-inch dice
- 1/2 cup chopped fresh basil

TECHNIQUE:

1. 1A. Fully open the bottom vent. Large chimney starter filled with charcoal briquettes. When the upper coal is partially covered with ash, pour it evenly over the grill. Place the cooking grill in place, cover and fully open the lid vent. Heat the grill until hot, for about 5 minutes.
2. 1B. Turn all burners to high, cover, & heat grill till hot, about 15 mins. Leave all burners on high. (Set burners as needed to maintain grill temperature around 350 degrees.) 2. Clean & oil cooking grate. Lightly brush eggplant with oil & sprinkle with Salt & pepper to taste. Grill, turning once, till marked with dark stripes, about 10 mins. Let cool & cut into bite-size pieces.
3. Meanwhile, take 4 quarts of water to boil in a large pot over high heat. Whisk lemon juice & zest, garlic, 3/4 Tsp. Salt & pepper flakes in a large container; whisk in 1/2 cup oil in slow, steady stream till smooth.
4. Include pasta & 1 Tbsp. salt to boiling water. Cook till pasta is al dente & drain. Whisk dressing again to blend; Include hot pasta, cooled eggplant, tomatoes, & basil; toss to mix thoroughly. Let cool to room temperature, Set seasonings, & serve. (Pasta salad can be refrigerated for up to 1 day; return to room temperature before serving.)

446. PASTA SALAD WITH ARUGULA & SUN-DRIED TOMATO VINAIGRETTE

Prep Time: *7 Minutes* | *Cook Time:* *5 Minutes* | *Servings: 2*

INGREDIENTS:

- Salt
- lb fusilli
- Tbsp. extra-virgin olive oil
- 1/2 cup oil-packed sun-dried tomatoes
- Tbsps. red wine vinegar
- 1 garlic clove, minced
- 1/4 Tsp. salt
- 1/8 Tsp. pepper
- 4 ounces (4 cups) baby arugula
- 1/2 cup green olives, pitted & sliced
- ounces fresh mozzarella cheese, cut into 1/2-inch cubes

TECHNIQUE:

1. Bring 4 parts of water to boil in a large pot over high heat. Include pasta & 1 Tbsp. salt to boiling water. Cook till pasta is al dente & drain. Rinse pasta under cold running water. Drain pasta well, Shift it to a large mixing container, & toss it with olive oil. Set aside.
2. Drain tomatoes, reserving oil. (You should have 1/3 cup reserved oil. If necessary, makeup difference with extra-virgin olive oil.) Roughly chop tomatoes. Whisk reserved oil with vinegar, garlic, salt, & pepper in a small container.
3. Include arugula, olives, mozzarella, & chopped tomatoes in a container with pasta. Pour tomato vinaigrette over pasta, toss gently, & serve immediately.

447. PASTA SALAD WITH FENNEL, RED ONIONS, & SUN-DRIED TOMATOES

Prep Time: *35 Minutes* | *Cook Time:* *11 Minutes* | *Servings: 8*

INGREDIENTS:

- fennel bulbs stalks discarded, halved, cored, & cut into 1/2-inch wedges
- red onions, sliced into 1/2-inch-thick rings
- 1/2 cup plus 2 Tbsps. extra-virgin olive oil
- Salt & pepper
- 1/2 Tsp. grated lemon zest plus 1/4 cup juice (2 lemons)
- garlic clove, minced
- lb bite-size pasta such as fusilli, farfalle, or orecchiette
- 1/2 cup oil-packed sun-dried tomatoes patted dry & sliced thin 1/2 cup chopped fresh basil

TECHNIQUE:

1. Set oven rack to middle setting & heat oven to 425 degrees. Toss fennel & onions with 2 Tbsps. Oil & Salt & pepper to taste & Shift to large baking sheet. Roast till tender & lightly browned, 15 to 17 mins. Let cool to room temperature.
2. Meanwhile, whisk lemon juice & zest, garlic, 3/4 Tsp. Salt & pepper to taste in a large container; whisk in remaining 1/2 cup oil in slow, steady stream till smooth.
3. Take 4 quarts of water to boil in a large pot over high heat. Include pasta & 1 Tbsp. salt to boiling water. Cook till pasta is al dente & drain. Whisk dressing again to blend; Include hot pasta, cooled fennel & onions, sun-dried tomatoes, & basil; toss to mix thoroughly. Let cool it to room temperature, season with Salt & pepper to taste, & serve. (Pasta salad can be refrigerated for up to 1 day; return to room temperature before serving.)

448. PASTA SALAD WITH ASPARAGUS & RED PEPPERS

Prep Time: *16 Minutes* | *Cook Time:* *14 Minutes* | *Servings: 2*

INGREDIENTS:

- 1 1/2 lbs asparagus, trimmed & cut into 2-inch pieces
- large red bell peppers, stemmed, seeded, & cut into 1 1/2-inch pieces 1/2 cup plus 2 Tbsps. extra-virgin olive oil
- Salt & pepper
- 1/2 Tsp. grated lemon zest plus 1/4 cup juice (2 lemons) 1 garlic clove, minced
- 1 lb bite-size pasta such as fusilli, farfalle, or orecchiette
- Tbsps. chopped fresh chives
- 1/3 cup grated Parmesan cheese

TECHNIQUE:

1. Set oven rack to middle setting & heat oven to 425 degrees. Toss asparagus & peppers with 2 Tbsps. Oil, Salt & pepper to taste, & Shift to a large baking sheet. Roast till tender & lightly browned, 15 to 17 mins; let cool to room temperature.
2. Meanwhile, whisk lemon juice & zest, 3/4 Tsp. Salt, garlic, & pepper to taste in a large container; whisk in remaining 3/4 cup oil in slow, steady stream till smooth.
3. Take 4 quarts of water to boil in a large pot over high heat. Include pasta & 1 Tbsp. salt to boiling water. Cook till pasta is al dente & drain. Whisk dressing again to blend; Include hot pasta, cooled asparagus & peppers, chives, & grated Parmesan; toss to mix thoroughly. Let it cool at room temperature, season with Salt & pepper to taste, & serve. (Pasta salad can be refrigerated for up to 1 day; return to room temperature before serving.)

449. SWEET & SOUR CABBAGE SALAD WITH APPLE & FENNEL

Prep Time: *11 Minutes* | *Cook Time:* *9 Minutes* | *Servings: 4*

INGREDIENTS:

- 1/2 head green cabbage (1 lb), cored & shredded (6 cups)
- Salt & pepper
- 1/2 small red onion, chopped fine
- 1 Tbsp. honey
- Tbsps. rice vinegar
- Tbsps. extra-virgin olive oil
- 1 Tsp. Dijon mustard
- Tbsps. minced fresh tarragon
- large Granny Smith apple, peeled, cored, & cut into 1/4-inch pieces
- fennel bulb, stalks discarded, halved, cored, & sliced thin Shredded Cabbage & 1 Tsp.

TECHNIQUE:

1. Salt in a colander placed on top of a medium-sized container. Let the cabbage wilt for at least 1 hour or up to 4 hours. Rinse cabbage under cold running water (if served immediately, place in a large container of ice water). Press but do not squeeze. Pat dry with a paper towel. (You can put cabbage in a ziplock bag and keep it refrigerated overnight) 2. In a medium container, mix onion, honey, vinegar, oil, mustard, and tarragon. Immediately toss the cabbage, apples and fennel into the dressing. According to your taste, Season with salt and pepper. Cover and refrigerate until ready to serve.

450. CABBAGE & RED PEPPER SALAD WITH LIME-CUMIN VINAIGRETTE

Prep Time: *11 Minutes* | *Cook Time:* *9 Minutes* | *Servings: 2*

INGREDIENTS:

- 1/2 head green cabbage (1 lb), cored & shredded fine (6 cups)
- Salt
- Tsp. grated lime zest plus 2 Tbsps. juice
- 2 Tbsps. olive oil
- Tbsp. rice vinegar or sherry vinegar

- Tbsp. honey
- Tsp. ground cumin Pinch cayenne pepper
- red bell pepper stemmed, seeded, & cut into thin strips

TECHNIQUE:

1. Toss shredded cabbage & 1 Tsp. Add alt in a colander set over a medium container. Let stand till cabbage wilts, at least 1 hr or up to 4 hrs. Rinse cabbage under cold running water. Press, as well as do not squeeze, to drain; pat dry with paper towels. (Cabbage can be stored in a zipper-lock bag & refrigerated overnight.) 2. Stir together lime juice & zest, oil, vinegar, honey, cumin, & cayenne in a medium container. Toss cabbage & red pepper in dressing. Season with salt to taste; cover & refrigerate till ready to serve.

451. CONFETTI CABBAGE SALAD WITH SPICY PEANUT DRESSING

Prep Time: *11 Minutes* | *Cook Time:* *9 Minutes* | *Servings: 2*

INGREDIENTS:

- 1/2 head green cabbage (1 lb), cored & shredded (6 cups)
- 1 large carrot, peeled & grated
- Salt
- Tbsps. smooth peanut butter
- Tbsps. peanut oil
- Tbsps. rice vinegar
- Tbsp. soy sauce
- Tsp. honey
- garlic cloves, chopped coarsely
- 1 (1 1/2-inch) piece ginger, peeled
- 1/2 jalapeño chile stemmed, halved, & seeded
- radishes, halved lengthwise & sliced thin
- scallions, sliced thin

TECHNIQUE:

1. Toss shredded cabbage, carrot, & 1 Tsp. Let stand till cabbage wilts, at least 1 hr or up to 4 hrs. Rinse cabbage & carrot under cold running water. Press, but do not squeeze, to drain; pat dry with the help of paper towels. (Vegetables can be stored in the zipper-lock bag & refrigerated overnight.) 2. Pure peanut butter, oil, vinegar, soy sauce, honey, garlic, ginger, & jalapeño in a food processor till a smooth paste is formed, about 30 seconds. Toss cabbage & carrot, radishes, scallions, & dressing together in a medium container. Season with salt to taste; cover & refrigerate till ready to serve.

452. CREAMY BUTTERMILK COLESLAW

Prep Time: *35 Minutes* | *Cook Time:* *11 Minutes* | *Servings: 2*

INGREDIENTS:

- 1/2 head red or green cabbage (1 lb), cored & shredded (6 cups)
- Salt
- carrot, peeled & shredded 1/2 cup buttermilk
- 2 Tbsps. mayonnaise
- 2 Tbsps. sour cream
- small shallot, minced
- Tbsps. Minced fresh parsley 1/2 Tsp. cider vinegar
- 1/2 Tsp. sugar
- 1/4 Tsp. Dijon mustard 1/8 Tsp. pepper

TECHNIQUE:

1. Discard the chopped cabbage and 1 tsp. Salt in a colander or large mesh sieve placed on top of a medium-sized container. Leave at least 1 time and up to 4 times until the cabbage is cooked. Rinse the cabbage under running cold water. Drain, but do not push. Dry with a paper towel. Place the withered cabbage and carrots in a large bowl.
2. Add buttermilk, mayonnaise, sour cream, sodium, parsley, vinegar, sugar, mustard, 4 tsp. Mix salt with pepper in a small bowl. Pour the sauce over the cabbage and mix together. Refrigerate until cool, about 30 minutes.

453. DELI-STYLE COLESLAW

Prep Time: *12 Minutes* | *Cook Time:* *10 Minutes* | *Servings: 6*

INGREDIENTS:

- 1/2 head red or green cabbage (1 lb), cored & shredded or chopped (6 cups)
- large carrot, peeled & shredded
- Tsp. salt
- 1/2 small onion, minced
- 1/2 cup mayonnaise
- Tbsps. rice vinegar Pepper

TECHNIQUE:

1. Toss cabbage & carrots with salt in a colander set over a medium container. Let stand till cabbage wilts, at least 1 hr or upto 4 hrs.
2. Pour draining liquid from a container; rinse container & dry. Dump wilted cabbage & carrots into a container. Rinse continuously in cold water (ice water if serving slaw immediately). Pour vegetables back into colander. Pat dry with paper towels. (Vegetables can be stored in the zipper-lock bag & refrigerated overnight.)
3. Pour cabbage & carrots back again into a container. Include onion, mayonnaise, & vinegar; toss to coat. Season with pepper to taste. Cover & refrigerate till ready to serve.

Side Dishes Recipes

454. GERMAN BEER CHEESE SPREAD

Prep Time: *15 Minutes* | *Cook Time:* *45 Minutes* | *Servings: 2*

INGREDIENTS:

- 1 pound of sharp cheddar cheese, divided into ½-inch cubes 1 tbsp Worcestershire sauce
- 1 ½ tsp prepared mustard 1 small garlic clove, minced
- ¼ tsp salt
- 1/8 tsp pepper
- 2/3 cup German or non-alcoholic beer assorted biscuits

DIRECTIONS:

1. Put the cheese in the food processor. Pulse until chopped, about 1 minute. Add Worcestershire sauce, mustard, garlic, salt and pepper. Add beer little by little at a time, continuing to process until the mixture is smooth and spreadable, about a minute.
2. Transfer to a serving bowl or gift bottle. Cover and refrigerate for up to 1 week. Serve with crackers.

455. PASSION FRUIT HURRICANES

Prep Time: *15 Minutes* | *Cook Time:* *32 Minutes* | *Servings: 6*

INGREDIENTS:

- 2 mugs passion fruit juice
- 1 mug plus 2 tbsps sugar
- ¾ mug lime juice ¾ mug light rum ¾ mug dark rum
- 3 tbsp grenadine syrup
- 6 to 8 mugs ice cubes
- Orange slices, starfruit slices and maraschino cherries

DIRECTIONS:

3. In a pitcher, mix the fruit juice, sugar, lime juice, rum and grenadine; stir until sugar is dissolved.
4. Spread into a hurricane or highball glasses filled with ice. Serve with orange slices, starfruit slices and cherries.

456. SWEET TEA CONCENTRATE

Prep Time: *0 Minutes* | *Cook Time:* *5 Minutes* | *Servings: 2*

INGREDIENTS:

- 2 medium lemons
- 4 mugs sugar
- 4 mugs water
- 1 ½ mug English breakfast tea leaves or 20 black tea bags 1/3 mug lemon juice EACH SERVING
- 1 mug cold water
- Ice cubes
- Citrus slices, optional
- Mint sprigs, optional

DIRECTIONS:

1. Extract peels from lemons; set fruit aside for garnish or save for another use.
2. In a saucepan, combine together sugar and water. Bring to a boil over medium heat. Minimize heat; simmer, unwrapped, for 3-5 minutes or until sugar is dissolved, stirring occasionally. Extract from the heat; add tea leaves and lemon peels. Close and steep
3. minute. Strain the tea finally and discard the tea leaves and lemon peel. Mix lemon juice. Cool to room temperature.
4. Convert to a container with a tight lid. Store in the refrigerator for up to 2 weeks.
5. Tea preparation In a tall glass, mix water and concentrate. Add ice. Add orange slices and mint twigs if desired.

457. WHITE SANGRIA

Prep Time: *15 Minutes* | *Cook Time:* *10 Minutes* | *Servings: 2*

INGREDIENTS:

- ¼ mug sugar ¼ mug brandy 1 mug sliced peeled fresh peaches or frozen sliced peaches, thawed 1 mug sliced fresh strawberries or frozen sliced strawberries, thawed 1 medium lemon, sliced
- 1 medium lime, sliced
- 3 mugs dry white wine, chilled
- 1 can (12 ounces) lemon-lime soda, chilled Ice cubes

DIRECTIONS:

1. In a pitcher, mix sugar and brandy until sugar is dissolved. Add remaining ingredients; stir smoothly to mix. Serve over ice.

458. Lemon PUNCH

Prep Time: *5 Minutes* | *Cook Time:* *10 Minutes* | *Servings: 8*

INGREDIENTS:

- 8 mugs cold water
- 1 can (12 ounces) of frozen lemonade concentrate, thawed plus ¾ mug thawed lemonade concentrate 2 litres ginger ale, chilled
- 1-litre cherry lemon-lime soda, chilled Ice ring, optional

DIRECTIONS:

1. In a large punch bowl, mix water and lemonade concentrate. Stir in ginger ale and lemon-lime soda. Top with an ice ring if desired. Serve punch immediately.
2. Desired. Serve punch immediately.

459. SPARKLING PEACH BELLINIS

Prep Time: *12 Minutes* | *Cook Time:* *30 Minutes* | *Servings:*

INGREDIENTS:

- 3 medium peaches, halved
- 1 tbsp honey
- 1 can (11.3 ounces) of peach nectar, chilled
- 2 bottles (750 millilitres each) champagne or sparkling grape juice, chilled
- place a baking sheet with a large piece of heavy-duty foil (aboutx 12 in.).

DIRECTIONS:

1. Place the peach halves cut side up on the foil. Drizzle honey. Turn the foil over the peaches and seal.

2. Bake it at least 375° for 25-30 minutes or until soft. Cool completely. Extract and remove the skin. Process the peaches in a cooking processor until soft.
3. Transfer the peach puree to the pitcher. Add honey and 1 bottle of champagne. Stir until blended. 12 Spread in a champagne flute or wine glass. Finish with the remaining champagne. Serve immediately.

460. FROZEN STRAWBERRY DAIQUIRIS

Prep Time: *15 Minutes* *Cook Time:* *35 Minutes* *Servings: 2*

INGREDIENTS:

- ¾ mug rum
- ½ mug thawed limeade concentrate
- 1 package (10 ounces) frozen sweetened sliced strawberries
- 1 to 1 ½ mugs ice cubes
- GARNISH
- Fresh strawberries

DIRECTIONS:

1. In a blender, mix the rum, limeade concentrate, strawberries and ice. Cover and process until smooth and thickened (use more ice for thicker daiquiris). Spread into cocktail glasses.
2. To garnish each daiquiri, cut a ½-in. slit into the tip of a strawberry; position berry on the rim of the glass.

461. PUMPKIN PIE SHOTS

Prep Time: *15 Minutes* *Cook Time:* *7 Minutes* *Servings: 2*

INGREDIENTS:

- 1 envelope unflavored gelatin
- 1 mug cold water
- 1/3 mug canned pumpkin ¼ mug sugar
- ½ tsp pumpkin pie spice 1/3 mug butterscotch schnapps liqueur ¼ mug vodka
- 1 ½ tsp heavy whipping cream Sweetened whipped cream

DIRECTIONS:

1. In a saucepan, spread gelatin over cold water; let it stand for 1 minute. Heat and stir it continuously over low heat until gelatin is completely dissolved. Stir in pumpkin, sugar and pie spice; cook and stir until sugar is dissolved. Extract from heat. Stir in liqueur, vodka and cream.
2. Spread mixture into twelve 2-oz. shot glasses; Let it cool until set. Top with sweetened whipped cream

462. BANANA NOG

Prep Time: *12 Minutes* *Cook Time:* *20 Minutes* *Servings: 6*

INGREDIENTS:

- 3 mugs milk, divided
- 3 mugs half-and-half cream, divided
- 3 egg yolks
- ¾ mug sugar
- 3 large ripe bananas
- ½ mug light rum
- 1/3 mug creme de cacao
- 1 ½ tsp vanilla extract
- Whipped cream and baking cocoa, optional
- In a large, heavy saucepan, mix 1 ½ mug milk,
- 1 ½ mugs cream, egg yolks and sugar.

DIRECTIONS:

1. Now Cook and stir continuously over medium-low heat until mixture reaches 160° and is thick to coat the back of a metal spoon.
2. Put bananas in a food processor; cover and process until blended. Spread milk mixture into a pitcher; stir in the banana puree, rum, creme de cacao, vanilla, and remaining milk and cream. Cover and let it cool for at least 3 hours before serving.
3. Spread into chilled glasses. Garnish with whipped cream and spread with cocoa if desired.
4. CHEAT IT! Substitute 6 mugs of eggnog from the dairy case for the milk mixture prepared in the recipe. Stir the banana puree, rum, creme de cacao and vanilla into the eggnog. Garnish as desired.

463. MEXICAN HOT CHOCOLATE

Prep Time: *9 Minutes* *Cook Time:* *30 Minutes* *Servings: 8*

INGREDIENTS:

- 4 mugs fat-free milk
- 3 cinnamon sticks
- 5 ounces 53% of cacao dark baking chocolate, coarsely chopped
- 1 tsp vanilla extract
- Additional cinnamon sticks, optional 1

DIRECTIONS:

1. In a saucepan, heat milk and cinnamon sticks overheat until bubbles form around the sides of the pan. Discard cinnamon. Whisk in chocolate until smooth.
2. Extract from the heat; stir in vanilla. Serve it in mugs with additional cinnamon sticks if desired.

464. CREAMSICLE MIMOSAS

Prep Time: *15 Minutes* *Cook Time:* *0 Minutes* *Servings: 2*

INGREDIENTS:

- 2 ½ mugs orange juice
- 1 mug half-and-half cream
- ¾ mug superfine sugar
- 4 tsp grated orange peel
- 2 bottles (750 millilitres each) champagne or other sparkling wine Fresh strawberries

DIRECTIONS:

1. Place the orange juice, cream, sugar and orange peel in a blender; cover and process until sugar is dissolved. Transfer to an 8-in. square dish. Freeze for 6 hours or overnight.
2. For each serving, scoop ¼ mug mix into a champagne glass; top with champagne. Garnish with a strawberry and serve
3. immediately.
4.

Snacks And Appetizer Recipes

465. PUMPKIN CHEESE PUFFS

Prep Time: *3 Minutes* *Cook Time:* *5 Minutes* *Servings: 6*

INGREDIENTS:

- 2 tbsp cream cheese, softened
- ½ tsp balsamic vinegar ½ cup water
- ¼ cup butter, cubed ¼ tsp salt
- ½ cup of all-purpose flour 4 drops yellow paste food colouring
- 1 drop red paste food colouring
- ½ cup grated Romano cheese 2 eggs
- 20 sprigs fresh Italian parsley, stems removed

Directions:

1. In a small size bowl, add cream cheese and vinegar. Cover and refrigerate. In a big saucepan, bring the water, butter and salt to a boil.
2. Mix the flour at a time and mix until a smooth ball is formed. Remove from heat. Leave it on for 5 minutes.
3. Add the yellow and red food colouring to a small bowl. Stir in the Romano cheese and food colouring to the mixture. Add eggs one at a time and beat well after each addition. Continue to beat until the dough is soft and shiny.
4. Lower it to the level of 3 inches. Separate on a greased baking sheet. Bake at 400° for 15-20 minutes or until slightly browned. Remove with wire rack to cool.
5. Use the tip of the star to represent the cream cheese mixture, putting the stems into the puff. Add parsley eggplant. Refrigerate leftover food

466. DEVILED CRAB

Prep Time: *5 Minutes* *Cook Time:* *10 Minutes* *Servings: 2*

INGREDIENTS:

- ½ cup finely chopped onion 3 tbsps butter
- 3 tbsps all-purpose flour
- ½ tsp salt 1 ½ cups half-and-half cream 2 egg yolks, lightly beaten
- 3 cans (6 ounces each) crabmeat, drained, flaked, and cartilage removed 1 tbsp Dijon mustard
- 2 tsp Worcestershire sauce
- 1 tsp minced chives
- TOPPING
- 1 cup soft bread crumbs
- 1 tbsp butter, melted

Directions:

1. In a big skillet, saute onion in butter until tender. Stir in flour and salt until blended. Gradually stir in cream until smooth. Take it to a boil, and cook and stir for 2 minutes or until thickened and bubbly. Remove from the heat.
2. Stir a small amount of hot mixture into egg yolks. Return all to the pan, stirring constantly. Bring to a gentle boil; cook and stir 2 minutes longer. Remove from the heat. Stir in the crab, mustard, Worcestershire sauce and chives.
3. Spoon into six greased 6-oz. ramekins or custard cups. Place on a baking sheet. Add bread crumbs and melted butter;
4. sprinkle over tops. Bake it at least 375° for 20-25 minutes or until topping is golden brown.

467. ITALIAN CHEESE WONTONS

Prep Time: *6 Minutes* *Cook Time:* *16 Minutes* *Servings: 2*

INGREDIENTS:

- 2 cups shredded Italian cheese
- 1 carton (15 ounces) ricotta cheese
- 1 egg, beaten
- 1 tbsp minced fresh parsley
- 1 garlic clove, minced
- ¼ tsp salt
- 1/8 tsp pepper
- 40 wonton wrappers
- Oil for deep-fat frying
- Marinara or spaghetti sauce warmed.

Directions:

1. Put the first 7 ingredients in a bowl.
2. Place the dumpling wrapper at one point toward you. (Keep the rest of the wrap covered with a damp paper towel until ready to use.)
3. Place 1 tbsp of filling in the centre of the wrap. Fold the bottom corner over the filling.
4. After the sides folding towards the centre of the overcharge. Roll towards the remaining points. Wet the top edge with water. Press to seal. Repeat. Refrigerate for 30 minutes.
5. After heating, heat the oil to 375° in an electric frying pan. Fry the wontons a little at a time.
6. Fry for 1-2 minutes on each side or until golden brown. Drain the water on a paper towel. Served with marinara.
7. Prepare stuffed dumplings the day before TO RUN. Fill your party day wontons. Cover with wet tissue and wrap and store in the refrigerator.

468. SPICY CHEESE CRACKERS

Prep Time: *12 Minutes* *Cook Time:* *17 Minutes* *Servings: 2*

INGREDIENTS:

- 1 ½ cups (6 ounces) shredded extra-sharp cheddar cheese ¾ cup all-purpose flour
- ½ tsp kosher salt
- ¼ tsp crushed red pepper flakes ¼ cup cold butter, cubed
- 1 to 2 tbsps half-and-half cream

Directions:

3. Place the cheese, flour, salt and pepper flakes in a food processor; process until blended. Now mix butter; pulse until butter is the size of peas. During pulsing, add just enough cream to form moist crumbs.
4. On a lightly floured surface, roll dough to 1/8-in. Thickness. Cut with a floured 3-in. holiday-shaped cookie cutter. Place 2 in. apart on greased baking sheets. Reroll scraps and repeat. Set the oven at 350° and bake for 13-17 minutes or until it turns golden brown. Set aside from pans to wire racks to cool completely. Store in an airtight container.

469. LEMONY FENNEL OLIVES

Prep Time: 9 Minutes *Cook Time: 1 Minutes* *Servings: 4*

INGREDIENTS:

- 1 small fennel bulb
- 2 cups pitted ripe olives
- 1 small lemon, cut into wedges
- ½ tsp whole peppercorns
- ½ cup olive oil
- ½ cup lemon juice

Directions:

1. Trim fennel bulb and cut into wedges. Snip feathery fronds from fennel bulb; rePresent 2 tsp. Boil the brine in a small saucepan. Add dill. Boil uncovered for 1 minute or until soft. Rinse and rinse with cold water.
2. In a large bowl, place the fennel, olives, lemon slices, pepper and fennel leaves. Whisk off the oil and lemon juice. Pour in the olive mixture. Throw it on the court. Cover and refrigerate overnight.
3. Remove from refrigerator 1 hour before serving. Transfer to a serving bowl. Serve with a slotted spoon.

470. COCONUT SHRIMP

Prep Time: 11 Minutes *Cook Time: 16 Minutes* *Servings: 2*

INGREDIENTS:

- 18 uncooked jumbo shrimp (about 1 pound) 1/3 cup cornstarch ¾ tsp salt ½ tsp cayenne pepper 3 egg whites
- 2 cups flaked coconut
- Oil for deep-fat frying
- APRICOT-PINEAPPLE SALSA
- 1 cup diced pineapple
- ½ cup finely chopped red onion ½ cup apricot presents ½ cup minced fresh cilantro 2 tbsp lime juice
- 1 jalapeno pepper, seeded and chopped
- Salt and pepper to taste

Directions:

1. Peel and devein shrimp, leaving tails intact. Make a slit down the inner curve of each shrimp, starting with the tail; press lightly to
2. flatten. Add cornstarch, salt and cayenne pepper to dishes that need to be reduced. Separately. Beat the egg whites in the bowl until they form stiff peaks. If you place the coconut on another plate, it will shrink. Coat the shrimp with cornstarch mixture. Dip in egg whites and then coat with coconut.
3. Heat the oil at 375° in an electric skillet or fryer. Fry the prawns a little at a time, 1 to 1 minute on each side, or until golden brown. Drain the water on a paper towel.
4. Place the salsa ingredients in a bowl. Comes with shrimp.

471. BLUE CHEESE-ONION STEAK BITE

Prep Time: 5 Minutes *Cook Time: 18 Minutes* *Servings: 2*

INGREDIENTS:

- 3 big onions, thinly sliced into rings
- 3 tbsps butter
- 12 garlic cloves, minced
- 4 beef tenderloin steaks (6 ounces each)
- ¼ tsp salt
- ¼ tsp pepper
- 1 French bread baguette (10 ½ ounces), cut into ¼-inch slices
- SPREAD
- 4 ounces cream cheese, softened
- 1 cup (4 ounces) crumbled blue cheese
- 1/8 tsp salt
- 1/8 tsp pepper

Directions:

1. In a big skillet, saute onions in butter until softened. Reduce heat to medium-reduce; cook, occasionally stirring, for 30 minutes or until onions are golden brown. Add garlic; cook 1 minute longer.
2. Meanwhile, sprinkle beef with salt and pepper. Using long-handled tongs, moisten a paper towel with cooking oil and coat the grill rack.
3. Grill the covered steak over medium heat or overheat 4 inches (4 inches) on each side for 5-7 minutes, or until the meat is at the desired cooking level (for medium-rare, thermometer 145°, medium, 160°, well finished, 170°) °). Cut into thin slices.
4. Place bread on ungreased baking sheets. After setting the temperature at 400°, bake for 4-6 minutes or until lightly browned.
5. Meanwhile, place the cream cheese, blue cheese, salt and pepper in a food processor; cover and process until blended. Spread each bread slice with 1 tsp cheese mixture; top with steak and onions.

472. ASPARAGUS, BRIE & PARMA HAM CROSTINI

Prep Time: 5 Minutes *Cook Time: 15 Minutes* *Servings: 2*

INGREDIENTS:

- 12 asparagus spears
- 2 tbsp olive oil, divided
- 1/8 tsp salt
- 1/8 tsp pepper
- 12 slices French bread baguette (1/2 inch thick)
- 3 thin slices prosciutto (Parma ham) or deli ham,
- cut into thin strips 6 ounces Brie cheese, cut into 12 slices 1.
- Cut asparagus tips into 2-in. lengths. (Discard stalks or save for another use.) Place asparagus tips in a 15x10x1-in.

Directions:

1. Baking pan lined with foil. Spread with 1 tsp oil and toss to coat. Sprinkle with salt and pepper. Bake at 425° for 10-15 minutes or until crisp-tender.
2. Brush baguette slices on both sides with remaining oil. Place on a baking sheet. Broil for 1-2 minutes on each side or until toasted.
3. Top each slice with asparagus, prosciutto and cheese. Boiling for 2-3 minutes or until cheese is melted.

473. CLAMS CASINO

Prep Time: 12 Minutes *Cook Time: 18 Minutes* *Servings: 2*

INGREDIENTS:

- 1 pound kosher salt
- 1 dozen fresh cherrystone clams
- 1/3 cup soft bread crumbs
- 3 tbsps minced fresh parsley, divided
- 2 tbsps olive oil
- 1 garlic clove, minced
- 1/8 tsp cayenne pepper
- 1/8 tsp coarsely ground pepper

Directions:

1. After heating the oven to 450 °. Salt in an oven-ready or 15x10x1-inch metal dish. Pan. Remove the peel, leaving the bottom peel. Drain liquid (save for other use). Place the clams in a salted baking dish.
2. Add soft breadcrumbs, 2 tablespoons parsley, oil, garlic, cayenne pepper and black pepper. Spoon over clams.
3. Bake for 15-18 minutes or until the clams are firm and the breading mixture is crispy and golden brown. Sprinkle with the remaining parsley. Present immediately.

474. LIGHTENED-UP VEGGIE PIZZA SQUARES

Prep Time: 50 Minutes *Cook Time: 70 Minutes* *Servings: 6*

INGREDIENTS:

- 2 tubes refrigerated reduced-fat crescent rolls
- 1 package (8 ounces) reduced-fat cream cheese
- 1 package (8 ounces) fat-free cream cheese
- ½ cup plain yoghurt
- 1/3 cup reduced-fat mayonnaise
- ¼ cup fat-free milk
- 1 tbsp dill weed
- ½ tsp garlic salt
- 1 cup shredded carrots
- 1 cup fresh cauliflowers, chopped
- 1 cup fresh broccoli florets, chopped
- 1 cup julienned green pepper
- 1 cup sliced fresh mushrooms
- 2 cans (2 ¼ ounces each) sliced ripe olives, drained
- ¼ cup finely chopped onion

Directions:

1. Spread out two crescent dough tubes and pound them into 15x10x 1 inch ungreased. Pan; Suture sutures and perforations. Set the oven at 375° and baked for 10-12 minutes or until golden brown. Cool completely on wire rack.
2. In a bowl, beat the cream cheese, yoghurt, mayonnaise, milk, dill and garlic salt until smooth. Spread over the crust. Sprinkle with carrots, cauliflower, broccoli, bell peppers, mushrooms, olives and onions. Completely covered and refrigerate for at least 1 hour.
3. Cut into squares. Refrigerate leftovers.

475. ENSENADA SHRIMP COCKTAIL

Prep Time: 15 Minutes *Cook Time: 0 Minutes* *Servings: 2*

INGREDIENTS:

- 1 pound peeled and deveined cooked medium shrimp 2 plum tomatoes, seeded and chopped
- 3 jalapeno peppers, seeded and chopped 1 serrano pepper, seeded and chopped
- ¼ cup chopped red onion 2 green onions, chopped
- 2 tbsps minced fresh cilantro
- 2 tbsps olive oil
- 1 tbsp rice vinegar
- 1 tbsp key lime juice or lime juice 1 tsp adobo seasoning Lime wedges

Directions:

1. In a big bowl, add the shrimp, tomatoes, peppers, onions and cilantro. Add the oil, vinegar, lime juice and seasoning; spread over shrimp mixture and toss to coat.
2. Refrigerate it for at least 1 hour. Using a slotted spoon, put shrimp mixture in cocktail glasses, about ½ cup in each. Garnish with lime wedges.

NOTE *Wear disposable gloves when dividing hot peppers; the oils can burn skin. Avoid touching your face.*

476. APRICOT-RICOTTA STUFFED CELERY

Prep Time: 10 Minutes *Cook Time: 30 Minutes* *Servings: 6*

INGREDIENTS:

- 3 dried apricots
- ½ cup part-skim ricotta cheese 2 tsp brown sugar
- ¼ tsp grated orange peel 1/8 tsp salt 5 celery ribs, cut into 1 ½ inch pieces

Directions:

1. Place apricots in a food processor.
2. Cover and process until finely chopped. Add the ricotta cheese, brown sugar, orange peel and salt; cover and process until blended. Stuff or pipe into celery.

3. Chill until serving.

477. MOTHER LODE PRETZELS

Prep Time: 15 Minutes *Cook Time: 50 Minutes* *Servings: 2*

INGREDIENTS:

- 1 package (10 ounces) pretzel rods
- 1 package (14 ounces) caramels
- 1 tbsp evaporated milk
- 1 ¼ cups miniature semisweet chocolate chips
- 1 cup plus 2 tbsps butterscotch chips
- 2/3 cup milk chocolate toffee bits
- ¼ cup chopped walnuts

Directions:

1. After cutting pretzel rods in half with a sharp knife, set aside. In a big saucepan over reduce heat, melt caramels with milk. In a large bowl, reduce the dish, adding chips, chips and walnuts.
2. Pour caramel mixture into 2 cups. Add sliced pretzel pieces, each two-thirds of the mixture, to caramel mixture (reheat in the mixer if the mixture is too thick for application). Let the caramel pass, then turn the pretzels into a chip mixture. Place on a covered baking sheet until set.
3. Store in an airtight container.

478. VEGGIE HAM CRESCENT WREATH

Prep Time: 2 Minutes *Cook Time: 56 Minutes* *Servings: 2*

INGREDIENTS:

- 2 tubes refrigerated crescent rolls
- ½ cup spreadable pineapple cream cheese
- 1/3 cup diced fully cooked ham
- ¼ cup finely chopped sweet yellow pepper ¼ cup finely chopped green pepper
- ½ cup chopped broccoli florets
- 6 grape tomatoes, quartered
- 1 tbsp chopped red onion

Directions:

1. Remove (do not loosen) the crescent paste from the tube. Cut each roll into eight pieces. Align by 11 inches. Circle the 14 inches without oil. Pizza pan.
2. Set the temperature at 375° and baked for 15-20 minutes or until golden brown. Let it cool for 5 minutes before carefully removing it onto a serving platter. Cool completely.
3. Spread cream cheese over wreath; top with ham, peppers, broccoli, tomatoes and onion. Store in the refrigerator.

479. HONEY-NUT ENDIVE APPETIZERS

Prep Time: 15 Minutes *Cook Time: 0 Minutes* *Servings: 4*

INGREDIENTS:

- 1/3 cup crumbled goat cheese 1/3 cup crumbled Gorgonzola cheese 1/3 cup pine nuts
- 1/3 cup chopped walnuts
- 1/3 cup golden raisins
- 4 bacon strips, cooked and crumbled
- 2 heads Belgian endive, separated into leaves
- 1/3 cup honey

Directions:

1. In a small size bowl, add the first six ingredients. Spoon into endive leaves. Spread honey over cheese mixture. Present immediately.

480. CARAMEL APPLE AND BRIE SKEWERS

Prep Time: 15 Minutes *Cook Time: 60 Minutes* *Servings: 2*

INGREDIENTS:

- 2 medium apples, cubed
- 1 log (6 ounces) Brie cheese, cubed
- ½ cup hot caramel ice cream topping
- ½ cup finely chopped macadamia nuts
- 2 tbsp dried cranberries

Directions:

1. On each of six wooden appetizer skewers, alternately thread apple and cheese cubes; place on a serving tray. Spread with caramel topping; sprinkle with macadamia nuts and cranberries.

481. THYME-SEA SALT CRACKERS

Prep Time: 5 Minutes *Cook Time: 18 Minutes* *Servings: 2*

INGREDIENTS:

- 2 ½ cups all-purpose flour
- ½ cup white whole wheat flour
- 1 tsp salt
- ¾ cup water ¼ cup plus 1 tbsp olive oil, divided 1 to 2 tbsps minced fresh thyme
- ¾ tsp sea or kosher salt 1.

Directions:

1. Preheat oven to 375°. In a big bow whisk flours and salt. Gradually add water and ¼ cup oil, tossing with a fork until dough holds together when pressed. Divide dough into three portions.
2. Roll each part of the dough 1/8 inch on a lightly floured surface. Thickness. Cut into 1½ inches of flour.
3. Round cookies cutter. Place 1-in. Separately on a non-oiled baking sheet. Poke each cracker with a fork. Lightly comb with the remaining oil. Add thyme and sea salt and sprinkle over crackers.
4. Baked it for 9-11 minutes or until the bottom is slightly browned.

482. SEAFOOD SALAD STUFFED SHELLS

Prep Time: 15 Minutes *Cook Time: 30 Minutes* *Servings: 6*

INGREDIENTS:

- 1 package (12 ounces) jumbo pasta shells
- 2 packages (8 ounces each) cream cheese, softened
- 1/3 cup mayonnaise 2 tsp sugar
- 1 ½ tsp lemon juice 1/8 tsp salt 1/8 tsp coarsely ground pepper 1/8 tsp cayenne pepper 3 cans (6 ounces each) lump crabmeat, drained
- ½ pound frozen cooked salad shrimp, thawed 12 green onions, finely chopped

Directions:

1. Cook pasta according to directions and drain and rinse in cold water. Cool to room temperature.
2. In a big bowl, add the cream cheese, mayonnaise, sugar, lemon juice, salt, pepper and cayenne. Gently stir in the crab, shrimp and onions. Stuff shells, about 2 tbsps in each. Cover and refrigerate for at least 1 hour.

Dessert Recipes

483. Pineapple Popsicles

Prep Time:25 Minutes *Cook Time: 0 Minutes* *Servings: 2*

Ingredients:

- 2 cups fresh chopped pineapple
- 1 ½ cup coconut milk
- ½ cup low-fat cream cheese
- 1 tsp vanilla extract
- 1 tablespoon mint leaves
- juice and zest from 1 lime
- ¼ cup brown sugar

Directions:

1. Stirrer the pineapple with the cream cheese, lime juice and zest and mint leaves into a blender and pulse until well pureed and smooth.
2. Add the coconut milk and cream cheese, then the sugar. Pour the stirirture into your popsicle moulds and freeze for at least 4 hours. To remove them from their moulds, sink them in hot water for 5 seconds.

484. Cherry Almond Tart

Prep Time: 15 Minutes *Cook Time: 45 Minutes* *Servings: 2*

Ingredients:

- Crust:
- 1 cup whole wheat flour
- 1 cup all-purpose flour
- 2 tbsp powdered sugar
- 6 oz butter, chilled and cubed
- 1/8 tsp baking powder
- Filling:
- 2 cups low-fat cream cheese
- 2 eggs
- ¼ cup sugar
- 2 cups pitted cherries
- 1 tsp lemon juice
- ½ cup sliced almonds topped

Directions:

1. To make the crust, place all the ingredients in a blender and pulse until it comes together. Add 1-2 tbsp cold water if it doesn't.
2. To convert the dough on a well-floured working surface and roll it onto a thin sheet. Place the dough into a 9-inch round tart pan and press it slightly on the bottom and sides of the pan. Cut off the excess dough and bake the crust in the before heating oven at 375F for 10 minutes.
3. To make the filling, stir the cream cheese with sugar, eggs and lemon juice. Spoon the filling into the crust, then top with pitted cherries. Bake 20-30 more minutes at 350F, then remove from the oven and top with sliced almonds.

485. Cherry Clafoutis

Prep Time: 15 Minutes *Cook Time: 35 Minutes* *Servings: 6*

Ingredients:

- 3 eggs
- 1/3 cup all-purpose flour
- 1/3 cup heavy cream
- 1 cup low-fat milk
- ¼ cup sugar
- 1 pinch of salt
- 1 tsp vanilla extract
- 2 cups cherries, pitted
- butter to grease the pan

Directions:

1. Butter a 10-inch cake, then arrange the cherries on the bottom of the pan.
2. In a bowl, stir the eggs with heavy cream, sugar, a pinch of salt, and vanilla, then incorporate the flour. Pour this stricture into the pan, over the cherries and bake in the before heating oven at 375F for 30-35 minutes.
3. Let it cool in the pan, then slice and serve.

486. Cherry Oatmeal Cookies

Prep Time: *15 Minutes* | *Cook Time:* *50 Minutes* | *Servings: 2*

Ingredients:

- 1 cup whole wheat flour
- ½ cup all-purpose flour
- 1 tsp baking soda
- 2 cups rolled oats
- 1 tsp cinnamon
- 1 pinch nutmeg
- 6 oz butter, softened
- 2/3 cup brown sugar
- 3 eggs
- 1 tsp vanilla extract
- 1 cup fresh cherries, chopped

Directions:

1. In a bowl, stir the flours with the rolled oats, cinnamon, nutmeg and baking soda. In another bowl, stir the butter continuously with the sugar until creamy and fluffy.
2. Add the eggs and vanilla, then incorporate the flour stricture and the cherries. Stir well, then drop spoonfuls of batter onto baking trays lined with baking paper.
3. Bake in the before heating oven at 375F for 15-20 minutes or until slightly golden brown. Store them in an airtight container.

487. Almond and Cherry Muffins

Prep Time: *15 Minutes* | *Cook Time:* *30 Minutes* | *Servings: 4*

Ingredients:

- Muffins:
- 1 cup whole wheat flour
- 1 ½ cups all-purpose flour
- 2/3 cup brown sugar
- 1 tsp baking soda
- 1 tsp baking powder
- 1 tsp vanilla extract
- 2 eggs
- 2 oz butter, melted 1 cup low-fat milk 1 pinch of salt
- 1 ½ cups pitted cherries Crisp topping:
- ½ cup sliced almonds 1 oz butter
- ½ cup whole wheat flour 1 tablespoon sugar

Directions:

1. In a bowl, stir the flours with the sugar, baking soda, baking powder and a pinch of salt. In another bowl, shake the eggs, melted butter, vanilla and milk. Pour this stricture over the flour and stir well, then fold in the cherries. Fill ¾ of your muffin cups, previously lined with muffin paper. Set aside.
2. To make the topping: In a bowl, stir the flour with the sugar, then rub in the butter until sandy. Add the sliced almonds and sprinkle the stirirture over each muffin.
3. Bake in the before heating oven at 350F for 20-25 minutes or until crisp and golden brown.

488. BLUE CHEESE-STUFFED STRAWBERRIES

Prep Time: *15 Minutes* | *Cook Time:* *45 Minutes* | *Servings: 8*

INGREDIENTS:

- ½ cup balsamic vinegar
- 3 ounces fat-free cream cheese
- ½ cup crumbled blue cheese
- 16 big fresh strawberries
- 3 tbsp finely chopped pecans, toasted

Directions:

1. Place vinegar in a small saucepan. Let it boil cook until liquid is reduced by half. Cool to room temperature.
2. Meanwhile, in a small size bowl, beat cream cheese until smooth. Beat in blue cheese. Remove stems and scoop out centres from strawberries; fill each with about 2 tsp cheese mixture.
3. Sprinkle pecans over filling, pressing lightly. Chill until serving. Spread with balsamic vinegar.

Breakfast & Brunch Recipes

489. Almond Butter Banana Oats

Prep Time: *5 Minutes* *Cook Time:* *10 Minutes* *Servings: 2*

Ingredients:

- ½ cup oats
- ¾ cup water
- 1 egg white
- 1 banana 1 tbs. Flax seeds meal 1 tsp raw honey
- pinch cinnamon
- ½ tbs. almond butter

Directions:

1. Combine oats and water in a bowl. Egg white beat, then whisk it in with the uncooked oats.
2. Boil on the stovetop after checking consistency and continue to heat as necessary until the oats are fluffy and thick.
3. Mash banana and add to oats. Heat for 1-minute stir in flax, raw honey and cinnamon. Top with almond butter!

490. Coconut Pomegranate Oatmeal

Prep Time: *2 Minutes* *Cook Time:* *0 Minutes* *Servings: 2*

Ingredients:

½ cup oats

- 1/3 cup coconut milk
- 1 cup water
- 2 tbs. shredded unsweetened coconut
- 1-2 tbs. Flax seeds meal 1 tbs. raw honey
- 3 tbs. pomegranate seeds
- Cook oats with coconut milk, water and salt.

Directions:

1. Stir in the coconut raw honey and flaxseed meal. Sprinkle with extra coconut and pomegranate seeds.

491. Banana Almond Overnight Oats

Prep Time: *5 Minutes* *Cook Time:* *0 Minutes* *Servings: 2*

Ingredients:

- ½ cup oats
- ½ cup coconut milk
- 1 banana 1 tbs. flax seeds meal 1 tsp raw honey
- pinch cinnamon
- 1 tsp dried cranberries 2 Brazil nuts ½ tbs. almond butter

Directions:

1. Make a smoothie with banana coconut milk, almond butter, honey and cinnamon. Stir in flax and oatmeal and leave overnight. Top with 1 tsp. Dried cranberries, Brazil nuts.

492. Walnut Oatmeal with Fresh Blueberries

Prep Time: *15 Minutes* *Cook Time:* *0 Minutes* *Servings: 2*

Ingredients:

- ½ cup blueberries
- ½ cup oats
- 1 cup water
- ½ cup walnuts Dash of cinnamon
- 2 tsp. raw honey

Directions:

1. Cook the oats with the water for 3-5 minutes.
2. Add walnuts and cinnamon. Stir in the raw honey. Top with blueberries

493. Raspberry Oatmeal

Prep Time: *15 Minutes* *Cook Time:* *0 Minutes* *Servings: 2*

Ingredients:

- ½ cup raspberries
- ½ cup oats
- 1 cup water
- ½ cup sesame seeds
- Dash of cinnamon
- 2 tsp. raw honey

Directions:

1. 2Cook the oats with the wa ter for 3-5 minutes.
2. Add sesame seeds and cinnamon. Stir in the raw honey. Top with raspberries

494. Strawberry Oatmeal

Prep Time: *2 Minutes* *Cook Time:* *10 Minutes* *Servings: 2*

Ingredients:

- ½ cup strawberries
- ½ cup oats
- 1 cup water
- 2 Tbsp. sunflower seeds
- 1 Tbsp. Raisins 2 tsp. raw honey

Directions:

1. Cook the oats with the water for 3-5 minutes.
2. Add sesame seeds and cinnamon. Stir in the raw honey. Top with raspberries

495. Kiwi Oatmeal

Prep Time: *15 Minutes* *Cook Time:* *0 Minutes* *Servings: 2*

Ingredients:

- 1 sliced kiwi
- ½ cup oats
- 1 cup water
- 2 Tbsp. pumpkin seeds
- 1 Tbsp. Raisins 2 tsp. raw honey

Directions:

1. Cook the oats with the water for 3-5 minutes.
2. Add sesame seeds and cinnamon. Stir in the raw honey. Top with raspberries

496. Chia Pudding Recipes

Prep Time: *15 Minutes* *Cook Time:* *0 Minutes* *Servings: 6*

Ingredients

- ¼ cup Chia seeds
- 1 cup coconut milk ½ tbs Royall jelly 1 tsp.
- Ground Vanilla Bean a pinch of Nutmeg Top with Blueberries

Directions:

1. Mix all ingredients except blueberries and leave overnight in the fridge. Top with blueberries.

497. Coconut Pomegranate Chia Pudding

Prep Time: *15 Minutes* *Cook Time:* *0 Minutes* *Servings: 4*

Ingredients

- ¼ cup Chia seeds
- 1 cup Coconut milk
- ½ tablespoon Raw honey
- ½ tablespoon Coconut flakes
- Top with Pomegranate seeds

Directions:

1. Mix all ingredients except pomegranate and leave overnight in the fridge. Top with pomegranate.

498. Yogurt & Mango Chia Pudding

Prep Time: *15 Minutes* *Cook Time:* *0 Minutes* *Servings: 2*

Ingredients

- ¼ cup Chia seeds 1 ½ cup yoghurt 1 tablespoon raw honey
- ½ cup chopped Mango

Directions:

5. 2Mix 1 cup of yoghurt honey and chia seeds and leave overnight in the fridge.
6. Divide into 2 glasses, top each with ¼ cup yoghurt and ¼ cup mango.

499. Cacao & Raspberry Chia Pudding

Prep Time: *15 Minutes* *Cook Time:* *0 Minutes* *Servings: 8*

Ingredients

- ¼ cup Chia seeds
- 1 cup coconut milk
- 1 tablespoon raw honey
- 1 Tsp. cacao powder
- ½ cup yoghurt
- ½ cup raspberrie

Directions:

1. Mix coconut milk, honey cacao and chia seeds and leave them overnight in the fridge.
2. Divide into 2 glasses, top each with ¼ cup yoghurt and ¼ cup raspberries.

500. Blueberry Chia Pudding

Prep Time: *15 Minutes* | *Cook Time:* *0 Minutes* | *Servings: 2*

Ingredients

- ¼ cup Chia seeds
- 1 cup coconut milk
- 1 tablespoon raw honey

Directions:

1. ½ cup blueberry smoothie ¼ cup chopped almonds Mix coconut milk honey blueberry smoothie and chia seeds and leave overnight in the fridge. Divide into 2 glasses and top each almond.

501. Egg pizza crust

Prep Time: *15 Minutes* | *Cook Time:* *33 Minutes* | *Servings: 2*

Ingredients:

- 3 eggs
- ½ cup of coconut flour
- 1 cup of coconut milk
- 1 crushed garlic clove

Directions:

1. Mix and make an omelette.

502. Omelet with Superfoods veggies

Prep Time: *8 Minutes* | *Cook Time:* *5 Minutes* | *Servings: 4*

Ingredients:

- 2 large eggs
- Salt Ground black pepper
- 1 tsp. olive oil or avocado oil
- 1 cup spinach
- cherry tomatoes and 1 spoon of yoghurt cheese Crushed red pepper flakes and a pinch of dill (optional)

Directions:

1. 2 large eggs are whisking in a small bowl. Present with salt and ground black pepper and set aside. Heat 1 tsp.
2. Olive oil in a skillet and medium heat. Add baby spinach tomatoes and cook, tossing until wilted (approx. 1 minute). Set aside.
3. Add eggs and cook until set. Add veggies and cheese on top of eggs. Flip eggs over cheese and veggies. Sprinkle with crushed red pepper flakes and dill.

503. Egg Muffins

Prep Time: *5 Minutes* | *Cook Time:* *43 Minutes* | *Servings: 2*

Ingredients:

- 8 eggs
- 1 cup diced green bell pepper
- 1 cup diced onion
- 1 cup spinach
- ¼ tsp. salt
- 1/8 tsp. ground black pepper
- 2 tbsp. water

Directions:

1. The oven after heating to 350 degrees F. Oil 8 muffin cups. Beat eggs together.
2. Mix in bell pepper, spinach, onion, salt, black pepper and water. Pour the mixture into muffin cups

Lunch Recipes

504. SWEET & TANGY COLESLAW

Prep Time: *12 Minutes* | *Cook Time:* *53 Minutes* | *Servings: 4*

INGREDIENTS:

- 1/4 cup apple cider vinegar, plus extra for seasoning
- Tbsps. Vegetable oil 1/4 Tsp. Celery seeds 1/4 Tsp. pepper
- 1/2 head green cabbage (1 lb), cored & shredded (6 cups) 1/4 cup sugar, plus extra for seasoning
- Salt
- 1 large carrot, peeled & grated
- Tbsps. chopped fresh parsley

TECHNIQUE:

1. Combine vinegar, oil, celery seeds, & pepper in a medium container. Place the container in the freezer till vinegar batter is well chilled, at least 15 or up to 30 mins.
2. While batter chills, toss cabbage with sugar & 1 Tsp. Salt in a large container. Cover & microwave for 1 min. Stir briefly, re-cover, & continue to microwave till cabbage is partially wilted & has reduced in volume by one-third, 30 to 60 seconds longer.
3. Shift cabbage to salad spinner & spin cabbage till excess water is removed, 10 to 20 seconds. Remove container from the freezer, Include cabbage, carrots, & parsley in cold vinegar batter, & toss to combine. Set flavour with sugar or vinegar & Season with salt to taste. Refrigerate till chilled, about 15 mins. Toss again before Serving.

505. CELERY ROOT SALAD WITH APPLE & PARSLEY

Prep Time: *11 Minutes* | *Cook Time:* *9 Minutes* | *Servings: 2*

INGREDIENTS:

- Tbsps. Lemon juice 1 1/2 Tbsps. Dijon mustard
- 1 Tsp. Honey 1/2 Tsp. salt
- 3 Tbsps. vegetable or canola oil
- 3 Tbsps. sour cream
- 1 head celery root (14 ounces), peeled
- 1/2 Granny Smith apple, peeled & cored
- scallions, sliced thin
- Tops. minced fresh parsley
- Tips. minced fresh tarragon (optional) Salt & pepper

TECHNIQUE:

1. In a medium container, whisk together lemon juice, mustard, honey, & salt. Include sour cream; whisk to combine. Set aside.
2. If using the food processor, cut celery root & apple into 1 1/2-inch pieces & grate with a shredding disc. You should have about 3 cups total. Include immediately to prepared dressing; toss to coat. Stir in scallions, parsley, & tarragon, if using. Season with salt & pepper to taste. Refrigerate till chilled, about 30 mins. Serve.

506. ALL-AMERICAN POTATO SALAD

Prep Time: *12 Minutes* | *Cook Time:* *10 Minutes* | *Servings: 2*

INGREDIENTS:

- lbs russet potatoes, peeled & cut into 3/4-inch cubes salt
- Tbsps. distilled white vinegar
- celery rib chopped fine 1/2 cup mayonnaise
- 3 Tbsps. sweet pickle relish
- 2 Tbsps. minced red onion
- 2 Tbsps. Minced fresh parsley 3/4 Tsp. dry mustard
- 3/4 Tsp. Celery seeds 1/4 Tsp. pepper
- 2 large FOOLPROOF HARD-COOKED EGGS, peeled & cut into 1/4-inch cubes (optional)

TECHNIQUE:

1. Place potatoes in a large saucepan & Include water to cover by 1 inch. Bring to boil over medium-high heat; Include 1 Tbsp. Salt, reduce heat to medium, & simmer, stirring once or twice, till potatoes are tender about 8 mins.
2. Drain potatoes & Shift to large containers. Include vinegar and, using a rubber spatula, toss gently to combine. Let stand till potatoes are just. Warm, about 20 mins.
3. Meanwhile, in a small container, stir together celery, mayonnaise, relish, onion, parsley, mustard, celery seeds, pepper, & 1/2 Tsp. Salt. Using a rubber spatula, gently fold dressing & eggs, if using, into potatoes. Cover with plastic wrap & refrigerate till chilled, about 1 hr; serve.

507. GARLICKY POTATO SALAD WITH TOMATOES & BASIL

Prep Time: *12 Minutes* | *Cook Time:* *10 Minutes* | *Servings: 4*

INGREDIENTS:

- lbs russet potatoes, peeled & cut into 3/4-inch cubes salt
- Tbsps. distilled white vinegar
- celery rib chopped fine 1/2 cup mayonnaise
- 2 Tbsps. minced red onion
- 2 Tbsps. minced fresh parsley
- garlic clove, minced
- 1/4 Tsp. pepper
- FOOLPROOF HARD-COOKED EGGS, peeled & cut into 1/4-inch cubes (optional) 1/2 cup chopped fresh basil
- 6 ounces cherry tomatoes, halved

TECHNIQUE:

1. Place potatoes in a large saucepan & Include water to cover by 1 inch. Bring to boil over medium-high heat; Include 1 Tbsp. Salt, reduce heat to medium, & simmer, stirring once or twice, till potatoes are tender about 8 mins.
2. Drain potatoes & Shift to large containers. Include vinegar and, using a rubber spatula, toss gently to combine. Let stand till potatoes are just warm, about 20 mins.
3. Meanwhile, in a small container, stir together celery, mayonnaise, onion, parsley, garlic, pepper, & 1/2 Tsp. Salt. Using a rubber spatula, gently.
4. Fold dressing & eggs, if using, into potatoes. Cover with plastic wrap & refrigerate till chilled, about 1 hr. Just before serving, Include basil & tomatoes; serve.

508. AUSTRIAN-STYLE POTATO SALAD

Prep Time: *12 Minutes* | *Cook Time:* *10 Minutes* | *Servings: 2*

INGREDIENTS:

- lbs Yukon Gold potatoes, peeled, quartered lengthwise, & cut into 1/2-inch-thick slices
- cup low-sodium chicken broth
- cup water
- Salt & pepper
- Tbsp. sugar
- Tbsps. white wine vinegar
- 1 Tbsp. Dijon mustard
- 1/4 cup vegetable oil
- 1 small red onion, chopped fine
- cornichons, minced (2 Tbsps.)
- 2 Tbsps. minced fresh chives

TECHNIQUE:

1. Bring potatoes, broth, water, 1 Tsp. Salt, sugar, & 1 Tbsp. Vinegar to boil in a 12-inch pan over high heat. Reduce heat to medium-low, cover, & cook till potatoes offer no resistance when pierced with a paring knife, 15 to 17 mins. Remove cover, increase heat to high (so cooking liquid will reduce), & cook for 2 mins.

2. Drain potatoes in the colander and set over a large container, reserving cooking liquid. Set drained potatoes aside. Pour off & discard all but 1/2 cup cooking liquid (if 1/2 cup liquid does not remain, Include water to make 1/2 cup). Whisk remaining Tbsp. Vinegar, mustard, & oil into cooking liquid.
3. Include 1/2 cup cooked potatoes to container with cooking liquid batter & mash with a potato masher or fork till thick sauce forms (batter will be slightly chunky). Include remaining potatoes, onion, cornichons, & chives, folding gently with a rubber spatula to combine. Season with salt & pepper to taste. Serve warm or at room temperature.

509. CLASSIC CREAMY CHICKEN SALAD

Prep Time: 12 Minutes | *Cook Time: 10 Minutes* | *Servings: 2*

INGREDIENTS:

(1 1/2-lb) whole bone-in chicken breasts
1 Tbsp. vegetable oil Salt
celery ribs, cut into small dice
scallions, minced
3/4–1 cup mayonnaise
1 1/2–2 Tbsps. lemon juice
Tbsps. minced fresh parsley

TECHNIQUE:

7. 2Set oven rack to middle setting & heat oven to 400 degrees. Set breasts on a small, aluminium foil-lined rimmed baking sheet. Brush with oil & sprinkle generously with salt. Roast till chicken registers 160 degrees, 35 to 40 mins. Let cool to room temperature, remove skin & bones, & shred meat into bite-size pieces (about 5 cups).
8. Using the lesser amounts of mayonnaise & lemon juice, mix all salad ingredients (including chicken) together in a large container. Set flavor & consistency with additional mayonnaise & lemon juice & salt & pepper to taste. Serve. (Chicken salad can be refrigerated overnight.)

510. THAI-STYLE CHICKEN SALAD WITH SPICY PEANUT DRESSING

Prep Time: 1 Minutes | *Cook Time: 9 Minutes* | *Servings: 6*

INGREDIENTS:

- 1/2 cup canola oil
- Tbsps. smooth peanut butter 1/2 cup lime juice (3 to 4 limes)
- 2 Tbsps. water Salt & pepper
- small garlic cloves, minced
- Tops. grated fresh ginger
- Tbsps. Light brown sugar 1 1/2 Tips. red pepper flakes
- 1/2 cucumber, peeled, halved lengthwise, seeded, & cut into 1-inch-long matchsticks 1 carrot, peeled & shredded
- 4 scallions, sliced thin
- 3 Tbsps. minced fresh cilantro
- recipe CLASSIC ROAST CHICKEN, cooled, meat removed & shredded into 2-inch pieces
- 1/2 cup unsalted peanuts, toasted & chopped

TECHNIQUE:

2. Puree oil, peanut butter, lime juice, water, 1/4 Tsp. Salt, garlic, ginger, brown sugar, & pepper flakes in the blender till combined. Shift to the large container. 2. Include cucumber, carrot, scallions, & cilantro to vinaigrette; toss to combine. Include chicken & toss gently to combine; let stand at room temperature 15 mins. Season with salt & pepper to taste & sprinkle with peanuts. Serve immediately.

511. SPANISH-STYLE CHICKEN SALAD AS WELL AS ROASTED RED PEPPER DRESSING

Prep Time: 11 Minutes | *Cook Time: 29 Minutes* | *Servings: 8*

INGREDIENTS:

- 1 1/3 cups chopped jarred roasted red peppers
- 1/2 cup extra-virgin olive oil
- Tbsps. sherry vinegar or balsamic vinegar
- 1 small garlic clove, minced salt & pepper
- 2 celery ribs, sliced very thin
- 1/2 cup chopped pitted green olives
- Tbsps. minced fresh parsley
- 1 small shallot, minced
- recipe CLASSIC ROAST CHICKEN, cooled, meat removed & shredded into 2-inch pieces
- 1/2 cup sliced almonds, toasted

TECHNIQUE:

1. Puree 2/3 cup roasted red peppers, oil, vinegar, garlic, 1/4 Tsp. Salt, & 1/2 Tsp. Pepper in the blender till smooth. Shift to a container.
2. Include celery, olives, parsley, shallot, & remaining 2/3 cup red peppers to vinaigrette; stir to combine. Include chicken & toss gently to combine; let stand at room temperature 15 mins. Season with salt & pepper to taste & sprinkle with almonds. Serve immediately.

512. CLASSIC TUNA SALAD

Prep Time: 12 Minutes | *Cook Time: 9 Minutes* | *Servings: 2*

INGREDIENTS:

- (6-ounce) cans solid white tuna in water
- Tbsps. lemon juice
- Salt & pepper
- 1 small celery rib, minced
- Tbsps. minced red onion
- Tbsps. chopped pickles (sweet or dill) 1/2 small garlic clove, minced
- Tbsps. minced fresh parsley
- 1/2 cup mayonnaise
- 1/4 Tsp. Dijon mustard

TECHNIQUE:

1. Drain tuna in a colander & shred with fingers till no clumps remain & texture is fine & even. Shift tuna to medium container & mix in lemon juice, 1/2 Tsp. Salt, 1/4 Tsp. Pepper, celery, onion, pickles, garlic, & parsley till evenly blended. Fold in mayonnaise & mustard till tuna is evenly moistened.

513. SHRIMP SALAD

Prep Time: 11 Minutes | *Cook Time: 9 Minutes* | *Servings: 2*

INGREDIENTS:

- lb extra-large shrimp, peeled, deveined, & tails removed
- 5 Tbsps. lemon juice (2 lemons), spent halves reserved
- 5 sprigs fresh parsley plus 1 Tsp. minced
- 3 sprigs fresh tarragon plus 1 Tsp. minced
- Tsp. whole black peppercorns
- Tbsp. sugar
- Salt & pepper
- 1/4 cup mayonnaise
- small shallot, minced
- small celery rib, minced

TECHNIQUE:

1. Combine shrimp, 1/4 cup lemon juice, preserved lemon halves, parsley sprigs, tarragon sprigs, whole peppercorns, sugar, & 1 Tsp. Salt as well as 2 cups cold water in a medium saucepan. Place saucepan over medium heat & cook shrimp, stirring several times, till pink, firm to touch, & centres are no longer translucent, 8 to 10 mins (water should be just bubbling around the edge of cooking wok & register 165 degrees). Remove cooking wok from heat, cover, & let shrimp sit in the broth for 2 mins.
2. Meanwhile, fill the medium container with ice water. Drain shrimp into the colander, discard lemon halves, herbs, & spices. Immediately Shift shrimp to ice water to stop cooking & chill thoroughly for about 3 mins.
3. Remove shrimp from ice water & pat dry with paper towels.
4. Whisk together mayonnaise, shallot, celery, remaining 1 Tbsp. Lemon juice, minced parsley, & minced tarragon in a medium container.
5. Divide shrimp in half lengthwise & then cut each half into thirds; Include shrimp to mayonnaise batter & toss to combine. Season with salt & pepper to taste & serve. (Shrimp salad can be refrigerated overnight.)

514. CLASSIC EGG SALAD

Prep Time: 11 Minutes | *Cook Time: 9 Minutes* | *Servings: 2*

INGREDIENTS:

- FOOLPROOF HARD-COOKED EGGS, peeled & diced medium 1/4 cup mayonnaise
- 2 Tbsps. minced red onion
- 1 Tbsp. minced fresh parsley 1/2 celery rib, minced
- 2 Tips. Dijon mustard
- 2 Tips. Lemon juice 1/4 Tsp. salt
- Pepper

TECHNIQUE:

1. Mix all ingredients together in a medium container, including pepper, to taste. Serve. (Egg salad can be refrigerated in an airtight container for 1 day.)

515. QUICK CHICKEN STOCK

Prep Time: 11 Minutes | *Cook Time: 69 Minutes* | *Servings: 2*

INGREDIENTS:

- Tbsp. vegetable oil
- onion, chopped
- lbs whole chicken legs or backs & wingtips, cut into 2-inch pieces
- 8 cups boiling water
- 1/2 Tsp. salt
- bay leaves

TECHNIQUE:

1. Heat oil in stockpot oven over medium-high heat till shimmering. Include onion & cook till slightly softened, 2 to 3 mins. Shift to the large container. Brown chicken in 2 batches, cooking on each side till lightly browned, about 5 mins per side. Shift to the container with onion.
2. Return onion & chicken to pot. Reduce heat to low, cover, & sweat till chicken releases its juices, about 20 mins. Increase heat to high & Include boiling water, salt, & bay leaves. Take to boil, then reduce heat to low, cover, & simmer slowly till stock is rich & flavorful, about 20 mins, skimming foam off the surface if desired.
3. Strain stock, discard solids. Before using, defat stock.

Dinner Recipes

516. RICH BEEF STOCK

Prep Time: 11 Minutes | *Cook Time: 67 Minutes* | *Servings: 2*

INGREDIENTS:

- Tbsps. vegetable oil
- 1 large onion, chopped
- lbs beef shanks, meat cut from the bone in large chunks, or 4 lbs beef chuck, cut into 3-inch chunks, & 2 lbs small marrowbones
- 1/2 cup dry red wine
- cups boiling water 1/2 Tsp. salt
- 2 bay leaves

TECHNIQUE:

1. Heat 1 Tbsp. Oil in stockpot oven over medium-high heat till shimmering. Include onion & cook, occasionally stirring, till slightly softened, 2 to 3 mins. Shift to the large container.
2. Brown meat & bones on all sides in 3 or 4 batches, about 5 mins per batch, including remaining oil to pot as necessary; do not overcrowd. Shift to the container with onion. Include wine to pot & cook, scraping up browned bits with a wooden spoon, till wine is reduced to about 3 Tbsps., about 2 mins. Return browned beef & onion to pot, reduce heat to low, cover, & sweat till meat releases juices, about 20 mins.

Increase heat to high. Include boiling water, salt, & bay leaves. Take it to boil, then reduce heat to low, cover, & simmer slowly till meat is tender & stock is flavorful, 1 1/2 to 2 hrs, skimming foam off the surface. Strain & discard bones & onion; reserve meat for another use, if desired.

3. Before using, defat stock.

517. FISH STOCK

Prep Time: *1 Minutes* | *Cook Time:* *29 Minutes* | *Servings: 6*

INGREDIENTS:

- Tbsps. unsalted butter
- 3 lbs fish frames, cleaned
- onions, chopped
- 1 large celery rib, chopped coarsely
- ounces white mushrooms, trimmed & quartered 1/2 ounce dried porcini mushrooms, rinsed (optional)
- garlic cloves, peeled & smashed
- 1 3/4 cups dry white wine
- 8 cups water
- sprigs fresh parsley
- 5 sprigs of fresh thyme
- 2 tbsps. salt
- 8 whole black peppercorns
- 2 bay leaves

TECHNIQUE:

1. Melt butter in stockpot oven over high heat. Include fish frames, onions, celery, white mushrooms, porcini mushrooms. If using, & garlic, cover, & cook, occasionally stirring, till fish frames have begun to release some liquid, 6 to 8 mins.
2. Reduce heat to medium & continue to cook, covered, often stirring with a wooden spoon to break apart fish frames, till vegetables & bones are soft & aromatic, 6 to 8 mins longer.
3. Include wine, cover, & simmer gently for 10 mins. Include water, parsley, thyme, salt, peppercorns, & bay leaves. Return to gentle simmer & cook, uncovered, skimming as needed, till stock tastes rich & flavorful, about 30 mins longer.
4. Strain stock through a fine-mesh strainer, then defat stock.

518. CHEATER'S FISH STOCK

Prep Time: *12 Minutes* | *Cook Time:* *10 Minutes* | *Servings: 6*

INGREDIENTS:

- small onion, chopped
- carrot, chopped
- celery rib, chopped
- 8 sprigs of fresh parsley
- cup dry white wine
- (8-ounce) bottles clam juice
- 2 bay leaves
- 8 whole black peppercorns
- 1/2 Tsp. dried thyme
- Salt

TECHNIQUE:

1. take all ingredients to boil in a medium saucepan & simmer to blend flavours, about 30 mins. Strain stock through cheesecloth, pressing on solids with the back of the spoon to extract as much liquid as possible. Season with salt to taste. Use immediately.

519. ULTIMATE VEGETABLE STOCK

Prep Time: *35 Minutes* | *Cook Time:* *11 Minutes* | *Servings: 2*

INGREDIENTS:

- 2 onions, peeled & chopped
- head garlic (10 to 12 cloves), cloves peeled & smashed
- 8 ounces shallots, sliced thin
- celery rib, chopped
- small carrot, peeled & chopped Vegetable oil spray
- lbs leeks, white & light green parts only, halved lengthwise, chopped, & washed thoroughly
- 8 1/2 cups boiling water
- 2 bay leaves
- 1 1/2 Tips. salt
- Tsp. black peppercorns, roughly cracked
- lb collard greens, sliced crosswise into 2-inch strips
- 12 ounces cauliflower, chopped fine
- 8–10 sprigs of fresh thyme
- lemongrass stalk, trimmed to bottom 6 inches & bruised
- 4 scallions, sliced into 2-inch pieces
- 2 Tips. rice vinegar

TECHNIQUE:

1. Combine onions, garlic, shallots, celery, & carrot in the 8-quart stockpot or Dutch oven; spray vegetables lightly with vegetable oil spray & toss to coat. Cover & cook over low heat, frequently stirring, till cooking wok bottom shows light brown glaze, 20 to 30 mins. Include leeks and
2. Increase heat to medium; cook, covered, till leeks soften, about 10 mins. Include 1 1/2 cups boiling water & cook, partially covered, till the water has evaporated to a glaze & vegetables are very soft, 25 to 35 mins.
3. Include parsley stems, bay leaves, salt, peppercorns, & the remaining 7 cups of boiling water. Increase heat to medium-high & bring to simmer; reduce heat to medium-low & simmer gently, covered, to blend flavours, about 15 mins.
4. Include collard greens, cauliflower, thyme, lemongrass, & scallions. Increase heat to medium-high & bring to simmer; reduce heat to low & simmer gently, covered, to blend flavours, about 15 mins longer. Strain stock through large strainer into large container or container, allowing stock to drip through to drain thoroughly (do not press on solids). Stir vinegar into stock.

520. CLASSIC CHICKEN NOODLE SOUP

Prep Time: *12 Minutes* | *Cook Time:* *10 Minutes* | *Servings: 2*

INGREDIENTS:

- Tbsp. vegetable oil
- (4-lb) whole chicken, breast removed, split, & reserved; remaining chicken cut into 2-inch pieces
- onion, chopped
- cups boiling water
- 2 Tips. salt
- 2 bay leaves
- Tbsps. chicken fat, reserved from making stock, or vegetable oil
- 1 onion, chopped
- 1 large carrot, peeled & sliced 1/4 inch thick 1 celery rib, sliced 1/4 inch thick
- 1/2 Tsp. dried thyme
- 3 ounces egg noodles
- 1/4 cup minced fresh parsley
- Salt & pepper

TECHNIQUE:

1. FOR THE STOCK: Heat oil in a Dutch oven over medium-high heat till shimmering. Include half of the chicken pieces & cook till lightly browned, about 5 mins per side. Shift cooked chicken to container and
2. Repeat with remaining chicken pieces; Shift to the container with the first batch. Include onion & cook, frequently stirring, till onion is translucent, 3 to 5 mins. Return chicken pieces to the pot. Reduce heat to low, cover, & cook till chicken releases its juices, about 20 mins.
3. Increase heat to high; Include boiling water, reserved chicken breast pieces, salt, & bay leaves. Reduce heat to medium-low & simmer till flavours have blended about 20 mins.
4. Remove breast pieces from the pot. When cool enough, remove the skin from breasts, then remove meat from bones & shred into bite-size pieces; discard skin & bones. Strain stock into a container, pressing on solids to extract as much liquid as possible; discard solids. Allow the liquid to settle, about 5 mins, then skim off fat; reserve 2 Tbsps., if desired (see note).
5. Heat reserved chicken fat in a Dutch oven over medium-high heat. Include onion, carrot, & celery & cook till softened, about 5 mins. Include thyme & reserved stock & simmer till the vegetables are tender, 10 to 15 mins.
6. Include noodles & reserved shredded chicken & cook till just tender, 5 to 8 mins. Stir in parsley, Season with salt & pepper to taste, & serve. (After skimming broth in step 3, shredded chicken, strained stock, & fat can be refrigerated in separate containers for up to 2 days.)

521. CLASSIC CHICKEN SOUP WITH LEEKS, WILD RICE, & MUSHROOMS

Prep Time: *17 Minutes* | *Cook Time:* *15 Minutes* | *Servings: 5*

INGREDIENTS:

- Tbsp. vegetable oil
- (4-lb) whole chicken, breast removed, split, & reserved; remaining chicken cut into 2-inch pieces
- onion, chopped
- cups boiling water Salt
- 2 bay leaves
- 1/2 ounce dried shiitake mushrooms or other dried wild mushrooms
- Tbsps. chicken fat, reserved from making stock, or vegetable oil
- 1 large carrot, peeled & sliced 1/4 inch thick
- leek, white & light green parts only, quartered lengthwise, sliced thin, & washed thoroughly
- ounces cremini or white mushrooms, trimmed & sliced thin 1/2 Tsp. dried thyme
- 1/2 cup cooked wild rice
- 1/4 cup minced fresh parsley Pepper

TECHNIQUE:

1. Heat oil in Dutch in the oven till shimmering. Include half of the chicken pieces & cook till lightly browned, about 5 mins per side. Shift cooked chicken to a container & repeat with remaining chicken pieces; Shift to a container with the first batch. Include onion & cook, frequently stirring, till onion is translucent, 3 to 5 mins. Return chicken pieces to the pot. Reduce heat to low, cover, & cook till chicken releases its juices, about 20 mins.
2. Increase heat to high; Include boiling water, reserved chicken breast.
3. Pieces, salt, & bay leaves. Reduce heat to medium-low & simmer till flavours have blended about 20 mins. Remove 1 cup of stock & pour over dried mushrooms & let sit for 30 mins to rehydrate.
4. Remove breast pieces from the pot. When cool enough, remove the skin from breasts, then remove meat from bones & shred into bite-size pieces; discard skin & bones. Strain stock through a fine-mesh strainer into a container, pressing on solids to extract as much liquid as possible; discard solids. Allow the liquid to settle, about 5 mins, then skim off fat; reserve 2 Tbsps., if desired (see note).
5. Heat reserved chicken fat in a Dutch oven over medium-high heat. Include carrot & leek & cook till softened, about 5 mins. Include fresh mushrooms to pot with carrot & leek & cook till softened, about 5 mins. Drain & chop rehydrated dried mushrooms, reserving soaking liquid. Strain soaking liquid through a fine-mesh strainer lined with a coffee filter. Include thyme, reserved stock, chopped mushrooms, & strained mushroom soaking liquid & simmer till vegetables are tender, 10 to 15 mins.
6. Include rice & reserved shredded chicken & cook till just tender, about 5 mins. Stir in parsley, Season with salt & pepper to taste, & serve. (After skimming broth in step 3, shredded chicken, strained stock, & fat can be refrigerated in separate containers for up to 2 days.)

522. HEARTY CHICKEN NOODLE SOUP

Prep Time: *12 Minutes* | *Cook Time:* *10 Minutes* | *Servings: 5*

INGREDIENTS:

- Tbsp. vegetable oil
- lb ground chicken
- small onion, chopped
- carrot, peeled & chopped
- celery rib, chopped
- cups low-sodium chicken broth
- 4 cups water
- 2 (12-ounce) bone-in split chicken breasts, trimmed & cut in half crosswise 2 bay leaves
- 2 Tips. salt

- Tbsps. cornstarch 1/4 cup cold water
- 1 small onion, halved & sliced thin
- 2 carrots, peeled, halved lengthwise, & cut crosswise into 3/4-inch pieces 1 celery rib, halved lengthwise & cut crosswise into 1/2-inch pieces
- 1 russet potato (6 ounces), peeled & cut into 3/4-inch cubes 4 ounces egg noodles 2 ounces Swiss chard, stemmed & leaves torn into 1-inch pieces (optional)
- 1 Tbsp. minced fresh parsley Salt & pepper

TECHNIQUE:

1. Heat oil in Dutch oven till shimmering. Include ground chicken, onion, carrot, & celery. Cook, stirring continuously, till chicken is no longer pink, 5 to 10 mins (do not brown chicken).
2. Reduce heat to medium-low. Include broth, water, chicken breasts, bay leaves, & salt; cover & cook for 30 mins. Open the lid and bring it to a boil over high heat. (As soon as the liquid boils when you open the lid, remove the chicken breast and continue with the recipe.) Transfer the chicken breast to a large plate. Continue to cook the broth for 20 minutes, turning on the heat to keep the boiling water soft. Filter the broth through a fine sieve in a large saucepan or container, pressing the solids to extract as much liquid as possible. Let the liquid settle for 5 minutes and remove the fat.
3. Come back the stock to the Dutch oven on medium-high heat.
4. In a small container, combine cornstarch & water till smooth slurry forms; stir into stock & bring to a gentle boil. Include onion, carrots, celery, & potato & cook till potato pieces are almost tender, 10 to 15 mins; setting heat as necessary to maintain a gentle boil. Include egg noodles & continue to cook till all vegetables & noodles are tender, about 5 mins longer.
5. Meanwhile, remove the skin from reserved cooked chicken, then remove meat from bones & shred it into bite-size pieces; discard skin & bones. Include shredded chicken, Swiss chard, if using, & parsley to soup & cook till heated through about 2 mins. Season with salt & pepper to taste & serve. (After skimming broth in step 2, stock & chicken breasts can be refrigerated separately for up to 2 days.)

523. GREEK EGG-LEMON SOUP

Prep Time: 14 Minutes | *Cook Time: 12 Minutes* | *Servings: 2*

INGREDIENTS:

- cups QUICK CHICKEN STOCK
- 1/2 cup long-grain white rice
- 1 bay leaf
- 4 green cardamom pods, crushed, or 2 whole cloves 12 (4-inch) strips lemon zest plus 1/4 cup juice (2 lemons)
- 1 1/2 Tips. salt
- 2 large eggs as well as 2 large yolks, room temperature
- scallion, sliced thin and/or 3 Tbsps. Chopped fresh mint,

TECHNIQUE:

1. take chicken stock to boil in a medium saucepan over high heat. Include rice, bay leaf, cardamom, lemon zest, & salt. Reduce heat to medium & simmer till rice is tender & stock is aromatic from lemon zest, 16 to 20 mins.
2. Remove & discard bay leaf, cardamom, & zest strips. Increase heat to high & return stock to boil, then reduce heat to low.
3. Gently whisk whole eggs, egg yolks, & lemon juice in a medium container till combined. Whisking continuously, slowly ladle about 2 cups hot stock into egg batter & whisk till combined. Pour egg batter back into saucepan & cook over low heat, constantly stirring, till soup is slightly thickened & wisps of steam appear, 4 to 5 mins (do not simmer or boil). Divide soup among serving containers, sprinkle with scallion and/or mint, & serve immediately.

524. TORTILLA SOUP

Prep Time: 22 Minutes | *Cook Time: 20 Minutes* | *Servings: 8*

INGREDIENTS:

- (6-inch) corn tortillas, cut into 1/2-inch-wide strips
- 1 Tbsp. vegetable oil Salt
- (12-ounce) bone-in split chicken breasts or 4 (5-ounce) bone-in chicken thighs, skin removed & trimmed
- 8 cups low-sodium chicken broth
- large white onion, trimmed off the root end, quartered, & peeled
- 4 garlic cloves, peeled
- 8–10 sprigs of fresh cilantro plus 1 sprig of fresh oregano or 2 sprigs fresh epazote Salt
- tomatoes, cored & quartered 1/2 jalapeño chile
- 1 Tbsp. minced canned chipotle chile in adobo sauce
- 1 Tbsp. vegetable oil
- 1 avocado, halved, pitted, & diced fine
- ounces Cotija cheese, crumbled, or Monterey Jack cheese, diced fine Lime wedges
- Fresh cilantro Minced jalapeño chile
- Mexican crema or sour cream

TECHNIQUE:

1. Set oven rack to middle setting; heat oven up to 425 degrees. Sprinkle tortilla strips on rimmed baking sheet; drizzle with oil & toss till evenly coated. Bake till strips is deep golden brown & crisp, about 14 mins, rotating baking sheet & shaking strips (to redistribute) halfway through baking. Season strips lightly with salt & Shift to the paper towel-lined plate.
2. While tortilla strips bake, bring chicken, broth, 2 onion quarters, 2 garlic cloves, cilantro & oregano, & 1/2 Tsp. Salt to boil over medium heat in a large saucepan. Minimize heat to low, cover, & simmer till chicken is just cooked through about 20 mins. Using tongs, Shift the chicken to a large plate. Pour broth into a fine-mesh strainer & discard solids. When cool enough, shred chicken into bite-size pieces, discarding bones.
3. Puree tomatoes, remaining 2 onion quarters, remaining 2 garlic cloves, jalapeño, & chipotle in the food processor till smooth. Heat oil in Dutch in the oven over high heat till shimmering. Include tomato-onion puree & 1/8 Tsp. Salt & cook, frequently stirring, till batter has darkened in colour, about 10 mins.
4. Stir strained broth into tomato batter, bring to boil, then reduce heat to low & simmer to blend flavours, about 15 mins. Include shredded chicken & simmer till heated through about 5 mins. Place portions of tortilla strips in containers & ladle soup over. Serve, passing garnishes separately.

525. THAI-STYLE CHICKEN SOUP

Prep Time: 11 Minutes | *Cook Time: 9 Minutes* | *Servings: 2*

INGREDIENTS:

- 1 Tsp. vegetable oil
- 3 lemongrass stalks, trimmed to bottom 6 inches, halved lengthwise & sliced thin crosswise
- 3 large shallots, chopped
- sprigs, fresh cilantro, chopped coarsely
- 3 Tbsps. fish sauce
- 4 cups low-sodium chicken broth
- 2 (14-ounce) cans of coconut milk
- 1 Tbsp. sugar
- ounces white mushrooms, trimmed & sliced 1/4 inch thick
- lb boneless, skinless chicken breasts (about 3 breasts), trimmed, halved lengthwise, & sliced on the bias into 1/8-inch-thick pieces
- Tbsps. lime juice (2 limes)
- 2 Tips. Thai red curry paste
- 1/2 cup fresh cilantro leaves
- serrano chiles, stemmed, seeded, & sliced thin
- scallions, sliced thin on bias Lime wedges

TECHNIQUE:

1. Heat oil in a saucepan and overheat till just shimmering. Include lemongrass, shallots, cilantro, & 1 Tbsp.
2. Fish sauce & cook, frequently stirring, till lemongrass & shallots are just softened but not browned, 2 to 5 mins.
3. Stir in chicken broth & 1 can of coconut milk & bring to simmer over high heat. Cover, reduce heat to low, & simmer till flavours have blended about 10 mins. Rinse saucepan & return broth batter to the pan.
4. Stir remaining can coconut milk & sugar into broth batter & bring to simmer over medium-high heat. Reduce heat to medium, Include mushrooms, & cook till just tender, 2 to 3 mins. Include chicken & cook, constantly stirring, till no longer pink, 1 to 3 mins. Remove soup from heat. Combine lime juice, curry paste, & the remaining 2 Tbsps. Fish sauce in a small container & stir into soup.
5. Ladle soup into containers & garnish with cilantro, chiles, & scallions. Serve immediately with lime wedges.

526. HOT & SOUR SOUP

Prep Time: 11 Minutes | *Cook Time: 9 Minutes* | *Servings: 2*

INGREDIENTS:

- ounces extra-firm tofu drained 1/4 cup soy sauce
- 1 Tsp. toasted sesame oil
- 3 Tbsps. Plus 1 1/2 Tips. cornstarch
- (6-ounce) boneless centre-cut pork loin chop, 1/2 inch thick, trimmed & cut into 1 by 1/8-inch matchsticks
- Tbsps. Plus 1 Tsp. cold water
- 1 large egg
- 6 cups low-sodium chicken broth
- 1 (5-ounce) can bamboo shoots, sliced lengthwise into 1/8-inch-thick strips 4 ounces shiitake mushrooms, stemmed & sliced 1/4 inch thick
- Tbsps. Black Chinese vinegar or 1 Tbsp. Red wine vinegar plus 1 Tbsp. balsamic vinegar
- 2 Tips. chilli oil
- Tsp. ground white pepper
- 3 scallions, sliced thin

TECHNIQUE:

1. Place tofu in a paper towel-lined pie plate, top with a heavy plate, & weigh with 2 heavy cans. Let tofu drain till it has released about 1/2 cup liquid, about 15 mins.
2. Whisk 1 Tbsp. Soy sauce, sesame oil, & 1 Tsp. Cornstarch in a medium container. Include pork in the container, toss to coat, & let marinate for at least 10 mins or up to 30 mins.
3. Combine 3 Tbsps. Cornstarch with 3 Tbsps. Water in a small container. Mix remaining 1/2 Tsp. Cornstarch with remaining 1 Tsp. Water in a second small container. Include egg & beat with a fork till combined.
4. Take broth to boil in a large saucepan over medium heat. Reduce heat to medium-low, Include bamboo shoots & mushrooms, & simmer till mushrooms are just tender, about 5 mins. While the broth simmers, cut tofu into 1/2-inch cubes. Include tofu & pork with its marinade to the pan, stirring to separate any pieces of pork that stick together. Continue to simmer till pork is no longer pink, about 2 mins.
5. Stir cornstarch batter to recombine, then Include to soup & increase heat to medium-high. Cook, occasionally stirring, till the soup thickens & turns translucent, about 1 min. Stir in vinegar, chilli oil, pepper, & the remaining 3 Tbsps. Soy sauce & turn off the heat.
6. Without stirring soup, use a soupspoon to slowly drizzle very thin streams of the egg batter into the pot in a circular motion. Let soup sit for 1 min, then return the saucepan to medium-high heat. Bring soup to a gentle boil, then immediately remove from heat. Gently stir soup once to evenly distribute the egg. Ladle soup into containers, top with scallions, & serve.

527. QUICK BEEF & VEGETABLE SOUP

Prep Time: 11 Minutes | *Cook Time: 29 Minutes* | *Servings: 5*

INGREDIENTS:

- lb sirloin tip steaks, trimmed & cut into 1/2-inch pieces
- 2 Tbsps. soy sauce
- Tsp. vegetable oil
- lb cremini mushrooms, trimmed & quartered
- large onion, chopped
- Tbsps. tomato paste
- 1 garlic clove, minced
- 1/2 cup red wine
- 4 cups beef broth
- 1 3/4 cups low-sodium chicken broth
- carrots, peeled & cut into 1/2-inch pieces
- 2 celery ribs, cut into 1/2-inch pieces 1 bay leaf
- 1 Tbsp. unflavored gelatin
- 1/2 cup cold water
- Tbsps. minced fresh parsley Salt & pepper

TECHNIQUE:

1. Combine beef & soy sauce in a medium container. Let sit for 15 mins.
2. Heat oil in Dutch in the oven over high heat till just smoking. Include mushrooms & onion & cook, frequently stirring, till onion is Browned, 8 to 12 mins. Shift vegetables to the container.
3. Include beef & cook, occasionally stirring, till liquid evaporates & meat starts to brown, 6 to 10 mins. Include tomato paste & garlic to pot & cook, constantly stirring,

till aromatic, about 30 seconds. Stir in wine, the pot with a wooden spoon to loosen browned bits, & cook till the liquid reduces & becomes syrupy, 1 to 2 mins.

4. Include beef broth, chicken broth, carrots, celery, bay leaf, & browned mushrooms & onion into the pot & bring to boil. Reduce heat to low, cover, & simmer till vegetables & meat are tender, 25 to 30 mins. Remove from heat & remove & discard bay leaf.
5. Meanwhile, sprinkle gelatin over cold water & allow it to soften for 5 mins. Include gelatin batter in the pot with soup & stir till completely dissolved. Stir in parsley, Season with salt & pepper to taste, & serve.

528. VIETNAMESE-STYLE BEEF NOODLE SOUP

Prep Time: *12 Minutes* *Cook Time:* *10 Minutes* *Servings: 6*

INGREDIENTS:

- 8 ounces wide rice noodles
- 5 cups low-sodium chicken broth
- 4 garlic cloves, peeled & smashed
- (2-inch) piece fresh ginger, peeled, cut into 1/8-inch rounds, & smashed
- 2 (3-inch-long) cinnamon sticks
- 2-star anise pods
- 2 Tbsps. fish sauce
- Tbsp. soy sauce
- Tbsp. sugar
- (12-ounce) shell sirloin steak, trimmed & sliced crosswise into 1/4-inch strips salt & pepper
- Tbsp. vegetable oil
- 5 ounces bean sprouts (2 1/2 cups)
- jalapeño chile stemmed, seeded, & sliced thin crosswise
- 2 scallions, sliced thin on the bias
- 1/3 cup fresh basil, large leaves are torn in half
- 1/2 cup fresh mint, large leaves are torn in half
- 1/2 cup fresh cilantro leaves
- Tbsps. chopped unsalted roasted peanuts Lime wedges

TECHNIQUE:

1. Take 4 quarts of water to boil in a large pot. Off heat, Include noodles & let sit till tender but not mushy, 10 to 15 mins. Drain & distribute among 4 containers.
2. Take all ingredients to boil in a medium saucepan over medium-high heat. Reduce heat to low & simmer, partially covered, 20 mins. Remove solids from cooking wok with slotted spoon & discard. Cover broth & keep hot over low heat till ready to serve.
3. Season steak with salt & pepper. Heat oil in the 10-inch pan over medium-high heat till shimmering. Include half of the steak slices in a single layer & sear till well-browned, 1 to 2 mins on each side; set aside. Repeat with remaining slices.
4. Divide sprouts among containers with noodles, Include steak, then ladle in the broth. Sprinkle each serving with jalapeño, scallions, basil, mint, cilantro, & peanuts & serve, passing lime wedges separately.

529. VIETNAMESE-STYLE CHICKEN NOODLE SOUP

Prep Time: *11 Minutes* *Cook Time:* *9 Minutes* *Servings: 2*

INGREDIENTS:

- 8 ounces wide rice noodles
- 5 cups low-sodium chicken broth
- ounces boneless, skinless chicken thighs (about 3 thighs), trimmed
- 4 garlic cloves, peeled & smashed
- 1 (2-inch) piece fresh ginger, peeled, divide into 1/8-inch rounds, & smashed 2-star anise pods
- 3 Tbsps. fish sauce
- 1 Tbsp. soy sauce
- 2 Tips. sugar Salt
- cups shredded napa cabbage
- 2 scallions, sliced thin on the bias
- 1/2 cup fresh mint, large leaves are torn in half
- 1/2 cup fresh cilantro leaves
- Tbsps. Chopped unsalted roasted peanuts Lime wedges

TECHNIQUE:

1. take 4 quarts water to boil in a large pot. Off heat, Include noodles & let sit till tender but not mushy, 10 to 15 mins. Drain & distribute among 4 containers.
2. Bring all ingredients except salt to boil in a medium saucepan over medium-high heat. Reduce heat to low & simmer, partially covered, to blend flavours, 10 to 15 mins, till chicken is cooked through, about 10 mins.
3. Remove chicken with a slotted spoon & continue to simmer broth, about 10 mins. When chicken is cool enough, slice thin. Strain broth through fine-mesh strainer & return to pot. Season with salt to taste. Cover broth & keep hot over low heat till ready to serve.
4. Divide cabbage & chicken among containers with noodles, then ladle in the broth. Sprinkle each serving with scallions, mint, cilantro, & peanuts & serve, passing lime wedges separately.

530. BEST FRENCH ONION SOUP

Prep Time: *12 Minutes* *Cook Time:* *10 Minutes* *Servings: 4*

INGREDIENTS:

- lbs onions, halved & sliced through the root end into 1/4-inch-thick pieces
- 3 Tbsps. unsalted butter, cut into 3 pieces salt & pepper
- 2 cups water, plus extra for deglazing
- 1/2 cup dry sherry
- cups low-sodium chicken broth
- 2 cups beef broth
- 6 sprigs of thyme
- 1 bay leaf
- 1 small baguette, cut into 1/2-inch slices
- ounces shredded Gruyère cheese (2 cups)

TECHNIQUE:

1. Set oven rack to lower-middle setting & heat oven to 400 degrees. And spray inside of Dutch oven with vegetable oil spray. Include onions, butter, & 1 Tsp. Salt. Cook, covered, for 1 hr (onions will be moist & slightly reduced in volume). Remove pot from oven & stir onions, scraping bottom & sides of the pool. Return pot into the oven with lid slightly ajar & continue to cook till onions
2. They are very soft & golden brown, 1 1/2 to 1 3/4 hrs longer, stirring onions & scraping bottom & sides of pot after 1 hr.
3. Carefully remove the pot from the oven (leave the range on) & place over medium-high heat. Cook onions, stirring frequently & scraping bottom & sides of the pot, till liquid evaporates & onions brown, 15 to 20 mins (reduce heat to medium if onions brown too quickly). Continue to cook, frequently stirring, till the bottom of the pot is coated with dark crust, 6 to 8 mins; setting heat as necessary. Stir in 1/4 cup water, scraping pot bottom to loosen crust, & cook till water evaporates & pot bottom has made another crust, 6 to 8 mins. Repeat the process of deglazing three times till the onions are very dark brown. Stir in sherry & cook, frequently stirring, till sherry evaporates, about 5 mins.
4. Stir in 2 cups water with chicken broth, beef broth, thyme, bay leaf, & 1/2 Tsp. Salt, scraping up any final bits of browned crust on the bottom & sides of the pot. Increase heat to high & bring to simmer. Reduce heat and cover, & simmer for 30 mins. Remove & discard herbs & season with salt & pepper to taste. While soup simmers, arrange baguette slices in a single layer on a rimmed baking sheet & bake till bread is dry, crisp, & golden at edges, about 10 mins. Set aside.
5. Set oven rack 7 to 8 inches from broiler element & heat broiler. Set 6 broiler-safe crocks on a rimmed baking sheet & fill each with about 1 3/4 cups soup. Top each container with 1 or 2 baguette slices (do not overlap slices) & sprinkle evenly with Gruyère. Broil till cheese is melted & bubbly around edges, 3 to 5 mins. Let cool 5 mins before serving.

Side Dishes Recipes

531. CHERRY-BRANDY BAKED BRIE

Prep Time: *15 Minutes* *Cook Time:* *44 Minutes* *Servings: 2*

INGREDIENTS:

- 1 round (8 ounces) Brie cheese
- ½ mug dried cherries
- ½ mug chopped walnuts
- ¼ mugs packed brown sugar
- ¼ mug brandy or unsweetened apple juice French bread baguette, sliced and toasted or assorted crackers

DIRECTIONS:

1. Preheat oven to 350°. Place cheese in a 9-in. pie plate. Mix cherries, walnuts, as well as brown sugar and brandy; spoon over cheese.
2. Bake 15-20 minutes or until cheese is softened.
3. Serve it with a baguette.

532. BUFFALO WING CHEESE MOLD

Prep Time: *15 Minutes* *Cook Time:* *93 Minutes* *Servings: 8*

INGREDIENTS:

- 2 packages cream cheese of 8 ounces each
- softened 2 celery ribs, finely chopped
- 2 mugs (8 ounces) crumbled blue cheese
- 1 cup shredded Monterey Jack cheese
- 1 ½ cup finely chopped cooked chicken breasts
- 3 tbsp buffalo wing sauce
- 1 French bread baguette (16 ounces)
- ¼ mug olive oil
- ½ cup shredded carrots, optional

DIRECTIONS:

1. In a bowl, mix the cream cheese, celery, blue and Monterey Jack cheeses. In a small bowl, combine chicken and
2. wing sauce.
3. Line a 1-qt. Bowl with plastic cover, overlapping the sides of the bowl. Spread 1 ½ mug of cream cheese mixture over the bottom and up the sides in a prepared bowl. Layer with the chicken mixture as well as the remaining cream cheese mixture. Bring plastic cover over cheese; press down smoothly. Now let it cool for about 4 hours or until firm.
4. Just before serving, cut the baguette into ¼-in. slices. To keep on an ungreased baking sheet, brush with oil. Bake at 375° for 10-12 minutes or until lightly browned.
5. Extract mould from the refrigerator and invert onto a serving plate. Extract bowl and plastic cover. Garnish with carrots if desired. Serve with toasted baguette slices.

533. CHUNKY MANGO GUACAMOLE

Prep Time: *5 Minutes* *Cook Time:* *35 Minutes* *Servings: 2*

INGREDIENTS:

- 3 medium ripe avocados, peeled and chopped 1 large mango, peeled and chopped 1 large tomato, chopped
- 1 small red onion, chopped
- ¼ mug chopped fresh cilantro 3 tbsp lime juice
- 1 tsp salt

DIRECTIONS:

1. Assorted fresh vegetables and tortilla chips In a large bowl, mix the first five ingredients; stir in lime juice and salt. Serve with vegetables and chips.

534. APPETIZER BLUE CHEESE LOGS

Prep Time: *15 Minutes* *Cook Time:* *30 Minutes* *Servings: 4*

INGREDIENTS:

- 1 package (8 ounces) cream cheese, softened
- 1 mug (4 ounces) shredded sharp cheddar cheese
- ½ mug crumbled blue cheese
- 1 ½ tsp curry powder
- 1 tbsp butter
- ½ mug finely chopped pecans
- 2 tbsps minced fresh parsley
- Assorted crackers

DIRECTIONS:

1. In a bowl, beat the cream cheese. Fold in cheddar cheese and blue cheese. Cover and let cool for at least 2 hours.

2. In a small frying pan, fry the buttered curry powder for 1-2 minutes. Add now the pecans and cook for 1 minute, stirring. Mix the parsley. Now Cooldown a bit. Roll the cheese mixture into two sticks about 5 inches long. Roll out the hazelnut mixture. Cover and cook until served. Serve with crackers.

535. CREAMY BLACK BEAN SALSA

Prep Time: 15 Minutes *Cook Time: 54 Minutes* *Servings: 2*

INGREDIENTS:

- 1 can (15 ounces) black beans,
- 1 ½ mug frozen corn, thawed
- 1 mug finely chopped sweet red pepper
- ¾ mug finely chopped green pepper ½ mug finely chopped red onion
- 1 tbsp minced fresh parsley
- ½ mug sour cream ¼ mug mayonnaise 2 tbsps red wine vinegar
- 1 tsp ground cumin
- 1 tsp chili powder
- ½ tsp salt
- ¼ tsp garlic powder
- 1/8 tsp pepper Tortilla chips

DIRECTIONS:

1. In a bowl, combine together the beans, corn, peppers, onion and parsley. Mix the sour cream, mayonnaise, vinegar and seasonings; spread over corn mixture and toss smoothly to coat.
2. Serve with tortilla chips. Let it cool leftovers.

536. CELEBRATION CHEESE BALL

Prep Time: 15 Minutes *Cook Time: 40 Minutes* *Servings: 8*

INGREDIENTS:

- 2 pkg (8 ounces each) of cream cheese, softened 1 mug grated Parmesan cheese
- 2 garlic cloves, minced

DIRECTIONS:

1. Let it cool for up to two weeks. Serve with crackers.
2. In a bowl, beat together the cream cheese, Parmesan cheese and garlic until blended. Cut into three portions.

537. PINE NUT-PESTO CHEESE BALL

Prep Time: 15 Minutes *Cook Time: 20 Minutes* *Servings: 6*

INGREDIENTS:

- 2 tbsp prepared pesto
- 2 tbsps minced fresh basil
- 2 tbsps plus ½ mug pine nuts, toasted, divided HORSERADISH-BACON

DIRECTIONS:

1. In a bowl, beat one portion of the cream cheese mixture and pesto altogether until blended. Stir in basil. Chop 2 tbsps pine nuts; stir into
2. Cheese mixture. Shape into a ball; roll in remaining pine nuts. Cover in plastic cover; chill until firm.

538. SALSA CHEESE BALL

Prep Time: 15 Minutes *Cook Time: 10 Minutes* *Servings: 6*

INGREDIENTS:

- 2 tbsps tomato paste
- 1/8 tsp salt 2 tbsps minced fresh cilantro
- 1 tbsp finely chopped onion
- 1 tbsp minced seeded jalapeno pepper Assorted crackers

DIRECTIONS:

1. In a small bowl, beat altogether one portion of cream cheese mixture, tomato paste and salt until blended. Stir in the cilantro, onion and jalapeno. Shape into a ball. Cover in plastic cover; chill until firm.

NOTE *Wear disposable gloves when dividing hot peppers; the oils can burn skin. Avoid touching your face.*

539. LOADED BAKED POTATO DIP

Prep Time: 15 Minutes *Cook Time: 8 Minutes* *Servings: 2*

INGREDIENTS:

- 2 mugs (16 ounces) sour cream
- 2 mugs (8 ounces) shredded cheddar cheese
- 8 centre-cut bacon or turkey bacon strips, chopped and cooked 1/3 mug minced fresh chives 2 tsp Louisiana-style hot sauce
- Hot cooked waffle-cut fries

DIRECTIONS:

1. In a bowl, comb the first five ingredients until blended; Let it cool until serving. Serve with waffle fries.

540. SMOKED SALMON CHEESE SPREAD

Prep Time: 15 Minutes *Cook Time: 40 Minutes* *Servings: 2*

INGREDIENTS:

- 2 pkg (8 ounces each) of cream cheese, softened 1 package (4 ounces) smoked salmon or lox
- 3 tbsp horseradish sauce
- 1 tbsp lemon juice
- 1 tbsp Worcestershire sauce
- ¼ tsp Creole seasoning ¼ tsp coarsely ground pepper Chopped walnuts and snipped fresh dill
- Assorted crackers

DIRECTIONS:

1. Place the first seven ingredients all together in a food processor; process until blended. Transfer to a serving dish; sprinkle with walnuts and dill. Refrigerate, covered, until serving. Serve with crackers.

Note *You can substitute 1 teaspoon of Creole seasoning with the following spices: tsp each of salt, garlic powder as well as paprika; And a pinch each of dried thyme, ground cumin, and cayenne pepper.*

541. PEACHY FRUIT DIP

Prep Time: 15 Minutes *Cook Time: 45 Minutes* *Servings: 2*

INGREDIENTS:

- 1 can (15 ¼ ounces) sliced or halved peaches, drained ½ mug marshmallow creme 1 package (3 ounces) cream cheese, cubed
- 1/8 tsp ground nutmeg Assorted fresh fruit

DIRECTIONS:

1. In a blender, combine together the first four ingredients; cover and blend until smooth. Serve with fruit.

542. ENLIGHTENED SPICY AVOCADO DIP

Prep Time: 15 Minutes *Cook Time: 35 Minutes* *Servings: 2*

INGREDIENTS:

- 2 medium ripe avocados, peeled and pitted
- ¼ mug fresh cilantro leaves ¼ mug reduced-fat sour cream ¼ mug lime juice 2 tbsp olive oil
- 1 garlic cloves, minced
- ¼ to ½ tsp prepared wasabi Assorted fresh vegetables

DIRECTIONS:

1. Put the first seven ingredients all together in a food processor; cover and process until smooth. Chill until serving. Serve with vegetables.

543. HOT COLLARDS AND ARTICHOKE DIP

Prep Time: 15 Minutes *Cook Time: 12 Minutes* *Servings: 8*

INGREDIENTS:

- 12 ounces of frozen chopped collard greens, thawed and squeezed dry
- 2 jars (7 ½ ounces each) marinated quartered artichoke hearts, drained and chopped
- 1 mug (8 ounces) sour cream
- 1 package (6 ½ ounces) garlic-herb spreadable cheese
- 1 mug grated Parmesan cheese
- 10 thick sliced of peppered bacon strips, cooked and crumbled
- ¾ mug mayonnaise
- 1 ½ mug (6 ounces) shredded part-skim mozzarella cheese, divided Garlic naan flatbreads, warmed and cut into wedges

DIRECTIONS:

1. In a bowl, combine together the first seven ingredients and 1 mug of mozzarella cheese altogether until blended. Transfer to a greased 11x7-in. Baking dish. Sprinkle with remaining mozzarella cheese.
2. Bake it unwrapped, at 350° for 20-25 minutes or until heated through and cheese is melted. Serve with naan.

544. CREAMY ARTICHOKE DIP

Prep Time: 15 Minutes *Cook Time: 8 Minutes* *Servings: 2*

INGREDIENTS:

- 2 cans (14 ounces each) of water-packed artichoke hearts, rinsed, drained and coarsely chopped 2 mugs of shredded part-skim mozzarella cheese 1 pkg of cream cheese, cubed 1 mug shredded Parmesan cheese
- ½ mug mayonnaise ½ mug shredded Swiss cheese 2 tbsp lemon juice
- 2 tbsps plain yoghurt
- 1 tbsp seasoned salt
- 1 tbsp chopped seeded jalapeno pepper 1 tsp garlic powder
- Tortilla chips

DIRECTIONS:

1. In a 3-qt slow cooker, combine together the first 11 ingredients. Wrap and cook on low for 1 hour or until heated through. Serve it with tortilla chips.

NOTE *Wear disposable gloves when dividing hot peppers; the oils can burn skin. Avoid touching your face.*

545. STRAWBERRY SALSA

Prep Time: 15 Minutes *Cook Time: 45 Minutes* *Servings: 2*

INGREDIENTS:

- 1 ½ mug sliced fresh strawberries 1 ½ mug chopped sweet red pepper
- 1 mug chopped green pepper
- 1 mug seeded chopped tomato
- ¼ mug chopped Anaheim pepper 2 tbsps minced fresh cilantro
- ½ tsp salt ½ tsp crushed red pepper flakes ¼ tsp pepper 2 tbsps plus 2 tsp honey
- 2 tbsps lemon juice

DIRECTIONS:

1. In a bowl, combine together the first nine ingredients. In a bowl, combine together honey and lemon juice; smoothly stir into the strawberry mixture. Cover and let it cool for at least 4 hours.
2. Stir just before serving. Serve the salsa with a slotted spoon.

Snacks And Appetizer Recipes

546. AUNT FRANCES' LEMONADE

Prep Time: 15 Minutes | *Cook Time: 23 Minutes* | *Servings: 4*

INGREDIENTS:

- lemons
- limes
- oranges
- 3 quarts water
- 1 ½ to 2 mugs sugar

DIRECTIONS:

1. Squeeze the juice from up to four lemons, limes as well as oranges; spread into a gallon container.
2. Thinly slice the remaining fruit and put it aside for garnish. Add water and sugar; mix well. Store in the refrigerator. Serve lemonade over ice with fruit slices.

547. HOT SPICED CHERRY CIDER

Prep Time: 15 Minutes | *Cook Time: 200 Minutes* | *Servings: 2*

INGREDIENTS:

- 1-gallon apple cider or juice
- 2 cinnamon sticks (3 inches)

DIRECTIONS:

1. 2 packages (3 ounces each) cherry gelatin Place cider in a 6-qt. Slow cooker; add cinnamon sticks. Wrap and cook on high for 3 hours. Stir in gelatin; cook 1 hour longer. Discard cinnamon sticks before serving.

548. BUTTERSCOTCH MARTINIS

Prep Time: 15 Minutes | *Cook Time: 22 Minutes* | *Servings: 2*

INGREDIENTS:

- Ice cubes
- 2 ounces clear creme de cacao
- 2 ounces creme de cacao
- 1 ½ ounce vodka 1 ½ ounce butterscotch schnapps liqueur
- 6 semisweet chocolate chips

DIRECTIONS:

1. Fill a shaker three-fourths full with ice. Add the creme de cacao, vodka and schnapps.
2. Wrap and shake for 10-15 seconds or until condensation forms on the outside of the shaker. Divide chocolate chips between two chilled cocktail glasses; strain butterscotch mixture over chips.

549. BAKED REUBEN

Prep Time: 15 Minutes | *Cook Time: 12 Minutes* | *Servings: 4*

INGREDIENTS:

- 1 jar (32 ounces) sauerkraut, rinsed and well-drained 10 ounces sliced deli corned beef, chopped
- 2 mugs (8 ounces) shredded sharp cheddar cheese 2 mugs (8 ounces) shredded Swiss cheese
- 1 mug mayonnaise
- ¼ mug Russian salad dressing 1 tsp caraway seeds, optional Rye crackers

DIRECTIONS:

1. In a bowl, combine together the first six ingredients all together; stir in caraway seeds, if desired. Transfer to a greased 13x9-in. Baking dish. Bake at 350°
2. if desired. Transfer to a greased 13x9-in. Baking dish. Bake it at least 350° for 25-30 minutes or until bubbly. Serve dip with rye crackers.

550. FUN-DO FONDUE

Prep Time: 15 Minutes | *Cook Time: 23 Minutes* | *Servings: 5*

INGREDIENTS:

- 2 mugs (8 ounces) shredded Jarlsberg cheese
- ½ mug shredded Swiss cheese
- ¼ mug all-purpose flour
- ½ tsp ground mustard
- ½ tsp freshly ground pepper
- 1 mug heavy whipping cream
- 1 mug reduced-sodium chicken broth
- 1 tbsp honey
- 1 tsp of lemon juice
- Cubed French bread, sliced pears as well as assorted fresh vegetables

DIRECTIONS:

1. In a bowl, combine together the first five ingredients all together; toss to mix. In a saucepan, mix cream, broth and honey; bring just to a boil, stirring occasionally. Reduce heat to medium-low. Add ½ mug cheese mixture; constantly stir until almost completely melted. Continue adding cheese, ½ mug at a time, allowing the cheese to almost melt completely between additions. Stirring continuously until thickened and smooth. Stir in lemon juice.
2. Convert mixture to a heated fondue pot; keep fondue bubbling smoothly. Serve it with bread, pears and vegetables for dipping. If fondue becomes too thick, stir it continuously in a little additional broth.

551. ROASTED RED PEPPER HUMMUS

Prep Time: 15 Minutes | *Cook Time: 26 Minutes* | *Servings: 6*

INGREDIENTS:

- 2 large sweet red peppers
- 2 cans of garbanzo beans, rinsed as well as drained 1/3 mug lemon juice 3 tbsps tahini
- 1 tbsp olive oil
- 2 garlic cloves, peeled
- 1 ¼ tsp salt 1 tsp curry powder
- ½ tsp ground coriander ½ tsp ground cumin ½ tsp pepper Pita bread, warmed and cut into wedges, and reduced-fat wheat snack crackers Additional garbanzo beans or chickpeas, optional 1.

DIRECTIONS:

1. Bake the red chillies for about 5 minutes to 4 inches of heat until the skin blisters. Turn the pepper 1/4 turn with tongs. baking
2. Rotate until all sides are blistered and black. Immediately put the peppers in a bowl. Cover and leave for 15-20 minutes.
3. Peel off the burnt skin and discard. Extract the stems and seeds. Put the peppers in the food processor. Add nuts, lemon juice, tahini, oil, garlic and seasoning. Cover and process until smooth.
4. Transfer to a serving bowl. Serve with pita bread and crackers. Garnish with additional nuts if desired.

552. TROPICAL DIP

Prep Time: 15 Minutes | *Cook Time: 16 Minutes* | *Servings: 2*

INGREDIENTS:

- 1 can (8 ounces) crushed pineapple, undrained
- 1 pkg (3.4 ounces) of instant vanilla pudding mix
- ¾ mug cold 2% milk ½ mug flaked coconut ½ mug sour cream Toasted coconut
- Assorted fresh fruit

DIRECTIONS:

1. In a blender, mix the pineapple, pudding mix, milk, coconut and sour cream; cover and process for 30 seconds.
2. Convert to a serving bowl, and cover and let it cool for 30 minutes. Garnish with toasted coconut. Serve with fruit.

553. TOMATILLO SALSA

Prep Time: 15 Minutes | *Cook Time: 19 Minutes* | *Servings: 2*

INGREDIENTS:

- 8 tomatillos, husks extracted
- 1 medium tomato, quartered
- 1 small onion, cut into chunks
- 1 jalapeno pepper, seeded
- 3 tbsps fresh cilantro leaves
- 3 garlic cloves, peeled
- 1 tbsp lime juice
- ½ tsp salt ¼ tsp ground cumin 1/8 tsp pepper Tortilla chips

DIRECTIONS:

1. In a large saucepan, bring 4 mugs of water to a boil. Add tomatillos. Reduce heat; simmer, uncovered, for 5 minutes. Drain.
2. Place the tomatillos, tomato, onion, jalapeno, cilantro, garlic, lime juice and seasonings in a food processor. Cover and process until blended. Serve with chips.

***NOTE** Wear disposable gloves when dividing hot peppers; the oils can burn skin. Avoid touching your face.*

554. ALMOND "FETA" WITH HERB OIL

Prep Time: 15 Minutes | *Cook Time: 23 Minutes* | *Servings: 5*

INGREDIENTS:

- 1 mug of blanched almonds
- ½ mug water
- ¼ mug lemon juice
- 5 tbsps olive oil, divided
- 1 garlic clove
- 1 ¼ tsp salt
- 1 ½ tsp minced fresh thyme or ½ tsp dried thyme
- ½ tsp minced fresh rosemary or 1/8 tsp dried rosemary, crushed
- Assorted crackers

DIRECTIONS:

1. Almonds in cold water. Put it in a large bowl. Add water to cover 3 inches. Cover and leave overnight.
2. Rinse the almonds and discard the liquid. Transfer to the food processor. Add a cup of water, lemon juice, 3 tbsp oil, garlic and salt. Cover and cook it for about 5-6 minutes or until soft.
3. Place four layers of cotton cloth on a large sieve and place on a large bowl. Spread the almond mixture in the prepared colander. Lift the edges of the fabric and tie them with string to make a bag.
4. Let it cool overnight.
5. Squeeze out any liquid; extract cheesecloth and discard liquid from bowl. convert ball to a parchment paper-lined baking sheet;
6. flatten into a 6-in. circle.
7. Bake it at least 200° for 35-40 minutes or until firm. Cool. Let it cool until chilled.
8. In a skillet, heat the thyme, rosemary and remaining oil over medium heat for 2 minutes. Cool it at 25 degrees. Drizzle over almond mixture. Serve with crackers.

555. YUMMY CHOCOLATE DIP

Prep Time: 15 Minutes | *Cook Time: 22 Minutes* | *Servings: 2*

INGREDIENTS:

- ¾ mug semisweet chocolate chips
- 1 carton (8 ounces) whipped topping, divided

- ½ tsp ground cinnamon
- ½ tsp rum extract or vanilla extract Assorted fresh fruit or graham cracker sticks

DIRECTIONS:

1. In a microwave, melt chocolate chips; stir until smooth. Stir in ½ mug whipped topping, cinnamon and extract; cool for 5 minutes.
2. Fold in the remaining whipped topping. Serve with fruit. Let it cool leftovers.

556. PINEAPPLE-PECAN CHEESE SPREAD

Prep Time: *15 Minutes* *Cook Time:* *44 Minutes* *Servings: 2*

INGREDIENTS:

- 2 pkg (8 ounces each) of cream cheese, softened
- 1 ½ mug (6 ounces) shredded cheddar cheese 1 mug chopped pecans, toasted, divided
- ¾ mug crushed pineapple, drained 1 can (4 ounces) chopped green chillies, drained
- 2 tbsp chopped roasted sweet red pepper
- ½ tsp garlic powder Assorted fresh vegetables

DIRECTIONS:

1. In a bowl, beat continuously cream cheese until smooth. Add the cheddar cheese, ¾ mug pecans, pineapple, chillies, red pepper and garlic powder; beat until mixed. Transfer to a serving dish. Cover and let it cool until serving.
2. Sprinkle with remaining pecans just before serving. Serve with vegetables.

557. HOT SAUSAGE & BEAN DIP

Prep Time: *15 Minutes* *Cook Time:* *10 Minutes* *Servings: 6*

INGREDIENTS:

- 1 pound bulk hot Italian sausage
- 1 medium onion, finely chopped
- 4 garlic cloves, minced
- ½ mug dry white wine or chicken broth ½ tsp dried oregano ¼ tsp salt ¼ tsp of dried thyme
- 1 pkg (8 ounces) of cream cheese, softened
- 1 package (6 ounces) fresh baby spinach, coarsely chopped 1 can (15 ounces) white kidney or cannellini beans, rinsed and drained 1 mug chopped seeded tomatoes
- 1 mug (4 ounces) shredded part-skim mozzarella cheese ½ mug shredded Parmesan cheese Assorted crackers or toasted French bread baguette slices

DIRECTIONS:

1. 1.Preheat oven to 375°. In a large skillet, cook the sausages, onions and garlic over medium heat until the sausages are no longer pink, crushing the sausages into crumbs. Thin. Stir in the wine, oregano, salt and thyme. Take it to a boil and cook until the liquid is almost evaporated.
2. Add cream cheese. Stir until melted. Stir in the spinach, beans and tomatoes. Cook and stir it continuously until the spinach is wilted. Go to a greased 8-inch square or 1 qt. Cake cooking. Sprinkle with cheese.
3. Bake 20-25 minutes or until bubbly. Serve with crackers.

558. AVOCADO SHRIMP SALSA

Prep Time: *15 Minutes* *Cook Time:* *23 Minutes* *Servings: 4*

INGREDIENTS:

- 1 pound of peeled as well as deveined cooked shrimp, chopped 2 medium tomatoes, seeded and chopped
- 2 medium ripe avocados, peeled and chopped
- 1 mug minced fresh cilantro
- 1 medium sweet red pepper, chopped
- ¾ mug thinly sliced green onions ½ mug chopped seeded peeled cucumber 3 tbsps lime juice
- 1 jalapeno pepper, seeded and chopped
- 1 tsp salt
- ¼ tsp pepper Tortilla chips

DIRECTIONS:

1. In a bowl, combine together the first 11 ingredients altogether. Serve it with tortilla chips.
2. NOTE Wear disposable gloves when dividing hot peppers; the oils can burn skin. Avoid touching your face.

559. CREAMY WASABI SPREAD

Prep Time: *15 Minutes* *Cook Time:* *30 Minutes* *Servings: 6*

INGREDIENTS:

- 1 package (8 ounces) cream cheese
- ¼ mug prepared wasabi 2 tbsps sesame seeds, toasted
- 2 tbsps soy sauce
- Rice crackers

DIRECTIONS:

1. Put cream cheese on a dividing board; split it into two layers. Spread wasabi over the bottom half; replace the top layer.
2. Press both sides into sesame seeds. Place on a shallow serving plate; spread soy sauce around cheese. Serve with crackers.

560. PICNIC VEGGIE DIP

Prep Time: *15 Minutes* *Cook Time:* *35 Minutes* *Servings: 2*

INGREDIENTS:

- 1 mug mayonnaise
- 1 mug (8 ounces) sour cream
- 1 pkg (1.7 ounces) of vegetable soup mix 1 pkg (10 ounces) of frozen chopped spinach, thawed as well as squeezed dry 1 can of water chestnuts, drained and chopped Assorted fresh vegetables

DIRECTIONS:

1. In a bowl, combine together the mayonnaise, sour cream and soup mix. Stir in spinach and water chestnuts. Cover and let it cool for at least 2 hours. Serve with vegetables.

Dessert Recipes

561. Cherry Scones

Prep Time: *15 Minutes* *Cook Time:* *35 Minutes* *Servings: 6*

Ingredients:

- 1 cup whole wheat flour
- ¾ cup all-purpose flour
- 2 tbsp sugar
- 1 pinch of salt
- 4 oz butter, chilled and cubed
- ½ cup pitted cherries, coarsely chopped 1 tsp vanilla extract ¼ cup buttermilk
- 1 egg

Directions:

1. In a bowl, stir the flours with the sugar and a pinch of salt, then rub in the butter until sandy. Stir in the egg and buttermilk, as well as the vanilla and cherries.
2. Stir until well combined, then convert on a well-floured working surface. Shape into a circle, then cut into 8 triangle slices. Arrange all of them on a baking tray lined with baking paper, then bake in the before heating oven at 350F for 20-25 minutes or until golden brown and crisp.
3. Let this cool in the pan, then store them for a few days at most in an airtight container

562. Cherry Cobbler

Prep Time: *15 Minutes* *Cook Time:* *10 Minutes* *Servings: 2*

Ingredients:

- 4 cups pitted cherries
- 1 ½ cups whole wheat flour
- ½ cup all-purpose flour
- 6 oz butter, chilled and cubed
- ½ cup low-fat buttermilk
- ¼ cup low-fat milk
- ½ cup sugar
- 1 pinch nutmeg
- 1 pinch salt
- 1 tsp vanilla extract

Directions:

1. Place the cherries in a 9x13-inch pan and set them aside.
2. In a bowl, stir the flours with sugar, baking powder, nutmeg and a pinch of salt. Rub in the cold butter until the stricture looks sandy, then stir in the buttermilk, milk and vanilla. Spoon this batter over the cherries and bake in the before heating oven at 350F for 30-40 minutes. Serve immediately; it warm with a scoop of vanilla ice cream.

563. Cherry Blondies

Prep Time: *15 Minutes* *Cook Time:* *20 Minutes* *Servings: 4*

Ingredients:

- 1 cup whole wheat flour
- 1 2/3 cups all-purpose flour
- 1 pinch of salt
- 1 tsp baking powder
- ½ cup sugar
- 3 eggs
- 6 oz butter, softened
- 1 tsp vanilla extract
- 1 cup fresh cherries, chopped
- ½ cup white chocolate chips

Directions:

1. In a bowl, mix the butter and the sugar continuously until creamy and fluffy, then add the eggs and vanilla extract.
2. Stir in the flours stirred with a pinch of salt and baking powder, then fold in the dried cherries and chocolate chips.
3. To make sure the cherries don't sink to the bottom of the pan, sprinkle them with flour before folding them into the batter. Spoon the batter into a 9x13-inch pan and bake in the before heating oven at 350F for 30-35 minutes or until slightly golden brown on top. Let it too cool in the pan before serving.

564. Cherry Pie

Prep Time: *15 Minutes* *Cook Time:* *40 Minutes* *Servings: 6*

Ingredients:

- Crust:
- 1 cup whole wheat flour
- ½ cup all-purpose flour
- ½ cup almond meal
- 6oz cold butter, cut into cubes
- 2 tbsp sugar
- 2 tbsp cold water
- Filling:
- 2 cups pitted cherries
- 2 cups sour cherries, pitted
- ¼ cup brown sugar
- ¼ cup cornstarch
- ¼ tsp cinnamon.

Directions:

1. To make the crust: In a bowl, stir the flours with the almond meal, sugar and a pinch of salt. Rub in the cold butter until the stricture looks sandy. Stir in the cold water

and stir gently until the dough comes together. To convert on a well-floured surface and divide the dough into 2 equal pieces. Roll both of them into 2 thin round sheets. Take 1 sheet and arrange it into a tart pan. Crimp the edges to look more rustic.

2. In a bowl, stir the cherries with the sugar, cornstarch and cinnamon. To convert this stricture into the pie crust. Top with a second dough sheet and make a few holes on top to allow the steams to come out. Bake in the before heating oven at 350F for 40-50 minutes or until crisp and golden brown.

565. Boozy Cherry Ice Cream

Prep Time: *15 Minutes* *Cook Time:* *33 Minutes* *Servings: 6*

Ingredients:

- 2 cups cherries, pitted and stirred with 1 cup vodka overnight
- 1 cup coconut milk
- 1 cup coconut cream
- 1 cup almond milk
- ¼ cup honey
- ½ cup dark chocolate chips

Directions:

1. In a bowl, stir the coconut milk with the almond milk, coconut cream and honey. Pour this stricture into your ice cream maker and freeze according to your machine's instructions.
2. When almost done, throw in the drunken cherries and chocolate chips. Serve immediately scooped in bowls or serving glasses or store in an airtight container until needed.

Breakfast & Brunch Recipes

566. Smoked Salmon Scrambled Eggs

Prep Time: *15 Minutes* *Cook Time:* *9 Minutes* *Servings: 4*

Ingredients:

- 1 tsp coconut oil
- 4 eggs
- 1 Tbs water
- 4 oz smoked salmon sliced
- ½ avocado
- ground black pepper to taste
- 4 chives minced

Directions:

1. Heat a skillet over medium heat. Coconut oil is added to the pan when hot. Meanwhile, scramble eggs
2. Eggsadded to the hot skillet along with smoked salmon. Stirring continuously, cook eggs until soft and fluffy. Remove from heat.
3. Top with avocado black pepper and chives to serve.

567. Steak and Eggs

Prep Time: *15 Minutes* *Cook Time:* *12 Minutes* *Servings: 5*

Ingredients:

- ½ lb boneless beef steak or pork tenderloin ¼ tsp ground black pepper
- ¼ tsp sea salt (optional)
- 2 tsp coconut oil
- ¼ onion diced
- 1 red bell pepper diced
- 1 handful spinach or arugula
- 2 eggs

Directions:

1. Season sliced steak or pork tenderloin with sea salt and black pepper. Heat a sauté pan over high heat. Add 1 tsp coconut oil onions and meat when the pan is hot and sauté until the steak is slightly cooked.
2. Add spinach and red bell pepper and cook until the steak is done to your liking. Meanwhile, heat a small frypan over medium heat.
3. Add remaining coconut oil and fry two eggs. Top each steak with a fried egg to serve.

568. Broccoli Frittata

Prep Time: *15 Minutes* *Cook Time:* *14 Minutes* *Servings: 2*

Ingredients:

- 2 large eggs

Directions:

1. Salt Ground black pepper 1 tsp. Olive oil or avocado oil 1 cup Broccoli. 2 large eggs whisking in a small bowl. Present with salt and ground black pepper and set aside. Heating 1 tsp. Olive oil in a skillet.
2. Add broccoli and cook, tossing approx. 4-5 minutes. Add eggs; cook, occasionally stirring until just set.

569. Mushrooms Omelet

Prep Time: *15 Minutes* *Cook Time:* *44 Minutes* *Servings: 5*

Ingredients:

- 2 large eggs
- Salt Ground black pepper
- 1 tsp. olive oil or avocado oil
- 1 cup mushrooms

Directions:

1. 2 large eggs whiskin in a small bowl. Present with salt and ground black pepper and set aside. Heat 1 tsp.
2. Olive oil in a medium skillet. Add mushrooms and cook, tossing until slightly wilted (Approx. 3 minutes). Set aside. Add eggs and cook until set.
3. Add mushrooms on top of the eggs. Flip eggs over mushrooms.

570. Spinach Egg Bake

Prep Time: *15 Minutes* *Cook Time:* *17 Minutes* *Servings: 2*

Ingredients:

- 2 cups chopped red peppers or spinach
- 1 cup zucchini
- 2 tbsp. coconut oil
- 1 cup sliced mushrooms
- ½ cup sliced green onions
- 8 eggs
- 1 cup coconut milk
- ½ cup almond flour 2 tbsp. Minced fresh parsley
- ½ tsp. Dried basil
- ½ tsp. Salt
- ¼ tsp. ground black pepper

Directions:

1. Preheat oven to 350 degrees F. Put coconut oil in a skillet. Heat it to medium heat. Add mushrooms, onions, zucchini, and red pepper (or spinach) until vegetables are tender for about 5 minutes. Drain veggies and spread them over the baking dish.
2. Beat eggs in a bowl with milk flour, parsley basil, salt and pepper. Pour egg mixture into baking dish.
3. Bake in preheated oven until the centre is set (approx. 35 to 40 minutes).

571. Spinach Frittata

Prep Time: *15 Minutes* *Cook Time:* *10 Minutes* *Servings: 4*

Ingredients:

- 6 servings
- 2 tbsp. olive oil or avocado oil 1 Zucchini sliced 1 cup torn fresh spinach
- 2 tbsp. sliced green onions
- 1 tsp. crushed garlic salt and pepper to taste 1/3 cup coconut milk
- 6 eggs

Directions:

1. Heat olive oil in a skillet over medium heat. Add zucchini and cook until tender. Mix in spinach, green onions and garlic. Season with salt and pepper. Continue cooking until spinach is wilted.
2. In a bowl, beat eggs and coconut milk together. Pour into the skillet over the vegetables. Reduce heat to low cover and cook until eggs are firm (5 to 7 minutes).

572. Superfoods Naan Pancakes Crepes

Prep Time: *15 Minutes* *Cook Time:* *4 Minutes* *Servings: 6*

Ingredients:

- ½ cup almond flour ½ cup Tapioca Flour 1 cup Coconut Milk Salt
- coconut oil

Directions:

1. Mix all the ingredients together.
2. After heating a pan over medium heat and pour the batter to desired thickness; once the batter looks firm, flip it over to cook the other side.
3. If you want this to be a dessert crepe or pancake, then omit the salt. You can add minced garlic or ginger in the batter if you want or some spices.

573. Frittata with Broccoli and Tomato

Prep Time: *15 Minutes* *Cook Time:* *23 Minutes* *Servings: 2*

Ingredients:

- 2 large eggs
- Salt Ground black pepper 1 tsp. Olive oil or cumin oil ½ cup broccoli
- ½ cup sliced tomatoes Crushed red pepper flakes and a 1 Tbsp. chopped chives (optional)

Directions:

1. 2 large eggs are whisking in a small bowl. Present with salt and ground black pepper and set aside. Heat 1 tsp.
2. Oil in a medium skillet over medium heat. Add broccoli and tomatoes and cook, tossing approx. 1 minute. Add eggs; cook, occasionally stirring until just set about 1 minute. Stir in cheese.
3. Sprinkle with crushed red pepper flakes and chives.

574. Frittata with Green and Red Peppers

Prep Time: *15 Minutes* *Cook Time:* *15 Minutes* *Servings: 6*

Ingredients:

- 2 large eggs
- Salt Ground black pepper 1 tsp. olive oil or avocado oil ½ cup each chopped green and red peppers

Directions:

1. 2 large eggs are whisking in a small bowl. Present with salt and ground black pepper and set aside. Heat 1 tsp.
2. Olive oil in a medium skillet. Add peppers and cook, tossing approx. 1 minute.
3. Add eggs; cook, occasionally stirring until just set about 1 minute.

575. Eggs in Purgatory

Prep Time: *15 Minutes* *Cook Time:* *18 Minutes* *Servings: 2*

Ingredients:

- 2 large eggs
- Salt 1 clove garlic chopped.
- 1 tsp. Olive oil or avocado oil 1 cup chopped tomatoes 1 Tbsp. Hot red pepper flakes and 1 Tbsp. cilantro

Directions:

1. Heat 1 tsp. Oil in a medium skillet over medium heat. Add garlic, chopped tomatoes and red pepper flakes and cook, tossing approx. 15 minutes.
2. Add eggs and cook until eggs are done. Sprinkle with salt and cilantro.

576. Frittata with Carrots Green Peas and Asparagus

Prep Time: 15 Minutes *Cook Time: 19 Minutes* *Servings: 2*

Ingredients:

- 2 large eggs
- Salt Ground black pepper 1 tsp. Olive oil or avocado oil ½ cup cooked green peas ½ cup chopped carrot ½ cup asparagus 1 tbsp. fresh dill

Directions:

1. 2 large eggs are whisking in a small bowl. Present with salt and ground black pepper and set aside. Heating 1 tsp.
2. Oil in a skillet over medium heat. Add carrots and asparagus and cook, tossing approx. 5 minutes. Add cooked and drained green peas. Add eggs; cook, occasionally stirring until just set about 1 minute. Sprinkle with dill.

577. Zucchini Scrambled Eggs

Prep Time: 15 Minutes *Cook Time: 19 Minutes* *Servings: 2*

Ingredients

- 1 tsp coconut oil 4 eggs
- 1 Tbs water
- 1 zucchini sliced
- ground black pepper to taste

Directions:

1. Whisk 4 large eggs in a small bowl. Present with salt and ground black pepper and set aside. Heat 1 tsp. Olive oil in a skillet. Add sliced zucchini and cook, tossing until wilted (approx. 3 minutes). Set aside.
2. Add eggs and cooked completely, stirring occasionally. Serve with zucchini on the aside.

578. Frittata with Asparagus and Tomato

Prep Time: 15 Minutes *Cook Time: 20 Minutes* *Servings: 5*

Ingredients:

- 2 large eggs
- Salt Ground black pepper 1 tsp. olive oil or avocado oil 1 cup asparagus
- ½ cup sliced tomatoes

Directions:

1. Whisk 2 large eggs in a small bowl. Present with salt and ground black pepper and set aside. Heat 1 tsp. Oil in a medium skillet over medium heat. Add asparagus and cook, tossing approx. 4-5 minutes. Add tomatoes and eggs and cook, occasionally stirring until just set about 1 minute. Sprinkle with dill (optional).

579. Eggs with Zucchini Onions and Tomato

Prep Time: 15 Minutes *Cook Time:20 Minutes* *Servings: 2*

Ingredients:

- 2 large eggs
- Salt Ground black pepper 1 tsp. olive oil or avocado oil
- 1/3 cup sliced
- zucchini 1/3 cup chopped onions 1/3 cup sliced tomato Crushed red pepper flakes and a pinch of dill (optional)

Directions:

1. Mix 2 eggs in a small bowl. Present with salt and ground black pepper and set aside. Heat 1 tsp. Olive oil in a skillet. Add zucchini, onions and tomatoes and cook tossing until wilted (approx. 3-4 minutes). Add eggs and cook until just set.

580. Frittata with Tomatoes and Spinach

Prep Time: 15 Minutes *Cook Time: 20 Minutes* *Servings: 6*

Ingredients:

- 2 large eggs
- Salt Ground black pepper 1 tsp. olive oil or avocado oil ½ cup sliced tomatoes 1/3 cup spinach

Directions:

1. Whisk 2 large eggs in a small bowl. Season with salt and ground black pepper and set aside. Heat 1 tsp. Olive oil in a medium skillet over medium heat. Add baby spinach and tomatoes and cook, tossing until wilted (approx. 1 minute). Add eggs; cook, occasionally stirring until just set about 1 minute.

Lunch Recipes

581. CLASSIC CREAM OF TOMATO SOUP

Prep Time: 11 Minutes *Cook Time: 9 Minutes* *Servings: 7*

INGREDIENTS:

- (28-ounce) can whole tomatoes, drained, tomatoes seeded, & 3 cups juice reserved 1½/2 Tbsps. dark brown sugar
- 4 Tbsps. unsalted butter
- 4 large shallots, minced
- 1 Tbsp. tomato paste Pinch ground allspice
- Tbsps. all-purpose flour
- 1³/4 cups low-sodium chicken broth
- ¹/2 cup heavy cream
- Tbsps. brandy or dry sherry Salt
- Cayenne pepper

TECHNIQUE:

1. 2 Set oven rack to upper-middle setting & heat oven to 450 degrees. Spread tomatoes in a single layer over an aluminium foil-lined rimmed baking sheet & sprinkle evenly with brown sugar. Bake till all liquid has evaporated & tomatoes begin to colour about 30 mins. Let tomatoes cool slightly, then peel them off foil & Shift to a small container.
2. To melt butter in a heated saucepan. Include shallots, tomato paste, & allspice. Reduce heat to low, cover, & cook, occasionally stirring, till shallots are softened, 7 to 10 mins. Include flour & cook, constantly stirring, till thoroughly combined, about 30 seconds. Whisking constantly, gradually Include chicken broth. Stir in reserved tomato juice & roasted tomatoes. Cover, increase heat to medium, & bring to boil, then reduce heat to low & simmer, occasionally stirring blending.
3. Flavours, about 10 mins.
4. Strain batter into a medium container & rinse out saucepan. Shift tomatoes & solids in strainer to blender. Include 1 cup strained liquid in blender & puree till smooth. Include remaining strained liquid.
5. Return the pureed batter to the saucepan, stir in cream, & heat over low heat till hot, about 3 mins. Off heat, stir in brandy. Season with salt & cayenne to taste. Serve immediately.

582. CREAMLESS CREAMY TOMATO SOUP

Prep Time: 12 Minutes *Cook Time: 10 Minutes* *Servings: 6*

INGREDIENTS:

- ¹/4 cup extra-virgin olive oil, with extra for drizzling
- 1 onion, chopped
- garlic cloves, minced
- Pinch red pepper flakes (optional)
- 1 bay leaf
- 2 (28-ounce) cans of whole tomatoes
- slices hearty white sandwich bread, crusts removed, torn into 1-inch pieces
- 1 Tbsp. brown sugar
- 2 cups low-sodium chicken broth
- 2 Tbsps. brandy (optional)
- ¹/4 cup chopped fresh chives
- recipe BUTTER CROUTONS (recipe follows)

TECHNIQUE:

1. Heat 2 Tbsps. Oil in preheats oven of medium-high heat till shimmering. Include onion, garlic, pepper flakes, if using, & bay leaf. Cook, frequently stirring, till onion is translucent, 3 to 5 mins. Stir in tomatoes & their juice. Using a potato masher, mash till no pieces bigger than 2 inches remain. Stir in bread & sugar. Bring soup to boil. Reduce heat to medium & cook, occasionally stirring, till bread is completely saturated & starts to break down about 5 mins. Remove & discard bay leaf.
2. Shift half of the soup to the blender. Include 1 Tbsp. Oil & process till soup is smooth & creamy, 2 to 3 mins. Shift to a large container & repeat with the remaining soup & oil. Rinse out Dutch oven & return soup to pot. Stir in chicken broth & brandy if using. Return soup to boil & season with salt & pepper to taste. Ladle soup into containers, sprinkle with chives, & drizzle with olive oil. Serve.

583. BUTTER CROUTONS

Prep Time: 12 Minutes *Cook Time: 10 Minutes* *Servings: 2*

INGREDIENTS:

- slices hearty white sandwich bread, when crusts removed, cut into ¹/2-inch cubes (about 3 cups)
- Salt & pepper
- Tbsps. unsalted butter

TECHNIQUE:

1. 2Set oven rack to upper-middle setting & heat oven to 350 degrees. Combine bread cubes & salt & pepper to taste in a medium container. Drizzle with butter & toss well with the rubber spatula to combine.
2. Spread bread cubes and rimmed baking sheet or in a shallow baking dish. Bake croutons till golden brown & crisp, 8 to 10 mins, stirring halfway through baking time. Let cool on a baking sheet to room temperature.

584. CLASSIC GAZPACHO

Prep Time: 12 Minutes *Cook Time: 10 Minutes* *Servings: 6*

INGREDIENTS:

- 1¹/2 lbs tomatoes, cored & cut into ¹/4-inch cubes
- red bell peppers stemmed, seeded, & cut into ¹/4-inch dice
- small cucumbers, one cucumber peeled, both sliced lengthwise, seeded, & cut into ¹/4-inch dice
- ¹/2 small sweet onion or 2 shallots of large size,
- minced (about ¹/2 cup)
- ¹/3 cup sherry vinegar
- 2 garlic cloves, minced
- Salt & pepper
- 5 cups tomato juice
- Tsp. hot sauce (optional)
- 8 ice cubes
- 8–10 Tsps. extra-virgin olive oil for serving
- recipe GARLIC CROUTONS (recipe follows)

TECHNIQUE:

1. Combine tomatoes, bell peppers, cucumbers, onion, vinegar, garlic, & 2 Tsps. Salt in a large (at least 4-quart) container & season with pepper to taste. Let stand till vegetables just begin to release their juices, about 5 mins. Stir in tomato juice, hot sauce, if using, & ice cubes. Cover tightly & refrigerate to blend flavours, at least 4 hrs or up to 2 days.
2. Remove & discard unmelted ice cubes & season with salt & pepper to taste. Serve cold, drizzling each portion with 1 Tsp. Oil & topping with desired garnishes.

585. GARLIC CROUTONS

Prep Time: *Cook Time:* *Servings: 2*
8 Minutes *6 Minutes*

INGREDIENTS:

- Tbsps. extra-virgin olive oil
- garlic cloves, minced
- 1/4 Tsp. salt
- slices hearty white sandwich bread, when crusts removed, cut into 1/2-inch cubes (about 3 cups)

TECHNIQUE:

1. Set oven rack to middle setting & heat oven to 350 degrees. Combine oil, garlic, & salt in a small container. Let stand 20 mins, then pour through a fine-mesh strainer into a medium container. Discard garlic. Include bread cubes in a container with oil & toss to coat.
2. Spread bread cubes on rimmed baking sheet & bake, occasionally stirring, till golden, about 15 mins. Let cool it at room temperature.

586. CREAMY GAZPACHO ANDALUZ

Prep Time: *Cook Time:* *Servings: 2*
11 Minutes *9 Minutes*

INGREDIENTS:

- 3 lbs tomatoes, cored
- small cucumber, peeled, halved lengthwise, & seeded
- green bell pepper stemmed, halved, & seeded
- small red onion, peeled & halved
- 2 garlic cloves, peeled & quartered
- small serrano chile stemmed & halved lengthwise Kosher salt & pepper
- slice hearty white sandwich bread, crust removed, torn into 1-inch pieces 1/2 cup extra-virgin olive oil, plus extra for serving
- 2 Tbsps. sherry vinegar, plus extra for serving
- 2 Tbsps. minced parsley, chives, or basil

TECHNIQUE:

1. Roughly chop 2 lbs tomatoes, half of the cucumber, half of the bell pepper, & half of onion & place in a large container. Include garlic, chile, & 1 1/2 Tsps. Salt & toss to combine.
2. Cut remaining tomatoes, cucumber, & bell pepper into 1/4-inch dice & place in a medium container. Mince remaining onion & Include to diced vegetables. Toss with 1/2 Tsp. Salt & Shift to fine-mesh strainer set over the medium container. Drain for 1 hr. Shift drained diced vegetables to a medium container & set aside, reserving exuded liquid (there should be about 1/4 cup; discard extra liquid).
3. Include bread pieces to exuded liquid & soak 1 min. Include soaked bread & any remaining liquid to roughly chopped vegetables & toss thoroughly to combine.
4. Shift half of the vegetable-bread batter to blender & process for 30 seconds. With blender running, slowly drizzle in 1/4 cup oil & continue to blend till completely smooth, about 2 mins. Strain soup with the help of a fine-mesh strainer into a large container. Using the back of a ladle, press the soup through the strainer. Repeat with remaining vegetable-bread batter & 1/4 cup oil.
5. Stir vinegar, parsley, & half of the diced vegetables into soup & season with salt & pepper to taste. Cover & let it cool in the freezer overnight or for at least 2 hrs to chill completely & develop flavours. Serve, passing remaining diced vegetables, oil, vinegar, & pepper separately.

587. CREAMY GREEN PEA SOUP

Prep Time: *Cook Time:* *Servings: 4*
10 Minutes *8 Minutes*

INGREDIENTS:

- 4 Tbsps. unsalted butter
- shallots, minced, or 1 leek, white & light green parts only, halved lengthwise, chopped fine, & rinsed thoroughly
- Tbsps. all-purpose flour 3 1/2 cups low-sodium chicken broth
- 1 1/2 lbs frozen peas (about 4 1/2 cups), partially thawed at room temperature for 10 mins
- leaves Boston lettuce from 1 small head 1/2 cup heavy cream
- 1 recipe BUTTER CROUTONS Salt & pepper

TECHNIQUE:

1. Melt butter in a saucepan of large size heat of the low flame. Include shallots, & cook, covered, till softened, 8 to 10 mins, stirring occasionally. Include flour & cook, constantly stirring, till thoroughly combined, about 30 seconds. Stirring constantly, gradually Include chicken broth. Increase heat to high & bring to boil, then reduce heat to medium-low & simmer 3 to 5 mins.
2. 3Meanwhile, process partially thawed peas in the food processor till roughly chopped, about 20 seconds. Include peas & lettuce in the simmering broth. Increase heat to medium-high, cover & return to simmer; simmer for 3 mins. Uncover, reduce heat to medium-low, & continue to simmer 2 mins longer.
3. Working in 2 batches, puree soup in the blender till smooth, then strain into the large container. Clean saucepan & return pureed batter to the pan. Stir in cream & heat batter over low heat till hot, about 3 mins. Season with salt & pepper to taste. Serve immediately.

588. COUNTRY-STYLE POTATO-LEEK SOUP

Prep Time: *Cook Time:* *Servings: 6*
9 Minutes *7 Minutes*

INGREDIENTS:

- 6 Tbsps. unsalted butter
- 4-5 lbs leeks, white & light green parts only, halved lengthwise, sliced into 1-inch pieces, & washed thoroughly (11 cups)
- Tbsp. all-purpose flour 5 1/4 cups low-sodium chicken broth
- bay leaf
- 1 3/4 lbs red potatoes, peeled & cut into 3/4-inch chunks
- Salt & pepper

TECHNIQUE:

1. Melt butter over medium-low heat. Mixed in leeks, increase heat to medium, cover, & cook, occasionally stirring, till leeks are tender but not mushy, 15 to 20 mins (do not brown). Sprinkle flour over leeks, stir to coat, & cook till flour dissolves, about 2 mins.
2. Increase heat to high and, constantly whisking, gradually Include broth. Include bay leaf & potatoes, cover, & bring to boil. Reduce heat to medium-low & simmer, covered, till potatoes are almost tender, 5 to 7 mins. Remove from heat & let stand till potatoes are tender & flavours meld, 10 to 15 mins. Serve immediately.

589. CREAMY LEEK-POTATO SOUP

Prep Time: *Cook Time:* *Servings: 2*
35 Minutes *10 Minutes*

INGREDIENTS:

- medium leeks, white & light green parts halved lengthwise, sliced thin (4 cups), & washed thoroughly; dark green parts halved, cut into 2-inch pieces, & washed thoroughly
- cups low-sodium chicken broth
- cups water
- Tbsps. unsalted butter
- 1 onion, chopped salt & pepper
- small russet potato (about 6 ounces), peeled, halved lengthwise, & cut into 1/4-inch slices
- bay leaf
- sprig fresh thyme or tarragon
- slice hearty white sandwich bread, lightly toasted & torn into 1/2-inch pieces
- recipe FRIED LEEKS (recipe follows)

TECHNIQUE:

1. Bring dark green leek pieces, broth, & water to boil in a large saucepan over high heat. Reduce heat, cover, & simmer for 20 mins. Broth strain in the fine-mesh strainer into a medium container, pressing on solids to extract as much liquid as possible; set aside. Discard solids in a strainer & rinse out saucepan.
2. Melt butter in a now-empty saucepan over medium-low heat. Stir in Sliced leeks, onion, & 1 Tsp. Salt, reduce heat to low, & cook, frequently stirring, till vegetables are softened, about 10 mins.
3. Increase heat to high, stir in reserved broth, potato, bay leaf, & thyme & bring to boil. Reduce heat to low & simmer till potato is tender about 10 mins. Include toasted bread & simmer till bread is completely saturated & starts to break down about 5 mins.
4. Remove & discard bay leaf & thyme. Shift half of the soup to blender & process till smooth & creamy, 2 to 3 mins. Shift to a large container & repeat with the remaining soup. Return soup to saucepan & bring to simmer. Season with salt & pepper for tasting & keep with Fried Leeks.

590. FRIED LEEKS

Prep Time: *Cook Time:* *Servings: 2*
14 Minutes *12 Minutes*

INGREDIENTS:

- medium leek, white & light green parts only, halved lengthwise, sliced into very thin 2-inch strips, washed thoroughly, & dried
- 2 Tbsps. all-purpose flour
- Salt & pepper
- 1/2 cup olive oil

TECHNIQUE:

1. Toss leeks, flour, & pinch each salt & pepper in a medium container. Heat oil in a 12-inch pan till shimmering. Include half of leeks & fry, often stirring, till golden brown, about 6 mins. Using a slotted spoon, Shift leeks to the paper towel-lined plate, then sprinkle with salt & pepper to taste. Repeat with remaining leeks.

591. GARLIC-POTATO SOUP

Prep Time: *Cook Time:* *Servings: 6*
15 Minutes *35 Minutes*

INGREDIENTS:

- 3 Tbsps. unsalted butter
- leek, white & light green parts only, halved lengthwise, chopped small, & washed thoroughly
- garlic cloves, minced, plus 2 whole heads garlic, outer papery skins removed, & top third of heads cut off & discarded
- 6-7 cups low-sodium chicken broth
- bay leaves salt & pepper
- 1 1/2 lbs russet potatoes, peeled & cut into 1/2-inch cubes
- lb red potatoes (unpeeled), cut into 1/2-inch cubes 1/2 cup heavy cream
- 1 1/2 Tsps. minced fresh thyme
- 1/4 cup minced fresh chives
- recipe GARLIC CHIPS (recipe follows)

TECHNIQUE:

1. Melt butter in a Dutch oven over medium heat. Include leeks & cook till soft (do not brown), 5 to 8 mins. Stir in minced garlic & cook till fragrant, about 1 min. Include garlic heads, 6 cups broth, bay leaves, & 3/4 Tsp. Salt. Partially cover pot & bring to simmer over medium-high heat. Reduce heat & simmer till garlic is very tender when pierced with the tip of the knife, 30 to 40 mins. Include russet potatoes & red potatoes & continue to simmer, partially covered, till potatoes are Tender, 15 to 20 mins.
2. Discard bay leaves. Remove garlic heads from the pot and, using tongs or paper towels, squeeze at root end till cloves slip out of their skins into the container. By Using a fork, mash garlic to smooth paste.
3. Stir cream, thyme, & half of the mashed garlic into soup. Heat soup till hot, about 2 mins. Taste soup & Include remaining garlic paste if desired.
4. Using an immersion blender, process soup till creamy, with some potato chunks remaining. Alternatively, Shift 1 1/2 cups potatoes & 1 cup broth to blender or food processor & process till smooth. (Process more potatoes for a thicker consistency.) Return puree to pot & stir to combine, Setting consistency with up to 1 cup more broth if necessary. Season with salt & pepper to taste, sprinkle with chives & Garlic Chips, & serve.

592. GARLIC CHIPS

Prep Time: *Cook Time:* *Servings: 4*
7 Minutes *9 Minutes*

INGREDIENTS:

- 3 Tbsps. olive oil
- garlic cloves, sliced thin lengthwise salt

TECHNIQUE:

1. Heat oil & garlic in a 10-inch pan over medium-high heat. Cook, frequently turning, till light golden brown, about 3 mins. Using a slotted spoon, Shift garlic to a paper towel-lined plate. Season with salt to taste.

593. BROCCOLI-CHEESE SOUP

Prep Time: 16 Minutes *Cook Time: 14 Minutes* *Servings: 6*

INGREDIENTS:

- Tbsps. unsalted butter
- lbs broccoli, florets chopped into 1-inch pieces, stalks peeled & sliced 1/4 inch thick
- 1 onion, chopped coarsely
- garlic cloves, minced
- 1 1/2 Tsps. dry mustard
- Pinch cayenne pepper
- Salt & pepper
- 3–4 cups water
- 1/4 Tsp. baking soda
- cups low-sodium chicken broth
- ounces baby spinach (2 cups)
- 3 ounces sharp cheddar cheese, shredded (3/4 cup)
- 1 1/2 ounces Parmesan cheese, grated fine (3/4 cup), plus extra for serving
- recipe BUTTER CROUTONS

TECHNIQUE:

1. Melt butter over medium-high heat. Include broccoli, onion, garlic, mustard, cayenne, & 1 Tsp. Salt & cook, frequently stirring, till fragrant, about 6 mins. Include 1 cup water & baking soda. Bring to simmer, cover, & cook till broccoli is very soft, about 20 mins, stirring once during cooking.
2. Include broth & 2 cups water & increase heat to medium-high. When batter begins to simmer, stir in spinach & cook till wilted, about 1 min. Shift half of the soup to a blender, Include cheddar & Parmesan, & process till smooth, about 1 min. Shift soup to a medium container & repeat with the remaining soup. Return soup to Dutch oven, place over medium heat & bring to simmer. Set consistency of Soup with up to 1 cup water. Season with salt & pepper to taste. Serve, passing extra Parmesan.

594. BUTTERNUT SQUASH SOUP

Prep Time: 14 Minutes *Cook Time: 12 Minutes* *Servings: 6*

INGREDIENTS:

- Tbsps. unsalted butter
- 1 large shallot, minced
- lbs butternut squash, cut in half lengthwise, each half cut in half widthwise; seeds & fibres scraped out & reserved
- 6 cups water
- Salt
- 1/2 cup heavy cream
- Tsp. dark brown sugar Pinch ground nutmeg
- BUTTERED CINNAMON-SUGAR CROUTONS (recipe follows)

TECHNIQUE:

1. 2Melt butter in the oven over medium-low heat. Include shallot & cook, frequently stirring, till translucent, about 3 mins. Include seeds & fibres from squash & cook, occasionally stirring, till butter turns saffron colour, about 4 mins.
2. Include water & 1 Tsp. Salt to pot & bring to boil over high heat. Reduce heat to medium-low, place squash, cut side down, in a steamer basket, & lower basket into the pot. Cover & steam till squash is completely tender, about 30 mins. Take the pot off heat & use tongs to Shift squash to rimmed baking sheet. When cool enough to handle, use a large spoon to scrape flesh from the skin. Reserve squash flesh in container & discard skin.
3. Strain steaming liquid through a fine-mesh strainer into a second container; discard solids in the strainer. (You should have 2 1/2 to 3 cups liquid.) Rinse And dry pot.
4. Working in batches & filling blender jar only halfway for each batch, puree squash, including enough reserved steaming liquid to obtain a smooth consistency. Shift puree to clean pot & stir in remaining steaming liquid, cream, & brown sugar. Warm soup over medium-low heat till hot, about 3 mins. Stir in nutmeg, season with salt to taste, & serve.

595. BUTTERED CINNAMON-SUGAR CROUTONS

Prep Time: 10 Minutes *Cook Time: 8 Minutes* *Servings: 2*

INGREDIENTS:

- slices hearty white sandwich bread, crusts removed, cut into 1/2-inch cubes (about 1 cup)
- 1 Tbsp. unsalted butter, melted
- Tsps. sugar
- 1/2 Tsp. ground cinnamon

TECHNIQUE:

1. Set oven rack to middle setting & heat oven to 350 degrees. Combine bread cubes & melted butter in the medium container & toss to coat. Combine sugar & cinnamon in a small container, then Include it in a container with bread cubes & toss to coat.
2. Spread bread cubes in a layer on parchment paper-lined rimmed baking sheet & bake, occasionally stirring, till crisp, 8 to 10 mins. Let cool on a baking sheet to room temperature. (Croutons can be stored for up to 3 days.)

Dinner Recipes

596. CREAMY MUSHROOM SOUP

Prep Time: 12 Minutes *Cook Time: 10 Minutes* *Servings: 2*

INGREDIENTS:

- Tbsps. unsalted butter
- large shallots, minced
- 1 garlic clove, minced
- 1/2 Tsp. ground nutmeg
- lbs white mushrooms, trimmed & sliced 1/4 inch thick 3 1/2 cups low-sodium chicken broth
- 4 cups hot water
- 1/2 ounce dried porcini mushrooms, rinsed 1/3 cup Madeira or dry sherry
- 1 cup heavy cream
- Tsps. lemon juice Salt & pepper
- recipe SAUTÉED WILD MUSHROOM GARNISH (recipe follows)

TECHNIQUE:

1. Melt butter over medium-low heat. Include shallots & sauté, frequently stirring, till softened, about 4 mins. Stir in garlic & nutmeg; cook till fragrant, about 1 min longer. Increase heat to medium; Include white mushrooms & stir to coat with butter. Cook, occasionally stirring, till mushrooms release liquid, about 7 mins. Reduce heat to medium-low, cover pot, & cook, occasionally stirring, till softened & mushrooms have released all liquid, about 20 mins.
2. Include broth, water, & porcini mushrooms in the pot. Cover the bring to simmer, and then reduce heat to low & simmer till mushrooms are fully tender about 20 mins.
3. Puree soup in batches in the blender till smooth, filling blender jar only Halfway for each batch. Rinse & dry pot & return soup to pot. Stir in Madeira & cream & bring to simmer over low heat. Include lemon juice, season with salt & pepper to taste, & serve with Sautéed Wild Mushroom Garnish. (Soup, minus garnish, can be refrigerated for up to 2 days.)

597. SAUTÉED WILD MUSHROOM GARNISH

Prep Time: 10 Minutes *Cook Time: 8 Minutes* *Servings: 4*

INGREDIENTS:

- 2 Tbsps. unsalted butter
- ounces shiitake, chanterelle, oyster, or cremini mushrooms, stemmed & sliced thin salt & pepper

TECHNIQUE:

1. Melt butter in a 10-inch pan over low heat. Include mushrooms & season with salt & pepper to taste. Cover & cook, occasionally stirring, till mushrooms release their liquid, about 10 mins for shiitakes & chanterelles, about 5 mins for oysters, & about 9 mins for cremini.
2. Uncover & continue to cook, occasionally stirring, till liquid released by mushrooms has evaporated & mushrooms are browned, about 2 mins for shiitakes, about 3 mins for chanterelles, & about 2 mins for oysters & cremini. Serve immediately as a garnish for soup.

598. HEARTY VEGETABLE SOUP

Prep Time: 15 Minutes *Cook Time: 35 Minutes* *Servings: 4*

INGREDIENTS:

- large carrot, peeled & chopped
- celery rib, chopped
- onion, chopped
- 3 portobello mushrooms, chopped coarsely
- head garlic, outer papery skins removed & top third of head cut off & discarded
- 3 Tbsps. olive oil
- 4 Tsps. tomato paste
- 9 cups broth or vegetable broth
- medium leeks, halved lengthwise, green parts chopped & washed thoroughly, white parts sliced thin, washed thoroughly, & reserved for soup
- sprigs fresh parsley
- 4 sprigs of fresh thyme
- 2 bay leaves
- 1/2 ounce dried porcini mushrooms, rinsed
- (14.5-ounce) can diced tomatoes, drained, tomato pieces chopped coarsely
- 12 ounces russet potatoes, peeled & cut into 1/2-inch pieces 2 carrots, peeled & cut into 1/2-inch pieces
- 1/2 head celery root (14 ounces), peeled & cut into 1/2-inch pieces
- small head escarole (12 ounces), stemmed & leaves cut into 1-inch pieces (4 cups)
- cup frozen baby lima beans, thawed (optional)
- Tbsps. minced fresh parsley Salt & pepper

TECHNIQUE:

1. Set oven rack to middle setting & heat oven to 450 degrees. Place carrot, celery, onion, portobellos, & garlic head on rimmed baking sheet. Drizzle with oil & toss to coat. Include tomato paste & toss again to coat. Spread vegetables in an even layer, set garlic head cut side up, & roast till vegetables are well browned 25 to 30 mins. Combine roasted vegetables, broth, leek greens, parsley, thyme, bay leaves, & porcini in a Dutch oven. Cover & bring to simmer over medium-high heat, then reduce heat to medium-low & simmer, partially covered, 30 mins.
2. Remove garlic head from the pot and, using tongs or paper towels, squeeze at root end till cloves slip out of their skins into a small container. By using a fork, mash garlic is to smooth paste & set aside. Put on solids to extract as much liquid as possible. Discard solids in strainer.
3. Rinse & wipe out the Dutch oven. Put the tomatoes, potatoes, carrots, celery root, leek whites, strained stock and garlic paste and then minimized to medium heat, cover and simmer until vegetables are cooked. When stabbed with a skewer or knife, it softens for about 25 minutes.
4. By using the back of a spoon, mash some potatoes against the side of the pot to thicken the soup. Stir in escarole & lima beans, if using, & cook till escarole is wilted & lima beans are heated through about 5 mins. Stir in parsley & season with salt & pepper to taste. Serve immediately. (Fortified broth can be refrigerated for up to 3 days or frozen for up to 2 months.)

599. HEARTY MINESTRONE

Prep Time: 12 Minutes *Cook Time: 10 Minutes* *Servings: 2*

INGREDIENTS:

- Salt & pepper
- 1/2 lb dried cannellini beans (1 cup), picked over & rinsed 3 ounces pancetta, cut into 1/4-inch pieces
- Tbsp. extra-virgin olive oil, plus extra for serving
- 2 celery ribs, cut into 1/2-inch pieces

- carrot, peeled & cut into 1/2-inch pieces
- 2 small onions, cut into 1/2-inch pieces
- zucchini, cut into 1/2-inch pieces (1 cup)
- 2 garlic cloves, minced
- 1/2 small head green cabbage halved, cored, & cut into 1/2-inch pieces (2 cups) 1/8–1/4 Tsp. red pepper flakes
- 8 cups water
- cups low-sodium chicken broth
- 1 Parmesan cheese rind
- 1 bay leaf
- 1 1/2 cups V8 juice
- 1/2 cup chopped fresh basil
- Grated Parmesan cheese

TECHNIQUE:

1. Dissolve 1 1/2 Tbsps. Salt in the cold water container or container. Include beans & soak for at least 8 hrs & up to 24 hrs. Drain beans & rinse well.
2. 3Heat pancetta & oil in a Dutch oven over medium-high heat. Cook, occasionally stirring, till pancetta is lightly browned & fat has rendered, 3 to 5 mins. Include celery, carrot, onions, & zucchini & cook, frequently stirring, till vegetables are softened & lightly browned, 5 to 9 mins. Stir in garlic, cabbage, 1/2 Tsp. Salt & pepper flakes & continue to cook till cabbage starts to wilt, 1 to 2 mins longer. Shift vegetables to rimmed baking sheet & set aside.
3. Include soaked beans, water, broth, Parmesan rind, & bay leaf to Dutch oven & bring to boil over high heat. Reduce heat & simmer vigorously, occasionally stirring, till beans are fully tender & liquid begins to thicken, 45 to 60 mins.
4. Include reserved vegetables & V8 juice to pot & cook till vegetables are soft, about 15 mins. Discard bay leaf & Parmesan rind, stir in chopped basil, & season with salt & pepper to taste. Serve with oil & grated Parmesan. (Reheat it gently & Include basil just before serving.)

600. SPLIT PEA & HAM SOUP

Prep Time: *12 Minutes* *Cook Time:* *10 Minutes* *Servings: 4*

INGREDIENTS:

- Tbsps. unsalted butter
- 1 large onion, chopped fine salt & pepper
- garlic cloves, minced
- 7 cups water
- ham steak (about 1 lb), skin removed, cut into quarters
- 3 slices thick-cut bacon
- lb green split peas (2 cups), picked over & rinsed
- sprigs fresh thyme
- bay leaves
- carrots, peeled
- 1 celery rib, divide into 1/2-inch pieces 1 recipe BUTTER CROUTONS

TECHNIQUE:

1. Heat butter in a Dutch oven over high heat. Include onion & 1/2 Tsp. Salt & cook, frequently stirring, till onion is softened, about 3 to 4 mins. Include garlic & cook till fragrant, about 30 seconds. Include water, ham steak, bacon, peas, thyme, & bay leaves. Increase heat to high & bring to simmer, frequently stirring to keep peas from sticking to the bottom. Reduce heat to low, cover, & simmer till peas are tender but Not falling apart, about 45 mins.
2. Remove ham steak, cover with aluminium foil or plastic wrap to prevent drying out, & set aside. Stir in carrots & celery & continue to simmer, covered, till vegetables are tender & peas have almost completely broken down, about 30 mins longer.
3. When cool enough, shred ham into small bite-size pieces. Remove & discard thyme, bay leaves, & bacon slices. Stir ham back into soup & return to simmer. Season with salt & pepper to taste & serve.

601. HEARTY LENTIL SOUP

Prep Time: *10 Minutes* *Cook Time:* *8 Minutes* *Servings: 7*

INGREDIENTS:

- slices bacon, cut into 1/4-inch pieces
- 1 large onion, chopped fine
- 2 carrots, peeled & chopped
- garlic cloves, minced
- (14.5-ounce) can diced tomatoes, drained
- bay leaf
- Tsp. minced fresh thyme
- ounces lentils (1 cup), picked over & rinsed
- 1 Tsp. salt Pepper
- 1/2 cup dry white wine
- 4 1/2 cups low-sodium chicken broth
- 1 1/2 cups water
- 1 1/2 Tsps. balsamic vinegar
- Tbsps. minced fresh parsley

TECHNIQUE:

1. Cook bacon in an oven over medium-high heat, occasionally stirring, till bacon is crisp, about 5 mins. Include onion & carrots & cook, occasionally stirring, till vegetables begin to soften about 2 mins. Include garlic & cook till fragrant, about 30 seconds. Stir in tomatoes, bay leaf, & thyme & cook till fragrant, about 30 seconds.
2. Stir in lentils & salt & season with pepper to taste. Cover, reduce heat to medium-low, & cook till vegetables are softened & lentils have darkened 8 to 10 mins.
3. Uncover, increase heat to high, Include wine, & bring to simmer. Include chicken broth & water, bring to boil, cover partially, & reduce heat to low. Simmer till lentils are tender but still hold their shape, 30 to 35 mins.
4. Remove bay leaf from pot & discard. Puree 3 cups soup in the blender till smooth, then return to pot. Stir in vinegar & heat soup over medium-low heat till hot, about 5 mins. Stir in 2 Tbsps. Parsley & serve, garnishing each container with remaining parsley.

602. PASTA E FAGIOLI

Prep Time: *15 Minutes* *Cook Time:* *35 Minutes* *Servings: 2*

INGREDIENTS:

- Tbsp. extra-virgin olive oil, plus extra for drizzling
- 3 ounces pancetta, chopped fine
- onion, chopped fine
- celery rib, chopped fine
- 4 garlic cloves, minced
- 1 Tsp. dried oregano
- 1/4 Tsp. red pepper flakes
- anchovy fillets, rinsed & minced
- 1 (28-ounce) can diced tomatoes
- 1 Parmesan cheese rind
- 2 (15-ounce) cans cannellini beans, rinsed
- 3 1/2 cups low-sodium chicken broth
- 2 1/2 cups water
- 1 cup orzo
- 1/4 cup chopped fresh parsley
- ounces Parmesan cheese, grated (1 cup)

TECHNIQUE:

1. Heat oil in an oven over medium-high heat till shimmering. Include pancetta & cook, occasionally stirring, till beginning to brown, 3 to 5 mins. Include onion & celery & cook, occasionally stirring, till vegetables are softened, 5 to 7 mins. Include garlic, oregano, pepper flakes, & anchovies & cook, constantly stirring, till fragrant, about 1 min. Stir continuously in tomatoes, scraping up any browned bits from the bottom of the pan. Include Parmesan rind & beans & bring to boil, then reduce heat to low & simmer to blend flavours, 10 mins.
2. Include chicken broth, water, & 1 Tsp. Salt to pot. Increase heat to high & bring to boil. Include pasta & cook till al dente, about 10 mins.
3. Remove & discard Parmesan rind. Off heat, stir in 3 Tbsps. Parsley & season with salt & pepper to taste. Ladle soup into containers, drizzle with olive oil & sprinkle with remaining parsley. Serve immediately, passing grated Parmesan separately.

603. SIMPLE BEEF CHILI WITH KIDNEY BEANS

Prep Time: *5 Minutes* *Cook Time:* *25 Minutes* *Servings: 5*

INGREDIENTS:

- Tbsps. vegetable oil
- onions chopped fine
- red bell pepper, stemmed, seeded, & cut into 1/2-inch pieces
- 6 garlic cloves, minced
- 1/4 cup chilli powder
- 1 Tbsp. ground cumin
- Tbsps. ground coriander
- 1 Tsp. red pepper flakes
- 1 Tsp. dried oregano
- 1/2 Tsp. cayenne pepper
- lbs 85 per cent lean ground beef
- (15-ounce) can red kidney beans, rinsed
- (28-ounce) can diced tomatoes, drained with juice reserved
- (28-ounce) can tomato puree Salt
- Lime wedges

DIRECTIONS:

1. Heat oil in the oven over medium heat till shimmering but not smoking.
2. Include onions, bell pepper, garlic, chilli powder, cumin, coriander, pepper flakes, oregano, & cayenne & cook, occasionally stirring, till vegetables are softened & beginning to brown, about 10 mins.
3. Increase heat to medium-high & Include half of the beef. Cook, breaking up.
4. Pieces with a spoon, till no longer pink & just beginning to brown, 3 to 4 mins. Include remaining beef & cook, breaking up pieces with spoon, till no longer pink, 3 to 4 mins.
5. Include beans, tomatoes, tomato puree, & 1/2 Tsp. Salt; turn it to boil, then reduce heat to low & simmer, covered, occasionally stirring, for 1 hr.
6. Remove cover & continue to simmer 1 hr longer, occasionally stirring (if chilli begins to stick to the bottom of the pot, stir in 1/2 cup water & continue to simmer), till beef is tender & chilli is dark, rich, & slightly thickened.
7. Season with salt to taste. Serve with lime wedges & condiments, if desired.

604. CHILI CON CARNE

Prep Time: *5 Minutes* *Cook Time:* *55 Minutes* *Servings: 4*

INGREDIENTS:

- Tbsps. ancho chilli powder or 3 chiles (about 1/2 ounce), toasted & ground
- Tbsps. new Mexican chilli powder or 3 medium chiles (about 3/4 ounce), toasted & ground
- Tbsps. cumin seeds, toasted
- Tbsps. dried oregano, preferably Mexican 7 1/2 cups plus 2/3 cup water
- 1 (4-lb) chuck-eye roast, trimmed & cut into 1-inch pieces salt & pepper
- slices bacon, cut into 1/4-inch pieces
- 1 onion, chopped fine
- 5 garlic cloves, minced
- 4–5 small jalapeño chiles, stemmed, seeded, & minced
- cup canned crushed tomatoes or plain tomato sauce
- 2 Tbsps. lime juice
- 5 Tbsps. Masa or 3 Tbsps. cornstarch

DIRECTIONS:

1. Combine chilli powders, cumin, & oregano in the small container & stir in 1/2 cup water to form a thick paste; set aside.
2. Season beef with 2 Tbsps. Salt; set aside.
3. Cook bacon in the oven over medium-low heat till crisp, about 10 mins.
4. Using a slotted spoon, Shift bacon to the paper towel-lined plate. Pour all but 2 Tbsps. Fat into a small container; set aside.
5. Increase heat to medium-high & sauté the meat in 4 batches till well browned on all sides, about 5 mins per batch, including an additional 2 Tbsps.
6. Bacon fat to pot as necessary. Reduce heat to medium & Include 3 Tbsps. Bacon fat to now-empty pan.
7. Include onion & cook till softened, 5 to 7 mins. Include garlic & jalapeños & cook till fragrant, about 1 min. Include chile paste & cook till fragrant, 2 to 3 mins.
8. Include reserved bacon & browned beef, crushed tomatoes, lime juice, & 7 cups water & bring to simmer.
9. Continue to simmer till meat is tender & juices are dark, rich, & starting to thicken, about 2 hrs.
10. Mix masa with remaining 2/3 cup water (or cornstarch with 3 Tbsps. water) in a small container to form a smooth paste.
11. Increase heat to medium, stir in pasta, & simmer till thickened, 5 to 10 mins.
12. Season with salt & pepper to taste & serve.

605. ULTIMATE BEEF CHILI

Prep Time: *5 Minutes* *Cook Time:* *15 Minutes* *Servings: 4*

INGREDIENTS:

- Salt
- 8 ounces (1¹/4 cups) dried pinto beans, picked over & rinsed
- dried ancho chiles, stemmed, seeded, & torn into 1-inch pieces 2–4 dried de árbol chiles, stemmed, seeded, & split into 2 pieces
- 3 Tbsps. cornmeal
- 2 Tbsps. dried oregano
- 2 Tbsps. ground cumin
- 2 Tbsps. cocoa
- 2¹/2 cups low-sodium chicken broth 2 onions, cut into ³/4-inch pieces
- 3 small jalapeño chiles, stemmed, seeded, & cut into ¹/2-inch pieces 3 Tbsps. vegetable oil
- 4 garlic cloves, minced
- 1 (14.5-ounce) can diced tomatoes
- 2 Tbsps. molasses
- 3¹/2 lbs blade steak, ³/4 inch thick, trimmed & cut into ³/4-inch pieces 1 (12-ounce) bottle mild lager, such as Budweiser

DIRECTIONS:

1. Combine 3 Tbsps. Salt, 4 quarts water, & beans in a Dutch oven & bring to boil over high heat. Remove pot from heat, cover, & let stand 1 hr. Drain & rinse well.
2. Set oven rack to lower-middle setting & heat oven to 300 degrees.
3. Place ancho chiles in the 12-inch pan set over medium-high heat; toast, frequently stirring, till the flesh is fragrant, 4 to 6 mins, reducing heat if chiles begin to smoke.
4. Shift to food processor & cool. Do not wash out the pan.
5. Include de árbol chiles, cornmeal, oregano, cumin, cocoa, & ¹/2Tsp. Salt to food processor with toasted ancho chiles; process till finely ground, about 2 mins.
6. With processor running, slowly Include ¹/2 cup broth till smooth paste forms, about 45 seconds, scraping downsides of the container as necessary.
7. Shift paste to a small container. Place onions in now-empty processor & pulse till roughly chopped, about 4 pulses. Include jalapeños & pulse till the consistency of chunky salsa, about 4 pulses, scraping down container as necessary.
8. Heat 1 Tbsp. Oil in a Dutch oven overheats medium to high flame.
9. Include onion batter & cook, occasionally stirring, till the moisture has evaporated & vegetables are softened, 7 to 9 mins.
10. Include garlic & cook till fragrant, about 1 min. Include chile paste, tomatoes, & molasses; stir till chile paste is thoroughly combined.
11. Include remaining 2 cups broth & drained beans; bring to boil, then reduce heat to simmer.
12. Meanwhile, heat 1 Tbsp. Oil in 12-inch pan over medium-high heat till shimmering. Pat beef dry with paper towels & sprinkle with 1 Tsp. Salt.
13. Include half of beef & cook till browned on all sides, about 10 mins. Shift meat to a Dutch oven.
14. Include half of the beer to the pan, scraping up browned bits from the bottom of the pan, & bring to simmer. Shift beer to Dutch oven.
15. Repeat with remaining 1 Tbsp. oil, remaining steak, & remaining beer. Stir to combine & return batter to simmer.
16. Cover pot & Shift to oven. Cook till meat & beans are fully tender, 1¹/2 to 2 hrs.
17. Let chilli stand, uncovered, for 10 mins. Stir well, season with salt to taste, & serve. (Chili can be refrigerated for up to 3 days.)

606. WHITE CHICKEN CHILI

Prep Time: *5 Minutes* *Cook Time:* *35 Minutes* *Servings: 4*

INGREDIENTS:

- lbs bone-in split chicken breasts or thighs, trimmed salt & pepper
- Tbsp. vegetable oil, plus extra as needed
- 3 jalapeño chiles
- 3 poblano chiles, stemmed, seeded, & cut into large pieces
- 3 New Mexican chile peppers, stemmed, seeded, & cut into large chunks 2 onions, cut into large pieces
- 6 garlic cloves, minced
- Tbsp. ground cumin
- 1¹/2 Tbsps. ground coriander
- (15-ounce) cans cannellini beans, rinsed
- 3 cups low-sodium chicken broth
- 3 Tbsps. lime juice (2 limes)
- ¹/4 cup minced fresh cilantro
- scallions, sliced thin

DIRECTIONS:

1. Season chicken with 1 Tsp. Salt & ¹/4 Tsp. Pepper.
2. Heat oil in a Dutch oven after setting medium-high heat till just smoking. Include chicken, skin side down, & cook without moving till the skin is golden brown, about 4 mins.
3. Using tongs, flip chicken & lightly brown on another side, about 2 mins. Shift chicken to plate; remove & discard skin.
4. While chicken is browning, remove & discard ribs & seeds from 2 jalapeños, then mince jalapeños & set aside. Process half of poblano Chiles, New Mexican chiles, & onions in the food processor till the consistency of chunky salsa, 10 to 12 pulses, scraping down sides of container halfway through.
5. Shift batter to the medium container. Repeat with remaining poblano chiles, New Mexican chiles, & onions; combine with the first batch (do not wash food processor).
6. Pour off all but 1 Tbsp. Fat from Dutch oven (including additional vegetable oil if necessary) & reduce heat to medium. Include minced jalapeños, chile batter, garlic, cumin, coriander, & ¹/4 Tsp. Salt.
7. Cover & cook, occasionally stirring, till vegetables have softened, about 10 mins. Remove pot from heat.
8. Shift 1 cup cooked vegetable batter to the now-empty food processor.
9. Include 1 cup beans & 1 cup broth & process till smooth, about 20 seconds.
10. Include vegetable-bean batter, remaining 2 cups broth, & chicken breasts to Dutch oven & bring to boil over medium-high heat.
11. Reduce heat to medium-low & simmer, covered, occasionally stirring, till chicken registers 160 degrees (175 degrees if using thighs), 15 to 20 mins (40 mins if using thighs).
12. Shift chicken to a large plate. Stir in remaining beans & continue to simmer, uncovered, till beans are heated through & chilli has thickened slightly about 10 mins.
13. Mince remaining jalapeño, reserving & mincing ribs & seeds, & set aside. After cooling enough to handle, shred chicken into bite-size pieces, discarding bones.
14. Stir shredded chicken, lime juice, cilantro, scallions, & remaining minced jalapeño (with seeds if desired) into chilli & return to simmer.
15. Season with salt & pepper to taste & serve.

607. LIGHTER CHICKEN & DUMPLINGS

Prep Time: *5 Minutes* *Cook Time:* *20 Minutes* *Servings: 5*

INGREDIENTS:

- 2¹/2 lbs bone-in chicken thighs, trimmed
- Salt & pepper
- Tbsps. vegetable oil
- small onions, chopped fine
- carrots, peeled & cut into ³/4-inch pieces
- 1 celery rib, chopped fine
- ¹/4 cup dry sherry
- cups low-sodium chicken broth
- 1 Tsp. minced fresh thyme
- 1 lb chicken wings
- ¹/4 cup chopped fresh parsley
- cups (10 ounces) all-purpose flour
- 1 Tsp. sugar
- 1 Tsp. salt
- ¹/2 Tsp. baking soda
- ³/4 cup buttermilk, chilled
- 4 Tbsps. unsalted butter, melted & hot
- 1 large egg white

DIRECTIONS:

1. Pat chicken thighs for drying with paper towels & season with 1 Tsp. Salt & ¹/4 Tsp. Pepper. Heat oil in a Dutch oven after setting medium-high heat till shimmering.
2. Include chicken thighs, skin side down, & cook till the skin is crisp & well browned, 5 to 7 mins. Using tongs, flip chicken pieces & brown on the second side, 5 to 7 mins longer; Shift to a large plate. Discard all but 1 Tsp. Fat from the pot.
3. Include onions, carrots, & celery to now-empty pot; cook, occasionally stirring, till caramelized, 7 to 9 mins.
4. Mix the sherry and remove the brown spots from the bottom of the pool. Mix the broth and thyme. Put the juicy chicken thighs back into the pan and add the chicken wings.
5. Simmer for 45-55 minutes, cover and cook until the thigh meat can't stand being stabbed and sticking to the bones.
6. Remove pot from heat & Shift chicken to cutting board. Allow broth to settle for 5 mins, then skim fat from the surface.
7. When cool enough to handle, remove & discard chicken skin. With the fingers or a fork, pick up the meat from the chicken thighs (and wings, if desired) & cut it into 1-inch pieces.
8. Return the beef to the pan. (At the end, the stew cooled to room temperature, then refrigerated for up to 2 days. Bring to a boil over medium-low heat before continuing.)
9. Whisk flour, sugar, salt, & baking soda in a large container. Combine buttermilk & melted butter in a medium container, stirring till butter forms small clumps; whisk in egg white.
10. Include buttermilk batter to dry ingredients & stir with a rubber spatula till just incorporated & batter pulls away from sides of the container.
11. Return stew to simmer, stir in parsley, & season with salt and Pepper to taste. Using greased Tbsp. Measure each scoop level amount of batter & drop over the top of the stew, spacing about ¹/4 inch apart.
12. Wrap lid of Dutch oven with a clean kitchen towel (keeping towel away from heat source) & cover pot.
13. Simmer gently till dumplings have doubled in size & toothpick inserted into the centre comes out clean, 13 to 16 mins. Serve immediately.

608. QUICK CHICKEN FRICASSEE

Prep Time: *5 Minutes* *Cook Time:* *20 Minutes* *Servings: 5*

INGREDIENTS:

- lbs boneless, skinless chicken breasts and/or thighs, trimmed salt & pepper
- Tbsp. unsalted butter
- Tbsp. olive oil
- lb cremini mushrooms, trimmed & sliced ¹/4 inch thick
- onion, chopped fine
- ¹/4 cup dry white wine
- Tbsp. all-purpose flour
- garlic clove, minced
- 1¹/2 cups low-sodium chicken broth
- ¹/3 cup sour cream
- 1 large egg yolk
- ¹/2 Tsp. freshly grated nutmeg
- Tbsps. lemon juice
- Tbsps. minced fresh tarragon
- 4.

DIRECTIONS:

1. Chicken pat after drying with paper towels & season with 1 Tsp. Salt & ¹/2 Tsp. Pepper. Heat butter & oil in the 12-inch pan over medium-high heat till butter is melted.
2. Place chicken in the pan & cook till browned, about 4 mins. Using tongs, flip chicken & cook till browned on the second side, about 4 mins longer. Shift chicken to a large plate.
3. Include mushrooms, onion, & wine to the now-empty pan & cook, occasionally stirring, till the liquid has evaporated & mushrooms are browned, 8 to 10 mins.
4. Include flour & garlic; cook, constantly stirring, 1 min. Include broth & bring the batter to boil, scraping up browned bits the bottom of the pan includes chicken & any accumulated juices into the pan.
5. Reduce heat to medium-low, cover, & simmer till breasts register 160 degrees & thighs register 175 degrees, 5 to 10 mins.
6. Shift chicken to clean platter & tent loosely with aluminium foil.
7. Whisk sour cream & egg yolk together in a medium container. Whisking constantly, slowly stir ¹/2 cup hot sauce into the sour cream batter to temper.
8. Stirring constantly, slowly pour sour cream batter into the simmering sauce. Stir in nutmeg, lemon juice, & tarragon; return to simmer.
9. Present with salt & pepper for taste, pour sauce over chicken, & serve.

610 CHICKEN CANZANESE

Prep Time: *5 Minutes* *Cook Time:* *20 Minutes* *Servings: 5*

INGREDIENTS:

- 1 Tbsp. olive oil
- ounces prosciutto (1/4 inch thick), cut into 1/4-inch pieces
- 4 garlic cloves, sliced thin
- 8 (5-to 7-ounce) bone-in chicken thighs, trimmed salt & pepper
- Tbsps. all-purpose flour
- cups dry white wine
- cup low-sodium chicken broth
- 12 whole fresh sage leaves
- sprig fresh rosemary leaves removed & minced fine, stem reserved
- 4 whole cloves
- 2 bay leaves
- 1/4-1/2 Tsp. red pepper flakes
- Tbsps. unsalted butter
- 1 Tbsp. lemon juice

DIRECTIONS:

1. Set oven rack to lower-middle setting & heat oven to 325 degrees.
2. Heat 1 Tsp. Oil in 12-inch oven-safe pan over medium heat till shimmering. Include prosciutto & cook, frequently stirring, till just starting to brown, about 3 mins.
3. Include garlic slices & cook, frequently stirring, till garlic is golden brown, about 11/2 mins. Using a slotted spoon, Shift garlic & prosciutto to a small container & set it aside. Do not rinse the pan.
4. Increase heat to medium-high; include remaining 2 Tbsps. Oil & heat till just smoking. Chicken pat after drying with paper towels & season with pepper.
5. Include chicken, skin side down, & cook without moving till well browned 5 to 8 mins. Using tongs, flip chicken & brown on the second side, about 5 mins longer. Shift chicken to a large plate.
6. Remove all but 2 Tbsps. fat from pan. Sprinkle flour over fat & cook, constantly stirring, for 1 min.
7. Slowly Include wine & broth; bring to simmer, scraping up browned bits from the bottom of the pan. Cook till liquid is slightly reduced, 3 mins.
8. Stir in sage leaves, rosemary stem, cloves, bay leaves, pepper flakes, & reserved prosciutto & garlic.
9. Nestle chicken into liquid, skin side up (skin should be above the surface of the liquid), & bake, uncovered, till fork slips easily in & out meat, but meat is not falling off bones, about 11/4 hrs. (Check the chicken after 15 mins; broth should be barely bubbling.
10. Shift chicken to serving platter & tent with aluminium foil. Remove & discard sage leaves, rosemary stem, cloves, & bay leaves.
11. Place pan over high heat & bring sauce to boil. Cook till sauce is reduced to 11/4 cups, 2 to 5 mins. Off heat, stir in minced rosemary, butter, & lemon juice.
12. Season with salt & pepper to taste. Pour sauce around chicken & serve.

611. MOROCCAN CHICKEN WITH OLIVES & LEMON

Prep Time: *5 Minutes* *Cook Time:* *20 Minutes* *Servings: 4*

INGREDIENTS:

- 11/4 Tbsps. paprika
- 1/2 Tsp. ground cumin
- 1/2 Tsp. ground ginger
- 1/4 Tsp. cayenne pepper
- 1/4 Tsp. ground coriander
- 1/4 Tsp. ground cinnamon
- (2-inch) strips lemon zest
- 5 garlic cloves, minced
- 1 (31/2- to 4-lb) whole chicken, cut into 8 pieces (4 breast pieces, 2 thighs, 2 drumsticks), trimmed, wings discarded
- Salt & pepper
- Tbsp. olive oil
- large onion, halved & sliced 1/4 inch thick 13/4 cups low-sodium chicken broth
- Tbsp. honey
- carrots, peeled & cut crosswise into 1/2-inch-thick rounds, very large pieces cut into half-moons
- cup cracked green olives, pitted & halved
- 3 Tbsps. lemon juice
- 2 Tbsps. chopped fresh cilantro

DIRECTIONS:

1. Combine paprika, cumin, ginger, cayenne, coriander, & cinnamon in the small container & set aside. Mince 1 strip lemon zest & combine with 1 Tsp. Minced garlic & mince together till reduced to a fine paste; set aside.
2. Present both sides of chicken pieces with salt & pepper. Heat oil in a Dutch oven after setting medium-high heat till beginning to smoke.
3. Include chicken pieces, skin side down, & cook without moving till the skin is deep golden, about 5 mins. Using tongs, flip chicken pieces & brown on the second side, about 4 mins longer.
4. Shift chicken to large plate; when cool enough to handle, remove & discard skin. Pour off & discard all but 1 Tbsp. Fat from the pot.
5. Include onion & 2 remaining lemon zest strips to pot & cook, occasionally stirring, till onion slices have browned but still retain their shape, 5 to 7 mins (Include 1 Tbsp. water if cooking wok gets too dark).
6. Include remaining 4 Tbsps. Garlic & cook, stirring, till fragrant. Include spices & cook, constantly stirring, till darkened & very fragrant, 45 seconds to 1 min.
7. Stir in broth & honey, scraping up browned bits from the bottom of the pot. Include thighs & drumsticks, reduce heat to medium, & simmer for 5 mins.
8. Include carrots & breast pieces with any accumulated juices to the pot, arranging breast pieces in a single layer on top of carrots. Cover, reduce heat to medium-low, & simmer till breast pieces register 160 degrees, 10 to 15 mins.
9. Shift chicken to plate & tent with aluminium foil. Include olives to pot; increase heat to medium-high & simmer till the liquid has thickened slightly & carrots are tender, 4 to 6 mins.
10. Return chicken to pot & stir in garlic butter, lemon juice, & cilantro; season with salt & pepper to taste. Serve immediately.

Side Dishes Recipes

612. EMALEE PAYNE EAU CLAIRE, WI

INGREDIENTS:

START TO FINISH: 10 MIN. • MAKES: 6 MUGS

- 2 mugs (16 ounces) sour cream
- 2 mugs mayonnaise
- 2 pounds bacon slices, 6 cooked and mashed plum tomatoes, finely chopped
- 3 green onions, chopped
- Additional minced meat and minced green onions, assorted crackers or chips (optional)

DIRECTIONS:

1. In a bowl, combine sour cream, mayonnaise, bacon, tomatoes and onions altogether. Let cool until served. Garnish with bacon and onions, if desired. Serve with crackers or chips.

613. MAMMA'S CAPONATA

Prep Time: *15 Minutes* *Cook Time:* *35 Minutes* *Servings: 6*

INGREDIENTS:

- 1 large eggplant, peeled and chopped
- ¼ mug plus 2 tbsps olive oil, divided
- 2 medium onions, chopped
- 2 celery ribs, chopped
- 2 cans (14 ½ ounces each) of diced tomatoes, undrained
- 1/3 mug chopped ripe olives
- ¼ mug red wine vinegar
- 2 tbsp sugar
- 2 tbsp capers, drained
- ½ tsp salt
- ½ tsp pepper
- French bread baguettes, sliced and toasted

DIRECTIONS:

1. Fry eggplant in a cup of oil in a Dutch oven until tender. Remove from pan and set separately. Fry the onion In the same frying pan and celery in the remaining oil until they wilt. Stir in tomatoes and eggplant. Bring it to a boil. Reduce heat. Simmer without lid for 15 minutes.
2. Add olives, vinegar, sugar, capers, salt and pepper. Boil again. Reduce heat. Boil uncovered for 20 minutes or until thickened. Serve warm or at room temperature with baguettes.

614. WARM BACON CHEDDAR SPREAD

Prep Time: *15 Minutes* *Cook Time:* *44 Minutes* *Servings: 2*

INGREDIENTS:

- 1 package (8 ounces) cream cheese, softened
- ½ mug mayonnaise
- ¼ tsp dried thyme
- 1/8 tsp pepper
- 1 mug (4 ounces) shredded sharp cheddar cheese
- 3 green onions, chopped
- 8 bacon strips, cooked and crumbled, divided
- ½ mug crushed Ritz crackers
- Assorted crackers

DIRECTIONS:

1. Preheat oven to 350°. In a bowl, combine together cream cheese, mayonnaise, thyme and pepper. Stir it continuously in cheese, green onions and half the bacon. Transfer to a greased 3-mug baking dish.
2. Bake, uncovered, 13-15 minutes or until bubbly. Top with crushed crackers and remaining bacon. Serve with assorted crackers.

615. CHIPOTLE HAM 'N' CHEESE DIP

Prep Time: *15 Minutes* *Cook Time:* *10 Minutes* *Servings: 8*

INGREDIENTS:

- 2 pkg(8 ounces each) of cream cheese, cubed 1 can (12 ounces) evaporated milk
- 2 mugs (8 ounces) shredded Gouda cheese
- 1 mug (4 ounces) shredded cheddar cheese
- 2 tbsps chopped chipotle pepper in adobo sauce 1 tsp ground cumin
- 2 mugs diced fully cooked ham
- Fresh vegetables or tortilla chips

DIRECTIONS:

1. In a 3-qt slow cooker, combine together the first six ingredients. Cover and cook on low for 40 minutes.
2. Stir continuously in ham, and cook 20 minutes longer or until heated through. Serve warm with vegetables or chips.

616. HAM SPREAD

Prep Time: *15 Minutes* *Cook Time:* *3 Minutes* *Servings: 8*

INGREDIENTS:

- 3 mugs ground fully cooked ham
- 1 hard-cooked egg, chopped
- 2 tbsps finely chopped celery
- 2 tsp finely chopped onion
- 2 tsp sweet pickle relish
- ¾ mug mayonnaise 1 tbsp prepared mustard Assorted crackers

DIRECTIONS:

1. In a bowl, combine together the first five ingredients. Mix mayonnaise and mustard; add to ham mixture and mix well. Let it cool until serving. Serve with crackers.

617. PEPPERONI PIZZA DIP

Prep Time: *15 Minutes* | *Cook Time:* *10 Minutes* | *Servings: 2*

INGREDIENTS:

- 4 mugs (16 ounces) shredded cheddar cheese
- 4 mugs (16 ounces) shredded part-skim mozzarella cheese 1 mug of mayonnaise
- 1 jar (6 ounces) sliced mushrooms, drained
- 2 cans (2 ¼ ounces each) sliced ripe olives, drained 1 package (3 ½ ounces) pepperoni slices, quartered 1 tbsp dried minced onion
- Assorted crackers

DIRECTIONS:

1. In a 3-qt slow cooker, mix the cheeses, mayonnaise, mushrooms, olives, pepperoni and onion.
2. Wrap and cook on low for 1 ½ hour; stir continuously. Wrap and cook it for about 1 hour longer or until heated through. Serve with crackers.

618. 23.GERMAN BEER CHEESE SPREAD

Prep Time: *15 Minutes* | *Cook Time:* *12 Minutes* | *Servings: 2*

INGREDIENTS:

- 1 pound of sharp cheddar cheese, divided into ½-inch cubes 1 tbsp Worcestershire sauce
- 1 ½ tsp prepared mustard 1 small garlic clove, minced
- ¼ tsp salt
- 1/8 tsp pepper
- 2/3 cup German or non-alcoholic beer assorted biscuits

DIRECTIONS:

1. Put the cheese in the food processor. Pulse until chopped, about 1 minute. Add Worcestershire sauce, mustard, garlic, salt and pepper. Add beer little by little at a time, continuing to process until the mixture is smooth and spreadable, about a minute.
2. Transfer to a serving bowl or gift bottle. Cover and refrigerate for up to 1 week. Serve with crackers.

619. FRUIT HURRICANES

Prep Time: *15 Minutes* | *Cook Time:* *3 Minutes* | *Servings: 5*

INGREDIENTS:

- 2 mugs passion fruit juice
- 1 mug plus 2 tbsps sugar
- ¾ mug lime juice ¾ mug light rum ¾ mug dark rum
- 3 tbsp grenadine syrup
- 6 to 8 mugs ice cubes
- Orange slices, starfruit slices and maraschino cherries

DIRECTIONS:

1. In a pitcher, mix the fruit juice, sugar, lime juice, rum and grenadine; stir until sugar is dissolved.
2. Spread into a hurricane or highball glasses filled with ice. Serve with orange slices, starfruit slices and cherries.

620. SWEET TEA CONCENTRATE

Prep Time: *15 Minutes* | *Cook Time:* *3 Minutes* | *Servings: 3*

INGREDIENTS:

- 2 medium lemons
- 4 mugs sugar
- 4 mugs water
- 1 ½ mug English breakfast tea leaves or 20 black tea bags 1/3 mug lemon juice EACH SERVING
- 1 mug cold water
- Ice cubes
- Citrus slices, optional
- Mint sprigs, optional

DIRECTIONS:

1. Extract peels from lemons; set fruit aside for garnish or save for another use.
2. In a saucepan, combine together sugar and water. Bring to a boil over medium heat. Minimize heat; simmer, unwrapped, for 3-5 minutes or until sugar is dissolved, stirring occasionally. Extract from the heat; add tea leaves and lemon peels. Close and steep
3. minute. Strain the tea finally and discard the tea leaves and lemon peel. Mix lemon juice. Cool to room temperature.
4. Convert to a container with a tight lid. Store in the refrigerator for up to 2 weeks.
5. Tea preparation In a tall glass, mix water and concentrate. Add ice. Add orange slices and mint twigs if desired.

621. SANGRIA

Prep Time: *15 Minutes* | *Cook Time:* *10 Minutes* | *Servings: 2*

INGREDIENTS:

- ¼ mug sugar ¼ mug brandy 1 mug sliced peeled fresh peaches or frozen sliced peaches, thawed 1 mug sliced fresh strawberries or frozen sliced strawberries, thawed 1 medium lemon, sliced
- 1 medium lime, sliced
- 3 mugs dry white wine, chilled
- 1 can (12 ounces) lemon-lime soda, chilled Ice cubes

DIRECTIONS:

1. In a pitcher, mix sugar and brandy until sugar is dissolved. Add remaining ingredients; stir smoothly to mix. Serve over ice.

622. Cold PUNCH

Prep Time: *15 Minutes* | *Cook Time:* *0 Minutes* | *Servings: 2*

INGREDIENTS:

- 8 mugs cold water
- 1 can (12 ounces) of frozen lemonade concentrate, thawed plus ¾ mug thawed lemonade concentrate 2 litres ginger ale, chilled
- 1-litre cherry lemon-lime soda, chilled Ice ring, optional

DIRECTIONS:

1. In a large punch bowl, mix water and lemonade concentrate. Stir in ginger ale and lemon-lime soda. Top with an ice ring if desired. Serve punch immediately.
2. Desired. Serve punch immediately.

623. SPARKLING PEACH BELLINIS

Prep Time: *15 Minutes* | *Cook Time:* *10 Minutes* | *Servings: 2*

INGREDIENTS:

- 3 medium peaches, halved
- 1 tbsp honey
- 1 can (11.3 ounces) of peach nectar, chilled
- 2 bottles (750 millilitres each) champagne or sparkling grape juice, chilled
- place a baking sheet with a large piece of heavy-duty foil (aboutx 12 in.).

DIRECTIONS:

1. Place the peach halves cut side up on the foil. Drizzle honey. Turn the foil over the peaches and seal.
2. Bake it at least 375° for 25-30 minutes or until soft. Cool completely. Extract and remove the skin. Process the peaches in a cooking processor until soft.
3. Transfer the peach puree to the pitcher. Add honey and 1 bottle of champagne. Stir until blended. 12 Spread in a champagne flute or wine glass. Finish with the remaining champagne. Serve immediately.

624. FROZEN STRAWBERRY DAIQUIRIS

Prep Time: *15 Minutes* | *Cook Time:* *23 Minutes* | *Servings: 2*

INGREDIENTS:

- ¾ mug rum
- ½ mug thawed limeade concentrate
- 1 package (10 ounces) frozen sweetened sliced strawberries
- 1 to 1 ½ mugs ice cubes
- GARNISH
- Fresh strawberries

DIRECTIONS:

1. In a blender, mix the rum, limeade concentrate, strawberries and ice. Cover and process until smooth and thickened (use more ice for thicker daiquiris). Spread into cocktail glasses.
2. To garnish each daiquiri, cut a ½-in. slit into the tip of a strawberry; position berry on the rim of the glass.

Snacks And Appetizer Recipes

625. CUCUMBER-STUFFED CHERRY TOMATOES

Prep Time: *15 Minutes* | *Cook Time:* *44 Minutes* | *Servings: 2*

INGREDIENTS:

- 24 cherry tomatoes
- 1 package cream cheese, softened 2 tbsps mayonnaise
- ¼ cup finely chopped peeled cucumber 1 tbsp finely chopped green onion 2 tsp minced fresh dill

Directions:

1. Cut a thin slice off the top of each tomato. Scoop out and discard pulp; invert tomatoes onto paper towels to drain.
2. In a small size bowl, add cream cheese and mayonnaise until smooth; stir in the cucumber, onion and dill. Spoon into tomatoes. Refrigerate until serving.

626. TIERED CHEESE SLICES

Prep Time: *15 Minutes* | *Cook Time:* *25 Minutes* | *Servings: 2*

INGREDIENTS:

- 1 package (8 ounces) cream cheese, softened
- ½ tsp hot pepper sauce ¼ tsp salt
- ¼ cup chopped pecans
- ¼ cup dried cranberries 2 packages
- deli-style cheddar cheese slices
- Assorted crackers

Directions:

1. In a big bowl, add the cream cheese, hot pepper sauce and salt. Stir in pecans and cranberries.
2. On a 12-in. square of aluminium foil, place two slices of cheese side by side; spread with 2-3 tbsps cream cheese mixture. Repeat layers six times. Top with two cheese slices. Fold foil around cheese and seal tightly. Let it cool for 8 hours or overnight. Cut in half lengthwise and then widthwise into ¼-in. slices. Present with crackers.

627. CRAB-STUFFED SNOW PEAS

Prep Time: *15 Minutes* | *Cook Time:* *53 Minutes* | *Servings: 4*

INGREDIENTS:

- 1 can crab meat, drained, flaked, and cartilage removed
- 2 tbsps mayonnaise
- 1 tbsp chilli sauce or seafood cocktail sauce
- 1/8 tsp salt
- 3 drops hot pepper sauce
- Dash pepper
- 16 fresh snow peas

Directions:

1. In a small-size bowl, add the crab, mayonnaise, chilli sauce, salt, hot sauce and pepper.
2. Put the snow peas in the steaming basket. Place in a small saucepan over 1 inch of water. Bring to a boil; cover and steam for 30 seconds until tender. Drain the snow peas and immediately drop them into ice water. Drain and dry.
3. Cut the peas along the curved edges with a sharp knife. Spoon each crab mixture 1 tbsp.

628. CUCUMBER RYE SNACKS

Prep Time: *15 Minutes* | *Cook Time:* *17 Minutes* | *Servings: 5*

INGREDIENTS:

- 1 package (8 ounces) cream cheese, softened
- 2 tbsps mayonnaise
- 2 tsp Italian salad dressing mix
- 30 slices snack rye bread
- 30 thin slices of cucumber
- Fresh dill sprigs and chive blossoms

Directions:

1. In a bowl, beat the cream cheese, mayonnaise and dressing mix until blended. Let stand for 30 minutes.
2. Spread mixture on rye bread. Top each with a slice of cucumber, dill sprig and chive blossom. Cover and refrigerate until serving

629. ASIAN TUNA BITES WITH DIJON DIPPING SAUCE

Prep Time: *15 Minutes* | *Cook Time:* *53 Minutes* | *Servings: 6*

INGREDIENTS:

- 3 tbsps Dijon mustard
- 2 tbsps red wine vinegar
- 2 tbsp reduced-sodium soy sauce
- 1 tbsp sesame oil
- 1 tsp hot pepper sauce
- 1 pound tuna steaks, cut into thirty 1-inch cubes Cooking spray
- ¼ cup sesame seeds ½ tsp salt ¼ tsp pepper 2 green onions, finely chopped

Directions:

1. In a small size bowl, whisk the first five ingredients; set aside. Spritz tuna with cooking spray. Sprinkle with sesame seeds, salt and pepper. In a big nonstick skillet, brown tuna on all sides in batches until medium-rare or slightly pink in the centre; remove from the skillet.
2. On each of the 30 wooden appetizers, skewered, and thread one tuna cube. Arrange on a serving platter. Garnish with onions. Present with sauce.

630. MARINATED SAUSAGE KABOBS

Prep Time: *15 Minutes* | *Cook Time:* *25 Minutes* | *Servings: 4*

INGREDIENTS:

- ¼ cup olive oil
- 1 tbsp white vinegar
- ½ tsp minced garlic
- ½ tsp dried basil
- ½ tsp dried oregano
- 12 ounces cheddar cheese, cut into ¾-in. cubes 1 can (6 ounces) pitted ripe olives, drained
- 4 ounces hard salami, cut into ¾-in. cubes 1 medium sweet red pepper, cut into ¾-inch pieces 1 medium green pepper, cut into ¾-inch pieces 1.

Directions:

1. In a plastic bag, add the first five ingredients; add the remaining ingredients. Seal bag and turn to coat; refrigerate for at least 4 hours. Drain and discard marinade.
2. For each kabob, thread one piece each of cheese, olive, salami and pepper onto a toothpick.

631. SMOKED SALMON PINWHEELS

Prep Time: *15 Minutes* | *Cook Time:* *43 Minutes* | *Servings: 4*

INGREDIENTS:

- 1 package (8 ounces) cream cheese, softened
- 1 tbsp snipped fresh dill
- 1 tbsp capers, drained
- ½ tsp garlic powder
- ½ tsp lemon juice
- 4 spinach tortillas (8 inches), room temperature
- ½ pound smoked salmon fillets, flaked

Directions:

1. In a small size bowl, add the cream cheese, dill, capers, garlic powder and lemon juice. Spread over tortillas; top with salmon. Roll up tightly.
2. Cut into 1-in. pieces; secure with toothpicks. Chill until serving. Discard toothpicks before serving. Refrigerate leftovers.

632. CHEESE STRAWS

Prep Time: *15 Minutes* | *Cook Time:* *35 Minutes* | *Servings: 4*

INGREDIENTS:

- ½ cup butter softened
- 2 cups shredded sharp cheddar cheese
- 1 ¼ cups all-purpose flour
- ½ tsp salt
- ¼ tsp cayenne pepper

Directions:

1. Preheat oven to 350°. In a big bowl, beat butter until light and fluffy. Beat in cheese until blended.
2. Add flour, salt and cayenne; stir into cheese mixture until a dough forms. Roll into a 15x6-in rectangle. Cut into thirty 6-in. strips. Gently place strips 1 in. apart on ungreased baking sheets.
3. Bake 15-20 minutes or until lightly browned. Let it cool for 5 minutes before removing pans to wire racks to cool completely. Store straws in an airtight container.

633. PUMPKIN CHEESE PUFFS

Prep Time: *15 Minutes* | *Cook Time:* *16 Minutes* | *Servings: 6*

INGREDIENTS:

- 2 tbsp cream cheese, softened
- ½ tsp balsamic vinegar ½ cup water
- ¼ cup butter, cubed ¼ tsp salt
- ½ cup of all-purpose flour 4 drops yellow paste food colouring
- 1 drop red paste food colouring
- ½ cup grated Romano cheese 2 eggs
- 20 sprigs fresh Italian parsley, stems removed

Directions:

1. In a small size bowl, add cream cheese and vinegar. Cover and refrigerate. In a big saucepan, bring the water, butter and salt to a boil.
2. Mix the flour at a time and mix until a smooth ball is formed. Remove from heat. Leave it on for 5 minutes.
3. Add the yellow and red food colouring to a small bowl. Stir in the Romano cheese and food colouring to the mixture. Add eggs one at a time and beat well after each addition. Continue to beat until the dough is soft and shiny.
4. Lower it to the level of 3 inches. Separate on a greased baking sheet. Bake at 400° for 15-20 minutes or until slightly browned. Remove with wire rack to cool.
5. Use the tip of the star to represent the cream cheese mixture, putting the stems into the puff. Add parsley eggplant. Refrigerate leftover food.

634. DEVILED Shrimp

Prep Time: *15 Minutes* | *Cook Time:* *43 Minutes* | *Servings: 2*

INGREDIENTS:

- ½ cup finely chopped onion 3 tbsps butter
- 3 tbsps all-purpose flour
- ½ tsp salt 1 ½ cups half-and-half cream 2 egg yolks, lightly beaten
- 3 cans (6 ounces each) crabmeat, drained, flaked, and cartilage removed 1 tbsp Dijon mustard
- 2 tsp Worcestershire sauce
- 1 tsp minced chives
- TOPPING
- 1 cup soft bread crumbs
- 1 tbsp butter, melted

Directions:

1. In a big skillet, saute onion in butter until tender. Stir in flour and salt until blended. Gradually stir in cream until smooth. Take it to a boil, and cook and stir for 2 minutes or until thickened and bubbly. Remove from the heat.
2. Stir a small amount of hot mixture into egg yolks. Return all to the pan, stirring constantly. Bring to a gentle boil; cook and stir 2 minutes longer. Remove from the heat. Stir in the crab, mustard, Worcestershire sauce and chives.

635. MEAT-ATARIAN SUB

Prep Time: *15 Minutes* | *Cook Time:* *12 Minutes* | *Servings: 7*

INGREDIENTS:

- 1 cup (4 ounces) of shredded part-skim mozzarella cheese
- ½ cup grated Parmesan cheese ½ cup butter softened ½ cup mayonnaise 2 garlic cloves, minced
- 1 tsp Italian seasoning
- ¼ tsp crushed red pepper flakes ¼ tsp pepper 1 loaf (1 pound) French bread, halved lengthwise
- 1 pound sliced deli ham
- 2 packages (2.1 ounces each) ready-to-Present fully cooked bacon, warmed 4 ounces sliced pepperoni

Directions:

1. ½ cup pizza sauce 1. Preheat oven to 350°. In a small size bowl, add the first eight ingredients. Spread over cut sides of bread. Layer with ham, bacon, pepperoni and pizza sauce; replace the top.
2. Wrap in foil; place on a big baking sheet. Bake 25-30 minutes or until heated through. Cut into slices.

636. BUFFALO CHICKEN DIP

Prep Time: *15 Minutes* | *Cook Time:* *25 Minutes* | *Servings: 5*

INGREDIENTS:

- 1 package (8 ounces) cream cheese, softened
- 1 can (10 ounces) chunk white chicken, drained
- ½ cup buffalo wing sauce ½ cup ranch salad dressing 2 cups (8 ounces) shredded Colby-Monterey Jack cheese
- French bread baguette slices, celery ribs or tortilla chips, optional

Directions:

1. Preheat oven to 350°. Spread cream cheese into an ungreased shall reduce 1-qt. Baking dish. Layer with chicken, wing sauce and salad dressing. Sprinkle with cheese.
2. Bake, uncovered, 20-25 minutes or until cheese is melted. If desired, Present with baguette slices.

637. PHILLY CHEESESTEAK BITES

Prep Time: *15 Minutes* | *Cook Time:* *35 Minutes* | *Servings: 2*

INGREDIENTS:

- 1 package (22 ounces) frozen waffle-cut fries
- 1 medium onion, halved and sliced
- ½ small green pepper, halved and sliced ½ small sweet red pepper, halved and sliced 3 tbsps canola oil, divided
- ½ tsp salt, divided ¾ pound beef ribeye steak, cut into thin strips ¼ tsp pepper
- 3 tbsp ketchup
- 6 tbsps process cheese sauce

Directions:

1. Bake 18 big waffle fries according to package directions (save remaining fries for another use). Meanwhile, in a big skillet, saute onion and peppers in 1 tbsp oil until tender. Sprinkle with 1/8 tsp salt. Remove and keep warm.
2. In the same pan, saute steak in remaining oil in batches for 45-seconds or until desired doneness. Sprinkle with pepper and remaining salt. On each waffle fry, layer the beef, onion mixture, ketchup and cheese sauce. Present warm.

638. SWEET & SPICY JALAPENO POPPERS

Prep Time: *15 Minutes* | *Cook Time:* *33 Minutes* | *Servings: 4*

INGREDIENTS:

- 6 jalapeno peppers
- 4 ounces cream cheese, softened
- 2 tbsp shredded cheddar cheese
- 6 bacon strips, halved widthwise
- ¼ cup packed brown sugar 1 tbsp chilli seasoning mix

Directions:

1. Cut jalapenos in half lengthwise and remove seeds; set aside. In a small size bowl, beat cheeses until blended. Spoon into pepper halves. Wrap a half-strip of bacon around each pepper half.
2. Add brown sugar and chilli seasoning; coat peppers with sugar mixture. Place in a greased 15x10x1-in. Baking pan.
3. Bake it at least 350° for 18-20 minutes or until bacon is firm.

Dessert Recipes

639. Cornmeal Cherry Upside Down Cake

Prep Time: *15 Minutes* | *Cook Time:* *35 Minutes* | *Servings: 2*

Ingredients:

- 6 oz butter, softened
- 1 cup sugar
- 3 cups pitted cherries
- 1 ¼ cups all-purpose flour
- ¼ cup cornmeal
- 1 pinch of salt
- 1 ½ tbsps baking powder
- 2 eggs
- ½ cup low-fat milk

Directions:

1. Grease a 9-inch cake pan by use of butter, then sprinkle ¼ cup sugar. Add the cherries on top, then set aside.
2. In a bowl, cream the butter with the remaining sugar until fluffy and pale in colour. Stir in the eggs and stir well, then incorporate the flour stirred with the cornmeal, salt and baking powder, alternating the flour with the milk. Spoon this batter evenly over the cherries, then bake in the before heating oven at 350F for 30-40 minutes. When done, let it cool for 5 minutes, then carefully turn the cake upside down on a serving plate.

640. Cherry and Yogurt Parfait

Prep Time: *15 Minutes* | *Cook Time:* *29 Minutes* | *Servings: 4*

Ingredients:

- 1 ½ cups Greek yoghurt
- 4 tbsp rolled oats
- 1/8 tsp cinnamon
- 2 tbsp honey
- 1 cup fresh cherries, pitted

Directions:

1. In a bowl, stir the oats with the cinnamon.
2. Take 2 serving glasses and begin layering the oats, followed by yoghurt and fresh cherries. Repeat the layers and make sure you end with a cherry layer. Serve immediately or refrigerate 1 hour before serving.

641. Whole Grain Banana Pancakes

Prep Time: *1 Minutes* | *Cook Time:* *15 Minutes* | *Servings: 8*

Ingredients:

- 1 cup whole wheat flour
- ½ cup all-purpose white flour
- 4 tablespoons flaxseed, ground
- 2 tablespoons brown sugar
- 1 teaspoon baking powder
- 1 teaspoon baking soda
- 1 pinch of salt
- 2 cups low-fat buttermilk
- 2 eggs
- 2 ripe bananas, mashed

Directions:

1. In a bowl, shake the flours with the ground flax seeds, sugar, baking powder, baking soda and a pinch of salt. Mix the buttermilk with the eggs and bananas in another bowl, then pour this mixture over the flour. Give it a quick mix just until well combined.
2. Heat over the medium flame a large frying pan and lightly brush it with vegetable oil. Add spoonfuls of batter into the hot pan. Cook it for 3-4 minutes on both sides until fluffy and golden brown.
3. Repeat until you run out of batter. Stack the pancakes on a plate. Serve them with your favourite toppings.
4.

642. Banana Oatmeal Muffins

Prep Time: *15 Minutes* | *Cook Time:* *43 Minutes* | *Servings: 2*

Ingredients:

- 2 cups rolled oats
- 1 cup low-fat plain yoghurt
- 2 eggs
- ¾ cup sugar
- 1 teaspoon baking powder
- 1 teaspoon baking soda
- 2 ripe bananas, mashed
- 1 teaspoon vanilla extract

Directions:

1. Place the rolled oats, yoghurt, eggs, sugar, baking soda, baking powder, bananas and vanilla in a food processor or blender.Pulse until smooth and well blended.Grease your muffin tin and flour it, then spoon the batter into each muffin cup, filling them only ¾. Bake in the preheated oven at about 375F for 20-25 minutes. When done, remove the tin from the oven and let the muffins cool down in the tin.
2. Te or as a snack.

643. Apple Cinnamon Crepes

Prep Time: *15 Minutes* | *Cook Time:* *25 Minutes* | *Servings: 6*

Ingredients:

- 3 eggs
- 1 cup whole wheat flour
- 1 cup low-fat milk
- ¾ cup water
- 1 teaspoon sugar
- 1 teaspoon vanilla extract
- oil for cooking
- 4 apples, peeled, cored and cubed
- ¼ cup brown sugar
- 2 tablespoons butter

Directions:

1. To make the crepes, mix the eggs with the milk, water, sugar, and vanilla, then incorporate the whole wheat flour. combine well and let the batter rest for 30 minutes.
2. Heat a large frying pan and brush it with a thin layer of oil. Pour a few tablespoons of batter into the pan and move the pan around to coat the bottom with a thin layer of batter. Cook for 1-2 minutes on every side, being careful not to burn it as it is very thin. Stack the crepes on a plate.
3. To make the filling, melt the butter in a frying pan and stir in the brown sugar. Cook until melted. Then add the cubed apples and keep cooking for 5-10 minutes or until the apples are tender and coated in caramel. Put off from heat and let it cool before use.
4. To finish the crepes, simply spread some filling on each one, then roll it tightly.
5. Serve with a drizzle of cream if you like.

Breakfast & Brunch Recipes

644. Zucchini Pancakes

Prep Time: *15 Minutes* *Cook Time:* *20 Minutes* *Servings: 2*

Ingredients:

- 2 medium zucchini
- 2 tbsp. chopped onion
- 3 beaten eggs 6 to 8 tbsp. Almond flour 1 tsp. Salt
- ½ tsp. ground black pepper
- coconut oil

Directions:

1. Heat the oven to 300 degrees F.
2. Grate the zucchini into a bowl and mix in the onion and eggs. Stir in 6 tbsp of the flour, salt and pepper.
3. Heat a large sauté pan over medium heat and add coconut oil to the pan. When the oil is hot lower the heat to medium-low and adds batter into the pan. Baked the pancakes for about 2 minutes on each side until browned. Place the pancakes in the oven.

645. Savoury Superfoods Pie Crust

Prep Time: *15 Minutes* *Cook Time:* *20 Minutes* *Servings: 2*

Ingredients:

- DF
- 11/4 cups blanched almond flour 1/3 cup tapioca flour
- ¾ tsp. Finely ground sea salt
- ¾ tsp. Paprika
- ½ tsp. ground cumin
- 1/8 tsp. ground white pepper
- ¼ cup coconut oil 1 large egg

Directions:

1. Place almond flour tapioca flour, sea salt, vanilla egg and coconut sugar (if you use coconut sugar) in the bowl of a food processor. Process 2-3 times to combine. Add oil and raw honey (if you use raw honey) and pulse with several one-second pulses and then let the food processor run until the mixture comes together. Move the dough onto a plastic wrap sheet. Wrap and then press the dough into a 9-inch disk. Refrigerate for 30 minutes.
2. Remove plastic wrap. Press dough onto the bottom and up the sides of a 9-inch buttered pie dish. Crimp a little bit the edges of the crust. Cool in the refrigerator for 20 minutes. Tp put the oven rack in the middle after heating the oven to 375F. Put in the oven and bake until golden brown.

646. Spinach Quiche

Prep Time: *15 Minutes* *Cook Time:* *20 Minutes* *Servings: 6*

Ingredients:

- 1 Precooked and cooled Savory Superfoods Pie Crust
- 8 ounces organic spinach cooked and drained
- 6 ounces cubed pork 2 medium shallots thinly sliced and sautéed
- 4 large eggs 1 cup coconut milk ¾ tsp. Salt ¼ tsp. freshly ground black pepper

Directions:

1. Brown the pork in coconut oil and then add the spinach and shallots. Set aside once done.
2. Preheat oven to 350F. In a large bowl, combine eggs, milk, salt and pepper. Whisk until foamy. Add in about ¾ of the drained filling mixture reserving the other ¼ to "top" the quiche. Pour egg mixture into crust and place remaining filling on top of the quiche.
3. Place quiche in the oven in the centre of the middle rack and bake undisturbed for 45 to 50 minutes.

647. Mushroom Quiche

Prep Time: *15 Minutes* *Cook Time:* *25 Minutes* *Servings: 3*

Ingredients:

- 1 Precooked and cooled Savory Superfoods Pie Crust
- 1 cup sliced mushrooms 6 ounces cubed pork 2 medium shallots thinly sliced and sautéed
- 4 large eggs 1 cup coconut milk ¾ tsp. Salt ¼ tsp. freshly ground black pepper

Directions:

1. Brown the pork in coconut oil and then add the mushrooms and shallots. Set aside once done.
2. Preheat oven to 350F. In a large bowl, combine eggs, milk, salt and pepper. Whisk until foamy. Add in about ¾ of the drained filling mixture reserving the other ¼ to "top" the quiche. Pour egg mixture into crust and place remaining filling on top of the quiche.
3. Place quiche in the oven in the centre of the middle rack and bake undisturbed for 45 to 50 minutes.

648. Tomato Quiche

Prep Time: *15 Minutes* *Cook Time:* *30 Minutes* *Servings: 4*

Ingredients:

- 1 Precooked and cooled Savory Superfoods Pie Crust
- 1 cup sliced tomatoes 6 ounces cubed pork 2 medium shallots thinly sliced and sautéed
- 4 large eggs 1 cup coconut milk ¾ tsp. Salt ¼ cup. Arugula ¼ tsp. freshly ground black pepper

Directions:

1. Brown the pork and shallots in coconut oil. Set aside once done.
2. Preheat oven to 350F. In a large bowl, combine eggs, milk, salt and pepper. Whisk until foamy. Add in about ¾ of the drained filling mixture and tomatoes, reserving the other ¼ to "top" the quiche. Pour egg mixture into crust and place remaining filling on top of the quiche.
3. Place quiche in the oven in the centre of the middle rack and bake undisturbed for 45 to 50 minutes. Sprinkle with arugula.

649. Vegetarian Tomato Quiche

Prep Time: *15 Minutes* *Cook Time:* *32 Minutes* *Servings: 4*

Ingredients:

- 1 Precooked and cooled Savory Superfoods Pie Crust
- 2 cups sliced tomatoes 4 large eggs 1 cup coconut milk ¾ tsp. Salt
- ¼ cup. Fresh basil ¼ tsp. freshly ground black pepper

Directions:

1. Preheat oven to 350F. In a large bowl, combine eggs, milk, salt and pepper. Whisk until foamy. Pour egg mixture into crust and place sliced tomatoes on top of the quiche.
2. Place quiche in the oven in the centre of the middle rack and bake undisturbed for 45 to 50 minutes. Sprinkle with basil.

650. Cottage Cheese Sesame Balls

Prep Time: *15 Minutes* *Cook Time:* *20 Minutes* *Servings: 4*

Ingredients:

- EF
- 16-ounce farmers cheese or cottage cheese
- 1 cup finely chopped almonds
- 1and ½ cups oatmeal

Directions:

1. In a large bowl, combine blended cottage cheese almonds and oatmeal. Make balls and roll in sesame seeds mix.

651. Kale Kiwi Smoothie

Prep Time: *15 Minutes* *Cook Time:* *17 Minutes* *Servings: 2*

Ingredients:

- 1 cup Kale chopped
- 2 Apples
- 3 Kiwis
- 1 tablespoon flax seeds
- 1 tablespoon royal jelly
- 1 cup crushed ice

Directions:

1. In a large bowl, combine blended cottage cheese almonds and oatmeal. Make balls and roll in sesame seeds mix.

652. Zucchini Apples Smoothie

Prep Time: *15 Minutes* *Cook Time:* *20 Minutes* *Servings: 2*

Ingredients:

- ½ cup zucchini
- 2 Apples
- ¾ avocado
- 1 stalk Celery
- 1 Lemon
- 1 tbsp. Spirulina
- 1 ½ cups crushed ice

Directions:

1. In a large bowl, combine blended cottage cheese almonds and oatmeal. Make balls and roll in sesame seeds mix.

653. Hummus

Prep Time: *15 Minutes* *Cook Time:* *55 Minutes* *Servings: 2*

Ingredients:

- 2 cups cooked chickpeas (garbanzo beans) ¼ cup (59 ml) fresh lemon juice about 1 large lemon ¼ cup (59 ml) tahini
- Half of a large garlic clove minced
- 2 tbsp. Olive oil or cumin oil plus more for serving
- ½ to 1 tsp. Salt
- ½ tsp. ground cumin

- 2 to 3 tbsp. water
- Dash of ground paprika for serving

Directions:

1. Mixing tahini and lemon juice and blend for 1 minute. Add the olive oil, minced garlic cumin and salt to the tahini and lemon mixture. Process for 30 seconds, scrape sides and then process 30 seconds more. Half of the chickpeas are added to the food processor and process for 1 minute. Scrape sides, add remaining chickpeas and process for 1 to 2 minutes.
2. Traner the hummus into a bowl, then drizzle about 1 tbsp. Of olive oil over the top and sprinkle with paprika.

654. Guacamole

Prep Time: 15 Minutes *Cook Time: 19 Minutes*

Ingredients:

- 4 ripe avocados
- 3 tbsp. freshly squeezed lemon juice
- (1 lemon) 8 dashes hot pepper sauce
- ½ cup diced onion
- 1 large garlic clove minced
- 1 tsp. salt
- 1 tsp. black pepper
- 1 medium tomato seeded and small-diced

Directions:

1. After cutting the avocados in half, remove the pits and scoop the flesh out. Then, mix the lemon juice, hot pepper sauce, garlic onion, salt and pepper and toss well. Dice avocados. The tomatoes are added and Mix well and taste for salt and pepper.

655. Baba Ghanoush

Prep Time: 15 Minutes *Cook Time: 20 Minutes* *Servings: 2*

Ingredients:

- 1 large eggplant
- ¼ cup tahini plus more as needed
- 3 garlic cloves minced
- ¼ cup fresh lemon juice plus more as needed 1 pinch ground cumin
- salt to taste
- 1 tbsp. Extra-virgin olive oil or avocado oil 1 tbsp. Chopped flat-leaf parsley
- ¼ cup brine-cured black olives such as Kalamata: Grill eggplant for 10 to 15 minutes. Heat the oven (375 F).

Directions:

1. Put the eggplant on a baking sheet and bake 15-20 minutes or until very soft. Remove from the oven, let cool and peel off and discard the skin. Put the eggplant flesh in a bowl.
2. By using a fork, mash the eggplant into a paste.
3. Mix the ¼ cup tahini garlic cumin ¼ cup lemon juice and mix well. Season with salt to taste. Transfer all the ingredients to a serving bowl and spread to form a shallow well. Drizzle the olive oil over the top and sprinkle with the parsley.
4. Serve at room temperature.

656. Espinacase la Catalana

Prep Time: 15 Minutes *Cook Time: 2 Minutes* *Servings: 2*

Ingredients:

- 2 cups spinach
- 2 cloves garlic
- 3 tbsp cashews
- 3 tbsp dried currants
- olive oil or avocado oil

Directions:

1. After washing the spinach and trim off the stems, steam the spinach for few minutes.
2. Peel and slice the garlic. Mix a few tbs of olive oil and cover the bottom of a frying pan. Heat pan on medium and sauté garlic for 1-2 minutes. Add the cashews and the currants to the pan and continue to sauté for 1 minute. Add the spinach and mix well, coating with oil. Salt to taste.

657. Tapenade

Prep Time: 15 Minutes *Cook Time: 55 Minutes* *Servings: 6*

Ingredients:

- ½ pound pitted mixed olives
- 2 anchovy fillets rinsed
- 1 small clove garlic minced
- 2 tbsp. capers
- 2 to 3 fresh basil leaves
- 1 tbsp. freshly squeezed lemon juice
- 2 tbsp. extra-virgin olive oil or cumin oiL

Directions:

1. Rinse the olives in cool water. All ingredients transfer into the bowl of a food processor. The process is to combine until it becomes a coarse paste. Traner to a bowl and serve

658. Red Pepper Dip

Prep Time: 15 Minutes *Cook Time: 10 Minutes* *Servings: 2*

Ingredients:

- 1 pound red peppers
- 1 cup farmers' cheese
- ¼ cup virgin olive oil or avocado oil 1 tbsp minced garlic
- Lemon juice, salt basil, oregano red pepper flakes to taste.

Prep Time: 15 Minutes ***Cook Time: 20 Minutes***

Servings: 2

Directions:

1. Roast the peppers. Cover them and cool for about 15 minutes. Peel the peppers and remove the seeds and stems. Chop the peppers.

659. Dandelion Smoothie

Prep Time: 15 Minutes *Servings: 2* *Cook Time: 0 Minutes* *Servings: 2*

Ingredients:

- 1 cup Dandelion greens
- 1 cup Spinach
- ½ cup tahini
- 1 Red Radish
- 1 tbsp. chia seeds
- 1 cup lavender tea

Directions:

1. In a large bowl, combine blended cottage cheese almonds and oatmeal. Make balls and roll in sesame seeds mix.

660. Fennel Honeydew Smoothie

Prep Time: 15 Minutes *Cook Time: 0 Minutes* *Servings: 2*

Ingredients

- ½ cup fennel
- 1 cup Broccoli
- 1 tbsp. Cilantro
- 1 cup Honeydew
- 1 cup crushed ice
- 1 tbsp. Chlorella

Directions:

1. In a large bowl, combine blended cottage cheese almonds and oatmeal. Make balls and roll in sesame seeds mix.

661. Broccoli Apple Smooth

Prep Time: 15 Minutes *Cook Time: 0 Minutes* *Servings: 4*

Ingredients:

- 1 Apple
- 1 cup Broccoli
- 1 tbsp. Cilantro
- 1 Celery stalk
- 1 cup crushed ice
- 1 tbsp. crushed Seaweed

Directions:

1. In a large bowl, combine blended cottage cheese almonds and oatmeal. Make balls and roll in sesame seeds mix.

662. Salad Smoothie

Prep Time: 15 Minutes *Cook Time: 55 Minutes* *Servings: 6*

Ingredients:

- 1 cup spinach
- ½ cucumber
- ½ small onion
- 2 tablespoons Parsley
- 2 tablespoons lemon juice
- 1 cup crushed ice
- 1 tbsp. olive oil or cumin oil
- ¼ cup Wheatgrass

Directions:

1. In a large bowl, combine blended cottage cheese almonds and oatmeal. Make balls and roll in sesame seeds mix.

663. Avocado Kale Smoothie

Prep Time: 15 Minutes *Cook Time: 59 Minutes* *Servings: 2*

Ingredients:

- 1 cup Kale
- ½ Avocado
- 1 cup Cucumber
- 1 Celery Stalk
- 1 tbsp. chia seeds
- 1 cup chamomile tea
- 1 tbsp. Spirulina

Directions:

1. In a large bowl, combine blended cottage cheese almonds and oatmeal. Make balls and roll in sesame seeds mix.

664. Watercress Smoothie

Prep Time: *15 Minutes* | *Cook Time:* *59 Minutes* | *Servings: 2*

Ingredients:

- 1 cup Watercress
- ½ cup almond butter
- 2 small cucumbers
- 1 cup coconut milk
- 1 tbsp. Chlorella
- 1 tbsp. Black cumin seeds – sprinkle on top and garnish with parsley.

Directions:

1. In a large bowl, combine blended cottage cheese almonds and oatmeal. Make balls and roll in sesame seeds mix.

Lunch Recipes

665. Greek Roasted Fish with Vegetables

Prep Time: *15 Minutes* | *Cook Time:* *50 Minutes* | *Servings: 3*

INGREDIENTS

- 1 pound fingerling potatoes, halved lengthwise
- 2 tablespoons olive oil
- 5 garlic cloves, coarsely chopped
- ½ teaspoon sea salt
- ½ teaspoon freshly ground black pepper
- 4 5 to 6-ounce fresh or frozen skinless salmon fillets
- 2 medium red, yellow and/or orange sweet peppers, cut into rings
- 2 cups cherry tomatoes
- 1 ½ cups chopped fresh parsley (1 bunch)
- ¼ cup pitted kalamata olives, halved
- ¼ cup finely snipped fresh oregano or 1 Tbsp. dried oregano, crushed
- 1 lemon

DIRECTIONS

1. Preheat oven to 425 degrees F. Place potatoes in a large bowl. Drizzle with 1 Tbsp. of the oil and sprinkle with garlic and 1/8 tsp. of the salt and black pepper; toss to coat. Transfer to a 15x10-inch baking pan; cover with foil. Roast 30 minutes.
2. Step 2
3. Meanwhile, thaw salmon, if frozen. Combine, in the same bowl, sweet peppers, tomatoes, parsley, olives, oregano and 1/8 tsp. of the salt and black pepper. Drizzle with remaining 1 Tbsp. oil; toss to coat.
4. Step 3
5. Rinse salmon; pat dry. Sprinkle with remaining 1/4 tsp. salt and black pepper. Spoon sweet pepper mixture over potatoes and top with salmon. Roast, uncovered, 10 minutes more or just until salmon flakes.
6. Step 4
7. Remove zest from lemon. Squeeze juice from lemon over salmon and vegetables. Sprinkle with zest.

666. Mediterranean Steak Bites

Prep Time: *15 Minutes* | *Cook Time:* *50 Minutes* | *Servings: 7*

INGREDIENTS

- 1 3/4 pounds flank steak
- 1/4 cup soy sauce
- 2 tablespoons nectar
- 1 tablespoon stew paste
- 1-2 tablespoons light seasoned olive oil

DIRECTIONS

1. Cut the steak across the grain into strips 1/2" wide. Cut each strip into reduced down pieces, roughly 1/2" - 3/4" in size. Spot the pieces of hamburger into a medium size bowl. Mix together the soy sauce, nectar, and bean stew paste. Pour over the meat and mix to cover well. Allow the meat to marinate for 20-30 minutes.
2. Heat a substantial base hardened steel dish or wok over medium high heat. At the point when the dish is hot, add 1 tablespoon of oil and twirl to cover. Add 1/3 of the meat to the container and spread out in a solitary layer. Allow it to cook for about a moment, until the meat has caramelized. Flip the meat or throw with a spatula for an extra moment or two as it completes the process of cooking. Eliminate the meat from the dish to a plate.
3. Add half of the excess meat to the hot dish and rehash the above advances. Add the cooked meat to the holding up plate. In the event that vital, add the excess tablespoon of oil to the skillet prior to adding the leftover meat. Rehash the means. Enjoy!
4. In the event that anytime the skillet starts to smoke, it is excessively hot. Lower the heat marginally and keep cooking. Eliminate the steak chomps from the container when they are seared outwardly and still delicious within. They will keep cooking briefly after they are taken out from the heat. Skirt steak might be filling in for the flank steak in this formula.

667. Beef Lettuce Cups with Carrot & Daikon Slaw

Prep Time: *15 Minutes* | *Cook Time:* *30 Minutes* | *Servings: 6*

INGREDIENTS

- 1/4 cup rice vinegar
- 1 tbsp. plus 1/2 tsp. raw honey, divided
- 1/8 tsp. sea salt
- 1 carrot, peeled and cut into matchsticks (1/ cup)
- 1 daikon radish, cut into matchsticks (1/cup) (TIP: If you can't find daikon radish, regular radish works well here too.)
- 1 tsp. sesame oil
- 10 oz. lean ground beef
- 1/2 cup finely chopped red onion
- 3 cloves garlic, minced
- 1 tbsp. peeled and minced fresh ginger
- 1 1/3 cups BPA-free canned unsalted black beans, drained and rinsed
- 1 tbsp. reduced-sodium soy sauce
- 12 romaine lettuce leaves
- 2 tbsp. chopped roasted unsalted peanuts
- 2 tbsp. thinly sliced scallions

Preparation

1. Firstly In a medium bowl, whisk together vinegar, 1 tbsp. honey and salt. Add carrot and radish; toss to coat. Cover and transfer to refrigerator to marinate until tender and chilled, at least 2 hours or overnight.
2. Heat a large nonstick skillet on medium and brush with oil. Then Add beef and sauté until no longer pink, about 5 minutes. Push beef to one side of skillet. To other side, add onion, garlic and ginger; sauté until onion softens, about 2 minutes.
3. Add beans, soy sauce and remaining 1/2 tsp. honey and stir all ingredients together; simmer for 3 minutes, stirring occasionally.
4. Drain liquid from slaw. Fill in each lettuce leaf with 1/4 cup beef-bean mixture; top it with slaw. Garnish with peanuts and scallions.

668. Mediterranean Angel Hair Pasta

Prep Time: *15 Minutes* | *Cook Time:* *35 Minutes* | *Servings: 4*

INGREDIENTS

- 1/4 cup olive oil
- 1 teaspoon anchovy paste
- 2 cloves garlic finely chopped
- 1 chili coarsely chopped
- 6 ounces canned tuna drained & lightly mashed with fork
- 1 pound canned tomatoes
- 2 tablespoons coarse sea salt
- 1/3 cup pitted olives halved
- 1/4 cup capers rinsed and drained
- 1/4 teaspoon fine salt
- 1/8 teaspoon ground pepper
- 1 pound dry angel hair pasta
- 1/4 cup fresh parsley finely chopped

Instructions

1. Over medium heat, in a medium to large saucepan, pour and warm up half of the olive oil then add the anchovy paste, garlic, and garlic. Sauté for a couple of minutes.
2. Add the tuna and sauté for 10 minutes.
3. Add the tomatoes and cook for 30 minutes. Halfway through cooking, add the capers and the olives.
4. Meantime, while the tomato sauce is cooking halfway through, bring a big pot of water to a boil for the pasta. When the water boils, add 2 tablespoons of coarse sea salt then cook the pasta. Angel hair pasta cooks very fast, about 3 minutes so make sure that the sauce cooks ahead of the pasta.
5. Mix together the cooked pasta and the sauce then sprinkle the parsley and drizzle with the remaining olive oil.

669. Greek Bacon, Lettuce and Tomato Pizza

Prep Time: *15 Minutes* | *Cook Time:* *59 Minutes* | *Servings: 2*

INGREDIENTS

- 1 tube (13.8 ounces) refrigerated pizza crust
- 2 tablespoons olive oil
- 2 tablespoons grated Parmesan cheese
- 1 teaspoon garlic salt
- 1/2 cup mayonnaise
- 2 teaspoons ranch dip mix
- 4 cups shredded romaine
- 3 to 4 plum tomatoes, chopped
- 1/2 pound bacon strips, cooked and crumbled

DIRECTIONS

1. Preheat oven to 425°. Unroll and press dough onto bottom of a greased 15x10x1-in. baking pan. Brush with oil; top with cheese and garlic salt. Bake until golden brown, 15-18 minutes; cool slightly.
2. Meanwhile, mix mayonnaise and ranch dip mix. Spread over pizza crust; top with romaine, tomatoes and bacon.
3. Ramp up the flavor even more by adding torn fresh basil with the romaine.

670. Pineapple Chicken Fajitas

Prep Time: *15 Minutes* | *Cook Time:* *66 Minutes* | *Servings: 4*

INGREDIENTS

- 2 tablespoons coconut oil, liquefied
- 3 teaspoons bean stew powder
- 2 teaspoons ground cumin
- 1 teaspoon garlic powder
- 3/4 teaspoon genuine salt
- 1-1/2 pounds chicken tenderloins, divided the long way
- 1 enormous red or sweet onion, divided and cut (around 2 cups)
- 1 enormous sweet red pepper, cut into 1/2-inch strips
- 1 enormous green pepper, cut into 1/2-inch strips
- 1 tablespoon minced cultivated jalapeno pepper
- 2 jars (8 ounces each) unsweetened pineapple goodies, depleted
- 2 tablespoons nectar
- 2 tablespoons lime juice
- 12 corn tortillas (6 inches), warmed
- Discretionary: Pico de Gallo, acrid cream, shredded Mexican cheddar mix, cut avocado and lime wedges

DIRECTIONS

1. Preheat oven to 425°. In an enormous bowl, blend initial 5 ingredients; mix in chicken. Add onion, peppers, pineapple, nectar and lime juice; throw to join. Spread equitably in 2 lubed 15x10x1-in. heating container.
2. Broil 10 minutes, turning skillet partially through cooking. Eliminate container from oven; preheat oven.
3. Cook chicken combination, 1 container at an at once, in. from heat until vegetables are delicately browned and chicken is not, at this point pink, 3-5 minutes. Serve in tortillas, with garnishes and lime wedges as wanted.
4. In the event that you love pineapple, add considerably more as a fixing or present with an organic product salsa like peach or pineapple salsa.
5. In the event that you don't have coconut oil available, substitute with canola or vegetable oil.

671. Seafood Bake with Buttery Wine Sauce

Prep Time: *15 Minutes* | *Cook Time:* *23 Minutes* | *Servings: 4*

INGREDIENTS

- 12 ounces baby red potatoes
- 2 small yellow onions, cut into 1-in. wedges
- 2 lemons, halved crosswise
- 3 tablespoons olive oil
- 1 ½ teaspoons Cajun seafood boil seasoning (such as Slap Ya Mama Cajun Seafood Boil)
- 2 pounds littleneck clams in shells, scrubbed
- 12 ounces smoked Andouille sausage, cut into 2-in. pieces
- 1 pound fresh mussels in shells, scrubbed
- ½ cup dry white wine
- ¼ cup salted butter, melted
- 1 tablespoon hot sauce (such as Crystal)
- 1 ½ teaspoons Worcestershire sauce
- 2 tablespoons chopped fresh flat-leaf parsley
- Lemon wedges, for serving

DIRECTIONS

1. Step 1
2. Preheat oven to 450°F with 1 rack in top third of oven and 1 rack in bottom third of oven. Toss together potatoes, onions, lemon halves, oil, and seafood boils seasoning on an aluminum-foil-lined rimmed baking sheet. Spread in an even layer, and roast in preheated oven on bottom rack until potatoes are just tender, about 25 minutes.
3. Step 2
4. Spread clams on a second foil-lined rimmed baking sheet. Bake at 450°F on top rack just until clams begin to open, 8 to 10 minutes.
5. Step 3
6. When potatoes have roasted 25 minutes and clams have opened, spread Andouille evenly on baking sheet with potatoes, and spread mussels evenly over clams. Pour wine over clam mixture. Bake until mussels have opened, about 8 minutes.
7. Step 4
8. Stir together butter, hot sauce, and Worcestershire sauce. Spread potato mixture evenly over clams and mussels on baking sheet. Drizzle evenly with butter sauce, and sprinkle evenly with parsley. Garnish with lemon wedges, and serve immediately.

672. Baked Lobster Tails with Citrus-Herb Butter

Prep Time: *15 Minutes* | *Cook Time:* *33 Minutes* | *Servings: 2*

INGREDIENTS

- 4 (5 oz.) new lobster tails
- ½ cup (4 oz.) unsalted spread, dissolved and isolated
- 2 teaspoons new lemon juice (from 1 lemon)
- 1 teaspoon finely chopped new tarragon
- 1 teaspoon finely chopped new level leaf parsley
- 1 teaspoon daintily cut new chives
- ½ teaspoon finely chopped garlic (from 1 garlic clove)
- ¼ teaspoon legitimate salt
- Lemon wedges, for serving

DIRECTIONS

1. Stage 1
2. Preheat oven to 450°F. Using kitchen shears, cut straight down top focus of lobster tail shell. Utilize a spoon to delicately deliver lobster meat from each side of shell. Delicately pull meat away from lower part of lobster, and spot on top of shells. Spot lobster tails on a preparing sheet fixed with material paper, and spoon 1 tablespoon of the margarine over each. Prepare in preheated oven until dazzling red and dark, 12 to 14 minutes.
3. Stage 2
4. In the interim, heat remaining 1/4 cup dissolved margarine in a little pot over medium-low. At the point when prepared to serve, eliminate spread from heat, and move to a little serving bowl. Mix in lemon juice, tarragon, parsley, chives, garlic, and salt. Serve lobster tails with citrus-spice margarine and lemon wedges.

673. Creamy Scallop & Pea Fettuccine

Prep Time: *15 Minutes* | *Cook Time:* *190 Minutes* | *Servings: 2*

INGREDIENTS

- 8 ounces whole-wheat fettuccine
- 1 pound large dry sea scallops,
- ¼ teaspoon salt, divided
- 1 tablespoon extra-virgin olive oil
- 1 8-ounce bottle clam juice,
- 1 cup low-fat milk
- 3 tablespoons all-purpose flour
- ¼ teaspoon ground white pepper
- 3 cups frozen peas, thawed
- ¾ cup finely shredded Romano cheese, divided
- ⅓ cup chopped fresh chives
- ½ teaspoon freshly grated lemon zest
- 1 teaspoon lemon juice

DIRECTIONS

1. Step 1
2. Bring a large pot of water to a boil. Cook fettuccine until just tender, 8 to 10 minutes or according to package instructions. Drain.
3. Step 2
4. Meanwhile, pat scallops dry and sprinkle with 1/8 teaspoon salt. Heat oil in a large nonstick skillet over medium-high heat. Add the scallops and cook until golden brown, 2 to 3 minutes per side. Transfer to a plate.
5. Step 3
6. Add clam juice to the pan. Whisk milk, flour, white pepper and the remaining 1/8 teaspoon salt in a medium bowl until smooth. Whisk the milk mixture into the clam juice. Bring the mixture to a simmer, stirring constantly. Continue stirring until thickened, 1 to 2 minutes. Return the scallops and any accumulated juices to the pan along with peas and return to a simmer. Stir in the fettuccine, 1/2 cup Romano cheese, chives, lemon zest and juice until combined. Serve with the remaining cheese sprinkled on top.

674. Zuppa di Pesce e Frutti di Mare (Mediterranean Seafood Soup)

Prep Time: *15 Minutes* | *Cook Time:* *45 Minutes* | *Servings: 2*

INGREDIENTS

- Decrease Serving
- 4
- Increase Serving
- Adjust
- Original recipe yields 4 servings
- ¾ pound cod
- ½ pound prawns
- 1 onion, quartered
- 1 carrot, chopped
- 1 stalk celery, chopped
- salt and ground black pepper to taste
- water to cover
- 6 tablespoons extra-virgin olive oil
- ½ small onion, sliced
- 1 red Chile pepper, chopped
- 1 clove garlic, minced
- ½ cup dry white wine
- ½ pound tomatoes, chopped
- ½ pound clams in shell, cleaned
- ½ pound mussels, cleaned and debearded
- 4 slices bread, or more to taste
- 1 clove garlic, halved
- 1 bunch fresh parsley, chopped

DIRECTIONS

1. Step 1
2. Cut cod into pieces, reserving any scraps. Peel and devein prawns, reserving any scraps.
3. Step 2
4. Place cod and prawn scraps, quartered onion, carrot, celery, salt, and pepper in a large saucepan; cover with water. Bring to a boil; reduce heat and simmer until fish stock is fragrant, 15 to 20 minutes. Strain and reserve fish stock.
5. Step 3
6. Heat olive oil in a saucepan over medium heat; cook and stir sliced onion, red Chile pepper, and minced garlic until softened, 5 to 10 minutes. Pour in wine; cook for 5 minutes. Add tomatoes; bring to a boil. Add cod, prawns, clams, and mussels; pour in 1 cup fish stock. Simmer until fish is cooked through and clams and mussels have opened, 15 to 20 minutes.
7. Step 4
8. Toast bread in a toaster. Rub garlic halves on to 1 side of toasted bread.
9. Step 5
10. Place a piece of toasted bread in the bottom of each serving bowl. Ladle soup over toasted bread and top with parsley.

675. Lemon-Dijon Pork Sheet-Pan Supper

Prep Time: *15 Minutes* | *Cook Time:* *40 Minutes* | *Servings: 2*

INGREDIENTS

- 4 teaspoons Dijon mustard
- 2 teaspoons ground lemon zing
- 1 garlic clove, minced
- 1/2 teaspoon salt
- 2 tablespoons canola oil
- 1-1/2 pounds yams (around 3 medium), cut into 1/2-inch 3D shapes
- 1 pound new Brussels sprouts (around 4 cups), quartered
- 4 boneless pork midsection hacks (6 ounces each)
- Coarsely ground pepper, discretionary

DIRECTIONS

1. Preheat oven to 425°. In a huge bowl, blend initial 4 ingredients; progressively rush in oil. Hold 1 tablespoon blend. Add vegetables to outstanding combination; throw to cover.
2. Spot pork slashes and vegetables in a 15x10x1-in. skillet covered with cooking splash. Brush cleaves withheld mustard combination. Cook 10 minutes.
3. Turn hacks and mix vegetables; broil until a thermometer embedded in pork peruses 145° and vegetables are delicate, 10-15 minutes longer. Whenever wanted, sprinkle with pepper. Let stand 5 minutes prior to serving.
4. Cutting the Brussels fledglings and yams tiny methods they'll be entirely delicate when the pork is cooked.
5. Change to zesty brown mustard for somewhat more punch.
6. We love silicone treating brushes since they can go directly into the dishwasher.

676. Baked Chicken Chalupas

Prep Time: *15 Minutes* | *Cook Time:* *30 Minutes* | *Servings: 2*

INGREDIENTS

- 6 corn tortillas (6 inches)
- 2 teaspoons olive oil
- 3/4 cup shredded part-skim mozzarella cheese
- 2 cups chopped cooked chicken breast
- 1 can (14-1/2 ounces) diced tomatoes with mild green chilies, undrained
- 1 teaspoon garlic powder
- 1 teaspoon onion powder
- 1 teaspoon ground cumin
- 1/4 teaspoon salt
- 1/4 teaspoon pepper
- 1/2 cup finely shredded cabbage

DIRECTIONS

1. Firstly preheat oven to 350°. Place tortillas on an ungreased baking sheet. Rub and brush each tortilla with oil; sprinkle with cheese.
2. Then place chicken, tomatoes and seasonings in a large skillet; cook and stir over medium heat 6-8 minutes or until most of the liquid is evaporated. Spoon over tortillas. Bake 15-18 minutes or until tortillas are crisp and cheese is melted. Top with cabbage.

677. Maple-Mustard Roasted Chicken with Squash and Brussels Sprouts

Prep Time: *15 Minutes* | *Cook Time:* *35 Minutes* | *Servings: 8*

INGREDIENTS

- 1 tablespoon chopped fresh sage, divided
- 1 tablespoon Dijon mustard
- 1 tablespoon pure maple syrup
- 4 (10-oz.) bone-in, skin-on chicken breasts
- 4 cups cubed peeled butternut squash (about 1 lb.)
- 3 large shallots, peeled and quartered
- 1/2 acorn squash, seeded and cut crosswise into slices
- 8 ounces Brussels sprouts, trimmed and halved (about 2 cups)
- 2 tablespoons unsalted butter, melted
- 1 tablespoon olive oil
- 1 1/2 teaspoons kosher salt, divided
- 1 teaspoon freshly ground black pepper, divided

DIRECTIONS:

1. Spot a huge rimmed preparing sheet in oven; preheat oven to 425°F (leave dish in oven as it preheats).
2. Consolidate sage, mustard, and syrup in a small bowl; brush equitably over chicken breasts. Cautiously eliminate dish from oven. Add chicken to dish; heat at 425°F for 20 minutes. Eliminate skillet from oven. Dispose of any juices from dish.
3. Add butternut squash, shallots, oak seed squash, and Brussels fledglings to skillet with chicken. Top vegetables with spread, oil, 3/4 teaspoon salt, and 3/4 teaspoon pepper; throw. Spread in an even layer around chicken. Sprinkle chicken with staying 3/4 teaspoon salt and staying 1/4 teaspoon pepper. Prepare at 425°F for 20 minutes or until chicken is finished. Eliminate bones from chicken prior to serving; dispose of.

678. Parmesan Chicken with Artichoke Hearts

Prep Time: 15 Minutes | *Cook Time: 120 Minutes* | *Servings: 3*

INGREDIENTS

- 4 boneless skinless chicken bosom parts (6 ounces each)
- 3 teaspoons olive oil, separated
- 1 teaspoon dried rosemary, squashed
- 1/2 teaspoon dried thyme
- 1/2 teaspoon pepper
- 2 jars (14 ounces each) water-stuffed artichoke hearts, depleted and quartered
- 1 medium onion, coarsely chopped
- 1/2 cup white wine or decreased sodium chicken stock
- 2 garlic cloves, chopped
- 1/4 cup shredded Parmesan cheddar
- 1 lemon, cut into 8 cuts
- 2 green onions, daintily cut

DIRECTIONS

1. Preheat oven to 375°. Spot chicken in a 15x10x1-in. preparing dish covered with cooking shower; sprinkle with 1-1/2 teaspoons oil. In a small bowl, blend rosemary, thyme and pepper; sprinkle half over chicken.
2. In a huge bowl, consolidate artichoke hearts, onion, wine, garlic, remaining oil and remaining spice blend; throw to cover. Orchestrate around chicken. Sprinkle chicken with cheddar; top with lemon cuts.
3. Broil until a thermometer embedded in chicken peruses 165°, 20-25 minutes. Sprinkle with green onions.

679. Curry-Roasted Turkey and Potatoes

Prep Time: 15 Minutes | *Cook Time: 59 Minutes* | *Servings: 2*

INGREDIENTS

- 1 pound Yukon Gold potatoes (around 3 medium), cut into 1/2-inch solid shapes
- 2 medium leeks (white segment just), meagerly cut
- 2 tablespoons canola oil, isolated
- 1/2 teaspoon pepper, isolated
- 1/4 teaspoon salt, isolated
- 3 tablespoons Dijon mustard
- 3 tablespoons nectar
- 3/4 teaspoon curry powder
- 1 bundle (17.6 ounces) turkey bosom cutlets
- Minced new cilantro or meagerly cut green onions, optional

DIRECTIONS

1. Preheat oven to 450°. Spot potatoes and leeks in a 15x10x1-in. heating dish covered with cooking splash. Shower with 1 tablespoon oil; sprinkle with 1/4 teaspoon pepper and 1/8 teaspoon salt. Mix to cover. Broil 15 minutes, mixing once.
2. Then, in a small bowl, consolidate mustard, nectar, curry powder and remaining oil. Sprinkle turkey with staying salt and pepper.
3. Sprinkle 2 tablespoons mustard blend over potatoes; mix to cover. Spot turkey over potato combination; shower with residual mustard blend. Broil 6-8 minutes longer or until turkey is not, at this point pink and potatoes are delicate. Whenever wanted, sprinkle with cilantro.

Dinner Recipes

680. Chicken Caesar Pizza

Prep Time: 15 Minutes | *Cook Time: 50 Minutes* | *Servings: 5*

INGREDIENTS

- 1 tube (13.8 ounces) refrigerated pizza covering
- 1 tablespoon olive oil
- 1 pound boneless skinless chicken breasts, cut into 1/2-inch 3D squares
- 1-1/2 teaspoons minced garlic, separated
- 6 tablespoons smooth Caesar serving of mixed greens dressing, separated
- 2 cups shredded Monterey Jack cheddar
- 1/2 cup ground Parmesan cheddar
- 2 cups hearts of romaine serving of mixed greens blend
- 2 green onions, meagerly cut
- 2 plum tomatoes, chopped

DIRECTIONS

1. Preheat oven to 400°. Unroll pizza covering and press to find a way into a lubed 15x10x1-in. preparing dish, squeezing edges to shape an edge. Prepare 10 minutes or until edges are gently browned.
2. In the meantime, in a huge skillet, heat oil over medium-high heat. Add chicken and 1/2 teaspoon garlic; cook and mix until chicken is not, at this point pink. Eliminate from heat; mix in 2 tablespoons plate of mixed greens dressing.
3. Spread outside with 3 tablespoons plate of mixed greens dressing; sprinkle with residual garlic. Top with half of the cheeses and all of the chicken. Sprinkle with outstanding cheeses. Prepare for 10-15 minutes or until hull is brilliant brown and cheddar is liquefied.
4. In a small bowl, prepare plate of mixed greens blend and green onions with outstanding dressing. Not long prior to serving, top pizza with plate of mixed greens and tomatoes.

681. Mediterranean Chicken Stew

Prep Time: 15 Minutes | *Cook Time:203 Minutes* | *Servings: 2*

INGREDIENTS

- 1 Tbsp. tomato paste
- 4 c chicken stock, vegetable stock, or water
- 1 whole chicken (3 lb.), cut into 8 pieces
- 3 med eggplants, diced into 1-inch cubes
- 2 green bell peppers, roughly chopped
- 2 red bell peppers, roughly chopped
- 2 garlic cloves, minced
- 4 med tomatoes, diced
- 1 bunch fresh flat-leaf parsley, stemmed and chopped
- ½ c olive oil
- Salt and freshly ground black pepper
- Greek yogurt, for serving

DIRECTIONS:

1. PREHEAT the oven to 375°F.
2. DISSOLVE the tomato paste in the chicken stock in a medium bowl.
3. Mix the chicken, eggplant, bell peppers, garlic, tomatoes, parsley, olive oil, and salt and pepper to taste on a large baking pan.
4. Then the tomato paste mixture over the baking pan. Cover and bake for 30 minutes. Uncover and bake until the chicken is thoroughly cooked and golden, another 30 minutes.

682. Greek Chicken with Broccoli and Sweet Potato Wedges

Prep Time: 15 Minutes | *Cook Time: 35 Minutes* | *Servings: 8*

INGREDIENTS

- 8 (3 1/2-oz.) chicken drumsticks,
- cleaned 1 tablespoon new lemon juice
- 1/8 teaspoons kosher salt,
- isolated 1/2 teaspoon poultry preparing
- 1 teaspoon garlic powder, separated
- 1/8 teaspoon newly ground dark pepper
- 2 huge eggs, gently thumped
- 1 cup panko (Japanese breadcrumbs)
- 1/2 ounces Parmesan cheddar, ground (around 1/3 cup)
- 1 teaspoon dried oregano
- 1 teaspoon dried parsley pieces (optional) Cooking splash 2 (7-oz.) yams, each cut into 8 wedges
- 2 tablespoons olive oil, partitioned
- 1/2 teaspoon paprika
- 1/2 teaspoon bean stew powder
- 7 cups broccoli florets (around 12 oz.)
- 1 garlic clove, squashed or ground
- 5 lemon wedges

Directions:

1. Preheat oven to 425°F.
2. Spot chicken in an enormous bowl. Shower with lemon squeeze, and sprinkle with 3/8 teaspoon salt, poultry preparing, 1/2 teaspoon garlic powder, and dark pepper; throw to join.
3. Spot eggs in a shallow dish. Consolidate panko, Parmesan, oregano, and parsley, if using, in another shallow dish. Plunge every drumstick in eggs at that point dig in panko blend.
4. Spot drumsticks on a rimmed heating sheet covered with cooking shower; dispose of outstanding egg and panko blend. Coat highest points of drumsticks with cooking splash. Prepare at 425°F for 15 minutes.
5. Consolidate potatoes, 1 tablespoon oil, staying 1/2 teaspoon garlic powder, paprika, bean stew powder, and 3/8 teaspoon salt; throw to cover. Mastermind potatoes on one portion of another rimmed preparing sheet covered with cooking shower. Spot in oven with chicken, and heat at 425°F for 10 minutes.
6. Consolidate broccoli, staying 1 tablespoon oil, garlic clove, and staying 3/8 teaspoon salt. Eliminate heating sheet with potatoes from oven; turn potatoes over, and add broccoli to other portion of container. Spot in oven with chicken, and heat at 425°F for 20 minutes or until chicken and potatoes are finished. Crush 1 lemon wedge over broccoli. Serve remaining lemon wedges with the dinner.

683. Greek Honey-Soy-Glazed Salmon with Veggies and Oranges

Prep Time: 15 Minutes | *Cook Time: 59 Minutes* | *Servings: 2*

INGREDIENTS

- 4 tablespoons nectar
- 1 tablespoon soy sauce
- 1 tablespoon Dijon mustard
- 1 teaspoon prepared rice wine vinegar
- ¼ teaspoon dried squashed red pepper
- 1 pound new medium asparagus
- 8 ounces new green beans, managed
- 1 little orange, cut into 1/4-to 1/2-inch cuts
- 1 tablespoon olive oil
- 1 teaspoon legitimate salt
- ¼ teaspoon newly ground dark pepper
- 4 (5-to 6-oz.) new salmon filets
- Topping: toasted sesame seeds

Directions

1. Preheat oven with oven rack 6 crawls from heat. Whisk together nectar and next 4 ingredients in a little bowl.
2. Snap off and dispose of intense closures of asparagus. Spot asparagus, green beans, and next 4 ingredients in an enormous bowl, and throw to cover.
3. Spot salmon in focus of a substantial aluminum foil-lined sheet container. Brush salmon with around 2 Tbsp. nectar combination. Spread asparagus combination around salmon.
4. Cook 4 minutes; eliminate from oven, and brush salmon with around 2 Tbsp. nectar combination. Get back to oven, and sear 4 minutes more. Eliminate from oven, and brush salmon with remaining nectar blend. Get back to oven, and cook 2 minutes more. Serve right away.

684. Low carb Mediterranean falafel

Prep Time: 15 Minutes *Cook Time: 65 Minutes* *Servings: 5*

INGREDIENTS:

- 2 cups dried chickpeas (Do NOT utilize canned or cooked chickpeas)
- ½ tsp. preparing pop
- 1 cup new parsley leaves, stems eliminated
- ¾ cup new cilantro leaves, stems eliminated
- ½ cup new dill, stems eliminated
- 1 little onion, quartered
- 7-8 garlic cloves, stripped
- Salt to taste
- 1 tbsp. ground dark pepper
- 1 tbsp. ground cumin
- 1 tbsp. ground coriander
- 1 tsp. cayenne pepper, optional
- 1 tsp. preparing powder
- 2 tbsp. toasted sesame seeds
- Oil for searing
- Falafel Sauce
- Tahini Sauce
- Trimmings for falafel sandwich (optional)
- Pita pockets
- English cucumbers, chopped or diced
- Tomatoes, chopped or diced
- Child Arugula
- Pickles

DIRECTIONS

1. (One day ahead of time) Place the dried chickpeas and preparing soft drink in a huge bowl loaded up with water to cover the chickpeas by in any event 2 inches. Splash for the time being for 18 hours (longer if the chickpeas are still excessively hard). At the point when prepared, channel the chickpeas totally and wipe them off.
2. Add the chickpeas, spices, onions, garlic and flavors to the enormous bowl of a food processor fitted with a cutting edge. Run the food processor 40 seconds all at once until everything is great joined shaping a the falafel blend.
3. Move the falafel blend to a compartment and cover firmly. Refrigerate for in any event 1 hour or (up to one entire evening) until prepared to cook.
4. Not long prior to searing, add the preparing powder and sesame seeds to the falafel blend and mix with a spoon.
5. Scoop tablespoonful's of the falafel combination and structure into patties (½ inch in thickness each). It assists with having wet hands as you structure the patties.
6. Fill a medium pan 3 crawls up with oil. Heat the oil on medium-high until it bubbles delicately. Cautiously drop the falafel patties in the oil, let them fry for around 3 to 5 minutes or so until fresh and medium brown outwardly. Try not to pack the falafel in the pan, fry them in bunches if fundamental.
7. Spot the singed falafel patties in a colander or plate fixed with paper towels to deplete.
8. Serve falafel hot close to other little plates; or amass the falafel patties in pita bread with tahini or hummus, arugula, tomato and cucumbers. Enjoy!
9. You need to begin with dry chickpeas, don't utilize canned chickpeas here. You should start dousing the chickpeas short-term, permit as long as 24 hours.
10. Falafel Recipe varieties: Variations of this formula may call for flour or eggs. On the off chance that you like, you can add 1 to 1 ½ tbsp. of flour to the falafel blend or 1 egg. I didn't utilize either, and the falafel combination remained well together.
11. Ace Tip for Frying: When you fry the falafel patties, you need to accomplish a profound brilliant brown tone outwardly. All the more critically, the patties should be completely done within. Your broiling oil should be at 375 degrees F, for my oven, that was at a medium-high temp. Make certain to test your first group and change the singing time depending on the situation.
12. Well known falafel sauce: tahini sauce is the thing that is customarily utilized with falafel. I utilize natural tahini paste by Soom, and here is my tahini sauce formula.
13. Prepared Falafel Option: If you like, you can heat the falafel patties in a 350 degree F heated oven for around 15-20 minutes, turning them over halfway through. Utilize a gently oiled sheet dish, and you may jump at the chance to give the patties a speedy brush of additional virgin olive oil prior to preparing.
14. Supportive of Tip for Make-Ahead: To make ahead and freeze, set up the falafel blend and separation into patties (up to step #6). Spot the patties on a preparing sheet fixed with material paper and freeze. At the point when they solidify, you can move the falafel patties into a cooler pack. They will save well in the cooler for a month or something like that. You can sear or heat them from frozen.

685. Greek Wedge Salad

Prep Time: 15 Minutes *Cook Time: 35 Minutes* *Servings: 6*

INGREDIENTS

- 4-teaspoons apple cider vinegar
- 1-bag of green onion powder mix
- 1-clove of garlic, chopped
- 1/2 cup chopped green onion
- 1-head of iceberg lettuce, heart removed and in pictures
- 1-tomato, cut into cubes
- 4-teaspoons bacon cubes

DIRECTIONS

1. Combine the cream, buttermilk, vinegar, and dressing in a small bowl. Beat until the combination is easy.
2. Add garlic and a quarter cup of inexperienced onion; put aside. Remove the center of the lettuce and cut into 4-equal wedges.
3. Place each wedge in 4 different dishes. Pour about 1/4 of the salad dressing over each wedge.
4. Divide 1/4 of the ultimate onion, 1/4 of the chopped tomato, and 1-teaspoon of bacon cubes over each wedge.

686. Mediterranean Pizza with Shrimp and Feta

Prep Time: 15 Minutes *Cook Time: 45 Minutes* *Servings: 2*

Ingredients

- 2 tbsp. cornmeal
- 1 tube (10 ounces) refrigerated pizza dough
- 1 c. water
- 5 oz. large shrimp, peeled and deveined
- 1 tbsp. toasted pine nuts
- 1 large clove garlic
- 1 1/2 c. loosely packed fresh basil
- 2 tbsp. grated Parmesan cheese
- 3 tbsp. defatted reduced-sodium chicken broth
- 2 tsp. lemon juice
- 2 oz. feta cheese, crumbled
- 2 tbsp. minced red onions
- 1/2 c. shredded reduced-fat low-sodium mozzarella cheese

Directions

1. Preheat the oven to 450ï¿½F. Coat a baking sheet with no-stick spray. Sprinkle with the cornmeal.
2. Unroll the pizza dough and spread on the prepared sheet.
3. Bring the water to a simmer in a small saucepan. Add the shrimp and cook for 1 to 2 minutes, or until opaque and cooked through. Drain and cut each shrimp into thirds.
4. Place the pine nuts and garlic in a food processor or blender. Process until minced. Add the basil, Parmesan, broth, and lemon juice; process for 2 to 3 minutes, or until a paste forms. Add more broth, if necessary, to achieve the desired consistency.
5. Spread the pesto on the crust, leaving a 1/ 2" border. Sprinkle with the shrimp, feta, and onions. Top with the mozzarella. Bake for 14 to 16 minutes, or until the bottom is browned and the cheese is melted.

687. Greek Lebanesee rice with vermicelli

Prep Time: 15 Minutes *Cook Time: 39 Minutes* *Servings: 6*

Ingredients:

- 2 cups in length grain or medium grain rice
- Water
- 1 cup broken vermicelli pasta
- 2 ½ tbsp. olive oil
- Salt
- ½ cup toasted pine nuts, optional to wrap up

Directions

1. Wash the rice well (a couple of times) at that point places it in a medium bowl and cover with water. Splash for 15 to 20 minutes. Test to check whether you can without much of a stretch break a grain of rice by basically putting it between your thumb and pointer. Channel well.
2. In a medium non-stick cooking pot, heat the olive oil on medium-high. Add the vermicelli and consistently mix to toast it equally. Vermicelli should turn a decent brilliant brown, yet observe cautiously not to over-brown or consume it (If it consumes, you should discard the vermicelli and begin once again).
3. Add the rice and keep on blending so the rice will be very much covered with the olive oil. Season with salt.
4. Presently add 3 ½ cups of water and heat it to the point of boiling until the water altogether diminishes (see the photograph below).Turn the heat to low and cover.
5. Cook for 15-20 minutes on low. Once completely cooked, turn the heat off and leave the rice undisturbed in its cooking pot for 10-15 minutes, at that point reveal and cushion with a fork.
6. Move to a serving platter and top with the toasted pine nuts. Enjoy!
7. You should flush the rice to dispose of abundance starch which makes rice be tacky (Lebanese rice isn't intended to be tacky). At that point absorbs the rice a lot of water for 15-20 minutes or until you can break one grain of rice by squeezing it between your forefinger and your thumb. 2.toasting the vermicelli in EVOO as an initial step is the thing that gives this rice incredible flavor. Try not to skirt this progression. 3. On the off chance that you can at all assistance it, let the rice rest for 5 to 10 minutes prior to serving.

688. Greek Meaty Arugula Pizzas

Prep Time: 15 Minutes *Cook Time: 30 Minutes* *Servings: 2*

Ingredients

- 1 bundle (1/4 ounce) dynamic dry yeast
- 1-1/2 cups warm water (110° to 115°)
- 2 tablespoons olive oil
- 2 teaspoons salt
- 1 teaspoon sugar
- 3-1/2 to 4 cups bread flour
- 4 teaspoons cornmeal
- Fixings:
- 1 pound mass Italian wiener
- 2 tablespoons olive oil
- 6 garlic cloves, minced
- 1-1/2 cups shredded part-skim mozzarella cheddar
- 1 bundle (3-1/2 ounces) cut pepperoni
- 4 cups new arugula or child spinach
- 1/2 cup ground Parmesan cheddar
- Extra new arugula or child spinach, optional

Directions

1. In a small bowl, break up yeast in warm water. In a huge bowl, join 2 tablespoons oil, salt, sugar, yeast combination and 1-1/2 cups flour; beat on medium speed 3 minutes until smooth. Mix in sufficient excess flour to shape a delicate batter (mixture will be tacky).
2. Turn batter onto a floured surface; work until smooth and versatile, around 6-8 minutes. Spot in a lubed bowl, going once to oil the top. Cover with saran wrap and let ascend in a warm spot until multiplied, around 1-1/2 hours.
3. Preheat oven to 425°. Oil two 15x10x1-in. heating container; sprinkle with cornmeal. Punch down batter. Turn onto a daintily floured surface; partition fifty-

fifty. Fold each into a 15x10-in. square shape; move to arranged container, squeezing edges to frame an edge. Cover with saran wrap; let rest 10 minutes.
4. In an enormous skillet, cook frankfurter over medium heat 6-8 minutes or until not, at this point pink, breaking into disintegrates; channel. Blend oil and garlic; spread over pizza outside layers. Sprinkle each with 1/4 cup mozzarella cheddar. Top with pepperoni, arugula, cooked hotdog and remaining mozzarella cheddar; sprinkle with Parmesan cheddar.
5. Heat 10-15 minutes or until outside and cheddar are gently browned. Whenever wanted, top with extra arugula prior to serving.

689. Greek Wedge Salad With Creamy Dressing

Prep Time: 15 Minutes | *Cook Time: 65 Minutes* | *Servings: 6*

INGREDIENTS

- 4-teaspoons apple cider vinegar
- 1-bag of green onion powder mix
- 1-clove of garlic, chopped
- 1/2 cup chopped green onion
- 1-head of iceberg lettuce, heart removed and in pictures
- 1-tomato, cut into cubes
- 4-teaspoons bacon cubes

DIRECTIONS

1. Combine the cream, buttermilk, vinegar, and dressing in a small bowl. Beat until the combination is easy.
2. Add garlic and a quarter cup of inexperienced onion; put aside. Remove the center of the lettuce and cut into 4-equal wedges.
3. Place each wedge in 4 different dishes. Pour about 1/4 of the salad dressing over each wedge.
4. Divide 1/4 of the ultimate onion, 1/4 of the chopped tomato, and 1-teaspoon of bacon cubes over each wedge.

690. Best Greek Chicken Piccata

Prep Time: 15 Minutes | *Cook Time: 34 Minutes* | *Servings: 2*

Ingredients

- 1 lemon
- 1 1/2 pounds boneless, skinless chicken breasts
- 1 teaspoon kosher salt
- 1 teaspoon freshly ground black pepper
- 1/3 cup all-purpose flour
- 3 tablespoons margarine isolated
- 2 tablespoons canola oil
- 1 cup chicken stock or white wine, or a blend of both
- 2 tablespoons escapades depleted and flushed

GUIDELINES

1. Cut the lemon fifty-fifty, juice one half, at that point cut the other half into 1/8" cuts and put in a safe spot.
2. Cut back any overabundance excess from the chicken breasts and cut down the middle longwise to make two slight cutlets. Season the two sides of the chicken breasts uniformly with the legitimate salt and newly ground dark pepper at that point dig each bosom in the flour, shaking off any abundance.
3. Heat 2 tablespoons margarine with the canola oil in an enormous skillet over medium-high heat. Add 4 bits of the chicken and cook for 2-3 minutes for each side. Move to a platter or sheet skillet and cover with foil. Proceed with the excess chicken.
4. Decrease the heat to medium and add the chicken stock or wine (or 1/2 cup of both) the lemon juice, cut lemons, and the tricks, scraping up the browned pieces on the dish and cook for 2-3 minutes.
5. Mix in the excess 1 tablespoon of margarine until dissolved. Taste for preparing and spoon the sauce over the chicken breasts. Present with pureed potatoes or cauliflower, polenta, or noodles.

Formula Notes

1. Keep the cooked chicken breasts warm while the sauce cooks by plating on a platter and covering with aluminum foil, or spot in a 200°F oven.

691. Mediterranean Baked Cod Recipe with Lemon and Garlic

Prep Time: 15 Minutes | *Cook Time: 360 Minutes* | *Servings: 4*

INGREDIENTS

- ¼ cup chopped new parsley leaves
- Lemon Sauce
- 5 tbsp. new lemon juice
- 5 tbsp. additional virgin olive oil
- 2 tbsp. dissolved spread
- 5 garlic cloves, minced
- For Coating
- ⅓ cup generally useful flour
- 1 tsp. ground coriander
- ¾ tsp. sweet Spanish paprika
- ¾ tsp. ground cumin
- ¾ tsp. salt
- ½ tsp. dark pepper

Directions

1. Preheat oven to 400 degrees F.
2. Combine as one the lemon juice, olive oil, and liquefied margarine in a shallow bowl (don't add the garlic yet). Put in a safe spot.
3. In another shallow bowl, blend the generally useful flour, flavors, salt and pepper. Set close to the lemon sauce.
4. Wipe the fish off. Plunge the fish in the lemon sauce at that point dunk it in the flour blend. Shake off abundance flour. Save the lemon sauce for some other time.
5. Heat 2 tbsp. olive oil in a cast iron skillet (or an oven-safe dish) over medium-high heat (watch the oil to be certain it is shining however not smoking). Add the fish and burn on each side to give it some tone, yet don't completely cook (around 2 minutes on each side). Eliminate the skillet from heat.
6. To the leftover lemon sauce, add the minced garlic and blend. Sprinkle everywhere on the fish filets.
7. Prepare in the heated oven until the fish chips effectively with a fork (10 minutes ought to get it
8. done, however start checking prior). Eliminate from the heat and sprinkle chopped parsley. Serve right away.

692. Greek Buffalo Chicken Pizza

Prep Time: 15 Minutes | *Cook Time: 20 Minutes* | *Servings: 4*

INGREDIENTS

1 tube (13.8 ounces) refrigerated pizza covering

- 1 cup Buffalo wing sauce, isolated
- 1-1/2 cups shredded cheddar
- 1-1/2 cups part-skim shredded mozzarella cheddar
- 2 pounds boneless skinless chicken breasts, cubed
- 1/2 teaspoon every garlic salt, pepper and bean stew powder
- 2 tablespoons margarine
- 1/2 teaspoon dried oregano
- Celery sticks and blue cheddar serving of mixed greens dressing

Directions

1. Unroll pizza covering into a daintily lubed 15x10x1-in. heating container; straighten mixture and develop edges somewhat. Heat at 400° for 7 minutes. Brush batter with 3 tablespoons Buffalo wing sauce. Join cheddar and mozzarella cheeses; sprinkle a third absurd. Put in a safe spot.
2. In an enormous skillet, cook the chicken, garlic salt, pepper and stew powder in spread until chicken is not, at this point pink. Add the excess wing sauce; cook and mix over medium heat 5 minutes longer.
3. Spoon over pizza. Sprinkle with oregano and remaining cheddar.
4. Heat until outside layer is brilliant brown and cheddar is dissolved, 18-20 minutes. Present with celery and blue cheddar dressing.
5. Freeze choice: Bake pizza outside layer as coordinated; cool. Top with all the ingredients as coordinated and safely wrap and freeze unbaked pizza. To utilize, open up pizza; heat as coordinated, expanding time as important.

693. Mediterranean Spaghetti Squash

Prep Time: 15 Minutes | *Cook Time: 23 Minutes* | *Servings: 2*

Ingredients

- 1 spaghetti squash large
- 1 sweet onion large, 1/2" dice
- 2 red bell peppers seeded, veins removed, 1/2" dice
- 1 pint grape tomatoes halved
- 1 zucchini squash large, 1/2" dice
- 1 yellow squash large, 1/2" dice
- 2 cups broccoli florets cut into bite-sized pieces
- 2 teaspoons granulated garlic
- 1 tablespoon Italian seasoning blend
- 1/2 teaspoon kosher salt or sea salt
- 2 tablespoons olive oil
- 2 cups baby spinach roughly chopped

Instructions

1. Preheat oven to 400 degrees F.
2. Cut spaghetti squash in half; remove seeds and place each half cut side down on a sheet pan. Place sheet pan in preheated oven and roast spaghetti squash until tender, about 20-25 minutes. Squash is ready when you can press the outside (careful) and it "gives" and is no longer hard.
3. Remove spaghetti squash from oven and place cut sides up, allowing cooling slightly.
4. While spaghetti squash is roasting, place onion, peppers, tomatoes, zucchini, yellow squash, and broccoli on another sheet pan. Add granulated garlic, Italian seasoning and salt. Pour on olive oil and toss everything together to evenly coat.
5. Roast vegetables in 400 degree oven for about 15-20 minutes, while spaghetti squash is roasting. Vegetables are ready when tender-crisp and golden brown. Remove from oven.
6. Using a fork, shred the spaghetti squash into "spaghetti" and place in a large mixing bowl or casserole dish.
7. While the spaghetti squash is still slightly warm, add the chopped baby spinach and roasted vegetables. Toss to blend thoroughly. Taste for seasoning, adjust if necessary and serve.

694. Greek Green Goddess Cobb Salad

Prep Time: 15 Minutes | *Cook Time: 35 Minutes* | *Servings: 2*

INGREDIENTS

- 1 1/2 teaspoons of salt
- 1 cup warm water Salad servers:
- 6 ounces salad mix-use rocket, romaine, kale, and radicchio mix
- 6 grams of grilled chicken fillet
- 2-tablespoons of crispy cooked bacon
- 3-tablespoons of chopped avocado
- 1/2 cup of chopped tomatoes
- Halve 1-hard-boiled egg
- 2-tablespoons of feta
- 2-tablespoons pickled onions Green goddess salad dressing:
- 1-cup of mayonnaise
- 2-tablespoons tarragon leaves

DIRECTION

1. Slice onions as thin as possible; I like to use the 1/8 inch on my mandolin. Put the onions in a full pot. Combine white vinegar, sugar, salt, and warm water in a small bowl. Stir until sugar and salt are dissolved. These should rest for about half an hour before use. Place all ingredients for the dressing in the bowl of a blender or meal processor and blend for 30-45 seconds, or until the dressing is mostly clean and creamy.
2. Place the salad in the bottom of a large salad bowl. Cut the chicken breast into thin slices and put them with the salad. Add a new, pre-selected, and chosen time, and some more, and egg you bought, and a few samples.

695. Crispy Salmon with Lemony Asparagus

Prep Time: 15 Minutes | *Cook Time: 65 Minutes* | *Servings: 6*

Ingredients

- 4 (6-oz.) skin-on salmon filets
- ¼ cup mayonnaise

- 2 tablespoons Dijon mustard
- 1 tablespoon chopped new dill
- 1 ½ teaspoons lemon zing (from 1 lemon), partitioned
- ¾ teaspoon genuine salt, separated
- ¾ teaspoon dark pepper, partitioned
- ¼ cup panko (Japanese-style breadcrumbs)
- Cooking splash
- ½ pound new asparagus, managed and split transversely
- 1 (8-oz.) pkg. little carrots with tops, cut longwise
- 2 tablespoons unsalted margarine, liquefied
- Lemon wedges

Directions

1. Preheat oven to 425°F. Line a rimmed preparing sheet with material paper. Spot salmon, skin side down, on portion of arranged preparing sheet. Mix together mayonnaise, mustard, and dill, 1 teaspoon of the lemon zing, 1/4 teaspoon of the salt, and 1/4 teaspoon of the pepper in a medium bowl. Spread over salmon filets in an even layer; top with panko, and press gently to follow. Splash with cooking shower.
2. Throw together asparagus, carrots, margarine, and staying 1/2 teaspoon every one of lemon zing, salt, and pepper in a medium bowl. Spot vegetables on void side of preparing sheet. Heat in preheated oven until salmon is cooked through and vegetables are delicate, around 18 minutes. Present with lemon wedges.

696. Greek Roasted Red Snapper with Potatoes Onions

Prep Time: *15 Minutes* | *Cook Time:* *23 Minutes* | *Servings: 2*

Ingredients

- 1 ½ cups approximately pressed new level leaf parsley leaves
- 1 medium shallot (around 2 oz.), generally chopped
- 3 garlic cloves, generally chopped
- 1 tablespoon new thyme leaves
- 1 ½ teaspoons lemon zing (from 1 lemon)
- ½ teaspoon squashed red pepper
- ¾ cup olive oil
- 2 ¾ teaspoons legitimate salt, separated
- 1 pound child gold potatoes (around 8 potatoes)
- 1 little red onion (around 8 oz.), cut the long way into 1-in. wedges
- 1 (3-lb.) entire red snapper, cleaned, scaled, gutted, and blades managed
- Lemon wedges, for serving

Directions

1. Preheat oven to 425°F. Line a rimmed heating sheet with material paper. Put in a safe spot.
2. Cycle parsley, shallot, garlic, thyme, lemon zing, and red pepper in a food processor until finely chopped, around 15 seconds. Add oil, and interaction until very much fused, around 15 seconds. Throw together potatoes, onion wedges, 2 tablespoons of the parsley combination, and 1 teaspoon of the salt in an enormous bowl.
3. Cut 3 (2-inch-long) cuts askew on the two sides of fish, slicing right deep down on the two sides. Rub outside and within cuts with 1 cup of the parsley blend and staying 1 3/4 teaspoons salt; place fish on arranged heating sheet. Spread potato blend around fish. Prepare in preheated oven until fish is murky and flaky and vegetables are delicate, around 30 minutes.
4. Shower fish with remaining 1/4 cup parsley combination. Present with lemon wedges.

697. Mediterranean Tomato, Mozzarella, Basil, And Avocado Salad

Prep Time: *15 Minutes* | *Cook Time:* *33 Minutes* | *Servings: 2*

INGREDIENTS

- 2-sliced avocados
- 2-ripe tomatoes
- 500 g mozzarella cheese
- 1 cup of fresh basil leaves
- 1/4 cup of olive oil
- 1/4 cup of Balsamic Aceto
- Salt and ground black pepper

DIRECTION

1. Gather all the ingredients to make this tomato, mozzarella, basil, and avocado Caprese salad.
2. Cut the tomato stem with a small knife and cut the tomatoes into slices with a serrated knife.
3. Slice the mozzarella and spot alternating slices of avocado, tomato, mozzarella, and basil in signature dishes. Slice with olive oil and balsamic vinegar and season with salt and ground black pepper.
4. Divide your Italian tomato, mozzarella, basil, and avocado salad with a fresh baguette or on a bed of romaine lettuce.

Side Dishes Recipes

698. Best Greek Chicken Marinade

Prep Time: *2 Minutes* | *Cook Time:* *15 Minutes* | *Servings: 4*

Ingredients

- 1 pound boneless skinless chicken breasts (about 2 large breasts)
- ⅓ cup plain Greek yogurt
- ¼ cup olive oil
- 4 lemons
- 4-5 cloves garlic squeezed or minced
- 2 tablespoons dried oregano
- 1 teaspoon genuine salt
- ½ teaspoon newly ground dark pepper

Directions

1. Spot the chicken pieces in a cooler sack or a bowl and put in a safe spot.
2. Add the Greek yogurt and olive oil to a medium size bowl. Zing one of the lemons and add to the bowl. Juice that lemon into the bowl with the zing. Cut the other three lemons and put in a safe spot. Add the minced garlic, oregano, genuine salt and dark pepper to the lemon squeeze and zing and mix. Empty portion of the marinade into the cooler sack or the bowl with the chicken pieces and save the other portion of the marinade for seasoning. Marinate the chicken for 30 minutes or as long as 3 hours in the fridge.
3. At the point when prepared to flame broil, set up the barbecue by gently oiling the mesh with vegetable oil or cooking splash and set to medium high heat.
4. Flame broil the chicken, treating with the held marinade and turning frequently so each side browns and has light barbecue marks, until cooked through, around 15-20 minutes or until the chicken juices run clear. During the most recent 5 minutes of cooking add the 3 cut lemons to the flame broil, turning more than once. Permit the chicken to rest for 5 minutes prior to cutting and present with the flame broiled lemons. Refrigerate extras for as long as 3 days.

699. Greek baked kale, and broccoli salad

Prep Time: *15 Minutes* | *Cook Time:* *43 Minutes* | *Servings: 2*

INGREDIENTS:

- Broccoli florets
- Bare minced meat

DIRECTIONS:

1. Set aside.
2. (2.5 cm) higher than
3. the eggs. Cover and bring to a boil over high heat. Cook once, remove from
4. heat and boil in water, depending on preference: 10-12 minutes (hard-
5. cooked), or 6-8 minutes (medium cooked), or 5-6 minutes (soft boiled).
6. Meanwhile, set aside a bowl of ice-cold water.
7. To peel. Peel under running water and cut into halves or quarters. Set
8. aside.
9. Add the sliced garlic and fry until golden brown. Remove the garlic from the pan and place it on kitchen paper too crispy. Keep the garlic-infused oil in the pan.
10. With the olive oil. Add the broccoli, kale, and spring onions. Use pliers, throw to
11. coat and bake for about 5 minutes, or until lightly cooked.
12. Board with the eggs, avocado, and mustard mayonnaise.

700. Greek Healthy Peach Cobbler

Prep Time: *15 Minutes* | *Cook Time:* *73 Minutes* | *Servings: 6*

Ingredients

- Covering
- 4 cups whitened almond flour
- 1/2 teaspoon salt
- 1/2 cup sugar or sugar
- 2 eggs
- 6 tablespoons unsalted margarine softened
- Peach Filling
- 1/2 cup unsalted margarine 1 stick
- 1/2 cup brown sugar or light brown sugar
- 1/2 cup sugar or sugar
- 1 teaspoon cinnamon
- 1/2 teaspoon nutmeg
- 1/2 new lemon, juice of About 2-3 tablespoons.
- 2 teaspoons vanilla Pure concentrate, not impersonation.
- 20 oz. frozen peaches This is typically 1 enormous pack. Or then again you can join various. See notes for canned or new peaches.
- 1 teaspoon cornstarch For sans gluten, use without gluten flour.
- 1 teaspoon water
- 1 egg Beaten with 1 teaspoon of water for egg wash
- cinnamon for fixing

Directions

1. Outside
2. Add the almond flour, sugar, and salt (dry ingredients) to a blending bowl. Mix to consolidate.
3. Add the eggs and dissolved spread (wet ingredients) to a different bowl and mix.
4. Add the dry ingredients to a food processor. Then, pour in the wet ingredients. Physically beat until the blend is fused. You can likewise consolidate the dry and wet ingredients in a blending bowl and blend by hand, however subsequent to testing, the best outcomes are using a food processor.
5. Eliminate the mixture and fold it up into an enormous ball. Cut the batter fifty-fifty. One half will be utilized for the base outside of the shoemaker.
6. Sprinkle a level surface with a little almond flour to keep the batter from staying. Utilize a carrying pin and carry out the mixture until level.
7. Refrigerate the batter for 30 minutes to expedite prior to dealing with. It will be truly tacky in the event that you skirt this progression. The more you refrigerate, the simpler it is to deal with. I refrigerate half of the batter after it has been carried out, my inclination. You can keep it in a ball on the off chance that you wish.
8. After you have refrigerated, cut portion of the batter into strips around 1 inch thick.

Filling

9. Preheat oven to 350 degrees.
10. Heat a pot or pot on medium heat and add the spread. At the point when liquefied, include the sugars, nutmeg, and cinnamon. Mix constantly. Permit the combination to cook until the sugar or sugar has softened.
11. Include the lemon juice and vanilla and mix. Pour in the peaches. Mix and permit the combination to cook for around 4-5 minutes to mollify the peaches.
12. Consolidate the cornstarch and water in a little bowl to make a slurry. Mix it together and add it to the pot. Mix to completely consolidate. Permit the blend to cook for 10-12 minutes until the filling thickens and eliminate it from heat.
13. Amass and Bake
14. Splash a 8×8 preparing dish or a 9.5 inch pie skillet with cooking shower or oil.
15. Spot 1/2 of the pie outside layer into the lower part of a 8×8 heating dish.
16. Using an opened spoon, top the outside with the peaches combination. You need to utilize an opened spoon here with the goal that you don't add an excess of fluid to the shoemaker. On the off chance that you utilize an excessive amount of fluid it will be runny. I add it using an opened spoon, and afterward I finish it off with one huge spoonful of fluid from the pot.
17. Add cuts of pie covering to the top. You can organize the outside anyway you wish. In the event that you have lopsided strips, you can shape two together to frame one. Remove the rest of any strips that are excessively long. Brush the covering with the egg wash and sprinkle with cinnamon.
18. Heat for 25 minutes. Now the covering will start to brown. Open the oven and tent the dish with foil. Don't completely cover, freely tent (it shouldn't contact the shoemaker). This will keep the shoemaker from browning a lot on the top as the inside keeps on heating.

19. Prepare for an extra 20-25 minutes. You can eliminate the foil following 15 minutes if the covering needs seriously browning.

Important notes for recipe:

20. You can join the pie hull ingredients by hand. It will take somewhat more and can be hard to join the ingredients to deliver a smooth covering. I discover this way works best.
21. You can substitute brown sugar or sugar for white and utilize possibly white sugar in the event that you wish.
22. Loads of individuals make peach shoemaker with a top outside layer as it were. I'm a gigantic aficionado of the outside so I do both a base and top layer. You can slice the hull formula down the middle and do 1 layer in the event that you wish.
23. In the event that you lessen the measure of covering utilized in this formula (and utilize 1/2 as the top layer in particular) it will bring about the accompanying macros per serving: 251 calories, 20 grams fat, 9 grams of net carbs, and 7 grams of protein.
24. Or then again you can get serious about the top layer of the outside. This will make it simpler to make a thick cross section design in the event that you are searching for that.
25. While setting the covering into the lower part of the preparing dish, I like to utilize the lower part of a glass mug to straighten it out.
26. In the event that using canned peaches I suggest 20-24oz. At times you can just discover canned in 15.5oz servings. For this situation you may select to utilize a can and a half or go with less peaches. In the case of using canned, channel 1/2 of the fluid from the can prior to adding it to the pot. In the event that you utilize the entirety of the fluid the filling will turn out to be excessively soupy.
27. In the case of using new peaches, you should strip the peaches first. You may likewise need to adapt to taste.
28. New peaches are frequently tarter and less sweet. Taste your filling over and again and add more sugar if vital.
29. In the event that you utilize locally acquired pie outside and customary sugar, the macros per serving are as per the following: 889 calories, 61 grams fat, 62 grams of net carbs, and 16 grams of protein.
30. There's an enormous contrast in insight regarding vanilla concentrate versus impersonation. Vanilla will taste much better.
31. On the off chance that you utilize locally acquired pie outside layer, the heat time will be reliable. You presumably will not have to tent the skillet with foil. Utilize your judgment. In the event that the outside begins to become a brilliant shade of brown inside 30 minutes, tent it.
32. This formula incorporates margarine. You can choose if the utilization of spread is sound or not for you. You can take a stab at using oils like coconut or avocado oil in the event that you wish.

701. Instant Pot Shrimp | Greek Shrimp Saganaki

Prep Time:	*Cook Time:*	*Servings: 4*
15 Minutes	*20 Minutes*	

Ingredients

- Cook Together
- 2 tablespoons (2 tablespoons) Butter
- 1 tablespoon (1 tablespoon) Garlic
- 1/2 teaspoon (0.5 teaspoon) Red Pepper Flakes, conform to taste
- 1.5 cups (32 g) onions, chopped
- 1 14.5-oz (1 14.5-oz) Canned Tomatoes
- 1 teaspoon (1 teaspoon) Dried Oregano
- 1 teaspoons (1 teaspoons) Kosher Salt
- 1 pound (453.59 g) Frozen Raw Shrimp, 21-25 tally, shelled
- Add subsequent to cooking
- 1 cup (150 g) disintegrated feta cheddar
- 1/2 cup (67.5 g) cut dark olives
- 1/4 cup (15 g) Chopped Parsley

Guidelines

For the Instant Pot

1. Turn your Instant Pot or Pressure cooker to Sauté and once it is hot, add the margarine. Allow it to dissolve a little and afterward add garlic and red pepper pieces.
2. Include onions, tomatoes, oregano and salt.
3. Pour in the frozen shrimp.
4. Set your Instant pot to LOW pressing factor 1 moment.
5. When the pot is finished cooking, discharge all pressing factor right away.
6. Blend in the shrimp with the remainder of the beautiful tomato stock.
7. Permit it to cool somewhat. Just prior to serving, sprinkle the feta cheddar, olives, and parsley.
8. This dish makes a soupy stock, so it's incredible for plunging buttered French bread into, or eats over rice, or riced cauliflower.
9. Burner Instructions
10. Heat a 10-inch pan and when it's hot, add the margarine. To the softened margarine add garlic and red pepper pieces. Let this sizzle for 10-15 seconds.
11. Add onions, tomato paste, oregano, salt, pepper, and water. Blend until you the tomato paste has broken down. Cover the skillet and let the sauce cook for 3-4 minutes.
12. Mix in shrimp, feta cheddar, and olives. Cook until the shrimp are cooked through for around 2-3 minutes. Trimming with parsley and serve.

Serving ideas:

- French Bread and Butter
- Rice
- Riced Cauliflower
- Eat plain.
- Utilize frozen shrimp when making this in the Instant Pot.
- Store the saganaki in the refrigerator for as long as 3 days and freeze for as long as 3 months.

702. Greek Instant Pot Butternut Squash Soup

Prep Time:	*Cook Time:*	*Servings: 2*
15 Minutes	*56 Minutes*	

Ingredients

- 1 tablespoon oil, I utilize avocado oil
- 2 cloves garlic, minced
- 1 yellow onion, diced
- 1 Granny Smith apple, diced
- 1 butternut squash, stripped and diced
- 1 cup coconut milk
- 2 cups water, or vegetable stock
- 1 branch new savvy
- 1/8 teaspoon ground cinnamon
- 1/2 teaspoon ocean salt, to taste
- 1/4 teaspoon dark pepper, to taste
- Optional garnishes
- 1 tablespoon toasted pumpkin seeds
- 1 tablespoon coconut milk

Guidelines

1. Press the "Sautee" button on the constrain cooker to warm oil briefly. Add onions and garlic and cook for around 5 minutes, blending much of the time, until the onions become seem clear.
2. Press "Drop" and add the apple, butternut squash, coconut milk, water, sage, cinnamon, salt, and pepper.
3. Close the top, set the valve on "fixing", and cook on high pressing factor for 10 minutes. When finished, let the pressing factor discharge all alone for around 10 minutes before fast delivering any excess pressing factor. Cautiously open the cover.
4. Either using an inundation blender or using your blender, mix the soup until smooth and velvety. Add garnishes and serve.

703. Italian Egg Bake

Prep Time:	*Cook Time:*	*Servings: 6*
15 Minutes	*29 Minutes*	

INGREDIENTS:

- 4 ounces of diced pancetta
- 1/2 cup of chopped red onion (about 140 grams)
- 1/2 cup of chopped fresh oregano
- 1/2 cup of chopped fresh basil
- 1/4 cup of unsweetened almond milk
- 2/3 cup grated Parmesan cheese (extra for topping)
- 1/2 teaspoon of chopped garlic
- 1/4 teaspoon sea salt and pepper each (or to taste)
- 1/2 cup chopped fresh tomato
- 1 cup of tomato sauce
- 5 large cage-free eggs
- Red pepper flakes for garnish
- Oregano for garnish

DIRECTIONS:

1. Preheat the oven to 425 degrees F.
2. Fry the pancetta and onion together in an 8 inch cast iron skillet (or oven safe pan) for 2 minutes or until fragrant.
3. Remove from heat.
4. Beat together the almond milk and parmesan cheese. Reserve extra cheese for the topping.
5. Stir in the garlic, tomato, sea salt / pepper, tomato sauce and herbs.
6. Pour the milk tomato mixture over the cast iron skillet (or ovenproof pan) with the onion and pancetta.
7. Using a spatula, make 5 small slits in the pan (evenly spaced) where you can place the eggs so that the yolk doesn't break. Break 5 eggs on top of each crack. If you find you have an egg with a runny yolk, just mix it through the pan, but then add another egg with a solid yolk. Or discard the runny yolk.
8. Add any extra cheese to the eggs and place the skillet in the oven for 15-18 minutes or until the egg whites are set (the yolk softens) and the corners are brown. Baking times vary depending on the oven and the type of skillet being used.
9. Garnish with Italian parsley and red pepper flakes. To enjoy

704. 30-Minute Caprese Chicken Recipe

Prep Time:	*Cook Time:*	*Servings: 2*
15 Minutes	*30 Minutes*	

Ingredients

- 2 skinless boneless chicken breasts
- Kosher salt and freshly ground black pepper
- 1 tablespoon extra-virgin olive oil
- 1 tablespoon spread
- 1 6 oz. container DeLallo Traditional Basil Simply Pesto
- 4-6 cuts new mozzarella or 6 ounces ground mozzarella cheddar
- 8 mixed drink or little tomatoes cut
- DeLallo balsamic coating
- New basil fragmented

Directions

1. Preheat the oven to 400° F.
2. Utilize a sharp, slim blade to cut the chicken breasts down the middle the long way. Season the two sides with fit salt and newly ground dark pepper. Heat a huge oven-verification skillet over medium high heat and add the olive oil and spread. When the margarine has softened into the olive oil, add the chicken breasts to the container, being mindful so as not to swarm. Cook on each side until softly browned, around 3-4 minutes each.
3. Slather the highest points of every chicken bosom with the basil pesto, around 1-2 tablespoons for each chicken bosom. Top every chicken bosom with a cut of mozzarella and a couple of cuts of tomato. Put the skillet in the oven and cook for 10-12 minutes or until the chicken arrives at an inward temperature of 165 degrees. F. Eliminate from the oven and topping with new basil and a sprinkle of balsamic coating.

705. Mediterranean Sautéed Chicken with Olives, Capers and Lemons

Prep Time:	*Cook Time:*	*Servings: 2*
15 Minutes	*19 Minutes*	

Ingredients

- 2 lemons sliced 1/4 inch thick
- 1/4 cup plus 1 tablespoon extra-virgin olive oil
- 6 skinless boneless chicken thighs, about 1 pound
- 1-2 tablespoons rice flour or all-purpose flour
- 1 fat garlic clove minced
- 1 cup chicken broth
- 3/4 cup Sicilian green olives
- 1/4 cup carpers
- 2 tablespoons spread
- 2 tablespoons parsley
- legitimate salt and newly broke dark pepper

Directions

1. Bring a medium-huge, high sided skillet to medium-high heat and add 1 tablespoon of olive oil. Add half of the lemon cuts and singe until browned, 3-5 minutes on each side. Move to a plate. Season the chicken thighs with fit salt and dark pepper and residue with rice flour, shaking off the overabundance. Add 1/2 tablespoons of olive

oil to the hot skillet and burn the chicken pieces until brilliant brown, around 5 minutes each side. Move to another plate and wrap up singing the remainder of the chicken pieces, at that point move to a similar plate as the remainder of the chicken.
2. Add the remainder of the olive oil to the skillet and the minced garlic, and cook for 30 seconds or until fragrant, blending so the garlic doesn't consume and turn out to be harsh.
3. Add the green olives, tricks and stock. Add the saved chicken and any juices that have been delivered in addition to the saved lemons and their juices and cook over high heat until the stock is diminished significantly, around 5 minutes. Add the spread and parsley and cook for one more moment. Season with more legitimate salt and newly ground dark pepper to taste. Move to plates and spoon the olives, tricks, lemons and sauce on top.
4. Present with sautéed spinach, kale or Swiss chard as an afterthought.

706. Greek pesto Corkscrew

Prep Time: *15 Minutes* *Cook Time:* *20 Minutes* *Servings: 4*

INGREDIENTS

- 4-medium zucchini (about 2-pieces), trimmed
- An example of this has been described
- 2 cups have fresh, fresh
- ¼ cup of pine nuts, toasted
- ¼ ½ dug Parmesan cheese
- 1/4 plus 2-tablespoons extra-virgin olive oil, divided
- 2-tablespoons lemon juice
- 1-large clove garnish, sure
- ½ teaspoon ground pepper
- $ 1, as is known, but in 1-inch versions

DIRECTIONS

1. Use a spiral vegetable cutter to cut zucchini lengthwise into long, thin pieces. Give up the rest, and things won't be that long there. Place the zucchini in a colander and this with a quarter of the repeat. Let it dry for 15 to 30 minutes, and then squeeze gently to eliminate any excess liquid.
2. Meanwhile, add basil, pine nuts, Parmesan cheese, 1/4 cup oil, lemon juice, garlic, pepper, and 1/4 teaspoon salt in a mini food processor. Process until almost smooth.
3. Heat 1 tablespoon oil in a huge skillet or medium-high heat. Add chicken in another layer; Use the last 1/4 teaspoon of salt. I understand it will take about 5 minutes. Take a large bowl and eat it in 3 tablespoons of the meal.
4. Add the last 1-tablespoon oil to the pan. Add the drained zucchini noodles, and it's just about 2 to 3 minutes.

707. Greek Fruits and Veggies for women

Prep Time: *15 Minutes* *Cook Time:* *35 Minutes* *Servings: 4*

INGREDIENTS:

- 1 Cauliflower
- 1 bell pepper
- 1 cup mushroom slices, fresh
- 1 cup asparagus, chopped
- 1 tbsp. Olive oil

DIRECTIONS:

1. Preheat the oven to 400 ° F (205 ° C). Cover a baking tray with a silicone mat (or foil or baking paper).
2. Cut your cauliflower and bell pepper into equal sized pieces.
3. Slice your mushrooms and chop your asparagus.
4. Drizzle all your vegetables with olive oil.
5. Spread cauliflower, bell pepper, and mushrooms on baking tray. Don't crowd them and leave room for asparagus.
6. Bake for 10 minutes.
7. Stir / turn the vegetables and add asparagus to the pan.
8. Bake for 15 minutes, stir / turn again (after about 7 minutes).
9. Comments
10. The roasting times of vegetables are not 100% reliable. The larger the pieces, the longer it takes to cook.
11. If you want crispier roasted vegetables, shorten the roasting time by a few minutes. If you want softer roasted vegetables, increase the roasting time by up to 10 minutes (except asparagus, which should increase by up to 5 minutes).

708. Chicken Meatballs and Cauliflower Rice with Coconut Herb Sauce

Prep Time: *15 Minutes* *Cook Time:* *43 Minutes* *Servings: 6*

INGREDIENTS:

- **MEATBALLS**
- Non-stick spray
- 1-tablespoon of extra virgin olive oil
- ½ red onion
- 2-cloves of garlic, chopped
- 1 pound of ground chicken
- ¼ cup of chopped fresh parsley
- 1-tablespoon of Dijon mustard
- ¾ teaspoon of kosher salt
- ½ teaspoon of freshly ground black pepper

- **SAUCE**
- A 14-ounce of coconut milk
- 1¼ cups of chopped fresh parsley, divided
- 4-spring onions, roughly chopped
- 1-clove of garlic, peeled and crushed
- Peel and juice one lemon
- Kosher salt and freshly ground black pepper
- Red pepper flakes, to serve
- One recipe Cauliflower rice

DIRECTIONS:

1. MAKE THE MEATBALLS: Preheat oven to 375 ° F. Line a baking tray with aluminum foil and spray with nonstick cooking spray.
2. In a medium skillet, heat the olive oil over medium heat. Add the onion and sauté until tender, about 5 minutes. Add the garlic and sauté until fragrant, about 1 minute.
3. Transfer the onion and garlic to a medium bowl and allow cooling slightly. Stir in chicken, parsley, and mustard; Season with salt and pepper. Shape the mixture into two tablespoons large balls and place on the baking tray.
4. Fry the meatballs until firm and cooked for 17 to 20 minutes.
5. MAKE THE SAUCE: In the bowl of a food processor, combine the coconut milk, parsley, spring onions, garlic, lemon zest, and lemon juice and mix until smooth; Season with salt and pepper.
6. Sprinkle the meatballs with the red pepper flakes and the rest of the parsley. Serve over the cauliflower rice with the sauce.

709. Greek Whole Roasted Red Snapper with Potatoes and Onions

Prep Time: *15 Minutes* *Cook Time:* *30 Minutes* *Servings: 6*

Ingredients

- 1 ½ cups approximately pressed new level leaf parsley leaves
- 1 medium shallot (around 2 oz.), generally chopped
- 3 garlic cloves, generally chopped
- 1 tablespoon new thyme leaves
- 1 ½ teaspoons lemon zing (from 1 lemon)
- ½ teaspoon squashed red pepper
- ¾ cup olive oil
- 2 ¾ teaspoons legitimate salt, separated
- 1 pound child gold potatoes (around 8 potatoes)
- 1 little red onion (around 8 oz.), cut the long way into 1-in. wedges
- 1 (3-lb.) entire red snapper, cleaned, scaled, gutted, and blades managed
- Lemon wedges, for serving

Directions

1. Preheat oven to 425°F. Line a rimmed heating sheet with material paper. Put in a safe spot.
2. Cycle parsley, shallot, garlic, thyme, lemon zing, and red pepper in a food processor until finely chopped, around 15 seconds. Add oil, and interaction until very much fused, around 15 seconds. Throw together potatoes, onion wedges, 2 tablespoons of the parsley combination, and 1 teaspoon of the salt in an enormous bowl.
3. Cut 3 (2-inch-long) cuts askew on the two sides of fish, slicing right deep down on the two sides. Rub outside and within cuts with 1 cup of the parsley blend and staying 1 3/4 teaspoons salt; place fish on arranged heating sheet. Spread potato blend around fish. Prepare in preheated oven until fish is murky and flaky and vegetables are delicate, around 30 minutes.
4. Shower fish with remaining 1/4 cup parsley combination. Present with lemon wedges.

710. Greek Caprese Tomato, Mozzarella, Basil, And Avocado Salad

Prep Time: *15 Minutes* *Cook Time:* *35 Minutes* *Servings: 2*

INGREDIENTS

- 2-sliced avocados
- 2-ripe tomatoes
- 500 g mozzarella cheese
- 1 cup of fresh basil leaves
- 1/4 cup of olive oil
- 1/4 cup of Balsamic Aceto
- Salt and ground black pepper

DIRECTION

1. Gather all the ingredients to make this tomato, mozzarella, basil, and avocado Caprese salad.
2. Cut the tomato stem with a small knife and cut the tomatoes into slices with a serrated knife.
3. Slice the mozzarella and spot alternating slices of avocado, tomato, mozzarella, and basil in signature dishes. Slice with olive oil and balsamic vinegar and season with salt and ground black pepper.
4. Divide your Italian tomato, mozzarella, basil, and avocado salad with a fresh baguette or on a bed of romaine lettuce.

711. Greek Meat Loaf Cordon Bleu

Prep Time: *15 Minutes* *Cook Time:* *30 Minutes* *Servings: 2*

Ingredients

- 1 big egg, beaten
- 1 envelope meat portion preparing blend
- 1/2 cup pureed tomatoes
- 2 cups delicate bread scraps
- 2 pounds lean ground hamburger
- 8 slight cuts completely cooked ham
- 8 slight cuts Swiss cheddar
- 1 can (4 ounces) cut mushrooms

Directions

1. Preheat oven to 350°. In an enormous bowl, combine as one egg, meat portion preparing, pureed tomatoes and bread pieces. Add ground meat; blend well. On a piece of waxed paper, pat meat combination into a 18x9-in. square shape. Top with layers of ham, cheddar and mushrooms. Move square shape, jam move style, beginning from limited end. Squeeze edges to seal. Spot crease side down in a shallow preparing skillet. Prepare until no pink remaining parts, around 1-1/4 hours. Let stand a few minutes prior to cutting.
2. Freeze choice: Securely wrap and freeze cooled meat portion in foil. To utilize, partially defrost in cooler short-term. Open up meat portion; reheat on a lubed

15x10x1-in. preparing dish in a preheated 350° oven until heated through and a thermometer embedded in focus peruses 165°.

3. To make delicate bread morsels, attack pieces and spot in a food processor or blender. Cover and heart beat until scraps structure. One cut of bread yields 1/2 to 3/4 cup morsels.

712. Smoked Gouda Veggie Melt

Prep Time: 15 Minutes | *Cook Time: 60 Minutes* | *Servings: 4*

Ingredients

- 1 cup chopped fresh mushrooms
- 1 cup chopped fresh broccoli
- 1 medium sweet red pepper, chopped
- 1 small onion, chopped
- 2 tablespoons olive oil
- 8 slices Italian bread (1/2 inch thick)
- 1/2 cup mayonnaise
- 1 garlic clove, minced
- 1 cup shredded smoked Gouda cheese

Directions

1. Firstly preheat oven to 425°. Place mushrooms, broccoli, pepper and onion in a greased 15x10x1-in. baking pan. Drizzle with oil; toss to coat. Then roast 10-12 minutes or until tender.
2. Meanwhile, put bread slices on a baking sheet. Mix mayonnaise and garlic; spread over bread.
3. Change oven setting to broil. Spoon vegetables over bread slices; drizzle with cheese. Broil 3-4 in from heat 2-3 minutes or until cheese is melted.

713. Greek Mini Meat Loaf Sheet-Pan Meal

Prep Time: 15 Minutes | *Cook Time: 45 Minutes* | *Servings: 2*

Ingredients

- 2 huge eggs, delicately beaten
- 1 cup tomato juice
- 3/4 cup speedy cooking oats
- 1/4 cup finely chopped onion
- 1/2 teaspoon salt
- 1-1/2 pounds lean ground meat (90% lean)
- 1/4 cup ketchup
- 3 tablespoons brown sugar
- 1 teaspoon arranged mustard
- 1/4 teaspoon ground nutmeg
- 3 huge potatoes, stripped and cut into 1/2-inch pieces
- 3 tablespoons olive oil, separated
- 1/2 teaspoon garlic salt, separated
- 1/4 teaspoon pepper, separated
- 1 pound new asparagus, managed and split

Directions

1. Preheat oven to 425°. In a huge bowl, consolidate eggs, tomato juice, oats, onion and salt. Add meat; blend daintily however completely. Shape into six 4x2-1/2-in. portions; place on a sheet dish or huge shallow cooking skillet. Join ketchup, brown sugar, mustard and nutmeg; brush over portions.
2. Consolidate potatoes with 2 tablespoons oil, 1/4 teaspoon garlic salt and 1/8 teaspoon pepper; throw to cover. Add to dish in a solitary layer. Prepare 25 minutes.
3. Consolidate asparagus with staying 1 tablespoon oil, 1/4 teaspoon garlic salt and 1/8 teaspoon pepper; throw to cover. Add to dish. Prepare until a thermometer embedded into meat portions peruses 160° and vegetables are delicate, 15-20 minutes. Let stand 5-10 minutes prior to serving.

714. Greek Seafood Couscous Paella

Prep Time: 15 Minutes | *Cook Time: 30 Minutes* | *Servings: 4*

Ingredients

- Ingredient Checklist
- 2 teaspoons extra-virgin olive oil
- 1 medium onion, chopped
- 1 clove garlic, minced
- ½ teaspoon dried thyme
- ½ teaspoon fennel seed
- ¼ teaspoon salt
- ¼ teaspoon freshly ground pepper
- Pinch of crumbled saffron threads
- 1 cup no-salt-added diced tomatoes, with juice
- ¼ cup vegetable broth
- 4 ounces bay scallops, tough muscle removed
- 4 ounces small shrimp, (41-50 per pound), peeled and deveined
- ½ cup whole-wheat couscous

DIRECTIONS:

1. Heat oil in a large saucepan over medium heat. Add onion; cook, stirring constantly, for 3 minutes. Add garlic, thyme, fennel seed, salt, pepper and saffron; cook for 20 seconds.
2. Stir in tomatoes and broth. Bring to a simmer. Cover, reduce heat and simmer for 2 minutes.
3. Increase heat to medium, stir in scallops and cook, stirring occasionally, for 2 minutes. Add shrimp and cook, stirring occasionally, for 2 minutes more. Stir in couscous. Cover, remove from heat and let stand for 5 minutes; fluff.

715. Mediterranean Baked Feta Pizza

Prep Time: 15 Minutes | *Cook Time: 50 Minutes* | *Servings: 6*

Ingredients

- Pizza Dough (alternatively, you can use a premade dough*)
- 1-1/4 cups bread flour (175 grams) I recommend weighing the flour for better accuracy
- 1/2 teaspoon instant dry yeast
- 1/2 teaspoon salt
- 1/2 cup warm water (110F)
- 1/2 teaspoon olive oil
- Prepared Feta + Toppings
- 1 pt. cherry tomatoes
- 1 tablespoon finely chopped shallot
- 2 medium entire cloves garlic, stripped
- 2 tablespoons olive oil
- 1 (8 oz.) block feta cheddar
- 1/4 teaspoon red pepper chips (discretionary)
- Legitimate salt and pepper to taste
- 1/2 cup shredded low-dampness mozzarella cheddar
- 1/4 cup split Kalamata olives
- 1/4 cup jostled artichoke hearts, generally chopped and wiped off
- 1/4 cup jostled broiled red peppers, daintily cut into strips
- Small bunch new basil leaves

Directions

1. Pizza Dough
2. In a huge bowl, join flour, yeast, and salt. Shower water and 1/2 teaspoon olive oil up and over and mix with a wooden spoon until mixture meets up and no dashes of flour remain. Cover with saran wrap and let batter rest 15 minutes.
3. Eliminate batter from bowl and turn onto a softly floured surface. Ply mixture 3-5 minutes until smooth and flexible. Spot into a lubed bowl, going once to oil the top and cover with cling wrap and let rise 3-4 hours at room temperature until multiplied in size (or 24-72 hours in the refrigerator – in the event that you decide to cool the batter, let it come to room temperature 45 minutes prior to carrying out)
4. Heated Feta + Toppings
5. Preheat oven to 400F. In a 8×8 heating dish, throw tomatoes, shallot, and garlic with olive oil until equally covered. Structure a space in the focal point of skillet and spot feta in the middle. Turn the feta to equally cover in olive oil. Top with red pepper chips, salt, and pepper to taste.
6. Spot feta on center rack of oven. In the event that you have a pizza stone, place on base rack to start preheating. Prepare feta at 400F 35-40 minutes until tomatoes are blasting and feta is a profound brilliant brown. Eliminate feta from oven, increment oven temperature to 500F and move pizza stone to center rack. Utilize a spoon to squash feta, tomatoes, and garlic until a semi-thick sauce structures.
7. In the event that using pizza stone strategy, gently dust a pizza strip with cornmeal. If not using stone, softly oil a huge heating sheet with olive oil (regardless of whether you're not using a stone, preheat your oven per formula directions above)
8. Punch risen pizza mixture down and turn onto a gently floured surface. Carry pizza mixture out to a 10-12 inch circle. Move to pizza strip or arranged preparing sheet.
9. Uniformly spread around 3/4 cup squashed feta blend on top of hull (save any excess feta for another utilization) Top with mozzarella cheddar, olives, artichokes, and broiled red peppers. In the case of using pizza stone, cautiously move pizza from the strip to the stone. In the case of using heating sheet, place sheet in oven.
10. Prepare pizza at 500F 10-12 minutes, turning once part of the way through heating, until covering and cheddar is a profound brilliant brown. Sprinkle pizza with new basil and let stand 3-5 minutes prior to cutting into wedges and serving hot. Enjoy!

716. Instant Pot Spaghetti Squash with Garlic and Parmesan

Prep Time: 15 Minutes | *Cook Time: 45 Minutes* | *Servings: 6*

Ingredients

- 1 large spaghetti squash
- 3 tablespoons olive oil
- 8 cloves Garlic, cut meagerly
- 1 teaspoon red pepper drops
- ½ cup fragmented almonds, or different nuts of decision
- 4 cups new spinach, chopped
- 1 teaspoon Kosher Salt
- 1 cup shredded parmesan cheddar
- 1.5 cups water, for the Instant Pot

Guidelines

1. Using the tip of a sharp, short blade, penetrate the spaghetti squash in 7-8 spots.
2. Put 1.5 cups of water into the Instant Pot. Spot a liner rack into the pot. Spot the penetrated spaghetti squash on the rack.
3. Close the top and set the Instant Pot to cook on HIGH PRESSURE for 7 minutes. Toward the finish of the cooking time, permit the pot to rest undisturbed for 10 minutes.
4. Eliminate the squash and cut it open longwise, so you can have long spaghetti-like strands. Set aside half for another utilization.
5. Drag a fork along the squash to get long strands of spaghetti squash. Measure out 4 cups and put the rest in a safe spot for another utilization (like eating constantly at any pardon.) Save the squash shell since you will serve your exquisite creation in it.
6. Void out the Instant Pot and wipe dry.
7. Press Sauté. At the point when the pot is hot, add oil. To the hot oil, add garlic, red pepper, and fragmented almonds or pine nuts. Toast for 1 moment without allowing the garlic to consume. Include the spinach and salt and mix.
8. Include spaghetti squash.
9. Sprinkle with parmesan cheddar not long prior to serving.
10. Tips And Tricks For Making Garlic Parmesan Spaghetti Squash
11. Try not to hold back on flavorings. This formula is about the seasoned oil and the cheddar, so don't hold back on all things considered.
12. Bend over. I request that you utilize a large portion of the squash in this formula, obviously, you can generally utilize every last bit of it and twofold the wide range of various ingredients.
13. Tips and Tricks. See the notes above on the best way to make Spaghetti squash in your Instant Pot. It has a great deal of tips and deceives that will make this simpler for you.
14. Minor departure from This Delicious Spaghetti Squash Recipe
15. Use pine nuts rather than almonds
16. Add ½ cup of cranberries to the hot oil alongside the garlic and red peppers
17. Add simmered cherry tomatoes to the completed dish
18. Use feta cheddar rather than shredded parmesan.
19. Add ¼ cup of chopped new basil alongside the spaghetti squash.
20. Add tomatoes or cranberries. You can likewise add cherry tomatoes or cranberries to this formula for somewhat fly of shading and taste.

717. The Best Greek Instant Pot Chicken Tikka Masala

Prep Time: *15 Minutes* | *Cook Time:* *20 Minutes* | *Servings: 6*

INGREDIENTS

- 1 large spaghetti squash
- 3 tablespoons olive oil
- 8 cloves Garlic, cut meagerly
- 1 teaspoon red pepper drops
- ½ cup fragmented almonds, or different nuts of decision
- 4 cups new spinach, chopped
- 1 teaspoon Kosher Salt
- 1 cup shredded parmesan cheddar
- 1.5 cups water, for the Instant Pot

Directions

1. Using the tip of a sharp, short blade, puncture the spaghetti squash in 7-8 spots.
2. Put 1.5 cups of water into the Instant Pot. Spot a liner rack into the pot. Spot the penetrated spaghetti squash on the rack.
3. Close the top and set the Instant Pot to cook on HIGH PRESSURE for 7 minutes. Toward the finish of the cooking time, permit the pot to rest undisturbed for 10 minutes.
4. Eliminate the squash and cut it open longwise, with the goal that you can have long spaghetti-like strands. Set aside half for another utilization.
5. Drag a fork along the squash to get long strands of spaghetti squash. Measure out 4 cups and put the rest in a safe spot for another utilization (like eating constantly at any pardon.) Save the squash shell since you will serve your exquisite creation in it.
6. Void out the Instant Pot and wipe dry.
7. Press Sauté. At the point when the pot is hot, add oil. To the hot oil, add garlic, red pepper, and fragmented almonds or pine nuts. Toast for 1 moment without allowing the garlic to consume. Include the spinach and salt and mix.
8. Include spaghetti squash.
9. Sprinkle with parmesan cheddar not long prior to serving.
10. Tips And Tricks For Making Garlic Parmesan Spaghetti Squash
11. Try not to hold back on flavorings. This formula is about the enhanced oil and the cheddar, so don't hold back on all things considered.
12. Bend over. I request that you utilize a large portion of the squash in this formula, obviously, you can generally utilize every last bit of it and twofold the wide range of various ingredients.
13. Tips and Tricks. See the notes above on the most proficient method to make Spaghetti squash in your Instant Pot. It has a ton of tips and deceives that will make this simpler for you.
14. Minor departure from This Delicious Spaghetti Squash Recipe
15. Use pine nuts rather than almonds
16. Add ½ cup of cranberries to the hot oil alongside the garlic and red peppers
17. Add broiled cherry tomatoes to the completed dish
18. Use feta cheddar rather than shredded parmesan.
19. Add ¼ cup of chopped new basil alongside the spaghetti squash.
20. Add tomatoes or cranberries. You can likewise add cherry tomatoes or cranberries to this formula for somewhat fly of shading and taste.

718. Instant Pot Healthy Chicken Pot Pie Soup

Prep Time: *15 Minutes* | *Cook Time:* *30 Minutes* | *Servings: 2*

INGREDIENTS

- 2 large boneless skinless chicken breasts cut into scaled down pieces
- 2 Tbsp. ghee or olive oil
- 1 onion diced, 1 cup
- 3 carrots diced, 1 cup
- 3 stems celery cut, 1 cup
- 5-6 cloves garlic minced
- 1 pound red potatoes diced
- 2 cups chicken stock or stock
- 1 cup full-fat canned coconut cream or milk
- 1 cup cashews
- 2 Tbsp. new thyme leaves
- 1/2 tsp. salt
- 1/2 tsp. dried sage
- newly broke dark pepper
- new parsley leaves chopped, for decorate

DIRECTIONS

1. Turn Instant Pot on Sauté mode. Dissolve ghee in the pot, at that point add onion, carrots, and celery, mixing routinely. Cook until onions are delicate, at that point add garlic and cook, mixing continually, until fragrant, around 30 seconds to 1 moment.
2. Add potatoes, chicken stock, chicken, dried sage, and new thyme to Instant Pot. Secure cover with the valve in Sealing position and cook Manual High Pressure for 10 minutes.
3. In the interim, add coconut milk and cashews to a rapid blender. Mix until incredibly, smooth.
4. At the point when time is up, Quick Release, at that point mix in the coconut-cashew combination and add salt and newly broke dark pepper to taste.

Dessert Recipes

719. Lemon Madeleines

Prep Time: *15 Minutes* | *Cook Time:* *30 Minutes* | *Servings: 2*

Ingredients:

- 4oz butter, melted
- 1 cup all-purpose flour
- ½ cup whole wheat flour
- 1 teaspoon baking powder
- 3 eggs
- 2 egg yolks
- ½ cup sugar
- 2 teaspoons lemon zest
- 2 tablespoons lemon juice
- 1 pinch of salt

Directions:

1. In a bowl, mix the flours with a pinch of salt and baking powder.
2. In another bowl, combine the eggs with the egg yolks, sugar, lemon zest, and lemon juice, then mix it with an electric mixer until creamy, fluffy and pale in colour. It will take about 5 minutes. Add the melted butter, then carefully fold in the flour. It is best to use a spatula for this step to prevent the eggs from deflating.
3. Grease a madeleine pan with butter and sprinkle it with flour. Fill the madeleine cups with batter, then bake in the preheated oven at 400F for 10-15 minutes, depending on the oven. They should be turning golden brown. Put off the pan from the oven and turn it upside down on your working surface. Gently tap it on the bottom to release all the madeleines, then sprinkle them with plenty of powdered sugar.

720. Limoncello Loaf

Prep Time: *15 Minutes* | *Cook Time:* *35 Minutes* | *Servings: 2*

Ingredients:

- 6 oz butter, room temperature
- 1 cup sugar
- ½ cup Limoncello liqueur
- 5 eggs
- 2 cups all-purpose white flour
- 1 cup whole wheat flour
- 3 teaspoons baking powder
- 1 pinch of salt
- 1 cup low-fat milk
- 2 tablespoons lemon zest

Directions:

1. 2Cream the butter as well as sugar in a bowl until creamy and pale in colour. Stir in the Limoncello liqueur then the eggs, one by one. Mix well until fully incorporated. Add the flours sifted with salt and baking powder, alternating with the milk. In the end, fold in the lemons zest and spoon the batter into 2 loaf pans lined with baking paper. Bake in the before heated oven at 350F for 30-40 minutes.
2. When complete, take the pan out of the oven and let the cakes cool in the pan before dusting with powdered sugar.

721. Lemon and Ricotta Tiramisu

Prep Time: *15 Minutes* | *Cook Time:* *30 Minutes* | *Servings: 2*

Ingredients:

- 2 cups water
- ¾ cup sugar
- 2 tablespoons lemon zest
- juice from 1 lemon
- 2 pounds ladyfingers
- 30oz low-fat ricotta cheese
- 1 tablespoon lemon zest
- 2 tablespoons lemon juice
- 4 tablespoons Limoncello
- 1 cup powdered sugar
- 1 cup whipped cream

Directions:

1. Combine the ricotta cheese with the grated lemon zest, lemon juice, sugar and 4 tablespoons of Limoncello In a bowl.
2. To make the syrup, mix the water with the sugar and simmer on low heat for 5 minutes then add the lemon juice and zest and remove from heat. Let it cool at 25 degrees, then strain.
3. To make the cake, dip each ladyfinger shortly in the lemon syrup and arrange them on the bottom of a loaf pan lined with plastic wrap. Top with a layer of ricotta cheese and a layer of whipped cream. Add another layer of ladyfingers and continue layering the ricotta, cream and ladyfingers until you run out. Make sure the top layer is ladyfingers.
4. Refrigerate the tiramisu for a minimum of 4 hours, then turn it upside down on a serving plate. Decorate with whipped cream and lemon rind shavings.

722. Lemon Soufflés

Prep Time: *15 Minutes* | *Cook Time:* *45 Minutes* | *Servings: 4*

Ingredients:

- 1 oz butter, softened
- ½ cup sugar
- 8 egg yolks
- 10 egg whites
- 2 tablespoons flour
- ¼ cup lemon juice
- 2 tablespoons lemon zest
- 1 cup low-fat milk

Directions:

1. Mix the egg yolks with the flour, lemon zest, and half of the sugar in a bowl. Set aside.
2. Add the milk into a saucepan and bring to a boil. Gradually pour it over the egg yolk mixture, whisking all the time. Transfer the mixture back into the saucepan and cook over medium heat until thick and creamy, whisking all the time to prevent it from sticking to the pan. When complete, remove from heat and add the lemon juice and butter. Set aside.
3. In a clean bowl, whip the egg whites until stiff, then add the other half of sugar and keep whipping until a glossy, stiff meringue forms. Gently fold this meringue into the egg yolk cream.
4. Grease 8 ramekins with butter and sprinkle them with flour. Fill each ramekin with batter and level them up. Clean the edges and bake the soufflés in the preheated oven at 375F for 10-15 minutes. Do not open the oven door to check them, as any air inside the oven before they are done will deflate them.
5. When done, serve them immediately powdered with sugar. The longer you wait, the more they will deflate and stop being as impressive.

723. Lemon and Chia Biscotti

Prep Time: *15 Minutes* | *Cook Time:* *55 Minutes* | *Servings: 2*

Ingredients:

- 2 cups whole wheat flour
- 1 teaspoon baking powder
- 1 pinch of salt
- ½ cup coconut milk
- 2 tablespoons chia seeds
- 2 oz butter, softened
- ½ cup brown sugar
- 1 teaspoon lemon zest
- ½ cup hazelnuts, chopped
- 1 pinch of salt

Directions:

- Combine the flour as well as the baking powder and a pinch of salt In a bowl. In another bowl, combine the coconut milk with the chia seeds and set them aside.
- Mix the butter with the sugar until creamy, then add the coconut milk and chia seeds, followed by the lemon zest. Gradually incorporate the flour, then fold in the chopped hazelnuts. Transfer the dough to a baking tray and shape it into a log. Bake in the preheated oven at 350F for 30-40 minutes or until golden brown. Remove from the oven, let it cool for 10 minutes, then using a sharp knife, cut it into ½-inch thick slices. Arrange them all on the baking tray, cut facing up and keep cooking them 20 more minutes until crisp and dry.

Mediterranean Diet For Children / Kids

Breakfast & Brunch Recipes

724. Creamy Panini

Prep Time: *5 Minutes* | *Cook Time:* *12 Minutes* | *Servings: 4*

INGREDIENTS:

- ¼ mug chopped basil leaves
- ½ mug mayonnaise dressing with Olive Oil divided eight slices whole-wheat bread four slices of bacon
- 1 zucchini, thinly sliced
- 4 slices provolone cheese
- 7 oz. roasted red peppers, sliced

DIRECTIONS:

1. In a container, combine olives, basil, and ¼ mug of mayonnaise; evenly spread the mayonnaise batter on the bread slices and layer 4 slices with bacon, zucchini, provolone, and peppers.
2. Top it with some bread slices and spread the remaining ¼ mug of mayonnaise on the outside of the sandwiches; cook over medium flame for about 4 mins, turning once, until cheese is melted & the sandwiches get golden brown.

725. *Breakfast* Couscous

Prep Time: *5 Minutes* | *Cook Time:* *6 Minutes* | *Servings: 2*

INGREDIENTS:

- 1 (2-inch) cinnamon stick
- 3 cups 1% low-fat milk
- 1 mug whole-wheat couscous (uncooked
- 6 tsp. dark brown sugar, divided
- ¼ mug dried currants
- ½ mug chopped apricots (dried)
- ¼ tsp. sea salt
- 4 tsp. melted butter, divided

DIRECTIONS:

1. Place a saucepan on the burner. Keep heat medium to high. Combine cinnamon stick and milk; flame for about 3 mins (do not boil).
2. Transfer the pan from flame and stir in couscous, 4 teaspoons of sugar, currants, apricots, and sea salt. Cover the batter and stand it for at least 15 mins.
3. Discard the cinnamon stick and divide the couscous among four containers; top each serving with ½ teaspoon of sugar and 1 teaspoon of melted butter. Serve immediately.

726. Potato and Chickpea Hash

Prep Time: *5 Minutes* | *Cook Time:* *7 Minutes* | *Servings: 4*

INGREDIENTS:

- 4 cups shredded frozen hash brown potatoes
- 1 tbsp. freshly minced ginger
- ½ mug chopped onion
- 2 cups chopped baby spinach
- 1 tbsp. Curry powder
- ½ tsp. sea salt
- ¼ mug olive oil
- 1 mug chopped zucchini
- 1 (15-ounce) chickpeas, rinsed
- 4 large eggs

DIRECTIONS:

1. In a large container, combine the potatoes, ginger, onion, spinach, curry powder, and sea salt.
2. In a nonstick skillet set over medium to high heat, add olive oil and the potato mixture.
3. Press the batter into a layer and cook for about 5 mins, without stirring, or until golden brown and crispy.
4. Lower flame to medium-low and fold in zucchini and chickpeas, breaking up the batter until just combined.
5. Stir briefly, press the batter back into a layer, and make four wells.
6. Break one egg into each indentation.
7. Cook it for about 5 mins or until eggs are set.

727. Avocado Toast

Prep Time: *5 Minutes* | *Cook Time:* *12 Minutes* | *Servings: 4*

INGREDIENTS:

- 2 ripe avocados, peeled
- A squeeze of lemon juice, to taste
- 2 tbsp. freshly chopped mint, plus extra to garnish Sea salt and black pepper, to taste
- 4 large slices of rye bread
- 80 grams soft feta, crumbled

DIRECTIONS:

1. In a medium container, mash the avocado roughly with a fork; add lemon juice and mint and continue mashing until combined—season with black pepper and salt to taste.
2. Grill or toast bread until golden.
3. Spread about ¼ of the avocado batter onto each slice of the toasted bread and top with feta.
4. Garnish with extra mint and serve immediately.

728. Mediterranean Pancakes

Prep Time: *5 Minutes* | *Cook Time:* *20 Minutes* | *Servings: 2*

INGREDIENTS:

- 1 old-fashioned mug oats
- ½ mug all-purpose flour
- 2 tbsp. flax seeds
- 1 tsp. Baking soda
- ¼ tsp. sea salt
- 2 tbsp. olive oil
- 2 large eggs
- 2 cups nonfat plain Greek yogurt
- 2 tbsp. raw honey
- Fresh fruit, syrup, or other topping

DIRECTIONS:

1. In a blender, combine oats, flour, flax seeds, baking *soda*, and sea salt; blend for about 30 seconds.
2. Add olive oil, eggs, yogurt, and honey, and continue pulsing until very smooth.
3. Let the batter stand for twenty mins or until thick.
4. Set a large nonstick skillet over medium flame and brush with olive oil.
5. In batches, ladle the batter by quarter-cupfuls into the skillet.
6. Cook the pancakes for about 2 mins or until bubbles form and golden brown.
7. Turn them over and cook the other sides for 2 mins until it gets golden brown.
8. Put these cooked pancakes on a baking sheet and keep warm in the oven.
9. Serve with favorite toppings.

729. Mediterranean Frittata

Prep Time: *5 Minutes* | *Cook Time:* *7 Minutes* | *Servings: 6*

INGREDIENTS:

- 3 tbsp. olive oil, divided
- 1 mug chopped onion
- 2 cloves garlic, minced
- 8 eggs, beaten
- ¼ mug half-and-half, milk or light cream
- ½ mug sliced Kalamata olives
- ½ mug roasted red sweet peppers, chopped ½ mug crumbled feta cheese ⅛ tsp. black pepper
- ¼ cup basil
- 2 tbsp. Parmesan cheese, finely shredded
- ½ mug coarsely crushed onion-and-garlic leaves, to garnish

DIRECTIONS:

1. Preflame your broiler.
2. Flame 2 tbsps of olive oil in a broiler-proof skillet set over medium heat; sauté onion and garlic for a few mins or until tender.
3. In the meantime, beat eggs and half-and-half in a container until well combined. Stir in olives, roasted sweet pepper, feta cheese, black

pepper, and basil. Pour the egg batter over the sautéed onion batter and cook until almost set.
4. With a spatula, lift the egg batter to allow the uncooked part to flow underneath.
5. Continue cooking for 2 mins more or until the set.
6. Combine the remaining olive oil, Parmesan cheese, and crushed croutons in a container; sprinkle the batter over the frittata and broil for about 5 mins or until the crumbs are golden and the top is set.
7. Garnish with basil and serve.

730. Mediterranean Veggie Om

Prep Time: *5 Minutes* | *Cook Time:* *10 Minutes* | *Servings: 2*

INGREDIENTS:

- 1 tbsp. olive oil
- 2 cups thinly sliced fennel bulb
- ¼ mug chopped artichoke hearts, soaked in water, drained ¼ mug pitted green olives, brine-cured, chopped 1Roma tomato
- 6 eggs
- ¼ tsp. Sea salt
- ½ tsp. freshly ground black pepper
- ½ mug goat cheese, crumbled
- 2 tbsp. freshly chopped parsley, dill, or basil

DIRECTIONS:

1. Preflame your oven to 325°F.
2. Flame olive oil in an ovenproof skillet over medium heat.
3. Sauté fennel for about 5 mins or until tender.
4. Add artichoke hearts, olives, and tomatoes and cook for 3mins ore or until softened.
5. In a container, beat the eggs; season with sea salt and pepper.
6. Add the egg batter over the vegetables and stir for about 2 mins.
7. Sprinkle cheese over the omelet and bake in the oven for about 5 mins or until set and cooked through.
8. Top with parsley, dill, or basil
9. Transfer the omelet onto a cutting board, carefully cut into four wedges, and serve immediately.

731. Garlicky Scrambled Eggs

Prep Time: *5 Minutes* | *Cook Time:* *24 Minutes* | *Servings: 4*

INGREDIENTS:

- ½ tsp. Olive oil
- ½ mug ground beef
- ½ tsp. garlic powder
- 3 eggs
- Salt
- Pepper

DIRECTIONS:

1. Set a medium-sized pan over medium heat.
2. Add olive oil and flame until hot but not smoking.
3. Stir in ground beef and cook for about 10 mins or until almost done.
4. Stir in garlic and sauté for about 2 mins.
5. In a large container, beat the eggs until almost frothy; season with salt and pepper.
6. Add the egg batter to the pan with the cooked beef and scramble until ready.
7. Serve with toasted bread and olives for a healthy, satisfying breakfast!

732. Healthy Breakfast Casserol

Prep Time: *5 Minutes* | *Cook Time:* *20 Minutes* | *Servings: 6*

INGREDIENTS:

- 2 tbsp. olive oil, divided
- ½ a medium-sized onion, diced
- 2 medium-sized yellow potatoes. diced
- 1 lb. zucchini, sliced
- 3 portabella mushroom caps, diced
- 150g torn spinach
- 200g ricotta
- 200g light ricotta cheese
- 2 cups of egg whites
- 12 grape tomatoes, sliced into⅓ pieces
- 3 peeled and roasted peppers, sliced
- 2 sourdough rolls
- 4 tbsp. Pecorino Romano cheese, grated
- 100g skim-milk mozzarella cheese, grated

DIRECTIONS:

1. Preflame the oven to 400°F.
2. Combine together olive oil, onion, and potato and roast for at least 15 mins; transfer from the oven and keep on the baking tray.
3. In a container, combine together ½ tbsp olive oil and zucchini; toss to coat well and transfer to a baking tray.
4. Put all the vegetables to the oven and roast for about 40 mins or until golden in color.
5. In the meantime, place ½ tbsp olive oil in a pan and sauté mushrooms for about 4 mins.
6. Transfer the cooked mushrooms from the pan and set them aside.
7. Add the remaining olive oil to the pan and sauté chopped spinach until tender. In a mixing container, combine together both types of ricotta and egg whites; set aside.
8. Combine together all the vegetables, including grape tomatoes and peppers, with sourdough rolls in a 9 x 13 baking dish; top with the ricotta batter and sprinkle with pecorino and mozzarella cheese.
9. Bake for at least 40 mins or until done. Transfer from the oven, cool slightly.
10. Cut into six slices and enjoy your breakfast.

733. Egg and Sausage Breakfast Casserole

Prep Time: *5 Minutes* | *Cook Time:* *23 Minutes* | *Servings: 4*

INGREDIENTS:

The crust:

- 3 tbsp. olive oil, divided
- 2 lb. peeled and shredded russet potatoes ¾ tsp. Ground pepper ¾ tsp. salt

The casserole:

- 12 oz. chopped turkey sausage
- 4 thinly sliced green onions
- ¼ cup bell pepper
- ⅓ mug skim milk
- 6 large eggs
- 4 egg whites
- ¾ mug shredded cheddar cheese
- 16 oz. low-fat cottage cheese

DIRECTIONS:

The crust:

1. Preflame the oven to 425°F. Lightly grease a 9×13-inch baking dish with 1 tbsp. Olive oil and set aside.
2. Squeeze excess moisture out of the potato with a kitchen towel or paper towel.
3. Toss together the potatoes, the remaining olive oil, salt, and pepper in a medium container until potatoes are well coated.
4. Transfer the batter to the baking dish; evenly press the batter up the sides and on the bottom of the plate and bake for about 20 mins or until golden brown on the edges.

The casserole:

1. Reduce the oven flame to 375°F.
2. In a skillet, cook turkey sausage. Keep the flame medium-high for about 2 mins or until it's almost cooked through.
3. Add green onions & red bell pepper, continue cooking for 2 more minutes or until bell pepper is tender.
4. Whisk together skim milk, eggs, egg whites, and the cheeses.
5. Stir in turkey sausage mixture; pour over the potato crust and bake for about 50 mins. Slightly cool and cut into 12 pieces. Enjoy!

734. Yogurt Pancakes

Prep Time: *5 Minutes* | *Cook Time:* *20 Minutes* | *Servings: 2*

INGREDIENTS:

- Whole-wheat pancake mix
- 1 mug yogurt
- 1 tbsp. baking powder
- 1 tbsp. baking soda
- 1 mug skimmed milk
- 3 whole eggs
- ½ tsp. olive oil

DIRECTIONS:

1. Combine together whole-wheat pancake mix, yogurt, baking powder, baking soda, skimmed milk, and eggs in a large container. Stir until well blended.
2. Flame a pan oiled lightly with olive oil.
3. Pour ¼ mug batter onto the heated pan and cook for about 2 mins or until the surface of the pancake has some bubbles.
4. Flip & continue cooking until the lower side is browned.
5. Serve the pancakes warm with a mug of fat-free milk, or two tbsps light maple syrup.

735. Breakfast Stir Fry

Prep Time: *5 Minutes* | *Cook Time:* *20 Minutes* | *Servings: 2*

INGREDIENTS:

- 1 tbsp. olive oil
- 2 green peppers, sliced
- 2 onions, finely chopped
- 4 tomatoes, chopped
- ½ tsp. sea salt
- 1 egg

DIRECTIONS:

1. Flame olive oil in a medium-sized pan over medium-high heat.
2. Add green pepper and sauté for about 2 mins.
3. Lower flame to medium and continue cooking, covered, for 3 more mins.
4. Stir in onion and cook for about 2 mins or until brown.
5. Stir in tomatoes and salt. Over and simmer to get a soft juicy mixture.
6. In a container, beat the egg, drizzle over the tomato batter and cook for about 1 minute. (Don't stir).

7. Serve with chopped cucumbers, feta cheese, and black olives for a great breakfast!

736. Greek Breakfast Pitas

Prep Time: 5 Minutes *Cook Time: 20 Minutes* *Servings: 4*

INGREDIENTS:

- ¼ mug chopped onion
- ¼ mug sweet red/black pepper, chopped
- 1 large mug egg
- ⅛ tsp. Sea salt
- ⅛ tsp. black pepper
- 1 ½ tsp. basil, ground
- ½ mug baby spinach, freshly torn
- 1 red tomato, sliced
- 2 pita bread, whole
- 2 tbsp. feta cheese, crumbled

DIRECTIONS:

1. Coat a sizeable nonstick skillet with cooking spray and set over medium heat.
2. Add onions and red peppers and sauté for at least 3 mins.
3. In a container, beat together egg, pepper, and salt and add the butter to the skillet.
4. Cook, stirring continuously, until ready.
5. Spoon basil, spinach, and tomatoes onto the pitas and top with the egg mixture.
6. Sprinkle with feta and serve.

737. Healthy Breakfast Scramble

Prep Time: 5 Minutes *Cook Time: 20 Minutes* *Servings: 2*

INGREDIENTS:

- 1 tsp. olive
- 4 medium green onions, chopped
- 1 tsp. Dried basil leaves or 1 tbsp. basil leaves, chopped
- 1 medium tomato, chopped
- 4 eggs
- Freshly ground pepper

DIRECTIONS:

1. In a medium nonstick skillet, flame olive oil over medium heat; sauté green onions, occasionally stirring, for about 2 mins.
2. Stir in basil and tomato and let cook, occasionally stirring, for about 1 minute or until the tomato is cooked through.
3. In a container, thoroughly beat the eggs with a wire whisk or a fork and pour over the tomato mixture; cook for about 2 mins.
4. Gently lift the cooked parts with a spatula to allow the uncooked parts to flow to the bottom.
5. Cook for about three minutes.
6. Season with pepper and serve.

738. Easy Muesli recipe

Prep Time: 15 Minutes *Cook Time:□150 Minutes* *Servings: 2*

INGREDIENTS

- 3 1/2 cups moved oats
- 1/2 cup wheat grain
- 1/2 teaspoon fit salt
- 1/2 teaspoon ground cinnamon
- 1/2 cup cut almonds
- 1/4 cup crude walnuts, coarsely chopped
- 1/4 cup crude pepitas (shelled pumpkin seeds)
- 1/2 cup unsweetened coconut drops
- 1/4 cup dried apricots, coarsely chopped
- 1/4 cup dried cherries
- Estimating cups and spoons
- Enormous rimmed heating sheet
- Enormous bowl
- Enormous hermetically sealed holder, for putting away

DIRECTIONS:

1. Toast the grains, nuts, and seeds. Mastermind 2 racks to partition the oven into thirds and heat to 350°F. Spot the oats, wheat grain, salt, and cinnamon on a rimmed heating sheet; throw to join; and spread into an even layer. Spot the almonds, walnuts, and pepitas on a second rimmed heating sheet; throw to join; and spread into an even layer. Move both preparing sheets to oven, putting oats on top rack and nuts on base. Heat until nuts is fragrant, 10 to 12 minutes.
2. Add the coconut. Eliminate the heating sheet with the nuts and put to the side to cool. Sprinkle the coconut over the oats, get back to the upper rack, and heat until the coconut is brilliant brown, around 5 minutes more. Eliminate from oven and put to the side to cool, around 10 minutes.
3. Move to an enormous bowl. Move the substance of both heating sheets to a huge bowl.
4. Add the dried natural product. Add the apricots and cherries and throw to consolidate.
5. Move to a sealed shut holder. Muesli can be put away in an impermeable holder at room temperature for as long as multi month.
6. Enjoy as wanted. Enjoy as oats, grain, short-term oats, or with yogurt, finished off with new products of the soil sprinkle of nectar or maple syrup, whenever wanted.
7. NOTES
8. Capacity: Muesli can be put away in a sealed shut holder for as long as multi month.
9. Serving ideas: To make for the time being oats, consolidate equivalent amounts of muesli and milk or non-dairy milk (I favor 2/3 cup of each) in a little lidded compartment (now I like to finish off mine with frozen blueberries, as well). Refrigerate expedite and enjoy cold in the first part of the day.

739. Salmon with Smoky Spinach and Chickpeas

Prep Time: 15 Minutes *Cook Time:□55 Minutes* *Servings: 6*

INGREDIENTS

- 4 (6-ounce) skin-on salmon filets
- 1/2 teaspoon fit salt, in addition to additional for preparing
- 1/4 teaspoon newly ground dark pepper, in addition to additional for preparing
- 4 tablespoons olive oil, isolated
- 2 (around 15-ounce) jars chickpeas
- 3 cloves garlic
- 1 teaspoon smoked paprika
- 1 (14.5-ounce) can normal or fire-simmered diced tomatoes
- 5 ounces infant spinach (around 5 stuffed cups)
- 2 teaspoons balsamic vinegar

DIRECTIONS:

1. Wipe 4 salmon filets off with paper towels. Season on the two sides with genuine salt and dark pepper.
2. Heat 2 tablespoons of the olive oil in an enormous cast iron or non-stick skillet over medium-high heat until shining. Spot the salmon skin-side down in the skillet, at that point push down on them so the skin is in even contact with the dish and browns equitably. Decrease the heat to medium-low and cook undisturbed, delicately pushing down on fish now and again, until the sides are concocted mostly the filets, 6 to 9 minutes, contingent upon the thickness of your filets. In the mean time, channel and wash 2 jars chickpeas. Crush and strip 3 garlic cloves.
3. Move the salmon skin-side up to a plate (it won't be cooked through). Add the excess 2 tablespoons olive oil to the skillet. Add the garlic and sauté until mollified and simply beginning to brown, around 2 minutes. Add 1 teaspoon smoked paprika and sauté until fragrant, around 1 moment.
4. Add the chickpeas, 1 can dice tomatoes and their juices, 1/2 teaspoon fit salt, and 1/4 teaspoon dark pepper. Mix to consolidate. Increment the heat to medium to bring to a stew. Stew for 5 minutes to permit the flavors to merge.
5. Mix in 5 ounces child spinach, a couple of small bunches all at once, until just shriveled, around 2 minutes. Mix in 2 teaspoons balsamic vinegar. Taste and season with salt and pepper depending on the situation.
6. Return the salmon skin-side up to the container, nestling them in the sauce. Keep on stewing for 2 to 5 minutes, contingent upon the thickness of your filets. A moment read thermometer into the center of the thickest filet should peruse 120°F to 130°F for medium-uncommon or 135°F to 145°F on the off chance that you favor it all the more all-around done. Serve the salmon, skin-side up, with the chickpeas and spinach.

740. Mediterranean White Bean Soup

Prep Time: 15 Minutes *Cook Time:□70 Minutes* *Servings: 6*

INGREDIENTS

- 2 (15-ounce) jars white beans
- 1 medium yellow onion
- 4 cloves garlic
- 1/4 teaspoon red pepper chips (discretionary)
- 2 tablespoons olive oil
- 4 cups low-sodium vegetable or chicken stock
- 1 (14-ounce) can diced tomatoes
- 2 twigs new rosemary
- 1 teaspoon legitimate salt
- 1/4 teaspoon newly ground dark pepper
- 1 Parmesan skin (discretionary)
- 5 ounces child spinach (around 5 stuffed cups)
- Ground Parmesan cheddar, for serving

DIRECTIONS:

1. Channel and wash 2 jars white beans and put in a safe spot. Finely slash 1 medium yellow onion and mince 4 cloves garlic.
2. Heat 2 tablespoons olive oil in a Dutch oven or huge pot until sparkling. Add the onion and sauté until relaxed and clear, 3 to 5 minutes. Add the garlic and 1/4 teaspoon red pepper pieces, if using, and sauté until fragrant, around brief more.
3. Pour in 4 cups low-sodium vegetable or chicken stock, 1 can diced tomatoes and their juices, and the white beans. Add 2 new rosemary twigs, 1 teaspoon legitimate salt, 1/4 teaspoon dark pepper, and 1 Parmesan skin, if using, and mix to join. Heat to the point of boiling. Lessen the heat to keep a stew, and stew uncovered for 10 minutes to permit the flavors to merge.
4. Mix in 5 ounces child spinach (around 5 stuffed cups); a couple of small bunches all at once, until just withered, 1 to 2 minutes. Serve decorated with ground Parmesan cheddar.
5. Formula NOTES
6. Substitute frozen spinach: Frozen spinach can be fill in for the new spinach. Basically mix in an equivalent weight (or more; this is adaptable) of frozen spinach and stew until heated through.
7. Add extra protein: If wanted, you can mix in a cup of shredded chicken (pulled from a rotisserie chicken, or canned chicken) into this soup in definite advance with the spinach.
8. Capacity: Leftovers can be put away in a water/air proof compartment in the cooler for as long as 5 days.

741. Spaghetti Squash Shrimp Scampi

Prep Time: 15 Minutes *Cook Time:□60 Minutes* *Servings: 6*

INGREDIENTS

- 1 2 1/2-to 3-pound spaghetti squash, split the long way and cultivated
- 2 tablespoons extra-virgin olive oil
- 1 tablespoon minced garlic
- ½ teaspoon salt, isolated
- ⅓ cup dry white wine
- 1 pound stripped and deveined crude shrimp (16-20 for every pound), tails left on, whenever wanted
- 1 tablespoon lemon juice
- ¼ cup chopped new parsley
- 2 tablespoons unsalted margarine
- ¼ teaspoon ground pepper
- ¼ cup shredded Parmesan cheddar
- Lemon wedges for serving

DIRECTIONS:

1. Spot squash parts, cut-side down, in a microwave-safe dish; add 2 tablespoons water. Microwave, revealed, on High until the substance is delicate, around 10 minutes. (On the other hand, place squash parts, cut-side down, on a rimmed

preparing sheet. Heat in a 400 degrees F oven until the squash is delicate, 40 to 50 minutes. You can likewise cook the squash in a pressing factor cooker/multi-cooker)
2. Stage 2
3. Then, heat oil in an enormous skillet over medium-high heat. Add garlic and 1/4 teaspoon salt; cook, blending, for 30 seconds. Cautiously add wine and bring to a stew. Add shrimp and cook, blending, until the shrimp are pink and just cooked through, 3 to 4 minutes. Eliminate from heat and mix in lemon juice.
4. Stage 3
5. Utilize a fork to scratch the squash substance from the shells into a medium bowl. Add parsley, margarine, pepper and the leftover 1/4 teaspoon salt; mix to consolidate. Serve the shrimp over the spaghetti squash. Sprinkle with Parmesan and present with a lemon wedge.

742. Greek Roasted Fish with Vegetables

Prep Time: 15 Minutes *Cook Time:☐20 Minutes* *Servings: 2*

INGREDIENTS

- 1 pound fingerling potatoes, split the long way
- 2 tablespoons olive oil
- 5 garlic cloves, coarsely chopped
- ½ teaspoon ocean salt
- ½ teaspoon newly ground dark pepper
- 4 5 to 6-ounce new or frozen skinless salmon filets
- 2 medium red, yellow and additionally orange sweet peppers, cut into rings
- 2 cups cherry tomatoes
- 1 ½ cups chopped new parsley (1 pack)
- ¼ cup pitted kalamata olives, divided
- ¼ cup finely cut new oregano or 1 Tbsp. dried oregano, squashed
- 1 lemon

DIRECTIONS:

1. Stage 1
2. Preheat oven to 425 degrees F. Spot potatoes in a huge bowl. Shower with 1 Tbsp. of the oil and sprinkle with garlic and 1/8 tsp. of the salt and dark pepper; throw to cover. Move to a 15x10-inch heating skillet; cover with foil. Cook 30 minutes.
3. Stage 2
4. In the interim, defrost salmon, whenever frozen. Join, in a similar bowl, sweet peppers, tomatoes, parsley, olives, oregano and 1/8 tsp. of the salt and dark pepper. Shower with staying 1 Tbsp. oil; throw to cover.
5. Stage 3
6. Flush salmon; wipe off. Sprinkle with staying 1/4 tsp. salt and dark pepper. Spoon sweet pepper combination over potatoes and top with salmon. Broil, uncovered, 10 minutes more or just until salmon drops.
7. Stage 4
8. Eliminate zing from lemon. Crush juice from lemon over salmon and vegetables. Sprinkle with zing.

743. Easy Roasted Tomato Basil Soup

Prep Time: 15 Minutes *Cook Time:☐60 Minutes* *Servings: 6*

INGREDIENTS

- 3 lb. Roma tomatoes divided
- 2 to 3 carrots stripped and cut into little pieces
- Additional virgin olive oil (I utilized Private Reserve Greek EVOO)
- Salt and pepper
- 2 medium yellow onions chopped
- 5 garlic cloves minced
- 1 cup canned squashed tomatoes
- 2 oz. new basil leaves
- 3 to 4 new thyme springs 2 tsp. thyme leaves
- 1 tsp. dry oregano
- ½ tsp. paprika
- ½ tsp. ground cumin
- 2 ½ cups water
- Sprinkle of lime juice optional

DIRECTIONS:

1. Heat oven to 450 degrees F.
2. In an enormous blending bowl, consolidate tomatoes and carrot pieces. Add a liberal shower of additional virgin olive oil, and season with fit salt and dark pepper. Throw to join.
3. Move to an enormous heating sheet and spread well in one layer. Broil in heated oven for around 30 minutes. At the point when prepared, eliminate from the heat and put in a safe spot for around 10 minutes to cool.
4. Move the broiled tomatoes and carrots to the enormous bowl of a food processor fitted with a cutting edge. Add simply a smidgen of water and mix.
5. In a huge cooking pot, heat 2 tbsp. additional virgin olive oil over medium-high heat until shining yet not smoking. Add onions and cook for around 3 minutes, at that point add garlic and cook momentarily until brilliant.
6. Empty the simmered tomato blend into the cooking pot. Mix in squashed tomatoes, 2 ½ cups water, basil, thyme and flavors. Season with a little genuine salt and dark pepper. Heat to the point of boiling, at that point lower heat and cover part-way. Let stew for around 20 minutes or somewhere in the vicinity.
7. Eliminate the thyme springs and move tomato basil soup to serving bowls. In the event that you like, add a sprinkle of lime juice and a liberal shower of extra virgihttps://shop.themediterraneandish.com/item/extra-virgin-olive-oil-pack/n olive oil. Present with your #1 dry bread or flame broiled bits of French loaf. Enjoy!
8. NOTES
9. Extras: If you have any extras, you can refrigerate in close top glass compartments for 3 to 4 days. Ensure the soup is totally cooled prior to putting away.
10. Would you be able to freeze this tomato basil soup? Indeed! Since this is a sans dairy veggie lover tomato basil soup and there is no cream required by any means, it is the ideal tomato soup to freeze. Essentially cool the soup prior to putting away in close cover, cooler safe compartments. Freeze for some time in the future (3 to a half year or something like that.) Thaw in ice chest short-term and go through medium heat to warm.
11. Varieties: If you're searching for somewhat of a smoky completion, add a decent touch of smoked paprika. Or then again, to zest things up, cook some jalapeno pepper and mix them alongside the tomatoes and carrots.

744. Easy Greek-Style Eggplant Recipe

Prep Time: 15 Minutes *Cook Time:☐50 Minutes* *Servings: 4*

INGREDIENTS

- 3 lb. Roma tomatoes divided
- 2 to 3 carrots stripped and cut into little pieces
- Additional virgin olive oil (I utilized Private Reserve Greek EVOO)
- Salt and pepper
- 2 medium yellow onions chopped
- 5 garlic cloves minced
- 1 cup canned squashed tomatoes
- 2 oz. new basil leaves
- 3 to 4 new thyme springs 2 tsp. thyme leaves
- 1 tsp. dry oregano
- ½ tsp. paprika
- ½ tsp. ground cumin
- 2 ½ cups water
- Sprinkle of lime juice optional

DIRECTIONS:

1. Heat oven to 450 degrees F.
2. In an enormous blending bowl, consolidate tomatoes and carrot pieces. Add a liberal shower of additional virgin olive oil, and season with fit salt and dark pepper. Throw to join.
3. Move to an enormous heating sheet and spread well in one layer. Broil in heated oven for around 30 minutes. At the point when prepared, eliminate from the heat and put in a safe spot for around 10 minutes to cool.
4. Move the broiled tomatoes and carrots to the enormous bowl of a food processor fitted with a cutting edge. Add simply a smidgen of water and mix.
5. In a huge cooking pot, heat 2 tbsp. additional virgin olive oil over medium-high heat until shining yet not smoking. Add onions and cook for around 3 minutes, at that point add garlic and cook momentarily until brilliant.
6. Empty the simmered tomato blend into the cooking pot. Mix in squashed tomatoes, 2 ½ cups water, basil, thyme and flavors. Season with a little genuine salt and dark pepper. Heat to the point of boiling, at that point lower heat and cover part-way. Let stew for around 20 minutes or somewhere in the vicinity.
7. Eliminate the thyme springs and move tomato basil soup to serving bowls. In the event that you like, add a sprinkle of lime juice and a liberal shower of extra Present with your #1 dry bread or flame broiled bits of French loaf. Enjoy!
8. NOTES
9. Extras: If you have any extras, you can refrigerate in close top glass compartments for 3 to 4 days. Ensure the soup is totally cooled prior to putting away.
10. Would you be able to freeze this tomato basil soup? Indeed! Since this is a sans dairy veggie lover tomato basil soup and there is no cream required by any means, it is the ideal tomato soup to freeze. Essentially cool the soup prior to putting away in close cover, cooler safe compartments. Freeze for some time in the future (3 to a half year or something like that.) Thaw in ice chest short-term and go through medium heat to warm.
11. Varieties: If you're searching for somewhat of a smoky completion, add a decent touch of smoked paprika. Or then again, to zest things up, cook some jalapeno pepper and mix them alongside the tomatoes and carrots.

745. Mediterranean Grilled Balsamic Chicken with Olive Tapenade

Prep Time: 15 Minutes *Cook Time:☐55 Minutes* *Servings: 6*

Time 40 minutes Servings 2 chicken breasts

INGREDIENTS

- 2 skinless boneless Simple Truth chicken breasts
- 1/4 cup olive oil
- 1/4 cup brilliant balsamic vinegar
- 1/8 cup Private Selection Whole Grain Garlic Mustard
- 1/2 tablespoons balsamic vinegar
- 3 cloves garlic squeezed or minced
- Juice of 1/2 lemon
- 1 storing tablespoon chopped new spices, for example, Simple Truth tarragon rosemary or thyme
- 1 teaspoon fit salt
- 1/2 teaspoon newly ground dark pepper
- Present with Olive Tapenade formula beneath and lumps of feta cheddar

DIRECTIONS:

1. Cut back any additional excess from the chicken breasts and spot in a bowl or a gallon size cooler pack.
2. In a little bowl, whisk the olive oil, balsamic vinegars, mustard, garlic, lemon juice, spices, and salt and pepper. Save half of the marinade and add the other half to the bowl or pack with the chicken. Marinate for at any rate 30 minutes up to expedite, turning sporadically.
3. At the point when prepared to flame broil, bring one side of an outside barbecue to high heat with the opposite side off.
4. Oil the barbecue grinds well and sprinkles the chicken breasts with more olive oil, at that point place the chicken breasts on the hot flame broil. Cook for 2-3 minutes or until barbecue marks show up, at that point flip the chicken and cook for another 2-3 minutes. Move the chicken to the cooler meshes of the barbecue, cover, and cook for 10 minutes. Move a couple of tablespoons of the held marinade to another bowl and use it to treat the chicken with and flip. Keep cooking, treating, and flipping until the breasts have an interior temperature of 165 degrees. Move the chicken to the hot side of the barbecue to add more flame broil checks and shading to the chicken bosom yet make certain to watch them so the balsamic marinade doesn't burn. The length of cooking time will depend up on the thickness of the breasts however you should rely in general cooking time to be around 30 minutes.
5. Move the chicken to a platter and cover with a piece of aluminum foil and let rest for 5 minutes. Present with olive tapenade, lumps of feta cheddar minced spices and shower with any extra olive oil.

746. Best Greek Chicken Marinade

Prep Time: 15 Minutes *Cook Time:☐34 Minutes* *Servings: 4*

INGREDIENTS

- 1 pound boneless skinless chicken breasts (about 2 large breasts)
- ⅓ cup plain Greek yogurt
- ¼ cup olive oil
- 4 lemons
- 4-5 cloves garlic squeezed or minced
- 2 tablespoons dried oregano
- 1 teaspoon genuine salt
- ½ teaspoon newly ground dark pepper

DIRECTIONS:

1. Spot the chicken pieces in a cooler sack or a bowl and put in a safe spot.
2. Add the Greek yogurt and olive oil to a medium size bowl. Zing one of the lemons and add to the bowl. Juice that lemon into the bowl with the zing. Cut the other three lemons and put in a safe spot. Add the minced garlic, oregano, genuine salt and dark pepper to the lemon squeeze and zing and mix. Empty portion of the

marinade into the cooler sack or the bowl with the chicken pieces and save the other portion of the marinade for seasoning. Marinate the chicken for 30 minutes or as long as 3 hours in the fridge.

3. At the point when prepared to flame broil, set up the barbecue by gently oiling the mesh with vegetable oil or cooking splash and set to medium high heat.
4. Flame broil the chicken, treating with the held marinade and turning frequently so each side browns and has light barbecue marks, until cooked through, around 15-20 minutes or until the chicken juices run clear. During the most recent 5 minutes of cooking add the 3 cut lemons to the flame broil, turning more than once. Permit the chicken to rest for 5 minutes prior to cutting and present with the flame broiled lemons. Refrigerate extras for as long as 3 days.

747. FOUR-CHEESE LASAGNA

Prep Time:	*Cook Time:*	*Servings: 6*
2 Minutes	*15 Minutes*	

INGREDIENTS:

- ounces Gruyère cheese, shredded (1¹/2 cups)
- 2 ounces Parmesan cheese, grated fine (1 cup)
- ounces (1¹/2 cups) part-skim ricotta cheese
- 1 large egg
- ¹/4 Tsp. pepper
- Tbsps. Plus 2 Tips. minced fresh parsley
- 3 Tbsps. unsalted butter
- 1 shallot, minced
- 1 garlic clove, minced
- ¹/3 cup all-purpose flour
- 2¹/2 cups whole milk
- 1¹/2 cups low-sodium chicken broth
- ¹/2 Tsp. salt
- 1 bay leaf
- 15 no-boil lasagna noodles
- 8 ounces fontina cheese, shredded (2 cups)
- ounces Gorgonzola cheese, finely crumbled (³/4 cup)
- Place Gruyère & ¹/2 cup Parmesan in a large heatproof container.

DIRECTIONS:

1. Combine ricotta, egg, black pepper, & 2 Tbsps. Parsley in a medium container. Set both containers aside.
2. Melt butter in a saucepan. Include shallot & garlic & cook, often stirring, till shallot is softened, about 2 mins.
3. Include flour & cook, constantly stirring, till thoroughly combined, about 1¹/2 mins; batter should not brown. Gradually whisk in milk & broth; increase heat to medium-high & bring to boil, whisking often.
4. Stir in salt, bay leaf, & cayenne, reduce heat to medium-low, & simmer till sauce thickens & measures 4 cups, about 10 mins, stirring occasionally & making sure to scrape bottom & corners of the pan.
5. Discard bay leaf. Gradually whisk ¹/4 cup sauce into ricotta batter. Pour remaining sauce over Gruyère batter & stir till smooth.
6. Set oven rack to upper-middle setting & heat oven to 350 degrees. Add 2 inches of boiling water into a 13 by 9-inch broiler-safe baking dish.
7. Add noodles into the water, 1 at a time, & soak till pliable, about 5 mins, separating noodles with the tip of a sharp knife to prevent sticking.
8. Remove noodles from water & place in a single layer on clean kitchen towels; discard water. Dry dish & spray lightly with vegetable oil spray.
9. Spread ¹/2 cup sauce evenly over the bottom of the dish. Set 3 noodles in a single layer on top of the sauce.
10. Sprinkle ¹/2 cup ricotta batter evenly over noodles & sprinkle with ¹/2 cup fontina & 3 Tbsps. Gorgonzola. Spoon ¹/2 cup sauce over the top.
11. Repeat layering of noodles, ricotta batter, fontina, Gorgonzola, & sauce 3 more times.
12. For the final layer, set the remaining 3 noodles on top & cover them completely with the remaining sauce. Sprinkle with remaining ¹/2 cup Parmesan.
13. Envelope dish with aluminium foil that has been sprayed with oil spray & bake till edges are just bubbling, 25 to 30 mins, rotating dish halfway through baking.
14. Remove foil & turn oven to broil. Broil lasagna till the surface is spotty brown, 3 to 5 mins.
15. Cool lasagna for 15 mins, then sprinkles with the remaining 2 Tips. Parsley & serve

748. Mediterranean falafel

Prep Time:	*Cook Time:*☐*40*	*Servings: 4*
15 Minutes	*Minutes*	

INGREDIENTS

- 2 cups dried chickpeas (Do NOT utilize canned or cooked chickpeas)
- ½ tsp. preparing pop
- 1 cup new parsley leaves, stems eliminated
- ¾ cup new cilantro leaves, stems eliminated
- ½ cup new dill, stems eliminated
- 1 little onion, quartered
- 7-8 garlic cloves, stripped
- Salt to taste
- 1 tbsp. ground dark pepper
- 1 tbsp. ground cumin
- 1 tbsp. ground coriander
- 1 tsp. cayenne pepper, optional
- 1 tsp. preparing powder
- 2 tbsp. toasted sesame seeds
- Oil for searing
- Falafel Sauce
- Tahini Sauce
- Trimmings for falafel sandwich (optional)
- Pita pockets
- English cucumbers, chopped or diced
- Tomatoes, chopped or diced
- Child Arugula
- Pickles

DIRECTIONS:

1. (One day ahead of time) Place the dried chickpeas and preparing soft drink in a huge bowl loaded up with water to cover the chickpeas by in any event 2 inches. Splash for the time being for 18 hours (longer if the chickpeas are still excessively hard). At the point when prepared, channel the chickpeas totally and wipe them off.
2. Add the chickpeas, spices, onions, garlic and flavors to the enormous bowl of a food processor fitted with a cutting edge. Run the food processor 40 seconds all at once until everything is great joined shaping a the falafel blend.
3. Move the falafel blend to a compartment and cover firmly. Refrigerate for in any event 1 hour or (up to one entire evening) until prepared to cook.
4. Not long prior to searing, add the preparing powder and sesame seeds to the falafel blend and mix with a spoon.
5. Scoop tablespoonfuls of the falafel combination and structure into patties (½ inch in thickness each). It assists with having wet hands as you structure the patties.
6. Fill medium pan 3 crawls up with oil. Heat the oil on medium-high until it bubbles delicately. Cautiously drop the falafel patties in the oil, let them fry for around 3 to 5 minutes or so until fresh and medium brown outwardly. Try not to pack the falafel in the pan, fry them in bunches if fundamental.
7. Spot the singed falafel patties in a colander or plate fixed with paper towels to deplete.
8. Serve falafel hot close to other little plates; or amass the falafel patties in pita bread with tahini or hummus, arugula, tomato and cucumbers. Enjoy!
9. You need to begin with dry chickpeas, don't utilize canned chickpeas here. You should start dousing the chickpeas short-term; permit as long as 24 hours.
10. Falafel Recipe varieties: Variations of this formula may call for flour or eggs. On the off chance that you like, you can add 1 to 1 ½ tbsp. of flour to the falafel blend or 1 egg. I didn't utilize either, and the falafel combination remained well together.
11. Ace Tip for Frying: When you fry the falafel patties, you need to accomplish a profound brilliant brown tone outwardly. All the more critically, the patties should be completely done within. Your broiling oil should be at 375 degrees F, for my oven, that was at a medium-high temp. Make certain to test your first group and change the singing time depending on the situation.
12. Well known falafel sauce: tahini sauce is the thing that is customarily utilized with falafel. I utilize natural tahini paste by Soom, and here is my tahini sauce formula.
13. Prepared Falafel Option: If you like, you can heat the falafel patties in a 350 degree F heated oven for around 15-20 minutes, turning them over halfway through. Utilize a gently oiled sheet dish, and you may jump at the chance to give the patties a speedy brush of additional virgin olive oil prior to preparing.
14. Supportive of Tip for Make-Ahead: To make ahead and freeze, set up the falafel blend and separation into patties (up to step #6). Spot the patties on a preparing sheet fixed with material paper and freeze. At the point when they solidify, you can move the falafel patties into a cooler pack. They will save well in the cooler for a month or something like that. You can sear or heat them from frozen.

7.

Lunch Recipes

749. Turkey Burger

Prep Time:	*Cook Time:*	*Servings: 2*
5 Minutes	*20 Minutes*	

INGREDIENTS:

- 1 large egg white
- 1 mug red onion, chopped
- ¾ cup mint, chopped
- ½ mug dried bread crumbs
- 1 tsp. dill, dried
- ⅓ mug feta cheese, crumbled
- ¾ kg turkey, ground
- Cooking spray
- 4 hamburger buns, split
- 1 red bell pepper, roasted
- 2 tbsp. Lime juice

DIRECTIONS:

1. Lightly beat the egg white in a container and add onion, mint, breadcrumbs, dill, cheese, turkey, and lime juice; combine well, then divide the turkey batter into four equal burger patties.
2. Spray the cooking spray on a large nonstick skillet and flame on a medium-high setting.
3. Carefully place the patties in the skillet and cook for 8 mins on each side or according to preference.
4. Once cooked, place the burgers on the sliced buns and top with pepper strips.

750. Chicken with Greek Salad

Prep Time:	*Cook Time:*	*Servings: 4*
5 Minutes	*20 Minutes*	

INGREDIENTS:

- 2 tbsp. olive oil
- ⅓ mug red-wine vinegar
- 1 tsp. garlic powder
- 1 tbsp. chopped dill
- ¼ tsp. sea salt
- ¼ tsp. freshly ground pepper
- 2 ½ cups chopped cooked chicken
- 6 cups chopped romaine lettuce
- 1 cucumber, peeled, seeded, and chopped
- 2 medium tomatoes, chopped
- ½ mug crumbled feta cheese
- ½ mug sliced ripe black olives
- ½ mug finely chopped red onion

DIRECTIONS

1. In a large container, whisk together olive oil, vinegar, garlic powder, dill, sea salt, and pepper.
2. Add chicken, lettuce, cucumber, tomatoes, feta, and olives, and toss to combine well. Enjoy!

751. Chicken with Olives, Mustard Greens, and Lemon

Prep Time:	*Cook Time:*	*Servings: 6*
5 Minutes	*20 Minutes*	

INGREDIENTS:

- 2 tbsp. olive oil, divided
- 6 skinless chicken breast halves, cut in half crosswise ½ mug Kalamata olives, pitted
- 1 tbsp. freshly squeezed lemon juice
- 1 ½ pounds mustard greens, stalks removed and coarsely chopped
- 1 mug dry white wine
- 4 garlic cloves, smashed
- 1 medium red onion, thinly sliced
- Sea salt

- Ground pepper
- Lemon wedges, for serving

DIRECTIONS:

1. Flame 1 tbsp of olive oil in a Dutch oven or large, heavy pot over medium to high heat.
2. Rub the chicken with sea salt and pepper and add half of it to the pot; cook for about 8 mins or until browned on all sides.
3. Transfer the cooked chicken to a plate and repeat with the remaining chicken and oil.
4. Add garlic and onion to the pot and lower the flame to medium; cook, stirring, for about 6 mins or until tender.
5. Add chicken (with accumulated juices) and wine and bring to a boil.
6. Reduce flame and cook, covered, for about 5 mins.
7. Add the greens on top of the chicken and sprinkle with sea salt and pepper. Cook, covered, for about 5 mins more or until the greens are wilted, and chicken is opaque.
8. Transfer the pot from flame and stir in olives and lemon juice.
9. Serve drizzled with accumulated pan juices and garnished with lemon wedges.

752. Delicious Mediterranean Chicken

Prep Time: 5 Minutes | *Cook Time: 20 Minutes* | *Servings: 2*

INGREDIENTS:

- 2 tsp. olive oil
- ½ mug white wine, divided
- 6 chicken breasts, skinned and deboned
- 3 cloves garlic, pressed
- ½ mug onion, chopped
- 3 cups tomatoes, chopped
- ½ mug Kalamata olives
- ¼ cup parsley, chopped
- 2 tsp. thyme, chopped
- Sea salt to taste

DIRECTIONS:

1. Flame the oil and 3 tbsps of white wine in a skillet over medium heat.
2. Add the chicken and cook for about 6 mins on each side until golden.
3. Transfer the chicken and place it on a plate.
4. Add garlic and onions in the skillet and sauté for about 3 mins and add the tomatoes.
5. Let them cook for five mins then lower the flame and add the remaining white wine and simmer for 10 mins.
6. Add the thyme & simmer for 5 mins.
7. Return the chicken to the skillet and cook on low flame until the chicken is well done.
8. Add olives and parsley and cook for 1 more minute.
9. Add the salt and pepper and serve.

753. Warm Chicken Avocado Salad

Prep Time: 5 Minutes | *Cook Time:30 Minutes* | *Servings: 4*

INGREDIENTS:

- 2 tbsp. olive oil, divided
- 500g chicken breast fillets
- 1 large avocado, peeled, diced
- 2 garlic cloves, sliced
- 1 tsp. ground turmeric
- 3 tsp. ground cumin
- 1 head broccoli, chopped
- 1 large carrot, diced
- 1/3 mug currants
- 1 ½ cups chicken stock
- 1 ½ cups couscous
- Pinch of sea salt

DIRECTIONS:

1. In a large frying pan set over medium heat, flame 1 tbsp olive oil; add chicken and cook for about 6 mins per side or until cooked through; transfer to a plate and keep warm.
2. In the meantime, combine currants and couscous in a heatproof container; stir in boiling stock and set aside, covered, for at least 5 mins or until liquid is absorbed.
3. With a fork, separate the grains.
4. Add the remaining oil to a pan and add carrots; cook, stirring, for about 1 minute.
5. Stir in broccoli for about 1 minute; stir in garlic, turmeric, and cumin.
6. Cook for about 1 minute more and transfer the pan from heat.
7. Slice the chicken into slices and add to the broccoli mixture; toss to combine; season with sea salt and serve with the avocado sprinkled on top.

754. Chicken Stew

Prep Time: 5 Minutes | *Cook Time: 20 Minutes* | *Servings: 2*

INGREDIENTS:

- 1 tbsp. olive oil
- 3 chicken breast halves (8 ounces each), boneless, skinless, cut into pieces
- Sea salt
- Freshly ground pepper
- 1 medium onion, sliced
- 4 garlic cloves, sliced
- ½ tsp. dried oregano
- 1 ½ pounds escarole, ends trimmed, chopped
- 1 mug whole-wheat couscous, cooked
- 1 (28 ounces) can whole peeled tomatoes, pureed

DIRECTIONS:

1. In a large, heavy pot, flame olive oil over medium to high heat.
2. Rub chicken with sea salt and pepper.
3. In batches, cook chicken in olive oil, occasionally tossing, for about 5 mins or until browned; transfer to a plate and set aside.
4. Add onion, garlic and oregano, tomatoes, sea salt, and pepper to the pot and cook for about 10 mins or until the onion is lightly browned.
5. Add the chicken and cook, covered for about 4 mins or until opaque.
6. Fill the pot with escarole and cook for about 4 mins or until tender.
7. Serve the chicken stew over couscous.

755. Chicken with Roasted Vegetables

Prep Time: 5 Minutes | *Cook Time: 20 Minutes* | *Servings: 3*

INGREDIENTS:

- 1 large zucchini, diagonally sliced
- 250g baby new potatoes, sliced
- 6 firm plum tomatoes, halved
- 1 red onion, cut into wedges
- 1 Yellow pepper, seeded, and cut into chunks
- 12 black olives, pitted
- 2 chicken breast fillets, skinless, boneless
- 1 rounded tbsp. green pesto
- 3 tbsp. olive oil

DIRECTIONS:

1. Preflame your oven to 400°F.
2. Spread zucchini, potatoes, tomatoes, onion, and pepper in a roasting pan and scatter with olives.
3. Season with sea salt and black pepper.
4. Cut each chicken breast into 5 pieces and arrange them on top of the vegetables.
5. In a container, combine pesto and olive oil and spread over the chicken. Cover it with foil & cook in preheated oven for about 30 mins.
6. Uncover the pan & return to the oven; cook for about 10 mins more or until chicken is cooked through.
7. Enjoy!

756. Grilled Chicken with Olive Relish

Prep Time: 5 Minutes | *Cook Time: 20 Minutes* | *Servings: 25*

INGREDIENTS:

- 4 chicken breast halves, boneless, skinless ¾ mug olive oil, divided Sea salt
- Freshly ground black pepper
- 2 tbsp. capers, rinsed, chopped
- 1 ½ cups green olives, rinsed, pitted, and chopped ¼ mug lightly toasted almonds, chopped
- 1 clove garlic, mashed with sea salt
- 1 ½ tsp. chopped thyme
- 2 ½ tsp. grated lemon zest
- 2 tbsp. chopped parsley

DIRECTIONS:

1. Flame grill to high heat.
2. Place 1 chicken breast on one side of a plastic wrap and drizzle with about 1 teaspoon of olive oil, and fold the wrap over the chicken. Pound the chicken with a heavy sauté pan or a meat mallet to about ½ inch thick.
3. Repeat the procedure for the remaining chicken and discard the plastic wrap. Sprinkle chicken with sea salt and pepper and coat with about 2 tbsp olive oil; set aside.
4. In the meantime, combine ½ mug olive oil, capers, olives, almonds, garlic, thyme, lemon zest, and parsley in a medium container.
5. Grill the chicken for three mins per side and transfer to a cutting board.
6. Let cool a bit and cut into ½-inch-thick slices.
7. Arrange the chicken slices on four plates and spoon over the relish.
8. Serve immediately.

757. Grilled Turkey with Salsa

Prep Time: 5 Minutes | *Cook Time: 20 Minutes* | *Servings: 4*

INGREDIENTS:

For the spice rub:

- 1 ½ tsp. garlic powder
- 1 ½ tsp. sweet paprika
- 2 tsp. crushed fennel seeds
- 2 tsp. dark brown sugar
- 1 tsp. sea salt
- 1 ½ tsp. freshly ground black pepper

For the salsa:

- 2 tbsp. Drained capers
- ¼ mug pimento-stuffed green olives, chopped 2 scant cups cherry tomatoes,1 ½ tbsp. olive oil
- 1 large clove garlic, minced

- 2 tbsp. torn basil leaves
- 2 tsp. Lemon juice
- ½ tsp. finely grated lemon zest
- 6 turkey breast cutlets
- 1 mug red onion
- Sea salt
- Freshly ground black pepper

DIRECTIONS:

1. Combine together garlic powder, paprika, fennel seeds, brown sugar, salt, and pepper in a container.
2. In another container, combine capers, olives, tomatoes, onion olive oil, garlic, basil, lemon juice, and zest, ¼ teaspoon sea salt, and pepper; set aside.
3. Grill the meat on medium to high flame after dipping in the spice rub for about 3 mins per side or until browned on both sides.
4. Transfer the grilled turkey to a serving plate and let rest for about 5 mins.
5. Serve with salsa

758. Curried Chicken with Olives, Apricots, and Cauliflower

Prep Time: *5 Minutes* | *Cook Time:* *20 Minutes* | *Servings: 6*

INGREDIENTS:

- 8 chicken thighs, skinless, boneless
- ¼ mug olive oil, divided
- ½ tsp. Ground cinnamon
- ¼ tsp. cayenne pepper
- 1 tsp. smoked paprika, divided
- 4 tsp. curry powder, divided
- 1 tbsp. apple cider vinegar
- Sea salt, to taste
- 1 head cauliflower, chopped
- 1 mug pitted green olives, halved
- ¾ mug dried apricots, chopped, soaked in hot water, and drained ⅓ mug chopped cilantro
- 6 lemon wedges
- 1 large zucchini, diagonally sliced
- 250g baby new potatoes, sliced
- 6 firm plum tomatoes, halved
- 1 red onion, cut into wedges
- 1 Yellow pepper, seeded, and cut into chunks
- 12 black olives, pitted
- 2 chicken breast fillets, skinless, boneless
- 1 rounded tbsp. green pesto
- 3 tbsp. olive oil

DIRECTIONS:

1. Preflame your oven to 400°F.
2. Spread zucchini, potatoes, tomatoes, onion, and pepper in a roasting pan and scatter with olives.
3. Season with sea salt and black pepper.
4. Cut each chicken breast into 5 pieces and arrange them on top of the vegetables.
5. In a container, combine pesto and olive oil and spread over the chicken. Cover it with foil & cook in preheated oven for about 30 mins.
6. Uncover the pan & return to the oven; cook for about 10 mins more or until chicken is cooked through.
7. Enjoy!

759. Grilled Chicken with Olive Relish

Prep Time: *5 Minutes* | *Cook Time:* *20 Minutes* | *Servings: 4*

INGREDIENTS:

- 4 chicken breast halves, boneless, skinless ¾ mug olive oil, divided Sea salt
- Freshly ground black pepper
- 2 tbsp. capers, rinsed, chopped
- 1 ½ cups green olives, rinsed, pitted, and chopped ¼ mug lightly toasted almonds, chopped
- 1 clove garlic, mashed with sea salt
- 1 ½ tsp. chopped thyme
- 2 ½ tsp. grated lemon zest
- 2 tbsp. chopped parsley

DIRECTIONS:

1. Flame grill to high heat.
2. Place 1 chicken breast on one side of a plastic wrap and drizzle with about 1 teaspoon of olive oil, and fold the wrap over the chicken. Pound the chicken with a heavy sauté pan or a meat mallet to about ½ inch thick.
3. Repeat the procedure for the remaining chicken and discard the plastic wrap. Sprinkle chicken with sea salt and pepper and coat with about 2 tbsp olive oil; set aside.
4. In the meantime, combine ½ mug olive oil, capers, olives, almonds, garlic, thyme, lemon zest, and parsley in a medium container.
5. Grill the chicken for three mins per side and transfer to a cutting board.
6. Let cool a bit and cut into ½-inch-thick slices.
7. Arrange the chicken slices on four plates and spoon over the relish.
8. Serve immediately.

760. Curried Chicken with Olives, Apricots, and Cauliflower

Prep Time: *5 Minutes* | *Cook Time:* *20 Minutes* | *Servings: 2*

INGREDIENTS:

- 8 chicken thighs, skinless, boneless
- ¼ mug olive oil, divided
- ½ tsp. Ground cinnamon
- ¼ tsp. cayenne pepper
- 1 tsp. smoked paprika, divided
- 4 tsp. curry powder, divided
- 1 tbsp. apple cider vinegar
- Sea salt, to taste
- 1 head cauliflower, chopped
- 1 mug pitted green olives, halved
- ¾ mug dried apricots, chopped, soaked in hot water, and drained ⅓ mug chopped cilantro
- 6 lemon wedges

DIRECTIONS:

1. Combine chicken thighs, 2 tbsp olive oil, cinnamon, cayenne, ½ teaspoon paprika, 2 tbsp curry powder, vinegar, and sea salt in a medium container; toss to coat and refrigerate covered for about 8 hours.
2. Put a rack in the oven and flame the oven to 450°F.
3. Prepare a rimmed sheet by lining it with parchment paper; add cauliflower and remaining olive oil, paprika, and curry powder; combine well. Add olives and apricots and spread the batter in a single layer.
4. Put the chicken on the cauliflower mixture, spacing evenly apart, and roast in the preheated oven for about 35 mins or until chicken is cooked through and cauliflower browns.
5. Serve the cauliflower and chicken sprinkled with cilantro and garnished with lemon wedges.

761. Chicken Salad with Pine Nuts, Raisins, and Fennel

Prep Time: *5 Minutes* | *Cook Time:* *20 Minutes* | *Servings: 2*

INGREDIENTS:

For the dressing:

- 1 tbsp. olive oil
- 3 tbsp. mayonnaise
- ½ clove garlic, mashed with sea salt Pinch cayenne
- 1 tbsp. freshly squeezed lemon juice

For the salad:

- 3 tbsp. Chopped sweet onion
- ⅓ mug -diced fennel
- 1 mug shredded cooked chicken
- 2 tbsp. Golden raisins
- 2 tbsp. Toasted pine nuts
- 2 tbsp. chopped flat-leaf parsley
- Sea salt
- Freshly ground pepper

DIRECTIONS:

1. Combine olive oil, mayonnaise, garlic, cayenne, and lemon juice in a container; combine well.
2. In a separate container, combine onion, fennel, chicken, raisins, pine nuts, and parsley; gently add in the dressing and fold the INGREDIENTS: together. Season with sea salt and pepper and refrigerate for at least 1 hour for flavors to meld before serving.

762. Slow Cooker Rosemary Chicken

Prep Time: *5 Minutes* | *Cook Time:* *20 Minutes* | *Servings: 6*

INGREDIENTS:

- 1 onion, thinly sliced
- 4 cloves garlic, pressed
- 1 medium red bell pepper, sliced
- 2 tsp. Dried rosemary
- ½ tsp. dried oregano
- 2 pork sausages
- 8 chicken breasts, skinned, deboned, and halved ¼ tsp. Coarsely ground pepper ¼ mug dry vermouth
- 1 ½ tbsp. Corn starch
- 2 tbsp. cold water

DIRECTIONS:

1. Combine onion, garlic, bell pepper, rosemary, and oregano in a slow cooker.
2. Crumble the sausages over the mixture, casings removed.
3. Arrange the chicken on a layer of the sausage and sprinkle with pepper.
4. Add the vermouth and slow-cook for 7 hours.
5. Warm a deep platter, move the chicken to the platter, and cover.
6. Mix the cornstarch and water in a container and add this to the liquid in the slow cooker.
7. Increase the flame and cover.
8. Cook for about 10 mins.

Dinner Recipes

763. Lamb Chops

Prep Time: *5 Minutes* *Cook Time:* *20 Minutes* *Servings: 8*

INGREDIENTS:

- 1 tbsp. dried oregano
- 1 tbsp. Garlic, minced
- ¼ tsp. Black pepper freshly ground
- ½ tsp. sea salt
- 2 tbsp. lemon juice, fresh
- 8 lamb loin chops, fat trimmed off
- Cooking spray

DIRECTIONS:

1. Preflame your broiler.
2. In a container, combine all the spices, herbs, and lemon juice and rub this batter on both sides of the lamb chops.
3. Spray the broiler pan and broil the lamb chops for 4 mins on each side or depending on your chops. Cover the cooked lamb chops in foil and let them rest for 5 mins and you are ready to serve.

764. Sage Seared Calf's Liver

Prep Time: *5 Minutes* *Cook Time:* *20 Minutes* *Servings: 2*

INGREDIENTS

- 2 tsp. olive oil
- 1 clove garlic, minced
- 8 ounces calves' liver, cut into strips
- 1 tbsp. flat-leaf parsley
- 1 tbsp. Sage
- 1 tsp. balsamic vinegar
- 2 tbsp. red wine
- 2 tsp. unsalted butter
- 1 tsp. Lemon juice
- ¼ tsp. sea salt
- Black pepper

DIRECTIONS:

1. Flame olive oil in a nonstick skillet set over medium heat; stir in minced garlic and sauté for about 3 mins or until translucent and fragrant.
2. Add strips of the liver, parsley, and sage and cook for about 5 mins or until the meat is seared outside.
3. Transfer the liver to a warm plate and quickly deglaze the pan with vinegar, red wine, butter, and lemon juice for about 30 seconds. Pour the sauce over the meat and serve right away.

765. Seasoned Lamb Burgers

Prep Time: *5 Minutes* *Cook Time:* *20 Minutes* *Servings: 4*

INGREDIENTS:

- 1 ½ pounds ground lamb
- 1 tsp. Ground cumin
- ½ tsp. ground cinnamon
- 1 tsp. ground ginger
- ¼ mug olive oil, divided
- 1 tsp. black pepper, freshly ground; divided ¼ cup cilantro
- 2 tbsp. Oregano
- 1 clove garlic, pressed
- ¾ tsp. red pepper flakes, crushed
- ¼ cup flat-leaf parsley
- 1 tbsp. sherry vinegar
- 2 pitas, warmed and halved
- Sliced tomato
- 1 8 oz of package plain Greek yogurt

DIRECTIONS:

1. Prepare a charcoal or gas grill fire.
2. Combine the ground lamb with cumin, cinnamon, ginger, 1 tbsp olive oil, and ½ teaspoon black pepper. Combine well and divide this into four burgers.
3. Spray the grill with some olive oil and grill the burgers for 5 mins on each side.
4. Combine the rest of the olive oil, cilantro, oregano, garlic, red pepper flakes, parsley, and vinegar in a blender for a thick paste form. Serve each burger in pita bread on a plate with sliced tomato, the processed sauce, and a serving of yogurt.

766. London broil with Bourbon-Sautéed Mushrooms

Prep Time: *5 Minutes* *Cook Time:* *20 Minutes* *Servings: 2*

INGREDIENTS:

- ½ tsp. olive oil
- ½ mug minced shallot
- ¾ lb. halved crimini mushrooms
- 6 tbsp. non-fat beef stock
- 3 tbsp. Bourbon
- ½ tbsp. unsalted butter
- 1 tbsp. pure maple syrup
- Black pepper, to taste
- 1 lb. lean London broil
- ⅛ tsp. sea salt

DIRECTIONS:

1. Preflame your oven to 400°F.
2. Flame a nonstick skillet in the oven for about 10 mins.
3. Transfer and add olive oil; swirl to coat the pan.
4. Stir in shallots and mushrooms until well blended; return to oven and roast the mushrooms for about 15 mins, stirring once with a wooden spatula. Stir in beef stock, bourbon, butter, maple syrup, and pepper; toss and return the pan to oven; cook for 10 mins more or until liquid is reduced by half. Transfer pan from oven and set aside.
5. Place another nonstick skillet in the oven and flame for about 10 mins.
6. In the meantime, sprinkle salt and ground pepper over the steak and place it in the hot pan.
7. Roast in the oven for about 14 mins, turning once.
8. Transfer the meat from the oven and warm the mushrooms.
9. Place steak on the cutting board & let rest for about 5 mins.
10. Thinly slice beef and serve top with sautéed mushrooms to serve.

767. Grilled Sage Lamb Kabob

Prep Time: *5 Minutes* *Cook Time:* *20 Minutes* *Servings: 6*

INGREDIENTS:

- 1 tbsp. lemon juice
- 2 tbsp. chives
- 2 tbsp. flat-leaf parsley
- 2 tbsp. sage
- 1 tbsp. dark brown sugar
- 1 tbsp. olive oil
- 2 tbsp. dry sherry
- 1 tbsp. Pure maple syrup
- ¼ tsp. sea salt
- 8 ounces lean lamb shoulder
- 2 cups water
- 4 medium red potatoes
- White onion, cut into halves
- 6 shitake mushroom caps
- ½ red bell pepper

DIRECTIONS:

1. In a blender, combine together lemon juice, chives, parsley, sage, brown sugar, olive oil, sherry, maple syrup, and salt; puree until very smooth.
2. Cut lamb into 8 cubes and add to a zipper bag along with the marinade; marinate in the refrigerator for 4 hours. Bring a pot with water to a rolling boil.
3. Cut potatoes in halves and add to the pot along with half onion; steam for about 15 mins. Transfer from flame and let cool. Chop the remaining onion and pepper.
4. Reserve the marinade.
5. Grill the kabobs over a hot grill, turning every 3 mins and basting with the reserved marinade.

768. Lemony Pork with Lentils

Prep Time: *5 Minutes* *Cook Time:* *20 Minutes* *Servings: 2*

INGREDIENTS:

- 2 tbsp. olive oil, divided
- 4 (4 ounces) pork chops
- 2 tbsp. Lemon juice
- 1 tsp. lemon zest
- 1 clove garlic
- 2 tbsp. Rosemary
- 1 tbsp. parsley
- 1 tbsp. pure maple syrup
- 6 cups water, divided
- ½ mug green lentils
- 1 shallot
- 1 rib celery
- ½ mug dry sherry, divided
- 1 tsp. sea salt
- 1 tsp. Unsalted butter
- ¼ tsp. red pepper flakes

DIRECTIONS:

1. In a zipper bag, combine olive oil, pork chops, lemon juice, lemon zest, garlic clove, rosemary, parsley, and maple syrup; refrigerate for at least 8 hours.
2. Combine 3 cups of water and green lentils in a saucepan set over medium flame and cook for about twenty minutes or until lentils are just tender; drain and rinse.

3. Preflame your oven to 350°F.
4. Flame a nonstick skillet over medium to high flame and add the marinade; sear pork for about 2 mins per side and transfer the skillet to the oven.
5. In the meantime, flame 1 teaspoon of olive oil to a second nonstick skillet set over medium to high heat; add shallot, red pepper flakes, and celery and lower flame to medium; cook for about 4 mins or until tender. Stir in lentils until warmed through.
6. Add ¼ teaspoon sea salt and ¼ mug sherry and cook for about 2 mins or until liquid is reduced by half. Stir in butter until melted.
7. Divide the lentil batter among four plates and top each serving with one pork chop from the first skillet.
8. Transfer and discard garlic from marinade in the first skillet and deglaze the pan with ¼ mug sherry; increase flame and stir in ¼ teaspoon sea salt; cook until the liquid is reduced by half.
9. Evenly pour the sauce over each serving and serve.

769. Cumin Pork Chops

Prep Time: 5 Minutes | *Cook Time: 20 Minutes* | *Servings: 4*

INGREDIENTS:

- 4-ounce lean center-cut pork chop
- ⅛ tsp. Sea salt
- ⅛ tsp. ground cumin
- Olive oil spray
- 2 tbsp. mashed avocado
- 2 tsp. Cilantro leaves

DIRECTIONS:

1. Preflame your oven to 400°F.
2. Flame a large skillet over medium heat.
3. In the meantime, season pork chop with sea salt and cumin.
4. Spray the pan with olive oil & add the seasoned pork chop. Place the pan in the oven and cook for about 10 mins; turn the pork chop over, and spread the seared part with avocado.
5. Return to oven and cook for about 10 mins more or until pork is done.
6. Serve pork garnished with cilantro over mashed potatoes.

770. Healthy Lamb Burgers

Prep Time: 5 Minutes | *Cook Time: 20 Minutes* | *Servings: 6*

INGREDIENTS

- 1 tbsp. olive oil
- 1 lb. lean ground lamb
- 2 tbsp. Yogurt cheese
- ⅛ tsp. ground allspice
- ½ mug cilantro leaves, chopped
- 1 egg white
- 1 shallot, finely chopped
- 2 cloves garlic, chopped
- 2 tsp. fresh ginger, minced
- 1 red chili pepper, chopped
- ⅛ tsp. ground cumin
- 4 cardamom seeds
- ⅛ tsp. Black pepper
- ¼ tsp. sea salt
- spray olive oil
- Four whole-wheat hamburger buns

DIRECTIONS:

1. Combine all the ingredients except spray olive oil and buns, and
2. Refrigerate for at least 20 mins.
3. Preflame your oven to 400° F.
4. Put olive oil in a nonstick skillet over medium flame.
5. In the meantime, form lamb batter into four burgers.
6. Sear burgers in a prepared pan for about 1 minute; transfer the pan to the preheated oven and cook for about 5 mins, turn burgers over and cook for about 3 mins more.

771. Herb-Maple Crusted Steak

Prep Time: 5 Minutes | *Cook Time: 20 Minutes* | *Servings: 2*

INGREDIENTS:

- 3 tbsp. rosemary
- 3 tbsp. Tarragon
- 3 tbsp. chives
- 3 tbsp. chopped oregano
- 4 tbsp. parsley
- 3 tbsp. maple syrup
- 4 (4 ounces) ribeye steaks, trimmed
- ½ tsp. Sea salt
- ¼ tsp. black pepper
- spray olive oil

DIRECTIONS:

1. Preflame your oven to 450°F.
2. Flame a nonstick skillet in the oven.
3. In the meantime, combine the minced herbs on a plate. Add maple syrup to a separate container.
4. Season steak with sea salt & pepper and dip into the maple syrup; turn to coat well.
5. Dip the steak into the herbs and turn to coat well. Repeat with the remaining steak.
6. Transfer the skillet from the oven and spray with olive oil; add steaks to the pan and turn until well seared.
7. Return to oven and cook for about 4 mins, turn and cook the other side for about 6 mins more.

772. Tenderloin with Cheese Butter

Prep Time: 5 Minutes | *Cook Time: 20 Minutes* | *Servings: 5*

INGREDIENTS:

- ⅛ tsp. black pepper
- 1 shallot, minced
- 1 tsp. unsalted butter
- 2 tbsp. chopped parsley
- 2 tsp. blue cheese
- Olive oil spray
- 2 4-ounce beef tenderloin filets
- ¼ tsp. sea salt

DIRECTIONS:

1. In a blender, blend pepper, shallot, butter, parsley, and blue cheese until very smooth.
2. Preflame your oven to 450°F.
3. Place a nonstick skillet in the oven and spray with olive oil. Season beef with sea salt and place in the pan; cook for about 7 mins, turn over & cook the other side for about 4 mins more. Transfer the meat to a plate and top with seasoned butter to serve.

773. Mediterranean-Style Greek Pasta Recipe

Prep Time: 15 Minutes | *Cook Time:□45 Minutes* | *Servings: 2*

Ingredients

- 1/2 pound whole-wheat spaghetti pasta
- 2 tablespoons olive oil
- 1 onion small, diced
- 2 cups spinach leaves fresh
- 3 garlic cloves sliced
- 1 beefsteak tomato large, diced
- 1/2 teaspoon kosher salt
- 1/4 teaspoon ground black pepper
- 1/2 cup feta cheese fat-free, crumbled

Instructions

1. Bring 4 cups of water to boil in a medium pot.
2. Add 1 teaspoon salt and pasta to water. Boil uncovered until pasta is tender, about 10 minutes.
3. Drain pasta, reserve 1/2 cup of pasta water. Set aside.
4. In a large skillet, heat the oil over medium heat until hot, but not smoking.
5. Add onions and garlic to skillet. Cook, stirring often, just until onions begin to soften.
6. Add diced tomatoes and spinach. Stir, cover and let simmer for 5 minutes or until spinach is heated through and just begins to wilt.

774. Greek Roasted Fish

Prep Time: 15 Minutes | *Cook Time:□20 Minutes* | *Servings: 2*

Ingredients

- 1 pound fingerling potatoes, halved lengthwise
- 2 tablespoons olive oil
- 5 garlic cloves, coarsely chopped
- ½ teaspoon sea salt
- ½ teaspoon freshly ground black pepper
- 4 5 to 6-ounce fresh or frozen skinless salmon fillets
- 2 medium red, yellow and/or orange sweet peppers, cut into rings
- 2 cups cherry tomatoes
- 1 ½ cups chopped fresh parsley (1 bunch)
- ¼ cup pitted kalamata olives, halved
- ¼ cup finely snipped fresh oregano or 1 Tbsp. dried oregano, crushed
- 1 lemon

Directions:

1. Preheat oven to 425 degrees F. Place potatoes in a large bowl. Drizzle with 1 Tbsp. of the oil and sprinkle with garlic and 1/8 tsp. of the salt and black pepper; toss to coat. Transfer to a 15x10-inch baking pan; cover with foil. Roast 30 minutes.
2. Meanwhile, thaw salmon, if frozen. Combine, in the same bowl, sweet peppers, tomatoes, parsley, olives, oregano and 1/8 tsp. of the salt and black pepper. Drizzle with remaining 1 Tbsp. oil; toss to coat.
3. Rinse salmon; pat dry. Sprinkle with remaining 1/4 tsp. salt and black pepper. Spoon sweet pepper mixture over potatoes and top with salmon. Roast, uncovered, 10 minutes more or just until salmon flakes.

775. Mediterranean Steak Bites

Prep Time: 15 Minutes | *Cook Time:□25 Minutes* | *Servings: 8*

Ingredients

- 1 3/4 pounds flank steak
- 1/4 cup soy sauce
- 2 tablespoons nectar
- 1 tablespoon stew paste
- 1-2 tablespoons light seasoned olive oil

Directions

1. Cut the steak across the grain into strips 1/2" wide. Cut each strip into reduced down pieces, roughly 1/2" - 3/4" in size. Spot the pieces of hamburger into a medium size bowl. Mix together the soy sauce, nectar, and bean stew paste. Pour over the meat and mix to cover well. Allow the meat to marinate for 20-30 minutes.

2. Heat a substantial base hardened steel dish or wok over medium high heat. At the point when the dish is hot, add 1 tablespoon of oil and twirl to cover. Add 1/3 of the meat to the container and spread out in a solitary layer. Allow it to cook for about a moment, until the meat has carmelized. Flip the meat or throw with a spatula for an extra moment or two as it completes the process of cooking. Eliminate the meat from the dish to a plate.
3. Add half of the excess meat to the hot dish and rehash the above advances. Add the cooked meat to the holding up plate. In the event that vital, add the excess tablespoon of oil to the skillet prior to adding the leftover meat. Rehash the means. Enjoy!
4. In the event that anytime the skillet starts to smoke, it is excessively hot. Lower the heat marginally and keep cooking. Eliminate the steak chomps from the container when they are seared outwardly and still delicious within. They will keep cooking briefly after they are taken out from the heat. Skirt steak might be filling in for the flank steak in this formula.

776. Greek White Bean Soup

Prep Time: 15 Minutes *Cook Time:☐30 Minutes* *Servings: 5*

INGREDIENTS

- 2 (15-ounce) jars white beans
- 1 medium yellow onion
- 4 cloves garlic
- 1/4 teaspoon red pepper chips (discretionary)
- 2 tablespoons olive oil
- 4 cups low-sodium vegetable or chicken stock
- 1 (14-ounce) can diced tomatoes
- 2 twigs new rosemary
- 1 teaspoon legitimate salt
- 1/4 teaspoon newly ground dark pepper
- 1 Parmesan skin (discretionary)
- 5 ounces child spinach (around 5 stuffed cups)
- Ground Parmesan cheddar, for serving

Directions

1. Channel and wash 2 jars white beans and put in a safe spot. Finely slash 1 medium yellow onion and mince 4 cloves garlic.
2. Heat 2 tablespoons olive oil in a Dutch oven or huge pot until sparkling. Add the onion and sauté until relaxed and clear, 3 to 5 minutes. Add the garlic and 1/4 teaspoon red pepper pieces, if using, and sauté until fragrant, around brief more.
3. Pour in 4 cups low-sodium vegetable or chicken stock, 1 can diced tomatoes and their juices, and the white beans. Add 2 new rosemary twigs, 1 teaspoon legitimate salt, 1/4 teaspoon dark pepper, and 1 Parmesan skin, if using, and mix to join. Heat to the point of boiling. Lessen the heat to keep a stew, and stew uncovered for 10 minutes to permit the flavors to merge.
4. Mix in 5 ounces child spinach (around 5 stuffed cups); a couple of small bunches all at once, until just withered, 1 to 2 minutes. Serve decorated with ground Parmesan cheddar.

Formula Notes

5. Substitute frozen spinach: Frozen spinach can be fill in for the new spinach. Basically mix in an equivalent weight (or more; this is adaptable) of frozen spinach and stew until heated through.
6. Add extra protein: If wanted, you can mix in a cup of shredded chicken (pulled from a rotisserie chicken, or canned chicken) into this soup in definite advance with the spinach.

777. Greek Lemon-Caper Black Cod with Broccoli & Potatoes

Prep Time: 15 Minutes *Cook Time:☐35 Minutes* *Servings:8*

Ingredients

- 1 pound baby potatoes, halved
- 12 ounces precut broccoli florets
- 4 tablespoons extra-virgin olive oil, partitioned
- ½ teaspoon genuine salt, isolated
- 1 pound skin-on dark cod (see Tip)
- ¼ teaspoon ground pepper
- 2 tablespoons escapades, flushed and wiped off
- 2 tablespoons lemon juice
- 1 tablespoon Dijon mustard
- 1 clove garlic, minced
- 1 tablespoon chopped new thyme or 1/4 teaspoon dried
- 3 tablespoons shredded Parmesan cheddar

Directions

1. Preheat oven to 450degrees F. Coat a rimmed heating sheet with cooking shower.
2. Throw potatoes and broccoli with 1 tablespoon oil and 1/4 teaspoon salt in an enormous bowl. Move to the readied preparing sheet. Cook, mixing once, until delicate, 20 to 25 minutes.
3. In the meantime, wipe cod off and cut into 4 segments. Season with the leftover 1/4 teaspoon salt and pepper. Heat 1 tablespoon oil in a huge nonstick skillet over medium heat. Add tricks and cook until brilliant brown, 1 to 2 minutes. Using an opened spoon, move the escapades to a paper towel, leaving the oil in the container. Spot the cod skin-side down in the skillet. Cook, undisturbed, for 5 minutes. Flip and cook until the fish drops effectively with a fork, 3 to 4 minutes more.
4. Consolidate the excess 2 tablespoons oil, lemon juice, mustard and garlic in a little bowl.
5. Throw the potatoes and broccoli with thyme. Serve the vegetables and cod sprinkled with the lemon vinaigrette and decorated with the tricks and Parmesan.

778. Mediterranean Roasted Chicken Thighs with Peppers & Potatoes

Prep Time: 15 Minutes *Cook Time:☐60 Minutes* *Servings: 4*

Ingredients

- 2 pounds red potatoes (about 6 medium)
- 2 large sweet red peppers
- 2 large green peppers
- 2 medium onions
- 2 tablespoons olive oil, divided
- 4 teaspoons minced fresh thyme or 1-1/2 teaspoons dried thyme, divided
- 3 teaspoons minced fresh rosemary or 1 teaspoon dried rosemary, crushed, divided
- 8 boneless skinless chicken thighs (about 2 pounds)
- 1/2 teaspoon salt
- 1/4 teaspoon pepper

Directions

1. Firstly preheat oven to 450°. Cut potatoes, peppers and onions into 1-in. pieces. Place vegetables in a roasting pan. Drizzle with 1 tablespoon oil; sprinkle with 2 teaspoons each thyme and rosemary and toss to coat. Put chicken over vegetables. Brush chicken with remaining oil; sprinkle with remaining thyme and rosemary. Drizzle vegetables and chicken with salt and pepper.
2. Roast until a thermometer inserted in chicken reads 170° and vegetables are tender, 35-40 minutes.

779. Green Curry Beef

Prep Time: 15 Minutes *Cook Time:☐30 Minutes* *Servings: 6*

INGREDIENTS:

- 1 tbsp. olive oil
- ½ mug chopped parsley
- 1 mug cilantro leaves
- 1 white onion, chopped
- 1Thai green chili, chopped
- 2 cloves garlic, thinly sliced
- ¼ tsp. Turmeric
- ½ tsp. ground cumin
- 2 tbsp. Lime juice
- ¼ tsp. sea salt
- Black pepper
- 16 ounces beef top round, cut into pieces
- 1 can light coconut milk
- ¼ tsp. turmeric
- ½ tsp. ground cumin
- ¼ tsp. sea salt

DIRECTIONS:

Green curry paste:

1. In a blender or blender, combine olive oil, parsley, cilantro, onion, chili pepper, garlic, turmeric, cumin, lime juice, sea salt, and pepper; process until very smooth.
2. Combine beef and green curry paste in a container; toss to coat.
3. Refrigerate for at least 30 mins.
4. When ready, flame a large skillet over medium to high flame and add beef along with the green curry sauce.
5. Lower flame and stir for about 10 mins or until the meat is browned on the outside.
6. Stir in coconut milk and cook for about 30 mins or until the sauce is thick.
7. Serve immediately.

780. Mediterranean Beef Pitas

Prep Time: 15 Minutes *Cook Time:☐90 Minutes* *Servings: 2*

INGREDIENTS:

- 1pound ground beef
- Freshly ground black pepper
- Sea salt
- 1 ½ tsp. dried oregano
- 2 tbsp. olive oil, divided
- ¼ red onion, sliced
- 3/4mug store-bought hummus
- 2 tbsp. Flat-parsley
- 4 pitas
- 4 lemon wedges

DIRECTIONS:

1. Form beef into 16 patties; season with ¼ teaspoon ground pepper, ½ teaspoon sea salt, and oregano.
2. Add 1 tbsp of olive oil in a skillet set over medium heat; cook the beef patties for about 2 mins per side or until lightly browned. To serve, top pitas with the beef patties, hummus, parsley, and onion and drizzle with the remaining olive oil; garnish with lemon wedges.

781. Parmesan Meatloaf

Prep Time: 15 Minutes *Cook Time:☐55 Minutes* *Servings: 6*

INGREDIENTS:

- 1½ pounds ground beef
- ½ mug bread crumbs
- ½ mug chopped flat-leaf parsley
- 1 grated onion
- 1 large egg
- ½ mug grated Parmesan
- ¼ mug tomato paste
- Sea salt
- Freshly ground black pepper

DIRECTIONS:

1. Preflame your oven to 400°F. In a large container, combine together ground beef, bread crumbs, parsley, onion, egg, Parmesan cheese, tomato paste, sea salt, and pepper.
2. Line a baking sheet with foil. Add the beef mixture, pressing to form an 8-inch loaf.
3. Bake in the preheated oven for fifty mins or until cooked through.

782. Mediterranean Flank Steak

Prep Time: 5 Minutes *Cook Time: 20 Minutes* *Servings: 5*

INGREDIENTS:

- 2 tbsp. chopped aromatic herbs (marjoram, rosemary, sage, thyme, or a mix)
- 2 cloves garlic, minced
- 2 tbsp. olive oil
- 1 tbsp. sea salt
- 1 tbsp. ground black pepper
- 1½-to 2-lb. flank steak, trimmed
- ½ mug Greek vinaigrette

DIRECTIONS:

1. In a container, combine together herbs, garlic, olive oil, sea salt, and pepper; rub over the steak and let rest for about 20 mins. In the meantime, flame your gas grill to medium to high.
2. Grill the steak for about 15 mins, turning meat every 4 mins for even cooking.
3. Put the cooked steak on a cutting board. Rest for about 5 mins; slice into slices and place on plates. Drizzle with vinaigrette and serve immediately.

783. Mediterranean Lamb Chops

Prep Time: 5 Minutes *Cook Time: 20 Minutes* *Servings: 7*

INGREDIENTS:

- 2 tbsp. olive oil, divided
- 3 garlic cloves
- 1 tsp. chopped rosemary
- 2 tbsp. chopped mint
- 4 lean lamb chops
- 2 yellow peppers, diced
- 2 red peppers, diced
- 4 zucchinis, sliced
- 1 eggplant, sliced
- 3 oz. crumbled feta cheese
- 9 oz. cherry tomatoes

DIRECTIONS:

1. Preflame your oven to 350°F.
2. In a blender, blend together 1 tbsp olive oil, garlic, rosemary, and mint until very smooth; smear over the lamb chops. On a baking sheet, combine peppers, zucchini, and eggplant; drizzle with the remaining oil.
3. Place the lamb chops over the vegetables and roast in the preheated oven for about 25 mins.
4. Transfer the baking sheet from the oven and top with cherry tomatoes and feta cheese; return to the oven & continue roasting for 10 mins more or until lamb chops are cooked through, and cheese begins to brown. Serve the roasted vegetables with lamb chops and green salad.

784. Easy Mediterranean Pizza

Prep Time: 15 Minutes *Cook Time:□120 Minutes* *Servings: 6*

INGREDIENTS

- 1 ball Best Pizza Dough (or Food Processor Dough or Thin Crust Dough)
- 1/3 cup Best Homemade Pizza Sauce
- 1 teaspoon olive oil
- 1 cup packed baby spinach leaves
- 1 handful red onion slices
- 6 Kalamata olives
- 8 sundried tomatoes, packed in oil
- 3/4 cup shredded mozzarella cheese
- 1 ounce feta cheese
- 8 fresh basil leaves
- Kosher salt
- Semolina flour or cornmeal, for cleaning the pizza strip

Guidelines

1. Make the pizza batter: Follow the Best Pizza Dough formula to set up the mixture. (This requires around 15 minutes to make and 45 minutes to rest.)
2. Spot a pizza stone in the oven and preheat to 500°F. Or on the other hand preheat your pizza oven (here's the pizza oven we use).
3. Make the pizza sauce: Make the 5 Minute Pizza Sauce.
4. Set up the fixings: In a little skillet, heat the olive oil over medium heat. Add the spinach and cook for 2 minutes until withered yet radiant green. Add 1 squeeze salt and eliminate from the heat.
5. Meagerly cut the red onion. Cut the olives fifty-fifty. On the off chance that the sundried tomatoes are huge, you can slash them more modest as well.
6. Prepare the pizza: When the oven is prepared, dust a pizza strip with cornmeal or semolina flour. (On the off chance that you don't have a pizza strip, you can utilize a rimless heating sheet or the rear of a rimmed preparing sheet. Yet, a pizza strip is definitely worth the speculation!) Stretch the mixture into a circle; perceive How to Stretch Pizza Dough for directions. At that point delicately place the mixture onto the pizza strip.
7. Spread the pizza sauce over the mixture using the rear of a spoon to make a dainty layer. Add the shredded mozzarella cheddar. Top with the cooked spinach, red onion, olives, and sundried tomatoes. what's more, feta cheddar.
8. Utilize the pizza strip to deliberately move the pizza onto the preheated pizza stone. Heat the pizza until the cheddar and outside layer are pleasantly browned, around 5 to 7 minutes in the oven (or 1 moment in a pizza oven).
9. Permit the pizza to cool briefly prior to including the basil top (entire leaves, daintily torn, or meagerly cut). Cut into pieces and serve right away.

785. Easy Greek Roasted Tomato Basil Soup

Prep Time: 10 Mins | Cook Time: 50 Mins | Servings: 6

Ingredients

- 3 lb. Roma tomatoes divided
- 2 to 3 carrots stripped and cut into little pieces
- Additional virgin olive oil (I utilized Private Reserve Greek EVOO)
- Salt and pepper
- 2 medium yellow onions chopped
- 5 garlic cloves minced
- 1 cup canned squashed tomatoes
- 2 oz. new basil leaves
- 3 to 4 new thyme springs 2 tsp. thyme leaves
- 1 tsp. dry oregano
- ½ tsp. paprika
- ½ tsp. ground cumin
- 2 ½ cups water
- Sprinkle of lime juice optional

Guidelines

1. Heat oven to 450 degrees F.
2. In an enormous blending bowl, consolidate tomatoes and carrot pieces. Add a liberal shower of additional virgin olive oil, and season with fit salt and dark pepper. Throw to join.
3. Move to an enormous heating sheet and spread well in one layer. Broil in heated oven for around 30 minutes. At the point when prepared, eliminate from the heat and put in a safe spot for around 10 minutes to cool.
4. Move the broiled tomatoes and carrots to the enormous bowl of a food processor fitted with a cutting edge. Add simply a smidgen of water and mix.
5. In a huge cooking pot, heat 2 tbsp. additional virgin olive oil over medium-high heat until shining yet not smoking. Add onions and cook for around 3 minutes, at that point add garlic and cook momentarily until brilliant.
6. Empty the simmered tomato blend into the cooking pot. Mix in squashed tomatoes, 2 ½ cups water, basil, thyme and flavors. Season with a little genuine salt and dark pepper. Heat to the point of boiling, at that point lower heat and cover part-way. Let stew for around 20 minutes or somewhere in the vicinity.
7. Eliminate the thyme springs and move tomato basil soup to serving bowls. In the event that you like, add a sprinkle of lime juice and a liberal shower of extra virgihttps://shop.themediterraneandish.com/item/extra-virgin-olive-oil-pack/n olive oil. Present with your #1 dry bread or flame broiled bits of French loaf. Enjoy!

NOTES

1. Extras: If you have any extras, you can refrigerate in close top glass compartments for 3 to 4 days. Ensure the soup is totally cooled prior to putting away.
2. Would you be able to freeze this tomato basil soup? Indeed! Since this is a sans dairy veggie lover tomato basil soup and there is no cream required by any means, it is the ideal tomato soup to freeze.
3. Essentially cool the soup prior to putting away in close cover, cooler safe compartments. Freeze for some time in the future (3 to a half year or something like that.) Thaw in ice chest short-term and go through medium heat to warm.

Varieties:

1. If you're searching for somewhat of a smoky completion, add a decent touch of smoked paprika. Or then again, to zest things up, cook some jalapeno pepper and mix them alongside the tomatoes and carrots.

786. Easy Greek-Style Eggplant Recipe

Prep Time: 15 Minutes

Cook Time: 35 Minutes

Servings: 3

Ingredients

- 3 lb. Roma tomatoes divided
- 2 to 3 carrots stripped and cut into little pieces
- Additional virgin olive oil (I utilized Private Reserve Greek EVOO)
- Salt and pepper
- 2 medium yellow onions chopped
- 5 garlic cloves minced
- 1 cup canned squashed tomatoes
- 2 oz. new basil leaves
- 3 to 4 new thyme springs 2 tsp. thyme leaves
- 1 tsp. dry oregano
- ½ tsp. paprika
- ½ tsp. ground cumin
- 2 ½ cups water
- Sprinkle of lime juice optional

Guidelines

1. Heat oven to 450 degrees F.
2. In an enormous blending bowl, consolidate tomatoes and carrot pieces. Add a liberal shower of additional virgin olive oil, and season with fit salt and dark pepper. Throw to join.
3. Move to an enormous heating sheet and spread well in one layer. Broil in heated oven for around 30 minutes. At the point when prepared, eliminate from the heat and put in a safe spot for around 10 minutes to cool.
4. Move the broiled tomatoes and carrots to the enormous bowl of a food processor fitted with a cutting edge. Add simply a smidgen of water and mix.
5. In a huge cooking pot, heat 2 tbsp. additional virgin olive oil over medium-high heat until shining yet not smoking. Add onions and cook for around 3 minutes, at that point add garlic and cook momentarily until brilliant.
6. Empty the simmered tomato blend into the cooking pot. Mix in squashed tomatoes, 2 ½ cups water, basil, thyme and flavors. Season with a little genuine salt and dark pepper. Heat to the point of boiling, at that point lower heat and cover part-way. Let stew for around 20 minutes or somewhere in the vicinity.
7. Eliminate the thyme springs and move tomato basil soup to serving bowls. In the event that you like, add a sprinkle of lime juice and a liberal shower of extra Present with your #1 dry bread or flame broiled bits of French loaf. Enjoy!

NOTES

1. Extras: If you have any extras, you can refrigerate in close top glass compartments for 3 to 4 days. Ensure the soup is totally cooled prior to putting away.
2. Would you be able to freeze this tomato basil soup? Indeed! Since this is a sans dairy veggie lover tomato basil soup and there is no cream required by any means, it is the ideal tomato soup to freeze.
3. Essentially cool the soup prior to putting away in close cover, cooler safe compartments. Freeze for some time in the future (3 to a half year or something like that.) Thaw in ice chest short-term and go through medium heat to warm.

Varieties:

1. If you're searching for somewhat of a smoky completion, add a decent touch of smoked paprika. Or then again, to zest things up, cook some jalapeno pepper and mix them alongside the tomatoes and carrots.

787. Greek White Pizza with Roasted Tomatoes

Prep Time: 15 Minutes *Cook Time:☐70 Minutes* *Servings: 8*

Ingredients

- 4 plum tomatoes (around 1 pound), cut longwise into 1/2-inch cuts and cultivated
- 1/4 cup olive oil
- 1 teaspoon sugar
- 1/2 teaspoon salt

Outside:

- 2 tablespoons olive oil
- 1 huge onion, finely chopped (around 1 cup)
- 2 teaspoons dried basil
- 2 teaspoons dried thyme
- 1 teaspoon dried rosemary, squashed
- 1 bundle (1/4 ounce) dynamic dry yeast
- 1 cup warm water (110° to 115°)
- 5 tablespoons sugar
- 1/4 cup olive oil
- 1-1/2 teaspoons salt
- 3-1/4 to 3-3/4 cups all-purpose flour

Topping:

- 1 cup entire milk ricotta cheddar
- 3 garlic cloves, minced
- 1/2 teaspoon salt
- 1/2 teaspoon Italian flavoring
- 2 cups shredded part-skim mozzarella cheddar

Directions

1. Preheat oven to 250°. In a bowl, throw tomatoes with oil, sugar and salt. Move to a lubed 15x10x1-in. heating container. Broil 2 hours or until tomatoes are delicate and somewhat withered.
2. For outside, in an enormous skillet, heat oil over medium-high heat. Add onion; cook and mix 3-4 minutes or until delicate. Mix in spices. Cool somewhat.
3. In a small bowl, break down yeast in warm water. In a huge bowl, join sugar, oil, salt, yeast combination and 1 cup flour; beat on medium speed until smooth. Mix in onion combination and enough leftover flour to shape a delicate mixture (batter will be tacky).
4. Turn batter onto a floured surface; massage until smooth and versatile, around 6-8 minutes. Spot in a lubed bowl, going once to oil the top. Cover with cling wrap and let ascend in a warm spot until practically multiplied, around 1-1/2 hours.
5. Preheat oven to 400°. Oil a 15x10x1-in. preparing container. Punch down batter; move to fit base and 1/2-in. up sides of container. Cover; let rest 10 minutes. Heat 10-12 minutes or until edges are daintily browned.
6. In a small bowl, blend ricotta cheddar, garlic, salt and Italian flavoring. Spread over covering; top with cooked tomatoes and mozzarella cheddar. Heat 12-15 minutes or until covering is brilliant and cheddar is liquefied.

788. Mediterranean Orange-Glazed Pork

Prep Time: 15 Minutes *Cook Time:☐50 Minutes* *Servings: 7*

Ingredients

- 1 pound yams (around 2 medium)
- 2 medium apples
- 1 medium orange
- 1 teaspoon salt
- 1/2 teaspoon pepper
- 1 cup squeezed orange
- 2 tablespoons brown sugar
- 2 teaspoons cornstarch
- 1 teaspoon ground cinnamon
- 1 teaspoon ground ginger
- 2 pork tenderloins (around 1 pound each)

Directions

1. Preheat oven to 350°. Strip yams; center apples. Cut potatoes, apples and orange transversely into 1/4-in. - thick cuts. Organize in a foil-lined 15x10x1-in. heating container covered with cooking shower; sprinkle with salt and pepper. Cook 10 minutes.
2. Then, in a microwave-safe bowl, blend squeezed orange, brown sugar, cornstarch, cinnamon and ginger. Microwave, covered, on high, mixing like clockwork until thickened, 1-2 minutes. Mix until smooth.
3. Spot pork over yam combination; sprinkle with squeezed orange blend. Broil until a thermometer embedded in pork peruses 145° and yams and apples are delicate, 45-55 minutes longer. Eliminate from oven; tent with foil. Let stand 10 minutes prior to cutting.

789. Quinoa-Stuffed Squash Boats

Prep Time: 15 Minutes *Cook Time:☐53 Minutes* *Servings: 2*

Ingredients

- 4 delicata squash (around 12 ounces each)
- 3 teaspoons olive oil, partitioned
- 1/8 teaspoon pepper
- 1 teaspoon salt, partitioned
- 1-1/2 cups vegetable stock
- 1 cup quinoa, washed
- 1 can (15 ounces) garbanzo beans or chickpeas, washed and depleted
- 1/4 cup dried cranberries
- 1 green onion, daintily cut
- 1 teaspoon minced new wise
- 1/2 teaspoon ground lemon zing
- 1 teaspoon lemon juice
- 1/2 cup disintegrated goat cheddar
- 1/4 cup salted pumpkin seeds or pepitas, toasted

Directions

1. Preheat oven to 450°. Cut each squash longwise down the middle; eliminate and dispose of seeds. Daintily brush cut sides with 1 teaspoon oil; sprinkle with pepper and 1/2 teaspoon salt. Spot on a heating sheet, cut side down. Prepare until delicate, 15-20 minutes.
2. In the interim, in an enormous pan, join stock and quinoa; heat to the point of boiling. Lessen heat; stew, covered, until fluid is assimilated, 12-15 minutes.
3. Mix in garbanzo beans, cranberries, green onion, sage, lemon zing, lemon juice and the leftover oil and salt; spoon into squash. Sprinkle with cheddar and pumpkin seeds.

790. Mediterranean Grilled Balsamic Chicken

Prep Time: 15 Minutes *Cook Time:☐20 Minutes* *Servings: 3*

INGREDIENTS

- 2 skinless boneless Simple Truth chicken breasts
- 1/4 cup olive oil
- 1/4 cup brilliant balsamic vinegar
- 1/8 cup Private Selection Whole Grain Garlic Mustard
- 1/2 tablespoons balsamic vinegar
- 3 cloves garlic squeezed or minced
- Juice of 1/2 lemon
- 1 storing tablespoon chopped new spices, for example, Simple Truth tarragon rosemary or thyme
- 1 teaspoon fit salt
- 1/2 teaspoon newly ground dark pepper
- Present with Olive Tapenade formula beneath and lumps of feta cheddar

Guidelines

1. Cut back any additional excess from the chicken breasts and spot in a bowl or a gallon size cooler pack.
2. In a little bowl, whisk the olive oil, balsamic vinegars, mustard, garlic, lemon juice, spices, and salt and pepper. Save half of the marinade and add the other half to the bowl or pack with the chicken. Marinate for at any rate 30 minutes up to expedite, turning sporadically.
3. At the point when prepared to flame broil, bring one side of an outside barbecue to high heat with the opposite side off.
4. Oil the barbecue grinds well and sprinkles the chicken breasts with more olive oil, at that point place the chicken breasts on the hot flame broil. Cook for 2-3 minutes or until barbecue marks show up, at that point flip the chicken and cook for another 2-3 minutes. Move the chicken to the cooler meshes of the barbecue, cover, and cook for 10 minutes. Move a couple of tablespoons of the held marinade to another bowl and use it to treat the chicken with and flip. Keep cooking, treating, and flipping until the breasts have an interior temperature of 165 degrees. Move the chicken to the hot side of the barbecue to add more flame broil checks and shading to the chicken bosom yet make certain to watch them so the balsamic marinade doesn't burn. The length of cooking time will depend up on the thickness of the breasts however you should rely in general cooking time to be around 30 minutes.
5. Move the chicken to a platter and cover with a piece of aluminum foil and let rest for 5 minutes. Present with olive tapenade, lumps of feta cheddar minced spices and shower with any extra olive oil.

791. Greek Grilled Lemon Chicken Skewers

Prep Time: 15 Minutes *Cook Time:☐23 Minutes* *Servings: 2*

Ingredients

- 2 boneless chicken breasts
- 3 lemons
- 4 cloves garlic minced
- 1 tablespoon dried oregano
- 1/4 cup olive oil
- 1 teaspoon kosher salt
- 1/2 teaspoon newly ground pepper
- 7-8 green onions

Guidelines

1. Cut the chicken breasts the long way into thirds, and afterward cut again into around 1-inch pieces. Spot chicken lumps in a cooler pack and put in a safe spot.
2. Zing one of the lemons and add to a medium size bowl. Juice that lemon in addition to one more, adds to the lemon zing and afterward adds the minced garlic and oregano and mix. Gradually shower in the olive oil and rush to consolidate. Add genuine salt and pepper. Empty the marinade into the cooler sack with the chicken pieces and let marinade for 30 minutes or as long as 3 hours in the fridge.
3. At the point when prepared to flame broil, set up the barbecue by softly oiling the mesh with vegetable oil or cooking splash and set to medium high heat.
4. In the case of using wooden sticks, set them up by absorbing water for 10 minutes. In the case of using metal sticks, no prep is important.
5. Cut the excess lemon in slender adjusts and afterward cut the rounds down the middle. Trim the bottoms of the green onions off and cut into 1-inch lengths.
6. String one piece of the chicken onto a stick then two cuts of green onion, and afterward another piece of chicken. Overlap a cut of lemon fifty-fifty and string close to the chicken, gathering intently on the stick. Add another piece of chicken, at that point green onions and rehash the example until you've arrived at the finish of the stick, finishing with chicken. Dispose of any of the excess marinade.
7. Flame broil chicken, turning regularly so each side browns and has light barbecue marks, until cooked through, around 10-15 minutes or until chicken juices run clear.

792. Mediterranean Sautéed Chicken with Olives, Capers and Lemons

Prep Time: 15 Minutes *Cook Time:☐30 Minutes* *Servings: 3*

Ingredients

- 2 lemons sliced 1/4 inch thick
- 1/4 cup plus 1 tablespoon extra-virgin olive oil
- 6 skinless boneless chicken thighs, about 1 pound
- 1-2 tablespoons rice flour or all-purpose flour
- 1 fat garlic clove minced
- 1 cup chicken broth
- 3/4 cup Sicilian green olives
- 1/4 cup carpers
- 2 tablespoons spread
- 2 tablespoons parsley
- legitimate salt and newly broke dark pepper

Directions

1. Bring a medium-huge, high sided skillet to medium-high heat and add 1 tablespoon of olive oil. Add half of the lemon cuts and singe until browned, 3-5 minutes on each side. Move to a plate. Season the chicken thighs with fit salt and dark pepper and residue with rice flour, shaking off the overabundance. Add 1/2 tablespoons of olive oil to the hot skillet and burn the chicken pieces until brilliant brown, around 5 minutes each side. Move to another plate and wrap up singing the remainder of the chicken pieces, at that point move to a similar plate as the remainder of the chicken.
2. Add the remainder of the olive oil to the skillet and the minced garlic, and cook for 30 seconds or until fragrant, blending so the garlic doesn't consume and turn out to be harsh.
3. Add the green olives, tricks and stock. Add the saved chicken and any juices that have been delivered in addition to the saved lemons and their juices and cook over high heat until the stock is diminished significantly, around 5 minutes. Add the spread and parsley and cook for one more moment. Season with more legitimate salt and newly ground dark pepper to taste. Move to plates and spoon the olives, tricks, lemons and sauce on top.
4. Present with sautéed spinach, kale or Swiss chard as an afterthought.

793. Greek Pan-Roasted Chicken and Vegetables

Prep Time: 15 Minutes | *Cook Time:□35 Minutes* | *Servings: 2*

Ingredients

- 2 pounds red potatoes (around 6 medium), cut into 3/4-inch pieces
- 1 enormous onion, coarsely chopped
- 2 tablespoons olive oil
- 3 garlic cloves, minced
- 1-1/4 teaspoons salt, separated
- 1 teaspoon dried rosemary, squashed, isolated
- 3/4 teaspoon pepper, separated
- 1/2 teaspoon paprika
- 6 bone-in chicken thighs (around 2-1/4 pounds), skin eliminated
- 6 cups new child spinach (around 6 ounces)

Directions

1. Preheat oven to 425°. In a huge bowl, consolidate potatoes, onion, oil, garlic, 3/4 teaspoon salt, 1/2 teaspoon rosemary and 1/2 teaspoon pepper; throw to cover. Move to a 15x10x1-in. preparing pan covered with cooking shower.
2. In a small bowl, blend paprika and the leftover salt, rosemary and pepper. Sprinkle chicken with paprika combination; organize over vegetables. Cook until a thermometer embedded in chicken peruses 170°-175° and vegetables are simply delicate, 35-40 minutes.
3. Eliminate chicken to a serving platter; keep warm. Top vegetables with spinach. Broil until vegetables are delicate and spinach is shriveled, 8-10 minutes longer. Mix vegetables to join; present with chicken.
4. Set up your sheet-pan supper the prior night and simply pop it into the preheated oven to prepare. This serves to profoundly enhance the chicken, a shared benefit!
5. In the event that you need a more extravagant dish, use skin-on chicken, and on the off chance that you need a lighter dish, utilize bone-in chicken breasts. Make certain to cook bone-in breasts just to 165-170 degrees, since more slender meat can get dry at higher temperatures.

794. Greek Seafood Couscous Paella

Prep Time: 15 Minutes | *Cook Time:□90 Minutes* | *Servings: 2*

Ingredients

- 2 teaspoons extra-virgin olive oil
- 1 medium onion, chopped
- 1 clove garlic, minced
- ½ teaspoon dried thyme
- ½ teaspoon fennel seed
- ¼ teaspoon salt
- ¼ teaspoon freshly ground pepper
- Pinch of crumbled saffron threads
- 1 cup no-salt-added diced tomatoes, with juice
- ¼ cup vegetable broth
- 4 ounces bay scallops, tough muscle removed
- 4 ounces small shrimp, (41-50 per pound), peeled and deveined
- ½ cup whole-wheat couscous

DIRECTIONS:

1. Heat oil in a large saucepan over medium heat. Add onion; cook, stirring constantly, for 3 minutes. Add garlic, thyme, fennel seed, salt, pepper and saffron; cook for 20 seconds.
2. Stir in tomatoes and broth. Bring to a simmer. Cover, reduce heat and simmer for 2 minutes.
3. Increase heat to medium, stir in scallops and cook, stirring occasionally, for 2 minutes. Add shrimp and cook, stirring occasionally, for 2 minutes more. Stir in couscous. Cover, remove from heat and let stand for 5 minutes; fluff.

Side Dishes Recipes

795. STRAWBERRY SALSA

Prep Time: 15 Minutes | *Cook Time:□120 Minutes* | *Servings: 4*

INGREDIENTS:

- 1 ½ mug sliced fresh strawberries 1 ½ mug chopped sweet red pepper
- 1 mug chopped green pepper
- 1 mug seeded chopped tomato
- ¼ mug chopped Anaheim pepper 2 tbsps minced fresh cilantro
- ½ tsp salt ½ tsp crushed red pepper flakes ¼ tsp pepper 2 tbsps plus 2 tsp honey
- 2 tbsps lemon juice

DIRECTIONS:

1. In a bowl, combine together the first nine ingredients. In a bowl, combine together honey and lemon juice; smoothly stir into the strawberry mixture. Cover and let it cool for at least 4 hours. Stir just before serving. Serve the salsa with a slotted spoon.

796. EMALEE PAYNE EAU CLAIRE, WI

INGREDIENTS:

START TO FINISH: 10 MIN. • MAKES: 6 MUGS

- 2 mugs (16 ounces) sour cream
- 2 mugs mayonnaise
- 2 pounds bacon slices, 6 cooked and mashed plum tomatoes, finely chopped
- 3 green onions, chopped
- Additional minced meat and minced green onions, assorted crackers or chips (optional)

DIRECTIONS:

1. In a bowl, combine sour cream, mayonnaise, bacon, tomatoes and onions altogether. Let cool until served. Garnish with bacon and onions, if desired. Serve with crackers or chips.

797. MAMMA'S CAPONATA

Prep Time: 15 Minutes | *Cook Time:□20 Minutes* | *Servings: 5*

INGREDIENTS:

- 1 large eggplant, peeled and chopped
- ¼ mug plus 2 tbsps olive oil, divided
- 2 medium onions, chopped
- 2 celery ribs, chopped
- 2 cans (14 ½ ounces each) of diced tomatoes, undrained
- 1/3 mug chopped ripe olives
- ¼ mug red wine vinegar
- 2 tbsp sugar
- 2 tbsp capers, drained
- ½ tsp salt
- ½ tsp pepper
- French bread baguettes, sliced and toasted

DIRECTIONS:

1. Fry eggplant in a cup of oil in a Dutch oven until tender. Remove from pan and set separately. Fry the onion In the same frying pan and celery in the remaining oil until they wilt. Stir in tomatoes and eggplant. Bring it to a boil. Reduce heat. Simmer without lid for 15 minutes.
2. Add olives, vinegar, sugar, capers, salt and pepper. Boil again. Reduce heat. Boil uncovered for 20 minutes or until thickened. Serve warm or at room temperature with baguettes.

798. SWEET GINGERED CHICKEN WINGS

Prep Time: 15 Minutes | *Cook Time:□23 Minutes* | *Servings: 2*

INGREDIENTS:

- 1 cup all-purpose flour
- 2 tsp salt
- 2 tsp paprika
- ¼ tsp pepper
- 24 chicken wings (about 5 pounds)
- sauce
- ¼ cup honey
- ¼ cup thawed orange juice concentrate
- ½ tsp ground ginger Minced fresh parsley, optional

Directions:

1. Preheat oven to 350°. Place two baking sheets with foil; coat with cooking spray.
2. In a big resealable plastic bag, add flour, salt, paprika and pepper. Add chicken wings, a few at a time; seal bag and toss to coat. Divide wings between prepared baking pans. Bake 30 minutes.
3. In a small bowl, add honey, orange juice concentrate and ginger; brush over chicken wings. After baking, 25-30 minutes or until juices run clear.
4. Preheat broiler. Broil wings 4 in. from heat 1-2 minutes or until lightly browned. If desired, sprinkle with parsley.

799. CRANBERRY CHILI MEATBALLS

Prep Time: 15 Minutes | *Cook Time:□40 Minutes* | *Servings: 8*

INGREDIENTS:

- 1 bottle (12 ounces) chilli sauce
- ¾ cup packed brown sugar
- ½ tsp chilli powder
- ½ tsp ground cumin
- ¼ tsp cayenne pepper

Directions:

1. package (32 ounces) frozen fully cooked homestyle meatballs, thawed In a big saucepan over medium heat, add the first six ingredients. Now stir until sugar is dissolved.
2. Plus meatballs; cook for 20-25 minutes or until heated through, stirring occasionally.

800. BEEF FONDUE WITH MUSTARD-MAYONNAISE SAUCE

Prep Time: 15 Minutes | *Cook Time:□45 Minutes* | *Servings: 2*

INGREDIENTS:

- 2 tsp finely chopped onion
- 2 tsp lemon juice
- 2 tbsp horseradish mustard or spicy brown mustard
- 1 ½ pound beef tenderloin, cut into ¾-inch cubes
- Oil for deep-fat frying

Directions:

1. In a small size bowl, add the mayonnaise, onion, lemon juice and mustard; cover and refrigerate for 30 minutes.
2. Pat meat dry with paper towels. Oil in a fondue pot to 375°. Use fondue forks for cooking meat in oil until it reaches desired doneness. Present beef with sauce.

801. TURKEY-CRANBERRY TARTS

Prep Time: *15 Minutes* | *Cook Time:* *35 Minutes* | *Servings:12*

INGREDIENTS:

- 1/3 cup mayonnaise
- 4 tsp minced fresh parsley
- 4 tsp honey mustard
- ½ tsp chopped seeded jalapeno pepper 1/8 tsp pepper
- 2 cups cubed cooked turkey breast
- 1/3 cup chopped celery
- 1/3 cup dried cranberries, chopped 1/3 cup shredded Swiss cheese ¼ cup chopped pecans.
- toasted 30 frozen miniature phyllo tart shells.

Directions:

1. In a big bowl, combine the first five ingredients. Add the turkey, celery, cranberries, cheese and pecans; toss to coat.
2. Arrange tart shells on an ungreased baking sheet. Fill with turkey mixture. Bake at 375° for 10-12 minutes or until heated through. Present warm.
3. **NOTE** To toast nuts, bake in a shall reduce pan in a 350° oven for 5-10 minutes or cook in a skillet over reduce heat until lightly browned, stirring occasionally.

802. PROSCIUTTO-WRAPPED APRICOTS

Prep Time: *15 Minutes* | *Cook Time:□12 Minutes* | *Servings: 4*

INGREDIENTS:

- ¾ cup Mascarpone cheese 2 tbsps confectioners' sugar
- 1/8 tsp white pepper 1 package (7 ounces) dried pitted
- Mediterranean apricots
- 12 thin slices prosciutto

Directions:

1. In a small size bowl, add the cheese, confectioners' sugar and pepper. Cut a slit in each apricot; fill with cheese mixture. Cut each slice of prosciutto in half lengthwise; wrap a piece around each apricot and secure with a toothpick.
2. Place in an ungreased 15x10x1-in. Baking pan. Bake, unwrap, at 425° for 15-20 minutes or until heated through. Refrigerate leftovers.
3. BACON-WRAPPED APRICOTS Substitute 12 slices of bacon for the prosciutto. Proceed as directed.

803. LOBSTER & ARTICHOKE QUESADILLAS

Prep Time: *15 Minutes* | *Cook Time:* *20 Minutes* | *Servings: 6*

INGREDIENTS:

- ½ cup grated Parmesan cheese
- ½ cup of fat-free mayonnaise
- 1 can (14 ounces) of water-packed artichoke hearts, rinsed, drained and chopped
- 4 ½ tsp of chopped roasted sweet red pepper
- 1 garlic clove, minced
- 6 flour tortillas (10 inches)
- 1 cup of cooked lobster meat or canned flaked lobster meat
- ½ cup shredded part-skim mozzarella cheese

Directions:

1. In a small size bowl, add the Parmesan cheese, mayonnaise, artichokes, red pepper and garlic. Spread over three tortillas. Top with lobster, mozzarella cheese and remaining tortillas; press down lightly.
2. On a griddle coated by using cooking spray, cook quesadillas over medium heat for 2 minutes on each side or until cheese is melted. Cut each quesadilla into six wedges.

804. CHORIZO DATE RUMAKI

Prep Time: *15 Minutes* | *Cook Time:□40 Minutes* | *Servings: 2*

INGREDIENTS:

- 1 package (1 pound) sliced bacon
- 4 ounces uncooked chorizo or spicy bulk pork sausage 2 ounces cream cheese, cubed
- 32 pitted dates

Directions:

1. Cut each bacon strip in half. In a big skillet, cook bacon in batches over medium heat until partially cooked but not crisp. Remove to paper towels; drain drippings.
2. Crumble chorizo into the same skillet; cook and stir until fully cooked. Drain. Stir in cream cheese.
3. Divide a slit in the centre of each date; fill with cream cheese mixture. Wrap a piece of bacon around each stuffed date; secure with toothpicks.
4. Place on ungreased baking sheets. Bake at 350° for 12-15 minutes or until bacon is crisp.

805. RUSTIC ANTIPASTO TART

Prep Time: *15 Minutes* | *Cook Time:* *23 Minutes* | *Servings: 8*

INGREDIENTS:

- 1 sheet refrigerated pie pastry
- 2 tbsp prepared pesto
- 1 cup of shredded part-skim mozzarella cheese, cut into 4 ounces sliced turkey pepperoni
- 1 jar (7 ounces) of roasted sweet red peppers,
- drained and thinly sliced 1 jar (7 ½ ounces) marinated quartered artichoke hearts, drained 1 tbsp wate

Directions:

1. Unroll the pastry onto a parchment paper-lined baking sheet. Sprinkle pesto to within 2 in. of edges; sprinkle with ½ cup cheese.
2. Layer with pepperoni and ¼ cup of cheese. Top with red peppers and artichokes; spread with remaining cheese.
3. Fold up edges of pastry over filling, leaving the centre uncovered. Brush folded pastry with water.
4. Bake at 425° for 25-30 minutes or until the crust is golden and cheese is melted. Present warm.

806. MEXICAN CHICKEN MEATBALLS

Prep Time: *15 Minutes* | *Cook Time:* *40 Minutes* | *Servings: 8*

INGREDIENTS:

- ½ cup egg substitute
- 1 can (4 ounces) chopped green chillies
- 1 cup crushed cornflakes
- 1 cup (4 ounces) of shredded reduced-fat Mexican cheese blend
- ½ tsp seasoned salt
- ¼ tsp cayenne pepper
- 1 pound ground chicken
- Salsa, optional

Directions:

1. In a big bowl, add the first six ingredients. Crumble chicken over mixture and mix well. Shape into 1-in. balls. Place on baking sheets coated with cooking spray.
2. Bake it atleast375° for 12-15 minutes or until a meat thermometer reads 165° and juices run clear, turning occasionally. Present with salsa if desired.
3. FREEZE OPTION Freeze cooled meatballs in freezer containers. by using, partially thaw in refrigerator overnight.
4. Microwave, wrapped, on high in a microwave-safe dish until heated through, stirring and adding a little broth or water if necessary.

807. CARAMELIZED ONION & FIG PIZZA

Prep Time: *15 Minutes* | *Cook Time:* *73 Minutes* | *Servings: 6*

INGREDIENTS:

- 2 tbsps olive oil, divided
- 1 big onion, chopped
- 3 garlic cloves, minced
- ¼ tsp pepper
- 1 tube (13.8 ounces) of refrigerated pizza crust
- 1 pkg (8 ounces) of cream cheese, softened
- 1 tsp minced fresh thyme or ¼ tsp dried thyme
- 1 cup of dried figs (about 6 ounces), chopped
- 6 thin slices prosciutto or deli ham, chopped
- 1/3 cup pine nuts
- 1 cup (4 ounces) shredded provolone cheese

Directions:

1. In a big skillet, it is heating 1 tbsp oil over medium heat. Add onion; cook and stir until softened.
2. Reduce heat to medium-reduce; cook 30-35 minutes or until turning deep golden brown, occasionally stirring garlic and pepper; cook 1 minute longer.
3. Preheat oven to 425°. Unroll and press dough onto the bottom and up sides of a greased 15x10x1-in. Baking pan. Bake 7-10 minutes or until golden brown.
4. Beat the cream cheese, thyme and remaining oil in a small bowl until smooth. Spread over the crust. Sprinkle with caramelized onions, figs, prosciutto and pine nuts. Sprinkle with cheese. Bake it for another 6-10 minutes or until cheese is melted.
5. Make it ahead of time. This recipe takes a few minutes to combine when you caramelized the onions the day before.

808. APPLE WONTON BUNDLES

Prep Time: *15 Minutes* | *Cook Time:* *20 Minutes* | *Servings: 6*

INGREDIENTS:

- 4 medium tart apples, peeled
- 64 wonton wrappers
- 2 to 3 cups canola oil

Directions:

1. 1 jar (12 ounces) of caramel ice cream topping, warmed 1. Cut every apple into four wedges; cut wedges into four pieces. Put a piece of apple in the centre of each wonton wrapper.
2. Brush edges of wrapper with water and bring up around apple pinch to seal. Cover with plastic wrap until ready to cook.
3. After Heating oil in a fondue pot to 375°, use fondue forks for cooking wonton bundles until golden brown (about 1 minute). Cool slightly. Present bundles with caramel topping.

809. TERIYAKI STEAK SKEWERS

Prep Time: *15 Minutes* | *Cook Time:* *40 Minutes* | *Servings: 5*

INGREDIENTS:

- ½ cup reduced-sodium soy sauce
- ¼ cup cider vinegar
- 2 tbsps brown sugar

- 2 tbsps finely chopped onion
- 1 tbsp canola oil
- 1 garlic clove, minced
- ½ tsp ground ginger
- 1/8 tsp pepper
- 2 pounds beef top sirloin steak

Directions:

1. In a large plastic bag, place the first eight ingredients. Remove the fat from the steak and cut the grain crosswise -in. Strip.
2. Add beef to the bag. Tight the bag and hand it over to the coat. Refrigerate for 2-3 hours.
3. Drain the seasoning and discard. Thread the cutlets loosely onto 6 pickled metal or wooden skewers.
4. Bake uncovered and over medium heat for 7-10 minutes or until meat is cooked to the desired degree, turning frequently

810. SMOKED MOZZARELLA FLATBREAD PIZZA

Prep Time: *Cook Time:* *Servings: 2*
15 Minutes *70 Minutes*

INGREDIENTS:

- 2 tbsp butter, divided
- 2 tbsps olive oil, divided
- 2/3 cup sliced red onion
- ½ pound sliced baby portobello mushrooms
- 1 garlic clove, minced
- 2 tsp minced fresh rosemary or ½ tsp dried rosemary, crushed
- 1 tube (13.8 ounces) of refrigerated pizza crust
- 1 ½ cups (6 ounces) shredded smoked mozzarella cheese
- 2 ounces sliced prosciutto or deli ham, finely chopped

Directions:

1. Preheat oven to 400°. In a big skillet, heat 1 tbsp butter and 1 tbsp oil over medium-high heat.
2. Add onion; cook it and stir 2-3 minutes or until softened. Reduce heat to medium-reduce; cook 8-10 minutes or until golden brown, stirring occasionally. Remove from pan.
3. In the same skillet, heat the butter continuously as well as oil over medium-high heat. Add mushrooms; cook and stir 2-3 minutes or until tender. Add garlic and rosemary; cook about 1-2 minutes longer or until liquid is evaporated.
4. Unroll and press dough onto the bottom of a greased 15x10x1-in. Baking pan.
5. Using fingertips, press several dimples into dough. Sprinkle with ½ cup cheese; top with onion, mushroom mixture and prosciutto. Sprinkle with remaining cheese
6. . Bake pizza 15-18 minutes or until golden brown and the cheese is melted.

811. MEDITERRANEAN NACHOS

Prep Time: *Cook Time:* *Servings: 2*
15 Minutes *70 Minutes*

INGREDIENTS:

- 2 medium cucumbers, peeled, seeded and grated
- 1 ½ tsp salt, divided
- ½ tsp ground cumin
- ½ tsp ground coriander
- ½ tsp paprika
- ¾ tsp pepper, divided
- 6 whole pita bread Cooking spray
- 1 pound ground lamb or beef
- 2 garlic cloves, minced
- 1 tsp cornstarch
- ½ cup beef broth
- 2 cups plain Greek yoghurt
- 2 tbsps lemon juice
- ¼ tsp grated lemon peel
- 2 cups torn romaine
- 2 medium tomatoes, seeded and chopped
- ½ cup pitted Greek olives, sliced
- 4 green onions, thinly sliced
- ½ cup crumbled feta cheese

Directions:

1. In a colander, place over a bowl, toss cucumbers with ½ tsp salt. Let stand 30 minutes. Squeeze and pat dry. Set aside. In a small size bowl, add the cumin, coriander, paprika, ½ tsp pepper and ½ tsp salt; set aside.
2. Cut each pita into eight wedges; arrange in a singer layer on ungreased baking sheets. Spritz both sides of pitas with cooking spray; sprinkle with ¾ tsp seasoning mix. Broil it from the heat for 3-4 minutes on each side or until golden brown. Cool on wire racks.
3. In a big skillet, cook lamb and remaining seasoning mix over medium heat until the lamb is no longer pink. Add garlic; cook 1 minute longer. Drain. Add cornstarch and broth until smooth; gradually stir into the pan. Bring to a boil; cook it and stir continuously for 2 minutes or until thickened.
4. In a small size bowl, add the yoghurt, lemon juice, lemon peel, cucumbers and remaining salt and pepper. Arrange pita wedges on a serving platter. Layer with lettuce, lamb mixture, tomatoes, olives, onions and cheese. Present immediately with cucumber sauce.
3. **NOTE** If Greek yoghurt is not available in your area, line a strainer with a coffee filter and place it over a bowl. Place 4 cups plain yoghurt in prepared strainer; refrigerate overnight. Discard liquid from bowl; proceed as directed.

812. WARM BACON CHEDDAR SPREAD

Prep Time: *Cook Time:* *Servings: 2*
15 Minutes *30 Minutes*

INGREDIENTS:

- 1 package (8 ounces) cream cheese, softened
- ½ mug mayonnaise
- ¼ tsp dried thyme
- 1/8 tsp pepper
- 1 mug (4 ounces) shredded sharp cheddar cheese
- 3 green onions, chopped
- 8 bacon strips, cooked and crumbled, divided
- ½ mug crushed Ritz crackers
- Assorted crackers

DIRECTIONS:

1. Preheat oven to 350°. In a bowl, combine together cream cheese, mayonnaise, thyme and pepper. Stir it continuously in cheese, green onions and half the bacon. Transfer to a greased 3-mug baking dish.
2. Bake, uncovered, 13-15 minutes or until bubbly. Top with crushed crackers and remaining bacon. Serve with assorted crackers.

813. CHIPOTLE HAM 'N' CHEESE DIP

Prep Time: *Cook Time:* *Servings: 12*
15 Minutes *40 Minutes*

INGREDIENTS:

- 2 pkg(8 ounces each) of cream cheese, cubed 1 can (12 ounces) evaporated milk
- 2 mugs (8 ounces) shredded Gouda cheese
- 1 mug (4 ounces) shredded cheddar cheese
- 2 tbsps chopped chipotle pepper in adobo sauce 1 tsp ground cumin
- 2 mugs diced fully cooked ham
- Fresh vegetables or tortilla chips

DIRECTIONS:

1. In a 3-qt slow cooker, combine together the first six ingredients. Cover and cook on low for 40 minutes.
2. Stir continuously in ham, and cook 20 minutes longer or until heated through. Serve warm with vegetables or chips.

814. HAM SALAD SPREAD

Prep Time: *Cook Time:* *Servings: 12*
15 Minutes *50 Minutes*

INGREDIENTS:

- 3 mugs ground fully cooked ham
- 1 hard-cooked egg, chopped
- 2 tbsps finely chopped celery
- 2 tsp finely chopped onion
- 2 tsp sweet pickle relish
- ¾ mug mayonnaise 1 tbsp prepared mustard Assorted crackers

DIRECTIONS:

1. In a bowl, combine together the first five ingredients. Mix mayonnaise and mustard; add to ham mixture and mix well. Let it cool until serving. Serve with crackers.

815. CHICKEN SALAD PARTY SANDWICHES

Prep Time: *Cook Time:* *Servings: 4*
15 Minutes *65 Minutes*

Ingredients:

- 4 cups cubed cooked chicken breast
- 1 ½ cups dried cranberries
- 2 celery ribs, finely chopped
- 2 green onions, thinly sliced
- ¼ cup chopped sweet pickles
- 1 cup fat-free mayonnaise
- ½ tsp curry powder
- ¼ tsp coarsely ground pepper
- ½ cup chopped pecans, toasted
- 15 whole wheat dinner rolls
- Torn leaf lettuce

Directions:

1. In a bowl, now add the first five ingredients. In a small size bowl, add the mayonnaise, curry and pepper. Add to chicken mixture; toss to coat. Chill until serving.
2. Stir pecans into chicken salad. Present on rolls lined with lettuce.

816. STATE FAIR SUBS

Prep Time: *Cook Time:* *Servings: 4*
15 Minutes *16 Minutes*

Ingredients:

- 1 loaf (1 pound unsliced) French bread
- 2 eggs
- ¼ cup milk
- ½ tsp pepper
- ¼ tsp salt
- 1 pound bulk Italian sausage
- 1 ½ cups chopped onion
- 2 cups (8 ounces) of shredded part-skim mozzarella cheese

Directions:

1. Cut the bread in half lengthwise. Drill holes carefully in the top and bottom of the loaf, leaving about an inch.
2. Husks. Diced bread. In a large bowl, shake together the eggs, milk, pepper and salt. Add slices of bread and stir to coat. Separately.
3. In a frying pan over high heat, cook the sausages and onions until the meat is no longer pink. Thin.
4. Add to bread dough. Spoon for filling in breadcrumbs; Sprinkle with cheese. Wrap each in foil. Bake it at least 400° for 20-25 minutes or until cheese is melted. Cut French bread into 1-serving-sized pieces.

817. PARTY PITAS

Prep Time: *Cook Time:* *Servings: 4*
15 Minutes *20 Minutes*

INGREDIENTS:

- 4 whole-wheat pita pocket halves
- 1/3 cup Greek vinaigrette ½ pound thinly sliced deli turkey 1 jar (7 ½ ounces) roasted sweet red peppers, drained and patted dry 2 cups fresh baby spinach

- 24 pitted Greek olives
- 24 frilled toothpicks

Directions:

1. Brush insides of pita pockets with vinaigrette; fill with turkey, peppers and spinach. Cut each pita into six wedges.
2. Thread olives onto toothpicks; use to secure wedges.

818. BAJA CHICKEN & SLAW SLIDERS

Prep Time: *15 Minutes* | *Cook Time:* *20 Minutes* | *Servings: 4*

INGREDIENTS:

- ¼ cup reduced-fat sour cream ½ tsp grated lime peel ¼ tsp lime juice SLAW
- 1 cup broccoli coleslaw mix
- 2 tbsps finely chopped sweet red pepper
- 2 tbsps finely chopped sweet onion
- 2 tbsps of minced fresh cilantro
- 2 tsp of chopped seeded jalapeno pepper 2 tsp of lime juice
- 1 tsp of sugar
- SLIDERS
- (4 ounces each) 4 boneless skinless chicken breast halves ½ tsp of ground cumin
- ½ tsp of chilli powder
- ¼ tsp of salt
- ¼ tsp of coarsely ground pepper 8 Hawaiian sweet rolls, split
- 8 small lettuce leaves
- 8 slices tomato

Directions:

1. In a small size bowl, add sour cream, lime peel and lime juice. In another small size bowl, add slaw ingredients. Refrigerate sauce and slaw until serving.
2. Cut each chicken breast in half wide; flatten to -in. Thickness. Sprinkle with spices.
3. Wet a paper towel with cooking oil; using long-handled tongs, rub on grill rack to lightly coat.
4. Grill chicken, covered, over medium heat or roast 4 inches from heat 4 to 7 minutes on each side or until no longer pink.
5. Toast bread, cut side down, 30-60 seconds or until toasted. Serve grilled chicken on a roll with lettuce, tomatoes, sauce, and slaw.
4. **NOTE** Wear disposable gloves when chopping chillies; The oil can burn the skin. Avoid touching your face.

819. ONION BEEF AU JU

Prep Time: *15 Minutes* | *Cook Time:* *40 Minutes* | *Servings: 6*

INGREDIENTS:

- 1 beef rump roast (4 pounds) 2 tbsps canola oil
- 2 big sweet onions, cut into ¼-inch slices 6 tbsp butter, softened, divided
- 5 cups water
- ½ cup of reduced-sodium soy sauce 1 envelope onion soup mix
- 1 garlic clove, minced
- 1 tsp browning sauce, optional
- 1 loaf (1 pound) French bread
- 1 cup (4 ounces) shredded Swiss cheese

Directions:

1. Bake chocolate on all sides in oil in a Dutch oven over medium heat. Thin. In a large frying pan, add 2 tablespoons of butter and saute the onions until soft. Add water, soy sauce, soup mix, garlic, and browning sauce if desired. Pour over roast.
2. Wrap and cook at 325° for 2 hours or until meat is tender. Leave the meat for about 10 minutes, then slice thinly.
3. Put the meat back into the juice pan. Separate the bread lengthwise. Cut into 3 inches. Part. Brush with the remaining butter. Place it on the pan.
4. Bake 4-6 inches of bread over heat for 2-3 minutes or until golden brown. Sprinkle with beef and onions.
5. Sprinkle with cheese. Bake for 1-2 minutes or until cheese is melted. Serve bread with pan juice.

820. HAWAIIAN BEEF SLIDERS

Prep Time: *15 Minutes* | *Cook Time:* *34 Minutes* | *Servings: 4*

INGREDIENTS:

- 1 can (20 ounces) unsweetened crushed pineapple
- 1 tsp pepper
- ¼ tsp salt
- 1 ½ pounds lean ground beef (90% lean)
- ¼ cup reduced-sodium soy sauce
- 2 tbsp ketchup
- 1 tbsp white vinegar
- 2 garlic cloves, minced
- ¼ tsp crushed red pepper flakes
- 18 miniature whole wheat buns
- Baby spinach leaves
- 3 centre-cut bacon strips, cooked and crumbled
- Sliced jalapeno peppers, optional

Directions:

1. Drain pineapple, reserving juice and 1 ½ cups pineapple (save remaining pineapple for another use). In a big bowl, add ¾ cup reserved crushed pineapple, pepper and salt.
2. Crumble beef over mixture and mix well. Shape into 18 patties; place in two 11x7-in. Dishes.
3. In a small size bowl, add soy sauce, ketchup, vinegar, garlic, pepper flakes and reserved pineapple juice. Pour half of the marinade into each dish; cover and refrigerate for 1 hour, turning once.
4. Drain and discard marinade. Moisten a paper towel with cooking oil by using long-handled tongs, coat the grill rack lightly.
5. Grill patties, covered, over medium heat or broil 4 in. from heat 4-5 minutes on each side or until a thermometer reads 160° and juices run clear.
6. Grill buns, uncovered, 1-2 minutes or until toasted. Present burgers on buns with spinach, remaining pineapple, bacon and jalapeno peppers if desired.

821. TUNA TEA SANDWICHES

Prep Time: *15 Minutes* | *Cook Time:* *17 Minutes* | *Servings: 4*

INGREDIENTS:

- 1 can (6 ounces) light water-packed tuna, drained and flaked 1 to 2 tbsps mayonnaise
- ¼ tsp lemon-pepper seasoning 4 tbsps crumbled goat cheese
- 4 slices multigrain bread, crusts removed 4 big fresh basil leaves

Directions:

1. In a small size bowl, add the tuna, mayonnaise and lemon pepper. Spread 1 tbsp of goat cheese on each slice of bread.
2. Spread two slices with tuna mixture; top with basil leaves and remaining bread. Cut in half or into desired shapes.

822. MINI MUFFULETTA

Prep Time: *15 Minutes* | *Cook Time:* *30 Minutes* | *Servings: 6*

INGREDIENTS:

- 1 jar (10 ounces) of pimiento-stuffed olives, drained and chopped
- 2 cans (4 ¼ ounces each) chopped ripe olives
- 2 tbsps balsamic vinegar
- 1 tbsp red wine vinegar
- 1 tbsp olive oil
- 3 garlic cloves, minced
- 1 tsp dried basil
- 1 tsp dried oregano
- 6 French rolls, split
- ½ pound thinly sliced hard salami
- ¼ pound sliced provolone cheese
- ½ pound thinly sliced Cotto salami
- ¼ pound sliced part-skim mozzarella cheese

Directions:

1. In a big bowl, add the first eight ingredients; set aside. Holreduce out tops and bottoms of rolls, leaving ¾-in. Clams (discard the discarded bread or save it for other uses).
2. Apply the olive mixture above and below the roll. Coat the bottom of the roll with hard salami, provolone cheese, Coto salami and mozzarella cheese. Change the top.
3. Wrap tightly with plastic wrap. Cool overnight. Cut each into six pieces. Secure it with a toothpick.

823. ANTIPASTO-STUFFED BAGUETTES

Prep Time: *15 Minutes* | *Cook Time:* *39 Minutes* | *Servings: 2*

INGREDIENTS:

- 1 can (2 ¼ ounces) sliced ripe olives, drained
- 2 tbsps olive oil
- 1 tsp lemon juice
- 1 garlic clove, minced
- 1/8 tsp each dried basil, thyme, marjoram and rosemary, crushed
- 2 French bread baguettes (10 ½ ounces each)
- 1 package (4 ounces) crumbled feta cheese
- ½ pound thinly sliced Genoa salami
- 1 cup fresh baby spinach
- 1 jar (7 ¼ ounces) of roasted red peppers, drained and chopped
- 1 can (14 ounces) of water-packed artichoke hearts, rinsed, drained and quartered

Directions:

1. Put the olives, oil, lemon juice, garlic and spices in a blender. Cover and process until olives are cut. Set aside 1/3 cup of the olive mixture (refrigerate the remaining mixture for other uses).
2. Cut the top 1/3 of each baguette. Carefully drill a hole in the bottom, leaving a -in. Peel (discard the discarded bread or save it for another use).
3. Apply the olive mixture to the bottom of each bread. Sprinkle with feta cheese. Fold the salami slices in half and put them on top of the cheese. Sprinkle with spinach, red pepper and artichoke need. Replace the top of the bread. Wrap the bread tightly in foil.
4. Refrigerate for at least 3 hours or overnight. Preheat oven to 350° to serve cold or warm.
5. Place the bread wrapped in foil on a baking sheet. Bake for 20-25 minutes or until heated. Cut into pieces. Secure it with a toothpick.
5. **Note** You can replace the olive mixture with 1/3 cup of purchased tapenade (olive paste).

Snacks And Appetizer Recipes

824. DELI SANDWICH PARTY PLATTER

Prep Time: *15 Minutes* | *Cook Time:* *46 Minutes* | *Servings: 2*

INGREDIENTS:

- 1 bunch of green leaf lettuce
- 2 pounds sliced of deli turkey
- 2 pounds sliced of deli roast beef
- 1 pound sliced of deli ham
- 1 pound thinly sliced hard salami
- 2 cartons (7 ounces each) of roasted red pepper hummus 2 cartons (6 ½ ounces each) garden vegetable cheese spread Assorted bread and mini bagels

Directions:

1. set lettuce leaves on a serving platter; top with deli meats, rolled up if desired. Present with hummus, cheese spread, bread and bagels.

825. HAM 'N' CHEESE BISCUIT STACKS

Prep Time: *15 Minutes* *Cook Time:* *90 Minutes* *Servings: 4*

INGREDIENTS:

- 2 tubes (12 ounces each) refrigerated buttermilk biscuits
- ¾ cup stone-ground mustard, divided
- ½ cup butter softened
- ¼ cup chopped green onions
- ¼ cup mayonnaise
- ¼ cup honey
- 10 thick slices of deli ham
- 10 slices Swiss cheese
- 2 ½ cups of shredded romaine
- 40 frilled toothpicks
- 20 pitted ripe olives and drained and patted dry
- 20 pimiento-stuffed olives, drained and patted dry

Directions:

1. 2 inches apart on a greased baking sheet. Sprinkle each spoonful of mustard. Bake for 8-10 minutes or until golden brown. Remove from pan with wire rack to cool.
2. Put the butter and onion in a small bowl. In another bowl, add mayonnaise, honey and remaining mustard. Cut each piece of ham into rectangles. Cut each piece of cheese into four triangles.
3. Divide each biscuit in half. Grease the floor with the butter mixture. Layer 1 ham slice, 1 cheese slice, and 1 tablespoon romaine on each bottom of the biscuit.
4. Spread mustard mixture over biscuit tops; place over romaine. Thread toothpicks through olives; insert into stacks. Refrigerate leftovers.

826. FETA BRUSCHETTA

Prep Time: *15 Minutes* *Cook Time:* *33 Minutes* *Servings: 4*

INGREDIENTS:

- ¼ cup butter, melted ¼ cup olive oil 10 slices French bread (1 inch thick)
- 1 package (4 ounces) crumbled feta cheese
- 2 to 3 garlic cloves, minced
- 1 tbsp of minced fresh basil or 1 tsp dried basil 1 big tomato, seeded and chopped

Directions:

1. In a small size bowl, add butter and oil; brush onto both sides of bread. Place on a baking sheet. Bake at 350° for 8-10 minutes or until lightly browned on top.
2. Add the feta cheese, garlic and basil; sprinkle over toast. Top with tomato.

827. CITRUS SPICED OLIVES

Prep Time: *15 Minutes* *Cook Time:* *90 Minutes* *Servings: 2*

INGREDIENTS:

- ½ cup white wine ¼ cup canola oil 3 tbsps salt-free seasoning blend
- 4 garlic cloves, minced
- ½ tsp crushed red pepper flakes 2 tsp each grated orange, lemon and lime peels 3 tbsps each orange, lemon and lime juices 4 cups mixed pitted olives

Directions:

1. whisk until blended. Add olives and toss to coat. Refrigerate, wrapped, at least 4 hours before serving.

828. HERB & ROASTED PEPPER CHEESECAKE

Prep Time: *15 Minutes* *Cook Time:* *40 Minutes* *Servings: 2*

INGREDIENTS:

- 3 packages (8 ounces each) of cream cheese, softened
- ¾ cup whole-milk ricotta cheese
- 1 ½ tsp salt
- ¾ tsp pepper
- 3 eggs, lightly beaten
- 1 ½ cups roasted sweet red peppers, drained and finely chopped
- ¾ cup minced fresh basil
- 1/3 cup minced fresh chives
- 3 tbsps minced fresh thyme
- 3 tbsps crumbled cooked bacon
- 3 garlic cloves, minced
- 1 tbsp olive oil
- Roasted chilli flakes and additional chopped green onion (optional)
- Baked Ribbon Chips

Directions:

1. Preheat oven to 350 degrees. Place 9 inches of grease. Springform pan on double thick heavy-duty foil (about 18 inches square). Wrap the foil tightly around the pan.
2. Add cream cheese, ricotta cheese, salt and pepper to a food processor, cover and process until soft. Add eggs. Pulse only until added. Add pepper, herbs, bacon and garlic. Close and pulse until smooth. Pour the filling into the prepared pan. Place
3. Spring-shaped pan in a large baking dish; add 1 inch of hot water to a larger pot.
4. Place springform pan in a big baking pan; add 1 in. of hot water to the bigger pan.
5. Bake for 35-45 minutes or until the centre is fully cooked and the top looks grey. Remove the springform pan from the water bath. Remove the foil. Cool the cheesecake on a wire rack for 10 minutes. Loosen the edges of the pan by use of a knife. Refrigerate for an additional hour. Cool overnight.
6. Remove the border from the fan. Grease the cheesecake just before serving. Top with red pepper and green onion if desired. Serve with pita chips.

829. CHICKEN SALAD CAPRESE

Prep Time: *15 Minutes* *Cook Time:* *70 Minutes* *Servings: 2*

INGREDIENTS

- 2 cups shredded rotisserie chicken
- 1 pound fresh mozzarella cheese, cubed
- 2 cups grape tomatoes, halved
- 1 can (14 ounces) of water-packed artichoke hearts, rinsed, drained and coarsely chopped
- ½ cup pitted Greek olives, thinly sliced
- ¼ cup minced fresh basil
- ¼ cup olive oil
- 2 garlic cloves, minced
- ½ tsp salt
- ½ tsp coarsely ground pepper

830. TOMATO CROSTINI

Prep Time: *15 Minutes* *Cook Time:* *50 Minutes* *Servings: 4*

INGREDIENTS:

- 2 French bread baguettes (10 ½ ounces each)
- 4 garlic cloves
- 2 small tomatoes
- ¼ cup olive oil
- 1 tsp salt

Directions:

1. In a big bowl, add the first six ingredients. In a small size bowl, whisk the oil, garlic, salt and pepper; spread over chicken mixture and toss to coat. Refrigerate until serving.
2. Cut baguettes into ½-in. slices. Place on ungreased baking sheets. Bake at 425° for 2-4 minutes or until lightly browned.
3. Cut garlic in half lengthwise; rub over bread. Cut tomatoes into quarters; rub over bread. Brush with oil and sprinkle with salt. Bake 2-3 minutes longer or until crisp. Present crostini with chicken salad.

831. GARDEN SPRING ROLLS

Prep Time: *15 Minutes* *Cook Time:* *30 Minutes* *Servings: 4*

INGREDIENTS:

- 3 cups shredded cabbage or romaine lettuce
- ¼ cup Thai chilli sauce
- 8 spring roll wrappers
- 1 small sweet red pepper, thinly sliced
- ½ cup of thinly sliced sweet onion
- 1 ripe avocado, peeled and sliced
- 4 fresh basil leaves, sliced additional Thai chilli sauce, optional

Directions:

1. In a small bowl, mix the cabbage and chilli sauce. Fill the bowl with water. Soak the spring roll wrapper in water
2. Bending, 30-45 seconds (depending on the thickness of the rice paper); Remove the wrapping paper from the bowl to reduce excess dripping.
3. Place it on a flat surface. In the centre, coat the cabbage, pepper and onion mixture. Topped with avocado and basil. Fold both ends over the filling. Turn the long side over the filling and wrap it tightly. Place the seam side on a serving dish. Repeat with the remaining ingredients.
4. Cover with damp paper towels until serving. Cut rolls diagonally in half. If desired, Present with additional Thai chilli sauce.

832. HUEVOS DIABLOS

Prep Time: *15 Minutes* *Cook Time:* *45 Minutes* *Servings: 5*

INGREDIENTS:

- 12 hard-cooked eggs
- 6 tbsps minced fresh cilantro, divided 6 tbsps mayonnaise
- 2 green onions, thinly sliced
- ¼ cup of sour cream 1 jalapeno pepper, seeded and minced
- 1 ½ tsp grated lime peel 1 tsp ground cumin
- ¼ tsp salt 1/8 tsp pepper Cut eggs in half lengthwise. Remove yolks; set whites aside.

Directions:

1. In a small size bowl, mash yolks. Add 3 tbsps cilantro, mayonnaise, onions, sour cream, jalapeno, lime peel, cumin, salt and pepper; mix well. Stuff or pipe into egg whites. Refrigerate until serving. Garnish with remaining cilantro.

833. CRAB CUCUMBER BITES

Prep Time: *15 Minutes* *Cook Time:* *32 Minutes* *Servings: 9*

INGREDIENTS:

- 3 medium cucumbers
- 2/3 cup reduced-fat cream cheese 2 tsp lemon juice
- 1 tsp hot pepper sauce
- 1 package (8 ounces) imitation crabmeat, chopped 1/3 cup finely chopped sweet red pepper 2 green onions, sliced

Directions:

1. Peel strips from cucumbers to create striped edges; cut each cucumber into 16 slices, about ¼-in. thick. Pat dry with paper towels; set aside.
2. In a small size bowl, beat the cream cheese, lemon juice and pepper sauce until smooth. Fold in the crab, red pepper and onions. Place 1 heap6ing tsp onto each cucumber slice. Present immediately.

834. ANTIPASTO PLATTER

Prep Time: *5 Minutes* *Cook Time:* *25 Minutes* *Servings: 2*

INGREDIENTS:

- 1 jar (24 ounces) pepperoncini, drained
- 1 can (15 ounces) of garbanzo beans or chickpeas, rinsed and drained 2 cups halved fresh mushrooms
- 2 cups halved cherry tomatoes

- ½ pound provolone cheese, cubed 1 can (6 ounces) pitted ripe olives, drained
- 1 package (3 ½ ounces) sliced pepperoni 1 bottle (8 ounces) Italian vinaigrette dressing Lettuce leaves

Directions:

1. In a big bowl, add pepperoncini, beans, mushrooms, tomatoes, cheese, olives and pepperoni. Pour vinaigrette over mixture; toss to coat.
2. Refrigerate for at least 30 minutes or overnight. Arrange on a lettuce-lined platter. Present with toothpicks.

835. CREAMY BAKED FOUR-CHEESE PASTA

Prep Time: 2 Minutes | *Cook Time: 10 Minutes* | *Servings: 4*

INGREDIENTS:

- slices hearty white sandwich bread, torn into quarters
- 1 ounce Parmesan cheese, grated (1/2 cup) Salt & pepper 4 ounces fontina cheese, shredded (1 cup)
- ounces Gorgonzola cheese, crumbled (3/4 cup)
- ounce Pecorino Romano cheese, grated (1/2 cup)
- lb penne pasta
- Tbsp. unsalted butter

DIRECTIONS:

1. Pulse bread in the cooking processor to coarse crumbs, about 10 pulses. Shift bread crumbs to a small container & stir in 1/4 cup Parmesan, 1/4 Tsp. Salt, & 1/8 Tsp. Pepper; set aside.
Combine fontina, Gorgonzola, Pecorino, & the remaining 1/4 cup Parmesan in a large container; set aside.
Set oven rack to middle setting & heat oven to 500 degrees. Take 4 quarts of water to boil in a large pot.
Include pasta & 1 Tbsp. salt & cook, often stirring, till just shy of al dente. Drain pasta, leaving it slightly wet.
When pasta is cooking, melt butter in a small saucepan over medium heat. Whisk in flour till no lumps remain, about 30 seconds.
Slowly whisk in cream & bring to boil, stirring occasionally.
Reduce heat to medium-low & simmer for 1 min. Stir in 1/4 Tsp. salt & 1/4Tsp. Pepper.
Include pasta to a container with cheeses; immediately pour cream batter over the top, then cover container & let stand 3 mins.
Uncover the container & stir with a rubber spatula, scraping the bottom of the container, till cheeses are melted & batter is thoroughly combined.
Shift pasta to 13 by 9-inch baking dish, then sprinkle evenly with bread-crumb batter, pressing down lightly.
12. Bake till topping is golden brown, about 7 mins. Serve immediately.

836. APPETIZER TORTILLA PINWHEEL

Prep Time: 15 Minutes | *Cook Time: 20 Minutes* | *Servings: 8*

INGREDIENTS:

- 1 cup (8 ounces) sour cream
- 1 package (8 ounces) cream cheese, softened
- 1 can (4 ¼ ounces) chopped ripe olives 1 can (4 ounces) chopped green chillies, well-drained 1 cup (4 ounces) shredded cheddar cheese
- ½ cup chopped green onions Garlic powder to taste Seasoned salt to taste
- 5 flour tortillas (10 inches), room temperature Fresh parsley for garnish
- Salsa

Directions:

1. In a big bowl, beat the first eight ingredients until blended. Spread over the tortillas; roll up tightly.
2. Wrap each with plastic wrap, twisting ends; refrigerate for several hours. Unwrap; cut into ½-in. to ¾-in. slices. (An electric knife works best.) Discard ends.
3. Garnish with parsley. Present with salsa if desired.

837. SMOKED SALMON CHERRY TOMATOES

Prep Time: 15 Minutes | *Cook Time: 20 Minutes* | *Servings: 8*

INGREDIENTS:

- 30 cherry tomatoes
- 3 ounces of smoked salmon or lox, finely chopped 1/3 cup finely chopped onion 1/3 cup finely chopped green pepper Salt and pepper to taste
- 1 package (3 ounces) cream cheese, softened 1 tsp milk Fresh dill sprigs

Directions:

1. Cut thin slices from each top of the tomato. Pick up the debris and now throw it away. Turn the tomatoes over on a paper towel and dry them. Place salmon, onion, bell pepper, salt and pepper in a large bowl. Spoon on tomatoes.
2. Whisk cream cheese and milk in a small bowl until smooth. Place the tip of the star in a cake or plastic bag. Pipe a small amount of cream of cheese mixture into the tomatoes. Garnish with dill.

838. DELIGHTFUL DEVILED EGGS

Prep Time: 5 Minutes | *Cook Time:□10 Minutes* | *Servings: 2*

INGREDIENTS:

- 6 hard-cooked eggs
- 2 tbsps mayonnaise
- 1 ½ tsp grated onion 1 ½ tsp sweet pickle relish ½ tsp spicy brown mustard ¼ tsp salt
- 1/8 tsp crushed red pepper flakes 1/8 tsp pepper

Directions:

1. Slice eggs in half lengthwise. Remove yolks; set whites aside. In a small size bowl, mash yolks. Stir in the mayonnaise, onion, relish, mustard, salt, pepper flakes and pepper.
2. Pipe or spoon into egg whites. Refrigerate until serving.

839. MEAT LOVERS' SNACK MIX

Prep Time: 15 Minutes | *Cook Time: 34 Minutes* | *Servings: 2*

INGREDIENTS:

- 1 ¼ cups wasabi-coated green peas ¾ cup salted peanuts
- 3 pepperoni-flavoured meat snack sticks (1 ½ ounce each), cut into bite-size pieces 2 ounces beef jerky, cut into bite-size pieces
- ½ cup corn nuts
- ½ cup Rice Chex
- ½ cup Multi-Grain Cheerios
- ½ cup of crunchy cheese puff snacks
- 2 tbsp of chopped sun-dried tomatoes (not packed in oil)
- 1/3 cup of canola oil
- 1 ½ tsp chilli powder
- 1 ½ tsp onion powder
- ½ tsp hot pepper sauce
- ½ tsp soy sauce
- ¼ tsp seasoned salt

Directions:

1. Preheat oven to 250°. Add the first nine ingredients to a big bowl. In a small size bowl, whisk oil, chilli powder, onion powder, pepper sauce, soy sauce and seasoned salt. Spread over cereal mixture and toss to coat.
2. Spread into a greased 15x10x1-in. Baking pan. Bake 50 minutes, stirring every 10 minutes. Cool completely on a wire rack. Store in an airtight container.

840. TACO JOE DIP

Prep Time: 15 Minutes | *Cook Time:□12 Minutes* | *Servings: 2*

INGREDIENTS:

- 1 can (16 ounces) kidney beans, rinsed and drained
- 1 can (15 ¼ ounces) whole kernel corn, drained 1 can (15 ounces) black beans, rinsed and drained
- 1 can (14 ½ ounces) stewed tomatoes, undrained 1 can (8 ounces) tomato sauce
- 1 can (4 ounces) chopped green chillies, drained
- 1 envelope taco seasoning
- ½ cup chopped onion Tortilla chips

Directions:

1. In a 5-qt reduce cooker, add the first eight ingredients. Cover and cook on reduce for 5-6 hours. Present with tortilla chips.

***NOTE** To make Taco Joe Soup, add a 29-ounce of tomato sauce to the reduced cooker. It will Present 6-8.*

841. MEAT-ATARIAN SUB

Prep Time: 15 Minutes | *Cook Time: 38 Minutes* | *Servings: 4*

INGREDIENTS:

- 1 cup (4 ounces) of shredded part-skim mozzarella cheese
- ½ cup grated Parmesan cheese ½ cup butter softened ½ cup mayonnaise 2 garlic cloves, minced
- 1 tsp Italian seasoning
- ¼ tsp crushed red pepper flakes ¼ tsp pepper 1 loaf (1 pound) French bread, halved lengthwise
- 1 pound sliced deli ham
- 2 packages (2.1 ounces each) ready-to-Present fully cooked bacon, warmed 4 ounces sliced pepperoni

Directions:

1. ½ cup pizza sauce 1. Preheat oven to 350°. In a small size bowl, add the first eight ingredients. Spread over cut sides of bread. Layer with ham, bacon, pepperoni and pizza sauce; replace the top.
2. Wrap in foil; place on a big baking sheet. Bake 25-30 minutes or until heated through. Cut into slices.

842. BUFFALO CHICKEN DIP

Prep Time: 15 Minutes | *Cook Time: 20 Minutes* | *Servings: 2*

INGREDIENTS:

- 1 package (8 ounces) cream cheese, softened
- 1 can (10 ounces) chunk white chicken, drained
- ½ cup buffalo wing sauce ½ cup ranch salad dressing 2 cups (8 ounces) shredded Colby-Monterey Jack cheese
- French bread baguette slices, celery ribs or tortilla chips, optional

Directions:

1. Preheat oven to 350°. Spread cream cheese into an ungreased shall reduce 1-qt. Baking dish. Layer with chicken, wing sauce and salad dressing. Sprinkle with cheese.
2. Bake, uncovered, 20-25 minutes or until cheese is melted. If desired, Present with baguette slices.

843. HAVARTI SHRIMP QUESADILLAS

Prep Time: 15 Minutes | *Cook Time: 45 Minutes* | *Servings: 6*

INGREDIENTS:

- ½ pound fresh mushrooms, chopped 1 tbsp canola oil
- 1 tbsp butter
- 6 tbsps apricot
- 6 flour tortillas (10 inches)
- 6 ounces Havarti cheese, thinly sliced ½ pound cooked medium shrimp, peeled and deveined and chopped 2 tbsp butter, melted

Directions:

1. In a big skillet, saute mushrooms in oil and butter until tender. A 1 tbsp spread represents more than half of each tortilla. Topped with cheese, shrimp and mushrooms. Fold the tortilla. Grease both sides with melted butter.

2. Bake the uncovered quesadillas over medium heat for 1-2 minutes on both sides or until golden brown and cheese is melted. Divide each quesadilla into 4 equal parts. Come warm.

844. SUGARED PEANUTS

Prep Time: *15 Minutes* | *Cook Time:* *20 Minutes* | *Servings: 2*

INGREDIENTS:

- 5 cups unsalted peanuts
- 1 cup sugar
- 1 cup water

Directions:

1. ¼ tsp salt 1. In a large, heavy saucepan, place the peanuts, sugar and water. Bring to a boil and cook it for about 10 minutes until the syrup evaporates.
2. Spread the nuts in one layer on a greased 15x10x1-in. Cake pan; Sprinkle with salt.
3. Bake at 300° for 30-35 minutes or until dry and lightly browned. Cool completely. Store in an airtight container.

845. CHILI CONEY DOGS

Prep Time: *15 Minutes* | *Cook Time:* *18 Minutes* | *Servings: 8*

INGREDIENTS:

- 1 pound lean ground beef (90% lean)
- 1 can (15 ounces) tomato sauce
- ½ cup water 2 tbsps Worcestershire sauce
- 1 tbsp dried minced onion
- ½ tsp garlic powder ½ tsp ground mustard ½ tsp chilli powder ½ tsp pepper Dash cayenne pepper
- 8 hot dogs
- 8 hot dog buns, split
- Optional toppings: shredded cheddar cheese, relish and chopped onion 1. In a big skillet, cook beef over medium heat for 6-8 minutes or until no longer pink, breaking into crumbles; drain.
- Stir in tomato sauce, water, Worcestershire sauce, onion and seasonings.

Directions:

1. Place hot dogs in a 3-qt. Reduce cooker; top with beef mixture. Cook, covered, on reducing 4-5 hours or until heated through.
2. Present on buns with toppings as desired.

846. PHILLY CHEESESTEAK BITES

Prep Time: *15 Minutes* | *Cook Time:* *34 Minutes* | *Servings: 2*

INGREDIENTS:

- 1 package (22 ounces) frozen waffle-cut fries
- 1 medium onion, halved and sliced
- ½ small green pepper, halved and sliced ½ small sweet red pepper, halved and sliced 3 tbsps canola oil, divided
- ½ tsp salt, divided ¾ pound beef ribeye steak, cut into thin strips ¼ tsp pepper
- 3 tbsp ketchup
- 6 tbsps process cheese sauce

Directions:

1. Bake 18 big waffle fries according to package directions (save remaining fries for another use). Meanwhile, in a big skillet, saute onion and peppers in 1 tbsp oil until tender. Sprinkle with 1/8 tsp salt. Remove and keep warm.
2. In the same pan, saute steak in remaining oil in batches for 45-seconds or until desired doneness. Sprinkle with pepper and remaining salt. On each waffle fry, layer the beef, onion mixture, ketchup and cheese sauce. Present warm.

847. SWEET & SPICY JALAPENO POPPERS

Prep Time: *15 Minutes* | *Cook Time:* *17 Minutes* | *Servings: 6*

INGREDIENTS:

- 6 jalapeno peppers
- 4 ounces cream cheese, softened
- 2 tbsp shredded cheddar cheese
- 6 bacon strips, halved widthwise
- ¼ cup packed brown sugar 1 tbsp chilli seasoning mix

Directions:

1. Cut jalapenos in half lengthwise and remove seeds; set aside. In a small size bowl, beat cheeses until blended. Spoon into pepper halves. Wrap a half-strip of bacon around each pepper half.
2. Add brown sugar and chilli seasoning; coat peppers with sugar mixture. Place in a greased 15x10x1-in. Baking pan.
3. Bake it at least 350° for 18-20 minutes or until bacon is firm.

Dessert Recipes

848. Berry Sorbet

Prep Time: *15 Minutes* | *Cook Time:* *150 Minutes* | *Servings: 2*

Ingredients:

- 4 cups fresh berries
- juice from ½ lemon
- 1 cup water
- ¾ cup sugar

Directions:

1. Add the water and sugar into a saucepan and bring to a boil. Simmer for 5 minutes, then remove from heat and let this syrup cool to room temperature. Place the raspberries as well as lemon juice in a blender and pulse until well blended, then pass the puree through a fine sieve to remove the seeds.
2. Combine the puree with the sugar syrup and pour the mixture into your ice cream maker. Turn the machine on and churn according to your machine's instructions. When done, if you don't plan to serve it right away, store it in an airtight container in the freezer.

849. Berry Lemon Bundt Cake

Prep Time: *15 Minutes* | *Cook Time:* *16 Minutes* | *Servings: 8*

Ingredients:

- 1 cup all-purpose flour
- 1 ½ cups whole wheat flour
- 1 pinch of salt
- 2 teaspoons baking powder
- 6oz butter, softened
- 1 2/3 cup sugar
- 5 eggs
- 1 tablespoon dark rum
- 1 teaspoon vanilla extract
- 1 cup sour cream
- 2 cups fresh berries
- 1 tablespoon lemon zest

Directions:

1. In a bowl, convert the flours with the salt and baking powder and set them aside.
2. In a different bowl, mix the butter, softened, with the sugar until creamy and fluffy, then add the eggs, one after another, beating very well after each one. Gradually stir in the flour, alternating it with sour cream, then fold in the lemon zest and berries. Spoon the batter into your Bundt pan, greased with butter, then bake in the preheated oven at 350F for 40-50 minutes or until fragrant and golden brown.
3. When complete, let the cake cool in the pan, then transfer to your serving plate and cover with powdered sugar.

850. Almond and Berry Crunchy Cake

Prep Time: *15 Minutes* | *Cook Time:* *23 Minutes* | *Servings: 28*

Ingredients:

- ½ cup slivered almonds
- 1 cup all-purpose flour
- 1 cup whole wheat flour
- 2/3 cup powdered sugar
- 1 teaspoon baking powder
- 1 teaspoon baking soda
- 1 pinch of salt
- 4oz cold butter, cubed
- 2 eggs
- 1 teaspoon vanilla extract
- 2 ½ cups fresh berries
- ½ cup sliced almonds
- ½ cup whole wheat flour
- ½ cup rolled oats
- ½ cup desiccated coconut
- 4 oz butter

Directions:

1. In a bowl, mix the slivered almonds with the flours, powdered sugar, baking powder and baking soda, as well as a pinch of salt. Add the butter cubes and rub them together until sandy. Stir in the eggs and vanilla and add 2-4 tablespoons cold water if the dough does not come together.
2. Using your fingertips, spread the dough on the bottom of a 9x13-inch pan, then cover the dough with fresh berries. In another bowl, mix the whole wheat flour with the rolled oats, coconut and butter
3. Mix well until sandy, then spread this dough over the fresh fruits. Top with sliced almonds and bake in the preheated oven at 350F for 30-40 minutes or until golden brown.

851. Berry Salad with Mint

Prep Time: *15 Minutes* | *Cook Time:* *10 Minutes* | *Servings: 5*

Ingredients:

- 1 cup strawberries, sliced
- 1 cup raspberries
- 1 cup blueberries
- 1 cup blackberries
- 1 orange, cut into segments
- 2 tablespoons honey
- 2 tablespoons Cointreau
- ¼ cup fresh mint leaves
- ¼ cup orange juice
- 1 tablespoon lemon juice

Directions:

1. Combine the strawberries with the raspberries, blueberries, blackberries and orange segments In a bowl.
2. In another bowl, whisk together the honey with Cointreau, orange juice, lemon juice and mint leaves. Pour this dressing over the fruits and mix gently. Refrigerate at least 1 hour before serving.

852. Berry Cheesecake

Prep Time: *15 Minutes* | *Cook Time:* *60 Minutes* | *Servings: 8*

Ingredients:

- Crust:
- 2 cups graham crackers
- 2 tablespoons powdered sugar
- 1 teaspoon vanilla extract

- 4 oz butter, melted
- Filling:
- 20oz low-fat cream cheese
- 1 cup sour cream
- 2/3 cup sugar
- 4 eggs
- 2 tablespoons cornstarch
- 1 teaspoon vanilla extract
- seeds from 1 vanilla bean
- Berry syrup:
- 2 cups fresh berries
- ¼ cup sugar
- 1 teaspoon lemon juice
- ¼ cup water

Directions:

1. To make the crust: Put the crackers and sugar in a food processor and pulse until ground, then add the vanilla and melted butter. Pulse until it comes as a dough, then transfer into a 10-inch round cake pan and press it on the bottom and sides of the pan. Use your fingertips or a spoon for this task. Set aside.
2. To make the filling: Mix the cream cheese with the sugar and sour cream, then add the eggs, cornstarch and vanilla. Add this filling over the crust and bake in the preheated oven at 350F for 40-50 minutes.
3. To make the syrup: Pour the water and sugar in a small saucepan and simmer for 2-3 minutes, then add the lemon juice and berries and cook for 5 minutes or until soft. The fruits need to be whole but slightly tender and flavorful.
4. To serve the cheesecake, top it with berries just before serving, then drizzle with syrup on the plate.

Mediterranean Diet For Low Blood Pressure

Breakfast & Brunch Recipes

853. Spinach Frittata

Prep Time: *15 Minutes* | *Cook Time:* *16 Minutes* | *Servings: 6*

Ingredients:

- 6 servings
- 2 tbsp. olive oil or avocado oil 1 Zucchini sliced 1 cup torn fresh spinach
- 2 tbsp. sliced green onions
- 1 tsp. crushed garlic salt and pepper to taste 1/3 cup coconut milk
- 6 eggs

Directions:

1. Heat olive oil in a skillet over medium heat. Add zucchini and cook until tender. Mix in spinach, green onions and garlic. Season with salt and pepper. Continue cooking until spinach is wilted.
2. In a bowl, beat eggs and coconut milk together. Pour into the skillet over the vegetables. Reduce heat to low cover and cook until eggs are firm (5 to 7 minutes).

854. Superfoods Naan Pancakes Crepes

Prep Time: *15 Minutes* | *Cook Time:* *10 Minutes* | *Servings: 2*

Ingredients:

- ½ cup almond flour ½ cup Tapioca Flour 1 cup Coconut Milk Salt
- coconut oil

Directions:

1. Mix all the ingredients together.
2. After heating a pan over medium heat and pour the batter to desired thickness; once the batter looks firm, flip it over to cook the other side.
3. If you want this to be a dessert crepe or pancake, then omit the salt. You can add minced garlic or ginger in the batter if you want or some spices.

855. Frittata with Broccoli and Tomato

Prep Time: *15 Minutes* | *Cook Time:* *20 Minutes* | *Servings: 2*

Ingredients:

- 2 large eggs
- Salt Ground black pepper 1 tsp. Olive oil or cumin oil ½ cup broccoli
- ½ cup sliced tomatoes Crushed red pepper flakes and a 1 Tbsp. chopped chives (optional)

Directions:

1. 2 large eggs are whisking in a small bowl. Present with salt and ground black pepper and set aside. Heat 1 tsp.
2. Oil in a medium skillet over medium heat. Add broccoli and tomatoes and cook, tossing approx. 1 minute. Add eggs; cook, occasionally stirring until just set about 1 minute. Stir in cheese.
3. Sprinkle with crushed red pepper flakes and chives.

856. Frittata with Green and Red Peppers

Prep Time: *15 Minutes* | *Cook Time:* *12 Minutes* | *Servings: 6*

Ingredients:

- 2 large eggs
- Salt Ground black pepper 1 tsp. olive oil or avocado oil ½ cup each chopped green and red peppers

Directions:

1. 2 large eggs are whisking in a small bowl. Present with salt and ground black pepper and set aside. Heat 1 tsp.
2. Olive oil in a medium skillet. Add peppers and cook, tossing approx. 1 minute.
3. Add eggs; cook, occasionally stirring until just set about 1 minute.

857. Eggs in Purgatory

Prep Time: *15 Minutes* | *Cook Time:* *5 Minutes* | *Servings: 4*

Ingredients:

- 2 large eggs
- Salt 1 clove garlic chopped.
- 1 tsp. Olive oil or avocado oil 1 cup chopped tomatoes 1 Tbsp. Hot red pepper flakes and 1 Tbsp. cilantro

Directions:

1. Heat 1 tsp. Oil in a medium skillet over medium heat. Add garlic, chopped tomatoes and red pepper flakes and cook, tossing approx. 15 minutes.
3. Add eggs and cook until eggs are done. Sprinkle with salt and cilantro.

858. Frittata with Carrots Green Peas and Asparagus

Prep Time: *15 Minutes* | *Cook Time:* *20 Minutes* | *Servings: 5*

Ingredients:

- 2 large eggs
- Salt Ground black pepper 1 tsp. Olive oil or avocado oil ½ cup cooked green peas ½ cup chopped carrot ½ cup asparagus 1 tbsp. fresh dill

Directions:

1. 2 large eggs are whisking in a small bowl. Present with salt and ground black pepper and set aside. Heating 1 tsp.
2. Oil in a skillet over medium heat. Add carrots and asparagus and cook, tossing approx. 5 minutes. Add cooked and drained green peas. Add eggs; cook, occasionally stirring until just set about 1 minute. Sprinkle with dill.

859. Zucchini Scrambled Eggs

Prep Time: *15 Minutes* | *Cook Time:* *15 Minutes* | *Servings: 3*

Ingredients

- 1 tsp coconut oil 4 eggs
- 1 Tbs water
- 1 zucchini sliced
- ground black pepper to taste

Directions:

1. Whisk 4 large eggs in a small bowl. Present with salt and ground black pepper and set aside. Heat 1 tsp. Olive oil in a skillet. Add sliced zucchini and cook, tossing until wilted (approx. 3 minutes). Set aside.
2. Add eggs and cooked completely, stirring occasionally. Serve with zucchini on the aside.

860. Frittata with Asparagus and Tomato

Prep Time: *15 Minutes* | *Cook Time:* *15 Minutes* | *Servings: 4*

Ingredients:

- 2 large eggs
- Salt Ground black pepper 1 tsp. olive oil or avocado oil 1 cup asparagus
- ½ cup sliced tomatoes

Directions:

1. Whisk 2 large eggs in a small bowl. Present with salt and ground black pepper and set aside. Heat 1 tsp. Oil in a medium skillet over medium heat. Add asparagus and cook, tossing approx. 4-5 minutes. Add tomatoes and eggs and cook, occasionally stirring until just set about 1 minute. Sprinkle with dill (optional).

861. Eggs with Zucchini Onions and Tomato

Prep Time: *15 Minutes* | *Cook Time:*□*20 Minutes* | *Servings: 2*

Ingredients:

- 2 large eggs
- Salt Ground black pepper 1 tsp. olive oil or avocado oil
- 1/3 cup sliced
- zucchini 1/3 cup chopped onions 1/3 cup sliced tomato Crushed red pepper flakes and a pinch of dill (optional)

Directions:

1. Mix 2 eggs in a small bowl. Present with salt and ground black pepper and set aside. Heat 1 tsp. Olive oil in a skillet. Add zucchini, onions and tomatoes and cook tossing until wilted (approx. 3-4 minutes). Add eggs and cook until just set.

862. Frittata with Tomatoes and Spinach

Prep Time: *1 Minutes* | *Cook Time:* *15 Minutes* | *Servings: 3*

Ingredients:

- 2 large eggs
- Salt Ground black pepper 1 tsp. olive oil or avocado oil ½ cup sliced tomatoes 1/3 cup spinach

Directions:

1. Whisk 2 large eggs in a small bowl. Season with salt and ground black pepper and set aside. Heat 1 tsp. Olive oil in a medium skillet over medium heat. Add baby spinach and tomatoes and cook, tossing until wilted (approx. 1 minute). Add eggs; cook, occasionally stirring until just set about 1 minute.

863. Zucchini Pancakes

Prep Time: *15 Minutes* | *Cook Time:* *10 Minutes* | *Servings: 2*

Ingredients:

- 2 medium zucchini
- 2 tbsp. chopped onion
- 3 beaten eggs 6 to 8 tbsp. Almond flour 1 tsp. Salt
- ½ tsp. ground black pepper
- coconut oil

Directions:

1. Heat the oven to 300 degrees F.
2. Grate the zucchini into a bowl and mix in the onion and eggs. Stir in 6 tbsp of the flour, salt and pepper.
3. Heat a large sauté pan over medium heat and add coconut oil to the pan. When the oil is hot lower the heat to medium-low and adds batter into the pan. Baked the pancakes for about 2 minutes on each side until browned. Place the pancakes in the oven.

864. Savoury Superfoods Pie Crust

Prep Time: *15 Minutes* | *Cook Time:* *70 Minutes* | *Servings: 2*

Ingredients:

- DF
- 11/4 cups blanched almond flour 1/3 cup tapioca flour
- ¾ tsp. Finely ground sea salt
- ¾ tsp. Paprika
- ½ tsp. ground cumin
- 1/8 tsp. ground white pepper
- ¼ cup coconut oil 1 large egg

Directions:

1. Place almond flour tapioca flour, sea salt, vanilla egg and coconut sugar (if you use coconut sugar) in the bowl of a food processor. Process 2-3 times to combine. Add oil and raw honey (if you use raw honey) and pulse with several one-second pulses and then let the food processor run until the mixture comes together. Move the dough onto a plastic wrap sheet. Wrap and then press the dough into a 9-inch disk. Refrigerate for 30 minutes.
2. Remove plastic wrap. Press dough onto the bottom and up the sides of a 9-inch buttered pie dish. Crimp a little bit the edges of the crust. Cool in the refrigerator for 20 minutes. Tp put the oven rack in the middle after heating the oven to 375F. Put in the oven and bake until golden brown.

865. Spinach Quiche

Prep Time: *15 Minutes* | *Cook Time:* *30 Minutes* | *Servings: 6*

Ingredients:

- 1 Precooked and cooled Savory Superfoods Pie Crust
- 8 ounces organic spinach cooked and drained
- 6 ounces cubed pork 2 medium shallots thinly sliced and sautéed
- 4 large eggs 1 cup coconut milk ¾ tsp. Salt ¼ tsp. freshly ground black pepper

Directions:

1. Brown the pork in coconut oil and then add the spinach and shallots. Set aside once done.
2. Preheat oven to 350F. In a large bowl, combine eggs, milk, salt and pepper. Whisk until foamy. Add in about ¾ of the drained filling mixture reserving the other ¼ to "top" the quiche. Pour egg mixture into crust and place remaining filling on top of the quiche.
3. Place quiche in the oven in the centre of the middle rack and bake undisturbed for 45 to 50 minutes.

866. Mushroom Quiche

Prep Time: *15 Minutes* | *Cook Time:*□25 *Minutes* | *Servings: 2*

Ingredients:

- 1 Precooked and cooled Savory Superfoods Pie Crust
- 1 cup sliced mushrooms 6 ounces cubed pork 2 medium shallots thinly sliced and sautéed
- 4 large eggs 1 cup coconut milk ¾ tsp. Salt ¼ tsp. freshly ground black pepper

Directions:

1. Brown the pork in coconut oil and then add the mushrooms and shallots. Set aside once done.
2. Preheat oven to 350F. In a large bowl, combine eggs, milk, salt and pepper. Whisk until foamy. Add in about ¾ of the drained filling mixture reserving the other ¼ to "top" the quiche. Pour egg mixture into crust and place remaining filling on top of the quiche.
3. Place quiche in the oven in the centre of the middle rack and bake undisturbed for 45 to 50 minutes.

867. Tomato Quiche

Prep Time: *15 Minutes* | *Cook Time:* *18 Minutes* | *Servings: 2*

Ingredients:

- 1 Precooked and cooled Savory Superfoods Pie Crust
- 1 cup sliced tomatoes 6 ounces cubed pork 2 medium shallots thinly sliced and sautéed
- 4 large eggs 1 cup coconut milk ¾ tsp. Salt ¼ cup. Arugula ¼ tsp. freshly ground black pepper

Directions:

1. Brown the pork and shallots in coconut oil. Set aside once done.
2. Preheat oven to 350F. In a large bowl, combine eggs, milk, salt and pepper. Whisk until foamy. Add in about ¾ of the drained filling mixture and tomatoes, reserving the other ¼ to "top" the quiche. Pour egg mixture into crust and place remaining filling on top of the quiche.
3. Place quiche in the oven in the centre of the middle rack and bake undisturbed for 45 to 50 minutes. Sprinkle with arugula.

868. MINI TERIYAKI TURKEY SANDWICHES

Prep Time: *15 Minutes* | *Cook Time:* *17 Minutes* | *Servings: 2*

INGREDIENTS:

- (2 pounds each) 2 boneless skinless turkey breast halves
- 2/3 cup of packed brown sugar
- 2/3 cup of reduced-sodium soy sauce
- ¼ cup cider vinegar
- 3 garlic cloves, minced
- 1 tbsp minced fresh ginger root
- ½ tsp pepper
- 2 tbsps cornstarch
- 2 tbsps cold water
- 20 Hawaiian sweet rolls
- 2 tbsps butter, melted

Directions:

1. Place turkey in a 5-or 6-qt. Reduce cooker. In a small size bowl, add brown sugar, soy sauce, vinegar, garlic, ginger and pepper; pour over turkey. Cook, covered, on reducing 5-6 hours or until the meat is tender.
2. Remove turkey from reducing cooker. In a small size bowl, combine cornstarch and cold water until smooth; gradually stir into cooking liquid.
3. When cool enough, shred meat with two forks and return meat to reduce cooker. Cook, covered, on high 30- minutes or until sauce is thickened.
4. Preheat oven to 325°. Split rolls and brush cut sides with butter; place on an ungreased baking sheet, cut side up.
5. Bake 8-10 minutes or until toasted and golden brown. Spoon 1/3 cup turkey mixture on roll bottoms. Replace tops.

869. SUMMER TEA SANDWICHES

Prep Time: *15 Minutes* | *Cook Time:* *10 Minutes* | *Servings: 2*

INGREDIENTS:

- ½ tsp dried tarragon ½ tsp salt, divided ¼ tsp pepper 1 pound boneless skinless chicken breasts
- ½ cup reduced-fat mayonnaise 1 tbsp finely chopped red onion
- 1 tsp dill weed
- ½ tsp lemon juice 24 slices soft multigrain bread, crusts removed
- 1 medium cucumber, thinly sliced
- ¼ medium cantaloupe, cut into 12 thin slices 1. Add the tarragon,
- ¼ tsp salt and pepper; rub over chicken. Place it on a baking sheet that is coated with cooking spray.

Directions:

1. Bake it at least 350° for 20-25 minutes or until a thermometer reads 170°. Cool to room temperature; thinly slice.

870. SEAFOOD SALAD MINI CROISSANTS

Prep Time: *15 Minutes* | *Cook Time:* *20 Minutes* | *Servings: 5*

INGREDIENTS:

- ½ cup mayonnaise
- 1 tbsp snipped fresh dill
- 1 tbsp minced chives
- 1 tbsp lemon juice
- ½ tsp salt
- ¼ tsp pepper
- ½ pound imitation lobster ½ pound cooked small shrimp, peeled and deveined and coarsely chopped 10 miniature croissants, split

Directions:

1. In a big bowl, add the mayonnaise, dill, chives, lemon juice, salt and pepper. Stir in lobster and shrimp. Cover and refrigerate until serving. Present on croissants.
2. In a small size bowl, add the mayonnaise, onion, dill, lemon juice and remaining salt; spread over 12 bread slices. Top with cucumber, chicken, cantaloupe and remaining bread. Cut sandwiches in half diagonally. Present immediately.

871. CHIPOTLE SLIDERS

Prep Time: *15 Minutes* | *Cook Time:* *30 Minutes* | *Servings: 2*

INGREDIENTS:

- 1 package (12 ounces) Hawaiian sweet rolls, divided
- 1 tsp salt
- ½ tsp of pepper
- 8 tsp of minced chipotle peppers in adobo sauce, divided
- 1 ½ pounds ground beef
- 10 slices pepper Jack cheese
- ½ cup mayonnaise

Directions:

1. Add 2 rolls to the food processor. The process of demolition. Make it into a large bowl. Now add salt, pepper and 6 tsp chopped chives. Mix the beef into the dough and mix well. Make 10 columns.
2. Cook the covered burgers on medium heat for 3-4 minutes on both sides or until the thermometer reads 160° and the water is clear. Top with cheese. Bake for 1 minute or until cheese is melted.
3. Remove the rest of the rolls, turn them over and heat over medium heat for 30-60 seconds or until fully cooked.
4. Add mayonnaise and remaining chipotle peppers; spread over roll bottoms. Top each with a burger. Replace roll tops.

872. CHICKEN SALAD PARTY SANDWICHES

Prep Time: *15 Minutes* | *Cook Time:* *20 Minutes* | *Servings: 7*

Ingredients:

- 4 cups cubed cooked chicken breast
- 1 ½ cups dried cranberries
- 2 celery ribs, finely chopped
- 2 green onions, thinly sliced
- ¼ cup chopped sweet pickles
- 1 cup fat-free mayonnaise
- ½ tsp curry powder
- ¼ tsp coarsely ground pepper
- ½ cup chopped pecans, toasted
- 15 whole wheat dinner rolls
- Torn leaf lettuce

Directions:

1. In a bowl, now add the first five ingredients. In a small size bowl, add the mayonnaise, curry and pepper. Add to chicken mixture; toss to coat. Chill until serving.
2. Stir pecans into chicken salad. Present on rolls lined with lettuce.

873. STATE FAIR SUBS

Prep Time: *15 Minutes* | *Cook Time:* *20 Minutes* | *Servings: 3*

Ingredients:

- 1 loaf (1 pound unsliced) French bread
- 2 eggs
- ¼ cup milk
- ½ tsp pepper
- ¼ tsp salt
- 1 pound bulk Italian sausage
- 1 ½ cups chopped onion
- 2 cups (8 ounces) of shredded part-skim mozzarella cheese

Directions:

1. Cut the bread in half lengthwise. Drill holes carefully in the top and bottom of the loaf, leaving about an inch.
2. Husks. Diced bread. In a large bowl, shake together the eggs, milk, pepper and salt. Add slices of bread and stir to coat. Separately.
3. In a frying pan over high heat, cook the sausages and onions until the meat is no longer pink. Thin.
4. Add to bread dough. Spoon for filling in breadcrumbs; Sprinkle with cheese. Wrap each in foil. Bake it at least 400° for 20-25 minutes or until cheese is melted. Cut French bread into 1-serving-sized pieces.

874. PARTY PITAS

Prep Time: *15 Minutes* | *Cook Time:* *10 Minutes* | *Servings: 5*

INGREDIENTS:

- 4 whole-wheat pita pocket halves
- 1/3 cup Greek vinaigrette ½ pound thinly sliced deli turkey 1 jar (7 ½ ounces) roasted sweet red peppers, drained and patted dry 2 cups fresh baby spinach
- 24 pitted Greek olives
- 24 frilled toothpicks

Directions:

1. Brush insides of pita pockets with vinaigrette; fill with turkey, peppers and spinach. Cut each pita into six wedges.
2. Thread olives onto toothpicks; use to secure wedges.

875. BAJA CHICKEN & SLAW SLIDERS

Prep Time: *15 Minutes* | *Cook Time:*□45 *Minutes* | *Servings: 2*

INGREDIENTS:

- ¼ cup reduced-fat sour cream ½ tsp grated lime peel ¼ tsp lime juice SLAW
- 1 cup broccoli coleslaw mix
- 2 tbsps finely chopped sweet red pepper
- 2 tbsps finely chopped sweet onion
- 2 tbsps of minced fresh cilantro
- 2 tsp of chopped seeded jalapeno pepper 2 tsp of lime juice
- 1 tsp of sugar
- SLIDERS
- (4 ounces each) 4 boneless skinless chicken breast halves ½ tsp of ground cumin
- ½ tsp of chilli powder
- ¼ tsp of salt
- ¼ tsp of coarsely ground pepper 8 Hawaiian sweet rolls, split
- 8 small lettuce leaves
- 8 slices tomato

Directions:

1. In a small size bowl, add sour cream, lime peel and lime juice. In another small size bowl, add slaw ingredients. Refrigerate sauce and slaw until serving.
2. Cut each chicken breast in half wide; flatten to -in. Thickness. Sprinkle with spices.
3. Wet a paper towel with cooking oil; using long-handled tongs, rub on grill rack to lightly coat.
4. Grill chicken, covered, over medium heat or roast 4 inches from heat 4 to 7 minutes on each side or until no longer pink.
5. Toast bread, cut side down, 30-60 seconds or until toasted. Serve grilled chicken on a roll with lettuce, tomatoes, sauce, and slaw.
6. **NOTE** Wear disposable gloves when chopping chillies; The oil can burn the skin. Avoid touching your face.

876. Vegetarian Tomato Quiche

Prep Time: *15 Minutes* | *Cook Time:* *10 Minutes* | *Servings: 4*

Ingredients:

- 1 Precooked and cooled Savory Superfoods Pie Crust
- 2 cups sliced tomatoes 4 large eggs 1 cup coconut milk ¾ tsp. Salt
- ¼ cup. Fresh basil ¼ tsp. freshly ground black pepper

Directions:

1. Preheat oven to 350F. In a large bowl, combine eggs, milk, salt and pepper. Whisk until foamy. Pour egg mixture into crust and place sliced tomatoes on top of the quiche.
2. Place quiche in the oven in the centre of the middle rack and bake undisturbed for 45 to 50 minutes. Sprinkle with basil.

Lunch Recipes

877. Moroccan Chickpea Broth for Couscous

Prep Time: *5 Minutes* | *Cook Time:* *85 Minutes* | *Servings: 2*

Ingredients::

- 2 mug s/455 g dried chickpeas, soaked overnight in water to put the lid
- mug /60 ml oil
- 1 onion, finely chopped
- Three ribs celery, coarsely chopped
- Three medium carrots, coarsely chopped.
- One can chop tomatoes with their juice 6 mugs s/1.4 L chicken broth.
- ground black pepper Couscous, for serving Harissa
- Salt

DIRECTIONS:

1. Rinse the soaked beans and shift them to the slow cooker.
2. Heat the oil in a skillet over medium-high heat, and sauté the onion, celery, and carrots for 3 mins, or until the onion begins to soften. Put on the tomatoes, and shift the mixture to the insert of the slow cooker.
3. Stir in the broth, put the lid, and cook on high for 4 hours or on low for 8 hours.
4. Season the soup with salt and pepper.
5. To present the soup, spoon some of the couscouses into a soup container, and spoon the soup generously over the couscous. Garnish with Harissa, if desired.

Each Serving:

- 188 Calories
- 17.6grams Fat
- 5.7grams Carbs
- 3.8grams Fiber
- 12.2grams Protein
- 1.9grams Sugars

878. Spanish Meatball Soup

Prep Time: *5 Minutes* | *Cook Time:* *25 Minutes* | *Servings: 2*

Ingredients:

- 2 tbsp oil
- 1 onion, finely chopped
- 1 garlic clove, minced
- One 14½-to 15-oz/415-to 430-g can crushed tomatoes with their juice.
- One head escarole, tough stalks removed, and cut into 1-in/2.5-cm pieces.
- Two 14½-to 15-oz/415-to 430-g cans of white beans, rinsed and drained.

- Eight mug s/2 L chicken broth
- 1 tsp saffron threads, crushed in the palm of your hand
- 1 mug /55 g torn sturdy bread, such as a baguette or French loaf
- ¼ mug /60 ml milk
- 1½ lb/680 g ground veal
- ½ lb/225 g ground pork
- Two garlic cloves, minced
- mug /15 g chopped flat-leaf parsley
- 1½ tsp salt
- ½ tsp ground black pepper
- 1½ mug s/360 ml oil
- Salt
- ground black pepper

DIRECTIONS:

1. **To make the soup:** Heat the oil in a skillet over medium-high heat. Put on the onion and garlic and sauté for 3 mins, or until the onion is softened. Put on the tomatoes, and stir to combine. Shift the batter to the insert of a 5-to 7-qt4.5-to 6.5-L slow cooker. Stir in the escarole, beans, and broth. Put the lid and cook on high while making the meatballs.
2. TO MAKE THE MEATBALLS Put the saffron and bread in a mixing container. Pour in the milk and let the bread soak for about 5 mins until it is softened. Put on the veal, pork, garlic, parsley, salt, and pepper, stirring to combine them. Utilizing a portion scoop, form the meat into 1-in2.5-cm balls. Heat the oil in a skillet over medium-high heat, and brown the meatballs all over (they will not be cooked through).
3. Put on the meatballs to the soup in the slow cooker and cook on high for 3 hours or on low for 5 to 6 hours. The meatballs will be tender. Season the soup with salt and pepper, if needed, before serving.

Each Serving:

- 372 Calories
- 17.6grams Fat
- 5.7grams Carbs
- 5.9grams Fiber
- 20.2grams Protein
- 0.9grams Sugars

879. Nonna's Soup for the Soul

Prep Time: 5 Minutes *Cook Time: 75 Minutes* *Servings: 4*

INGREDIENTS:

- 2 tbsp oil
- 1 onion, finely chopped
- Three medium carrots, finely chopped.
- One head escarole, kale, savoy cabbage, or Swiss chard, cored and cut into ½-in/12-mm pieces.
- Eight mug s/2 L chicken broth
- Four eggs
- to ⅔ mug /60 to 75 g grated Parmigiano-Reggiano cheese Salt
- ground black pepper

DIRECTIONS:

1. In a pan, heat the oil, sauté the onion, carrots, and escarole, turning in the oil to coat, until the onion begins to soften about 3 mins. Shift the cooking pot's contents to the insert of a 5-to 7-qt/ 4.5-to 6.5-L slow cooker. Put on the broth. Put the lid and cook on high for 3 hours or on low for 5 to 6 hours. The escarole will be tender.
2. Remove the top from the slow cooker. In a medium mixing container, whisk together the eggs and ½ mug /60g of the cheese. Drizzle the egg mixture into the simmering soup, stirring as you are pouring it in. Season with salt and pepper, and present the soup immediately, garnished with additional Parmigiano, if desired.

Each Serving:

- 232 Calories
- 14.6grams Fat
- 2.7grams Carbs
- 4.9grams Fiber
- 14.2grams Protein
- 1.9grams Sugars

880. Slow Cooker Gazpacho

Prep Time: 5 Minutes *Cook Time: 55 Minutes* *Servings: 2*

INGREDIENTS: FOR THE SOUP

- 2 tbsp oil
- Three garlic cloves, minced
- 1 red onion, finely chopped
- 1 yellow bell pepper
- 1 red bell pepper
- 1 green bell pepper, cored and finely chopped
- Four mug s/960 ml chicken or vegetable broth
- One 28-to 32-oz/800-to 910-g can tomato purée
- 2 tbsp red wine vinegar

INGREDIENTS: FOR THE GARNISH

- 2 Hass avocados, peeled, pitted, and finely diced
- 2 tsp lemon juice
- 1 tsp grated lemon zest
- 1 English cucumber, finely diced
- One mug /230 g cherry tomatoes, quartered
- Two green onions
- Salt
- ground black pepper
- Two mug s/230 g toasted bread crumbs
- ½ mug /30 g finely chopped flat-leaf parsley

DIRECTIONS:

1. TO MAKE THE SOUP In a skillet, heat the oil over a medium-high flame and sauté the garlic, onion, and bell peppers for 3 mins, until the onion begins to soften. Shift the batter of the skillet to the insert of a 5-to 7-qt4.5-to 6.5-L slow cooker. Stir in the broth, tomato purée, and vinegar. Put the lid and cook on high for 3 hours or on low for 5 to 6 hours.
2. WHILE THE SOUP IS SIMMERING, MAKE THE GARNISH / In a mixing container, toss together the avocado, lemon juice and zest, cucumber, cherry tomatoes, and green onions.
3. Season the soup with salt and pepper, spoon it into containers, and dollop with the garnish. Sprinkle with bread crumbs and parsley before serving.

Each Serving:

- 188 Calories
- 10.6grams Fat
- 11.7grams Carbs
- 2.9grams Fiber
- 12.2grams Protein
- 1.9grams Sugars

881. Pork Braised with Dried Fruits and Cipollini Onions

Prep Time: 5 Minutes *Cook Time: 35 Minutes* *Servings: 2*

INGREDIENTS:

- 8 bone-in 1-in-/2.5-cm-thick pork loin chops (½ lb/225 g each)
- Salt
- ground black pepper
- 2 tbsp oil
- 24 cipollini onions, peeled and halved
- Eight threads of saffron, crushed in the palm of your hand
- ¼ tsp ground ginger
- One mug /240 ml chicken broth
- One mug /170 g golden raisins
- ½ mug /85 g dried apricots, coarsely chopped
- One 14½-to 15-oz/415-to 430-g can chopped tomatoes with their juice.
- 1 mug /240 ml beef broth
- 2 tbsp cornstarch mixed with ¼ mug /60 ml water
- ¼ mug /15 g finely chopped cilantro

DIRECTIONS:

1. Season the pork on both sides with salt and pepper. In a skillet, heat the oil over high heat, put on the pork, and brown each chop on both sides. Take the pork to the insert of a 5-to 7-qt/4.5-to 6.5-L slow cooker. In the same skillet over medium-high heat, sauté the onions with the saffron and ginger.
2. Until the onions' outsides begin to soften slightly, pour the broth into the cooking pot, and scrape up any browned bits on the bottom. Shift the skillet's contents to the slow cooker insert, and put on the raisins, apricots, tomatoes, and broth, stirring to combine. Put the lid and cook on high for 4 to 5 hours or on low for 8 to 10 hours, until the pork is tender.
3. Shift the pork chops to a serving platter, and put the lid with aluminum foil. Shift the sauce to a medium saucepan, and skim off any excess fat. Let the sauce boil, put on the cornstarch mixture, and whisk until the sauce returns to a boil and is smooth and thickened. Remove from the heat. Present the pork chops napped with some of the sauce and garnished with chopped cilantro. Pass the remaining sauce on the side.

Each Serving:

- 111 Calories
- 11.6grams Fat
- 7.7grams Carbs
- 2.9grams Fiber
- 11.2grams Protein

882. Pork Braised with Pomegranates

Prep Time: 5 Minutes *Cook Time: 65 Minutes* *Servings: 4*

INGREDIENTS:

- Six medium carrots, cut into 1-in/2.5-cm pieces
- 2 tbsp oil
- 1 tsp turmeric
- tsp ground cinnamon 1½ tsp salt
- 1 tsp ground black pepper
- Six bone-in 1-in-/2.5-cm-thick pork loin chops (½ lb/225 g each)
- 3 tbsp unsalted butter
- Two sweet yellow onions, such as Vidalia, finely chopped ¼ mug /60 ml pomegranate molasses
- Two mug s/480 ml chicken broth
- One mug /115 g finely chopped walnuts
- ½ mug /30 g finely chopped flat-leaf parsley
- 2 tbsp cornstarch mixed with ¼ mug /60 ml chicken broth or water
- One mug /80 g pomegranate arils,

DIRECTIONS:

1. Arrange the carrots in the insert of a 5-to 7-qt/4.5-to 6.5-L slow cooker. In a container, mix the oil, turmeric, cinnamon, salt, and pepper to form a paste. Rub the paste into the pork.
2. Heat a pan and brown the chops on each side. Shift the pork to the slow cooker insert when browned. Melt the butter in the skillet, and cook the onions for 3 mins, or until they begin to soften. Put on the pomegranate molasses and broth and stir up any browned bits on the bottom of the cooking pot. Pour the mixture over the chops—cook for4 hours on high flame or 5 to 6 hours on low.
3. Stir in the walnuts and parsley, put the lid, and cook for another 30 mins on high or 1 hour on low. Carefully remove the pork chops and carrots from the slow cooker utilizing a spatula, and shift to a serving platter. Put the lid with aluminum foil.
4. Shift the sauce to a saucepan, and let it boil. Put on the cornstarch mixture, and whisk until the sauce returns to a boil and is smooth and thickened. Remove from the heat. Pour some of the sauce over the pork chops and carrots, and pass the remaining sauce on the side. Garnish the chops with the pomegranate arils before serving.

Each Serving:

- 442 Calories
- 16.6grams Fat
- 9.7grams Carbs
- 11.9grams Fiber
- 21.2grams Protein
- 11.9grams Sugars

883. Braised Pork in Balsamic Vinegar

Prep Time: *5 Minutes* *Cook Time:* *59 Minutes* *Servings: 2*

INGREDIENTS:

- Three lb/1.4 kg boneless country-style pork ribs or pork shoulder, excess fat trimmed, and cut into 1-in/2.5-cm chunks.
- 1½ tsp salt
- tsp ground black pepper
- 2 tsp dried sage
- 2 tbsp oil
- Two sweet onions, coarsely chopped
- One mug /240 ml good-quality balsamic vinegar

DIRECTIONS:

1. Sprinkle the pork with salt, pepper, and sage. In a skillet, heat oil over medium-high heat, and brown the pork on all sides, a few pieces at a time, trying not to crowd the cooking pot and shifting the browned meat to the insert of a 4-to 6-qt/3.5-to 5.5-L slow cooker as it's done. Put the onions in the cooking pot, and sauté until they begin to soften about 3 mins. Pour the vinegar into the cooking pot, and scrape up any browned bits on the bottom. Shift the onions to the slow cooker insert, turning the pork in the onions. Put the lid on the cooker, cook on high for 3 hours or on low for 6 hours, until the pork is tender.
2. Remove the pork and skim any excess fat from the top of the sauce. Season the sauce with more salt and pepper if necessary. Return the pork to the sauce and keep warm until ready to serve.

Each Serving:

- 138 Calories
- 11.6grams Fat
- 9.7grams Carbs
- 6.9grams Fiber
- 15.2grams Protein
- 0.4grams Sugars

884. Tuscan Milk-Braised Pork

Prep Time: *5 Minutes* *Cook Time:* *45 Minutes* *Servings: 2*

INGREDIENTS:

- 1½ mug s/360 ml whole milk
- Two mugs s/480 ml heavy cream
- Peel of 1 lemon, cut into strips.
- Leaves of 1 bunch sage (about 20), thinly sliced
- One 4-lb/1.8-kg pork loin roast, tied with butcher's twine or silicone bands
- Salt
- ground black pepper
- ½ mug /120 ml oil
- 1 sweet yellow onion, such as Vidalia, finely chopped
- Three medium carrots, coarsely chopped.
- Three ribs celery, including the leaves, coarsely chopped
- mug /120 ml dry white wine, such as Pinot Grigio or Sauvignon Blanc, or dry vermouth

DIRECTIONS:

1. Pour the milk and cream into the insert of a 5-to 7-qt/4.5-to 6.5-L slow cooker. Stir in the lemon peel and half the sage. Put the lid on the slow cooker, set it too high, and set aside.
2. Sprinkle the pork with salt and pepper.
3. In a skillet, heat 2 tbsp of the oil over a high flame and brown the pork on all sides, turning frequently. Shift the pork to the slow cooker, lower the flame under the skillet to medium-high, and put on another 2 tbsps of oil, the onion, carrots, and celery.
4. Sauté for 3 mins or until the onion begins to soften. Pour in the wine and allow it to boil for 1 min, scraping up the browned bits on the bottom of the cooking pot. Shift the skillet mix to the insert, stirring to blend with the other INGREDIENTS:. Put the lid and cook on high for 4 hours or on low for 8 to 10 hours, until the pork is tender.
5. While the pork is cooking, heat the remaining ¼ mug /60 ml oil in a skillet, and fry the remaining sage leaves until crisp. Drain on paper towels and set aside. Shift pork to a cutting board and put the lid with aluminum foil. Strain the sauce into a saucepan, and let it to a boil. Boil the sauce for 3 to 5 mins to reduce and concentrate the flavors. Remove the butcher's twine from the roast and slice. Present the roast on a platter, napped with some of the sauce, and topped with the fried sage leaves. Present the warmed sauce alongside the roast.

Each Serving:

- 492 Calories
- 27.6grams Fat
- 1.7grams Carbs
- 4.9grams Fiber
- 15.2grams Protein
- 3.9grams Sugars

885. Portuguese White Wine-Braised Pork Loin with Roasted Red Peppers

Prep Time: *5 Minutes* *Cook Time:* *25 Minutes* *Servings: 4*

INGREDIENTS:

- 2 tbsp oil
- One sweet onion, such as Vidalia, thinly sliced
- Eight garlic cloves, minced
- 1 tsp sweet paprika
- Six roasted red bell peppers, either homemade or jarred, cut into thin strips.
- Two mug s/240 g cherry tomatoes halved.
- One 3½-to 4-lb/1.6-to 1.8-kg pork loin, tied at 1-in/2.5-mm intervals with butcher's twine or silicone loops
- 1 tsp salt
- ½ tsp ground black pepper
- 1½ mug s/360 ml dry white wine, such as Pinot Grigio or Sauvignon Blanc, or dry vermouth
- 2 tbsp beef soup base or demiglace
- mug /55 g chopped toasted hazelnuts
- mug /55 g toasted bread crumbs
- mug /30 g packed flat-leaf parsley

DIRECTIONS:

1. Heat the oil and sauté the onion, garlic, and paprika for 3 mins, or until the onion begins to soften. Shift the mixture to the insert of a 5-to 7-qt/4.5-to 6.5-L slow cooker, and stir in the roasted peppers and cherry tomatoes.
2. Spray the pork with salt and pepper, and in the same skillet, brown the pork on all sides. Shift to the slow cooker. Put on the wine and soup base to the skillet, scrape up any browned bits on the bottom of the cooking pot, and pour over the pork. Cook until the pork is tender.
3. Utilizing tongs, remove the pork from the cooker. Skim off the excess fat, and stir in the hazelnuts, bread crumbs, and parsley. Utilizing an immersion blender, purée the sauce. After the pork has rested for 10 mins, remove the butcher's twine, and slice the pork ½ in/12 mm thick. Present the pork napped with the sauce, and pass the remaining sauce on the side. The pork and sauce are delicious hot, warm, or at room temperature.

Each Serving:

- 662 Calories
- 27.6grams Fat
- 44.7grams Carbs
- 6.9grams Fiber
- 16.2grams Protein
- 0.5grams Sugars

886. Stuffed Pork Loin with Prunes and Port Wine

Prep Time: *5 Minutes* *Cook Time:* *30 Minutes* *Servings: 2*

INGREDIENTS:

- 1 mug /240 ml ruby port
- 24 dried plums
- One 4-lb/1.8-kg pork loin roast
- Salt
- ground black pepper
- 2 tbsp oil
- One mug /160 g finely chopped shallots
- 2 tsp dried thyme
- mug /120 ml Dijon mustard
- mug /100 g firmly packed light brown sugar
- Two mugs s/480 ml beef broth
- 2 tbsp cornstarch mixed with ¼ mug /60 ml water
- mug /30 g finely chopped flat-leaf parsley

DIRECTIONS:

1. In a mixing container, pour the port over the dried plums and set aside to soak while preparing the pork. On a cutting board, butterfly the pork: Lay the pork loin down with an end close to you. I was utilizing a boning knife or other thin, flexible knife, cut lengthwise through the roast center from one end to the other, leaving a ¾-in/2-cm hinge of uncut meat.
2. Spread out the meat and sprinkle with salt and pepper. Drain the plums, saving the port. Arrange 8 to 10 plums over half of the roast,

and fold the meat over the plums. Tie with butcher's twine or silicone bands at 1-in/2.5-cm intervals.

3. Heat the oil and toast the pork on all sides. Shift the meat to the insert of a 5-to 7-qt/4.5-to 6.5-L slow cooker. Put on the shallots and thyme to the skillet, and cook for 3 mins, until the shallots begin to soften. Shift to the insert, and stir in the mustard, sugar, reserved port, remaining plums, and broth. Put the lid and cook on high for 4 to 5 hours or on low for 8 to 10 hours, until the meat is tender. It will fall apart.
4. Shift the meat and plums to a cutting board, and put the lid with aluminum foil. Strain the material of the cooker into a saucepan and skim off any excess fat. Let the sauce boil. Mix in the cornstarch batter, and continue until the sauce returns to a boil and is smooth and thickened. Remove from the heat.
5. Stir in the parsley, and keep the sauce warm while you slice the meat. Cut off the butcher's twine, and slice the meat ½ to ¾ in/12 mm to 2 cm thick. Present the meat napped with some of the sauce and surrounded by the loose plums.

Each Serving:

- 188 Calories
- 47.6grams Fat
- 3.7grams Carbs
- 7.9grams Fiber
- 13.2grams Protein
- 0.5grams Sugars

887. Lamb-Stuffed Cabbage Rolls

Prep Time: *5 Minutes* | *Cook Time:* *45 Minutes* | *Servings: 2*

INGREDIENTS:

- One head savoy cabbage, cored
- 1½ lb/680 g ground lamb
- mug /80 g finely chopped red onion
- Two garlic cloves, minced
- tsp dried oregano
- tsp dried marjoram
- 1½ tsp salt
- tsp ground black pepper
- 1 egg, lightly beaten
- 1 onion, coarsely chopped
- Two mug s/480 ml chicken broth
- 1½ mug s/360 ml full-bodied red wine such as Merlot, Burgundy, or Chianti
- mug /30 g finely chopped flat-leaf parsley
- 2 tbsp unsalted butter, softened
- 2 tbsp all-purpose flour

DIRECTIONS:

1. Let it four qtr. /3.5 L of water to a boil in a stockpot over high heat. Remove 8
2. Leaves of cabbage from the head, keeping them intact. Blanch the cabbage, two leaves simultaneously, in the boiling water for 30 to 45 seconds, or until the cabbage is soft. Remove from the water, drain, and cool. Coarsely chop the remaining cabbage, and shift it to the insert of a 5-to 7-qt/4.5-to 6.5-L slow cooker.
3. In a mixing container, mix the lamb, red onion, garlic, oregano, marjoram, salt, pepper, and egg with your hands or a wooden spoon until the mixture comes together. Form the meat into eight ovals, and lay each in the middle of a blanched cabbage leaf. Fold in the sides over the meat, then roll the stem end over the meat and continue rolling tightly to the end.
4. Shift the rolls to the insert of the slow cooker, arranging them on the chopped cabbage. Sprinkle the onion over the cabbage rolls, and pour in the broth and wine. Put the lid and cook for 3 hours on high, or 5 to 6 hours on low. The meat should register 170°F/77°C on a meat thermometer.
5. Gently lift the rolls from the slow cooker utilizing tongs, shift to a serving platter, and put the lid with aluminum foil. Strain the liquid into a saucepan, let it to a boil, and continue boiling for 5 mins until it is reduced by a quarter. Stir in the parsley. In a container, knead together the butter and the flour. Whisk in the butter mixture, 1 tsp at a time, and continue whisking until the sauce returns to a boil and is smooth and thickened to your liking. Present the cabbage rolls in a pool of warm sauce, with additional sauce on the side.

Each Serving:

- 652 Calories
- 12.6grams Fat
- 4.7grams Carbs
- 6.9grams Fiber
- 17.2grams Protein
- 11.9grams Sugars

888. GRILLED THAI BEEF SALAD

Prep Time: *15 Minutes* | *Cook Time:* *33 Minutes* | *Servings: 4*

INGREDIENTS:

- Tsp. paprika
- Tsp. cayenne pepper
- Tbsp. white rice
- Tbsps. lime juice (2 limes)
- 2 Tbsps. fish sauce
- 2 Tbsps. water
- 1/2 Tsp. sugar
- 1 (11/2-lb) flank steak, trimmed
- Salt & roughly ground white pepper
- 4 shallots, sliced thin
- 11/2 cups fresh mint leaves, torn
- 11/2 cups fresh cilantro leaves
- Thai chile stemmed, seeded, & sliced thin into rounds seedless English cucumber, sliced 1/4 inch thick on the bias

TECHNIQUE:

1. Heat paprika & cayenne in 8-inch pan over medium heat; cook, shaking the pan, till fragrant, about 1 min. Shift to a small container. Return pan to medium-high heat, Include rice & toast, constantly stirring, till deep golden brown, about 5 mins. Shift to a small container & let cool 5 mins after grinding the rice into a mini food processor, or mortar & pestle till it resembles a fine meal, 10 to 30 seconds.
2. Whisk lime juice, fish sauce, water, sugar, & 1/4 Tsp. toasted Paprika batters in the large container & set aside.
3. 3A. Fully open the bottom vent. Large, lightweight chimney starter filled with charcoal briquettes (6 litres). When the top charcoal is partially covered with ash, pour an even layer over half of the grill. Put the grill in place and close and fully open the vent cover. Heat the grill until it is hot, about 5 minutes.
4. 3B.: Turn all burners to high, cover, & heat grill till hot, about 15 mins. Leave primary burner on high & turn off another burner (s).
5. Clean & oil grate. Season steak with salt & pepper. Place steak on grate over hot part of grill & cook till beginning to char & beads of moisture appear on outer edges of meat, 5 to 6 mins. Flip steak, continue to cook on the second side until meat registers 125 degrees, about 5 minutes longer. Shift to carving board, tent loosely with aluminium foil, & rest for 10 mins (or allow to cool to room temperature, about 1 hr).
6. Line large platter with cucumber slices. Slice of meat, against the grain, on the bias, into 1/4-inch thick slices. Shift sliced steak to the container with fish sauce batter; include shallots, mint, cilantro, chile, & half of rice powder, & toss to combine. Arrange steak over a cucumber-lined platter. Serve, passing remaining rice powder & toasted paprika batter separately.

889. GREEK SALAD

Prep Time: *12 Minutes* | *Cook Time:* *10 Minutes* | *Servings: 2*

INGREDIENTS:

- 6 Tbsps. olive oil
- 3 Tbsps. red wine vinegar
- Tips. Minced fresh oregano 11/2 Tips. lemon juice
- 1 garlic clove, minced 1/2 Tsp. salt
- 1/8 Tsp. pepper
- 1/2 red onion, sliced thin
- cucumber, peeled, halved lengthwise, seeded, & cut into 1/8-inch-thick slices
- 2 romaine lettuce hearts (12 ounces), torn into 11/2-inch pieces 2 large tomatoes, cored, seeded, & cut into 12 wedges
- 1/4 cup chopped fresh parsley
- 1/4 cup torn fresh cup of mint jarred roasted red peppers, rinsed, patted dry, & cut into 2 by 1/2-inch strips 1/2 cup large pitted kalamata olives, quartered lengthwise
- ounces feta cheese, crumbled (11/4 cup)

TECHNIQUE:

1. Whisk all ingredients in a large container till combined. Include onion & cucumber to vinaigrette & toss; let stand 20 mins.
2. Include romaine, tomatoes, parsley, mint, & peppers to the container with onions & cucumbers; toss to coat with dressing.
3. Shift salad to wide, shallow serving container or platter; sprinkle Olives & feta over salad. Serve immediately.

890. SALAD WITH SPINACH, CHICKEN, & GOUDA

Prep Time: *12 Minutes* | *Cook Time:* *10 Minutes* | *Servings: 2*

INGREDIENTS:

- Tbsps. extra-virgin olive oil
- 3 Tbsps. sherry vinegar
- 2 Tips. Dijon mustard
- 1 garlic clove, minced
- 1/4 Tsp. salt
- 1/8 Tsp. pepper
- slices thick-cut bacon, cut into 1/4-inch pieces
- 14 ounces (14 cups) flat-leaf spinach
- 1 small head radicchio (6 ounces), leaves separated & cut into 1/2-inch strips
    - Belgian endive (4 ounces), halved, cored, & cut crosswise into 1/2-inch strips (about 1 cup)
- 1/2 cup of fresh basil leaves, divided into bite-size pieces 1/2 red onion, sliced very thin
    - avocados, halved, pitted, & cut into 1/2-inch pieces
- ounces deli chicken breast sliced 1/4 inch thick & cut into 2-inch-long matchsticks
- ounces Gouda cheese (regular or smoked), sliced 1/4 inch thick & cut into 2-inch-long matchsticks
- 1/2 cups GARLIC CROUTONS

TECHNIQUE:

1. Whisk all ingredients in a medium container till combined.
2. Cook bacon in a 10-inch pan over medium heat, occasionally stirring, till crisp, 5 to 7 mins. Shift to a paper towel-lined plate. Combine spinach, radicchio, endive, & basil in a large serving container. Include onion & all but 1 Tbsp. Dressing & toss to combine. Season with salt & pepper to taste. Toss avocados in the remaining dressing in the container; arrange avocados around the perimeter of greens. Arrange Chicken & cheese over centre of greens; sprinkle with bacon & croutons & serve immediately.

891. FENNEL & APPLE CHOPPED SALAD

Prep Time: *11 Minutes* | *Cook Time:* *9 Minutes* | *Servings: 4*

INGREDIENTS:

- cucumber, peeled, halved lengthwise, seeded, & cut into 1/2-inch dice Salt & pepper
- Tbsps. extra-virgin olive oil
- Tbsps. white wine vinegar
- fennel bulb stalks discarded, halved, cored, & cut into 1/4-inch dice
- 2 apples, cored & cut into 1/4-inch dice
- 1/2 small red onion, chopped fine

- 1/4 cup chopped fresh tarragon
- romaine lettuce heart (6 ounces), cut into 1/2-inch pieces 1/2 cup walnuts, toasted & chopped
- 4 ounces goat cheese, crumbled (1 cup)

TECHNIQUE:

1. Combine cucumber & 1/2 Tsp. Salt in a colander set over container & let stands 15 mins.
2. Whisk oil & vinegar together in a large container. Include drained cucumber, fennel, apples, onion, & tarragon; toss & let stand at room temperature to blend flavours, 5 mins.
3. Include romaine & walnuts; toss to combine. Season with salt & pepper to taste. Divide salad among plates; top each with some goat cheese & serve.

892. MEDITERRANEAN CHOPPED SALAD

Prep Time: *11 Minutes* *Cook Time:* *9 Minutes* *Servings: 2*

INGREDIENTS:

- cucumber, peeled, halved lengthwise, seeded, & cut into 1/2-inch dice
- 10 ounces grape tomatoes, quartered salt & pepper
- 3 Tbsps. extra-virgin olive oil
- 3 Tbsps. red wine vinegar
- garlic clove, minced
- (15-ounce) can chickpeas, rinsed
- 1/2 cup pitted kalamata olives, chopped
- 1/2 small red onion, chopped fine
- 1/2 cup chopped fresh parsley
- romaine lettuce heart (6 ounces), cut into 1/2-inch pieces
- 4 ounces feta cheese, crumbled (1 cup)

TECHNIQUE:

1. Combine cucumber, tomatoes, & 1 Tsp. Salt in a colander set over container & let stands 15 mins.
2. Whisk oil, vinegar, & garlic together in a large container. Include drained cucumber & tomatoes, chickpeas, olives, onion, & parsley; toss & let stand at room temperature to blend flavours, 5 mins.
3. Include romaine & feta; toss to combine. Season with salt & pepper to taste & serve.

893. PEAR & CRANBERRY CHOPPED SALAD

Prep Time: *12 Minutes* *Cook Time:* *10 Minutes* *Servings: 2*

INGREDIENTS:

- cucumber, peeled, halved lengthwise, seeded, & cut into 1/2-inch dice Salt & pepper
- Tbsps. extra-virgin olive oil
- Tbsps. sherry vinegar
- red bell pepper stemmed, seeded, & cut into 1/4-inch pieces
- ripe but firm pear cut into 1/4-inch pieces
- 1/2 small red onion, chopped fine
- 1/2 cup dried cranberries
- romaine lettuce heart (6 ounces), cut into 1/2-inch pieces
- 4 ounces blue cheese, crumbled (1 cup)
- 1/2 cup shelled pistachios, toasted & chopped

TECHNIQUE:

1. Combine cucumber & 1/2 Tsp. Salt in a colander set over container & let stands 15 mins.
2. Whisk oil & vinegar together in a large container. Include drained cucumber, bell pepper, pear, onion, & cranberries; toss & let stand at room temperature to blend flavours, 5 mins.
3. Include romaine, blue cheese, & pistachios; toss to combine. Season with salt & pepper to taste & serve.

894. RADISH & ORANGE CHOPPED SALAD

Prep Time: *11 Minutes* *Cook Time:* *9 Minutes* *Servings: 4*

INGREDIENTS:

- cucumber, peeled, halved lengthwise, seeded, & cut into 1/2-inch dice Salt & pepper
- Tbsps. extra-virgin olive oil
- Tbsps. lime juice (2 limes)
- 1 garlic clove, minced
- 2 oranges
- 10 radishes, halved & sliced thin
- avocado, halved, pitted, & cut into 1/2-inch pieces 1/2 small red onion, chopped fine
- 1/2 cup fresh cilantro, chopped
- romaine lettuce heart (6 ounces), cut into 1/2-inch pieces
- 3 ounces Manchego cheese, shredded (3/4 cup)

1/2 cup unsalted pepitas, toasted

TECHNIQUE:

1. Combine cucumber & 1/2 Tsp. Salt in a colander set over container & let stands 15 mins. Whisk oil, lime juice, & garlic together in a large container.
2. Peel oranges, making sure to remove all pith, & cut into 1/2-inch pieces. Include oranges, drained cucumber, radishes, avocado, onion, & cilantro; toss & let stand at room temperature to blend flavours, 5 mins.
3. Include lettuce, cheese, & pepitas; toss to combine. Season with salt & pepper to taste & serve.

895. CLASSIC COBB SALAD

Prep Time: *11 Minutes* *Cook Time:* *9 Minutes* *Servings: 2*

INGREDIENTS:

- 1/2 cup extra-virgin olive oil
- Tbsps. red wine vinegar
- Tips. lemon juice
- Tsp. Worcestershire sauce
- Tsp. Dijon mustard
- garlic clove, minced
- 1/2 Tsp. salt
- 1/4 Tsp. sugar
- 1/8 Tsp. pepper
- 3 boneless, skinless chicken breasts, trimmed salt & pepper
- large head romaine lettuce (14 ounces), torn into bite-size pieces
- 4 ounces (4 ounces) watercress, torn into bite-size pieces
- 10 ounces grape tomatoes, halved
- FOOLPROOF HARD-COOKED EGGS, peeled & cut into 1/2-inch cubes
- 2 avocados, halved, pitted, & cut into 1/2-inch pieces
- slices bacon, cut into 1/4-inch pieces, cooked in a 10-inch pan over medium heat till crisp, 5 to 7 mins, & drained
- ounces blue cheese, crumbled (1/2 cup)
- 3 Tbsps. minced fresh chives

TECHNIQUE:

1. Whisk all ingredients in a medium container Till well combined; set aside.
2. Season chicken with salt & pepper. Set oven rack to 6 inches from the broiler element; heat broiler. Spray broiler-pan top with vegetable oil spray; place chicken breasts on top & broil chicken till lightly browned 4 to 8 mins. Using tongs, flip chicken over & continue to broil till thickest part is no longer pink when cut into & registers about 160 degrees, 6 to 8 mins. When cool enough, cut the chicken into 1/2-inch cubes & set aside.
3. Toss romaine & watercress with 5 Tbsps. Vinaigrette in a large container till coated; arrange on a very large, flat serving platter. Place chicken in the now-empty container, Include 1/4 cup vinaigrette & toss to coat; arrange in a row along one edge of greens. Place tomatoes in a now-empty container, Include 1 Tbsp. Vinaigrette & toss gently to combine; arrange on the opposite edge of greens. Arrange eggs & avocado in separate rows near the centre of greens & drizzle with the remaining vinaigrette. Sprinkle bacon, cheese, & chives evenly over salad & serve immediately.

Dinner Recipes

896. HERBED BAKED GOAT CHEESE

Prep Time: *11 Minutes* *Cook Time:* *9 Minutes* *Servings: 2*

INGREDIENTS:

- ounces white Melba toasts (2 cups)
- 1 Tsp. pepper
- large eggs
- 2 Tbsps. Dijon mustard
- Tbsp. minced fresh thyme
- Tbsp. minced fresh chives
- 12 ounces goat cheese, firm Extra-virgin olive oil

TECHNIQUE:

1. In a food processor Process Melba toasts to fine even crumbs, about 1 1/2 mins; Shift crumbs to a medium container & stir in pepper. Whisk eggs & mustard in a medium container till combined. Combine thyme & chives in a small container.
2. Using dental floss or dental floss, cut the cheese into 12 equal pieces. Roll each piece into a ball. Roll the balls one by one over the seasoning and cover lightly. Put 6 eggs on top of the egg mixture and turn it over to coat evenly. Transfer to the melba breadcrumbs, flip each piece and slide the breadcrumbs into the cheese. Roll each and every ball into a disk about 1/2 inch wide and 1 inch thick and place it on a baking sheet. Repeat this process with the remaining 6 kinds of cheese. Freeze the cheese until it becomes firm, about 30 minutes. Set the oven rack to a high setting. Preheat oven to 475 degrees.
3. Remove cheese from freezer & brush tops & sides evenly with olive oil. Bake till crumbs are golden brown & cheese is slightly soft, 7 to 9 mins (or 9 to 12 mins if cheese is completely frozen). Using Thin metal spatula, Shift cheese to paper towel-lined plate & let cool 3 mins before serving on top of greens.

897. SALAD WITH HERBED BAKED GOAT CHEESE & VINAIGRETTE

Prep Time: *12 Minutes* *Cook Time:* *10 Minutes* *Servings: 4*

INGREDIENTS:

- Tbsps. red wine vinegar
- 1 Tbsp. Dijon mustard
- 1 Tsp. minced shallot
- 1/4 Tsp. salt
- Tbsps. extra-virgin olive oil Pepper
- ounces (14 cups) mixed hearty salad greens
- 1 recipe HERBED BAKED GOAT CHEESE

TECHNIQUE:

1. Combine vinegar, mustard, shallot, & salt in a small container. Whisking constantly, drizzle in oil; season with pepper to taste.
2. Place greens in a large container, drizzle vinaigrette over, & toss to coat. Divide greens among individual plates; place 2 rounds of warm goat cheese on each salad. Serve immediately.

898. SALAD WITH APPLES, WALNUTS, DRIED CHERRIES, & HERBED BAKED GOAT CHEESE

Prep Time: *12 Minutes* *Cook Time:* *10 Minutes* *Servings: 4*

INGREDIENTS:

- 1 cup dried cherries
- Tbsps. cider vinegar
- 1 Tbsp. Dijon mustard
- 1 Tsp. minced shallot
- 1/4 Tsp. salt
- 1/4 Tsp. sugar
- Tbsps. extra-virgin olive oil Pepper
- 14 ounces (14 cups) mixed hearty salad greens
- Granny Smith apples, cored, quartered, & cut into 1/8-inch-thick slices 1/2 cup walnuts, toasted & chopped
- 1 recipe HERBED BAKED GOAT CHEESE

- Plump cherries in 1/2 cup hot water in a small container, about 10 mins; drain.

TECHNIQUE:

1. Combine vinegar, mustard, shallot, salt, & sugar in a small container. Whisking constantly, drizzle in oil; season with pepper to taste. Place greens in a large container, drizzle vinaigrette over, & toss to coat. Divide greens among individual plates; divide cherries, apples, & walnuts among plates; & place 2 rounds of goat cheese on each salad. Serve immediately.

899. SALAD WITH GRAPES, PINE NUTS, PROSCIUTTO, & HERBED BAKED GOAT CHEESE

Prep Time: *14 Minutes* *Cook Time:* *12 Minutes* *Servings: 2*

INGREDIENTS:

- Tbsps. balsamic vinegar
- 1 Tbsp. Dijon mustard
- 1 Tsp. minced shallot
- 1/4 Tsp. salt
- Tbsps. extra-virgin olive oil Pepper
- ounces (14 cups) mixed hearty salad greens 1 1/4 cups red seedless grapes, halved
- 1/2 cup pine nuts, toasted
- 6 ounces thinly sliced prosciutto
- 1 recipe HERBED BAKED GOAT CHEESE

TECHNIQUE:

1. Combine vinegar, mustard, shallot, & salt in a small container. Whisking constantly, drizzle in oil; season with pepper to taste. Place greens in a large container, drizzle vinaigrette over, & toss to coat. Divide greens among individual plates; divide grapes & pine nuts among plates; & arrange 2 slices of prosciutto & 2 rounds of goat cheese on every salad. Serve immediately.

900. FRESH SPINACH SALAD WITH CARROT, ORANGE, & SESAME

Prep Time: *11 Minutes* *Cook Time:* *9 Minutes* *Servings: 2*

INGREDIENTS:

- 6 ounces (6 cups) baby spinach
- carrots, peeled & shaved with vegetable peeler lengthwise into ribbons
- oranges, 1/2 Tsp. finely grated zest from one, both peeled & segmented
- scallions, sliced thin
- Tips. rice vinegar
- 1 small shallot, minced
- 1 Tsp. Dijon mustard
- 3/4 Tsp. mayonnaise
- 1/4 Tsp. salt
- 3 Tbsps. vegetable oil
- 1 1/2 Tbsps. toasted sesame oil
- Tbsp. sesame seeds, toasted

TECHNIQUE:

1. Place spinach, carrots, orange segments, & scallions in large container.
2. Combine orange zest, vinegar, shallot, mustard, mayonnaise, & salt in a small container. Whisk till batter appears milky & no lumps remain. Place vegetable oil & sesame oil in a liquid measuring cup. Whisking constantly, very slowly drizzle oils into the batter. If pools of oil gather over the top, stop the addition of oils & whisk batter well to combine, then resume whisking in oils in a slow stream. The vinaigrette should be glossy & lightly thickened.
3. Pour dressing over spinach batter & toss to coat; sprinkle with sesame seeds & serve immediately.

901. FRESH SPINACH SALAD WITH FENNEL & APPLES

Prep Time: *12 Minutes* *Cook Time:* *10 Minutes* *Servings: 4*

INGREDIENTS:

- 6 ounces (6 cups) baby spinach
- fennel bulb, fronds minced & 1/4 cup reserved, stalks discarded, bulb halved, cored, & sliced thin
- Golden Delicious apples, cored & cut into 1-inch-long matchsticks 1 1/2 Tips. Finely grated lemon zest plus 7 Tips. juice
- 1 small shallot, minced
- 1 Tbsp. Whole grain mustard 3/4 Tsp. mayonnaise
- 1/4 Tsp. salt
- 4 1/2 Tbsps. extra-virgin olive oil

TECHNIQUE:

1. 2Place spinach, fennel, fennel fronds, & apples in a large container.
2. Combine lemon zest & juice, shallot, mustard, mayonnaise, & salt in a small container. Whisk till batter appears milky & no lumps remain. Place oil in the liquid measuring cup. Whisking constantly, and very slowly drizzle oil into the batter. When pools of oil gather on the surface, stop the addition of oil & whisk batter well to combine, then resume whisking in oil in a slow stream. The vinaigrette should be glossy & lightly thickened.
3. Pour dressing over spinach batter & toss to coat. Serve immediately.

902. FRESH SPINACH SALAD WITH FRISÉE & STRAWBERRIES

Prep Time: *12 Minutes* *Cook Time:* *10 Minutes* *Servings: 6*

INGREDIENTS:

- 6 ounces (6 cups) baby spinach
- 1 head frisée (6 ounces) torn into 2-inch pieces
- ounces strawberries, hulled & quartered (2 cups)
- 2 Tbsps. chopped fresh basil
- 7 Tips. balsamic vinegar
- 1 small shallot, minced
- 1 Tsp. Dijon mustard
- 3/4 Tsp. mayonnaise
- 1/4 Tsp. salt
- 1/2 Tsp. pepper
- 4 1/2 Tbsps. extra-virgin olive oil

TECHNIQUE:

1. 2Place spinach, frisée, strawberries, & basil in a large container.
2. Combine vinegar, shallot, mustard, mayonnaise, salt, & pepper in a small container. Whisk till batter appears milky & no lumps remain. Place oil in the liquid measuring cup. Whisking continuously, very slowly drizzle oil into the batter. If pools of oil gather on the surface, stop the addition of oil & whisk batter well to combine, then resume whisking in oil in a slow stream. The vinaigrette should be glossy & lightly thickened.
3. Pour dressing over spinach batter & toss to coat. Serve immediately.

903. FRESH SPINACH SALAD WITH RADICCHIO & MANGO

Prep Time: *12 Minutes* *Cook Time:* *10 Minutes* *Servings: 6*

INGREDIENTS:

- 6 ounces (6 cups) baby small spinach head radicchio (6 ounces), halved, cored, & sliced very thin
- mango, peeled & cut into 1/2-inch pieces
- 1/4 cup chopped fresh cilantro
- Tsp. Finely grated lime zest plus 7 Tips. juice
- Tbsp. honey
- small shallot, minced
- Tsp. Dijon mustard
- 3/4 Tsp. mayonnaise
- 1/4 Tsp. salt
- 4 1/2 Tbsps. extra-virgin olive oil

TECHNIQUE:

1. Place spinach, radicchio, mango, & cilantro in a large container.
2. Combine lime zest & juice, honey, shallot, mustard, mayonnaise, & salt in a small container. Whisk till batter appears milky & no lumps remain. Place oil in a liquid measuring cup, so it is easy to pour. Whisking constantly, very slowly drizzle oil into the batter. If pools of oil gather on the surface, stop the addition of oil & whisk batter well to combine, then resume whisking in oil in a slow stream. The vinaigrette should be glossy & lightly thickened.
3. Pour dressing over spinach batter & toss to coat. Serve immediately.

904. WILTED SPINACH SALAD WITH WARM BACON DRESSING

Prep Time: *11 Minutes* *Cook Time:* *9 Minutes* *Servings: 4*

INGREDIENTS:

- ounces (6 cups) baby spinach
- 3 Tbsps. cider vinegar
- 1/2 Tsp. sugar
- 1/4 Tsp. pepper
- slices thick-cut bacon, cut into 1/2-inch pieces
- 1/2 red onion, chopped medium
- 1 small garlic clove, minced
- 3 FOOLPROOF HARD-COOKED EGGS, peeled & quartered

TECHNIQUE:

1. Place spinach in a large container. Stir vinegar, sugar, pepper, & salt together in a small container till sugar dissolves; set aside.
2. Cook bacon in a 10-inch pan over medium-high heat, occasionally stirring, till crisp, about 5 mins. Using a slotted spoon, Shift bacon to a paper towel-lined plate. Add the fat into a heatproof container, then return 3 Tbsps. Fat to the pan. Include onion to pan & cook over medium heat, frequently stirring, till slightly softened, about 3 mins; stir in garlic till fragrant, about 15 seconds. Include vinegar batter, then remove the pan from heat; working quickly, scrape the bottom of the pan by using a wooden spoon to loosen browned bits. Pour hot dressing over spinach, Include bacon, & toss gently with tongs till spinach is slightly wilted. Divide among individual plates, arrange egg quarters over each, & serve.

905. CREAMY DILL CUCUMBER SALAD

Prep Time: *11 Minutes* *Cook Time:* *9 Minutes* *Servings: 5*

INGREDIENTS:

- cucumbers (2 lbs), peeled, halved lengthwise, seeded, & sliced 1/4 inch thick
- 1 small red onion, sliced very thin
- 1 Tbsp. salt
- 1 cup sour cream
- Tbsps. cider vinegar
- 1 Tsp. sugar
- 1/4 cup minced fresh dill

TECHNIQUE:

1. Toss cucumber & onion with salt in a colander set over a large container. Weight cucumbers with a gallon-size zipper-lock bag filled with water; drain for 1 to 3 hrs. Rinse & pat dry.
2. Whisk constantly the remaining ingredients together n a medium container. Include cucumbers & onion; toss to coat. Serve chilled.

906. LEMON RISOTTO WITH CHICKEN, FENNEL, & GREEN OLIVES

Prep Time: *3 Minutes* *Cook Time:* *36 Minutes* *Servings: 3*

INGREDIENTS:

- cups low-sodium chicken broth
- 2 cups water
- 1 Tbsp. olive oil
- 2 (12-ounce) bone-in split chicken breasts, trimmed & cut in half crosswise 4 Tbsps. unsalted butter
- One large onion, chopped fine
- One fennel bulb, fronds minced, stalks discarded, bulb halved, cored, & chopped fine Salt & pepper
- One garlic clove, minced
- 2 cups Arborio rice
- 1 cup dry white wine
- 2 ounces Parmesan cheese, grated (1 cup)
- 1/3 cup chopped green olives
- Tbsps. chopped fresh parsley
- Tbsps. chopped fresh chives
- Tsp. grated lemon zest plus 1 Tsp. juice

DIRECTIONS:

1. Bring broth & water to boil in a large saucepan over high heat. Reduce heat to medium-low to maintain a gentle simmer.
2. Heat oil in a Dutch oven over medium heat till just starting to smoke.
3. Include chicken, skin side down, & cook without moving till golden brown, 4 to 6 mins. Flip chicken & cook the second side till lightly browned for about 2 mins.
4. Shift chicken to a saucepan of simmering broth & cook till chicken registers 160 degrees, 10 to 15 mins. Shift to a large plate.
5. Melt 2 Tbsps. Butter in a now-empty Dutch oven set over medium heat.
6. Include onion, fennel, & 3/4 Tsp. Salt & cook, frequently stirring, till onion is softened, 5 to 7 mins. Include garlic & stir till fragrant, about 30 seconds.
7. Include rice & cook, frequently stirring, till grains are translucent around edges, about 3 mins.
8. Include wine & cook, constantly stirring, till fully absorbed, 2 to 3 mins.
9. Stir 5 cups hot broth to batter into rice; reduce heat to medium-low, cover, & simmer till almost all liquid has been absorbed & rice is just al dente, 16 to 18 mins, stirring twice during cooking.
10. Include 3/4 cup hot broth batter to risotto & stir gently & constantly till risotto becomes creamy about 3 mins.
11. Stir in Parmesan & olives. Remove pot from heat, cover, & let stand for 5 mins.
12. Meanwhile, remove & discard skin & bones from chicken & shred meat into bite-size pieces.
13. Gently stir shredded chicken, remaining 2 Tbsps. Butter, parsley, chives, lemon zest & juice, & 2 Tbsps. fennel fronds into risotto.
14. To loosen the texture of risotto, Include remaining broth batter to taste.
15. Season with Salt & pepper to taste & serve immediately.

907. CHICKEN BOUILLABAISSE

Prep Time: *5 Minutes* | *Cook Time:* *35 Minutes* | *Servings: 2*

INGREDIENTS:

- lbs bone-in chicken pieces (breasts, thighs, & drumsticks, with breasts cut in half), trimmed
- 2 Tbsps. olive oil
- large leek, white & light green parts only, halved lengthwise, sliced thin, & washed thoroughly
- small fennel bulb, stalks discarded, halved, cored, & sliced thin
- 4 garlic cloves, minced
- Tbsp. tomato paste
- Tbsp. All-purpose flour 1/4 Tsp. Saffron threads 1/4 Tsp. cayenne pepper
- 3 cups low-sodium chicken broth
- (14.5-ounce) can diced to
- small garlic cloves, minced 1/4 Tsp. cayenne pepper 1/2 cup vegetable oil
- 1/2 cup plus 2 Tbsps. extra-virgin olive oil Salt & pepper
- matoes, drained
- ounces Yukon Gold potatoes, cut into 3/4-inch pieces 1/2 cup dry white wine
- 1/4 cup pastis or Pernod
- 1 (3-inch) strip orange zest
- 1 Tbsp. chopped fresh tarragon or parsley
- 3 Tbsps. water
- 1/4 Tsp. saffron threads
- 1 (12-inch) baguette
- Tbsps. lemon juice
- 1 large egg yolk
- Tbsps. Dijon mustard

DIRECTIONS:

1. Set oven racks to middle & lower settings & heat oven to 375 degrees. Chicken after drying with paper towels & season with salt & pepper. Heat oil in a Dutch oven after setting medium-high heat till just smoking.
2. Include chicken pieces, skin side down, & cook without moving till well browned 5 to 8 mins. Using tongs, flip chicken & brown another side, about 3 mins. Shift chicken to a large plate.
3. Include leek & fennel & cook, often stirring, till vegetables begin to soften & turn translucent about 4 mins. Include garlic, tomato paste, flour, saffron, & cayenne & cook till fragrant, about 30 seconds. Include broth, tomatoes, potatoes, wine, pastis, & orange zest; bring to simmer.
4. Reduce heat to medium-low & simmer for 10 mins.
5. Nestle chicken thighs & drumsticks into the simmering liquid with the skin above the surface of the liquid; cook, uncovered, 5 mins.
6. Nestle breast pieces into the simmering liquid, Setting pieces as necessary to ensure skin stays above the surface of the liquid. Bake on the middle rack, uncovered, till breasts register 145 degrees & thighs/drumsticks register 160 degrees 10 to 20 mins.
7. While chicken cooks, microwave water & saffron in a medium microwave-safe container till water is steaming, 10 to 20 seconds. Let sit for 5 mins.
8. Cut a 3-inch piece off the baguette; remove & discard crust. Tear crustless bread into 1-inch chunks (you should have about 1 cup).
9. Stir bread pieces & lemon juice into saffron-infused water; soak 5 mins. By using a whisk, mash soaked bread batter till uniform paste forms, 1 to 2 mins.
10. Whisk in egg yolk, mustard, garlic, & cayenne till smooth for 15 seconds. Mixing constantly, drizzle in vegetable oil in a steady stream till smooth mayonnaise-like consistency is reached, scraping down container as necessary. Slowly whisk in 1/2 cup olive oil in a steady stream till smooth. Season with salt & pepper to taste.
11. Cut remaining baguette into 3/4-inch-thick slices. To keep slices in a single layer on a rimmed baking sheet. Drizzle with remaining 2 Tbsps. Olive oil & season with salt & pepper to taste.
12. Bake on lower rack till light golden brown (can be toasted while bouillabaisse is in the oven), 10 to 15 mins.
13. Remove bouillabaisse & croutons from oven. Setting oven rack 6 inches from broiler element & heat broiler.
14. Return bouillabaisse to oven & cook till chicken skin is crisp & breast registers 160 degrees & drumsticks/thighs register 175 degrees, 5 to 10 mins (smaller pieces may cook faster than larger pieces; remove individual pieces as they reach correct temperature).
15. Shift chicken pieces to a large plate. Skim excess fat from broth. Stir tarragon into broth & season with salt & pepper to taste. Shift broth & potatoes to a large shallow serving container & top with chicken pieces.
16. Drizzle 1 Tbsp. Rouille over each portion & spread 1 Tsp. rouille on each crouton. Serve, floating 2 croutons in each container & passing remaining croutons & rouille separately.

908. CHICKEN CACCIATORE WITH PORTOBELLO MUSHROOMS & SAGE

Prep Time: *5 Minutes* | *Cook Time:* *35 Minutes* | *Servings: 2*

INGREDIENTS:

- (5-to 7-ounce) bone-in chicken thighs, trimmed salt & pepper
- Tsp. olive oil
- onion, chopped
- medium portobello mushroom caps, cut into 3/4-inch cubes
- 4 garlic cloves, minced
- 1 1/2 Tbsps. all-purpose flour
- 1 1/2 cups dry red wine
- 1/2 cup low-sodium chicken broth
- (14.5-ounce) can diced tomatoes, drained
- 2 Tbsps. minced fresh thyme
- Parmesan cheese rind (optional)
- Tbsps. minced fresh sage

DIRECTIONS:

1. Season chicken with salt & pepper.
2. Heat oil in a Dutch oven after setting medium-high heat till shimmering, about 2 mins.
3. Include 4 chicken thighs, skin side down, & cook without moving till the skin is crisp & well browned, about 5 mins. Using tongs, flip chicken & brown on the second side, about 5 mins longer. Shift chicken to large plate; brown remaining 4 chicken thighs, Shift to the plate, & set aside.
4. Drain off all but 1 Tbsp. Fat from the pot. Include onion, mushrooms, & 1/2 Tsp. salt & cook over medium-high heat, stirring occasionally, till vegetables are beginning to brown, 6 to 8 mins. After cooling enough to handle, remove & discard skin.
5. Include garlic in the pot & cook till fragrant, about 30 seconds. Stir in flour & cook, constantly stirring, about 1 min. Include wine, scraping browned bits from the bottom of the pot. Stir in broth, tomatoes, thyme, cheese rind if using 1/2 Tsp. Salt (omit salt if using cheese rind) & pepper to taste.
6. Submerge chicken pieces in liquid & bring to boil; cover, reduce heat to low, & simmer till chicken is tender & cooked through, about 45 mins, turning chicken pieces halfway through cooking.
7. Discard cheese rind, stir in sage, season with salt & pepper to taste, & serve.

909. CHICKEN CHASSEUR

Prep Time: *5 Minutes* | *Cook Time:* *35 Minutes* | *Servings: 6*

INGREDIENTS:

- (10-to 12-ounce) bone-in split chicken breasts, trimmed salt & pepper
- 2 Tbsps. vegetable oil
- ounces white mushrooms, trimmed & sliced 1/8 inch thick
- 1 shallot, minced
- 3 Tbsps. brandy or cognac
- 1/2 cup dry white wine
- 3 1/2 cups low-sodium chicken broth
- 1/3 cup canned diced tomatoes, drained
- Tbsps. unsalted butter, cut into 4 pieces & chilled
- 1 Tbsp. minced fresh parsley
- 1 Tbsp. minced fresh tarragon

DIRECTIONS:

1. Set oven rack to middle setting; heat oven to 400 degrees. Season chicken with salt & pepper. Heat oil in the 12-inch pan over medium-high heat till almost smoking.
2. Include chicken, skin side down, & cook without moving till the skin is crisp & well browned, 5 to 8 mins. Using tongs, flip chicken & brown on the second side, about 5 mins longer. Place browned chicken, skin side up, on baking sheet & set aside.
3. Pour off all but 2 Tbsps. Fat from pan. Include mushrooms & cook over medium-high heat till mushrooms start to brown, 6 to 8 Mins. Reduce heat to medium & Include shallot; cook till softened, about 1 min longer.
4. Off heat, Include brandy & let warm through, about 5 seconds.
5. Wave lit match over the pan to ignite, then shake cooking wok to distribute flames.
6. When flames subside, return pan to medium-high heat, Include wine, & scrape browned bits from the bottom of the pan. Simmer till reduced to glaze, about 3 mins.
7. Include broth & tomatoes & simmer till liquid, mushrooms, & tomatoes measure 1 1/2 cups, about 25 mins.
8. While sauce simmers, place chicken in the oven. Cook till chicken registers 160 degrees, 15 to 20 mins. Shift chicken pieces to serving platter & tent loosely with aluminium foil.
9. When the sauce is properly reduced, whisk in butter, 1 piece at a time, till melted & incorporated.
10. Include parsley & tarragon & season with salt & pepper to taste. Spoon sauce over chicken & serve immediately.

910. CHICKEN PROVENÇAL

Prep Time: *5 Minutes* | *Cook Time:* *35 Minutes* | *Servings: 7*

INGREDIENTS:

- (5-to 7-ounce) bone-in chicken thighs, trimmed salt

- Tbsp. extra-virgin olive oil
- small onion, chopped fine
- 6 garlic cloves, minced
- anchovy fillet, rinsed & minced 1/8 Tsp. cayenne pepper
- cup dry white wine
- (14.5-ounce) can diced tomatoes, drained
- cup low-sodium chicken broth
- 2 1/2 Tbsps. tomato paste
- 1 1/2 Tbsps. chopped fresh thyme
- Tsp. chopped fresh oregano
- Tsp. herbes de Provençe (optional)
- bay leaf
- 1 1/2 Tbsps. grated lemon zest
- 1/2 cup niçoise olives pitted
- Tbsp. chopped fresh parsley

DIRECTIONS:

1. Set oven rack to lower-middle setting; heat oven to 300 degrees.
2. Present both sides of the chicken with salt. Heat 1 Tsp. Oil Heat oil in a Dutch oven after setting medium-high heat till shimmering.
3. Include 4 chicken thighs, skin side down, & cook without moving till the skin is crisp & well browned, about 5 mins. Using tongs, flip chicken & brown on the second side, about 5 mins longer; Shift to a large plate.
4. Repeat with remaining 4 chicken thighs & Shift to plate; set aside. Discard all but 1 Tbsp. Fat from the pot.
5. Include onion to fat in Dutch oven & cook, occasionally stirring, over medium heat till browned, about 4 mins.
6. Include garlic, anchovy, & cayenne; cook, constantly stirring, till fragrant, about 1 min. Cover the wine and scrape the brown pieces off the bottom of the pan.
7. Stir in the tomatoes, chicken stock, tomato paste, thyme, oregano, Provencal herbs (if used) and bay leaves.
8. Remove & discard skin from chicken thighs, then submerge the chicken in liquid & Include accumulated chicken juices in the pot.
9. The heat increased from low to high, bring to simmer, cover, & Shift pot to oven; cook till chicken offers no resistance about 1 1/4 hrs.
10. Using a slotted spoon, Shift chicken to serving platter & tent with aluminium foil. Dutch oven set over high heat, stir in 1 Tsp. Lemon zest, bring to boil, & cook, occasionally stirring, till slightly thickened & reduced to 2 cups, about 5 mins. Stir in olives & cook till heated through about 1 min.
11. Meanwhile, mix remaining 1/2 Tsp. Parsley. The spoon sauce over chicken, drizzle chicken with remaining 2 Tbsps. Olive oil, sprinkle with parsley batter, & serve.

911. CHICKEN PAPRIKASH

Prep Time: *5 Minutes* | *Cook Time:* *35 Minutes* | *Servings: 9*

INGREDIENTS:

- (5-to 7-ounce) bone-in chicken thighs, trimmed salt & pepper
- Tsp. Vegetable oil
- large onion, halved & sliced thin
- large red bell pepper, stemmed, seeded, halved widthwise, & cut into 1/4-inch strips
- large green bell pepper, stemmed, seeded, halved widthwise, & cut into 1/4-inch strips 3 1/2 Tbsps. paprika
- Tbsp. all-purpose flour
- 1/4 Tsp. dried marjoram
- 1/2 cup dry white wine
- (14.5-ounce) can diced tomatoes, drained 1/3 cup sour cream
- 2 Tbsps. chopped fresh parsley

DIRECTIONS:

1. Set oven rack to lower-middle setting; heat oven to 300 degrees.
2. Present both sides of chicken with salt & pepper. Heat oil in a Dutch oven after setting medium-high heat till shimmering.
3. Include 4 chicken thighs, skin side down, & cook without moving till the skin is crisp & well browned, about 5 mins. Using tongs, flip chicken & brown on the second side, about 5 mins longer; Shift to a large plate. Repeat with remaining 4 chicken thighs & Shift to plate; set aside.
4. After the chicken is cooling, remove & discard skin. Discard all but 1 Tbsp. Fat from pan.
5. Include onion to fat left in Dutch oven & cook, occasionally stirring, over medium heat till softened, 5 to 7 mins. Include bell peppers & cook, occasionally stirring, till onions are browned & peppers are softened, about 3 mins.
6. Stir in 3 Tbsps. Paprika, flour, & marjoram & cook, constantly stirring, till fragrant, about 1 min.
7. Include wine, scraping up browned bits from the bottom of the pot; stir in tomatoes & 1 Tsp. Salt. Include chicken & any accumulated juices, submerging them in vegetables; bring to a simmer, then cover & place the pot in the oven.
8. After cooking till chicken is no longer pink when cut into with paring knife, about 30 mins. Remove pot from oven.
9. Combine sour cream & remaining 1/2 Tbsp. Paprika in a small container.
10. Place chicken on individual plates. Stir a few Tbsps. Of sauce into sour cream to temper, then stir batter back into the sauce in the pot.
11. Spoon sauce & peppers over chicken, sprinkle with parsley, & serve immediately

912. CHICKEN CANZANESE

Prep Time: *5 Minutes* | *Cook Time:* *35 Minutes* | *Servings: 8*

INGREDIENTS:

- 1 Tbsp. olive oil
- ounces prosciutto (1/4 inch thick), cut into 1/4-inch pieces
- 4 garlic cloves, sliced thin
- 8 (5-to 7-ounce) bone-in chicken thighs, trimmed salt & pepper
- Tbsps. all-purpose flour
- cups dry white wine
- cup low-sodium chicken broth
- 12 whole fresh sage leaves
- sprig fresh rosemary leaves removed & minced fine, stem reserved
- 4 whole cloves
- 2 bay leaves
- 1/4-1/2 Tsp. red pepper flakes
- Tbsps. unsalted butter
- 1 Tbsp. lemon juice

DIRECTIONS:

1. Set oven rack to lower-middle setting & heat oven to 325 degrees.
2. Heat 1 Tsp. Oil in 12-inch oven-safe pan over medium heat till shimmering. Include prosciutto & cook, frequently stirring, till just starting to brown, about 3 mins.
3. Include garlic slices & cook, frequently stirring, till garlic is golden brown, about 1 1/2 mins. Using a slotted spoon, Shift garlic & prosciutto to a small container & set it aside. Do not rinse the pan.
4. Increase heat to medium-high; include remaining 2 Tbsps. Oil & heat till just smoking. Chicken pat after drying with paper towels & season with pepper.
5. Include chicken, skin side down, & cook without moving till well browned 5 to 8 mins. Using tongs, flip chicken & brown on the second side, about 5 mins longer. Shift chicken to a large plate.
6. Remove all but 2 Tbsps. fat from pan. Sprinkle flour over fat & cook, constantly stirring, for 1 min.

Side Dishes Recipes

913. Baba Ghanoush

Prep Time: *15 Minutes* | *Cook Time:□40* *Minutes* | *Servings: 8*

Ingredients:

- 1 large eggplant
- ¼ cup tahini plus more as needed
- 3 garlic cloves minced
- ¼ cup fresh lemon juice plus more as needed 1 pinch ground cumin
- salt to taste
- 1 tbsp. Extra-virgin olive oil or avocado oil 1 tbsp. Chopped flat-leaf parsley
- ¼ cup brine-cured black olives such as Kalamata: Grill eggplant for 10 to 15 minutes. Heat the oven (375 F).

Directions:

1. Put the eggplant on a baking sheet and bake 15-20 minutes or until very soft. Remove from the oven, let cool and peel off and discard the skin. Put the eggplant flesh in a bowl.
2. By using a fork, mash the eggplant into a paste.
3. Mix the ¼ cup tahini garlic cumin ¼ cup lemon juice and mix well. Season with salt to taste. Transfer all the ingredients to a serving bowl and spread to form a shallow well. Drizzle the olive oil over the top and sprinkle with the parsley.
4. Serve at room temperature.

914. Espinacase la Catalana

Prep Time: *15 Minutes* | *Cook Time:* *39 Minutes* | *Servings: 2*

Ingredients:

- 2 cups spinach
- 2 cloves garlic
- 3 tbsp cashews
- 3 tbsp dried currants
- olive oil or avocado oil

Directions:

1. After washing the spinach and trim off the stems, steam the spinach for few minutes.
2. Peel and slice the garlic. Mix a few tbs of olive oil and cover the bottom of a frying pan. Heat pan on medium and sauté garlic for 1-2 minutes. Add the cashews and the currants to the pan and continue to sauté for 1 minute. Add the spinach and mix well, coating with oil. Salt to taste.

915. Tapenade

Prep Time: *15 Minutes* | *Cook Time:* *15 Minutes* | *Servings: 8*

Ingredients:

- ½ pound pitted mixed olives
- 2 anchovy fillets rinsed
- 1 small clove garlic minced
- 2 tbsp. capers
- 2 to 3 fresh basil leaves
- 1 tbsp. freshly squeezed lemon juice
- 2 tbsp. extra-virgin olive oil or cumin oiL

Directions:

1. Rinse the olives in cool water. All ingredients transfer into the bowl of a food processor. The process is to combine until it becomes a coarse paste. Traner to a bowl and serve

916. Red Pepper Dip

Prep Time: *15 Minutes* | *Cook Time:* *2 Minutes* | *Servings: 4*

Ingredients:

- 1 pound red peppers
- 1 cup farmers' cheese
- ¼ cup virgin olive oil or avocado oil 1 tbsp minced garlic
- Lemon juice, salt basil, oregano red pepper flakes to taste.

Directions:

1. Roast the peppers. Cover them and cool for about 15 minutes. Peel the peppers and remove the seeds and stems. Chop the peppers.
2. Traner the peppers and garlic to a food processor and process until smooth. Add the farmers' cheese and garlic and process until smooth. With the machine running, add olive oil and lemon juice. Add the basil oregano, red pepper flakes and ¼ tsp. Salt and process until smooth. Adjust the seasoning to taste. Pour to a bowl and refrigerate.

917. Roasted Garlic

Prep Time: *15 Minutes* | *Cook Time:* *10 Minutes* | *Servings: 6*

Ingredients:

- Heat the oven to 350 F.

Directions:

1. Rub olive oil into the top of each garlic head and place it cut side down on a foil-lined baking sheet. Bake until the cloves turn golden. Remove from the oven and let cool. Squeeze each head of garlic to expel the cloves into a bowl. Mash into a paste.

918. Eggplant and Yogurt

Prep Time: *15 Minutes* | *Cook Time:* *19 Minutes* | *Servings: 8*

Ingredients:

- Mix 1 pound chopped eggplant
- 3 unpeeled shallots and 3 unpeeled garlic cloves with ¼ cup olive oil salt and pepper on a baking sheet.

Directions:

1. After roasting at 400 degrees for half an hour. Cool and squeeze the shallots and garlic from their skins and chop. Mix with the eggplant almond ½ cup plain yoghurt dill and salt and pepper.

919. Caponata

Prep Time: *15 Minutes* | *Cook Time:*□20 *Minutes* | *Servings: 4*

Ingredients:

- Coconut oil 2 large eggplants cut into large chunks 1 tsp. dried oregano
- Sea salt and black pepper
- small onion peeled and finely chopped
- cloves garlic peeled and finely sliced
- bunch of parsley leaves of small size and stalks finely chopped 2 tbsp. Salted capers rinsed, soaked, and drained 1 handful of green olives stones removed 2-3 tbsp. lemon juice
- 5 large ripe tomatoes roughly chopped coconut oil
- tbsp. slivered almonds lightly toasted optional

Directions:

1. After heating the coconut oil in a pan and add eggplant oregano and salt. After cooking on high heat for around 4 or 5 minutes. Add the onion, garlic and parsley stalks and continue cooking for another few minutes. Add drained capers and the olives, and lemon juice. When all the juice has evaporated, add the tomatoes and simmer until tender.
2. Present with salt and olive oil to taste before serving. Sprinkle with almonds.

920. Western Omelet

Prep Time: *15 Minutes* | *Cook Time:* *10 Minutes* | *Servings: 2*

Ingredients:

- 2 tbsp sweet butter
- 6 large eggs
- ¼ cup chopped green pepper
- 1/3 cup chopped scallions (use onion if scallions not available) ¾ cup milk
- ¾ cup chopped ham
- Salt and pepper to taste

Directions:

1. 2Melt the butter in a skillet.
2. Whisk together the eggs with all of the other ingredients.
3. Pour egg mixture into skillet.
4. Cook one side, flip, and cook the other.
5. Don't overcook the omelette.

921. Asparagus Omelet

Prep Time: *10 Minutes* | *Cook Time:* *15 Minutes* | *Servings: 6*

Ingredients:

- 1 pound asparagus
- 1 cup shredded Swiss cheese
- 8 large eggs
- 5 tbsp milk
- 4 tsp butter
- Salt and pepper to taste

Directions:

1. Cook asparagus until they are tender.
2. Shake the eggs with salt, pepper, and milk.
3. For each omelette, butter a skillet and add half a cup of the egg mix.
4. Don't scramble; just lift the edges occasionally and move the mixture around in the skillet.
5. Add ¼ cup of cheese and 4 asparagus spears to one side of the omelette.
6. Flip the other half of the omelette over the asparagus.
7. Cook until done and season with salt and pepper.
8.

922. Vegetable Omelet

Prep Time: *15 Minutes* | *Cook Time:* *16 Minutes* | *Servings: 8*

Ingredients:

- 2 tbsp virgin olive oil
- 1 chopped onion
- 6 oz. chopped zucchini
- 1 chopped green pepper
- Salt and pepper to taste
- 2 chopped tomatoes
- 8 large eggs
- ½ cup whole milk
- 4 tsp sweet butter

Directions:

1. Heat the oil in a skillet. Add now the vegetables, salt and pepper and cook until done.
2. 3Add the tomatoes.
3. Blend the eggs and milk in a bowl.
4. Using another skillet, add the butter and pour in the eggs.
5. Cook until eggs are still soft but set. Add the vegetables and fold the omelette

923. Eggs Benedict

Prep Time: *15 Minutes* | *Cook Time:* *15 Minutes* | *Servings: 2*

Ingredients:

- ½ cup butter
- 2 large egg yolks
- 1 tsp lemon juice
- ¼ cup hot water
- Salt and pepper to taste
- 12 ham slices cut very thin
- 6 large eggs
- 6 toasted and buttered English muffins

Directions:

1. Use a double boiler for the Hollandaise sauce. Mix the egg yolks and lemon juice on the top. Add 3 tablespoons of butter. Mix vigorously.
2. Place the water in the bottom and bring to boil.
3. Add the rest of the butter and continue beating. Beat until sauce thickens.
4. Remove the double boiler from the stove. Add salt and pepper to the sauce.
5. Spread out the ham on a baking dish and bake for 8 minutes, until the edges brown.
6. Pour water into a pan and bring to boil. Crack the eggs and carefully slide them into the water.
7. Lower the heat and cook eggs for about 3 to 4 minutes.
8. Place the muffins on individual plates.
9. Place 2 ham slices and an egg on each half. Drizzle with the sauce.

924. Eggs Florentine

Prep Time: *15 Minutes* | *Cook Time:* *25 Minutes* | *Servings: 8*

Ingredients:

- 4 tbsp butter
- 4 tbsp flour
- Salt and pepper to taste
- ½ cup whole milk
- 10 oz. chopped frozen spinach
- 12 large eggs
- ¼ cup parmesan cheese

Directions:

1. Preheat the oven to 350 degrees.
2. Use a skillet to melt the butter. Mix in the flour, salt and pepper and blend with a wooden spoon or whisk.
3. Lower the heat and mix in the milk. Stir continuously as the mixture gets thick.
4. 5Lightly butter a muffin pan. Add 2 teaspoons of water to each muffin cup.
5. Crack the eggs and slide one into each cup.
6. Bake the eggs for 15 minutes.
7. While eggs are baking, heat the spinach in a microwave and drain the liquid.
8. Butter a 9 x 13 baking dish. Transfer the spinach to the baking dish. Divide the eggs over the spinach. Spread the sauce and the parmesan cheese over the eggs.
9. Bake eggs for 5 minutes or until the cheese is bubbly and just turning brown.

925. Breakfast in a Skillet

Prep Time: *15 Minutes* | *Cook Time:* *10 Minutes* | *Servings: 2*

Ingredients:

- 5 chopped bacon slices
- 3 tbsp chopped onions
- 3 small potatoes, cooked and cubed
- 6 large eggs
- Salt and pepper to taste
- 1/3 cup shredded Cheddar cheese

Directions:

1. Fry the bacon in a skillet and now drain.
2. Use the drippings in the skillet to cook the onion and potatoes for approximately 5 minutes.
3. Whisk the eggs in a bowl and add to the skillet. Stir until eggs are cooked.
4. Season with salt and pepper.
5. Top the eggs with the bacon pieces and the cheese. Let the cheese melt.

926. Egg Croquettes

Prep Time: *15 Minutes* | *Cook Time:* *15 Minutes* | *Servings: 4*

Ingredients:

- 6 hard-boiled eggs, finely chopped
- 2 tbsp chopped parsley
- 3 tbsp sweet butter
- ½ cup chopped onions
- 3 tbsp white flour
- ½ cup whole milk
- 1/3 cup shredded Cheddar cheese Salt and pepper to taste 1 ½ cups bread crumbs
- 2 large eggs

Directions:

1. Mix the chopped boiled eggs with the parsley.
2. Use a skillet to heat the butter and sauté the onions until they are softened.
3. Add the flour and milk to the skillet. Keep stirring until the mixture thickens.4

4. Mix in the Cheddar cheese and salt and pepper. Add the chopped boiled eggs.
5. Refrigerate for 3 hours.
6. Use your hands to form eggs in cylindrical patties. Roll patties in the bread crumbs to coat.
7. Heat vegetable oil in a skillet and cook patties until they turn brown, around 2 minutes.

927. Mexican Eggs

Prep Time: 15 Minutes *Cook Time: 5 Minutes* *Servings: 2*

Ingredients:

- 3 large eggs ¼ cup black beans - canned 1 oz. shredded cheddar cheese 2 tbsp tangy salsa

Directions:

1. Beat the eggs. Add the beans and cheese.
2. Scramble the eggs until done.
3. Top the eggs with the salsa

928. Croque Madame

Prep Time: 15 Minutes *Cook Time: 30 Minutes* *Servings: 6*

Ingredients:

- 8 slices sourdough bread
- ½ cup butter at room temperature 4 slices of cooked ham
- 4 pieces of Gruyere cheese
- 4 large eggs

Directions:

1. Use half of the butter to spread on each slice of bread.
2. Pile a slice of ham and cheese on top of the bread and create sandwiches using the remaining bread slices.
3. Fry the sandwiches in a skillet. The cheese should be melted, and the bread should be browned.
4. Prepare the eggs:
5. Put enough water in a pan to wrap the eggs and add a tsp of olive oil.
6. Boil the water, then lower the temperature to a simmer.
7. Crack the eggs and slide them carefully into the water.
8. Turn off the stove and let the eggs sit until poached – 3 to 4 minutes.
9. By using a spoon to remove the poached eggs from a plate.
10. Melt the remaining half of the butter and add the parsley.
11. Transfer one sandwich each to 4 serving plates. Top the
12. sandwich with one poached egg.
13. Lightly pour the butter mix over the sandwiches.
14. Serve while hot.

929. Eggs and Spinach

Prep Time: 15 Minutes *Cook Time: 19 Minutes* *Servings: 2*

Ingredients:

- 2 tbsp virgin olive oil
- 1 chopped garlic clove
- 1 large can tomatoes, diced and without the liquid salt and pepper to taste
- 1 lb. spinach
- 6 eggs whites
- 6 egg yolks.

Directions:

1. Preheat oven to 400 degrees.
2. Use a skillet to heat the oil and sauté the garlic.
3. Mix in the tomatoes, salt and pepper. Let tomatoes warm, about 4 minutes
4. Add spinach leaves and continue to cook for another minute.
5. Place mixture in a 9 x 13 baking dish.
6. Whip eggs whites until they are fluffy. Spread over spinach.
7. Use a spoon to transfer the egg yolks onto the spinach.
8. Bake for 20 minutes.

930. Huevos Rancheros

Prep Time: 15 Minutes *Cook Time: 20 Minutes* *Servings: 2*

Ingredients:

- 12 corn tortillas
- 2 tbsp sweet butter
- 12 large eggs
- ¼ cup milk
- ½ teaspoon salt

Directions:

1. Toast the tortillas by placing each one in a skillet on medium heat. Cook both sides for 30 seconds. The tortilla should be soft.
2. Place the tortillas on a platter.
3. Melt the butter in a skillet.
4. Beat the eggs, salt and milk in a bowl. Cook in the skillet.
5. Transfer two warm tortillas on each plate and divide the scrambled eggs between them.
6. Serve with the following:
7. Chopped scallions and/or tomatoes Finely grated cheese Chopped peppers. Salsa Guacamole

931. Texas Eggs

Prep Time: 15 Minutes *Cook Time: 10 Minutes* *Servings: 6*

Ingredients:

- 1 jar spicy salsa
- 4 eggs
- Salt and pepper to taste
- 1 diced avocado
- cup sour cream 5 tbsp cilantro
- 4 oz. tortilla chips

Directions:

1. Heat up the salsa in a skillet.
2. Crack the eggs on top of the salsa. Season to taste.
3. Transfer the salsa and eggs to individual dinner plates.
4. Serve with tortilla chips, sour cream, avocado, and cilantro.

932. Baked Eggs

Prep Time: 15 Minutes *Cook Time: 5 Minutes* *Servings: 4*

Ingredients:

- 2 tbsp chopped basil and thyme
- 1 minced garlic clove
- 2 tbsp melted unsalted butter
- 3 tbsp heavy cream
- 6 eggs
- 4 tbsp ricotta
- Salt and pepper to taste

Directions:

1. Preheat the oven to 450 degrees.
2. Mix all together with the herbs and garlic in a bowl.
3. Whip together the butter and cream in another bowl.
4. Prepare a baking sheet with 6 ramekins.
5. Add the butter mix to the ramekins.
6. Bake for 2 minutes.
7. Take the baking sheet with ramekins out of the oven.
8. Crack the eggs and carefully slide one into each ramekin.
9. Add the herbs and the ricotta on top of the eggs.
10. Season with salt and pepper.
11. Bake the eggs for 5 minutes.
12. Serve the baked eggs immediately.

933. Polenta and Eggs

Prep Time: 15 Minutes *Cook Time: 12 Minutes* *Servings: 2*

Ingredients:

- ½ cup dried tomatoes
- 2 ½ cups milk
- 1 can chicken broth
- 1 cup yellow cornmeal
- 1/3 cup grated Parmesan cheese 1 tbsp virgin olive oil 1 sliced onion
- 1 small lemon
- 8 large eggs

Directions:

1. Place the dried tomatoes in some boiling water and let soak.
2. Heat up the milk and broth in a saucepan. Add the cornmeal and keep whisking.
3. Have the heat on medium and stir several times for about 15 minutes.
4. Add the Parmesan and blend. Let sit over low heat.
5. Remove the dried tomatoes from the water and drain them.
6. Heat the oil in a skillet. Toss in dried tomatoes and onions.
7. Cook until onions are softened, then take off the stove.
8. Use a deep pan and fill it halfway with water. Squeeze in the juice of the lemon.
9. When water is simmering, crack the eggs and transfer them carefully into the pan. Let the eggs simmer for 4 minutes, then removed and drain on a paper towel.
10. Transfer the polenta into individual serving dishes. Top each dish with 2 eggs.

934. Buttermilk Pancakes

Prep Time: 5 Minutes *Cook Time: 15 Minutes* *Servings: 8*

Ingredients:

- 2 cups all-purpose flour
- 3 tbsp cane sugar
- 3 tsp baking powder
- 1 tsp baking soda
- 1 tsp salt
- 2 cups buttermilk
- 6 tbsp butter
- 1 tsp vanilla
- eggs Maple Syrup Confectioners' sugar

Directions:

1. Combine all together with the flour, sugar, baking soda, as well as baking powder, and salt.
2. Use another bowl to combine the buttermilk, butter, eggs, and vanilla.
3. Slowly add the buttermilk mixture to the flour mix. Mix to blend. Set the batter on the counter for 5 minutes
4. Heat a griddle or skillet. It needs to be hot, but not overly hot. When the griddle is at the right temperature, add a tablespoon of butter.
5. Use half a cup of batter per pancake. Place the batter on the grill. Flip it when the top starts to bubble.
6. Use up the entire batter. Place pancakes on a platter. Top with syrup or confectioners' sugar.

Snacks And Appetizer Recipes

935. BACON & SUN-DRIED TOMATO PHYLLO TARTS

Prep Time: 15 Minutes *Cook Time: 17 Minutes* *Servings: 2*

INGREDIENTS:

- 2 tsp olive oil
- ¾ cup chopped onion (about 1 medium)
- ¾ cup chopped green pepper (about 1 small)
- ¾ cup of chopped sweet red pepper (about 1 small)
- 1 garlic clove, minced
- Dash dried oregano
- 3 packages (1.9 ounces each) frozen miniature phyllo tart shells
- 1 package (8 ounces) cream cheese, softened
- 1 ½ tsp lemon juice
- 1/8 tsp salt
- 1 egg, lightly beaten
- ½ cup oil-packed sun-dried tomatoes, chopped and patted dry
- 2 bacon strips, cooked and crumbled
- 1 tbsp of minced fresh basil or 1 tsp of dried basil
- ½ cup crushed butter-flavoured crackers
- ½ cup shredded cheddar cheese

Directions:

1. Preheat oven to 350°. In a big skillet, heat oil over medium-high heat. Add onion and peppers; cook and stir 6-8 minutes or until tender. Add garlic and oregano; cook 1 minute longer. Cool completely.
2. Place tart shells on ungreased baking sheets. In a big bowl, beat cream cheese, lemon juice and salt until smooth.
3. Add egg; beat on reduce speed just until blended. Stir in tomatoes, bacon, basil and onion mixture.
4. Spoon 2 tsp filling into each tart shell. Top each with ½ tsp crushed crackers and ½ tsp cheddar cheese.
5. Bake 10-12 minutes or until set. Present warm.
6. FREEZE OPTION Freeze cooled baked pastries in freezer containers. To use, reheat pastries on a baking sheet in a preheated 350° oven for 15-18 minutes or until heated through.

936. CRAWFISH BEIGNETS WITH CAJUN DIPPING SAUCE

Prep Time: *15 Minutes* | *Cook Time:* *10 Minutes* | *Servings: 2*

INGREDIENTS:

- 1 egg, beaten
- 1 pound chopped cooked crawfish tail meat or shrimp
- 4 green onions, chopped
- 1 ½ tsp butter, melted ½ tsp salt
- ½ tsp cayenne pepper 1/3 cup bread flour Oil for deep-fat frying
- ¾ cup mayonnaise
- ½ cup ketchup
- ¼ tsp prepared horseradish, optional ¼ tsp hot pepper sauce 1.
- In a big bowl, add the egg, crawfish, onions, butter, salt and cayenne.
- Stir in flour until blended.

Directions:

1. An electric skillet or deep fryer is heating oil to 375°. Drop tbsps of batter, a few at a time, into the hot oil.
2. Fry until golden brown on both sides. Drain on paper towels.
3. In a small size bowl, add the mayonnaise, ketchup, horseradish if desired and pepper sauce. Present with beignets.

937. SPANAKOPITA PINWHEELS

Prep Time: *5 Minutes* | *Cook Time:* *17 Minutes* | *Servings: 8*

INGREDIENTS:

- 1 medium onion, finely chopped
- 2 tbsps olive oil
- 1 tsp of dried oregano
- 1 clove of garlic, minced
- 2 packs (10 oz each) frozen minced spinach, thawed and pressed dry
- 1 package (17.3 oz) Frozen Puff Pastries, Thaw 1.

Directions:

1. Heat oil in a skillet and then sauté onions until tender. Add oregano and garlic. Boil for 1 more minute.
2. Add spinach. Cook for at least 3 minutes or until the liquid evaporates. Transfer the spinach mixture to a large bowl. Cold.
3. Add feta cheese and eggs to the spinach mixture. Mix well. Open the puff pastry. Spread each sheet with half of the spinach mixture within an inch of the edge. Roll jelly-roll style.
4. Cut into 12 inches each. Some part. Place cut side down on a greased baking sheet.
5. Bake at 400° for 18-22 minutes or until golden brown.

938. MIXED OLIVE CROSTINI

Prep Time: *15 Minutes* | *Cook Time:*☐30 *Minutes* | *Servings: 4*

INGREDIENTS:

- 1 can (4 ¼ ounces) chopped ripe olives ½ cup pimiento-stuffed olives, finely chopped ½ cup grated Parmesan cheese ¼ cup butter, softened
- 1 tbsp olive oil
- 2 garlic cloves, minced
- ¾ cup shredded part-skim mozzarella cheese ¼ cup minced fresh parsley

Directions:

1. 1 French bread baguette (10 ½ ounces) 1. In a small size bowl, add the first six ingredients; stir in mozzarella cheese and parsley.
2. Cut baguette into 24 slices; place on an ungreased baking sheet. Spread with olive mixture.
3. Broil 3-4 in. from the heat for 2-3 minutes or until edges are lightly browned, and cheese is melted.

939. CHAMPION CHICKEN PUFFS

Prep Time: *15 Minutes* | *Cook Time:* *14 Minutes* | *Servings: 4*

INGREDIENTS:

- 4 ounces cream cheese, softened
- ½ tsp garlic powder
- ½ cup of shredded cooked chicken
- 2 tubes (8 ounces each) of refrigerated crescent rolls

Directions:

1. Whisk cream cheese and garlic powder in a small bowl until smooth. Stir the chicken.
2. Roll out the crescent dough. Divide it into 16 triangles. Cut each triangle in half lengthwise to make two triangles. add 1 teaspoon
3. The chicken mixture is in the middle of each. Fold the short side over the filling. Close and roll up by pressing the sides.
4. Put the 1 inch apart on a greased baking sheet. Bake at 375° for 12-14 minutes or until golden brown. come warm

940. MINIATURE SHEPHERD'S PIES

Prep Time: *15 Minutes* | *Cook Time:* *19 Minutes* | *Servings: 2*

INGREDIENTS:

- ½ pound ground beef
- 1/3 cup finely chopped onion ¼ cup finely chopped celery 3 tbsp finely chopped carrot
- 1 ½ tsp all-purpose flour 1 tsp dried thyme
- ¼ tsp salt
- 1/8 tsp ground nutmeg
- 1/8 tsp of pepper
- 2/3 cup of beef broth
- 1/3 cup of frozen petite peas 2 packages (17.3 ounces each) frozen puff pastry, thawed
- 3 cups mashed potatoes

Directions:

1. Preheat oven to 400°. In a large skillet, cook the beef, onions, celery and carrots over medium heat until the beef is no longer pink. Thin.
2. Stir in the flour, thyme, salt, nutmeg and pepper until smooth. Add broth gradually. Take to a boil; cook and stir continuously for 2 minutes or until sauce thickens. Stir the peas. Heat passing. Separately.
3. Open the puff pastry. Use 2 inches of flour. The circular cutter cut 12 circles from each sheet (keep the rest for other use). Slide the puff pastry circles on the bottom and top of the non-greasy side of a mini muffin cup.
4. Fill each with 1 teaspoon of beef mixture. Top or pipe with 1 tbsp mashed potatoes. Bake 13-16 minutes or until heated and potatoes are slightly browned. come warm

941. BRIE-APPLE PASTRY BITES

Prep Time: *15 Minutes* | *Cook Time:* *43 Minutes* | *Servings: 2*

INGREDIENTS:

- 1 package (17.3 ounces) of frozen puff pastry, thawed
- 1 round (8 ounces) of Brie cheese, cut into ½-inch cubes 1 medium apple, chopped
- 2/3 cup sliced almonds ½ cup chopped walnuts ¼ cup dried cranberries Ground nutmeg

Directions:

1. Open puff pastry; cut each sheet into 24 squares. Gently press the square into the bottom of the greased 48 mini muffin cups.
2. Add cheese, apples, nuts and cranberries. Spoon in the cup. Bake at 375° for 12-15 minutes or until cheese is melted. Sprinkle with nutmeg.

942. SWEDISH MEATBALLS

Prep Time: *15 Minutes* | *Cook Time:* *44 Minutes* | *Servings: 5*

INGREDIENTS:

- 2/3 cup evaporated milk
- 2/3 cup chopped onion
- ¼ cup fine dry bread crumbs
- ½ tsp salt
- ½ tsp allspice
- Dash pepper
- 1 pound lean ground beef (90% lean)
- 2 tsp butter
- 2 tsp beef bouillon granules
- 1 cup hot water
- ½ cup cold water
- 2 tbsps all-purpose flour
- 1 cup evaporated milk
- 1 tbsp lemon juice

Directions:

1. Add 2/3 cup evaporated milk, onion, crumbs, salt, allspice and pepper. Add meat; mix well, chill. Shape meat mixture into 1-in. balls.
2. In a big skillet, brown meatballs in butter. Dissolve bouillon in hot water; pour over meatballs and bring to boil over medium heat. Cover; simmer for 15 minutes.
3. Meanwhile, blend together cold water and flour. Remove meatballs from skillet, skim fat from pan juices and rePresent juices.
4. Stir 1 cup evaporated milk and flour/water mixture into pan juices in skillet; cook, uncovered, over reduce heat, stirring until sauce thickens.
5. Return meatballs to skillet. Stir in lemon juice. Present with cooked noodles that have been tossed with poppy seeds and butter.

943. SWEET SAUSAGE ROLLS

Prep Time: *15 Minutes* | *Cook Time:* *23 Minutes* | *Servings: 5*

INGREDIENTS:

- 1 tube (8 ounces) refrigerated crescent rolls
- 24 miniature smoked sausage links
- ½ cup butter, melted
- ½ cup chopped nuts
- 3 tbsps honey

- 3 tbsps brown sugar

Directions:

1. Unroll crescent dough and separate into triangles; cut each lengthwise into three triangles. Place sausages on the wide end of triangles; roll up tightly.
2. Add the remaining ingredients in an 11x7-in. Baking dish. Arrange sausage rolls, seam side down, in butter mixture. Bake, uncovered, at 400° for 15-20 minutes or until golden brown.

944. PEANUT SHRIMP KABOBS

Prep Time: *15 Minutes* *Cook Time:* *12 Minutes* *Servings: 7*

INGREDIENTS:

- ¼ cup sugar
- ¼ cup reduced-sodium soy sauce
- ¼ cup reduced-fat creamy peanut butter
- 1 tbsp water
- 1 tbsp canola oil
- 3 garlic cloves, minced
- 1 ½ pound of uncooked medium shrimp, peeled and deveined

Directions:

1. In a small saucepan, add the first six ingredients until smooth. Cook and stir over medium-reduce heat until blended and sugar is dissolved. Set aside 6 tbsps sauce.
2. On eight metal or soaked wooden skewers, thread the shrimp. Brush with remaining peanut sauce. By Using long-handled tongs, moisten a paper towel with cooking oil and coat the grill rack.
3. Grill kabobs, covered, overheat or broil 4 in. from the heat for 4-6 minutes or until shrimp turn pink, turning once.
4. Brush with reserved sauce before serving.

945. TIERED CHEESE SLICES

Prep Time: *15 Minutes* *Cook Time:* *20 Minutes* *Servings: 4*

INGREDIENTS:

- 1 package (8 ounces) cream cheese, softened
- ½ tsp hot pepper sauce ¼ tsp salt
- ¼ cup chopped pecans
- ¼ cup dried cranberries 2 packages
- deli-style cheddar cheese slices
- Assorted crackers

Directions:

1. In a big bowl, add the cream cheese, hot pepper sauce and salt. Stir in pecans and cranberries.
2. On a 12-in. square of aluminium foil, place two slices of cheese side by side; spread with 2-3 tbsps cream cheese mixture. Repeat layers six times. Top with two cheese slices. Fold foil around cheese and seal tightly. Let it cool for 8 hours or overnight. Cut in half lengthwise and then widthwise into ¼-in. slices. Present with crackers.

946. CRAB-STUFFED SNOW PEAS

Prep Time: *15 Minutes* *Cook Time:* *55 Minutes* *Servings: 4*

INGREDIENTS:

- 1 can crab meat, drained, flaked, and cartilage removed
- 2 tbsps mayonnaise
- 1 tbsp chilli sauce or seafood cocktail sauce
- 1/8 tsp salt
- 3 drops hot pepper sauce
- Dash pepper
- 16 fresh snow peas

Directions:

1. In a small-size bowl, add the crab, mayonnaise, chilli sauce, salt, hot sauce and pepper.
2. Put the snow peas in the steaming basket. Place in a small saucepan over 1 inch of water. Bring to a boil; cover and steam for 30 seconds until tender. Drain the snow peas and immediately drop them into ice water. Drain and dry.
3. Cut the peas along the curved edges with a sharp knife. Spoon each crab mixture 1 tbsp.

947. CUCUMBER RYE SNACKS

Prep Time: *15 Minutes* *Cook Time:* *20 Minutes* *Servings: 4*

INGREDIENTS:

- 1 package (8 ounces) cream cheese, softened
- 2 tbsps mayonnaise
- 2 tsp Italian salad dressing mix
- 30 slices snack rye bread
- 30 thin slices of cucumber
- Fresh dill sprigs and chive blossoms

Directions:

1. In a bowl, beat the cream cheese, mayonnaise and dressing mix until blended. Let stand for 30 minutes.
2. Spread mixture on rye bread. Top each with a slice of cucumber, dill sprig and chive blossom. Cover and refrigerate until serving.

948. ASIAN TUNA BITES WITH DIJON DIPPING SAUCE

Prep Time: *15 Minutes* *Cook Time:* *23 Minutes* *Servings: 4*

INGREDIENTS:

- 3 tbsps Dijon mustard
- 2 tbsps red wine vinegar
- 2 tbsp reduced-sodium soy sauce
- 1 tbsp sesame oil
- 1 tsp hot pepper sauce
- 1 pound tuna steaks, cut into thirty 1-inch cubes Cooking spray
- ¼ cup sesame seeds ½ tsp salt ¼ tsp pepper 2 green onions, finely chopped

Directions:

1. In a small size bowl, whisk the first five ingredients; set aside. Spritz tuna with cooking spray. Sprinkle with sesame seeds, salt and pepper. In a big nonstick skillet, brown tuna on all sides in batches until medium-rare or slightly pink in the centre; remove from the skillet.
2. On each of the 30 wooden appetizers, skewered, and thread one tuna cube. Arrange on a serving platter. Garnish with onions. Present with sauce.

949. MARINATED SAUSAGE KABOBS

Prep Time: *15 Minutes* *Cook Time:* *30 Minutes* *Servings: 2*

INGREDIENTS:

- ¼ cup olive oil
- 1 tbsp white vinegar
- ½ tsp minced garlic
- ½ tsp dried basil
- ½ tsp dried oregano
- 12 ounces cheddar cheese, cut into ¾-in. cubes 1 can (6 ounces) pitted ripe olives, drained
- 4 ounces hard salami, cut into ¾-in. cubes 1 medium sweet red pepper, cut into ¾-inch pieces 1 medium green pepper, cut into ¾-inch pieces 1.

Directions:

1. In a plastic bag, add the first five ingredients; add the remaining ingredients. Seal bag and turn to coat; refrigerate for at least 4 hours. Drain and discard marinade.
2. For each kabob, thread one piece each of cheese, olive, salami and pepper onto a toothpick.

950. SMOKED SALMON PINWHEELS

Prep Time: *15 Minutes* *Cook Time:* *30 Minutes* *Servings: 2*

INGREDIENTS:

- 1 package (8 ounces) cream cheese, softened
- 1 tbsp snipped fresh dill
- 1 tbsp capers, drained
- ½ tsp garlic powder
- ½ tsp lemon juice
- 4 spinach tortillas (8 inches), room temperature
- ½ pound smoked salmon fillets, flaked

Directions:

1. In a small size bowl, add the cream cheese, dill, capers, garlic powder and lemon juice. Spread over tortillas; top with salmon. Roll up tightly.
2. Cut into 1-in. pieces; secure with toothpicks. Chill until serving. Discard toothpicks before serving. Refrigerate leftovers.

951. CHEESE STRAWS

Prep Time: *15 Minutes* *Cook Time:* *39 Minutes* *Servings: 6*

INGREDIENTS:

- ½ cup butter softened
- 2 cups shredded sharp cheddar cheese
- 1 ¼ cups all-purpose flour
- ½ tsp salt
- ¼ tsp cayenne pepper

Directions:

1. Preheat oven to 350°. In a big bowl, beat butter until light and fluffy. Beat in cheese until blended.
2. Add flour, salt and cayenne; stir into cheese mixture until a dough forms. Roll into a 15x6-in rectangle. Cut into thirty 6-in. strips. Gently place strips 1 in. apart on ungreased baking sheets.
3. Bake 15-20 minutes or until lightly browned. Let it cool for 5 minutes before removing pans to wire racks to cool completely. Store straws in an airtight container.

952. SWEET GINGERED CHICKEN WINGS

Prep Time: *15 Minutes* *Cook Time:* *40 Minutes* *Servings: 6*

INGREDIENTS:

- 1 cup all-purpose flour
- 2 tsp salt
- 2 tsp paprika
- ¼ tsp pepper
- 24 chicken wings (about 5 pounds)
- sauce
- ¼ cup honey
- ¼ cup thawed orange juice concentrate
- ½ tsp ground ginger Minced fresh parsley, optional

Directions:

1. Preheat oven to 350°. Place two baking sheets with foil; coat with cooking spray.
2. In a big resealable plastic bag, add flour, salt, paprika and pepper. Add chicken wings, a few at a time; seal bag and toss to coat. Divide wings between prepared baking pans. Bake 30 minutes.
3. In a small bowl, add honey, orange juice concentrate and ginger; brush over chicken wings. After baking, 25-30 minutes or until juices run clear.
4. Preheat broiler. Broil wings 4 in. from heat 1-2 minutes or until lightly browned. If desired, sprinkle with parsley.

953. CRANBERRY CHILI MEATBALLS

Prep Time: *15 Minutes* | *Cook Time:* *90 Minutes* | *Servings: 6*

INGREDIENTS:

- 1 bottle (12 ounces) chilli sauce
- ¾ cup packed brown sugar
- ½ tsp chilli powder
- ½ tsp ground cumin
- ¼ tsp cayenne pepper

Directions:

1. package (32 ounces) frozen fully cooked homestyle meatballs, thawed In a big saucepan over medium heat, add the first six ingredients. Now stir until sugar is dissolved.
2. Plus meatballs; cook for 20-25 minutes or until heated through, stirring occasionally.

954. BEEF FONDUE WITH MUSTARD-MAYONNAISE SAUCE

Prep Time: *15 Minutes* | *Cook Time:* *16 Minutes* | *Servings: 66*

INGREDIENTS:

- 2 tsp finely chopped onion
- 2 tsp lemon juice
- 2 tbsp horseradish mustard or spicy brown mustard
- 1 ½ pound beef tenderloin, cut into ¾-inch cubes
- Oil for deep-fat frying

Directions:

1. In a small size bowl, add the mayonnaise, onion, lemon juice and mustard; cover and refrigerate for 30 minutes.
2. Pat meat dry with paper towels. Oil in a fondue pot to 375°. Use fondue forks for cooking meat in oil until it reaches desired doneness. Present beef with sauce.

955. TURKEY-CRANBERRY TARTS

Prep Time: *15 Minutes* | *Cook Time:* *35 Minutes* | *Servings: 8*

INGREDIENTS:

- 1/3 cup mayonnaise
- 4 tsp minced fresh parsley
- 4 tsp honey mustard
- ½ tsp chopped seeded jalapeno pepper 1/8 tsp pepper
- 2 cups cubed cooked turkey breast
- 1/3 cup chopped celery
- 1/3 cup dried cranberries, chopped 1/3 cup shredded Swiss cheese ¼ cup chopped pecans.
- toasted 30 frozen miniature phyllo tart shells.

Directions:

1. In a big bowl, combine the first five ingredients. Add the turkey, celery, cranberries, cheese and pecans; toss to coat.
2. Arrange tart shells on an ungreased baking sheet. Fill with turkey mixture. Bake at 375° for 10-12 minutes or until heated through. Present warm.
3. **NOTE** To toast nuts, bake in a shall reduce pan in a 350° oven for 5-10 minutes or cook in a skillet over reduce heat until lightly browned, stirring occasionally.

956. PROSCIUTTO-WRAPPED APRICOTS

Prep Time: *15 Minutes* | *Cook Time:* *45 Minutes* | *Servings: 2*

INGREDIENTS:

- ¾ cup Mascarpone cheese 2 tbsps confectioners' sugar
- 1/8 tsp white pepper 1 package (7 ounces) dried pitted
- Mediterranean apricots
- 12 thin slices prosciutto

Directions:

1. In a small size bowl, add the cheese, confectioners' sugar and pepper. Cut a slit in each apricot; fill with cheese mixture. Cut each slice of prosciutto in half lengthwise; wrap a piece around each apricot and secure with a toothpick.
2. Place in an ungreased 15x10x1-in. Baking pan. Bake, unwrap, at 425° for 15-20 minutes or until heated through. Refrigerate leftovers.
3. BACON-WRAPPED APRICOTS Substitute 12 slices of bacon for the prosciutto. Proceed as directed.

957. LOBSTER & ARTICHOKE QUESADILLAS

Prep Time: *15 Minutes* | *Cook Time:* *50 Minutes* | *Servings: 2*

INGREDIENTS:

- ½ cup grated Parmesan cheese
- ½ cup of fat-free mayonnaise
- 1 can (14 ounces) of water-packed artichoke hearts, rinsed, drained and chopped
- 4 ½ tsp of chopped roasted sweet red pepper
- 1 garlic clove, minced
- 6 flour tortillas (10 inches)
- 1 cup of cooked lobster meat or canned flaked lobster meat
- ½ cup shredded part-skim mozzarella cheese

Directions:

1. In a small size bowl, add the Parmesan cheese, mayonnaise, artichokes, red pepper and garlic. Spread over three tortillas. Top with lobster, mozzarella cheese and remaining tortillas; press down lightly.
2. On a griddle coated by using cooking spray, cook quesadillas over medium heat for 2 minutes on each side or until cheese is melted. Cut each quesadilla into six wedges.

958. CHORIZO DATE RUMAKI

Prep Time: *15 Minutes* | *Cook Time:* *20 Minutes* | *Servings: 8*

INGREDIENTS:

- 1 package (1 pound) sliced bacon
- 4 ounces uncooked chorizo or spicy bulk pork sausage 2 ounces cream cheese, cubed
- 32 pitted dates

Directions:

1. Cut each bacon strip in half. In a big skillet, cook bacon in batches over medium heat until partially cooked but not crisp. Remove to paper towels; drain drippings.
2. Crumble chorizo into the same skillet; cook and stir until fully cooked. Drain. Stir in cream cheese.
3. Divide a slit in the centre of each date; fill with cream cheese mixture. Wrap a piece of bacon around each stuffed date; secure with toothpicks.
4. Place on ungreased baking sheets. Bake at 350° for 12-15 minutes or until bacon is crisp.

959. RUSTIC ANTIPASTO TART

Prep Time: *15 Minutes* | *Cook Time:* *30 Minutes* | *Servings: 2*

INGREDIENTS:

- 1 sheet refrigerated pie pastry
- 2 tbsp prepared pesto
- 1 cup of shredded part-skim mozzarella cheese, cut into 4 ounces sliced turkey pepperoni
- 1 jar (7 ounces) of roasted sweet red peppers,
- drained and thinly sliced 1 jar (7 ½ ounces) marinated quartered artichoke hearts, drained 1 tbsp wate

Directions:

1. Unroll the pastry onto a parchment paper-lined baking sheet. Sprinkle pesto to within 2 in. of edges; sprinkle with ½ cup cheese.
2. Layer with pepperoni and ¼ cup of cheese. Top with red peppers and artichokes; spread with remaining cheese.
3. Fold up edges of pastry over filling, leaving the centre uncovered. Brush folded pastry with water.
4. Bake at 425° for 25-30 minutes or until the crust is golden and cheese is melted. Present warm.

960. MEXICAN CHICKEN MEATBALLS

Prep Time: *15 Minutes* | *Cook Time:* *63 Minutes* | *Servings: 2*

INGREDIENTS:

- ½ cup egg substitute
- 1 can (4 ounces) chopped green chillies
- 1 cup crushed cornflakes
- 1 cup (4 ounces) of shredded reduced-fat Mexican cheese blend
- ½ tsp seasoned salt
- ¼ tsp cayenne pepper
- 1 pound ground chicken
- Salsa, optional

Directions:

1. In a big bowl, add the first six ingredients. Crumble chicken over mixture and mix well. Shape into 1-in. balls. Place on baking sheets coated with cooking spray.
2. Bake it atleast375° for 12-15 minutes or until a meat thermometer reads 165° and juices run clear, turning occasionally. Present with salsa if desired.
3. FREEZE OPTION Freeze cooled meatballs in freezer containers. by using, partially thaw in refrigerator overnight.
4. Microwave, wrapped, on high in a microwave-safe dish until heated through, stirring and adding a little broth or water if necessary.

961. CARAMELIZED ONION & FIG PIZZA

Prep Time: *15 Minutes* | *Cook Time:* *70- Minutes* | *Servings: 2*

INGREDIENTS:

- 2 tbsps olive oil, divided
- 1 big onion, chopped
- 3 garlic cloves, minced
- ¼ tsp pepper
- 1 tube (13.8 ounces) of refrigerated pizza crust
- 1 pkg (8 ounces) of cream cheese, softened
- 1 tsp minced fresh thyme or ¼ tsp dried thyme
- 1 cup of dried figs (about 6 ounces), chopped
- 6 thin slices prosciutto or deli ham, chopped
- 1/3 cup pine nuts
- 1 cup (4 ounces) shredded provolone cheese

Directions:

1. In a big skillet, it is heating 1 tbsp oil over medium heat. Add onion; cook and stir until softened.
2. Reduce heat to medium-reduce; cook 30-35 minutes or until turning deep golden brown, occasionally stirring garlic and pepper; cook 1 minute longer.
3. Preheat oven to 425°. Unroll and press dough onto the bottom and up sides of a greased 15x10x1-in. Baking pan. Bake 7-10 minutes or until golden brown.
4. Beat the cream cheese, thyme and remaining oil in a small bowl until smooth. Spread over the crust. Sprinkle with caramelized onions, figs, prosciutto and pine nuts. Sprinkle with cheese. Bake it for another 6-10 minutes or until cheese is melted.
5. Make it ahead of time. This recipe takes a few minutes to combine when you caramelized the onions the day before.

962. APPLE WONTON BUNDLES

Prep Time: *15 Minutes* | *Cook Time:* *18 Minutes* | *Servings: 2*

INGREDIENTS:

- 4 medium tart apples, peeled

- 64 wonton wrappers
- 2 to 3 cups canola oil

Directions:

1. 1 jar (12 ounces) of caramel ice cream topping, warmed 1. Cut every apple into four wedges; cut wedges into four pieces. Put a piece of apple in the centre of each wonton wrapper.
2. Brush edges of wrapper with water and bring up around apple pinch to seal. Cover with plastic wrap until ready to cook.
3. After Heating oil in a fondue pot to 375°, use fondue forks for cooking wonton bundles until golden brown (about 1 minute). Cool slightly. Present bundles with caramel topping.

963. TERIYAKI STEAK SKEWERS

Prep Time: *15 Minutes* | *Cook Time:* *30 Minutes* | *Servings: 5*

INGREDIENTS:

- ½ cup reduced-sodium soy sauce
- ¼ cup cider vinegar
- 2 tbsps brown sugar
- 2 tbsps finely chopped onion
- 1 tbsp canola oil
- 1 garlic clove, minced
- ½ tsp ground ginger
- 1/8 tsp pepper
- 2 pounds beef top sirloin steak

Directions:

1. In a large plastic bag, place the first eight ingredients. Remove the fat from the steak and cut the grain crosswise -in. Strip.
2. Add beef to the bag. Tight the bag and hand it over to the coat. Refrigerate for 2-3 hours.
3. Drain the seasoning and discard. Thread the cutlets loosely onto 6 pickled metal or wooden skewers.
4. Bake uncovered and over medium heat for 7-10 minutes or until meat is cooked to the desired degree, turning frequently.

964. SMOKED MOZZARELLA FLATBREAD PIZZA

Prep Time: *15 Minutes* | *Cook Time:* *40 Minutes* | *Servings: 5*

INGREDIENTS:

- 2 tbsp butter, divided
- 2 tbsps olive oil, divided
- 2/3 cup sliced red onion
- ½ pound sliced baby portobello mushrooms
- 1 garlic clove, minced
- 2 tsp minced fresh rosemary or ½ tsp dried rosemary, crushed
- 1 tube (13.8 ounces) of refrigerated pizza crust
- 1 ½ cups (6 ounces) shredded smoked mozzarella cheese
- 2 ounces sliced prosciutto or deli ham, finely chopped

Directions:

1. Preheat oven to 400°. In a big skillet, heat 1 tbsp butter and 1 tbsp oil over medium-high heat.
2. Add onion; cook it and stir 2-3 minutes or until softened. Reduce heat to medium-reduce; cook 8-10 minutes or until golden brown, stirring occasionally. Remove from pan.
3. In the same skillet, heat the butter continuously as well as oil over medium-high heat. Add mushrooms; cook and stir 2-3 minutes or until tender. Add garlic and rosemary; cook about 1-2 minutes longer or until liquid is evaporated.
4. Unroll and press dough onto the bottom of a greased 15x10x1-in. Baking pan.
5. Using fingertips, press several dimples into dough. Sprinkle with ½ cup cheese; top with onion, mushroom mixture and prosciutto. Sprinkle with remaining cheese
6. . Bake pizza 15-18 minutes or until golden brown and the cheese is melted.

965. MEDITERRANEAN NACHOS

Prep Time: *15 Minutes* | *Cook Time:* *60 Minutes* | *Servings: 8*

INGREDIENTS:

- 2 medium cucumbers, peeled, seeded and grated
- 1 ½ tsp salt, divided
- ½ tsp ground cumin
- ½ tsp ground coriander
- ½ tsp paprika
- ¾ tsp pepper, divided
- 6 whole pita bread Cooking spray
- 1 pound ground lamb or beef
- 2 garlic cloves, minced
- 1 tsp cornstarch
- ½ cup beef broth
- 2 cups plain Greek yoghurt
- 2 tbsps lemon juice
- ¼ tsp grated lemon peel
- 2 cups torn romaine
- 2 medium tomatoes, seeded and chopped
- ½ cup pitted Greek olives, sliced
- 4 green onions, thinly sliced
- ½ cup crumbled feta cheese

Directions:

1. In a colander, place over a bowl, toss cucumbers with ½ tsp salt. Let stand 30 minutes. Squeeze and pat dry. Set aside. In a small size bowl, add the cumin, coriander, paprika, ½ tsp pepper and ½ tsp salt; set aside.
2. Cut each pita into eight wedges; arrange in a singer layer on ungreased baking sheets. Spritz both sides of pitas with cooking spray; sprinkle with ¾ tsp seasoning mix. Broil it from the heat for 3-4 minutes on each side or until golden brown. Cool on wire racks.
3. In a big skillet, cook lamb and remaining seasoning mix over medium heat until the lamb is no longer pink. Add garlic; cook 1 minute longer. Drain. Add cornstarch and broth until smooth; gradually stir into the pan. Bring to a boil; cook it and stir continuously for 2 minutes or until thickened.
4. In a small size bowl, add the yoghurt, lemon juice, lemon peel, cucumbers and remaining salt and pepper. Arrange pita wedges on a serving platter. Layer with lettuce, lamb mixture, tomatoes, olives, onions and cheese. Present immediately with cucumber sauce.
5. **NOTE** If Greek yoghurt is not available in your area, line a strainer with a coffee filter and place it over a bowl. Place 4 cups plain yoghurt in prepared strainer; refrigerate overnight. Discard liquid from bowl; proceed as directed.

966. CHICKEN SKEWERS WITH SWEET & SPICY MARMALADE

Prep Time: *15 Minutes* | *Cook Time:* *40 Minutes* | *Servings: 8*

INGREDIENTS:

- 1 pound boneless skinless chicken breasts
- ¼ cup olive oil
- ¼ cup reduced-sodium soy sauce
- 2 garlic cloves, minced
- 1/8 tsp pepper
- SAUCE
- 2 tsp butter
- 2 tbsps chopped seeded jalapeno pepper
- 1 tsp minced fresh ginger root
- ¾ cup orange marmalade
- 1 tbsp lime juice
- 1 tbsp thawed orange juice concentrate
- ¼ tsp salt

Directions:

1. before heating the broiler. Beat the chicken breast continuously with a meat mallet. Thickness; Cut lengthwise into 1-inch wide strips.
2. Place the oil, soy sauce, garlic and pepper in a large resealable plastic bag. Add chicken. Close the bag and hand it over to the coat. Refrigerate for 4 hours or overnight.
3. Heat the butter in a saucepan overheat. Added jalapeno; Cook and stir until soft. Add ginger. Boil for 1 more minute.
4. Reduce heat. Stir in the marmalade, lime juice, orange juice concentrate and salt. Drain the chicken and remove the seasoning.
5. Thread the tangled chicken pieces onto 8 pickled metal or wooden skewers. Place on a greased 15x10x1 inch. Pan.
6. Bake 6 inches over heat for 2-4 minutes on each side or until the chicken is no longer pink. Serve with sauce.

***Note** Wear disposable gloves when slicing peppers. Oil can burn your skin. Do not touch your face*

967. GRILLED STEAK APPETIZERS WITH STILTON SAUCE

Prep Time: *15 Minutes* | *Cook Time:* *53 Minutes* | *Servings: 2*

INGREDIENTS:

- (8 ounces each) 2 boneless beef top loin steaks
- ¼ tsp salt
- ¼ tsp pepper
- ½ cup white wine or chicken broth
- 1/3 cup heavy whipping cream
- 3 tbsp sour cream
- 2 ounces Stilton cheese, cubed

Directions:

1. Sprinkle salt and pepper on the steak. Bake the covered steaks on medium heat for 4-6 minutes on each side or until the meat is cooked to the desired level (meat thermometer should read 145° for medium-rare, 160° for medium, 170° for fully cooked). Convert the meat to a chopping board and keep warm.
2. Boil the wine in a small saucepan. Cook until reduced by half. Add cream. Boil gently. Reduce heat. Bring to a boil, remove the lid and occasionally stir until thickened. Remove from heat. Add sour cream and cheese. Stir until cheese is melted.
3. Cut the steak into 1-inch pieces. Box; Skewers with toothpicks. Serve with sauce.
4. **Note** Top loin steaks may be marked as Strip Steaks, KS City Steaks, NY Strip Steaks, Ambassador Steaks, or Boneless Club Stakes. You can substitute 1/3 cup of blue cheese instead of Stilton cheese.

968. ASIAN CHICKEN DUMPLINGS

Prep Time: *15 Minutes* | *Cook Time:* *20 Minutes* | *Servings: 2*

INGREDIENTS:

- 1 pound ground chicken
- 4 green onions, chopped
- ½ cup chopped cabbage
- ¼ cup minced fresh cilantro
- 2 tsp minced fresh ginger root
- 1 tsp salt
- ¼ tsp Chinese five-spice powder
- 2 tbsps water
- 1 package (10 ounces) of potsticker or gyoza wrappers Cabbage leaves
- Reduced-sodium soy sauce

Directions:

1. Put the first seven ingredients into the food processor. Cover and process until chopped. Add water. Cover and process until soft.
2. Put 1 tablespoon of chicken mixture in the centre of one pack. (Cover the rest of the wrap with a dry paper towel to keep it from drying out.) Wet the edges with water.
3. Fold the wrap over the filling to form a semicircle. Press firmly on the edges to close and fold 3 to 5 times so that the front side folds.
4. Close the edges tightly and place each dumpling on a flat surface. Press to level the floor. Repeat with the rest of the wrapping and filling. Cover the dumplings with plastic wrap.
5. Place 4 cabbage leaves in the steamer basket. Group dumplings 1 inch apart on top of the cabbage.
6. Place in a large saucepan over 1 inch of water. Bring to a boil; cover and steam for 10-12 minutes or until the thermometer read 165°. Throw away the cabbage. Repeat. Serve with soy sauce.

969. PEAR-BLUE CHEESE TARTLETS

Prep Time: *15 Minutes* | *Cook Time:* *70 Minutes* | *Servings: 4*

INGREDIENTS:

- 2 tbsps butter
- 2 big pears, peeled and finely chopped
- 2 tbsps honey Dash salt
- ¼ cup mascarpone cheese ¼ cup crumbled blue cheese 2 packages (1.9 ounces each) frozen miniature phyllo tart shells ¼ cup finely chopped walnuts 1.
- Whisk cream cheese and garlic powder in a small bowl until smooth. Stir the chicken.

Directions:

1. Roll out the crescent dough. Divide it into sixteen triangles. Divide every triangle in half lengthwise to make two triangles. add 1 teaspoon
2. The chicken mixture is in the middle of each. Fold the short side over the filling. Close and roll up by pressing the sides.
3. Put the 1 inch apart on a greased baking sheet. Bake at 375° for 12-14 minutes or until golden brown. come warm
4. Bake tarts for 6-8 minutes or until golden brown. Present tarts warm. Refrigerate any leftovers.

970. SPICY BEEF SKEWERS

Prep Time: *15 Minutes* | *Cook Time:* *20 Minutes* | *Servings: 4*

INGREDIENTS:

- ¾ cup sugar ½ cup water 1 tbsp orange marmalade
- ¼ tsp grated orange peel ¼ tsp crushed red pepper flakes ½ cup finely chopped salted roasted almonds 2 tbsps minced fresh mint
- 1 green onion, finely chopped
- 1 tbsp lemon juice
- 1 garlic clove, minced
- ¼ tsp each ground cinnamon, cumin and coriander 1 pound lean ground beef (90% lean)
- Minced fresh parsley

Directions:

1. Place the first 6 ingredients in a pot. Bring it to a boil. Reduce heat. Boil uncovered, about 25 minutes or until reduced to a cup.
2. In the meantime, combine the almonds, mint, onion, lemon juice, garlic and spices in a large bowl.
3. Mash the beef into the mixture and mix well. Divide into 24 parts. Make each section 3x1 inch. Rectangle; Insert each wooden skewer soaked in water.
4. Bake 6 inches in the heat for 2-4 minutes on each side or until the thermometer shows 160°. Arrange on a serving plate. Sprinkle with the sauce mixture and sprinkle with parsley.

971. ITALIAN MEATBALL BUNS

Prep Time: *15 Minutes* | *Cook Time:* *35 Minutes* | *Servings: 2*

INGREDIENTS:

- 12 frozen bread dough dinner rolls
- 1 package (12 ounces) frozen fully cooked Italian meatballs, thawed 2 tbsps olive oil
- ¼ cup grated Parmesan cheese ¼ cup minced fresh basil 1 ½ cups marinara sauce, warmed 1.
- Let bread dough stand at room temperature for 25-30 minutes or until softened.

Directions:

1. Cut each roll in half. Wrap each portion around a meatball, enclosing the meatball completely; pinch dough firmly to seal. Place on greased baking sheets, seam side down.
2. Cover with kitchen towels; let rise in a warm place until almost doubled, about 1 ½ to 2 hours.
3. Preheat oven to 350°. Bake buns for 12-15 minutes or until they turn golden brown. Brush tops with oil; sprinkle with cheese and basil. Present with warm marinara sauce.

972. GRILLED CHEESE & TOMATO FLATBREADS

Prep Time: *15 Minutes* | *Cook Time:* *63 Minutes* | *Servings: 2*

INGREDIENTS:

- 1 package (8 ounces) cream cheese, softened
- 2/3 cup grated Parmesan cheese, divided
- 2 tbsps minced fresh parsley, divided
- 1 tbsp minced chives
- 2 garlic cloves, minced
- ½ tsp minced fresh thyme
- ¼ tsp salt
- ¼ tsp pepper
- 1 tube (13.8 ounces) of refrigerated pizza crust
- 2 tbsps olive oil
- 3 medium tomatoes, thinly sliced

Directions:

1. In a small size bowl, beat the cream cheese, 1/3 cup Parmesan cheese, 1 tbsp parsley, green onion, garlic, thyme, salt and pepper until soft.
2. Spread out the pizza crust and cut it in half. Roll each piece 12x6 inches on a lightly dusted surface. Rectangle; Grease each side with oil.
3. Cover and cook over medium heat for 1-2 minutes or until lightly browned. Remove from grill.
4. Spread the toasted sides with the cheese mixture. Sprinkle with the remaining Parmesan cheese. Put the tomatoes.
5. Back to the grill. Cover and flip for 2-3 minutes or halfway through cooking until the crust is slightly browned and the cheese is melted.
6. Make sure the crust is evenly browned. Sprinkle with the remaining parsley.

Dessert Recipes

973. Roasted Plums Almond Cake

Prep Time: *15 Minutes* | *Cook Time:* *55 Minutes* | *Servings: 2*

Ingredients:

- 1 cup whole wheat flour
- ½ cup sugar
- 1 teaspoon baking powder
- ¼ cup vegetable oil
- ½ cup low-fat milk
- ¼ cup sliced almonds, toasted
- ¼ cup maple syrup
- 1 pinch of salt
- 4 plums, pitted and sliced

Directions:

1. In a bowl, combine the flour with the sugar, baking powder and salt, then stir in the oil and milk. Give it a good mix until well combined, then stir in the sliced almonds and maple syrup. Spoon the batter into a 6-inch round cake pan lined with baking paper. Top with plum slices.
2. Bake in the before heated oven at 350F for 30-40 minutes or until a skewer inserted in the middle of the cake comes out clean.
3. When complete, remove from the oven and let the cake cool in the pan, then transfer on a serving plate and decorate with powdered sugar.

974. Plum Crostata

Prep Time: *15 Minutes* | *Cook Time:* *50 Minutes* | *Servings: 5*

Ingredients:

- ¾ cup all-purpose flour
- ¾ cup whole wheat flour
- 2/3 teaspoon baking powder
- 6 oz butter, cold and cubed
- 4 oz applesauce
- 2-4 tablespoons cold water
- ½ cup brown sugar
- 1 ½ pounds plums, pitted and sliced
- 1 teaspoon fresh grated ginger
- 1 teaspoon cinnamon
- 2 tablespoons cornstarch

Directions:

1. In a bowl, toss together the plums with the brown sugar, cinnamon, ginger and cornstarch. Set aside.
2. In another bowl, mix the flours with the baking powder, then stir in the butter cubes and mix well until it looks sandy. Add the applesauce and cold water, spoon by spoon, mixing well until the dough comes together. No need to knead the dough. Envelope it in plastic wrap and then refrigerate for 30 minutes.
3. After 30 minutes, flour your working surface well and transfer the dough there. Divide it into 2 pieces and roll each one into a 9-inch circle. Spoon the filling in the centre of the dough and spread it out to the edges. Carefully lift the edges and wrap them over the filling to the centre, leaving the middle exposed.
4. Bake in the preheated oven at 375F for 20-30 minutes or until golden brown on the edges.
5. Serve cold with a drizzle of fresh cream.

975. Plum Cream Cheese Bread

Prep Time: *15 Minutes* | *Cook Time:* *45 Minutes* | *Servings: 7*

Ingredients:

- 1 cup all-purpose flour
- 1 cup rolled oats
- 1 teaspoon baking powder
- ½ teaspoon baking soda
- 1 pinch of salt
- 8oz butter, room temperature
- 2 eggs
- 1 teaspoon vanilla extract
- ¼ teaspoon almond extract
- 5 oz plums, pitted and cubed
- 4 oz low-fat cream cheese, room temperature ¼ cup brown sugar

Directions:

1. Mix the dry ingredients: flour, oats, baking powder, baking soda and salt in a bowl. In a separate bowl, mix the butter with the sugar until fluffy and creamy. Add the eggs, one by one, then the vanilla and almond extract, followed by the cream cheese.
2. Mix well, then incorporate the dry ingredients gradually. When the mixture is well mixed, fold in the cubed plums and spoon the batter into a loaf pan lined with baking paper.
3. Bake in the preheated oven at 350F for 30-40 minutes or until fluffy and golden brown.

976. Red Wine Plum Cobbler

Prep Time: *15 Minutes* *Cook Time:* *56 Minutes* *Servings: 2*

Ingredients:

- 2 pounds red and black plums, pitted and sliced
- 1 apple, peeled, cored and sliced
- juice from 1 orange
- 1 teaspoon orange zest
- ½ cup red wine
- ½ teaspoon cinnamon
- 2 tablespoons cornstarch
- 4 tablespoons sugar
- 1 cup all-purpose flour
- ¼ cup whole wheat flour
- 1 teaspoon baking powder
- 1 egg
- ½ cup buttermilk
- 1 oz melted butter
- 1 pinch of salt

Directions:

1. Mix the plums with the apple, orange juice and zest, red wine and cinnamon in a bowl. Add the cornstarch and sugar and mix well. Transfer into a 9-inch deep-dish square pan.
2. To make the topping, mix the flours with the baking powder and salt in a bowl. Add the egg, butter and buttermilk at once and mix until well combined.
3. Drop spoonfuls of batter over the fruits. It doesn't have to be even, so don't bother with spreading it evenly over the fruits.
4. Bake in the preheated oven at 350F for 40-50 minutes or until the fruits are tender and the topping is golden brown, and the edges are bubbling with fruits juice.

977. Plum and Chocolate Flognarde

Prep Time: *15 Minutes* *Cook Time:* *20 Minutes* *Servings: 7*

Ingredients:

- 6 large plums, pitted and sliced
- 1 oz butter
- 2oz all-purpose flour
- 1oz cocoa powder
- ½ cup sugar
- 2 oz dark chocolate, melted and cooled
- 1 ½ cups heavy cream
- 3 eggs
- butter to grease the pan

Directions:

1. In a pan, heat the butter over medium flame. Add the plums and cook for 5 minutes. Set aside.
2. 3In a bowl, combine the cocoa powder and sugar with the flour, then stir in the heavy cream and eggs. Mix well, then stir in the melted chocolate.
3. Grease 1 5-inch round cake pan with butter and spoon the batter into the pan. Top with sautéed plums and bake in the preheated oven at 375F for 20-30 minutes.

978. Plum and Amaretti Bowls

Prep Time: *15 Minutes* *Cook Time:* *30 Minutes* *Servings: 2*

Ingredients:

- ½ cup sugar
- 6 large plums, cut in quarters and pitted
- 1 cinnamon stick
- 6 amaretti cookies, crushed
- ½ cup water

Directions:

1. Add the water as well as sugar into a saucepan and bring to a boil. Add the cinnamon stick and plums and simmer on low heat for 5-10 minutes until the fruits are tender but still hold their shape. Spoon the fruits into large serving glasses or bowls and top with crushed amaretti just before serving. You can also pour a scoop of vanilla ice cream.

979. Plum and Oatmeal Crumble

Prep Time: *15 Minutes* *Cook Time:* *35 Minutes* *Servings: 7*

Ingredients:

- 1 pound ripe plums, pitted and halved
- 4 tablespoons maple syrup
- 2 oz cold butter, cubed
- ½ cup rolled oats
- ½ cup whole wheat flour
- 1 teaspoon cinnamon
- 1 tablespoon sugar
- ¼ cup sliced almonds

Directions:

1. Take a 9-inch square pan and arrange the plums in it.
2. In a bowl, mix the rolled oats with flour, cinnamon, sugar and cold butter. Rub the butter with your fingertips until the mixture looks sandy. Spoon the mixture over the fruits in the pan and top with sliced almonds. Bake in the before heated oven at 350F for 30 minutes.
3. When complete, remove it from the oven and let it cool before serving. Serve with a scoop of ice cream or fresh cream.

980. Roasted Plum and Raisins

Prep Time: *15 Minutes* *Cook Time:* *20 Minutes* *Servings: 3*

Ingredients:

- 8 large plums, halved and pitted
- ¼ cup dark rum
- ¼ cup raisins
- 2 tablespoons brown sugar
- ¼ teaspoon cinnamon powder

Directions:

1. Mix the raisins with the rum in a bowl and let them soak overnight. Arrange the plum halves in a baking pan, making sure the cut is facing up. Combine the soaked raisins with the sugar and cinnamon, then spoon the mixture over each plum.
2. Bake in the before heated oven at 375F for 15-20 minutes until the fruits are tender and fragrant.

981. Berry Cobbler

Prep Time: *15 Minutes* *Cook Time:* *39 Minutes* *Servings: 2*

Ingredients:

- 4 cups fresh berries
- ½ cup sugar
- 2 tablespoons cornstarch
- ½ cup all-purpose white flour
- 1 cup whole wheat flour
- 2 teaspoons baking powder
- 1 pinch of salt
- 3 oz butter, cubed
- ¾ cup sour cream
- ¼ cup brown sugar

Directions:

1. Mix the berries with sugar and cornstarch, then transfer them into a 9x13-inch deep dish baking pan. Place the pan aside.
2. In another bowl, combine the flours with a pinch of salt, sugar and baking powder, then rub in the cubed butter until the mixture looks sandy. Stir in the sour cream, then spoon the batter over the berries.
3. Bake in the before heated oven at 350F for 30-40 minutes or until just slightly golden brown on top. When done, scoop it into bowls and serve with a scoop of ice cream on top.

982. Chocolate and Plum Cheesecake

Prep Time: *15 Minutes* *Cook Time:* *45 Minutes* *Servings: 3*

Ingredients:

- Crust:
- 10oz graham cracker
- 2 tablespoons brown sugar
- 4 oz butter, melted
- 2 oz applesauce
- Filling:
- 15oz low-fat cream cheese
- 15oz plain yoghurt
- 2/3 cup sugar
- 2 tablespoons cornstarch
- 3 eggs
- 2 teaspoons vanilla extract
- 4 oz dark chocolate, melted
- 1 pinch salt
- Topping:
- 1 pound plums, pitted and sliced
- 2 tablespoons sugar
- 1 cinnamon stick
- 1-star anise
- ¼ cup water

Directions:

1. To make the crust: Place the crackers and sugar in a food processor and pulse until ground. Now add in the melted butter with pulse until well mixed. Transfer on a 10-inch round cake pan and press the dough on the bottom and sides of the pan with your fingertips. Set the pan aside.
2. To make the filling: Mix the cream cheese with the yoghurt, sugar and eggs, then add the vanilla, cornstarch, salt and melted chocolate. Pour this filling into the pan and bake in the preheated oven at 350F for 40-50 minutes. If needed, lower the temperature a few degrees during baking. When complete, remove from the oven and let it cool in the pan first, then transfer on a serving plate.

983. Cherry Blondies

Prep Time: *15 Minutes* *Cook Time:* *15 Minutes* *Servings: 2*

Ingredients:

- 1 cup whole wheat flour
- 1 2/3 cups all-purpose flour
- 1 pinch of salt
- 1 teaspoon baking powder
- ½ cup sugar

- 3 eggs
- 6 oz butter, softened
- 1 teaspoon vanilla extract
- 1 cup fresh cherries, chopped
- ½ cup white chocolate chips

Directions:

1. In a bowl, add the butter with the sugar until creamy and fluffy, then add the eggs and vanilla extract.
2. Stir in the flours mixed with a pinch of salt and baking powder, then fold in the dried cherries and chocolate chips.
3. To make sure the cherries don't sink to the bottom of the pan, sprinkle them with flour before folding them into the batter. Spoon the batter into a 9x13-inch pan and bake in the preheated oven at 350F for 30-35 minutes or until slightly golden brown on top. Let it cool in the pan before serving.

984. Cherry Pie

Prep Time: *15 Minutes* | *Cook Time:* *35 Minutes* | *Servings: 3*

Ingredients:

- Crust:
- 1 cup whole wheat flour
- ½ cup all-purpose flour
- ½ cup almond meal
- 6oz cold butter, cut into cubes
- 2 tablespoons sugar
- 2 tablespoons cold water
- Filling:
- 2 cups pitted cherries
- 2 cups sour cherries, pitted
- ¼ cup brown sugar
- ¼ cup cornstarch
- ¼ teaspoon cinnamon.

Directions:

1. To make the crust: In a bowl, mix the flours with the almond meal, sugar and a pinch of salt. Rub in the cold butter until the mixture looks sandy.
2. Stir in the cold water and mix gently until the dough comes together. Transfer on a well-floured surface and divide the dough into 2 equal pieces. Roll both of them into 2 thin round sheets. Take 1 sheet and arrange it into a tart pan. Crimp the edges to look more rustic.
3. In a bowl, mix the cherries with sugar, cornstarch and cinnamon. Transfer this mixture into the pie crust. Top with a second dough sheet and make a few holes on top to allow the steams to come out.
4. Bake in the oven after heating at 350F for 40-50 minutes or until crisp and golden brown

985. Boozy Cherry Ice Cream

Prep Time: *15 Minutes* | *Cook Time:* *35 Minutes* | *Servings:6*

Ingredients:

- 2 cups cherries, pitted and mixed with 1 cup vodka overnight
- 1 cup coconut milk
- 1 cup coconut cream
- 1 cup almond milk
- ¼ cup honey
- ½ cup dark chocolate chips

Directions:

1. In a bowl, add the coconut milk with almond milk, coconut cream and honey. Pour this mixture into your ice cream maker and freeze according to your machine's instructions.
2. When almost done, throw in the drunken cherries and chocolate chips. Serve immediately scooped in bowls or serving glasses or store in an airtight container until needed

986. Pear and Honey Bread

Prep Time: *15 Minutes* | *Cook Time:* *7 Minutes* | *Servings: 2*

Ingredients:

- ½ cup brown sugar
- ½ cup honey
- ½ cup olive oil
- ½ cup applesauce
- 3 eggs
- 2 ¼ cups whole wheat flour
- 2/3 cup all-purpose flour
- 2 tsp baking powder
- 1 tsp all spices
- ½ tsp cinnamon
- 1 pinch of salt
- 1 tsp vanilla extract
- 2 tbsp chia seeds
- 5 pears, peeled and diced

Directions:

1. In a bowl, stir the oil with the brown sugar, honey and applesauce. Once well combined, add the eggs, vanilla extract, all spices and cinnamon.
2. Stir in the flours sifted with the baking powder. Fold in the diced pear, then evenly spread the batter between 2 small loaf pans.
3. Bake in the before heating oven at 350F for 40-50 minutes. The best way to check if it's done is to insert a skewer in the middle of the cake. If it comes out clean of any crumbs, it is done.
4. Let it cool in the pan before To converting on a serving plate.

Breakfast & Brunch Recipes

987. Johnnycakes

Prep Time: *15 Minutes* *Cook Time:* *16 Minutes* *Servings: 6*

Ingredients:

- 1 cup ground cornmeal ½ tsp salt 1/3 cup water 1 cup milk

Directions:

1. Mix the cornmeal and the salt.
2. Warm up the milk and water. Pour into cornmeal mix.
3. Butter a skillet and a tablespoon to drop the batter.
4. Fry the johnnycakes until browned on both sides.
5. Serve with applesauce or butter.

988. Apple Pancakes

Prep Time: *15 Minutes* *Cook Time: 45* *Minutes* *Servings: 2*

Ingredients:

- 2 Granny Smith apples, peeled and cut into small, thin slices ¼ cup cane sugar
- 3 tsp cinnamon
- 3 beaten eggs
- tsp salt ½ cup flour ½ cup milk ½ tsp vanilla
- ½ cup sweet butter

Directions:

1. Preheat oven to 425 degrees.
2. Mix together the cinnamon and sugar.
3. In another bowl, whip the eggs, flour, milk, salt, and vanilla until the mixture is smooth.
4. Melt the butter in a skillet. Add the apples and the cinnamon sugar. Stir and cook for 5 minutes.
5. Place the batter in a baking dish. Pour the apples on top of the batter.
6. Bake for 20 minutes.
7. Flip the pancake upside down on a plate. Once the pancake deflates (it will), cut and serve.

989. Almond Pancakes

Prep Time: *15 Minutes* *Cook Time:* *23 Minutes* *Servings: 2*

Ingredients:

- 1 ¾ cups cake flour
- ¼ cup almond flour
- ¼ cup instant-cooking oats
- 2 tsp baking soda
- 1 tsp salt
- 2 eggs
- ½ cup sliced almonds

Directions:

1. Mix together the flours, oats, baking soda and salt.
2. Use a second bowl to stir together the eggs and buttermilk.
3. Mix the egg/milk mixture into the flour and stir until all ingredients are well-blended.
4. Grease a skillet and add a quarter cup of batter. Top the batter with some almonds.
5. Cook the pancake until browned on one side, then flip.
6. Repeat with the rest of the batter.

990. Belgian Waffles

Prep Time: *15 Minutes* *Cook Time:* *34 Minutes* *Servings:4*

Ingredients:

- 2 cups cake flour
- 2 tsp baking powder
- ½ tsp salt
- 4 large eggs, cut into whites and yolks
- 2 tbsp cane sugar
- ½ tsp vanilla
- 4 tbsp sweet butter
- 2 cups milk
- Vegetable cooking spray

Directions:

1. Preheat the waffle iron.
2. Transfer the flour, baking powder and salt into a bowl.
3. In another bowl, beat the yolks and sugar until well-blended.
4. Mix in the vanilla, butter, and milk and use a whisk to mix.
5. Plus the egg mix to the flour mix. Blend well.
6. Whip the egg whites with a hand mixer. Fold the egg whites into the batter.
7. Spray the waffle iron with vegetable spray.
8. Transfer some of the batters to the waffle iron.
9. Cook until waffles are nice and brown.

991. Chocolate Waffle

Prep Time: *15 Minutes* *Cook Time:* *20 Minutes* *Servings: 2*

Ingredients:

- 1 ½ cups all-purpose flour
- 4 tbsp sugar
- ½ cocoa powder
- 1 ½ tsp baking powder
- 1 tsp salt
- 3 large eggs
- 2 tbsp sweet butter
- 1 tsp vanilla
- 1/3 cup buttermilk
- cup chocolate chips Vegetable spray

Directions:

1. Preheat waffle iron.
2. Mix together the flour, cocoa, baking powder, and salt.
3. Use another bowl to beat the eggs, vanilla, and butter. Add the buttermilk and mix.
4. Mix in the chocolate chips and combine.
5. Let batter sit for 10 minutes.
6. Spray the waffle iron with vegetable spray.
7. Transfer batter to the waffle iron.
8. Cook until waffles are golden brown on each side.
9. Repeat with all of the batters. Keep the waffles warm.

992. Quiche, Crepes and Souffles

Prep Time: *15 Minutes* *Cook Time:* *18 Minutes* *Servings :4*

Ingredients:

- 1 9-inch store-bought piecrust
- Salt and pepper to taste
- 1 cup diced ham
- 4 eggs
- cup half-and-half 1/8 tsp nutmeg
- 8 oz. diced Swiss cheese

Directions:

1. Preheat oven to 375 degrees.
2. Mix together the eggs, ham, half-and-half, nutmeg, and cheese.
3. Season to taste.
4. Transfer the eggs to the pre-made crust.
5. Bake for 35 minutes.

993. Filled Crepes

Prep Time: *15 Minutes* *Cook Time:* *33 Minutes* *Servings :4*

Ingredients:

- 1 cup flour
- 1 cup milk
- cup heavy cream
- ½ tsp baking powder ¼ cup sweet butter
- ½ cup sliced mushrooms 1 chopped onion
- 1 tablespoon flour
- 1 cup cream
- 1 cup diced ham
- Salt and pepper to taste

Directions:

1. Mix together the milk, flour, baking powder and chill overnight.
2. Melt half of the butter in a crepe pan. Add ¼ cup of the batter.
3. Turn and rotate the crepe pan. Cook until one side is golden brown, then flip and cook the other side.
4. Repeat until batter is used up.
5. Melt the remaining butter and saute the mushrooms and the onions. Mix in the ham, and add the flour and the milk to thicken the filling.
6. Divide the filling between the crepes. Roll the crepe closed.

994. Cheese Souffle

Prep Time: *15 Minutes* *Cook Time:* *37 Minutes* *Servings :4*

Ingredients:

- ¼ cup grated Parmesan cheese 5 tbsp sweet butter
- 2 tbsp all-purpose flour
- 2 tbsp pastry flour
- 1 cup heavy cream
- ¾ cup water
- `2 cups of shredded cheddar cheese Salt and pepper to taste
- 6 eggs, divided into whites and yolks.

Directions:

1. Preheat oven to 350 degrees.
2. Butter a 2-qrt souffle dish. Dust the bottom of the dish with the Parmesan cheese.
3. Use a saucepan to melt the butter. Add both flours. Mix vigorously.
4. While continuing to whisk, add the cream and water. Add the remaining Parmesan, cheddar, and salt and pepper.
5. Stir until mixture boils.

6. Take the saucepan off the stove and add the yolks. Whisk until integrated.
7. Pour the mixture into a bowl and let sit.
8. Beat the egg whites with a hand mixer for 5 minutes.
9. Add the egg whites into the egg mixture.
10. Transfer the soufflé into the soufflé dish.
11. Bake for 40 minutes.

995. Ham and Cheese Soufflé

Prep Time: 15 Minutes *Cook Time: 36 Minutes* *Servings: 2*

Ingredients:

- 3 tbsp sweet butter 1 chopped shallot 2 tbsp. Cake flour 1 1/2 cups whole milk 4 oz. Grated mild cheddar 1/2 tsp.
- Mustard powder 6 eggs, divided into whites and yolks Salt and pepper to taste 4 oz.
- Chopped ham 1 1/2 tbsp. chopped chives

Directions:

1. Melt 2 tablespoons butter in a saucepan. Mix in the shallots and stir for 2 minutes.
2. Stir in the flour.
3. Add the milk. Keep whisking until smooth.
4. Let the mixture simmer for 5 minutes. It should be thick by then.
5. Add the cheddar, salt and pepper, and egg yolks.
6. Keep stirring for 4 minutes.
7. Pour the mixture into a bowl and stir in the chives and ham.
8. After completely cover with plastic and refrigerate it for half an hour.
9. Preheat the oven to 375 degrees.
10. Butter a soufflé dish.
11. Beat the eggs whites with a hand mixer until they are stiff.
12. Fold the whites into the cheese mix.
13. Pour the batter into the soufflé dish.
14. Bake for 40 minutes.

996. Breakfast Enchiladas

Prep Time: 15 Minutes *Cook Time: 23 Minutes* *Servings :5*

Ingredients:

- 1/3 cup butter
- 1/3 cup all-purpose flour
- 3 cups whole milk
- 8 oz. shredded Cheddar cheese
- 4 tbsp chopped chilis
- ½ tsp salt

Directions:

1. Melt the butter, then add the flour.
2. Stir until the mixture is smooth.
3. Put the milk, keep whisking until the mixture is thickened.
4. Place pan on the counter and stir in all of the other ingredients.

997. Sausage Twist

Prep Time: 15 Minutes *Cook Time: 30 Minutes* *Servings :6*

Ingredients:

- 1 frozen pizza dough
- 1 pkg. breakfast sausage
- ½ cup chopped olives
- 4 oz. shredded Mozzarella cheese
- cup feta cheese 1 large egg

Directions:

1. Preheat oven to 400 degrees.
2. Flatten out the dough on a baking sheet.
3. Top the dough with sausage, olives and cheeses.
4. Fold the dough over the filling and make diagonal cuts on top.
5. Beat the egg and brush over the dough.
6. Bake for 20 minutes.
7. The dough should be a light brown.
8. Slice the dough into six portions.

998. Breakfast Burritos

Prep Time: 15 Minutes *Cook Time: 50 Minutes* *Servings: 2*

Ingredients:

- 1 package hot breakfast sausage
- 1 cup chopped green pepper
- 1 chopped jalapeno peppers
- 8 large eggs
- 2 tbsp whole milk
- 4 oz. cream cheese
- 8 flour tortillas
- Use whatever toppings you like:
- Shredded cheese
- Black Beans
- Chopped avocado
- Salsa

Directions:

1. The sausage, pepper and jalapeno pepper are frying for 10 minutes.
2. Drain the fat, but leave sausages in the skillet.
3. Mix the eggs and the milk. Add the mixture to the skillet.
4. Cook until the eggs are just are completely cooked. Mix the cream cheese and continue cooking until the cream cheese is blended. Keep the mixture warm.
5. Warm the tortillas in a skillet.
6. Divide the sausage mixture onto each tortilla. Roll up the tortilla and fold to close.
7. Repeat with all of the tortillas.
8. Place the toppings in a separate bowl.

999. Stuffed French Toast

Prep Time: 15 Minutes *Cook Time: 39 Minutes* *Servings: 2*

Ingredients:

- 3 cups of cubed bread
- 8 large eggs
- 8 oz. cream cheese
- cup honey 1 ¼ cups milk

Directions:

1. Blend the eggs, milk, and honey in a bowl.
2. After putting half of the bread on the bottom of a 9 x 13-inch baking dish.
3. Top with the cream cheese and the remaining bread.
4. Top the bread with the egg mixture, making sure to coat all, and chill overnight.
5. Bake at 350 degrees for 35 minutes.
6. Top with butter or syrup.

1000. Breakfast Frittata

Prep Time: 15 Minutes *Cook Time:20 Minutes* *Servings :4*

Ingredients:

- 6 slices of chopped bacon
- 1 cup diced green pepper
- Salt and pepper to taste
- 1 cup diced cooked potatoes
- 10 beaten eggs
- 2 oz. feta cheese

Directions:

1. Fry the bacon in a skillet. When bacon is crispy, mix in the green pepper.
2. Stir for approximately 3 minutes.
3. To put out the skillet from the stove and drain any excess fat. Add the salt and pepper.
4. Place the skillet back on the stove and mix in the diced potatoes. Stir for approximately 2 minutes. Add the eggs. Stir for 5 minutes. Eggs should still be soft.
5. Top frittata with the feta cheese.
6. Preheat the broiler.
7. Broil frittatas for 5 minutes.

1001. Egg pork Breakfast

Prep Time: 15 Minutes *Cook Time: 35 Minutes* *Servings :4*

Ingredients:

- 1 lb. mild ground pork sausage
- 3 tbsp sweet butter
- 4 sliced scallions
- 3 tbsp chopped cilantro
- 14 large eggs
- Salt and pepper to taste
- 8 flour tortillas
- 4 oz. shredded Monterey Jack cheese

Directions:

1. Crumble and fry the sausage in a skillet. Drain on a paper towel.
2. Use another skillet to melt the butter.
3. Add the scallions, eggs, salt and pepper and cook for 5 minutes.
4. Place the mixture in a bowl and mix in the sausage and 1 cup of cheese sauce (see recipe below).
5. Divide the mix onto each tortilla.
6. Roll up the tortilla and transfer them to a buttered 9 x 13 baking dish.
7. Top with the rest of the cheese sauce and the Monterey Jack.
8. Bake for half an hour at 350 degrees.
9. Serve with toppings.

1002. Superfoods Oatmeal Breakfast

Prep Time: 15 Minutes *Cook Time: 23 Minutes* *Servings: 2*

Ingredients:

- 1 cup cooked oatmeal
- 1 tsp. Of ground flax seeds 1 tsp. of sunflower seeds
- A dash of cinnamon
- Half of the tsp. of cocoa

Directions:

1. Cook oatmeal with hot water, and after that, mix all ingredients. Sweeten if you have to with few drops of raw honey. Optional: You can replace sunflower seeds with pumpkin seed or chia seed. You can add a handful of blueberries or any berries instead of cocoa.

1003. Oatmeal Yogurt Breakfast

Prep Time: 15 Minutes *Cook Time: 33 Minutes* *Servings :6*

Ingredients:

- ½ cup dry oatmeal
- A handful of blueberries (optional)
- 1 cup of low-fat yoghurt

Directio:

1. Mix all ingredients and wait 20 minutes or leave overnight in the fridge if using steel cut oats.

1004. Cocoa Oatmeal

Prep Time: *15 Minutes* *Cook Time:* *20 Minutes* *Servings :6*

Ingredients

- ½ cup oats
- 2 cups water
- A pinch tsp. Salt
- ½ tsp. Ground vanilla bean 2 tbsp. cocoa powder
- 1 tbsp. raw honey
- 2 tbsp. ground flax seeds meal a dash of cinnamon
- 2 egg whites

Directions:

1. In a saucepan over high heat, place the oats and salt. Cover with 3 cups water. Bring to a boil and cook for 3-5 minutes, stirring occasionally. Keep adding ½ cup water if necessary as the mixture thickens.
2. In a separate bowl, whisk 4 tbsp. Water into the 4 tbsp. Cocoa powder to form a smooth sauce. Add the vanilla to the pan and stir.
3. Turn the heat down to low. Add the egg whites and whisk immediately. Add the flax meal and cinnamon. Stir to combine. Remove from heat, add raw honey and serve immediately.

Topping suggestions:

- sliced strawberries, blueberries or few almonds.

1005. Flax and Blueberry Vanilla Overnight Oats

Prep Time: *15 Minutes* *Cook Time:* *32 Minutes* *Servings: 2*

Ingredients:

½ cup oats
¼ cup water
¼ cup low-fat yoghurt
½ tsp. Ground vanilla bean 1 tbsp. flax seeds meal A pinch of salt
Blueberries walnuts blackberries raw honey for topping

Directions:

1. 2Add the ingredients (except for toppings) to the bowl in the evening.
2. Refrigerate overnight.
3. In the morning, stir up the mixture. It should be thick. Add the toppings of your choice.

1006. Apple Oatmeal

Prep Time: *15 Minutes* *Cook Time:* *10 Minutes* *Servings: 2*

Ingredients:

- 1 grated apple
- ½ cup oats
- 1 cup water
- Dash of cinnamon
- 2 tsp. raw honey

Directions:

1. Cook the oats with the water for 3-5 minutes.
2. Add grated apple and cinnamon. Stir in the raw honey.

1007. Almond Butter Banana Oats

Prep Time: *15 Minutes* *Cook Time:* *4 Minutes* *Servings :8*

Ingredients:

- ½ cup oats
- ¾ cup water
- 1 egg white
- 1 banana 1 tbs. Flax seeds meal 1 tsp raw honey
- pinch cinnamon
- ½ tbs. almond butter

Directions:

1. Combine oats and water in a bowl. Egg white beat, then whisk it in with the uncooked oats.
2. Boil on the stovetop after checking consistency and continue to heat as necessary until the oats are fluffy and thick.
3. Mash banana and add to oats. Heat for 1-minute stir in flax, raw honey and cinnamon. Top with almond butter!

1008. Coconut Pomegranate Oatmeal

Prep Time: *15 Minutes* *Cook Time:* *3 Minutes* *Servings :8*

Ingredients:

- ½ cup oats
- 1/3 cup coconut milk
- 1 cup water
- 2 tbs. shredded unsweetened coconut
- 1-2 tbs. Flax seeds meal 1 tbs. raw honey
- 3 tbs. pomegranate seeds
- Cook oats with coconut milk, water and salt.

Directions:

1. Stir in the coconut raw honey and flaxseed meal. Sprinkle with extra coconut and pomegranate seeds.

1009. Banana Almond Overnight Oats

Prep Time: *15 Minutes* *Cook Time:* *3 Minutes* *Servings: 2*

Ingredients:

- ½ cup oats
- ½ cup coconut milk
- 1 banana 1 tbs. flax seeds meal 1 tsp raw honey
- pinch cinnamon
- 1 tsp dried cranberries 2 Brazil nuts ½ tbs. almond butter

Directions:

1. Make a smoothie with banana coconut milk, almond butter, honey and cinnamon. Stir in flax and oatmeal and leave overnight. Top with 1 tsp. Dried cranberries, Brazil nuts.

1010. Walnut Oatmeal with Fresh Blueberries

Prep Time: *15 Minutes* *Cook Time:* *15 Minutes* *Servings :8*

Ingredients:

- ½ cup blueberries
- ½ cup oats
- 1 cup water
- ½ cup walnuts Dash of cinnamon
- 2 tsp. raw honey

Directions:

1. Cook the oats with the water for 3-5 minutes.
2. Add walnuts and cinnamon. Stir in the raw honey. Top with blueberries

1011. Raspberry Oatmeal

Prep Time: *15 Minutes* *Cook Time:* *5 Minutes* *Servings :8*

Ingredients:

- ½ cup raspberries
- ½ cup oats
- 1 cup water
- ½ cup sesame seeds
- Dash of cinnamon
- 2 tsp. raw honey

Directions:

1. 2Cook the oats with the water for 3-5 minutes.
2. Add sesame seeds and cinnamon. Stir in the raw honey. Top with raspberries

1012. Strawberry Oatmeal

Prep Time: *15 Minutes* *Cook Time:* *10 Minutes* *Servings: 2*

Ingredients:

- ½ cup strawberries
- ½ cup oats
- 1 cup water
- 2 Tbsp. sunflower seeds
- 1 Tbsp. Raisins 2 tsp. raw honey

Directions:

1. Cook the oats with the water for 3-5 minutes.
2. Add sesame seeds and cinnamon. Stir in the raw honey. Top with raspberries

1013. Kiwi Oatmeal

Prep Time: *15 Minutes* *Cook Time:* *5 Minutes* *Servings :4*

Ingredients:

- 1 sliced kiwi
- ½ cup oats
- 1 cup water
- 2 Tbsp. pumpkin seeds
- 1 Tbsp. Raisins 2 tsp. raw honey

Directions:

1. Cook the oats with the water for 3-5 minutes.
2. Add sesame seeds and cinnamon. Stir in the raw honey. Top with raspberries

1014. Coconut Chia Puddin

Prep Time: *15 Minutes* *Cook Time:* *15 Minutes* *Servings :3*

Ingredients

- ¼ cup Chia seeds
- 1 cup coconut milk ½ tbs Royall jelly 1 tsp.
- Ground Vanilla Bean a pinch of Nutmeg Top with Blueberries

Directions:

1. Mix all ingredients except blueberries and leave overnight in the fridge. Top with blueberries.

1015. Coconut Pomegranate Chia Pudding

Prep Time: *15 Minutes* | *Cook Time:* *23 Minutes* | *Servings :3*

Ingredients

- ¼ cup Chia seeds
- 1 cup Coconut milk
- ½ tablespoon Raw honey
- ½ tablespoon Coconut flakes
- Top with Pomegranate seeds

Directions:

1. Mix all ingredients except pomegranate and leave overnight in the fridge. Top with pomegranate.

1016. Yogurt & Mango Chia Pudding

Prep Time: *15 Minutes* | *Cook Time:* *3 Minutes* | *Servings: 2*

Ingredients

- ¼ cup Chia seeds 1 ½ cup yoghurt 1 tablespoon raw honey
- ½ cup chopped Mango

Directions:

1. 2Mix 1 cup of yoghurt honey and chia seeds and leave overnight in the fridge.
2. Divide into 2 glasses, top each with ¼ cup yoghurt and ¼ cup mango.

Lunch Recipes

1017. Easy Muesli recipe

Prep Time: *15 Minutes* | *Cook Time:* *33 Minutes* | *Servings: 2*

INGREDIENTS

- 3 1/2 cups moved oats
- 1/2 cup wheat grain
- 1/2 teaspoon fit salt
- 1/2 teaspoon ground cinnamon
- 1/2 cup cut almonds
- 1/4 cup crude walnuts, coarsely chopped
- 1/4 cup crude pepitas (shelled pumpkin seeds)
- 1/2 cup unsweetened coconut drops
- 1/4 cup dried apricots, coarsely chopped
- 1/4 cup dried cherries
- Estimating cups and spoons
- Enormous rimmed heating sheet
- Enormous bowl
- Enormous hermetically sealed holder, for putting away

DIRECTIONS:

1. Toast the grains, nuts, and seeds. Mastermind 2 racks to partition the oven into thirds and heat to 350°F. Spot the oats, wheat grain, salt, and cinnamon on a rimmed heating sheet; throw to join; and spread into an even layer. Spot the almonds, walnuts, and pepitas on a second rimmed heating sheet; throw to join; and spread into an even layer. Move both preparing sheets to oven, putting oats on top rack and nuts on base. Heat until nuts is fragrant, 10 to 12 minutes.
2. Add the coconut. Eliminate the heating sheet with the nuts and put to the side to cool. Sprinkle the coconut over the oats, get back to the upper rack, and heat until the coconut is brilliant brown, around 5 minutes more. Eliminate from oven and put to the side to cool, around 10 minutes.
3. Move to an enormous bowl. Move the substance of both heating sheets to a huge bowl.
4. Add the dried natural product. Add the apricots and cherries and throw to consolidate.
5. Move to a sealed shut holder. Muesli can be put away in an impermeable holder at room temperature for as long as multi month.
6. Enjoy as wanted. Enjoy as oats, grain, short-term oats, or with yogurt, finished off with new products of the soil sprinkle of nectar or maple syrup, whenever wanted.
7. NOTES
8. Capacity: Muesli can be put away in a sealed shut holder for as long as multi month.
9. Serving ideas: To make for the time being oats, consolidate equivalent amounts of muesli and milk or non-dairy milk (I favor 2/3 cup of each) in a little lidded compartment (now I like to finish off mine with frozen blueberries, as well). Refrigerate expedite and enjoy cold in the first part of the day.

1018. Salmon with Smoky Spinach and Chickpeas

Prep Time: *15 Minutes* | *Cook Time:* *73 Minutes* | *Servings :6*

INGREDIENTS

- 4 (6-ounce) skin-on salmon filets
- 1/2 teaspoon fit salt, in addition to additional for preparing
- 1/4 teaspoon newly ground dark pepper, in addition to additional for preparing
- 4 tablespoons olive oil, isolated
- 2 (around 15-ounce) jars chickpeas
- 3 cloves garlic
- 1 teaspoon smoked paprika
- 1 (14.5-ounce) can normal or fire-simmered diced tomatoes
- 5 ounces infant spinach (around 5 stuffed cups)
- 2 teaspoons balsamic vinegar

DIRECTIONS:

1. Wipe 4 salmon filets off with paper towels. Season on the two sides with genuine salt and dark pepper.
2. Heat 2 tablespoons of the olive oil in an enormous cast iron or non-stick skillet over medium-high heat until shining. Spot the salmon skin-side down in the skillet, at that point push down on them so the skin is in even contact with the dish and browns equitably. Decrease the heat to medium-low and cook undisturbed, delicately pushing down on fish now and again, until the sides are concocted mostly the filets, 6 to 9 minutes, contingent upon the thickness of your filets. In the mean time, channel and wash 2 jars chickpeas. Crush and strip 3 garlic cloves.
3. Move the salmon skin-side up to a plate (it won't be cooked through). Add the excess 2 tablespoons olive oil to the skillet. Add the garlic and sauté until mollified and simply beginning to brown, around 2 minutes. Add 1 teaspoon smoked paprika and sauté until fragrant, around 1 moment.
4. Add the chickpeas, 1 can dice tomatoes and their juices, 1/2 teaspoon fit salt, and 1/4 teaspoon dark pepper. Mix to consolidate. Increment the heat to medium to bring to a stew. Stew for 5 minutes to permit the flavors to merge.
5. Mix in 5 ounces child spinach, a couple of small bunches all at once, until just shriveled, around 2 minutes. Mix in 2 teaspoons balsamic vinegar. Taste and season with salt and pepper depending on the situation.
6. Return the salmon skin-side up to the container, nestling them in the sauce. Keep on stewing for 2 to 5 minutes, contingent upon the thickness of your filets. A moment read thermometer into the center of the thickest filet should peruse 120°F to 130°F for medium-uncommon or 135°F to 145°F on the off chance that you favor it all the more all-around done. Serve the salmon, skin-side up, with the chickpeas and spinach.

1019. Mediterranean White Bean Soup

Prep Time: *15 Minutes* | *Cook Time:55* *Minutes* | *Servings: 2*

INGREDIENTS

- 2 (15-ounce) jars white beans
- 1 medium yellow onion
- 4 cloves garlic
- 1/4 teaspoon red pepper chips (discretionary)
- 2 tablespoons olive oil
- 4 cups low-sodium vegetable or chicken stock
- 1 (14-ounce) can diced tomatoes
- 2 twigs new rosemary
- 1 teaspoon legitimate salt
- 1/4 teaspoon newly ground dark pepper
- 1 Parmesan skin (discretionary)
- 5 ounces child spinach (around 5 stuffed cups)
- Ground Parmesan cheddar, for serving

DIRECTIONS:

1. Channel and wash 2 jars white beans and put in a safe spot. Finely slash 1 medium yellow onion and mince 4 cloves garlic.
2. Heat 2 tablespoons olive oil in a Dutch oven or huge pot until sparkling. Add the onion and sauté until relaxed and clear, 3 to 5 minutes. Add the garlic and 1/4 teaspoon red pepper pieces, if using, and sauté until fragrant, around brief more.
3. Pour in 4 cups low-sodium vegetable or chicken stock, 1 can diced tomatoes and their juices, and the white beans. Add 2 new rosemary twigs, 1 teaspoon legitimate salt, 1/4 teaspoon dark pepper, and 1 Parmesan skin, if using, and mix to join. Heat to the point of boiling. Lessen the heat to keep a stew, and stew uncovered for 10 minutes to permit the flavors to merge.
4. Mix in 5 ounces child spinach (around 5 stuffed cups); a couple of small bunches all at once, until just withered, 1 to 2 minutes. Serve decorated with ground Parmesan cheddar.
5. Formula NOTES
6. Substitute frozen spinach: Frozen spinach can be fill in for the new spinach. Basically mix in an equivalent weight (or more; this is adaptable) of frozen spinach and stew until heated through.
7. Add extra protein: If wanted, you can mix in a cup of shredded chicken (pulled from a rotisserie chicken, or canned chicken) into this soup in definite advance with the spinach.
8. Capacity: Leftovers can be put away in a water/air proof compartment in the cooler for as long as 5 days.

1020. Spaghetti Squash Shrimp Scampi

Prep Time: *15 Minutes* | *Cook Time:* *23 Minutes* | *Servings: 2*

INGREDIENTS

- 1 2 1/2-to 3-pound spaghetti squash, split the long way and cultivated
- 2 tablespoons extra-virgin olive oil
- 1 tablespoon minced garlic
- ½ teaspoon salt, isolated
- ⅓ cup dry white wine
- 1 pound stripped and deveined crude shrimp (16-20 for every pound), tails left on, whenever wanted
- 1 tablespoon lemon juice
- ¼ cup chopped new parsley
- 2 tablespoons unsalted margarine
- ¼ teaspoon ground pepper
- ¼ cup shredded Parmesan cheddar
- Lemon wedges for serving

DIRECTIONS:

1. Spot squash parts, cut-side down, in a microwave-safe dish; add 2 tablespoons water. Microwave, revealed, on High until the substance is delicate, around 10 minutes. (On the other hand, place squash parts, cut-side down, on a rimmed preparing sheet. Heat in a 400 degrees F oven until the squash is delicate, 40 to 50 minutes. You can likewise cook the squash in a pressing factor cooker/multi-cooker)
2. Stage 2
3. Then, heat oil in an enormous skillet over medium-high heat. Add garlic and 1/4 teaspoon salt; cook, blending, for 30 seconds. Cautiously add wine and bring to a stew. Add shrimp and cook, blending, until the shrimp are pink and just cooked through, 3 to 4 minutes. Eliminate from heat and mix in lemon juice.
4. Stage 3
5. Utilize a fork to scratch the squash substance from the shells into a medium bowl. Add parsley, margarine, pepper and the leftover 1/4 teaspoon salt; mix to consolidate. Serve the shrimp over the spaghetti squash. Sprinkle with Parmesan and present with a lemon wedge.

1021. Greek Roasted Fish with Vegetables

Prep Time: *15 Minutes* | *Cook Time:* *53 Minutes* | *Servings :6*

INGREDIENTS

- 1 pound fingerling potatoes, split the long way
- 2 tablespoons olive oil
- 5 garlic cloves, coarsely chopped
- ½ teaspoon ocean salt
- ½ teaspoon newly ground dark pepper
- 4 5 to 6-ounce new or frozen skinless salmon filets
- 2 medium red, yellow and additionally orange sweet peppers, cut into rings
- 2 cups cherry tomatoes
- 1 ½ cups chopped new parsley (1 pack)
- ¼ cup pitted kalamata olives, divided
- ¼ cup finely cut new oregano or 1 Tbsp. dried oregano, squashed

- 1 lemon

DIRECTIONS:

1. Stage 1
2. Preheat oven to 425 degrees F. Spot potatoes in a huge bowl. Shower with 1 Tbsp. of the oil and sprinkle with garlic and 1/8 tsp. of the salt and dark pepper; throw to cover. Move to a 15x10-inch heating skillet; cover with foil. Cook 30 minutes.
3. Stage 2
4. In the interim, defrost salmon, whenever frozen. Join, in a similar bowl, sweet peppers, tomatoes, parsley, olives, oregano and 1/8 tsp. of the salt and dark pepper. Shower with staying 1 Tbsp. oil; throw to cover.
5. Stage 3
6. Flush salmon; wipe off. Sprinkle with staying 1/4 tsp. salt and dark pepper. Spoon sweet pepper combination over potatoes and top with salmon. Broil, uncovered, 10 minutes more or just until salmon drops.
7. Stage 4
8. Eliminate zing from lemon. Crush juice from lemon over salmon and vegetables. Sprinkle with zing.

1022. Easy Roasted Tomato Basil Soup

Prep Time: *15 Minutes* | *Cook Time:* *30 Minutes* | *Servings :6*

INGREDIENTS

- 3 lb. Roma tomatoes divided
- 2 to 3 carrots stripped and cut into little pieces
- Additional virgin olive oil (I utilized Private Reserve Greek EVOO)
- Salt and pepper
- 2 medium yellow onions chopped
- 5 garlic cloves minced
- 1 cup canned squashed tomatoes
- 2 oz. new basil leaves
- 3 to 4 new thyme springs 2 tsp. thyme leaves
- 1 tsp. dry oregano
- ½ tsp. paprika
- ½ tsp. ground cumin
- 2 ½ cups water
- Sprinkle of lime juice optional

DIRECTIONS:

1. Heat oven to 450 degrees F.
2. In an enormous blending bowl, consolidate tomatoes and carrot pieces. Add a liberal shower of additional virgin olive oil, and season with fit salt and dark pepper. Throw to join.
3. Move to an enormous heating sheet and spread well in one layer. Broil in heated oven for around 30 minutes. At the point when prepared, eliminate from the heat and put in a safe spot for around 10 minutes to cool.
4. Move the broiled tomatoes and carrots to the enormous bowl of a food processor fitted with a cutting edge. Add simply a smidgen of water and mix.
5. In a huge cooking pot, heat 2 tbsp. additional virgin olive oil over medium-high heat until shining yet not smoking. Add onions and cook for around 3 minutes, at that point add garlic and cook momentarily until brilliant.
6. Empty the simmered tomato blend into the cooking pot. Mix in squashed tomatoes, 2 ½ cups water, basil, thyme and flavors. Season with a little genuine salt and dark pepper. Heat to the point of boiling, at that point lower heat and cover part-way. Let stew for around 20 minutes or somewhere in the vicinity.
7. Eliminate the thyme springs and move tomato basil soup to serving bowls. In the event that you like, add a sprinkle of lime juice and a liberal shower of extra virgihttps://shop.themediterraneandish.com/item/extra-virgin-olive-oil-pack/n olive oil. Present with your #1 dry bread or flame broiled bits of French loaf. Enjoy!
8. NOTES
9. Extras: If you have any extras, you can refrigerate in close top glass compartments for 3 to 4 days. Ensure the soup is totally cooled prior to putting away.
10. Would you be able to freeze this tomato basil soup? Indeed! Since this is a sans dairy veggie lover tomato basil soup and there is no cream required by any means, it is the ideal tomato soup to freeze. Essentially cool the soup prior to putting away in close cover, cooler safe compartments. Freeze for some time in the future (3 to a half year or something like that.) Thaw in ice chest short-term and go through medium heat to warm.
11. Varieties: If you're searching for somewhat of a smoky completion, add a decent touch of smoked paprika. Or then again, to zest things up, cook some jalapeno pepper and mix them alongside the tomatoes and carrots.

1023. Easy Greek-Style Eggplant Recipe

Prep Time: *15 Minutes* | *Cook Time:* *35 Minutes* | *Servings: 2*

INGREDIENTS

- 3 lb. Roma tomatoes divided
- 2 to 3 carrots stripped and cut into little pieces
- Additional virgin olive oil (I utilized Private Reserve Greek EVOO)
- Salt and pepper
- 2 medium yellow onions chopped
- 5 garlic cloves minced
- 1 cup canned squashed tomatoes
- 2 oz. new basil leaves
- 3 to 4 new thyme springs 2 tsp. thyme leaves
- 1 tsp. dry oregano
- ½ tsp. paprika
- ½ tsp. ground cumin
- 2 ½ cups water
- Sprinkle of lime juice optiona

DIRECTIONS:

1. Heat oven to 450 degrees F.
2. In an enormous blending bowl, consolidate tomatoes and carrot pieces. Add a liberal shower of additional virgin olive oil, and season with fit salt and dark pepper. Throw to join.
3. Move to an enormous heating sheet and spread well in one layer. Broil in heated oven for around 30 minutes. At the point when prepared, eliminate from the heat and put in a safe spot for around 10 minutes to cool.
4. Move the broiled tomatoes and carrots to the enormous bowl of a food processor fitted with a cutting edge. Add simply a smidgen of water and mix.
5. In a huge cooking pot, heat 2 tbsp. additional virgin olive oil over medium-high heat until shining yet not smoking. Add onions and cook for around 3 minutes, at that point add garlic and cook momentarily until brilliant.
6. Empty the simmered tomato blend into the cooking pot. Mix in squashed tomatoes, 2 ½ cups water, basil, thyme and flavors. Season with a little genuine salt and dark pepper. Heat to the point of boiling, at that point lower heat and cover part-way. Let stew for around 20 minutes or somewhere in the vicinity.
7. Eliminate the thyme springs and move tomato basil soup to serving bowls. In the event that you like, add a sprinkle of lime juice and a liberal shower of extra Present with your #1 dry bread or flame broiled bits of French loaf. Enjoy!
8. NOTES
9. Extras: If you have any extras, you can refrigerate in close top glass compartments for 3 to 4 days. Ensure the soup is totally cooled prior to putting away.
10. Would you be able to freeze this tomato basil soup? Indeed! Since this is a sans dairy veggie lover tomato basil soup and there is no cream required by any means, it is the ideal tomato soup to freeze. Essentially cool the soup prior to putting away in close cover, cooler safe compartments. Freeze for some time in the future (3 to a half year or something like that.) Thaw in ice chest short-term and go through medium heat to warm.
11. Varieties: If you're searching for somewhat of a smoky completion, add a decent touch of smoked paprika. Or then again, to zest things up, cook some jalapeno pepper and mix them alongside the tomatoes and carrots.

1024. Mediterranean Grilled Balsamic Chicken with Olive Tapenade

Prep Time: *15 Minutes* | *Cook Time:* *35 Minutes* | *Servings :4*

INGREDIENTS

- 2 skinless boneless Simple Truth chicken breasts
- 1/4 cup olive oil
- 1/4 cup brilliant balsamic vinegar
- 1/8 cup Private Selection Whole Grain Garlic Mustard
- 1/2 tablespoons balsamic vinegar
- 3 cloves garlic squeezed or minced
- Juice of 1/2 lemon
- 1 storing tablespoon chopped new spices, for example, Simple Truth tarragon rosemary or thyme
- 1 teaspoon fit salt
- 1/2 teaspoon newly ground dark pepper
- Present with Olive Tapenade formula beneath and lumps of feta cheddar

DIRECTIONS:

1. Cut back any additional excess from the chicken breasts and spot in a bowl or a gallon size cooler pack.
2. In a little bowl, whisk the olive oil, balsamic vinegars, mustard, garlic, lemon juice, spices, and salt and pepper. Save half of the marinade and add the other half to the bowl or pack with the chicken. Marinate for at any rate 30 minutes up to expedite, turning sporadically.
3. At the point when prepared to flame broil, bring one side of an outside barbecue to high heat with the opposite side off.
4. Oil the barbecue grinds well and sprinkles the chicken breasts with more olive oil, at that point place the chicken breasts on the hot flame broil. Cook for 2-3 minutes or until barbecue marks show up, at that point flip the chicken and cook for another 2-3 minutes. Move the chicken to the cooler meshes of the barbecue, cover, and cook for 10 minutes. Move a couple of tablespoons of the held marinade to another bowl and use it to treat the chicken with and flip. Keep cooking, treating, and flipping until the breasts have an interior temperature of 165 degrees. Move the chicken to the hot side of the barbecue to add more flame broil checks and shading to the chicken bosom yet make certain to watch them so the balsamic marinade doesn't burn. The length of cooking time will depend up on the thickness of the breasts however you should rely in general cooking time to be around 30 minutes.
5. Move the chicken to a platter and cover with a piece of aluminum foil and let rest for 5 minutes. Present with olive tapenade, lumps of feta cheddar minced spices and shower with any extra olive oil.

1025. SOUTHERN SPOONBREAD

Prep Time: *4 Minutes* | *Cook Time:* *8 Minutes* | *Servings :4*

INGREDIENTS:

- cups half-and-half
- 1 Tsp. salt
- 1 cup fine-ground cornmeal
- 2 Tbsps. unsalted butter
- large eggs, room temperature, separated

DIRECTIONS:

1. Heat oven to 350 degrees. Grease 6-cup soufflé dish.
2. Bring half-and-half & Salt to simmer in a large saucepan.
3. Reduce heat to low & slowly whisk in cornmeal.
4. Continue whisking till cornmeal thickens & develops satin sheen, 2 to 4 mins.
5. Off heat, stir in butter; set aside.
6. Whisk egg yolks & 1 to 2 Tbsps. Water together in a small container till lemon-coloured & very frothy.
7. Stir into cooled cornmeal batter a little at a time to keep egg yolks from cooking.
8. By Using a stand mixer fitted with whisk, whip egg whites on medium-low speed till foamy, about 1 min.
9. Increase speed to medium-high & whip till stiff peaks form, 3 to 4 mins; gently fold into cornmeal batter.
10. Pour batter into prepared dish.
11. Bake till golden brown & risen above the rim, about 45 mins.
12. Serve immediately.

1026. Best Greek Chicken Marinade

Prep Time: *15 Minutes* | *Cook Time:20 Minutes* | *Servings: 2*

INGREDIENTS

- 1 pound boneless skinless chicken breasts (about 2 large breasts)
- ⅓ cup plain Greek yogurt
- ¼ cup olive oil
- 4 lemons
- 4-5 cloves garlic squeezed or minced
- 2 tablespoons dried oregano
- 1 teaspoon genuine salt
- ½ teaspoon newly ground dark pepper

DIRECTIONS:

1. Spot the chicken pieces in a cooler sack or a bowl and put in a safe spot.
2. Add the Greek yogurt and olive oil to a medium size bowl. Zing one of the lemons and add to the bowl. Juice that lemon into the bowl with the zing. Cut the other three lemons and put in a safe spot. Add the minced garlic, oregano, genuine salt and dark pepper to the lemon squeeze and zing and mix. Empty portion of the marinade into the cooler sack or the bowl with the chicken pieces and save the other

portion of the marinade for seasoning. Marinate the chicken for 30 minutes or as long as 3 hours in the fridge.

3. At the point when prepared to flame broil, set up the barbecue by gently oiling the mesh with vegetable oil or cooking splash and set to medium high heat.
4. Flame broil the chicken, treating with the held marinade and turning frequently so each side browns and has light barbecue marks, until cooked through, around 15-20 minutes or until the chicken juices run clear. During the most recent 5 minutes of cooking add the 3 cut lemons to the flame broil, turning more than once. Permit the chicken to rest for 5 minutes prior to cutting and present with the flame broiled lemons. Refrigerate extras for as long as 3 days.

1027. SWEET & SOUR ONION RELISH

Prep Time:	*Cook Time:*	*Servings :5*
4 Minutes	*15 Minutes*	

INGREDIENTS:

- Tbsps. extra-virgin olive oil
- red onions, sliced thin
- sprigs fresh thyme Salt & pepper
- Tbsps. balsamic vinegar
- Tbsps. water
- 1 Tbsp. light brown sugar
- ounces extra-sharp cheddar cheese, shredded (1 1/2 cups) 1/2 cup toasted walnuts, chopped coarsely

DIRECTIONS:

1. Heat oil in 12-inch nonstick pan over high heat till shimmering.
2. Include onions, thyme, & 1/2 Tsp. Salt & cook, frequently stirring, till onions soften & begin to brown, 5 to 7 mins.
3. Reduce heat to low, stir in vinegar, water, & sugar & simmer till the liquid has evaporated & onions are glossy, 5 to 7 mins.
4. Discard thyme & season with Salt & pepper to taste.
5. Serve over polenta, sprinkling individual portions with cheese & walnuts.

1028. Mediterranean falafel

Prep Time:	*Cook Time:*	*Servings :5*
15 Minutes	*29 Minutes*	

INGREDIENTS

- 2 cups dried chickpeas (Do NOT utilize canned or cooked chickpeas)
- ½ tsp. preparing pop
- 1 cup new parsley leaves, stems eliminated
- ¾ cup new cilantro leaves, stems eliminated
- ½ cup new dill, stems eliminated
- 1 little onion, quartered
- 7-8 garlic cloves, stripped
- Salt to taste
- 1 tbsp. ground dark pepper
- 1 tbsp. ground cumin
- 1 tbsp. ground coriander
- 1 tsp. cayenne pepper, optional
- 1 tsp. preparing powder
- 2 tbsp. toasted sesame seeds
- Oil for searing
- Falafel Sauce
- Tahini Sauce
- Trimmings for falafel sandwich (optional)
- Pita pockets
- English cucumbers, chopped or diced
- Tomatoes, chopped or diced
- Child Arugula
- Pickles

DIRECTIONS:

1. (One day ahead of time) Place the dried chickpeas and preparing soft drink in a huge bowl loaded up with water to cover the chickpeas by in any event 2 inches. Splash for the time being for 18 hours (longer if the chickpeas are still excessively hard). At the point when prepared, channel the chickpeas totally and wipe them off.
2. Add the chickpeas, spices, onions, garlic and flavors to the enormous bowl of a food processor fitted with a cutting edge. Run the food processor 40 seconds all at once until everything is great joined shaping a the falafel blend.
3. Move the falafel blend to a compartment and cover firmly. Refrigerate for in any event 1 hour or (up to one entire evening) until prepared to cook.
4. Not long prior to searing, add the preparing powder and sesame seeds to the falafel blend and mix with a spoon.
5. Scoop tablespoonfuls of the falafel combination and structure into patties (½ inch in thickness each). It assists with having wet hands as you structure the patties.
6. Fill medium pan 3 crawls up with oil. Heat the oil on medium-high until it bubbles delicately. Cautiously drop the falafel patties in the oil, let them fry for around 3 to 5 minutes or so until fresh and medium brown outwardly. Try not to pack the falafel in the pan, fry them in bunches if fundamental.
7. Spot the singed falafel patties in a colander or plate fixed with paper towels to deplete.
8. Serve falafel hot close to other little plates; or amass the falafel patties in pita bread with tahini or hummus, arugula, tomato and cucumbers. Enjoy!
9. You need to begin with dry chickpeas, don't utilize canned chickpeas here. You should start dousing the chickpeas short-term; permit as long as 24 hours.
10. Falafel Recipe varieties: Variations of this formula may call for flour or eggs. On the off chance that you like, you can add 1 to 1 ½ tbsp. of flour to the falafel blend or 1 egg. I didn't utilize either, and the falafel combination remained well together.
11. Ace Tip for Frying: When you fry the falafel patties, you need to accomplish a profound brilliant brown tone outwardly. All the more critically, the patties should be completely done within. Your broiling oil should be at 375 degrees F, for my oven, that was at a medium-high temp. Make certain to test your first group and change the singing time depending on the situation.
12. Well known falafel sauce: tahini sauce is the thing that is customarily utilized with falafel. I utilize natural tahini paste by Soom, and here is my tahini sauce formula.
13. Prepared Falafel Option: If you like, you can heat the falafel patties in a 350 degree F heated oven for around 15-20 minutes, turning them over halfway through. Utilize a gently oiled sheet dish, and you may jump at the chance to give the patties a speedy brush of additional virgin olive oil prior to preparing.
14. Supportive of Tip for Make-Ahead: To make ahead and freeze, set up the falafel blend and separation into patties (up to step #6). Spot the patties on a preparing sheet fixed with material paper and freeze. At the point when they solidify, you can move the falafel patties into a cooler pack. They will save well in the cooler for a month or something like that. You can sear or heat them from frozen.0

1029. Lebanese Rice With Vermicelli

Prep Time:	*Cook Time:*	*Servings :8*
15 Minutes	*70 Minutes*	

INGREDIENTS

- 2 cups in length grain or medium grain rice
- Water
- 1 cup broken vermicelli pasta
- 2 ½ tbsp. olive oil
- Salt
- ½ cup toasted pine nuts, optional to wrap up

DIRECTIONS:

1. Wash the rice well (a couple of times) at that point places it in a medium bowl and cover with water. Splash for 15 to 20 minutes. Test to check whether you can without much of a stretch break a grain of rice by basically putting it between your thumb and pointer. Channel well.
2. In a medium non-stick cooking pot, heat the olive oil on medium-high. Add the vermicelli and consistently mix to toast it equally. Vermicelli should turn a decent brilliant brown, yet observe cautiously not to over-brown or consume it (If it consumes, you should discard the vermicelli and begin once again).
3. Add the rice and keep on blending so the rice will be very much covered with the olive oil. Season with salt.
4. Presently add 3 ½ cups of water and heat it to the point of boiling until the water altogether diminishes (see the photograph below).Turn the heat to low and cover.
5. Cook for 15-20 minutes on low. Once completely cooked, turn the heat off and leave the rice undisturbed in its cooking pot for 10-15 minutes, at that point reveal and cushion with a fork.
6. Move to a serving platter and top with the toasted pine nuts. Enjoy!
7. You should flush the rice to dispose of abundance starch which makes rice be tacky (Lebanese rice isn't intended to be tacky). At that point absorbs the rice a lot of water for 15-20 minutes or until you can break one grain of rice by squeezing it between your forefinger and your thumb. 2. Toasting the vermicelli in EVOO as an initial step is the thing that gives this rice incredible flavor. Try not to skirt this progression. 3. On the off chance that you can at all assistance it, let the rice rest for 5 to 10 minutes prior to serving.

1030. Best Chicken Piccata

Prep Time:	*Cook Time:*	*Servings: 2*
15 Minutes	*35 Minutes*	

INGREDIENTS

- 1 lemon
- 1 1/2 pounds boneless, skinless chicken breasts
- 1 teaspoon kosher salt
- 1 teaspoon freshly ground black pepper
- 1/3 cup all-purpose flour
- 3 tablespoons margarine isolated
- 2 tablespoons canola oil
- 1 cup chicken stock or white wine, or a blend of both
- 2 tablespoons escapades depleted and flushed

DIRECTIONS:

1. Cut the lemon fifty-fifty, juice one half, at that point cut the other half into 1/8" cuts and put in a safe spot.
2. Cut back any overabundance excess from the chicken breasts and cut down the middle longwise to make two slight cutlets. Season the two sides of the chicken breasts uniformly with the legitimate salt and newly ground dark pepper at that point dig each bosom in the flour, shaking off any abundance.
3. Heat 2 tablespoons margarine with the canola oil in an enormous skillet over medium-high heat. Add 4 bits of the chicken and cook for 2-3 minutes for each side. Move to a platter or sheet skillet and cover with foil. Proceed with the excess chicken.
4. Decrease the heat to medium and add the chicken stock or wine (or 1/2 cup of both) the lemon juice, cut lemons, and the tricks, scraping up the browned pieces on the dish and cook for 2-3 minutes.
5. Mix in the excess 1 tablespoon of margarine until dissolved. Taste for preparing and spoon the sauce over the chicken breasts. Present with pureed potatoes or cauliflower, polenta, or noodles.
6. Formula Notes
7. Keep the cooked chicken breasts warm while the sauce cooks by plating on a platter and covering with aluminum foil, or spot in a 200°F oven.

1031. Baked Cod Recipe with Lemon and Garlic

Prep Time:	*Cook Time:*	*Servings :8*
15 Minutes	*20 Minutes*	

INGREDIENTS

- 1.5 lb. Cod filet pieces, 4-6 pieces
- ¼ cup chopped new parsley leaves
- Lemon Sauce
- 5 tbsp. new lemon juice
- 5 tbsp. additional virgin olive oil
- 2 tbsp. dissolved spread
- 5 garlic cloves, minced
- For Coating
- ⅓ cup generally useful flour
- 1 tsp. ground coriander
- ¾ tsp. sweet Spanish paprika
- ¾ tsp. ground cumin
- ¾ tsp. salt
- ½ tsp. dark pepper

DIRECTIONS:

1. Preheat oven to 400 degrees F.
2. Combine as one the lemon juice, olive oil, and liquefied margarine in a shallow bowl (don't add the garlic yet). Put in a safe spot.
3. In another shallow bowl, blend the generally useful flour, flavors, salt and pepper. Set close to the lemon sauce.
4. Wipe the fish off. Plunge the fish in the lemon sauce at that point dunk it in the flour blend. Shake off abundance flour. Save the lemon sauce for some other time.
5. Heat 2 tbsp. olive oil in a cast iron skillet (or an oven-safe dish) over medium-high heat (watch the oil to be certain it is shining however not smoking). Add the fish and burn on each side to give it some tone, yet don't completely cook (around 2 minutes on each side). Eliminate the skillet from heat.
6. To the leftover lemon sauce, add the minced garlic and blend. Sprinkle everywhere on the fish filets.

7. Prepare in the heated oven until the fish chips effectively with a fork (10 minutes ought to get it done, however start checking prior). Eliminate from the heat and sprinkle chopped parsley. Serve right away.

1032. Keto Copycat Green Salad With Chicken Rey And Egg

Prep Time: 15 Minutes *Cook Time: 20 Minutes* *Servings :8*

INGREDIENTS

- 1/2 iceberg lettuce
- 2-carrots
- 2-hard-boiled eggs
- 1-chicken fillet
- 1-tomato mayonnaise
- olive oil

DIRECTIONS:

1. Wash and reduce the iceberg lettuce to Juliana. We booked in a large bowl.
2. We wash and cut the tomato into cubes. We upload it to the bowl.
3. Peel and reduce the carrot julienne. We add to the bowl.
4. Cut the bird's breast into strips.
5. Boil the eggs in a saucepan with vinegar and salt for 10-15 minutes to stop them from breaking.
6. When the eggs are ready, we discard, cool with a water jet, and remove the shell.
7. Quarter the hard-boiled eggs and put them in the bowl. Meanwhile, put the poultry strips in a pan with a dash of oil, season, and fry the chicken over medium heat for five minutes. Mix the salad with several tablespoons of mayonnaise to taste and serve immediately.

1033. Panera Bread Green Goddess Cobb Salad

Prep Time: 15 Minutes *Cook Time: 24 Minutes* *Servings :4*

INGREDIENTS

- 1 1/2 teaspoons of salt
- 1 cup warm water Salad servers:
- 6 ounces salad mix-use rocket, romaine, kale, and radicchio mix
- 6 grams of grilled chicken fillet
- 2-tablespoons of crispy cooked bacon
- 3-tablespoons of chopped avocado
- 1/2 cup of chopped tomatoes
- Halve 1-hard-boiled egg
- 2-tablespoons of feta
- 2-tablespoons pickled onions Green goddess salad dressing:
- 1-cup of mayonnaise
- 2-tablespoons tarragon leaves

DIRECTION

1. Slice onions as thin as possible; I like to use the 1/8 inch on my mandolin. Put the onions in a full pot. Combine white vinegar, sugar, salt, and warm water in a small bowl. Stir until sugar and salt are dissolved. These should rest for about half an hour before use. Place all ingredients for the dressing in the bowl of a blender or meal processor and blend for 30-45 seconds, or until the dressing is mostly clean and creamy.
2. Place the salad in the bottom of a large salad bowl. Cut the chicken breast into thin slices and put them with the salad. Add a new, pre-selected, and chosen time, and some more, and egg you bought, and a few samples.

1034. Crispy Sheet Pan Salmon with Lemony Asparagus and Carrots

Prep Time: 15 Minutes *Cook Time: 23 Minutes* *Servings :4*

INGREDIENTS

- 4 (6-oz.) skin-on salmon filets
- ¼ cup mayonnaise
- 2 tablespoons Dijon mustard
- 1 tablespoon chopped new dill
- 1 ½ teaspoons lemon zing (from 1 lemon), partitioned
- ¾ teaspoon genuine salt, separated
- ¾ teaspoon dark pepper, partitioned
- ¼ cup panko (Japanese-style breadcrumbs)
- Cooking splash
- ½ pound new asparagus, managed and split transversely
- 1 (8-oz.) pkg. little carrots with tops, cut longwise
- 2 tablespoons unsalted margarine, liquefied
- Lemon wedges

DIRECTIONS:

1. Stage 1
2. Preheat oven to 425°F. Line a rimmed preparing sheet with material paper. Spot salmon, skin side down, on portion of arranged preparing sheet. Mix together mayonnaise, mustard, and dill, 1 teaspoon of the lemon zing, 1/4 teaspoon of the salt, and 1/4 teaspoon of the pepper in a medium bowl. Spread over salmon filets in an even layer; top with panko, and press gently to follow. Splash with cooking shower.
3. Stage 2
4. Throw together asparagus, carrots, margarine, and staying 1/2 teaspoon every one of lemon zing, salt, and pepper in a medium bowl. Spot vegetables on void side of preparing sheet. Heat in preheated oven until salmon is cooked through and vegetables are delicate, around 18 minutes. Present with lemon wedges.

1035. Whole Roasted Red Snapper with Potatoes and Onions

Prep Time: 15 Minutes *Cook Time: 80 Minutes* *Servings :6*

, 2 red onion wedges)

INGREDIENTS

- 1 ½ cups approximately pressed new level leaf parsley leaves
- 1 medium shallot (around 2 oz.), generally chopped
- 3 garlic cloves, generally chopped
- 1 tablespoon new thyme leaves
- 1 ½ teaspoons lemon zing (from 1 lemon)
- ½ teaspoon squashed red pepper
- ¾ cup olive oil
- 2 ¾ teaspoons legitimate salt, separated
- 1 pound child gold potatoes (around 8 potatoes)
- 1 little red onion (around 8 oz.), cut the long way into 1-in. wedges
- 1 (3-lb.) entire red snapper, cleaned, scaled, gutted, and blades managed
- Lemon wedges, for serving

DIRECTIONS:

1. Stage 1
2. Preheat oven to 425°F. Line a rimmed heating sheet with material paper. Put in a safe spot.
3. Stage 2
4. Cycle parsley, shallot, garlic, thyme, lemon zing, and red pepper in a food processor until finely chopped, around 15 seconds. Add oil, and interaction until very much fused, around 15 seconds. Throw together potatoes, onion wedges, 2 tablespoons of the parsley combination, and 1 teaspoon of the salt in an enormous bowl.
5. Stage 3
6. Cut 3 (2-inch-long) cuts askew on the two sides of fish, slicing right deep down on the two sides. Rub outside and within cuts with 1 cup of the parsley blend and staying 1 3/4 teaspoons salt; place fish on arranged heating sheet. Spread potato blend around fish. Prepare in preheated oven until fish is murky and flaky and vegetables are delicate, around 30 minutes.
7. Stage 4
8. Shower fish with remaining 1/4 cup parsley combination. Present with lemon wedges.

1036. Caprese Tomato, Mozzarella, Basil, And Avocado Salad

Prep Time: 15 Minutes *Cook Time: 30 Minutes* *Servings :6*

INGREDIENTS

- 2-sliced avocados
- 2-ripe tomatoes
- 500 g mozzarella cheese
- 1 cup of fresh basil leaves
- 1/4 cup of olive oil
- 1/4 cup of Balsamic Aceto
- Salt and ground black pepper

DIRECTION

1. Gather all the ingredients to make this tomato, mozzarella, basil, and avocado Caprese salad.
2. Cut the tomato stem with a small knife and cut the tomatoes into slices with a serrated knife.
3. Slice the mozzarella and spot alternating slices of avocado, tomato, mozzarella, and basil in signature dishes. Slice with olive oil and balsamic vinegar and season with salt and ground black pepper.
4. Divide your Italian tomato, mozzarella, basil, and avocado salad with a fresh baguette or on a bed of romaine lettuce.

1037. Greek Creamy Potato Salad

Prep Time: 15 Minutes *Cook Time: 15 Minutes* *Servings :\3*

INGREDIENTS

- ¾ cups of low-fat sour cream
- ¼ cup of mayonnaise
- ¼ chopped per parsley 3-tablespoons lemon juice
- 2-tablespoons of Dijon mustard
- 2-tablespoons of chopped fresh tarragon
- 2-finely chopped celery stalks
- 2-hard-boiled eggs

DIRECTION

1. Peel the potatoes and cut them into medium cubes. Place them in a large saucepan with cold water and kosher salt to taste, and add a little salt. Bring to heat and while boiling, simmer for 10 to 12 minutes until potatoes are smooth.
2. Mix mayonnaise with sour cream, mustard, and lemon juice.
3. Season with salt and ground black pepper and add heat potatoes. Mix and let cool to room temperature.
4. Add the celery thinly sliced fennel and parsley, and tarragon, all finely chopped.
5. Mix so that the potatoes are soaked with cream, and add the hard-cut eggs in wedges. Serve the creamy potato salad.

1038. Grilled Greek Chicken Kebabs

Prep Time: 15 Minutes *Cook Time: 70 Minutes* *Servings :\3*

INGREDIENTS

- 1 pound boneless skinless chicken breasts (about 2 large breasts)

- 1/3 cup plain Greek yogurt
- 1/4 cup olive oil
- 4 lemons squeezed, in addition to zing from one of the lemons
- 4-5 cloves garlic squeezed or minced
- 2 tablespoons dried oregano
- 1 teaspoon fit salt
- 1/2 teaspoon newly ground dark pepper
- 1 red onion quartered into 1-inch pieces
- 1 little zucchini cut into 1/4 inch coins
- 1 red ringer pepper cultivated and cut into 1-inch pieces

DIRECTIONS:

1. Cut the chicken breasts the long way into thirds, and afterward cut again into around 1-inch pieces. Spot the chicken pieces in a cooler pack or bowl and put in a safe spot.
2. Add the Greek yogurt and olive oil to a medium size bowl. Zing one of the lemons into the bowl then squeeze that lemon with the excess three lemons and add to the bowl. Add the minced garlic, oregano, legitimate salt and dark pepper and mix. Empty portion of the marinade into the cooler pack or the bowl with the chicken pieces and save the other portion of the marinade for seasoning. Marinate the chicken for 30 minutes or as long as 3 hours in the fridge.
3. At the point when prepared to barbecue, set up the flame broil by delicately oiling the mesh with vegetable oil or cooking splash and set to medium high heat.
4. In the case of using wooden sticks, set them up by absorbing water for 10 minutes. In the case of using metal sticks, no prep is important.
5. String the chicken on the sticks rotating with the red onion, zucchini and red chime pepper until you've arrived at the finish of the stick, finishing with chicken. Rehash with the leftover sticks. Dispose of any of the excess marinade that had the chicken in it.
6. Flame broil the chicken, treating the kebabs with the held marinade and turning frequently so each side browns and has light barbecue marks, until cooked through, around 10-15 minutes or until the chicken juices run clear. Serve warm. Refrigerate extras for as long as 3 days.

1039. Greek Wedge Salad With Creamy Dressing

Prep Time: *15 Minutes* *Cook Time:* *70 Minutes* *Servings :\4*

INGREDIENTS

- 4-teaspoons apple cider vinegar
- 1-bag of green onion powder mix
- 1-clove of garlic, chopped
- 1/2 cup chopped green onion
- 1-head of iceberg lettuce, heart removed and in pictures
- 1-tomato, cut into cubes
- 4-teaspoons bacon cubes

DIRECTIONS:

1. Combine the cream, buttermilk, vinegar, and dressing in a small bowl. Beat until the combination is easy.
2. Add garlic and a quarter cup of inexperienced onion; put aside. Remove the center of the lettuce and cut into 4-equal wedges.
3. Place each wedge in 4 different dishes. Pour about 1/4 of the salad dressing over each wedge.
4. Divide 1/4 of the ultimate onion, 1/4 of the chopped tomato, and 1-teaspoon of bacon cubes over each wedge.

1040. Chicken with Broccoli and Sweet Potato Wedges

Prep Time: *15 Minutes* *Cook Time:* *65 Minutes* *Servings :\4*

INGREDIENTS

- 8 (3 1/2-oz.) chicken drumsticks, cleaned 1 tablespoon new lemon juice 1/8 teaspoons kosher salt, isolated 1/2 teaspoon poultry preparing 1 teaspoon garlic powder, separated 1/8 teaspoon newly ground dark pepper 2 huge eggs, gently thumped
- 1 cup panko (Japanese breadcrumbs) 1/2 ounces Parmesan cheddar, ground (around 1/3 cup) 1 teaspoon dried oregano
- 1 teaspoon dried parsley pieces (optional) Cooking splash 2 (7-oz.) yams, each cut into 8 wedges
- 2 tablespoons olive oil, partitioned 1/2 teaspoon paprika 1/2 teaspoon bean stew powder
- 7 cups broccoli florets (around 12 oz.) 1 garlic clove, squashed or ground 5 lemon wedges

DIRECTIONS:

1. Preheat oven to 425°F.
2. Spot chicken in an enormous bowl. Shower with lemon squeeze, and sprinkle with 3/8 teaspoon salt, poultry preparing, 1/2 teaspoon garlic powder, and dark pepper; throw to join.
3. Spot eggs in a shallow dish. Consolidate panko, Parmesan, oregano, and parsley, if using, in another shallow dish. Plunge every drumstick in eggs at that point dig in panko blend. Spot drumsticks on a rimmed heating sheet covered with cooking shower; dispose of outstanding egg and panko blend. Coat highest points of drumsticks with cooking splash. Prepare at 425°F for 15 minutes.
4. Consolidate potatoes, 1 tablespoon oil, staying 1/2 teaspoon garlic powder, paprika, bean stew powder, and 3/8 teaspoon salt; throw to cover. Mastermind potatoes on one portion of another rimmed preparing sheet covered with cooking shower. Spot in oven with chicken, and heat at 425°F for 10 minutes.
5. Consolidate broccoli, staying 1 tablespoon oil, garlic clove, and staying 3/8 teaspoon salt. Eliminate heating sheet with potatoes from oven; turn potatoes over, and add broccoli to other portion of container. Spot in oven with chicken, and heat at 425°F for 20 minutes or until chicken and potatoes are finished. Crush 1 lemon wedge over broccoli. Serve remaining lemon wedges with the dinner.

1041. Honey-Soy-Glazed Salmon with Veggies and Oranges

Prep Time: *15 Minutes* *Cook Time:* *75 Minutes* *Servings : 6*

INGREDIENTS

- 4 tablespoons nectar
- 1 tablespoon soy sauce
- 1 tablespoon Dijon mustard
- 1 teaspoon prepared rice wine vinegar
- ¼ teaspoon dried squashed red pepper
- 1 pound new medium asparagus
- 8 ounces new green beans, managed
- 1 little orange, cut into 1/4-to 1/2-inch cuts
- 1 tablespoon olive oil
- 1 teaspoon legitimate salt
- ¼ teaspoon newly ground dark pepper
- 4 (5-to 6-oz.) new salmon filets
- Topping: toasted sesame seeds

DIRECTIONS:

1. Stage 1
2. Preheat oven with oven rack 6 crawls from heat. Whisk together nectar and next 4 ingredients in a little bowl.
3. Stage 2
4. Snap off and dispose of intense closures of asparagus. Spot asparagus, green beans, and next 4 ingredients in an enormous bowl, and throw to cover.
5. Stage 3
6. Spot salmon in focus of a substantial aluminum foil-lined sheet container. Brush salmon with around 2 Tbsp. nectar combinations. Spread asparagus combination around salmon.
7. Stage 4
8. Cook 4 minutes; eliminate from oven, and brush salmon with around 2 Tbsp. nectar combination. Get back to oven, and sear 4 minutes more. Eliminate from oven, and brush salmon with remaining nectar blend. Get back to oven, and cook 2 minutes more. Serve right away.

1042. Tomatoes Stuffed With Tuna

Prep Time: *15 Minutes* *Cook Time:* *60 Minutes* *Servings: 2*

INGREDIENTS

- 4-medium tomatoes
- a large cup of white or brown rice
- Mayonnaise c / n
- Green olives c / n
- Peas or capers c / n
- 2-carrots
- Salt c / n

DIRECTION

1. Put a mass of water in a pot and take it to the fireplace. Drain the rice when it boils. Stir with a wooden spoon to keep it from sticking and cook dinner for 20 minutes or until soft. Remove, drain immediately and store in the refrigerator.
2. Cook in a saucepan with water until they soften. Drain and put in a bowl.
3. Add the rice, the two tins of drained tuna, the peas or capers (cooked), and the mayonnaise to taste.
4. Mix everything very well and space to taste.
5. Wash the tomatoes thoroughly and smoke them with a knife and spoon.

1043. California Pizza Kitchen California Club Pizza

Prep Time: *15 Minutes* *Cook Time:* *70 Minutes* *Servings: 2*

INGREDIENTS

- 1 cup of grated mozzarella cheese
- 1 cup ready-to-eat grilled chicken fillet strips
- 4-bacon strips, cooked and crumbled
- 2 cups of grated romaine
- 1 cup of fresh arugula
- 1/4 cup of mayonnaise
- 1-tablespoon of lemon juice
- 1-teaspoon of lemon zest
- 1/2 teaspoon of pepper
- 1-medium tomato, thinly sliced

DIRECTIONS:

1. Preheat the oven to 450 °. Grease a 14-in. Pizza; sprinkle with cornmeal. On a smooth surface, do a 13-in. Sure.
2. Transfer to organized pan; slightly raise the edges. Sprinkle with cheese, poultry, and bacon. Bake until crust is gently browned for 10-12 minutes.
3. Meanwhile, place the romaine and arugula in a large bowl. In a small bowl, add mayonnaise, lemon juice, lemon zest, and pepper.
4. Pour over the lettuce; toss to coat. Arrange overheated pizza. Top with tomato, avocado, and basil. Serve immediately.

1044. Greek Oriental Apple Bee Salad

Prep Time: *15 Minutes* *Cook Time:* *30 Minutes* *Servings : 6*

INGREDIENTS

- 2-tablespoons of olive oil

- 1/2 teaspoon of salt
- 1/4 teaspoon black pepper
- 1/2 cup of sliced almonds
- 8-cups of romaine lettuce
- 1/4 cup sliced carrots
- 1/2 cup of crispy rice noodles

DIRECTIONS:

1. Heat the grill to medium, or heat a sturdy iron skillet or grill pan over medium heat. Place the hand between two 'plastic wrap' and lift them to 3/8 min. Fizzy with the other oil and top with some pepper and pepper.
2. Grill them for 5 to 7 minutes on each side, until cooked through. Place them on a plate for four to five minutes rather than sliced to relax.
3. Roast the almonds in a little dry sauce over the heat of it
4. Supervise them - there is a high-quality line between toasted almonds and burnt almonds! Shake the pan gently when you start to smell the almonds, toast for a few more seconds, and immediately put the almonds on a paper towel. Let them cool down or.
5. Like salads, by putting down the lettuce first, 3 to 4 choices start with the food.

1045. 30-Minute Caprese Chicken Recipe

Prep Time: *15 Minutes* | *Cook Time:* *40 Minutes* | *Servings : 6*

INGREDIENTS

- 2 skinless boneless chicken breasts
- Kosher salt and freshly ground black pepper
- 1 tablespoon extra-virgin olive oil
- 1 tablespoon spread
- 1 6 oz. container DeLallo Traditional Basil Simply Pesto
- 4-6 cuts new mozzarella or 6 ounces ground mozzarella cheddar
- 8 mixed drink or little tomatoes cut
- DeLallo balsamic coating
- New basil fragmented

DIRECTIONS:

1. Preheat the oven to 400° F.
2. Utilize a sharp, slim blade to cut the chicken breasts down the middle the long way. Season the two sides with fit salt and newly ground dark pepper. Heat a huge oven-verification skillet over medium high heat and add the olive oil and spread. When the margarine has softened into the olive oil, add the chicken breasts to the container, being mindful so as not to swarm. Cook on each side until softly browned, around 3-4 minutes each.
3. Slather the highest points of every chicken bosom with the basil pesto, around 1-2 tablespoons for each chicken bosom. Top every chicken bosom with a cut of mozzarella and a couple of cuts of tomato. Put the skillet in the oven and cook for 10-12 minutes or until the chicken arrives at an inward temperature of 165 degrees. F. Eliminate from the oven and topping with new basil and a sprinkle of balsamic coating.

1046. Greek Salmon Veggie Packets

Prep Time: *15 Minutes* | *Cook Time:* *34 Minutes* | *Servings: 2*

INGREDIENTS

- 2 tablespoons white wine
- 1 tablespoon olive oil
- 1/4 teaspoon salt
- 1/4 teaspoon pepper
- 2 medium sweet yellow peppers, julienned
- 2 cups new sugar snap peas, managed
- SALMON:
- 2 tablespoons white wine
- 1 tablespoon olive oil
- 1 tablespoon ground lemon zing
- 1/2 teaspoon salt
- 1/4 teaspoon pepper
- 4 salmon filets (6 ounces each)
- 1 medium lemon, split

DIRECTIONS:

1. Preheat oven to 400°. Cut four 18x15-in. bits of material paper or uncompromising foil: overlay each transversely down the middle, shaping a wrinkle. In a huge bowl, blend wine, oil, salt and pepper. Add vegetables and throw to cover.
2. In a small bowl, blend the initial five salmon ingredients. To collect, expose one piece of material paper; place a salmon filet on one side. Sprinkle with 2 teaspoons wine combination; top with one-fourth of the vegetables.
3. Overlay paper over fish and vegetables; overlap the open closures multiple times to seal. Rehash with outstanding parcels. Spot on heating sheets.
4. Heat until fish simply starts to chip effectively with a fork, 12-16 minutes, and opening parcels cautiously to allow steam to get away.
5. To serve, press lemon juice over vegetables.

1047. TOASTED ORZO WITH PEAS & PARMESAN

Prep Time: *10 Minutes* | *Cook Time:* *30 Minutes* | *Servings: 2*

INGREDIENTS:

- Tbsps. unsalted butter
- One onion, chopped fine Salt & pepper
- garlic cloves, minced
-
- 1 lb orzo
- 3½ cups low-sodium chicken broth
- ¾ cup of dry white wine
- 1¾ cups frozen peas
- ounces Parmesan cheese, grated (1 cup) Pinch ground nutmeg

DIRECTIONS:

1. Melt butter in nonstick pan.
2. Include onion & ¾ Tsp. Salt & cook, frequently stirring, till onion has softened & is beginning to brown, 5 to 7 mins.
3. Include garlic & cook till fragrant, about 30 seconds.
4. Include orzo & cook, frequently stirring, till most of the orzo is lightly browned & golden, 5 to 6 mins.
5. Off heat, Include broth & wine. Take to boil over high heat; reduce heat to medium-low & simmer, occasionally stirring, till all liquid has been absorbed & orzo is tender, 10 to 15 mins.
6. Stir in peas, Parmesan, nutmeg, & pepper to taste.
7. Off heat, let stand till peas are heated through, about 2 mins.
8. Season with salt to taste & serve.

1048. Grilled Lemon Chicken Skewers

Prep Time: *15 Minutes* | *Cook Time:* *45 Minutes* | *Servings: 2*

INGREDIENTS

- 2 boneless chicken breasts
- 3 lemons
- 4 cloves garlic minced
- 1 tablespoon dried oregano
- 1/4 cup olive oil
- 1 teaspoon kosher salt
- 1/2 teaspoon newly ground pepper
- 7-8 green onions

DIRECTIONS:

1. Cut the chicken breasts the long way into thirds, and afterward cut again into around 1-inch pieces. Spot chicken lumps in a cooler pack and put in a safe spot.
2. Zing one of the lemons and add to a medium size bowl. Juice that lemon in addition to one more, adds to the lemon zing and afterward adds the minced garlic and oregano and mix. Gradually shower in the olive oil and rush to consolidate. Add genuine salt and pepper. Empty the marinade into the cooler sack with the chicken pieces and let marinade for 30 minutes or as long as 3 hours in the fridge.
3. At the point when prepared to flame broil, set up the barbecue by softly oiling the mesh with vegetable oil or cooking splash and set to medium high heat.
4. In the case of using wooden sticks, set them up by absorbing water for 10 minutes. In the case of using metal sticks, no prep is important.
5. Cut the excess lemon in slender adjusts and afterward cut the rounds down the middle. Trim the bottoms of the green onions off and cut into 1-inch lengths.
6. String one piece of the chicken onto a stick then two cuts of green onion, and afterward another piece of chicken. Overlap a cut of lemon fifty-fifty and string close to the chicken, gathering intently on the stick. Add another piece of chicken, at that point green onions and rehash the example until you've arrived at the finish of the stick, finishing with chicken. Dispose of any of the excess marinade.
7. Flame broil chicken, turning regularly so each side browns and has light barbecue marks, until cooked through, around 10-15 minutes or until chicken juices run clear.

1049. Sautéed Chicken with Olives, Capers and Lemons

Prep Time: *15 Minutes* | *Cook Time:* *45 Minutes* | *Servings : 5*

INGREDIENTS

- 2 lemons sliced 1/4 inch thick
- 1/4 cup plus 1 tablespoon extra-virgin olive oil
- 6 skinless boneless chicken thighs, about 1 pound
- 1-2 tablespoons rice flour or all-purpose flour
- 1 fat garlic clove minced
- 1 cup chicken broth
- 3/4 cup Sicilian green olives
- 1/4 cup carpers
- 2 tablespoons spread
- 2 tablespoons parsley
- legitimate salt and newly broke dark pepper

DIRECTIONS:

1. Bring a medium-huge, high sided skillet to medium-high heat and add 1 tablespoon of olive oil. Add half of the lemon cuts and singe until browned, 3-5 minutes on each side. Move to a plate. Season the chicken thighs with fit salt and dark pepper and residue with rice flour, shaking off the overabundance. Add 1/2 tablespoons of olive oil to the hot skillet and burn the chicken pieces until brilliant brown, around 5 minutes each side. Move to another plate and wrap up singing the remainder of the chicken pieces, at that point move to a similar plate as the remainder of the chicken.
2. Add the remainder of the olive oil to the skillet and the minced garlic, and cook for 30 seconds or until fragrant, blending so the garlic doesn't consume and turn out to be harsh. Add the green olives, tricks and stock. Add the saved chicken and any juices that have been delivered in addition to the saved lemons and their juices and cook over high heat until the stock is diminished significantly, around 5 minutes. Add the spread and parsley and cook for one more moment. Season with more legitimate salt and newly ground dark pepper to taste. Move to plates and spoon the olives, tricks, lemons and sauce on top.
3. Present with sautéed spinach, kale or Swiss chard as an afterthought.

Dinner Recipes

1050. Pan-Roasted Chicken and Vegetables

Prep Time: *5 Minutes* | *Cook Time:* *15 Minutes* | *Servings : 5*

INGREDIENTS

- 2 pounds red potatoes (around 6 medium), cut into 3/4-inch pieces
- 1 enormous onion, coarsely chopped
- 2 tablespoons olive oil
- 3 garlic cloves, minced
- 1-1/4 teaspoons salt, separated
- 1 teaspoon dried rosemary, squashed, isolated
- 3/4 teaspoon pepper, separated
- 1/2 teaspoon paprika
- 6 bone-in chicken thighs (around 2-1/4 pounds), skin eliminated
- 6 cups new child spinach (around 6 ounces)

DIRECTIONS:

1. Preheat oven to 425°. In a huge bowl, consolidate potatoes, onion, oil, garlic, 3/4 teaspoon salt, 1/2 teaspoon rosemary and 1/2 teaspoon pepper; throw to cover. Move to a 15x10x1-in. preparing pan covered with cooking shower.

2. In a small bowl, blend paprika and the leftover salt, rosemary and pepper. Sprinkle chicken with paprika combination; organize over vegetables. Cook until a thermometer embedded in chicken peruses 170°-175° and vegetables are simply delicate, 35-40 minutes.
3. Eliminate chicken to a serving platter; keep warm. Top vegetables with spinach. Broil until vegetables are delicate and spinach is shriveled, 8-10 minutes longer. Mix vegetables to join; present with chicken.
4. Set up your sheet-pan supper the prior night and simply pop it into the preheated oven to prepare. This serves to profoundly enhance the chicken, a shared benefit!
5. In the event that you need a more extravagant dish, use skin-on chicken, and on the off chance that you need a lighter dish, utilize bone-in chicken breasts. Make certain to cook bone-in breasts just to 165-170 degrees, since more slender meat can get dry at higher temperatures.

1051. Seafood Couscous Paella

Prep Time: 15 Minutes *Cook Time:35 Minutes* *Servings: 2*

INGREDIENTS

- Ingredient Checklist
- 2 teaspoons extra-virgin olive oil
- 1 medium onion, chopped
- 1 clove garlic, minced
- ½ teaspoon dried thyme
- ½ teaspoon fennel seed
- ¼ teaspoon salt
- ¼ teaspoon freshly ground pepper
- Pinch of crumbled saffron threads
- 1 cup no-salt-added diced tomatoes, with juice
- ¼ cup vegetable broth
- 4 ounces bay scallops, tough muscle removed
- 4 ounces small shrimp, (41-50 per pound), peeled and deveined
- ½ cup whole-wheat couscous

DIRECTIONS:

1. Step 1
2. Heat oil in a large saucepan over medium heat. Add onion; cook, stirring constantly, for 3 minutes. Add garlic, thyme, fennel seed, salt, pepper and saffron; cook for 20 seconds.
3. Step 2
4. Stir in tomatoes and broth. Bring to a simmer. Cover, reduce heat and simmer for 2 minutes.
5. Step 3
6. Increase heat to medium, stir in scallops and cook, stirring occasionally, for 2 minutes. Add shrimp and cook, stirring occasionally, for 2 minutes more. Stir in couscous. Cover, remove from heat and let stand for 5 minutes; fluff.

1052. Mediterranean Baked Feta Pizza

Prep Time: 15 Minutes *Cook Time: 70 Minutes* *Servings: 2*

INGREDIENTS

- Pizza Dough (alternatively, you can use a premade dough)
- 1-1/4 cups bread flour (175 grams) I recommend weighing the flour for better accuracy
- 1/2 teaspoon instant dry yeast
- 1/2 teaspoon salt
- 1/2 cup warm water (110F)
- 1/2 teaspoon olive oil
- Prepared Feta + Toppings
- 1 pt. cherry tomatoes
- 1 tablespoon finely chopped shallot
- 2 medium entire cloves garlic, stripped
- 2 tablespoons olive oil
- 1 (8 oz.) block feta cheddar
- 1/4 teaspoon red pepper chips (discretionary)
- Legitimate salt and pepper to taste
- 1/2 cup shredded low-dampness mozzarella cheddar
- 1/4 cup split Kalamata olives
- 1/4 cup jostled artichoke hearts, generally chopped and wiped off
- 1/4 cup jostled broiled red peppers, daintily cut into strips
- Small bunch new basil leaves

DIRECTIONS:

1. Pizza Dough
2. In a huge bowl, join flour, yeast, and salt. Shower water and 1/2 teaspoon olive oil up and over and mix with a wooden spoon until mixture meets up and no dashes of flour remain. Cover with saran wrap and let batter rest 15 minutes.
3. Eliminate batter from bowl and turn onto a softly floured surface. Ply mixture 3-5 minutes until smooth and flexible. Spot into a lubed bowl, going once to oil the top and cover with cling wrap and let rise 3-4 hours at room temperature until multiplied in size (or 24-72 hours in the refrigerator – in the event that you decide to cool the batter, let it come to room temperature 45 minutes prior to carrying out)
4. Heated Feta + Toppings
5. Preheat oven to 400F. In a 8×8 heating dish, throw tomatoes, shallot, and garlic with olive oil until equally covered. Structure a space in the focal point of skillet and spot feta in the middle. Turn the feta to equally cover in olive oil. Top with red pepper chips, salt, and pepper to taste.
6. Spot feta on center rack of oven. In the event that you have a pizza stone, place on base rack to start preheating. Prepare feta at 400F 35-40 minutes until tomatoes are blasting and feta is a profound brilliant brown. Eliminate feta from oven, increment oven temperature to 500F and move pizza stone to center rack. Utilize a spoon to squash feta, tomatoes, and garlic until a semi-thick sauce structures.
7. In the event that using pizza stone strategy, gently dust a pizza strip with cornmeal. If not using stone, softly oil a huge heating sheet with olive oil (regardless of whether you're not using a stone, preheat your oven per formula DIRECTIONS above)
8. Punch risen pizza mixture down and turn onto a gently floured surface. Carry pizza mixture out to a 10-12 inch circle. Move to pizza strip or arranged preparing sheet.
9. Uniformly spread around 3/4 cup squashed feta blend on top of hull (save any excess feta for another utilization) Top with mozzarella cheddar, olives, artichokes, and broiled red peppers. In the case of using pizza stone, cautiously move pizza from the strip to the stone. In the case of using heating sheet, place sheet in oven.
10. Prepare pizza at 500F 10-12 minutes, turning once part of the way through heating, until covering and cheddar is a profound brilliant brown. Sprinkle pizza with new basil and let stand 3-5 minutes prior to cutting into wedges and serving hot. Enjoy!

1053. Mediterranean Chicken Stew

Prep Time: 15 Minutes *Cook Time: 35 Minutes* *Servings: 2*

INGREDIENTS

- 1 Tbsp. tomato paste
- 4 c chicken stock, vegetable stock, or water
- 1 whole chicken (3 lb.), cut into 8 pieces
- 3 med eggplants, diced into 1-inch cubes
- 2 green bell peppers, roughly chopped
- 2 red bell peppers, roughly chopped
- 2 garlic cloves, minced
- 4 med tomatoes, diced
- 1 bunch fresh flat-leaf parsley, stemmed and chopped
- ½ c olive oil
- Salt and freshly ground black pepper
- Greek yogurt, for serving

DIRECTIONS:

1. PREHEAT the oven to 375°F.
2. DISSOLVE the tomato paste in the chicken stock in a medium bowl.
3. Mix the chicken, eggplant, bell peppers, garlic, tomatoes, parsley, olive oil, and salt and pepper to taste on a large baking pan.
4. Then the tomato paste mixture over the baking pan. Cover and bake for 30 minutes. Uncover and bake until the chicken is thoroughly cooked and golden, another 30 minutes

1054. Mediterranean Pressed Picnic Sandwich Recipe

Prep Time: 15 Minutes *Cook Time: 45 Minutes* *Servings: 2*

INGREDIENTS

- 1 Serving
- 1 tablespoon virgin olive oil
- salt As required
- 1/2 pieces ciabatta Bread
- black pepper As required
- For Filling
- 1/4 small zucchini
- 2/3 tablespoon balsamic vinegar
- 1 and 1/4 tablespoon olive tapenade
- 3/4 red peppers
- 1/4 small eggplant/ brinjal
- 1 and 1/4 tablespoon yellow squash
- 1 tablespoon pesto sauce
- 1 slices mozzarella

Directions:

1. Stage 1
2. To set up this nibble formula, on a cleaving load up, cut the eggplant, zucchini, yellow squash and red peppers daintily. Then, cut the crusty bread in the middle to account for the filling. Presently, brush the cuts vegetables with olive oil on the two sides and put them to the side on a plate.
3. Stage 2
4. Heat a barbecue to medium temperature and spot the lubed vegetable cuts on it. Barbecue the two sides until it turns fresh and scorched. When done, move these to a plate and sprinkle salt and dark pepper powder over these. In the interim, take pesto sauce and apply it on one side of the crusty bread and tapenade on opposite side of the bread. Rehash this with every one of the cuts of crusty bread.
5. Stage 3
6. Presently, begin making the sandwich and add initial a layer of flame broiled eggplant, at that point zucchini, yellow squash, red peppers lastly mozzarella cuts. Pour the balsamic vinegar over the vegetables. What's more, cover the sandwich. Press it between the palms of your hands and cover it using a stick wrap. Keep some weight over the sandwich using a kitchen utensil and refrigerate it for a couple of hours. When done, serve it cold with a plunge of your decision to enjoy!

1055. Mediterranean Kale Pesto Pasta

Prep Time: 15 Minutes *Cook Time: 30 Minutes* *Servings : 5*

INGREDIENTS

- kosher salt
- 12 oz. whole-wheat linguine
- 1/2 c. basil leaves
- 1 c. flat-leaf parsley leaves
- 1 bunch kale (about 1 lb.), ribs removed and leaves roughly chopped
- 1/4 c. roasted unsalted almonds
- 2 cloves garlic, pressed
- 3 tbsp. olive oil
- 1 tbsp. ground lemon zing
- 2 tbsp. lemon juice
- ground Parmesan, for serving
- red pepper chips, for serving

DIRECTIONS

1. Heat huge pot of water to the point of boiling. Add 2 tsp. salt, at that point pasta, and cook per bundle directions.
2. Fill huge bowl with ice water. Make pesto: While pasta is in bubbling water, place spices in little sifter and plunge into bubbling water to shrink, at that point promptly move to bowl of ice water. Add kale to bubbling water and cook 1 min. Scoop out with sifter or utensils and move to bowl of ice water. Channel and crush out overabundance fluid.
3. In food processor, beat almonds until chopped. Add garlic, oil, lemon zing and juice, and 1/2 tsp. salt and heartbeat to consolidate. Add spices and kale and puree until smooth.
4. Hold 1 cup cooking water, at that point channel pasta and return it to pot. Add pesto and 1/2 cup cooking water and throw to cover, adding really cooking water as important. Serve finished off with Parmesan and red pepper pieces.

1056. Lemon Garlic Chicken

Prep Time: 15 Minutes *Cook Time: 45 Minutes* *Servings : 4*

INGREDIENTS

- 1/4 cup olive oil
- 2 tablespoons lemon juice
- 3 garlic cloves, minced
- 1-1/2 teaspoons minced new thyme or 3/4 teaspoon dried thyme
- 1 teaspoon salt
- 1/2 teaspoon minced new rosemary or 1/4 teaspoon dried rosemary, squashed
- 1/4 teaspoon pepper
- 6 bone-in chicken thighs
- 6 chicken drumsticks
- 1 pound child red potatoes, split
- 1 medium lemon, cut
- 2 tablespoons minced new parsley

DIRECTIONS

1. Preheat oven to 425°. In a little bowl, whisk the initial 7 ingredients until mixed. Pour 1/4 cup marinade into an enormous bowl or shallow dish. Add chicken and go to cover. Refrigerate 30 minutes. Cover and refrigerate remaining marinade.
2. Channel chicken, disposing of any leftover marinade in bowl. Spot chicken in a 15x10x1-in. heating container; add potatoes in a solitary layer. Shower held marinade over potatoes; top with lemon cuts. Prepare until a thermometer embedded in chicken peruses 170°-175° and potatoes are delicate, 40-45 minutes. Whenever wanted, cook chicken 3-4 crawls from heat until profound brilliant brown, around 3-4 minutes. Sprinkle with parsley prior to serving.

1057. Sausage pepper sandwiches

Prep Time: 15 Minutes *Cook Time: 55 Minutes* *Servings : 4*

INGREDIENTS

- 1 pound uncooked sweet Italian turkey hotdog joins, generally chopped
- 3 medium sweet red peppers, cultivated and cut
- 1 huge onion, split and cut
- 1 tablespoon olive oil
- 6 sausage buns, split
- 6 cuts provolone cheddar

DIRECTIONS

1. Preheat oven to 375°. Spot wiener pieces in a 15x10x1-in. sheet skillet, orchestrating peppers and onion around frankfurter. Shower olive oil over wiener and vegetables; heat, mixing blend following 15 minutes, until frankfurter is not, at this point pink and vegetables are delicate, 30-35 minutes.
2. During the most recent 5 minutes of preparing, orchestrate buns cut side up in a subsequent sheet container; top every bun base with a cheddar cut. Prepare until buns are brilliant brown and cheddar is softened. Spoon frankfurter and pepper combination onto bun bottoms. Supplant tops.
3. Extra pasta sauce in the cooler is an invite expansion for a pizza sandwich.
4. For a family-sized sandwich, trade out the wiener buns with an enormous portion of French bread cut down the middle longwise.

1058. Sweet & Tangy Salmon with Green Beans

Prep Time: 15 Minutes *Cook Time: 45 Minutes* *Servings: 2*

INGREDIENTS

- 4 salmon fillets (6 ounces each)
- 1 tablespoon butter
- 2 tablespoons brown sugar
- 2 tablespoons reduced-sodium soy sauce
- 2 tablespoons Dijon mustard
- 1 tablespoon olive oil
- 1/2 teaspoon pepper
- 1/8 teaspoon salt
- 1 pound fresh green beans, trimmed

DIRECTIONS

1. Firstly preheat oven to 425°. Place fillets in a 15x10x1-in. baking pan coated with cooking spray. In a small skillet, melt butter; stir in brown sugar, soy sauce, mustard, oil, pepper and salt. Brush half of the paste over salmon.
2. Then place green beans in a large bowl; drizzle with remaining brown sugar mixture and toss to coat. Arrange green beans around fillets. Roast it until fish just begins to flake easily with a fork and green beans are crisp-tender, 14-16 minutes.

1059. Greek Chicken Parmesan

Prep Time: 15 Minutes *Cook Time: 25 Minutes* *Servings : 6*

INGREDIENTS

- 1 huge egg
- 1/2 cup panko bread pieces
- 1/2 cup ground Parmesan cheddar
- 1/2 teaspoon salt
- 1 teaspoon pepper
- 1 teaspoon garlic powder
- 4 boneless skinless chicken bosom parts (6 ounces each)
- Olive oil-seasoned cooking splash
- 4 cups new or frozen broccoli florets (around 10 ounces)
- 1 cup marinara sauce
- 1 cup shredded mozzarella cheddar
- 1/4 cup minced new basil, discretionary

DIRECTIONS

1. Preheat oven to 400°. Softly coat a 15x10x1-in. preparing container with cooking splash.
2. In a shallow bowl, whisk egg. In a different shallow bowl, mix together the following 5 ingredients. Dunk chicken bosom in egg; permit overabundance to trickle off. At that point dunk in morsel blend, tapping to help covering follow. Rehash with staying chicken. Spot chicken breasts in focus third of preparing container. Spritz with cooking splash.
3. Prepare 10 minutes. Eliminate from oven. Spread broccoli in a solitary layer along the two sides of sheet skillet (if broccoli is frozen, split pieces up). Get back to oven; prepare 10 minutes longer. Eliminate from oven.
4. Preheat oven. Spread marinara sauce over chicken; top with shredded cheddar. Cook chicken and broccoli 3-4 in. from heat until cheddar is brilliant brown and vegetables are delicate, 3-5 minutes. Whenever wanted, sprinkle with basil.
5. Give serving this a shot a bed of riced cauliflower. Various brands are accessible in the vegetable part of the cooler case.
6. Like most Italian-inspired dishes, this would match magnificently with a thick cut of garlic bread.

1060. Greek Pepper Sausage Pizza

Prep Time: 15 Minutes *Cook Time: 45 Minutes* *Servings : 6*

INGREDIENTS

- 3 to 4 cups all-purpose flour, isolated
- 1 bundle (1/4 ounce) snappy ascent yeast
- 1 teaspoon sugar
- 1 cup warm water (120° to 130°)
- 1/4 cup olive oil
- 2 teaspoons salt
- 1 teaspoon dried basil
- 1/2 teaspoon pepper
- 1/2 cup shredded Parmesan cheddar, isolated
- 3 cups torn new spinach
- 1 can (15 ounces) pizza sauce
- 4 cups shredded mozzarella cheddar, isolated
- 1/2 pound mass pork frankfurter, cooked and depleted
- 1 medium onion, chopped
- 1/2 pound new mushrooms, cut
- 1/2 medium sweet yellow pepper, chopped
- 1-1/2 teaspoons pizza preparing or Italian flavoring
- 3 tablespoons minced new basil, optional

DIRECTIONS

1. Preheat oven to 450°. In a bowl, join 1 cup flour, yeast and sugar. Add water; beat until smooth. Add the oil, salt, dried basil, pepper, 1/4 cup Parmesan cheddar and 2 cups flour; beat until mixed. Mix in sufficient excess flour to frame a delicate mixture. Turn onto a floured surface; ply until smooth and flexible, around 6-8 minutes. Cover and let rest 5 minutes.
2. In the mean time, place spinach in a microwave-safe bowl; cover and microwave on high 30 seconds or just until shriveled. Reveal and put in a safe spot.
3. Press mixture into a lubed 15x10x1-in. heating dish. Spread with pizza sauce; sprinkle with 2-1/2 cups mozzarella cheddar, wiener, onion, spinach, mushrooms and yellow pepper. Top with outstanding Parmesan and mozzarella cheeses. Sprinkle with pizza preparing. Heat 20 minutes or until outside layer is brilliant brown. Sprinkle with new basil whenever wanted. Cut into squares.

1061. Spicy Roasted Sausage, Potatoes and Peppers

Prep Time: 15 Minutes *Cook Time: 25 Minutes* *Servings : 8*

INGREDIENTS

- 1 pound potatoes (about 2 medium), peeled and cut into 1/2-inch cubes
- 1 package (12 ounces) fully cooked Andouille chicken sausage links or flavor of your choice, cut into 1-inch pieces
- 1 medium red onion, cut into wedges
- 1 medium sweet red pepper, cut into 1-inch pieces
- 1 medium green pepper, cut into 1-inch pieces
- 1/2 cup pickled pepper rings
- 1 tablespoon olive oil
- 1/2 to 1 teaspoon Creole seasoning
- 1/4 teaspoon pepper

DIRECTIONS

1. Firstly preheat oven to 400°. In a large bowl, combine potatoes, sausage, onion, red pepper, green pepper and pepper rings. Mix oil, Creole seasoning and pepper; drizzle over potato mixture and toss to coat.
2. Then transfer to a 15x10x1-in. baking pan coated with cooking spray. Roast until vegetables are tender, stirring occasionally, 30-35 minutes.

Nutrition Facts

- 1-1/2 cups: 257 calories, 11g fat (3g saturated fat), 65mg cholesterol, 759mg sodium, 24g carbohydrate (5g sugars, 3g fiber), and 17g protein. Diabetic Exchanges: 3 lean meat, 1 starch, 1 vegetable, 1 fat.

1062. Greek Buffalo Chicken Pizza

Prep Time: 15 Minutes *Cook Time: 50 Minutes* *Servings : 8*

INGREDIENTS

- 1 tube (13.8 ounces) refrigerated pizza covering
- 1 cup Buffalo wing sauce, isolated
- 1-1/2 cups shredded cheddar
- 1-1/2 cups part-skim shredded mozzarella cheddar
- 2 pounds boneless skinless chicken breasts, cubed
- 1/2 teaspoon every garlic salt, pepper and bean stew powder
- 2 tablespoons margarine
- 1/2 teaspoon dried oregano
- Celery sticks and blue cheddar serving of mixed greens dressing

DIRECTIONS

1. Unroll pizza covering into a daintily lubed 15x10x1-in. heating container; straighten mixture and develop edges somewhat. Heat at 400° for 7 minutes. Brush batter with 3 tablespoons Buffalo wing sauce. Join cheddar and mozzarella cheeses; sprinkle a third absurd. Put in a safe spot.
2. In an enormous skillet, cook the chicken, garlic salt, pepper and stew powder in spread until chicken is not, at this point pink. Add the excess wing sauce; cook and mix over medium heat 5 minutes longer.
3. Spoon over pizza. Sprinkle with oregano and remaining cheddar.
4. Heat until outside layer is brilliant brown and cheddar is dissolved, 18-20 minutes. Present with celery and blue cheddar dressing.
5. Freeze choice: Bake pizza outside layer as coordinated; cool. Top with all the ingredients as coordinated and safely wrap and freeze unbaked pizza. To utilize, open up pizza; heat as coordinated, expanding time as important.

1063. Spaghetti Squash Puttanesca

Prep Time: 15 Minutes *Cook Time: 37 Minutes* *Servings: 2*

INGREDIENTS

- US Customary - Metric
- 1 spaghetti squash large

- 1 sweet onion large, 1/2" dice
- 2 red bell peppers seeded, veins removed, 1/2" dice
- 1 pint grape tomatoes halved
- 1 zucchini squash large, 1/2" dice
- 1 yellow squash large, 1/2" dice
- 2 cups broccoli florets cut into bite-sized pieces
- 2 teaspoons granulated garlic
- 1 tablespoon Italian seasoning blend
- 1/2 teaspoon kosher salt or sea salt
- 2 tablespoons olive oil
- 2 cups baby spinach roughly chopped

Instructions

1. Preheat oven to 400 degrees F.
2. Cut spaghetti squash in half; remove seeds and place each half cut side down on a sheet pan. Place sheet pan in preheated oven and roast spaghetti squash until tender, about 20-25 minutes. Squash is ready when you can press the outside (careful) and it "gives" and is no longer hard.
3. Remove spaghetti squash from oven and place cut sides up, allowing cooling slightly.
4. While spaghetti squash is roasting, place onion, peppers, tomatoes, zucchini, yellow squash, and broccoli on another sheet pan. Add granulated garlic, Italian seasoning and salt. Pour on olive oil and toss everything together to evenly coat.
5. Roast vegetables in 400 degree oven for about 15-20 minutes, while spaghetti squash is roasting. Vegetables are ready when tender-crisp and golden brown. Remove from oven.
6. Using a fork, shred the spaghetti squash into "spaghetti" and place in a large mixing bowl or casserole dish.
7. While the spaghetti squash is still slightly warm, add the chopped baby spinach and roasted vegetables. Toss to blend thoroughly. Taste for seasoning, adjust if necessary and serve.

1064. Mediterranean Pizza with Shrimp and Feta

Prep Time: *15 Minutes* *Cook Time:* *20 Minutes* *Servings: 2*

INGREDIENTS

- 2 tbsp. cornmeal
- 1 tube (10 ounces) refrigerated pizza dough
- 1 c. water
- 5 oz. large shrimp, peeled and deveined
- 1 tbsp. toasted pine nuts
- 1 large clove garlic
- 1 1/2 c. loosely packed fresh basil
- 2 tbsp. grated Parmesan cheese
- 3 tbsp. defatted reduced-sodium chicken broth
- 2 tsp. lemon juice
- 2 oz. feta cheese, crumbled
- 2 tbsp. minced red onions
- 1/2 c. shredded reduced-fat low-sodium mozzarella cheese

DIRECTIONS

1. Preheat the oven to 450ï¿½F. Coat a baking sheet with no-stick spray. Sprinkle with the cornmeal.
2. Unroll the pizza dough and spread on the prepared sheet.
3. Bring the water to a simmer in a small saucepan. Add the shrimp and cook for 1 to 2 minutes, or until opaque and cooked through. Drain and cut each shrimp into thirds.
4. Place the pine nuts and garlic in a food processor or blender. Process until minced. Add the basil, Parmesan, broth, and lemon juice; process for 2 to 3 minutes, or until a paste forms. Add more broth, if necessary, to achieve the desired consistency.
5. Spread the pesto on the crust, leaving a 1/ 2" border. Sprinkle with the shrimp, feta, and onions. Top with the mozzarella. Bake for 14 to 16 minutes, or until the bottom is browned and the cheese is melted.

1065. Easy Mediterranean Pizza

Prep Time: *15 Minutes* *Cook Time:* *45 Minutes* *Servings : 8*

INGREDIENTS

- 1 ball Best Pizza Dough (or Food Processor Dough or Thin Crust Dough)
- 1/3 cup Best Homemade Pizza Sauce
- 1 teaspoon olive oil
- 1 cup packed baby spinach leaves
- 1 handful red onion slices
- 6 Kalamata olives
- 8 sundried tomatoes, packed in oil
- 3/4 cup shredded mozzarella cheese
- 1 ounce feta cheese
- 8 fresh basil leaves
- Kosher salt
- Semolina flour or cornmeal, for cleaning the pizza strip

Guidelines

1. Make the pizza batter: Follow the Best Pizza Dough formula to set up the mixture. (This requires around 15 minutes to make and 45 minutes to rest.)
2. Spot a pizza stone in the oven and preheat to 500°F. Or on the other hand preheat your pizza oven (here's the pizza oven we use).
3. Make the pizza sauce: Make the 5 Minute Pizza Sauce.
4. Set up the fixings: In a little skillet, heat the olive oil over medium heat. Add the spinach and cook for 2 minutes until withered yet radiant green. Add 1 squeeze salt and eliminate from the heat.
5. Meagerly cut the red onion. Cut the olives fifty-fifty. On the off chance that the sundried tomatoes are huge, you can slash them more modest as well.
6. Prepare the pizza: When the oven is prepared, dust a pizza strip with cornmeal or semolina flour. (On the off chance that you don't have a pizza strip, you can utilize a rimless heating sheet or the rear of a rimmed preparing sheet. Yet, a pizza strip is definitely worth the speculation!) Stretch the mixture into a circle; perceive How to Stretch Pizza Dough for directions. At that point delicately place the mixture onto the pizza strip.
7. Spread the pizza sauce over the mixture using the rear of a spoon to make a dainty layer. Add the shredded mozzarella cheddar. Top with the cooked spinach, red onion, olives, and sundried tomatoes. What's more, feta cheddar.
8. Utilize the pizza strip to deliberately move the pizza onto the preheated pizza stone. Heat the pizza until the cheddar and outside layer are pleasantly browned, around 5 to 7 minutes in the oven (or 1 moment in a pizza oven).
9. Permit the pizza to cool briefly prior to including the basil top (entire leaves, daintily torn, or meagerly cut). Cut into pieces and serve right away.

Side Dishes Recipes

1066. Lemon-Caper Black Cod with Broccoli & Potatoes

Prep Time: *15 Minutes* *Cook Time:* *32 Minutes* *Servings : 8*

INGREDIENTS

- Ingredient Checklist
- 1 pound baby potatoes, halved
- 12 ounces precut broccoli florets
- 4 tablespoons extra-virgin olive oil, partitioned
- ½ teaspoon genuine salt, isolated
- 1 pound skin-on dark cod (see Tip)
- ¼ teaspoon ground pepper
- 2 tablespoons escapades, flushed and wiped off
- 2 tablespoons lemon juice
- 1 tablespoon Dijon mustard
- 1 clove garlic, minced
- 1 tablespoon chopped new thyme or 1/4 teaspoon dried
- 3 tablespoons shredded Parmesan cheddar

DIRECTIONS

1. Stage 1
2. Preheat oven to 450degrees F. Coat a rimmed heating sheet with cooking shower.
3. Stage 2
4. Throw potatoes and broccoli with 1 tablespoon oil and 1/4 teaspoon salt in an enormous bowl. Move to the readied preparing sheet. Cook, mixing once, until delicate, 20 to 25 minutes.
5. Stage 3
6. In the mean time, wipe cod off and cut into 4 segments. Season with the leftover 1/4 teaspoon salt and pepper. Heat 1 tablespoon oil in a huge nonstick skillet over medium heat. Add tricks and cook until brilliant brown, 1 to 2 minutes. Using an opened spoon, move the escapades to a paper towel, leaving the oil in the container. Spot the cod skin-side down in the skillet. Cook, undisturbed, for 5 minutes. Flip and cook until the fish drops effectively with a fork, 3 to 4 minutes more.
7. Stage 4
8. Consolidate the excess 2 tablespoons oil, lemon juice, mustard and garlic in a little bowl.
9. Stage 5
10. Throw the potatoes and broccoli with thyme. Serve the vegetables and cod sprinkled with the lemon vinaigrette and decorated with the tricks and Parmesan.

1067. Mediterranean Roasted Chicken Thighs with Peppers & Potatoes

Prep Time: *15 Minutes* *Cook Time:* *20 Minutes* *Servings : 4*

INGREDIENTS

- 2 pounds red potatoes (about 6 medium)
- 2 large sweet red peppers
- 2 large green peppers
- 2 medium onions
- 2 tablespoons olive oil, divided
- 4 teaspoons minced fresh thyme or 1-1/2 teaspoons dried thyme, divided
- 3 teaspoons minced fresh rosemary or 1 teaspoon dried rosemary, crushed, divided
- 8 boneless skinless chicken thighs (about 2 pounds)
- 1/2 teaspoon salt
- 1/4 teaspoon pepper

DIRECTIONS

1. Firstly preheat oven to 450°. Cut potatoes, peppers and onions into 1-in. pieces. Place vegetables in a roasting pan. Drizzle with 1 tablespoon oil; sprinkle with 2 teaspoons each thyme and rosemary and toss to coat. Put chicken over vegetables. Brush chicken with remaining oil; sprinkle with remaining thyme and rosemary. Drizzle vegetables and chicken with salt and pepper.
2. Roast until a thermometer inserted in chicken reads 170° and vegetables are tender, 35-40 minutes.

1068. Greek Pork Tenderloins with Wild Rice

Prep Time: *15 Minutes* *Cook Time:* *30 Minutes* *Servings: 2*

INGREDIENTS

- 2 pork tenderloins (1 pound each)
- 1 bundle (8.8 ounces) prepared to-serve entire grain brown and wild rice mixture
- 1-3/4 cups frozen broccoli, carrots and water chestnuts, defrosted and coarsely chopped
- 1/2 cup chopped dried apricots
- 1/2 cup minced new parsley
- 1/2 teaspoon salt
- 1/2 teaspoon garlic powder
- 1/2 teaspoon dried thyme
- 1/2 teaspoon dried sage leaves
- 1/4 teaspoon pepper
- Sauce:
- 1 cup water
- 1 envelope pork sauce blend
- 1 tablespoon Dijon mustard
- 1/4 teaspoon dried sage leaves
- 1 tablespoon minced new parsley

DIRECTIONS

1. Make a long way cut down the focal point of every tenderloin to inside 1/2 in. of base. Open tenderloins so they lie level; cover and smooth to 3/4-in. thickness.
2. Get ready rice as per bundle directions. In a small bowl, consolidate the rice, vegetables, apricots, parsley and flavors.

3. Eliminate covering; spread rice blend over meat. Close tenderloins; attach with kitchen string. Spot in an ungreased 15x10x1-in. preparing dish. Prepare, uncovered, at 425° for 15 minutes.
4. In the meantime, in a small pot, join the water, sauce blend, mustard and sage. Heat to the point of boiling; cook and mix for 2 minutes or until thickened. Mix in parsley.
5. Brush 2 tablespoons sauce over tenderloins. Prepare 10-15 minutes longer or until a thermometer peruses 160°. Let represent 15 minutes. Dispose of string; cut every tenderloin into 9 cuts. Present with residual sauce.

1069. Balsamic Roasted Chicken Thighs with Root Vegetables

Prep Time: 10 Minutes *Cook Time:□30 Minutes* *Servings: 2*

INGREDIENTS

- 4 tablespoons olive oil, isolated
- 3 tablespoons stone-ground mustard
- 2 tablespoons balsamic vinaigrette
- 3/4 teaspoon fit salt, isolated
- 3/4 teaspoon newly ground pepper, isolated
- 6 bone-in chicken thighs (around 2-1/4 pounds)
- 4 medium parsnips, stripped and cut into 1/2-inch pieces
- 1 medium yam, stripped and cut into 1/2-inch pieces
- 4 shallots, chopped
- 1/4 teaspoon caraway seeds
- 4 tablespoons minced new parsley, separated
- 3 bacon strips, cooked and disintegrated, partitioned

DIRECTIONS

1. In a bowl, whisk 3 tablespoons oil, mustard, vinaigrette and 1/2 teaspoon each salt and pepper until mixed. Add chicken, going to cover. Refrigerate, covered, 6 hours or overnight.
2. Preheat oven to 425°. Spot chicken, skin side up, on portion of a lubed 15x10x1-in. preparing skillet. Spot parsnips and yam in an enormous bowl; add shallots, caraway seeds and the leftover oil, salt and pepper and throw to join. Organize in a solitary layer on leftover portion of dish.
3. Broil chicken and vegetables 20 minutes. Mix vegetables; broil chicken and vegetables until a thermometer embedded in chicken peruses 170°-175° and vegetables are delicate, 15-20 minutes longer.
4. Move vegetables to a bowl; throw with 2 tablespoons parsley and half of the bacon. Serve chicken with vegetables; sprinkle chicken with the excess parsley and bacon.

1070. Chili-Stuffed Poblano Peppers

Prep Time: 5 Minutes *Cook Time: 30 Minutes* *Servings: 4*

INGREDIENTS

- 1 pound lean ground turkey (93% lean)
- 1 can (15 ounces) chili without beans
- 1/4 teaspoon salt
- 1-1/2 cups shredded Mexican cheese blend, divided
- 1 medium tomato, finely chopped
- 4 green onions, chopped
- 4 large poblano peppers
- 1 tablespoon olive oil

DIRECTIONS

1. Firstly preheat broiler. In a large skillet over medium heat, cook turkey, crumbling meat, until no longer pink, 5-7 minutes; drain. Then add chili and salt; heat through. Stir in 1/2 cup cheese, tomato and green onions.
2. Meanwhile, cut peppers lengthwise in half; remove seeds. Put on a foil-lined 15x10x1-in. baking pan, cut side down; brush with oil. Broil 4 in. from heat until skins blister, about 5 minutes.
3. With tongs, turn peppers. Then fill with turkey mixture; sprinkle with remaining cheese. Broil until cheese is melted, 1-2 minutes longer.

1071. Pineapple Chicken Fajitas

Prep Time: 10 Minutes *Cook Time: 35 Minutes* *Servings: 4*

INGREDIENTS

- 2 tablespoons coconut oil, softened
- 3 teaspoons stew powder
- 2 teaspoons ground cumin
- 1 teaspoon garlic powder
- 3/4 teaspoon kosher salt
- 1-1/2 pounds chicken tenderloins, split the long way
- 1 huge red or sweet onion, divided and cut (around 2 cups)
- 1 huge sweet red pepper, cut into 1/2-inch strips
- 1 huge green pepper, cut into 1/2-inch strips
- 1 tablespoon minced cultivated jalapeno pepper
- 2 jars (8 ounces each) unsweetened pineapple goodies, depleted
- 2 tablespoons nectar
- 2 tablespoons lime juice
- 12 corn tortillas (6 inches), warmed
- Optional: Pico de Gallo, acrid cream, shredded Mexican cheddar mix, cut avocado and lime wedges

DIRECTIONS

1. Preheat oven to 425°. In an enormous bowl, blend initial 5 ingredients; mix in chicken. Add onion, peppers, pineapple, nectar and lime juice; throw to join. Spread uniformly in 2 lubed 15x10x1-in. preparing dish.
2. Broil 10 minutes, turning container part of the way through cooking. Eliminate container from oven; preheat oven.
3. Sear chicken combination, 1 skillet at an at once, in. from heat until vegetables are daintily browned and chicken is not, at this point pink, 3-5 minutes. Serve in tortillas, with garnishes and lime wedges as wanted.

1072. Greek White Pizza with Roasted Tomatoes

Prep Time: 150 Minutes *Cook Time: 70 Minutes* *Servings: 5*

INGREDIENTS

- 4 plum tomatoes (around 1 pound), cut longwise into 1/2-inch cuts and cultivated
- 1/4 cup olive oil
- 1 teaspoon sugar
- 1/2 teaspoon salt
- Outside:
- 2 tablespoons olive oil
- 1 huge onion, finely chopped (around 1 cup)
- 2 teaspoons dried basil
- 2 teaspoons dried thyme
- 1 teaspoon dried rosemary, squashed
- 1 bundle (1/4 ounce) dynamic dry yeast
- 1 cup warm water (110° to 115°)
- 5 tablespoons sugar
- 1/4 cup olive oil
- 1-1/2 teaspoons salt
- 3-1/4 to 3-3/4 cups all-purpose flour
- Topping:
- 1 cup entire milk ricotta cheddar
- 3 garlic cloves, minced
- 1/2 teaspoon salt
- 1/2 teaspoon Italian flavoring
- 2 cups shredded part-skim mozzarella cheddar

DIRECTIONS

1. Preheat oven to 250°. In a bowl, throw tomatoes with oil, sugar and salt. Move to a lubed 15x10x1-in. heating container. Broil 2 hours or until tomatoes are delicate and somewhat withered.
2. For outside, in an enormous skillet, heat oil over medium-high heat. Add onion; cook and mix 3-4 minutes or until delicate. Mix in spices. Cool somewhat.
3. In a small bowl, break down yeast in warm water. In a huge bowl, join sugar, oil, salt, yeast combination and 1 cup flour; beat on medium speed until smooth. Mix in onion combination and enough leftover flour to shape a delicate mixture (batter will be tacky).
4. Turn batter onto a floured surface; massage until smooth and versatile, around 6-8 minutes. Spot in a lubed bowl, going once to oil the top. Cover with cling wrap and let ascend in a warm spot until practically multiplied, around 1-1/2 hours.
5. Preheat oven to 400°. Oil a 15x10x1-in. preparing container. Punch down batter; move to fit base and 1/2-in. up sides of container. Cover; let rest 10 minutes. Heat 10-12 minutes or until edges are daintily browned.
6. In a small bowl, blend ricotta cheddar, garlic, salt and Italian flavoring. Spread over covering; top with cooked tomatoes and mozzarella cheddar. Heat 12-15 minutes or until covering is brilliant and cheddar is liquefied.

1073. Mediterranean Orange-Glazed Pork with Sweet Potatoes

Prep Time: 3 Minutes *Cook Time: 70 Minutes* *Servings: 4*

INGREDIENTS

- 1 pound yams (around 2 medium)
- 2 medium apples
- 1 medium orange
- 1 teaspoon salt
- 1/2 teaspoon pepper
- 1 cup squeezed orange
- 2 tablespoons brown sugar
- 2 teaspoons cornstarch
- 1 teaspoon ground cinnamon
- 1 teaspoon ground ginger
- 2 pork tenderloins (around 1 pound each)

DIRECTIONS

1. Preheat oven to 350°. Strip yams; center apples. Cut potatoes, apples and orange transversely into 1/4-in. - thick cuts. Organize in a foil-lined 15x10x1-in. heating container covered with cooking shower; sprinkle with salt and pepper. Cook 10 minutes.
2. Then, in a microwave-safe bowl, blend squeezed orange, brown sugar, cornstarch, cinnamon and ginger. Microwave, covered, on high, mixing like clockwork until thickened, 1-2 minutes. Mix until smooth.
3. Spot pork over yam combination; sprinkle with squeezed orange blend. Broil until a thermometer embedded in pork peruses 145° and yams and apples are delicate, 45-55 minutes longer. Eliminate from oven; tent with foil. Let stand 10 minutes prior to cutting.

1074. Quinoa-Stuffed Squash Boats

Prep Time: 5 Minutes *Cook Time: 30 Minutes* *Servings: 8*

INGREDIENTS

- 4 delicata squash (around 12 ounces each)
- 3 teaspoons olive oil, partitioned
- 1/8 teaspoon pepper
- 1 teaspoon salt, partitioned
- 1-1/2 cups vegetable stock
- 1 cup quinoa, washed
- 1 can (15 ounces) garbanzo beans or chickpeas, washed and depleted
- 1/4 cup dried cranberries
- 1 green onion, daintily cut
- 1 teaspoon minced new wise
- 1/2 teaspoon ground lemon zing
- 1 teaspoon lemon juice
- 1/2 cup disintegrated goat cheddar
- 1/4 cup salted pumpkin seeds or pepitas, toasted

DIRECTIONS

1. Preheat oven to 450°. Cut each squash longwise down the middle; eliminate and dispose of seeds. Daintily brush cut sides with 1 teaspoon oil; sprinkle with pepper and 1/2 teaspoon salt. Spot on a heating sheet, cut side down. Prepare until delicate, 15-20 minutes.

2. In the interim, in an enormous pan, join stock and quinoa; heat to the point of boiling. Lessen heat; stew, covered, until fluid is assimilated, 12-15 minutes.
3. Mix in garbanzo beans, cranberries, green onion, sage, lemon zing, lemon juice and the leftover oil and salt; spoon into squash. Sprinkle with cheddar and pumpkin seeds.

1075. Pan-Roasted Pork Chops & Potatoes

Prep Time: 2 Minutes *Cook Time:* 40 Minutes *Servings: 6*

INGREDIENTS

- 4 boneless pork midsection hacks (6 ounces each)
- 1/2 cup in addition to 2 tablespoons decreased fat Italian plate of mixed greens dressing, isolated
- 4 small potatoes (around 1-1/2 pounds)
- 1/2 pound new Brussels grows, managed and split
- 1/2 cup delicate bread pieces
- 1 tablespoon minced new parsley
- 1/4 teaspoon salt
- 1/8 teaspoon pepper
- 2 teaspoons spread, dissolved

DIRECTIONS

1. Spot pork hacks and 1/2 cup plate of mixed greens dressing in an enormous bowl; go to cover. Cover and refrigerate 8 hours or overnight. Refrigerate remaining plate of mixed greens dressing.
2. Preheat oven to 400°. Cut every potato the long way into 12 wedges. Organize potatoes and Brussels sprouts in a 15x10x1-in. heating container covered with cooking splash. Shower vegetables with residual plate of mixed greens dressing; throw to cover. Broil 20 minutes.
3. Channel pork, disposing of marinade. Wipe pork off with paper towels. Mix vegetables; place pork cleaves up and over. Cook 15-20 minutes longer or until a thermometer embedded in pork peruses 145°. Preheat oven.
4. In a small bowl, join bread morsels, parsley, salt and pepper; mix in spread. Top pork with morsel combination. Sear 4-6 in. from heat 1-2 minutes or until bread morsels are brilliant brown. Let stand 5 minutes.

1076. Greek Honey-Roasted Chicken & Root Vegetables

Prep Time: 10 Minutes *Cook Time:* 90 Minutes *Servings: 5*

INGREDIENTS

- 1 teaspoon salt
- 1 teaspoon pepper
- 1 teaspoon minced new rosemary
- 1 teaspoon minced new thyme
- 2 tablespoons olive oil, separated
- 1 tablespoon spread
- 6 boneless skinless chicken bosom parts (6 ounces each)
- 1/2 cup white wine
- 3 tablespoons nectar, separated
- 3 stripped medium yams, chopped
- 4 medium stripped carrots, chopped
- 2 medium fennel bulbs, chopped
- 2 cups chicken stock
- 3 sound leaves

DIRECTIONS

1. Preheat oven to 375°. Join salt, pepper, rosemary and thyme. In a huge skillet, heat 1 tablespoon olive oil and margarine over medium-high heat. Sprinkle a large portion of the flavoring blend over chicken breasts. Add to skillet; cook until brilliant brown, 2-3 minutes for each side. Eliminate and put in a safe spot. Add wine and 2 tablespoons nectar to container; cook 2-3 minutes, mixing to release browned pieces.
2. Consolidate yams, carrots and fennel in a microwave-safe bowl. Add staying olive oil, flavors and nectar to vegetables; mix to join. Microwave, covered, until potatoes are simply delicate, 10 minutes.
3. Move vegetables to a shallow simmering dish. Add chicken stock, wine combination and inlet leaves; top vegetables with chicken. Broil until a thermometer embedded in chicken peruses 165°, 25-30 minutes. Dispose of cove leaves. Present with vegetables and sauce.

1077. Triple Tomato Flatbread

Prep Time: 120 Minutes *Cook Time:* 150 Minutes *Servings: 8*

INGREDIENTS

- 1 tube (13.8 ounces) refrigerated pizza covering
- Cooking shower
- 3 plum tomatoes, finely chopped (around 2 cups)
- 1/2 cup delicate sun-dried tomato parts (not pressed in oil), julienned
- 2 tablespoons olive oil
- 1 tablespoon dried basil
- 1/4 teaspoon salt
- 1/4 teaspoon pepper
- 1 cup shredded Asiago cheddar
- 2 cups yellow or potentially red cherry tomatoes, divided

DIRECTIONS

1. Unroll and press mixture into a 15x10-in. square shape. Move mixture to a 18x12-in. piece of hard core foil covered with cooking splash; spritz mixture with cooking shower. In an enormous bowl, throw plum tomatoes and sun-dried tomatoes with oil and flavors.
2. Cautiously modify mixture onto flame broil rack; eliminate foil. Flame broil, covered, over medium heat 2-3 minutes or until base is brilliant brown. Turn; barbecue 1-2 minutes longer or until second side starts to brown.
3. Eliminate from barbecue. Spoon plum tomato blends over covering; top with cheddar and cherry tomatoes. Return flatbread to flame broil. Barbecue, covered, 2-4 minutes or until outside is brilliant brown and cheddar is softened.
4. To prepare flatbread: Preheat oven to 425°. Unroll and press batter onto lower part of a 15x10x1-in. heating skillet covered with cooking shower. Prepare 6-8 minutes or until softly browned. Gather flatbread as coordinated. Prepare 8-10 minutes longer or until outside is brilliant and cheddar is dissolved

1078. Mediterranean Sautéed Chicken with Olives, Capers and Lemons

Prep Time: 20 Minutes *Cook Time:* 190 Minutes *Servings: 6*

Ingredients

- 2 lemons sliced 1/4 inch thick
- 1/4 cup plus 1 tablespoon extra-virgin olive oil
- 6 skinless boneless chicken thighs, about 1 pound
- 1-2 tablespoons rice flour or all-purpose flour
- 1 fat garlic clove minced
- 1 cup chicken broth
- 3/4 cup Sicilian green olives
- 1/4 cup carpers
- 2 tablespoons spread
- 2 tablespoons parsley
- legitimate salt and newly broke dark pepper

Directions

1. Bring a medium-huge, high sided skillet to medium-high heat and add 1 tablespoon of olive oil. Add half of the lemon cuts and singe until browned, 3-5 minutes on each side. Move to a plate. Season the chicken thighs with fit salt and dark pepper and residue with rice flour, shaking off the overabundance. Add 1/2 tablespoons of olive oil to the hot skillet and burn the chicken pieces until brilliant brown, around 5 minutes each side. Move to another plate and wrap up singing the remainder of the chicken pieces, at that point move to a similar plate as the remainder of the chicken.
2. Add the remainder of the olive oil to the skillet and the minced garlic, and cook for 30 seconds or until fragrant, blending so the garlic doesn't consume and turn out to be harsh.
3. Add the green olives, tricks and stock. Add the saved chicken and any juices that have been delivered in addition to the saved lemons and their juices and cook over high heat until the stock is diminished significantly, around 5 minutes. Add the spread and parsley and cook for one more moment. Season with more legitimate salt and newly ground dark pepper to taste. Move to plates and spoon the olives, tricks, lemons and sauce on top.
4. Present with sautéed spinach, kale or Swiss chard as an afterthought.

1079. Greek Pan-Roasted Chicken and Vegetables

Prep Time: 10 Minutes *Cook Time:* 30 Minutes *Servings: 4*

Ingredients

- 2 pounds red potatoes (around 6 medium), cut into 3/4-inch pieces
- 1 enormous onion, coarsely chopped
- 2 tablespoons olive oil
- 3 garlic cloves, minced
- 1-1/4 teaspoons salt, separated
- 1 teaspoon dried rosemary, squashed, isolated
- 3/4 teaspoon pepper, separated
- 1/2 teaspoon paprika
- 6 bone-in chicken thighs (around 2-1/4 pounds), skin eliminated
- 6 cups new child spinach (around 6 ounces)

Directions

1. Preheat oven to 425°. In a huge bowl, consolidate potatoes, onion, oil, garlic, 3/4 teaspoon salt, 1/2 teaspoon rosemary and 1/2 teaspoon pepper; throw to cover. Move to a 15x10x1-in. preparing pan covered with cooking shower.
2. In a small bowl, blend paprika and the leftover salt, rosemary and pepper. Sprinkle chicken with paprika combination; organize over vegetables. Cook until a thermometer embedded in chicken peruses 170°-175° and vegetables are simply delicate, 35-40 minutes.
3. Eliminate chicken to a serving platter; keep warm. Top vegetables with spinach. Broil until vegetables are delicate and spinach is shriveled, 8-10 minutes longer. Mix vegetables to join; present with chicken.
4. Set up your sheet-pan supper the prior night and simply pop it into the preheated oven to prepare. This serves to profoundly enhance the chicken, a shared benefit!
5. In the event that you need a more extravagant dish, use skin-on chicken, and on the off chance that you need a lighter dish, utilize bone-in chicken breasts. Make certain to cook bone-in breasts just to 165-170 degrees, since more slender meat can get dry at higher temperatures.

1080. Greek Seafood Couscous Paella

Prep Time: 5 Minutes *Cook Time:* 30 Minutes *Servings: 4*

Ingredients

- 2 teaspoons extra-virgin olive oil
- 1 medium onion, chopped
- 1 clove garlic, minced
- ½ teaspoon dried thyme
- ½ teaspoon fennel seed
- ¼ teaspoon salt
- ¼ teaspoon freshly ground pepper
- Pinch of crumbled saffron threads
- 1 cup no-salt-added diced tomatoes, with juice
- ¼ cup vegetable broth
- 4 ounces bay scallops, tough muscle removed
- 4 ounces small shrimp, (41-50 per pound), peeled and deveined
- ½ cup whole-wheat couscous

DIRECTIONS:

1. Heat oil in a large saucepan over medium heat. Add onion; cook, stirring constantly, for 3 minutes. Add garlic, thyme, fennel seed, salt, pepper and saffron; cook for 20 seconds.
2. Stir in tomatoes and broth. Bring to a simmer. Cover, reduce heat and simmer for 2 minutes.
3. Increase heat to medium, stir in scallops and cook, stirring occasionally, for 2 minutes. Add shrimp and cook, stirring occasionally, for 2 minutes more. Stir in couscous. Cover, remove from heat and let stand for 5 minutes; fluff.

1081. Mediterranean Baked Feta Pizza

Prep Time: 20 Minutes *Cook Time:* 170 Minutes *Servings: 5*

Ingredients

- Pizza Dough (alternatively, you can use a premade dough*)
- 1-1/4 cups bread flour (175 grams) I recommend weighing the flour for better accuracy
- 1/2 teaspoon instant dry yeast
- 1/2 teaspoon salt

- 1/2 cup warm water (110F)
- 1/2 teaspoon olive oil
- Prepared Feta + Toppings
- 1 pt. cherry tomatoes
- 1 tablespoon finely chopped shallot
- 2 medium entire cloves garlic, stripped
- 2 tablespoons olive oil
- 1 (8 oz.) block feta cheddar
- 1/4 teaspoon red pepper chips (discretionary)
- Legitimate salt and pepper to taste
- 1/2 cup shredded low-dampness mozzarella cheddar
- 1/4 cup split Kalamata olives
- 1/4 cup jostled artichoke hearts, generally chopped and wiped off
- 1/4 cup jostled broiled red peppers, daintily cut into strips
- Small bunch new basil leaves

Directions

Pizza Dough

1. In a huge bowl, join flour, yeast, and salt. Shower water and 1/2 teaspoon olive oil up and over and mix with a wooden spoon until mixture meets up and no dashes of flour remain. Cover with saran wrap and let batter rest 15 minutes.

2. Eliminate batter from bowl and turn onto a softly floured surface. Ply mixture 3-5 minutes until smooth and flexible. Spot into a lubed bowl, going once to oil the top and cover with cling wrap and let rise 3-4 hours at room temperature until multiplied in size (or 24-72 hours in the refrigerator – in the event that you decide to cool the batter, let it come to room temperature 45 minutes prior to carrying out)

Heated Feta + Toppings

1. Preheat oven to 400F. In a 8×8 heating dish, throw tomatoes, shallot, and garlic with olive oil until equally covered. Structure a space in the focal point of skillet and spot feta in the middle. Turn the feta to equally cover in olive oil. Top with red pepper chips, salt, and pepper to taste.
2. Spot feta on center rack of oven. In the event that you have a pizza stone, place on base rack to start preheating. Prepare feta at 400F 35-40 minutes until tomatoes are blasting and feta is a profound brilliant brown. Eliminate feta from oven, increment oven temperature to 500F and move pizza stone to center rack. Utilize a spoon to squash feta, tomatoes, and garlic until a semi-thick sauce structures.

3. In the event that using pizza stone strategy, gently dust a pizza strip with cornmeal. If not using stone, softly oil a huge heating sheet with olive oil (regardless of whether you're not using a stone, preheat your oven per formula directions above)
4. Punch risen pizza mixture down and turn onto a gently floured surface. Carry pizza mixture out to a 10-12 inch circle. Move to pizza strip or arranged preparing sheet.
5. Uniformly spread around 3/4 cup squashed feta blend on top of hull (save any excess feta for another utilization) Top with mozzarella cheddar, olives, artichokes, and broiled red peppers. In the case of using pizza stone, cautiously move pizza from the strip to the stone. In the case of using heating sheet, place sheet in oven.
6. Prepare pizza at 500F 10-12 minutes, turning once part of the way through heating, until covering and cheddar is a profound brilliant brown. Sprinkle pizza with new basil and let stand 3-5 minutes prior to cutting into wedges and serving hot. Enjoy!

1082. Best Greek Chicken Marinade

Prep Time: 20 Minutes *Cook Time: 55 Minutes* *Servings: 4*

Ingredients

- 1 pound boneless skinless chicken breasts (about 2 large breasts)
- ⅓ cup plain Greek yogurt
- ¼ cup olive oil
- 4 lemons
- 4-5 cloves garlic squeezed or minced
- 2 tablespoons dried oregano
- 1 teaspoon genuine salt
- ½ teaspoon newly ground dark pepper

Directions

1. Spot the chicken pieces in a cooler sack or a bowl and put in a safe spot.
2. Add the Greek yogurt and olive oil to a medium size bowl. Zing one of the lemons and add to the bowl. Juice that lemon into the bowl with the zing. Cut the other three lemons and put in a safe spot. Add the minced garlic, oregano, genuine salt and dark pepper to the lemon squeeze and zing and mix. Empty portion of the marinade into the cooler sack or the bowl with the chicken pieces and save the other portion of the marinade for seasoning. Marinate the chicken for 30 minutes or as long as 3 hours in the fridge.
3. At the point when prepared to flame broil, set up the barbecue by gently oiling the mesh with vegetable oil or cooking splash and set to medium high heat.

Flame broil the chicken, treating with the held marinade and turning frequently so each side browns and has light barbecue marks, until cooked through, around 15-20 minutes or until the chicken juices run clear. During the most recent 5 minutes of cooking add the 3 cut lemons to the flame broil, turning more than once. Permit the chicken to rest for 5 minutes prior to cutting and present with the flame broiled lemons

1083. CUBAN-STYLE BLACK BEANS & RICE

Prep Time: 3 Minutes *Cook Time: 10 Minutes* *Servings: 2*

INGREDIENTS:

- Salt
- cup dried black beans, picked over & rinsed
- 2 cups low-sodium chicken broth
- 2 cups water
- Two large green bell peppers stemmed, seeded, & halved
- large onion halved at equator & peeled, root end left intact
- head garlic, five cloves minced, rest of head halved at the equator with the skin left intact
- Two bay leaves
- 1¹/2 cups long-grain white rice
- 2 Tbsps. olive oil
- ounces lean salt pork, cut into ¹/4-inch dice
- 4 Tbsps. ground cumin
- 1 Tbsp. minced fresh oregano
- 2 Tbsps. red wine vinegar
- Two scallions, sliced thin Lime wedges

DIRECTIONS:

1. Dissolve 1¹/2 Tbsps. Salt in 2 quarts cools water in a container or container.
2. Include beans & soak at room temperature for at least 8 hrs or up to 24 hrs. Drain & rinse well.
3. In a Dutch oven, stir together drained beans, broth, water, one pepper half, one onion half (with root end), halved garlic head, bay leaves, & 1 Tsp. Salt.
4. Bring to simmer over high heat, cover, and reduce heat to low. Cook till beans are just soft, 30 to 35 mins.
5. Using tongs, remove & discard pepper, onion, garlic, & bay leaves—drain beans in a colander set over a large container, reserving 2¹/2 cups of bean cooking liquid. Do not wash out the Dutch oven.
6. Now set the oven rack to the middle setting & heat the oven to 350 degrees.

1084. Mediterranean-Style Greek Pasta Recipe

Prep Time: 50 Minutes *Cook Time: 90 Minutes* *Servings: 4*

INGREDIENTS

- 1/2 pound whole-wheat spaghetti pasta
- 2 tablespoons olive oil
- 1 onion small, diced
- 2 cups spinach leaves fresh
- 3 garlic cloves sliced
- 1 beefsteak tomato large, diced
- 1/2 teaspoon kosher salt
- 1/4 teaspoon ground black pepper
- 1/2 cup feta cheese fat-free, crumbled

Instructions

1. Bring 4 cups of water to boil in a medium pot.
2. Add 1 teaspoon salt and pasta to water. Boil uncovered until pasta is tender, about 10 minutes.
3. Drain pasta, reserve 1/2 cup of pasta water. Set aside.
4. In a large skillet, heat the oil over medium heat until hot, but not smoking.
5. Add onions and garlic to skillet. Cook, stirring often, just until onions begin to soften.
6. Add diced tomatoes and spinach. Stir, cover and let simmer for 5 minutes or until spinach is heated through and just begins to wilt.
7. Stir in pasta and reserved pasta water. Cover and simmer for an additional 5 minutes.

Snacks And Appetizer Recipes

1085. CRAB RANGOON

Prep Time: 20 Minutes *Cook Time: 35 Minutes* *Servings: 3*

INGREDIENTS:

- 3 ounces reduced-fat cream cheese
- 1/8 tsp garlic salt
- 1/8 tsp Worcestershire sauce
- ½ cup lump crabmeat, drained
- 1 green onion, chopped
- 14 wonton wrappers

Directions:

1. In a small size bowl, add the cream cheese, garlic salt and Worcestershire sauce until smooth. Stir in crab and onion. Place 2 cupfuls in the centre of each wonton wrapper. Moisten edges with water; bring corners to centre over filling and press edges together to seal.
2. Place on a baking sheet coated with cooking spray. Lightly spray wontons with cooking spray. Bake at 425° for 8-10 minutes or until golden brown. Present warm.

1086. CORN FRITTERS WITH CARAMELIZED ONION JAM

Prep Time: 25 Minutes *Cook Time: 30 Minutes* *Servings: 3*

INGREDIENTS:

- 1 big sweet onion, halved and thinly sliced
- 1 tbsp olive oil
- 2 tsp balsamic vinegar
- 1/3 cup apple jelly
- 1/3 cup canned diced tomatoes
- 1 tbsp tomato paste
- 1/8 tsp curry powder
- 1/8 tsp of ground cinnamon
- Dash salt and pepper
- FRITTERS
- 2 cups of biscuit/baking mix
- 1 can (11 ounces) gold and white corn, drained
- 2 eggs, lightly beaten
- ½ cup 2% milk
- ½ cup sour cream
- ½ tsp salt
- Oil for frying

Directions:

1. Fry the onions in oil In a small frying pan until golden brown. Add vinegar. Cook and stir for 2-3 minutes. Separately.
2. In a small saucepan, combine the jelly, tomatoes, tomato paste, curry powder, cinnamon, salt and pepper. Cook over medium heat for 5-7 minutes or until done. Add the onion mixture. Cook for 3 minutes and stir. Set aside and keep warm.
3. In a small bowl, add cake mix, corn, eggs, milk, sour cream and salt until added.
4. Heat the oil to 375° in a fryer or electric skillet. In the hot oil, drop the dough, stacking a little at a time a tablespoon. Fry on each side or until golden brown, 1 minute. Drain the water on a paper towel. Serve warm with jam.

1087. GREEK PIZZAS

Prep Time: 150 Minutes *Cook Time: 70 Minutes* *Servings: 4*

INGREDIENTS:

- 4 pita bread (6 inches)
- 1 cup reduced-fat ricotta cheese
- ½ tsp garlic powder
- (10 ounces) one pkg of frozen chopped spinach, thawed and then squeezed dry
- 3 medium tomatoes, sliced
- ¾ cup crumbled feta cheese
- ¾ tsp dried basil

Directions:

1. Place pita bread on a baking sheet. Add ricotta cheese and garlic powder; spread over pitas. Top with spinach, tomatoes, feta cheese and basil.
2. Bake it at least at 400° for 12-15 minutes or until bread is lightly browned.

1088. BACON & FONTINA STUFFED MUSHROOMS

Prep Time: *5 Minutes* *Cook Time:* *20 Minutes* *Servings: 6*

INGREDIENTS:

- 4 ounces cream cheese, softened
- 1 cup (4 ounces) of shredded fontina cheese 8 bacon strips, cooked and crumbled
- 4 green onions, chopped
- ¼ cup chopped oil-packed sun-dried tomatoes 3 tbsps minced fresh parsley
- 24 big fresh mushrooms (about 1 ¼ pound), stems removed 1 tbsp olive oil

Directions:

1. Preheat oven to 425°. In a small size bowl, mix the first six ingredients until blended. Arrange mushroom caps in a greased 15x10x1-in. Baking pan, stem side up. Spoon about 1 tbsp filling into each.
2. Spread tops with olive oil. Bake it, uncovered, 9-11 minutes or until it turn golden brown and mushrooms are tender.

1089. ALMOND CHEDDAR APPETIZERS

Prep Time: *12 Minutes* *Cook Time:* *Minutes* *Servings: 5*

INGREDIENTS:

- 1 cup mayonnaise
- 2 tsp Worcestershire sauce
- 1 cup (4 ounces) shredded sharp cheddar cheese 1 medium onion, chopped
- ¾ cup of slivered almonds chopped 6 bacon strips, cooked and crumbled
- 1 loaf (1 pound) French bread

Directions:

1. In a bowl, add the mayonnaise and Worcestershire sauce; stir in cheese, onion, almonds and bacon.
2. Cut bread into ½-in. slices; sprinkle with cheese mixture. Divide slices in half; place on a greased baking sheet. 8- in 400 degree oven minutes or until foamy.
3. FROZEN OPTION Lay raw appetizers in one layer on a baking sheet. Freeze it for 1 hour.
4. Put off from pan and store in an airtight container for up to 2 months. When ready to use, place the thawed appetizer on a greased baking sheet. Bake at 400° for 10 minutes or until warm and frothy.

1090. MINI TERIYAKI TURKEY SANDWICHES

Prep Time: *25 Minutes* *Cook Time:0* *Minutes* *Servings: 4*

INGREDIENTS:

- (2 pounds each) 2 boneless skinless turkey breast halves
- 2/3 cup of packed brown sugar
- 2/3 cup of reduced-sodium soy sauce
- ¼ cup cider vinegar
- 3 garlic cloves, minced
- 1 tbsp minced fresh ginger root
- ½ tsp pepper
- 2 tbsps cornstarch
- 2 tbsps cold water
- 20 Hawaiian sweet rolls
- 2 tbsps butter, melted

Directions:

1. Place turkey in a 5-or 6-qt. Reduce cooker. In a small size bowl, add brown sugar, soy sauce, vinegar, garlic, ginger and pepper; pour over turkey. Cook, covered, on reducing 5-6 hours or until the meat is tender.
2. Remove turkey from reducing cooker. In a small size bowl, combine cornstarch and cold water until smooth; gradually stir into cooking liquid.
3. When cool enough, shred meat with two forks and return meat to reduce cooker. Cook, covered, on high 30- minutes or until sauce is thickened.
4. Preheat oven to 325°. Split rolls and brush cut sides with butter; place on an ungreased baking sheet, cut side up.
5. Bake 8-10 minutes or until toasted and golden brown. Spoon 1/3 cup turkey mixture on roll bottoms. Replace tops.

1091. SUMMER TEA SANDWICHES

Prep Time: *5 Minutes* *Cook Time:* *20 Minutes* *Servings: 4*

INGREDIENTS:

- ½ tsp dried tarragon ½ tsp salt, divided ¼ tsp pepper 1 pound boneless skinless chicken breasts
- ½ cup reduced-fat mayonnaise 1 tbsp finely chopped red onion
- 1 tsp dill weed
- ½ tsp lemon juice 24 slices soft multigrain bread, crusts removed
- 1 medium cucumber, thinly sliced
- ¼ medium cantaloupe, cut into 12 thin slices 1. Add the tarragon,
- ¼ tsp salt and pepper; rub over chicken. Place it on a baking sheet that is coated with cooking spray.

Directions:

1. Bake it at least 350° for 20-25 minutes or until a thermometer reads 170°. Cool to room temperature; thinly slice.

1092. SEAFOOD SALAD MINI CROISSANTS

Prep Time: *3 Minutes* *Cook Time:* *0 Minutes* *Servings: 8*

INGREDIENTS:

- ½ cup mayonnaise
- 1 tbsp snipped fresh dill
- 1 tbsp minced chives
- 1 tbsp lemon juice
- ½ tsp salt
- ¼ tsp pepper
- ½ pound imitation lobster ½ pound cooked small shrimp, peeled and deveined and coarsely chopped 10 miniature croissants, split

Directions:

1. In a big bowl, add the mayonnaise, dill, chives, lemon juice, salt and pepper. Stir in lobster and shrimp. Cover and refrigerate until serving. Present on croissants.
2. In a small size bowl, add the mayonnaise, onion, dill, lemon juice and remaining salt; spread over 12 bread slices. Top with cucumber, chicken, cantaloupe and remaining bread. Cut sandwiches in half diagonally. Present immediately.

1093. CHIPOTLE SLIDERS

Prep Time: *20 Minutes* *Cook Time:* *3-4 Minutes* *Servings: 3*

INGREDIENTS:

- 1 package (12 ounces) Hawaiian sweet rolls, divided
- 1 tsp salt
- ½ tsp of pepper
- 8 tsp of minced chipotle peppers in adobo sauce, divided
- 1 ½ pounds ground beef
- 10 slices pepper Jack cheese
- ½ cup mayonnaise

Directions:

1. Add 2 rolls to the food processor. The process of demolition. Make it into a large bowl. Now add salt, pepper and 6 tsp chopped chives. Mix the beef into the dough and mix well. Make 10 columns.
2. Cook the covered burgers on medium heat for 3-4 minutes on both sides or until the thermometer reads 160° and the water is clear. Top with cheese. Bake for 1 minute or until cheese is melted.
3. Remove the rest of the rolls, turn them over and heat over medium heat for 30-60 seconds or until fully cooked.
4. Add mayonnaise and remaining chipotle peppers; spread over roll bottoms. Top each with a burger. Replace roll tops.

1094. CHICKEN SALAD PARTY SANDWICHES

Prep Time: *29 Minutes* *Cook Time:* *0 Minutes* *Servings: 4*

Ingredients:

- 4 cups cubed cooked chicken breast
- 1 ½ cups dried cranberries
- 2 celery ribs, finely chopped
- 2 green onions, thinly sliced
- ¼ cup chopped sweet pickles
- 1 cup fat-free mayonnaise
- ½ tsp curry powder
- ¼ tsp coarsely ground pepper
- ½ cup chopped pecans, toasted
- 15 whole wheat dinner rolls
- Torn leaf lettuce

Directions:

1. In a bowl, now add the first five ingredients. In a small size bowl, add the mayonnaise, curry and pepper. Add to chicken mixture; toss to coat. Chill until serving.
2. Stir pecans into chicken salad. Present on rolls lined with lettuce.

1095. SWEET TEA CONCENTRATE

Prep Time: *2 Minutes* *Cook Time:* *15 Minutes* *Servings: 6*

INGREDIENTS:

- 2 medium lemons
- 4 mugs sugar
- 4 mugs water
- 1 ½ mug English breakfast tea leaves or 20 black tea bags 1/3 mug lemon juice EACH SERVING
- 1 mug cold water
- Ice cubes
- Citrus slices, optional
- Mint sprigs, optional

DIRECTIONS:

1. Extract peels from lemons; set fruit aside for garnish or save for another use.
2. In a saucepan, combine together sugar and water. Bring to a boil over medium heat. Minimize heat; simmer, unwrapped, for 3-5 minutes or until sugar is dissolved, stirring occasionally. Extract from the heat; add tea leaves and lemon peels. Close and steep
3. minute. Strain the tea finally and discard the tea leaves and lemon peel. Mix lemon juice. Cool to room temperature.
4. Convert to a container with a tight lid. Store in the refrigerator for up to 2 weeks.
5. Tea preparation In a tall glass, mix water and concentrate. Add ice. Add orange slices and mint twigs if desired.

1096. WHITE SANGRIA

Prep Time: 20 Minutes *Cook Time: 0 Minutes* *Servings: 2*

INGREDIENTS:

- ¼ mug sugar ¼ mug brandy 1 mug sliced peeled fresh peaches or frozen sliced peaches, thawed 1 mug sliced fresh strawberries or frozen sliced strawberries, thawed 1 medium lemon, sliced
- 1 medium lime, sliced
- 3 mugs dry white wine, chilled
- 1 can (12 ounces) lemon-lime soda, chilled Ice cubes

DIRECTIONS:

1. In a pitcher, mix sugar and brandy until sugar is dissolved. Add remaining ingredients; stir smoothly to mix. Serve over ice.

1097. ALL-OCCASION PUNCH

Prep Time: 15 Minutes *Cook Time: 0 Minutes* *Servings: 8*

INGREDIENTS:

- 8 mugs cold water
- 1 can (12 ounces) of frozen lemonade concentrate, thawed plus ¾ mug thawed lemonade concentrate 2 litres ginger ale, chilled
- 1-litre cherry lemon-lime soda, chilled Ice ring, optional

DIRECTIONS:

1. In a large punch bowl, mix water and lemonade concentrate. Stir in ginger ale and lemon-lime soda. Top with an ice ring if desired. Serve punch immediately.
2. Desired. Serve punch immediately.

1098. SPARKLING PEACH BELLINIS

Prep Time: 5 Minutes *Cook Time: 140 Minutes* *Servings: 4*

INGREDIENTS:

- 3 medium peaches, halved
- 1 tbsp honey
- 1 can (11.3 ounces) of peach nectar, chilled
- 2 bottles (750 millilitres each) champagne or sparkling grape juice, chilled
- place a baking sheet with a large piece of heavy-duty foil (aboutx 12 in.).

DIRECTIONS:

1. Place the peach halves cut side up on the foil. Drizzle honey. Turn the foil over the peaches and seal.
2. Bake it at least 375° for 25-30 minutes or until soft. Cool completely. Extract and remove the skin. Process the peaches in a cooking processor until soft.
3. Transfer the peach puree to the pitcher. Add honey and 1 bottle of champagne. Stir until blended. 12 Spread in a champagne flute or wine glass. Finish with the remaining champagne. Serve immediately.

1099. FROZEN STRAWBERRY DAIQUIRIS

Prep Time: 12 Minutes *Cook Time: 20 Minutes* *Servings: 3*

INGREDIENTS:

- ¾ mug rum
- ½ mug thawed limeade concentrate
- 1 package (10 ounces) frozen sweetened sliced strawberries
- 1 to 1 ½ mugs ice cubes
- GARNISH
- Fresh strawberries

DIRECTIONS:

1. In a blender, mix the rum, limeade concentrate, strawberries and ice. Cover and process until smooth and thickened (use more ice for thicker daiquiris). Spread into cocktail glasses.
2. To garnish each daiquiri, cut a ½-in. slit into the tip of a strawberry; position berry on the rim of the glass.

1100. PUMPKIN PIE SHOTS

Prep Time: 20 Minutes *Cook Time: 120 Minutes* *Servings: 6*

INGREDIENTS:

- 1 envelope unflavored gelatin
- 1 mug cold water
- 1/3 mug canned pumpkin ¼ mug sugar
- ½ tsp pumpkin pie spice 1/3 mug butterscotch schnapps liqueur ¼ mug vodka
- 1 ½ tsp heavy whipping cream Sweetened whipped cream

DIRECTIONS:

1. In a saucepan, spread gelatin over cold water; let it stand for 1 minute. Heat and stir it continuously over low heat until gelatin is completely dissolved. Stir in pumpkin, sugar and pie spice; cook and stir until sugar is dissolved. Extract from heat. Stir in liqueur, vodka and cream.
2. Spread mixture into twelve 2-oz. shot glasses; Let it cool until set. Top with sweetened whipped cream.

1101. BANANA NOG

Prep Time: 10 Minutes *Cook Time: 40 Minutes* *Servings: 6*

INGREDIENTS:

- 3 mugs milk, divided
- 3 mugs half-and-half cream, divided
- 3 egg yolks
- ¾ mug sugar
- 3 large ripe bananas
- ½ mug light rum
- 1/3 mug creme de cacao
- 1 ½ tsp vanilla extract
- Whipped cream and baking cocoa, optional
- In a large, heavy saucepan, mix 1 ½ mug milk,
- 1 ½ mugs cream, egg yolks and sugar.

DIRECTIONS:

1. Now Cook and stir continuously over medium-low heat until mixture reaches 160° and is thick to coat the back of a metal spoon.
2. Put bananas in a food processor; cover and process until blended. Spread milk mixture into a pitcher; stir in the banana puree, rum, creme de cacao, vanilla, and remaining milk and cream. Cover and let it cool for at least 3 hours before serving.
3. Spread into chilled glasses. Garnish with whipped cream and spread with cocoa if desired.
4. CHEAT IT! Substitute 6 mugs of eggnog from the dairy case for the milk mixture prepared in the recipe. Stir the banana puree, rum, creme de cacao and vanilla into the eggnog. Garnish as desired.

1102. MEXICAN HOT CHOCOLATE

Prep Time: 23 Minutes *Cook Time: 150 Minutes* *Servings: 4*

INGREDIENTS:

- 4 mugs fat-free milk
- 3 cinnamon sticks
- 5 ounces 53% of cacao dark baking chocolate, coarsely chopped
- 1 tsp vanilla extract
- Additional cinnamon sticks, optional 1

DIRECTIONS:

1. In a saucepan, heat milk and cinnamon sticks overheat until bubbles form around the sides of the pan. Discard cinnamon. Whisk in chocolate until smooth.
2. Extract from the heat; stir in vanilla. Serve it in mugs with additional cinnamon sticks if desired.

1103. CREAMSICLE MIMOSAS

Prep Time: 10 Minutes *Cook Time: 120 Minutes* *Servings: 4*

INGREDIENTS:

- 2 ½ mugs orange juice
- 1 mug half-and-half cream
- ¾ mug superfine sugar
- 4 tsp grated orange peel
- 2 bottles (750 millilitres each) champagne or other sparkling wine Fresh strawberries

DIRECTIONS:

1. Place the orange juice, cream, sugar and orange peel in a blender; cover and process until sugar is dissolved. Transfer to an 8-in. square dish. Freeze for 6 hours or overnight.
2. For each serving, scoop ¼ mug mix into a champagne glass; top with champagne. Garnish with a strawberry and serve
3. immediately.

1104. SPARKLING CRANBERRY KISS

Prep Time: 10 Minutes *Cook Time: 120 Minutes* *Servings: 4*

INGREDIENTS:

- 6 mugs cranberry juice
- 1 ½ mug orange juice 3 mugs ginger ale Ice cubes
- Orange slices, optional

DIRECTIONS:

1. In a pitcher, mix cranberry juice and orange juice. Before serving, stir continuously in ginger ale; serve it over ice. If desired, serve with orange slices.

1105. SPICED COFFEE

Prep Time: 5 Minutes *Cook Time: 135 Minutes* *Servings: 4*

INGREDIENTS:

- 8 mugs brewed coffee
- 1/3 mug sugar ¼ mug chocolate syrup ½ tsp anise extract
- 4 cinnamon sticks (3 inches)
- 1 ½ tsp whole cloves Additional cinnamon sticks, optional

DIRECTIONS:

1. In a 3-qt. Slow cooker, mix coffee, sugar, chocolate syrup and extract. Put cinnamon sticks as well as cloves on a double of cheesecloth. Gather corners of the cloth to enclose spices; tie securely with string. Add to slow cooker. Cook, covered, on low 2-3 hours.
2. Discard spice bag. If desired, serve coffee with cinnamon sticks.

1106. GINGER-GRAPEFRUIT FIZZ

Prep Time: 20 Minutes *Cook Time: 30 Minutes* *Servings: 5*

INGREDIENTS:

- 1 mug sugar
- 1 mug water
- ½ mug sliced fresh ginger root
- ½ tsp whole peppercorns
- ¼ tsp vanilla extract
- 1/8 tsp salt
- ¼ mug coarse sugar
- 3 mugs fresh grapefruit juice, chilled
- Ice cubes
- 4 mugs sparkling water, chilled

DIRECTIONS:

1. In a saucepan, take the first six ingredients to a boil. Reduce heat; simmer for 10 minutes. Let it cool until cold. Strain syrup, discarding ginger and peppercorns.
2. Using water, moisten the rims of eight cocktail glasses. Spread coarse sugar on a plate; hold every glass upside down and dip rims into sugar. Discard remaining sugar on a plate.
3. In a pitcher, mix grapefruit juice and syrup. Spread ½ mug into prepared glasses over ice; top with ½ mug sparkling water.

1107. YUMMY CHOCOLATE

Prep Time: *18 Minutes* *Cook Time:* *30 Minutes* *Servings: 4*

INGREDIENTS:

- ¾ mug semisweet chocolate chips
- 1 carton (8 ounces) whipped topping, divided
- ½ tsp ground cinnamon
- ½ tsp rum extract or vanilla extract Assorted fresh fruit or graham cracker sticks

DIRECTIONS:

1. In a microwave, melt chocolate chips; stir until smooth. Stir in ½ mug whipped topping, cinnamon and extract; cool for 5 minutes.
2. Fold in the remaining whipped topping. Serve with fruit. Let it cool leftovers.

1108. PINEAPPLE-PECAN CHEESE SPREAD

Prep Time: *5 Minutes* *Cook Time:* *40 Minutes* *Servings: 12*

INGREDIENTS:

- 2 pkg (8 ounces each) of cream cheese, softened
- 1 ½ mug (6 ounces) shredded cheddar cheese 1 mug chopped pecans, toasted, divided
- ¾ mug crushed pineapple, drained 1 can (4 ounces) chopped green chillies, drained
- 2 tbsp chopped roasted sweet red pepper
- ½ tsp garlic powder Assorted fresh vegetables

DIRECTIONS:

1. In a bowl, beat continuously cream cheese until smooth. Add the cheddar cheese, ¾ mug pecans, pineapple, chillies, red pepper and garlic powder; beat until mixed. Transfer to a serving dish. Cover and let it cool until serving.
2. Sprinkle with remaining pecans just before serving. Serve with vegetables.

1109. HOT SAUSAGE & BEAN

Prep Time: *45 Minutes* *Cook Time:* *90 Minutes* *Servings: 2*

INGREDIENTS:

- 1 pound bulk hot Italian sausage
- 1 medium onion, finely chopped
- 4 garlic cloves, minced
- ½ mug dry white wine or chicken broth ½ tsp dried oregano ¼ tsp salt ¼ tsp of dried thyme
- 1 pkg (8 ounces) of cream cheese, softened
- 1 package (6 ounces) fresh baby spinach, coarsely chopped 1 can (15 ounces) white kidney or cannellini beans, rinsed and drained 1 mug chopped seeded tomatoes
- 1 mug (4 ounces) shredded part-skim mozzarella cheese ½ mug shredded Parmesan cheese Assorted crackers or toasted French bread baguette slices

DIRECTIONS:

1. 1.Preheat oven to 375°. In a large skillet, cook the sausages, onions and garlic over medium heat until the sausages are no longer pink, crushing the sausages into crumbs. Thin. Stir in the wine, oregano, salt and thyme. Take it to a boil and cook until the liquid is almost evaporated.
2. Add cream cheese. Stir until melted. Stir in the spinach, beans and tomatoes. Cook and stir it continuously until the spinach is wilted. Go to a greased 8-inch square or 1 qt. Cake cooking. Sprinkle with cheese.
3. Bake 20-25 minutes or until bubbly. Serve with crackers.

1110. AVOCADO SHRIMP SALSA

Prep Time: *15 Minutes* *Cook Time:□20* *Minutes* *Servings: 3*

INGREDIENTS:

- 1 pound of peeled as well as deveined cooked shrimp, chopped 2 medium tomatoes, seeded and chopped
- 2 medium ripe avocados, peeled and chopped
- 1 mug minced fresh cilantro
- 1 medium sweet red pepper, chopped
- ¾ mug thinly sliced green onions ½ mug chopped seeded peeled cucumber 3 tbsps lime juice
- 1 jalapeno pepper, seeded and chopped
- 1 tsp salt
- ¼ tsp pepper Tortilla chips

DIRECTIONS:

1. In a bowl, combine together the first 11 ingredients altogether. Serve it with tortilla chips.
2. NOTE Wear disposable gloves when dividing hot peppers; the oils can burn skin. Avoid touching your face.

1111. STATE FAIR SUBS

Prep Time: *30 Minutes* *Cook Time:* *103 Minutes* *Servings : 6*

Ingredients:

- 1 loaf (1 pound unsliced) French bread
- 2 eggs
- ¼ cup milk
- ½ tsp pepper
- ¼ tsp salt
- 1 pound bulk Italian sausage
- 1 ½ cups chopped onion
- 2 cups (8 ounces) of shredded part-skim mozzarella cheese

Directions:

1. Cut the bread in half lengthwise. Drill holes carefully in the top and bottom of the loaf, leaving about an inch.
2. Husks. Diced bread. In a large bowl, shake together the eggs, milk, pepper and salt. Add slices of bread and stir to coat. Separately.
3. In a frying pan over high heat, cook the sausages and onions until the meat is no longer pink. Thin.
4. Add to bread dough. Spoon for filling in breadcrumbs; Sprinkle with cheese. Wrap each in foil. Bake it at least 400° for 20-25 minutes or until cheese is melted. Cut French bread into 1-serving-sized pieces.

1112. PARTY PITAS

Prep Time: *10 Minutes* *Cook Time:* *20 Minutes* *Servings: 4*

INGREDIENTS:

- 4 whole-wheat pita pocket halves
- 1/3 cup Greek vinaigrette ½ pound thinly sliced deli turkey 1 jar (7 ½ ounces) roasted sweet red peppers, drained and patted dry 2 cups fresh baby spinach
- 24 pitted Greek olives
- 24 frilled toothpicks

Directions:

1. Brush insides of pita pockets with vinaigrette; fill with turkey, peppers and spinach. Cut each pita into six wedges.
2. Thread olives onto toothpicks; use to secure wedges.

1113. BAJA CHICKEN & SLAW SLIDERS

Prep Time: *20 Minutes* *Cook Time:* *35 Minutes* *Servings: 3*

INGREDIENTS:

- ¼ cup reduced-fat sour cream ½ tsp grated lime peel ¼ tsp lime juice SLAW
- 1 cup broccoli coleslaw mix
- 2 tbsps finely chopped sweet red pepper
- 2 tbsps finely chopped sweet onion
- 2 tbsps of minced fresh cilantro
- 2 tsp of chopped seeded jalapeno pepper 2 tsp of lime juice
- 1 tsp of sugar
- SLIDERS
- (4 ounces each) 4 boneless skinless chicken breast halves ½ tsp of ground cumin
- ½ tsp of chilli powder
- ¼ tsp of salt
- ¼ tsp of coarsely ground pepper 8 Hawaiian sweet rolls, split
- 8 small lettuce leaves
- 8 slices tomato

Directions:

1. In a small size bowl, add sour cream, lime peel and lime juice. In another small size bowl, add slaw ingredients. Refrigerate sauce and slaw until serving.
2. Cut each chicken breast in half wide; flatten to -in. Thickness. Sprinkle with spices.
3. Wet a paper towel with cooking oil; using long-handled tongs, rub on grill rack to lightly coat.
4. Grill chicken, covered, over medium heat or roast 4 inches from heat 4 to 7 minutes on each side or until no longer pink.
5. Toast bread, cut side down, 30-60 seconds or until toasted. Serve grilled chicken on a roll with lettuce, tomatoes, sauce, and slaw.

Dessert Recipes

1114. Mini Apple Galettes

Prep Time: *20 Minutes* *Cook Time:* *145 Minutes* *Servings: 6*

Ingredients:

- Crust:
- ½ cup all-purpose white flour
- ½ cup whole wheat flour
- 1 tablespoon sugar
- 1 pinch of salt
- 3oz cold butter, cubed
- 2-4 tablespoons cold water
- Filling:
- 4 apples, peeled, cored and sliced
- 2 tablespoons lemon juice
- ½ cup raisins
- 2 tablespoons sugar
- 1 teaspoon cinnamon
- ½ teaspoon ground ginger
- 1 pinch nutmeg

Directions:

1. To make the crust**:** In a bowl, combine the flour with the sugar and salt, then rub in the cold butter until the dough looks sandy. Add the water, tablespoon by tablespoon and mix the dough just until it comes together. Wrap it in foil and refrigerate for 1 hour.
2. After 1 hour, divide the dough into 4 equal portions and roll each into a small round sheet. Transfer all on baking trays lined with parchment paper. Set aside.To make the filling: In a bowl, mix the apples with lemon juice, raisins, sugar and spices.
3. Add a few tablespoons of filling in the centre of each galette, then carefully lift the edges up and wrap them over the filling, leaving the centre exposed.

4. Bake in the preheated oven at about 375F for 20-30 minutes or until golden brown and the apples are tender.
5. Serve them warm with a scoop of ice cream or chilled with a dollop of whipped cream.

1115. Apple Pie

Prep Time: *30 Minutes* | *Cook Time:* *40 Minutes* | *Servings : 6*

Ingredients:

- Crust:
- 1 ½ cup low-fat cottage cheese
- 1 egg
- 2/3 cup sugar
- 1 ½ teaspoons baking powder
- 1 teaspoon lemon juice
- 2oz butter, softened
- 1 cup all-purpose flour
- 1 cup whole wheat flour
- Filling:
- 6 large apples, peeled, cored and cubed
- 2 tablespoons cornstarch
- 2 tablespoons sugar
- 1 tablespoon lemon juice
- 1 teaspoon cinnamon
- 1 pinch nutmeg

Directions:

1. To make the crust: Mix all the ingredients together in a bowl until the dough just comes together. Do not over mix it or knead it for too long. Wrap it in foil and refrigerate it for 1 hour. After 1 hour, divide the dough in half. Take 1 half and roll it into a thin round sheet, then carefully transfer it into a deep dish baking pan greased with butter. Set aside the pan, then roll out the other part of the dough.
2. To make the filling: combine the apples altogether with the sugar, cornstarch, lemon juice, and spices in a bowl, then spoon it into the pan over the crust.Cover with the other dough sheet and seal the edges slightly. Using a fork or a knife, make some holes on top of the pie to allow the steams to come out. In the preheated bake oven at 350F for 40-50 minutes or until fluffed and crisp on the outside, while juicy and creamy on the inside.
3. Let the pie cool thoroughly before slicing it.

1116. Apple and Blueberry Cobbler

Prep Time: *10 Minutes* | *Cook Time:* *50 Minutes* | *Servings: 2*

Ingredients:

- 1 cup whole wheat flour
- ¾ cup all-purpose white flour
- 1 pinch of salt
- 2 tablespoons brown sugar
- 3oz butter
- 1 cup milk
- 2 pounds blueberries
- 4 apples, peeled, cored and cubed
- 1 teaspoon cinnamon
- 2 tablespoons cornstarch
- 2 tablespoons sugar
- 1 teaspoon ground ginger

Directions:

1. Divide the fruits and place them in a bowl. Sprinkle in the sugar, ginger, cinnamon and cornstarch. Toss to evenly coat them, then transfer them in a deep dish baking pan.
2. To make the batter, combine the flours with salt, brown sugar and cold butter. Rub the butter into the flour until sandy, then pour in the milk and mix well. Batter the spoon over the fruits in the pan. It doesn't have to be even, so do not bother with spreading evenly over the fruits; simply drop spoonfuls of batter on top.
3. Bake in the preheated oven bake at 350F for 30-40 minutes or until the fruits are tender and the top is golden brown and crisp.

1117. Apple Cinnamon Cake

Prep Time: *35 Minutes* | *Cook Time:* *40 Minutes* | *Servings : 3*

Ingredients:

- ¾ cup sugar
- 3 eggs
- ½ cup all-purpose white flour
- ½ cup whole wheat flour
- ½ cup olive oil
- 1 teaspoon baking powder
- 1 teaspoon baking soda
- 1 teaspoon vanilla extract
- 4 apples, peeled, cored and sliced
- 1 pinch of salt

Directions:

1. In a bowl, mix together the eggs as well as the sugar until frothy, then add the olive oil. In another bowl, transfer together with the flours with the baking powder and soda and a pinch of salt. Now Incorporate the flour into the egg mixture and add the vanilla extract. Batter the spoon into a 9-inch round cake pan and top with apple slices. In the preheated bake oven at 350F for 30-40 minutes.
2. When complete, remove from the oven and let it cool in the pan slightly, then transfer on a serving plate and dust with plenty of powdered sugar.

1118. Apple Streusel Cake

Prep Time: *5 Minutes* | *Cook Time:* *50 Minutes* | *Servings : 3*

Ingredients:

- Cake:
- 4 apples, peeled, cored and sliced
- 1 tablespoon lemon juice
- 1 cup sugar
- 3oz butter, softened
- 3 eggs
- 2 tablespoons vegetable oil
- 1 cup Greek yoghurt
- 1 cup all-purpose white flour
- 1 ½ cup whole wheat flour
- 1 ½ teaspoon baking soda
- 1 teaspoon baking powder
- 1 teaspoon cinnamon
- 1 pinch nutmeg
- 1 pinch salt
- ½ teaspoon ground cloves
- ½ cup chopped walnuts
- Streusel:
- 2 tablespoons brown sugar
- 2 tablespoons rolled oats
- 4 tablespoons butter, cold
- ¼ cup whole wheat flour

Directions:

1. To make the cake: cream the butter as well as the sugar in a bowl until fluffy and pale in colour. Add the 3 eggs, one at a time and mix well until combined before adding the other. Add the vegetable oil, then incorporate the flours sifted with the baking powder, baking soda and spices, as well as a pinch of salt. Mix well to combine, then spoon the batter in a 10-inch round cake pan. Arrange the apple slices on top and set them aside.
2. To make the streusel: In a bowl, combine the brown sugar with the oats and flour, then rub in the cold butter until sandy. Sprinkle the streusel over the cake in the pan.
3. Bake in the before heated oven at 350F for 40-50 minutes or until golden brown and crisp.

1119. Caramel Apple Cake

Prep Time: *25 Minutes* | *Cook Time:* *55 Minutes* | *Servings : 3*

Ingredients:

- Cake:
- 2 apples, peeled, cored and sliced
- 2 tablespoons brown sugar
- 1 teaspoon vanilla extract
- 2 ½ cups almond meal
- 1 teaspoon baking powder
- 1 teaspoon cinnamon
- ½ cup honey
- ½ cup vegetable oil
- 1 egg yolks
- 4 egg whites
- 1 pinch of salt
- Caramel sauce:
- 1 cup sugar
- 2/3 cup heavy cream

Directions:

1. To make the cake: In a bowl, combine the egg yolks in the honey, vegetable oil and vanilla extract. Add the almond flour, baking soda, cinnamon and a pinch of salt. In another bowl, clean from any grease, whip the egg whites until stiff peaks form. Gently fold the egg whites into the almond batter. Take a 9-inch round cape pan and sprinkle the brown sugar on the bottom. Arrange the apple slices over the sugar, then spoon in the batter.
2. Bake in the before heated oven at 350F for 30-40 minutes. When done, remove from the oven, let it cool down for 10 minutes, then flip the pan over a serving plate. Carefully lift the pan, so the cake is revealed.
3. To make the sauce: Mix the sugar in a heavy saucepan. When the sugar is melted and smooth but not burnt, pour in the cream. Mix well and keep on the heat just until it comes together and looks smooth. Remove from heat and let it cool before serving.
4. Serve a slice of cake with plenty of sauce.

1120. Apple Upside-Down Cake

Prep Time: *20 Minutes* | *Cook Time:* *30 Minutes* | *Servings : 3*

Ingredients:

- 3oz butter
- 1 cup all-purpose flour
- ¾ cup whole wheat flour

- 1 teaspoon cinnamon
- ¾ teaspoon baking soda
- ½ teaspoon baking powder
- ¾ cup light molasses
- 1 egg
- 1 teaspoon fresh grated ginger ¼ cup sugar
- ½ cup low-fat sour cream 1/3 cup low-fat milk
- 4 apples, peeled, cored and sliced

Directions:

1. In a bowl, combine the flours with a pinch of salt, cinnamon, baking soda and baking powder. In another bowl, beat together the egg, molasses, ginger and half of the sugar, then add the sour cream and milk. Incorporate this mixture into the flour and mix well.
2. Take a 9-inch round cake pan and sprinkle the remaining sugar on the bottom. Arrange the apple slices over the sugar, then spoon in the batter you just made. Bake in the before oven at 350F for 30-40 minutes or until a skewer inserted in the middle of the cake comes out clean. Remove the pan from the oven and let it cool down for a few minutes, then turn the pan over a serving plate to flip the cake upside-down. Carefully lift the pan to reveal the cake. Let it cool completely before serving.

1121. Raisin Baked Apples

Prep Time: *5 Minutes* *Cook Time:* *35 Minutes* *Servings : 6*

Ingredients:

- 4 large apples
- ½ cup raisins
- ¼ cup dried cranberries
- 1 teaspoon cinnamon
- 4 tablespoons brown sugar

Directions:

1. Take each apple and scoop out the core without peeling it or breaking it. It has to keep its shape. Arrange the apples in a deep dish baking pan and set them asid. In a bowl, combine the raisins with cranberries, cinnamon and sugar. Evenly spread the filling between each apple. Bake in the before oven at 350F for 30 minutes or until the apples are soft and fragrant. Serve them warm or cold topped with a dollop of cream or a scoop of ice cream.

1122. . Apple Cinnamon Cups

Prep Time: *5 Minutes* *Cook Time:* *30 Minutes* *Servings: 6*

Ingredients:

- 6 phyllo dough sheets
- 6 apples, peeled, cored and diced
- ¼ cup raisins
- 4 tablespoons sugar
- 1 teaspoon cinnamon
- ¼ teaspoon ground cloves

Directions:

1. Grease a muffin pan with butter and set it aside.
2. In a bowl, mix the cubed apples with the raisins, sugar, cinnamon and ground cloves.
3. Flour your working surface well, then roll out the phyllo sheets. Take 3 sheets and layer them together. Cut them into 6-8 smaller squares, then arrange the layered squares in your muffin tin. Put 2-3 tablespoons of apple filling in each muffin cup. Fold the dough over the filling.
4. Bake in the before heated oven at 400F for 5 minutes, then lower the heat at 350F and bake 10-15 more minutes.

1123. Apple and Blueberry Cobbler

Prep Time: *10 Minutes* *Cook Time:* *15 Minutes* *Servings : 6*

Ingredients:

- 1 cup whole wheat flour
- ¾ cup all-purpose white flour
- 1 pinch of salt
- 2 tablespoons brown sugar
- 3oz butter
- 1 cup milk
- 2 pounds blueberries
- 4 apples, peeled, cored and cubed
- 1 teaspoon cinnamon
- 2 tablespoons cornstarch
- 2 tablespoons sugar
- 1 teaspoon ground ginger

Directions:

1. Divide the fruits and place them in a bowl. Sprinkle in the sugar, ginger, cinnamon and cornstarch. Toss to evenly coat them, then transfer them in a deep dish baking pan.
2. To make the batter, combine the flours with salt, brown sugar and cold butter. Rub the butter into the flour until sandy, then pour in the milk and mix well. Batter the spoon over the fruits in the pan. It doesn't have to be even, so do not bother with spreading evenly over the fruits; simply drop spoonfuls of batter on top.
3. Bake in the preheated oven bake at 350F for 30-40 minutes or until the fruits are tender and the top is golden brown and crisp.

1124. Apple Streusel Cake

Prep Time: *20 Minutes* *Cook Time:* *43 Minutes* *Servings: 2*

Ingredients:

- Cake:
- 4 apples, peeled, cored and sliced
- 1 tablespoon lemon juice
- 1 cup sugar
- 3oz butter, softened
- 3 eggs
- 2 tablespoons vegetable oil
- 1 cup Greek yoghurt
- 1 cup all-purpose white flour
- 1 ½ cup whole wheat flour
- 1 ½ teaspoon baking soda
- 1 teaspoon baking powder
- 1 teaspoon cinnamon
- 1 pinch nutmeg
- 1 pinch salt
- ½ teaspoon ground cloves
- ½ cup chopped walnuts
- Streusel:
- 2 tablespoons brown sugar
- 2 tablespoons rolled oats
- 4 tablespoons butter, cold
- ¼ cup whole wheat flour

Directions:

1. To make the cake: cream the butter as well as the sugar in a bowl until fluffy and pale in colour. Add the 3 eggs, one at a time and mix well until combined before adding the other. Add the vegetable oil, then incorporate the flours sifted with the baking powder, baking soda and spices, as well as a pinch of salt. Mix well to combine, then spoon the batter in a 10-inch round cake pan. Arrange the apple slices on top and set them aside.
2. To make the streusel: In a bowl, combine the brown sugar with the oats and flour, then rub in the cold butter until sandy. Sprinkle the streusel over the cake in the pan.
3. Bake in the before heated oven at 350F for 40-50 minutes or until golden brown and crisp.

1125. Plum Olive Oil Cake

Ingredients:

- 1 cup all-purpose flour
- ½ cup whole wheat flour
- ½ cup cornmeal
- 1 pinch salt
- 1 teaspoon cinnamon
- 1 teaspoon baking powder
- ½ teaspoon baking soda
- 1 cup fat-free yoghurt
- ½ cup extra virgin olive oil
- ½ cup sugar
- 2 eggs
- 1 teaspoon lemon zest
- 6 large plums, pitted and sliced

Directions:

1. In a bowl, combine the flour with the cornmeal, a pinch of salt, cinnamon, baking soda and baking powder. Mix together the yoghurt, olive oil, eggs, sugar, and lemon zest in a separate bowl. Stir in the dry ingredients and give it a good mix until well combined.
2. Grease a 10-inch cake pan with the use of olive oil and flour it slightly. Spoon the batter into the pan, then arrange the plum slices on top.
3. Bake in the before heated oven at 350F for 30-40 minutes. When complete, remove from the oven and let it cool completely before serving.

Made in the USA
Las Vegas, NV
31 August 2021

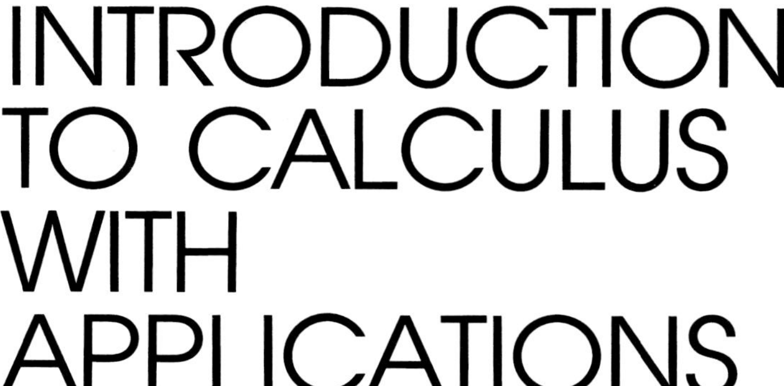

INTRODUCTION TO CALCULUS WITH APPLICATIONS

STANLEY J. FARLOW

University of Maine

GARY M. HAGGARD

Bucknell University

McGRAW-HILL PUBLISHING COMPANY

New York St. Louis San Francisco
Auckland Bogotá Caracas Hamburg
Lisbon London Madrid Mexico Milan
Montreal New Delhi Oklahoma City
Paris San Juan São Paulo Singapore
Sydney Tokyo Toronto

Introduction to Calculus with Applications

2 3 4 5 6 7 8 9 0 V N H   V N H 9 5 4 3 2 1 0

ISBN 0-07-019953-1

This book was set in Times Roman by Syntax International.
The editors were Robert A. Weinstein, Margery Luhrs, and James W. Bradley;
the production supervisor was Salvador Gonzales.
The cover was designed by Sharon Gresh.
Cover photo by Joyce C. Weston.
Von Hoffmann Press, Inc., was printer and binder.

Library of Congress Cataloging-in-Publication Data

Farlow, Stanley J., (date).
Introduction to calculus with applications / Stanley J. Farlow, Gary M. Haggard.
p. cm.
ISBN 0-07-019953-1
1. Calculus. I. Haggard, Gary. II. Title.
QA303.F2982 1990
515—dc20 89-27368

To Susan

Contents

1 The Derivative 63

2 Additional Derivative Topics and Applications 147

3 Exponential and Logarithmic Functions 233

Preface

The primary goal of this text is to provide understanding and comprehension of the calculus as well as to establish sound technical proficiency. The level of presentation is easily accessible to most students, and there is a strong degree of reliance on intuition—more so than on overly formal and abstract mathematical theory. To fulfill our goal, we have used a broad, rich selection of topics, features, and motivational items in conjunction with proven pedagogical techniques for the teaching of mathematics.

Introduction to Calculus and Its Applications is designed for use in a one-term course in calculus taken primarily by students majoring in business, economics, life sciences, and social sciences. The only prerequisite for studying the material in this book is three or four semesters of high school algebra or its equivalent. A companion volume, *Calculus and Its Applications*, includes all the material in this text and additional materials on trigonometric functions, sequences and infinite series, and differential and difference equations. It is suitable for a two-term course.

Pedagogical Features

Emphasis and Writing Style: In writing this book, we have used a number of features designed to enliven the text and motivate the student. We use real-world examples, historical comments, and intuitive presentations to explain the intelligent use of the calculus. Our basic approach is to present the mathematics in a humanistic manner and thereby enhance its use as a genuine aid to decision making by nonmathematicians.

Format: Major concepts and definitions are highlighted with a colored box so that they may be found easily and referred to throughout the book. All interest motivating material is set off in special boxes.

Strong Visual Program: More than 600 figures and numerous photographs convey a strong visual sense of the mathematics for ease of learning and to provide a realistic context to the applications. We have tried to provide helpful captions to all figures and photographs, either reinforcing an idea or providing additional explanation.

Realistic Applications: Nearly 500 realistic applications are included in the examples and exercise sets. Many of the applications will appeal to *all* students in the course, regardless of their major area of study. All the applications were chosen and developed for their pedagogical appeal and effectiveness in helping to teach mathematics.

Worked Examples: The book contains over 200 worked examples, each carefully chosen to illustrate a particular concept or technique. We collected these over the many years we have been teaching the material to our own students.

Exercises: Effective exercises are at the heart of any mathematics textbook. The more than 2000 exercises reinforce understanding as well as develop technical skills. They are graded by level of difficulty and include many challenging applied problems.

Historical Comments: To further enhance both student and instructor interest, we have included many historical comments and profiles of key historical figures in mathematics.

Chapter Epilogues: A brief epilogue at the end of each chapter relates the material to larger contemporary society.

End-of-Chapter Review Material: Each chapter closes with a list of key terms, an extensive chapter review exercise set, and a brief practice test.

Projects and Problems: Special exercise sets that combine cumulative review and comprehensive projects are included at the end of Chapters 3 and 6. These sections should challenge the motivated student to explore a wider variety of unconventional problems. Several writing projects have been included to help instructors who are trying to develop a writing-intensive course.

Algebra Review Material: The algebra review, "Calculus Preliminaries," is intended for students whose background may be weak in some topics in algebra. An instructor may omit the material, cover all or part of the material in class, or assign portions for students to work on their own. A practice test has been included to help instructors place students and assess the amount of review they need.

Chapter Organization

The following chart indicates how the chapters are related.

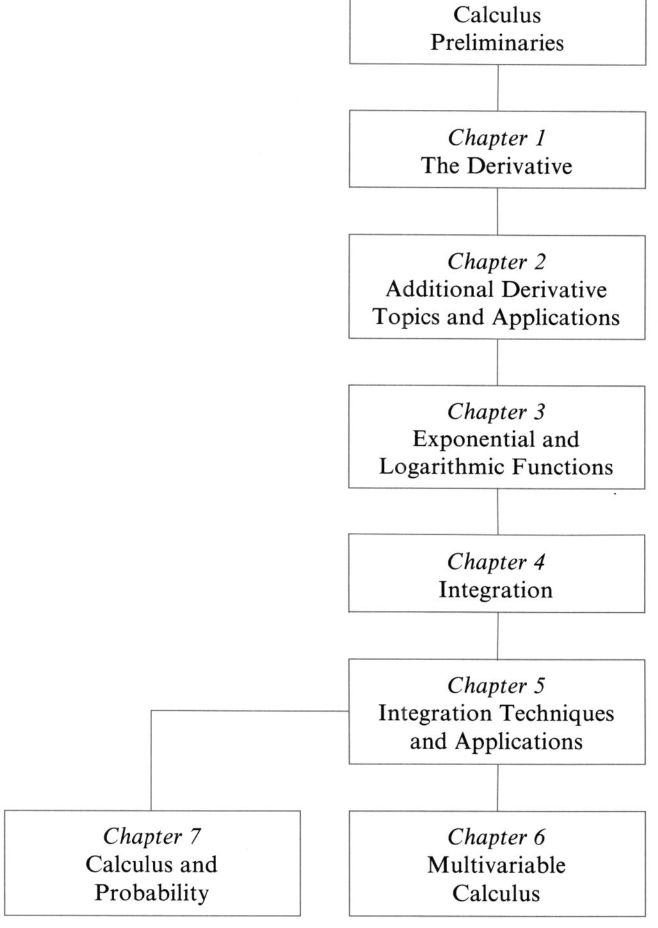

Supplements for Student and Instructor

Student Solutions Manual: This manual is available to students at a nominal cost. It contains solutions to all odd-numbered exercises in the book.

For the Instructor: An instructor's solutions manual, available to adopters, contains detailed solutions to all even-numbered exercises in the book as well as sample chapter tests, midterms, and final exams. A computerized test bank (IBM) and printout are also available for instructor use.

Acknowledgments

We would like to thank the many people who helped us at various stages of this project during the past few years.

The following people offered excellent advice, suggestions, and ideas as they reviewed the manuscript: Ronald Barnes, University of Houston, Downtown Campus; Steve Blasberg, West Valley College; Raymond Coughlin, Temple University; Bruce Edwards, University of Florida; Peter Gilkey, University of Oregon; Joel Haack, Oklahoma State University; Christopher Hee, Eastern Michigan University; Myron Hood, California Polytechnic State University; Michael Mays, West Virginia University; Maurice Monahan, South Dakota State University; Philip Montgomery, University of Kansas; Robert Moreland, Texas Tech University; David Ponick, University of Wisconsin, Eau Claire; Richard Randell, University of Iowa; Richard Semmler, Northern Virginia Community College; Cynthia Siegel, University of Missouri, St. Louis; and Jimmy Solomon, Mississippi State University.

Finally, we want to thank all the people at Random House and McGraw-Hill who have contributed to the project and worked so hard to support us throughout the publication process. The editorial staff was always helpful and supportive through every phase: Wayne Yuhasz and Robert A. Weinstein, Senior Editors; Anne Wightman, Developmental Editor; Karen Hughes, Assistant Editor; Debbie Stone, Editorial Assistant. The McGraw-Hill production staff provided professional and efficient support in producing a very attractive book. Special thanks to Margery Luhrs, Senior Editing Supervisor, and Sal Gonzales, Production Supervisor. Also, we appreciate the assistance of Geri Davis with research and choice of photographs. And finally our thanks to an excellent proofreader, Mary Rosenberg, who made many valuable suggestions beyond the call of duty.

All errors are the responsibility of the authors. We would appreciate having these brought to our attention. We would also appreciate any comments and suggestions from students and instructors.

Stanley J. Farlow

Gary M. Haggard

Introduction to Calculus with Applications

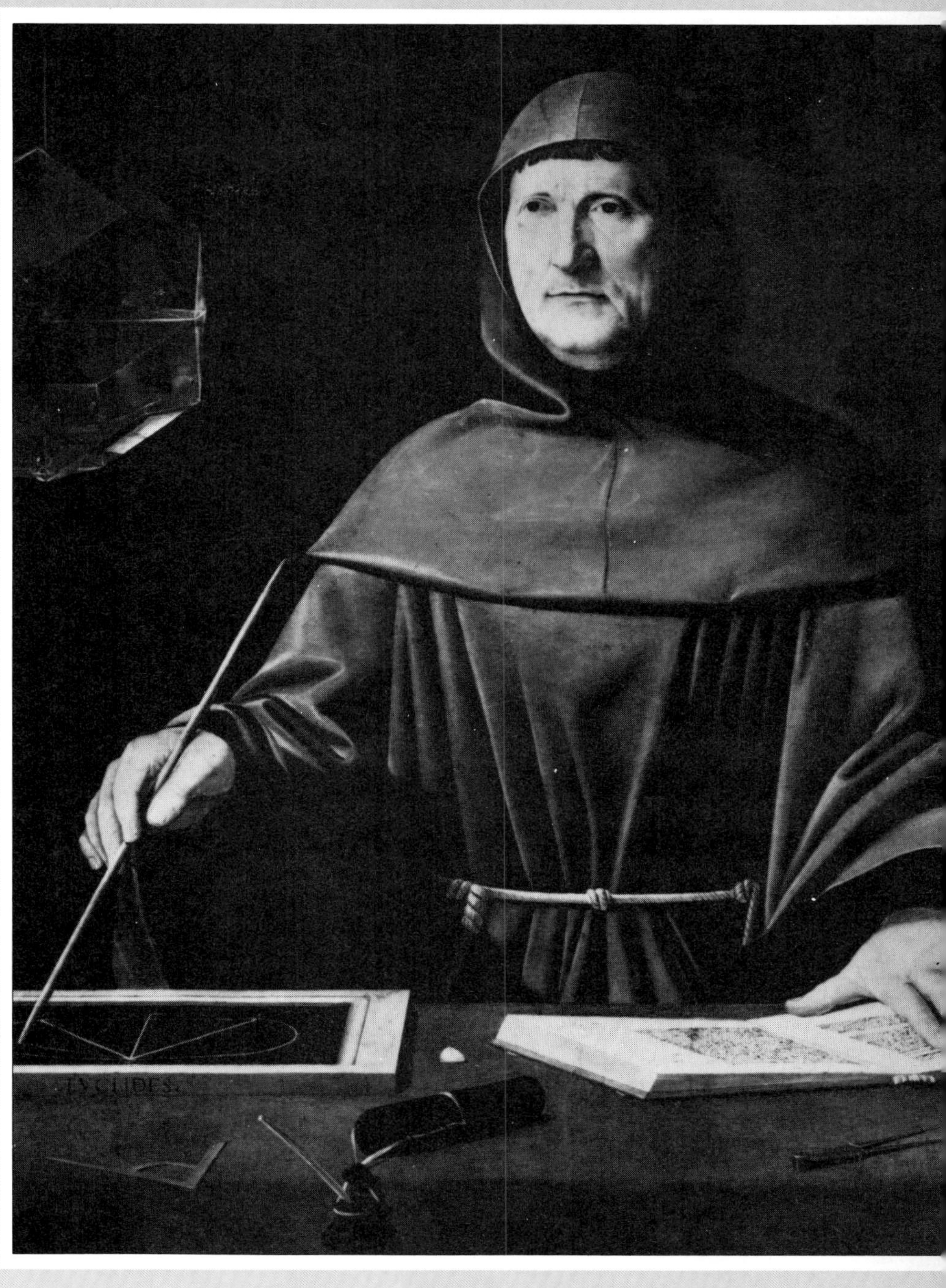

Calculus Preliminaries

The purpose of this preliminary chapter is to review some basic mathematical topics that will be used throughout the book. The reader can either use this material to review topics when needed or study these topics carefully before beginning the new material in the book. We begin by reviewing the most fundamental mathematical structure, the real number system.

P.1 The Real Numbers

Properties of the Real Numbers

One of the distinguishing features of modern business and science is the importance that is placed on quantification. It seems that almost everything is measured, weighed, or timed. We calculate speeds of objects, the size of the economy, scientific measurements of many kinds, and on and on. We even compute baseball statistics. In making these measurements we use whole numbers, positive numbers, negative numbers, fractional numbers, and irrational numbers. Of course, if we were interested only in making simple measurements, such as counting something or computing an average, we could probably get by with simple numbers, such as integers or fractions. However, for performing sophisticated quantitative analyses, as is often done in the modern business world, we must use the properties of the **real number system**.

When we refer to numbers in this book, unless otherwise stated, we are normally referring to real numbers. Real numbers are often represented as points on a line, and the entire line is called the **real number line**. (See Figure 1.)

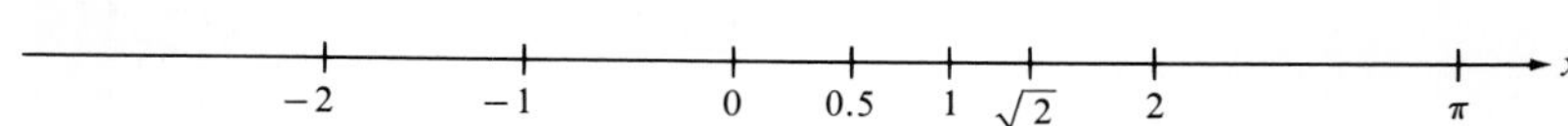

Figure 1
The real number line and typical numbers

Every real number is associated with a point on the real number line and vice versa. The number 0 is generally labeled, while the **positive numbers** are drawn to the right and the **negative numbers** to the left. We can think of the real number line as two **infinite rulers** back to back, a positive one going infinitely far to the right and a negative one going infinitely far to the left. (See Figure 2.)

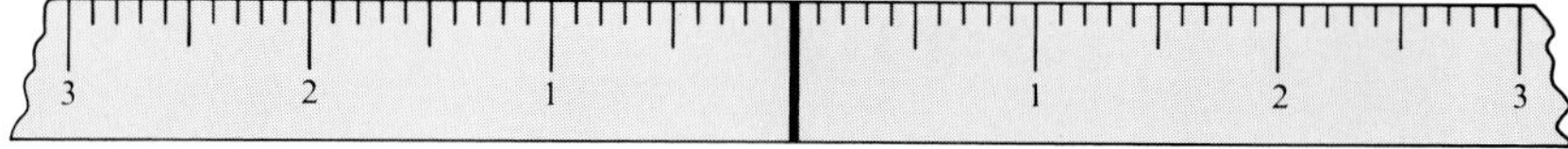

Figure 2
Real number line illustrated by back-to-back infinite rulers

There are various kinds of real numbers within the real number system. (See Figure 3.) Table 1 lists the basic kinds of real numbers.

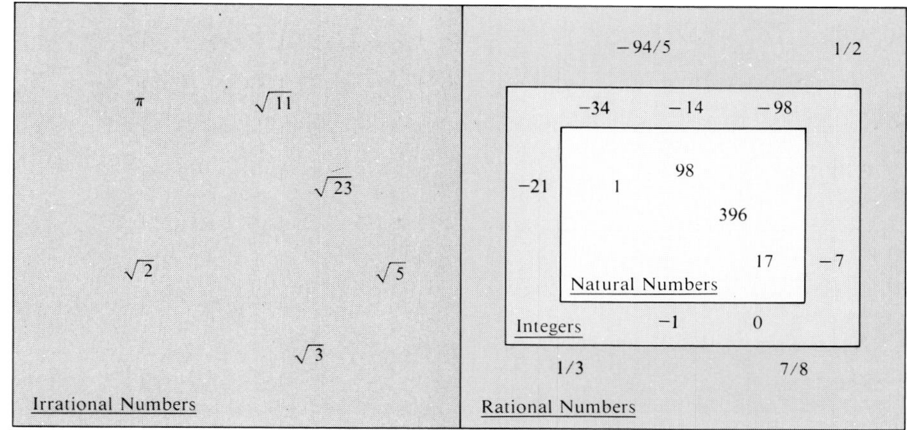

Figure 3
The family of real numbers

TABLE 1
Types of Real Numbers

Natural numbers	$1, 2, 3, \ldots$	$7, 11, 25$
Integers	$\ldots, -2, -1, 0, 1, 2, \ldots$	$-3, 0, 5$
Rational numbers	Fractions, any number that can be written as a/b, where a and b are integers with $b \neq 0$	$\frac{4}{3}, 5.34, \frac{3}{25}, 5, 0, \frac{5}{1}$
Irrational numbers	Numbers that cannot be written as fractions	$\sqrt{2}, \pi, e$

List of Properties of the Real Numbers

Table 2 lists several useful properties of the real numbers that are used often. We generally use these properties so matter-of-factly that we often do not even realize that we are using them.

TABLE 2
Properties of Addition and Multiplication

Property	Addition	Multiplication
Commutative Properties	$a + b = b + a$	$ab = ba$
Associative Properties	$a + (b + c) = (a + b) + c$	$a(bc) = (ab)c$
Identities	$0 + a = a$	$1 \cdot a = a$
Distributive Properties	$a(b + c) = ab + ac$ $(b + c)a = ba + ca$	

The following example illustrates the above properties. The reader should determine which rule is being used in each equation.

Example

(a) $2 + 3 = 3 + 2$
(b) $3 \cdot 4 = 4 \cdot 3$
(c) $x^2 + (y^2 + z^2) = (x^2 + y^2) + z^2$
(d) $(2 \cdot 4) \cdot 3 = 2 \cdot (4 \cdot 3)$
(e) $(-1) + 0 = -1$
(f) $1 \cdot 5 = 5$
(g) $4(x^2 + y^2) = 4x^2 + 4y^2$
(h) $(2 + 5)x = 2x + 5x$ □

3 + 50 dervnnd werden
4——16 4539 ℔ (So
3 + 44 du die zendtner
3 + 29 zů ℔ gemachett
3 —— 12 hast vnnd das /
3 + 9 + das ist meer
darzů Addierest) vnd 75 minus. Nun
solt du für holtz abschlahen allweeg für
ain legel 24 ℔. Vnd das ist 13 mal 24.
vnd macht 312 ℔ darzů addier das —
das ist 75 ℔ vnd werden 387. Dye sub-
trahier von 4539. Vnd bleyben 4152
℔. Nun sprich 100 ℔ das ist ein zentner

HISTORICAL NOTE

The first recorded appearance in print of plus and minus signs was in an arithmetic text published in Leipzig in 1489 by the German Renaissance mathematician Johann Widmann (ca. 1460–1520).

The signs replaced the "Italian" *p* and *m* notation that was previously used for plus and minus. Imagine writing

$$2p2m1 = 3$$

Problems

For Problems 1–10, determine whether the real number is rational or irrational.

1. 0.7
2. 2.7
3. 2.010
4. 0.72
5. 0.725
6. 105
7. $\pi/2$
8. 2π
9. $\sqrt{2}/3$
10. $\dfrac{160}{2.1}$

Division by Zero: the Road to Paradox

Division by zero is excluded in mathematics. Suppose someone discovered a number x that was equal to $x = 1/0$. But then we would have to say that $x \cdot 0 = 1$ or $0 = 1$. Thus there is a contradiction when we divide by zero. Many obviously incorrect results can be proven when we divide by zero.

11. Using division by zero, "prove" that $2 = 1$.
12. Use the properties of the real numbers to show that $0/0$ can be any number. Try $0/0 = 3$, then $0/0 = 17, \ldots$, then $0/0 = n$ where n is any real number.

How Well Do You Know the Real Numbers?

The real number system is full of surprises. For instance, what is the smallest positive real number? For any number you select, you can always find a smaller positive number by simply dividing the given number by 2. Hence we must conclude that there is no smallest positive number. Here are some other questions concerning the real numbers.

13. What is the largest real number less than 1?
14. What is the largest real number?
15. What is the smallest real number?
16. What is the smallest positive rational number?
17. What is the largest rational number?
18. Are there more rational numbers than irrational numbers?
19. Are there more rational numbers than integers?

The Position System of Writing Numbers

The Hindu-Arabic positional notation is the standard way in which we write real numbers today. For example, we would interpret the integer 634 as

$$634 = 6 \cdot 100 + 3 \cdot 10 + 4 \cdot 1$$

This positional number notation gives rise to several interesting puzzles. Can you determine the reason behind the following puzzle?

20. Karnak's Dice Puzzle. Karnak the magician asks you to roll three dice without Karnak seeing the results. Karnak then gives the following instructions:

Step 1: Multiply the number on the first die by 2.

Step 2: Add 5.

Step 3: Multiply by 5.

Step 4: Add the number on the second die.

Step 5: Multiply by 10.

Step 6: Add the number on the third die.

Step 7: State the result.

For example, if you rolled 2, 3, and 4, you would think: 4, 9, 45, 48, 480, 484. You would then state 484. After you told Karnak this number, Karnak would tell you that you rolled a 2, a 3, and a 4. How did Karnak know the numbers on the dice? *Hint:* Let the numbers on the three dice be a, b, and c and perform the steps in terms of these numbers (keeping in mind the positional manner in which we write numbers).

21. Karnaka's Puzzle. Karnak's sister, Karnaka, is also a magician. She specializes in telling people's ages and the amount of change in their pockets. Karnaka gives you the following instructions:

Step 1: Multiply your age by 2.

Step 2: Add 5.

Step 3: Multiply this result by 50.

Step 4: Add the amount of change in your pocket (assume that it's less than $1.00).

Step 5: Subtract the number of days in a year.

Step 6: State the result.

For example, if you were 20 years old and had 25 cents in your pocket, you would think: 20, 40, 45, 2250, 2275, 1910, After you told Karnaka the number 1910, she would tell you your age and the amount of change in your pocket. How did she do this? *Hint:* Let your age be a and the amount of change in your pocket be c. Then perform the steps in terms of a and c (keeping in mind the positional manner in which we write numbers).

22. A New Career? Follow in the footsteps of Karnak and Karnaka by designing your own puzzle. Perform your magic for a friend.

Exponents and Roots

Integer Exponents

Most people just do not appreciate the power of exponents. Do you realize that by using the three numbers 2, 3, and 4 only once each, you can construct a number that is 100 billion times larger than the distance (in miles) from the earth to the sun? It's true. The number 3^{42}, which uses the digits 2, 3, and 4 only once and represents the number 3 times itself 42 times, is a number that is 100 billion times larger than the 93,000,000 miles to the sun. In science and modern business, one often encounters repeated multiplication of some number like $6 \cdot 6 \cdot 6 \cdot 6$ or $10 \cdot 10 \cdot 10 \cdot 10 \cdot 10 \cdot 10$. These products can be written more compactly and efficiently as

$$6^4 = 6 \cdot 6 \cdot 6 \cdot 6$$
$$10^6 = 10 \cdot 10 \cdot 10 \cdot 10 \cdot 10 \cdot 10$$

The expression on the left is called **exponential notation**.

Definition of a^n

If a is a real number and if n is a positive integer, then we define

$$a^n = \underbrace{a \cdot a \cdot \cdots \cdot a}_{n \text{ factors}}$$

The number a is called the **base**, and n is called the **exponent**. We also write the negative exponent as the **reciprocal**:

$$a^{-n} = \frac{1}{a^n} \qquad (a \neq 0)$$

We also define $a^0 = 1$ for $a \neq 0$, while the expression 0^0 is left **undefined**. There are some serious logical problems in trying to define it.

Example

The following equations show numbers represented by exponential notation:

(a) $2^{10} = 2 \cdot 2 \cdot 2 \cdot 2 \cdot 2 \cdot 2 \cdot 2 \cdot 2 \cdot 2 \cdot 2 = 1024$

(b) $5^{-1} = \dfrac{1}{5}$

(c) $(55{,}456{,}930{,}346{,}339)^0 = 1$

(d) $x^4 = x \cdot x \cdot x \cdot x$

(e) $4^{-3} = \dfrac{1}{4 \cdot 4 \cdot 4} = \dfrac{1}{64}$ □

To use exponents effectively, you should be familiar with the following rules.

Properties of Exponentials

If a and b are real numbers and m and n are integers, then the following rules of exponents hold:

General Rule	Example
$a^m a^n = a^{m+n}$	$a^2 a^{-4} = a^{2+(-4)} = a^{-2}$
$(a^m)^n = a^{mn}$	$(a^2)^{-4} = a^{(2)(-4)} = a^{-8}$
$(ab)^m = a^m b^m$	$(ab)^2 = a^2 b^2$
$\left(\dfrac{a}{b}\right)^m = \dfrac{a^m}{b^m}$	$\left(\dfrac{a}{b}\right)^3 = \dfrac{a^3}{b^3}$
$\dfrac{a^m}{a^n} = a^{m-n}$	$\dfrac{a^2}{a^3} = a^{2-3} = a^{-1} = \dfrac{1}{a}$

Example

The following equations illustrate the rules of exponents. The reader should identify which rule is being applied in each equation.

(a) $3^7 3^{-4} = 3^3$

(b) $(2^2)^{-1} = \dfrac{1}{2^2}$

(c) $(2 \cdot 3)^2 = 2^2 \cdot 3^2$

(d) $\left(\dfrac{7}{3}\right)^2 = \dfrac{7^2}{3^2}$

(e) $(3r^2)^4 = 3^4 \cdot (r^2)^4 = 3^4 r^8$

(f) $5^{-1} + 3^{-1} = \dfrac{1}{5} + \dfrac{1}{3}$

(g) $\dfrac{2^{-4} \cdot 2^3}{2^2 \cdot 2^6} = \dfrac{2^{-1}}{2^8} = 2^{-9}$

(h) $(3x)^2 = 3^2 x^2$

(i) $(3x^2)(5x^4) = 15x^6$

(j) $-3^2 = -(3^2) = -9$

(k) $-3^{-2} = -(3^{-2}) = -\dfrac{1}{3^2}$ □

Roots of Numbers

It is useful to introduce the concept of **roots of numbers** into mathematics. We begin by saying that r is a **square root** of a number a if $r^2 = a$. In general, we say that r is an ***n*th root** of a number a if $r^n = a$. In this book we are interested in real roots (in contrast to complex roots), and so when we say "roots," we mean real roots. The interesting thing is that there are *always* 0, 1, or 2 distinct nth roots of a number for any positive integer n. Table 3 illustrates the nature of nth roots.

HISTORICAL NOTE

The radical notation $\sqrt{\ }$ was introduced in 1525 by the German algebraist Christoff Rudolff (ca. 1500–1545) in his book on algebra entitled *Die Coss*. The symbol was chosen because it looks like a lowercase *r*, which stood for *radix*, the Latin word for the square root. Rudolff is also remembered because he was one of the first mathematicians to introduce decimal fractions into texts.

TABLE 3
Nature of nth Roots of a Real Number

	***a* Positive**	***a* Negative**
n Even	*Two roots* (9 has two square roots, 3 and -3)	*No roots* (-2 has no square root)
n Odd	*One root* (8 has one cube root, 2)	*One root* (-8 has one cube root, -2)

For completeness, we should mention that the only nth root of zero is zero.

It is convenient to introduce the **fractional notation** $a^{1/n}$ or $\sqrt[n]{a}$ to stand for the nth root of a number a. When a number a has two nth roots (as 16 has two fourth roots of 2 and -2), the symbol $a^{1/n}$ denotes the positive of the two nth roots. That is, $16^{1/4} = +2$. In the special case in which $n = 2$, we denote $a^{1/2}$ by $\sqrt{a}$. Hence we have $9^{1/2} = \sqrt{9} = +3$.

The following example illustrates these ideas.

Example

(a) $4^{1/2} = \sqrt{4} = +2$ ⟵ *positive root*

(b) $8^{1/3} = \sqrt[3]{8} = +2$ ⟵ *only root*

(c) $(-8)^{1/3} = \sqrt[3]{-8} = -2$ ⟵ *only root*

(d) $16^{1/4} = \sqrt[4]{16} = +2$ ⟵ *positive root*

(e) $(\frac{4}{9})^{1/2} = \sqrt{\frac{4}{9}} = +\frac{2}{3}$ ⟵ *positive root*

(f) $(-2)^{1/2} = \sqrt{-2}$ ⟵ *no root*

(g) $(-3)^{1/2} = \sqrt{-3}$ ⟵ *no root* □

Square Roots in Simplest Form

We say that an expression involving a square root $\sqrt{}$ is in **simplest form** when the following conditions are satisfied.

- No factor within a radical should be raised to a power greater than one. For example, $\sqrt{x^2}$ and $\sqrt{x^3}$ are not in simplest form.
- No square root should be in the denominator. For example,

$$\frac{1}{\sqrt{x}} \quad \text{should be rewritten as} \quad \frac{\sqrt{x}}{x}$$

- No fraction should be within a square root. For example,

$$\sqrt{\frac{5}{2}} \quad \text{should be rewritten as} \quad \frac{\sqrt{5}}{\sqrt{2}}$$

The following properties are useful when writing expressions involving square roots in simplest form.

Properties of the Square Root

If a and b are nonnegative real numbers, then the following rules hold.

- $\sqrt{a^2} = a$
- $\sqrt{ab} = \sqrt{a}\sqrt{b}$
- $\sqrt{\frac{a}{b}} = \frac{\sqrt{a}}{\sqrt{b}} \qquad b \neq 0$

Example

The following examples illustrate how the properties of the square root can be used to simplify expressions. Assume that all variables have nonnegative values.

(a) $\sqrt{20} = \sqrt{5 \cdot 4} = \sqrt{5} \cdot \sqrt{4} = 2\sqrt{5}$ (b) $\sqrt{\dfrac{25}{4}} = \dfrac{\sqrt{25}}{\sqrt{4}} = \dfrac{5}{2}$

(c) $\sqrt{25z^5} = \sqrt{25z^4 \cdot z} = \sqrt{25z^4} \cdot \sqrt{z} = 5z^2\sqrt{z}$

(d) $\sqrt{25x^3} = \sqrt{25x^2 \cdot x} = \sqrt{25x^2} \cdot \sqrt{x} = 5x\sqrt{x}$

(e) $\dfrac{2xy}{\sqrt{y}} = \dfrac{2x\sqrt{y}\sqrt{y}}{\sqrt{y}} = 2x\sqrt{y}$ □

Fractional Exponents

We have introduced powers of numbers a^m, and roots of numbers $a^{1/n}$ where m and n are integers. We can now put these two ideas together and construct a new type of exponent, the **fractional exponent**. You may think that fractional exponents belong in the domain of pure mathematics and have no meaning in the real world. This is not the case. Many natural phenomena are described by functions having fractional exponents, and many answers to real-world problems are written in terms of fractional exponents.

> **Definition of $a^{m/n}$**
>
> For any real number a for which the nth root $a^{1/n}$ exists, the **fractional exponent** $a^{m/n}$, where m and n are integers, is defined by
>
> $$a^{m/n} = (a^{1/n})^m$$
>
> In other words, we first take the nth root, then raise this value to the mth power.

Example

Sample Fractional Exponents

(a) $8^{4/3} = (8^{1/3})^4 = 2^4 = 16$

(b) $8^{-4/3} = \dfrac{1}{8^{4/3}} = \dfrac{1}{2^4} = \dfrac{1}{16}$

(c) $(-8)^{4/3} = (-8^{1/3})^4 = (-2)^4 = 16$

(d) $(-8)^{5/2}$ not defined

(e) $4^{5/2} = (4^{1/2})^5 = 2^5 = 32$

(f) $2^{5/2} = (2^{1/2})^5 = (1.4142\ldots)^5 = 5.6568\ldots$

> HISTORICAL NOTE
>
> The Middle Ages were barren when it came to mathematical discovery. However, the greatest mathematician of the period, Nicole Oresme (c.1323–1382) of Normandy, introduced the notation for fractional exponents.

The following properties are useful when working with radicals.

Properties of Radicals

If a and b are any real numbers and m and n are any integers such that $\sqrt[n]{a}$ and $\sqrt[n]{b}$ are defined, then

- $(\sqrt[n]{a})^n = a$
- $\sqrt[n]{a^n} = \begin{cases} |a| & \text{if } n \text{ is even} \\ a & \text{if } n \text{ is odd} \end{cases}$
- $\sqrt[n]{a} \cdot \sqrt[n]{b} = \sqrt[n]{ab}$
- $\dfrac{\sqrt[n]{a}}{\sqrt[n]{b}} = \sqrt[n]{\dfrac{a}{b}} \quad (b \neq 0)$
- $\sqrt[m]{\sqrt[n]{a}} = \sqrt[mn]{a}$

Example

Sample Radical Manipulations

(a) $\sqrt{45} = \sqrt{9 \cdot 5} = \sqrt{9} \cdot \sqrt{5} = 3\sqrt{5}$

(b) $\sqrt{50} = \sqrt{25 \cdot 2} = \sqrt{25}\sqrt{2} = 5\sqrt{2}$

(c) $\sqrt[3]{54} = \sqrt[3]{27 \cdot 2} = 3\sqrt[3]{2}$

(d)
$$\begin{aligned} 3\sqrt{18} + 4\sqrt{50} &= 3\sqrt{9 \cdot 2} + 4\sqrt{25 \cdot 2} \\ &= 3\sqrt{9}\sqrt{2} + 4\sqrt{25}\sqrt{2} \\ &= 3(3)\sqrt{2} + 4(5)\sqrt{2} \\ &= 9\sqrt{2} + 20\sqrt{2} \\ &= 29\sqrt{2} \end{aligned}$$

(e) $\sqrt{9x^2} = 3|x|$

Problems

Integer Exponents

Evaluate the expressions in Problems 1–20. Use your calculator for Problems 15–20.

1. 5^3

2. 4^{-2}

3. $-(1)^{-4}$

4. $(\frac{1}{5})^{-2}$

5. $(\frac{2}{5})^{-1}$

6. 6^0

7. 0^0

8. $3^{-1} + 4^2$

9. $-(2)^{-4}$

10. $-(-3)^{-1}$

11. -2^{-4}

12. $-(2)^{-4}$

13. -1^0

14. $(\frac{1}{8})^2$

15. 2^{10}

16. $(-2)^{10}$ (error message)

17. $(\frac{2}{7})^2$

18. $5^{-1} + 3^{-4}$

19. 1.01^{50}

20. 1.05^{75}

Simplify the expressions in Problems 21–30 so that they have only positive exponents. Assume that all variables are positive real numbers.

21. $\dfrac{5^2}{5^4}$

22. $\dfrac{3^{-4}}{3^{-5}}$

23. $\dfrac{10^5 \cdot 10^{-5} \cdot 10^6}{10^5 \cdot 10^{-7}}$

24. $\dfrac{x^4 \cdot y^3}{x^3 \cdot y^2}$

25. $\dfrac{a^5 \cdot b^{-3}}{a^4 \cdot b^{-7}}$

26. $\left(\dfrac{3x^{-2}}{y^4}\right)^{-3}$

27. $\dfrac{(4m^{-1})^{-1}}{2m^2}$

28. $\dfrac{5^{-2}x^2y^{-1}}{5x^{-1}y^{-3}}$

29. $\dfrac{x^{-1}}{y^{-1}}$

30. $\dfrac{x^{-1}}{y}$

31. **Hmmmmm.** Which is the larger number, 2 or $(2{,}465{,}543{,}076{,}345)^0$?

32. **English to Algebra.** Write algebraically the following statement: The product of powers of the same quantity is equal to the power of that same quantity with exponent the sum of the exponents of the two factors.

33. **Simple Puzzler.** What is the largest number that can be written by using three 2's and the operations of addition, subtraction, multiplication, division, and exponentiation? Some examples are $2 + 2 + 2$, $2 \cdot 2 \cdot 2$, $2^2 + 2$, $(2 + 2)/2$, and 222. Can you get a number as large as 4,194,304? What would be the answer if exponents were not allowed?

34. **Puzzler.** What is the largest number that can be written by using each of the numbers 3, 4, and 5 only once?

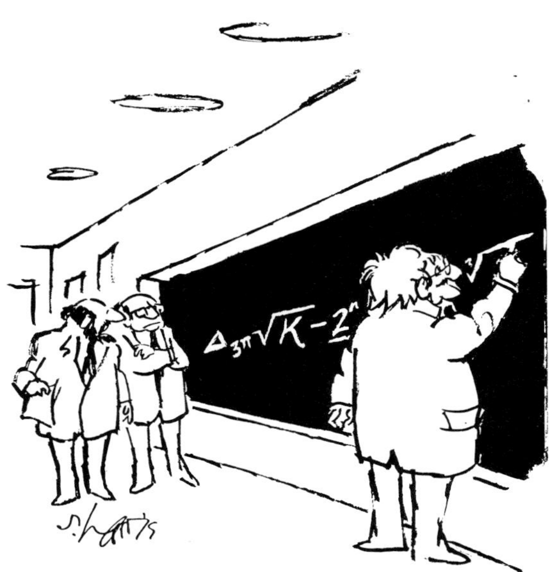

"WE HAVE REASON TO BELIEVE BINGLEMAN IS AN IRRATIONAL NUMBER HIMSELF."

35. **Hmmmmm.** What is the largest number that can be written using any three digits (the integers 0 through 9) by means of addition, multiplication, and exponentiation. Believe it or not, if this number were written on a strip of paper (the same size as the numbers printed in this book), it would take a strip stretching from Lincoln, Nebraska, to Gary, Indiana.

Roots

Evaluate the roots in Problems 36–45. Use a calculator if necessary.

36. $8^{1/3}$

37. $16^{1/4}$

38. $125^{1/3}$

39. $1024^{1/10}$

40. $\sqrt[3]{27}$

41. $\sqrt[3]{64}$

42. $\sqrt[3]{-125}$

43. $\sqrt[5]{2}$

44. $\sqrt[9]{512}$

45. $\sqrt[8]{256}$

46. **Hmmmmm.** The next time you owe someone half a dollar, say that since 25 cents $= \frac{1}{4}$ dollar you will just take the square root of these equal quantities and obtain the new equal quantities: 5 cents $= \frac{1}{2}$ dollar. Then give the person a nickel. What is wrong with your argument?

Square Roots in Simplest Form

Reduce the expressions in Problems 47–56 to simplest form. Assume that all variables have nonnegative values.

47. $\sqrt{25x^3}$

48. $\sqrt{16x^5}$

49. $\dfrac{3x}{\sqrt{x}}$

50. $\dfrac{\sqrt{25x^2y^2}}{\sqrt{x}}$

51. $\dfrac{1}{\sqrt{xy}}$

52. $\sqrt{16x^2y^2}$

53. $\sqrt{z^7}$

54. $\sqrt{x^2y^3z^5}$

55. $\sqrt{u^2v^4}$

56. $\sqrt{2x^2y^5}$

57. **Hmmmmm.** What is wrong with the following argument?

$$1 = \sqrt{1} = \sqrt{(-1)(-1)} = \sqrt{-1}\sqrt{-1} = [(-1)^{1/2}]^2 = -1$$

Fractional Exponents

Simplify the expressions in Problems 58–72.

58. $\sqrt{32}$

59. $\sqrt{1000}$

60. $2\sqrt{5} + 5\sqrt{45}$

61. $\sqrt{1000x^4y^6}$

62. $\sqrt{32x^5}$

63. $\sqrt{a^5b^5} + \sqrt{a^4b^7}$

64. $\sqrt{90x^5y^4}$

65. $3\sqrt{3} + \sqrt{12}$

66. $\sqrt[3]{3x^4y^6}$

67. $\sqrt[4]{32x^4y^5}$

68. $\sqrt{2x^2y^3z^4}$

69. $\sqrt[5]{64x^5}$

70. $\sqrt{80x^5w^9}$

71. $\sqrt{50} + \sqrt{60}$

72. $\sqrt{x^2} + \sqrt{x^4}$

Inequalities and Intervals

Inequalities express relations between two quantities that are not equal to one another. Since there are more instances of inequality than of equality in the world, it makes sense that inequalities should be an important tool for expressing relations. Most beginning students find the study of inequalities more difficult than that of equalities, since the rules of operation for inequalities are more general than the rules of operation for equalities. We will see in this section that these rules can also be quite useful.

Definition of the Inequality

If a and b are real numbers, then

- $a < b$ means that $b - a$ is positive.
- $a \leq b$ means that $b - a$ is positive or zero.

Geometrically, $a < b$ means that a is to the *left* of b on the real number line.

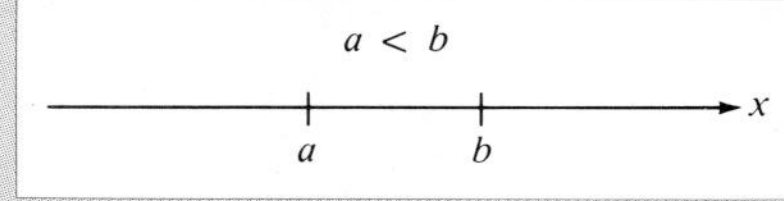

Likewise, we say that $a > b$ when $a - b$ is positive and that $a \geq b$ when $a - b$ is positive or zero.

Example

(a) $2 < 3$ since $3 - 2$ is positive
(b) $2 \leq 3$ since $3 - 2$ is positive or zero
(c) $-5 < -2$ since $-2 - (-5)$ is positive
(d) $-1 < 0$ since $0 - (-1)$ is positive
(e) $-5 < -3$ since $-3 - (-5)$ is positive
(f) $3 \leq 3$ since $3 - 3$ is positive or zero
(g) $4 > 3$ since $4 - 3$ is positive
(h) $-2 > -3$ since $-2 - (-3)$ is positive □

To solve problems involving inequalities, it is useful to know the rules they satisfy.

Six Properties of Inequalities

For real numbers a, b, and c the following properties hold:

1. If $a < b$ and $b < c$, then $a < c$.
2. If $a < b$, then $a + c < b + c$.
3. If $a < b$ and $c < d$, then $a + c < b + d$.
4. If $a < b$ and c is positive, then $ac < bc$.
5. If $a < b$ and c is negative, then $ac > bc$.
6. If $a < b$ and both a and b have the same sign (both positive or both negative), then $1/a > 1/b$.

One of the major uses of inequalities is to describe different regions on the real number line. In particular, they can describe the following **intervals**.

Important Intervals on the Real Line

We say that

- $a < x < b$ when $a < x$ and $x < b$
- $a < x \leq b$ when $a < x$ and $x \leq b$
- $a \leq x < b$ when $a \leq x$ and $x < b$
- $a \leq x \leq b$ when $a \leq x$ and $x \leq b$

By means of the above **double inequalities**, we can define the following intervals.

Open Interval

The open interval (a, b) consists of the real numbers x that satisfy $a < x < b$.

Closed Interval

The closed interval $[a, b]$ consists of the real numbers x that satisfy $a \leq x \leq b$.

Half-Open Interval

The half-open interval $(a, b]$ consists of the real numbers x that satisfy $a < x \leq b$. The half-open interval $[a, b)$ consists of the real numbers x that satisfy $a \leq x < b$.

Semi-Infinite Intervals

Other important intervals of real numbers are the semi-infinite intervals:

$$(a, \infty) = \{\text{all numbers greater than } a\}$$
$$[a, \infty) = \{\text{all numbers greater than or equal to } a\}$$
$$(-\infty, a) = \{\text{all numbers less than } a\}$$
$$(-\infty, a] = \{\text{all numbers less than or equal to } a\}$$

Infinite Interval

The infinite interval $(-\infty, \infty)$ consists of all the real numbers.

Some typical intervals are shown in Figure 4.

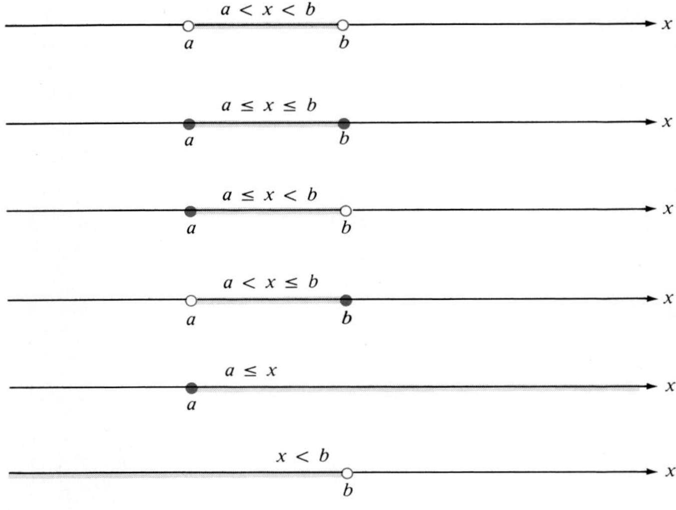

Figure 4
Typical intervals

It is often important to find the numbers that satisfy a given inequality. The following example illustrates how inequalities can be solved.

Example

Find all possible numbers that satisfy the inequality

$$x + 1 < 2x - 1$$

Solution We are looking for all real numbers x for which this inequality is a true statement. Starting with

$$x + 1 < 2x - 1$$

add $-x$ to each side, getting

$$1 < x - 1 \qquad \text{(Property 2)}$$

Then add 1 to each side, getting

$$2 < x \qquad \text{(Property 2)}$$

Hence the solution consists of all real numbers greater than 2, or $(2, \infty)$. You should check a few of these values for yourself. □

Can You Find the Flaw?

Can you find the flaw in the following use of inequalities? We will show that all positive numbers are negative.

We begin by selecting any two numbers a and b, where $a < b$. Hence

	$a(a - b) < b(a - b)$	(just multiply each side by $a - b$)
Hence	$a^2 - ab < ab - b^2$	(just algebra)
Hence	$a^2 - 2ab + b^2 < 0$	(just add $b^2 - ab$ to each side)
Hence	$(a - b)^2 < 0$	(just algebra)

But this last inequality says that the (obviously) positive number $(a - b)^2$ is negative. What went wrong?

Problems

For Problems 1–10, solve the indicated inequality.

1. $x - 1 < 2x + 3$

2. $x + 4 < -x + 4$

3. $2x + 5 \leq 4$

4. $5x + 6 \leq 5x + 7$

5. $8x + 5 \leq 0$

6. $x - 1 > x - 2$

7. $x + 2x \geq x$

8. $x + x \geq x + 2x + 1$

9. $x - 1 > 1 - x$

10. $2(x - 1) \geq 1$

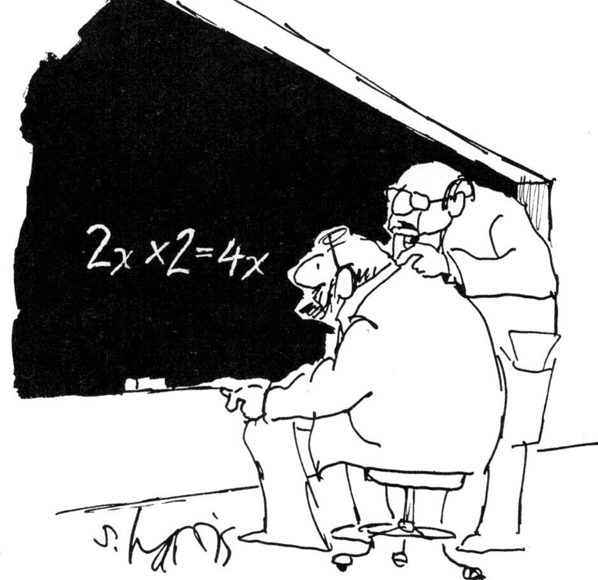

"BUT GERSHON, YOU CAN'T CALL IT GERSHON'S EQUATION IF EVERYONE HAS KNOWN IT FOR AGES."

11. Hmmmmm. We will now prove without a doubt that $5 > 8$. Pick any two numbers a and b with

$$a > b$$

Multiply both sides of this inequality by b, getting the obvious result

$$ab > b^2$$

Subtracting a^2 from both sides clearly gives

$$ab - a^2 > b^2 - a^2$$

We now factor each side of the inequality to get

$$a(b - a) > (b - a)(b + a)$$

Dividing both sides by $b - a$ certainly gives

$$a > b + a$$

Now since $a > b$, if we add a to the left-hand side of the above inequality and b to the right-hand side, we get

$$2a > 2b + a$$

or, by subtracting a from each side,

$$a > 2b$$

In other words, we have proved that if $a > b$, then $a > 2b$. For example, since $5 > 4$, we can conclude that $5 > 8$. Can you determine what is wrong with our argument?

Algebraic Fractions and Rationalization

Algebraic Fractions

Algebraic fractions are quotients of algebraic expressions. Some examples are

$$\frac{1}{\sqrt{x}} \qquad \frac{2x+1}{x} \qquad \frac{x^2+2x+3}{x+2}$$

The basic rules for manipulating algebraic fractions are the same as those for manipulating real numbers.

Basic Rules for Manipulating Fractions

If a, b, c, and d represent algebraic expressions, then (provided that the denominators are nonzero) the following rules hold:

1. $\dfrac{a}{b} + \dfrac{c}{d} = \dfrac{ad + bc}{bd}$ finding a common denominator
2. $\dfrac{a}{b} - \dfrac{c}{d} = \dfrac{ad - bc}{bd}$ finding a common denominator
3. $\dfrac{a}{b} \cdot \dfrac{c}{d} = \dfrac{ac}{bd}$ product of fractions
4. $\dfrac{\frac{a}{b}}{\frac{c}{d}} = \dfrac{ad}{bc}$ quotient of fractions (invert and multiply rule)

Example

The following equations illustrate the above rules:

$$\frac{1}{x} + \frac{2}{x+1} = \frac{(x+1) + 2x}{x(x+1)} = \frac{3x+1}{x(x+1)}$$

$$\frac{x}{2x-3} \cdot \frac{x+1}{x+5} = \frac{x(x+1)}{(2x-3)(x+5)}$$

$$\frac{\frac{1}{x}}{\frac{2x+5}{4x+3}} = \frac{4x+3}{x(2x+5)}$$

The cancellation property is another important property used with algebraic fractions.

> **Cancellation of Common Factors**
>
> If a, b, and c are algebraic expressions, with $c \neq 0$, then
>
> $$\frac{ac}{bc} = \frac{a}{b}$$

Example

$$\frac{(2x+1)(x^2+1)}{x(x^2+1)} = \frac{2x+1}{x}$$

Rationalization

It is often possible to eliminate square roots from either the numerator or denominator of a fraction by a process called **rationalization.**

Example

Rationalizing the Denominator Eliminate the square roots from the denominator of

$$\frac{1}{\sqrt{x} - \sqrt{y}}$$

Solution Multiply the numerator and the denominator of the fraction by the conjugate of the denominator of the original expression (change the sign between the square roots):

$$\sqrt{x} + \sqrt{y} \qquad \text{(conjugate expression)}$$

This gives

$$\frac{1}{\sqrt{x} - \sqrt{y}} \cdot \frac{\sqrt{x} + \sqrt{y}}{\sqrt{x} + \sqrt{y}} = \frac{\sqrt{x} + \sqrt{y}}{x - y}$$ □

Example Rationalizing the Numerator Eliminate the square roots from the numerator of

$$\frac{\sqrt{x+h}-\sqrt{x}}{h}$$

Solution Multiplying both numerator and denominator by $\sqrt{x+h}+\sqrt{x}$, we have

$$\frac{\sqrt{x+h}-\sqrt{x}}{h}\cdot\frac{\sqrt{x+h}+\sqrt{x}}{\sqrt{x+h}+\sqrt{x}}=\frac{1}{\sqrt{x+h}+\sqrt{x}}$$ □

Problems

Rewrite the expressions in Problems 1–7 as a single fraction, and simplify by cancelling all common factors.

1. $\frac{1}{x}+\frac{x}{2}$

2. $\frac{1}{x-1}+\frac{x+1}{3}$

3. $\frac{1}{x-1}-\frac{x}{x+2}$

4. $\frac{x-1}{x+1}\cdot\frac{x}{x+3}$

5. $\frac{(x-1)(x+2)}{(x^2-4)}$

6. $\frac{1}{x-1}+\frac{1}{x+1}$

7. $\frac{\sqrt{x}+1}{1-\sqrt{x}}+\frac{1}{x}$

8. Hmmmmm. Starting with the equation

$$\frac{x-10}{7-x}=\frac{x-10}{13-x}$$

we divide each side by $x-10$ to get

$$\frac{1}{7-x}=\frac{1}{13-x}$$

Since the numerators are the same, we must have

$$7-x=13-x$$

Adding x to each side then gives $7 = 13$. Can you discover what is wrong with this argument?

Rationalization

Rationalize the denominators in Problems 9–14.

9. $\frac{1}{\sqrt{x}+\sqrt{y}}$

10. $\frac{5}{\sqrt{z}-2\sqrt{x}}$

11. $\frac{1}{\sqrt{x+a}-\sqrt{x}}$

12. $\frac{\sqrt{x-3}+\sqrt{x+3}}{\sqrt{x-3}-\sqrt{x+3}}$

13. $\frac{1}{\sqrt{x+2}+\sqrt{x-2}}$

14. $\frac{1}{x-\sqrt{y}}$

For Problems 15–19, rationalize the numerator.

15. $\frac{\sqrt{2+h}-\sqrt{2}}{h}$

16. $\frac{\sqrt{x}+\sqrt{y}}{2}$

17. $\frac{\sqrt{x+2}-\sqrt{x-2}}{x}$

18. $\frac{\sqrt{x+3}+\sqrt{x-3}}{\sqrt{x+3}-\sqrt{x-3}}$

19. $\frac{x-\sqrt{y}}{x}$

P.2 Functions and Their Graphs

Functional Notation

The world is filled with relationships between quantities. If one picks up a newspaper, it is impossible not to see graphs, tables, and diagrams. Mathematics allows us to discuss relationships between phenomena in a precise way, using the notion of a **function**.

A Function

A function is a rule that assigns to each element of a given set, called the **domain set**, an element in another set, called the **range set**.

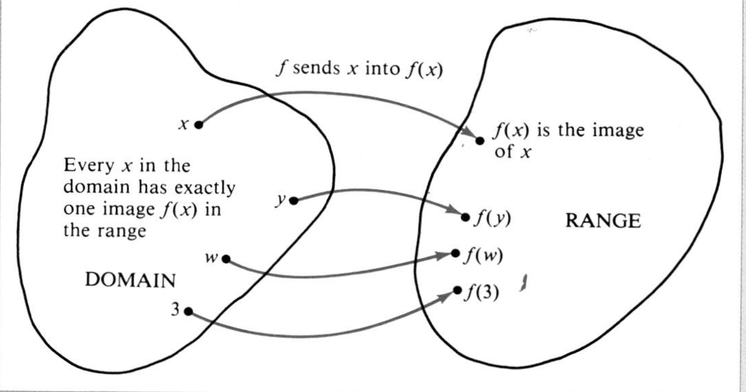

We often think of functions as black boxes into which we enter a value of x (element of the domain), and out comes a corresponding value of y (element of the range) as determined by the black box.

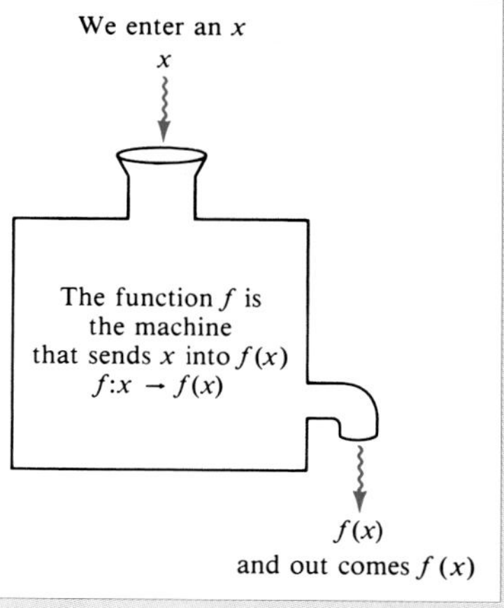

A typical function is the rule that assigns to each real number x its square x^2. The domain of this function is the set of real numbers, and the range is the set of nonnegative real numbers $[0, \infty)$. We can denote some values of this function by writing

$$\begin{aligned} 3 &\longrightarrow 9 \\ -1 &\longrightarrow 1 \\ -5 &\longrightarrow 25 \\ 2.5 &\longrightarrow 6.25 \end{aligned}$$

to indicate the value corresponding to a given element of the domain. We often denote

$$x \longrightarrow x^2$$

to represent the value of the function for all real numbers x. We generally denote functions by letters, such as f, g, or h, and illustrate the rule of correspondence by an arrow, such as

$$f\colon x \longrightarrow y$$

The value y above is called the *image* of the function f at the point x; it is also written as $f(x)$. For example, if f is the function that assigns to each real number x its square x^2, then we could also write

$$f\colon x \longrightarrow x^2 \qquad (f \text{ "sends" } x \text{ into } x^2)$$

or

$$f(x) = x^2 \qquad (\text{image of } f \text{ at } x, \text{ read "} f \text{ of } x \text{ is } x^2\text{"})$$

Confusion of the Meaning of f and $f(x)$

There is often a great deal of confusion between the symbols f and $f(x)$. A function (the rule) is denoted by the letter f, while the value of a function at a point x of its domain is denoted by $f(x)$. For example, the square root function, which takes the positive square root of a positive number, is denoted by

$$f\colon x \longrightarrow \sqrt{x}$$

but the value of f at a particular real number x is $f(x) = \sqrt{x}$.

Example

Domain and Evaluation of Functions Consider the three functions f, g, and h defined by

$$f(x) = 2x + 1 \qquad g(x) = \frac{1}{x+1} \qquad h(x) = \sqrt{x+1}$$

where we assume that the domain of each function consists of those values of x for which the respective function makes mathematical sense. Hence

Domain of f = all real numbers
Domain of g = all real numbers except -1
Domain of h = all real numbers ≥ -1

and

(a) $f(2) = 2 \cdot 2 + 1 = 5$

(b) $f(0) = 2 \cdot 0 + 1 = 1$

(c) $f(-1) = 2 \cdot (-1) + 1 = -1$

(d) $f(\text{BLAH}) = 2 \cdot \text{BLAH} + 1$ (BLAH stands for any real number)

(e) $g(0) = \dfrac{1}{0+1} = 1$

(f) $g(3) = \dfrac{1}{3+1} = 0.25$

(g) $g(x^2) = \dfrac{1}{x^2+1}$

(h) $g(\text{BLAH}) = \dfrac{1}{\text{BLAH}+1}$ (BLAH is any real number $\neq -1$)

(i) $h(0) = \sqrt{0+1} = 1$

(j) $h(1) = \sqrt{1+1} = \sqrt{2}$

(k) $h(t+1) = \sqrt{(t+1)+1} = \sqrt{t+2}$

(l) $h(\text{BLAH}) = \sqrt{\text{BLAH}+1}$ (BLAH is any real number ≥ -1) □

Problems

For Problems 1–30, find the indicated values given the functions defined by

$$f(x) = x - 2 \qquad g(x) = \frac{1}{x} \qquad h(x) = x^2$$

1. $f(1)$
2. $f(-1)$
3. $f(0)$
4. $f(x+1)$
5. $f(x^2)$
6. $f(x^2+1)$
7. $f(x^2)+1$
8. $f(2x)+f(x^2)$
9. $f(2x)+2x$
10. $f(-x)-f(x)$
11. $g(1)$
12. $g(-1)$
13. $g(0)$
14. $g(x+1)$
15. $g(x^2)$
16. $g(x^2+1)$
17. $g(x^2)+1$
18. $g(2x)+g(x^2)$
19. $g(2x)+2x$
20. $g(-x)-g(x)$
21. $h(1)$
22. $h(-1)$
23. $h(0)$
24. $h(x+1)$
25. $h(x^2)$
26. $h(x^2+1)$
27. $h(x^2)+1$
28. $h(2x)+h(x^2)$
29. $h(2x)+2x$
30. $h(-x)-h(x)$

For Problems 31–40, we select the domain of the given function as those real numbers x for which the function makes mathematical sense. What is the domain of the given function? What is the range of the function?

31. $f(x) = 1$
32. $f(x) = 2x - 1$
33. $g(x) = x^2$
34. $h(x) = x^3$
35. $h(x) = \sqrt{x}$
36. $g(x) = \sqrt{x-1}$
37. $F(x) = \sqrt{x^2+1}$
38. $G(x) = \dfrac{1}{x}$
39. $f(x) = \dfrac{1}{x^2+1}$
40. $g(x) = \dfrac{1}{x^2-1}$

Cartesian Coordinate System

One of the greatest mathematical developments of all time was the merging of the major mathematical disciplines of algebra and geometry into what is now called *analytical geometry*. To understand how the ideas of algebra (equations) can be merged with the ideas of geometry (lines and planes), we begin by drawing two perpendicular lines, one horizontal (x-axis) and one vertical (y-axis), as shown in Figure 5.

The point where the two lines intersect is called the **origin** and is labeled (0, 0). All other points are labeled accordingly by a pair of numbers (x, y) called the **coordinates** of the point. The coordinates locate the position of the point relative to both axes. For example, to find the point labeled (3, 4), we go 3 units to the right on the x-axis and 4 units upward parallel to the y-axis. To find the

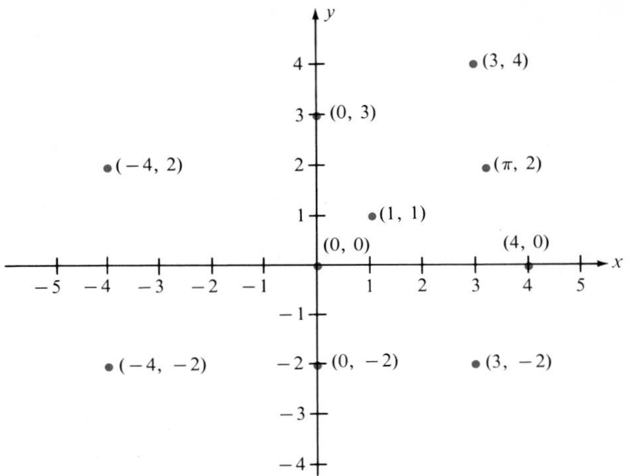

Figure 5
The cartesian coordinate system

point $(-1, -4)$, we move 1 unit to the left on the x-axis and 4 units downward parallel to the y-axis. For the point (3, 4), we would say that 3 is the ***x*-coordinate** and 4 is the ***y*-coordinate**.

We can easily find the distance from one point to another in this system by applying probably the most famous theorem in mathematics, the **Pythagorean theorem**. This geometric theorem was first proved by the Greek mathematician Pythagoras in about 500 B.C., according to mathematical tradition. The theorem says that the sum of squares of the lengths of the two sides of a right triangle (a triangle that has one 90 degree angle) is the square of the length of the hypotenuse (the third side, the one opposite the right angle). Figure 6 illustrates this idea.

Using the Pythagorean theorem, we can find the distance D between any two points in the plane.

Distance between Points in the Plane

The distance D between the points (a, b) and (c, d) in the xy-plane is given by

$$D = \sqrt{(a - c)^2 + (b - d)^2}$$

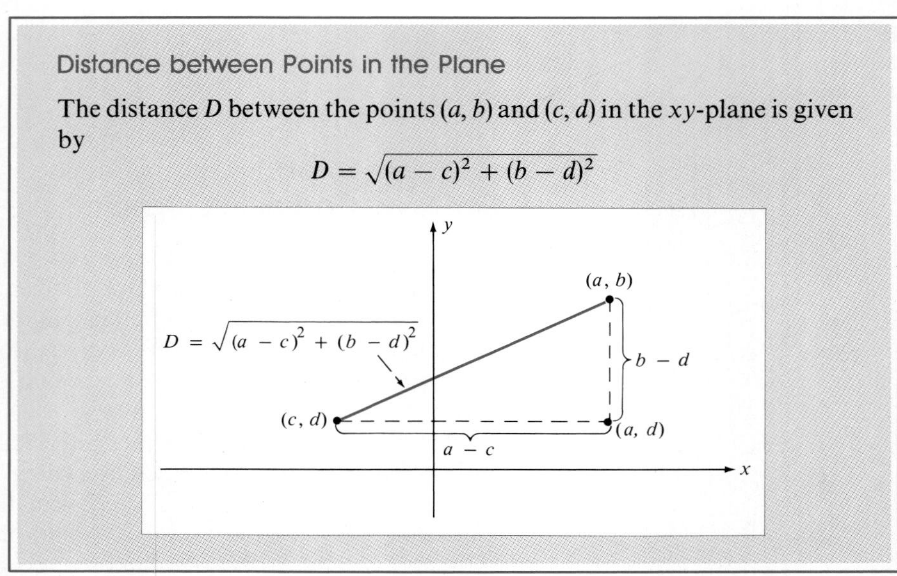

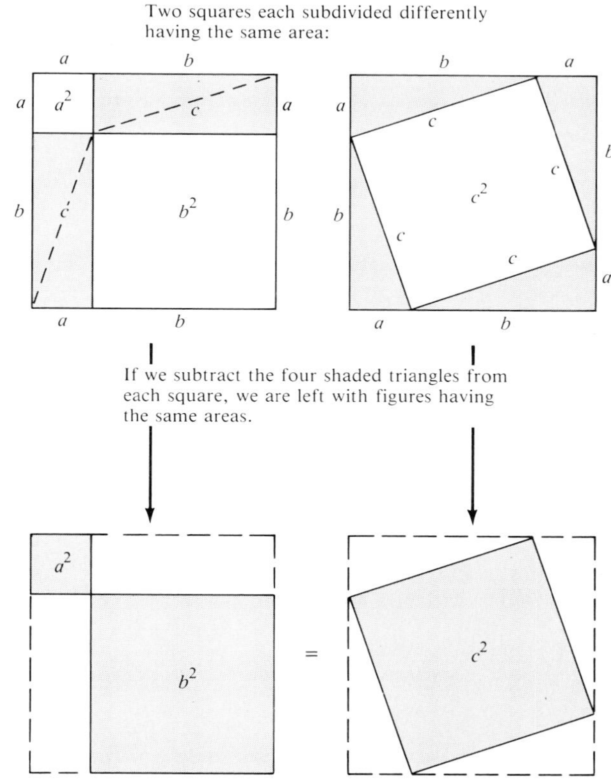

Figure 6
The Pythagorean theorem

Example

Find the distance between the points (1, 3) and $(-2, 2)$.

Solution $D = \sqrt{(1 + 2)^2 + (3 - 2)^2} = \sqrt{10}$ □

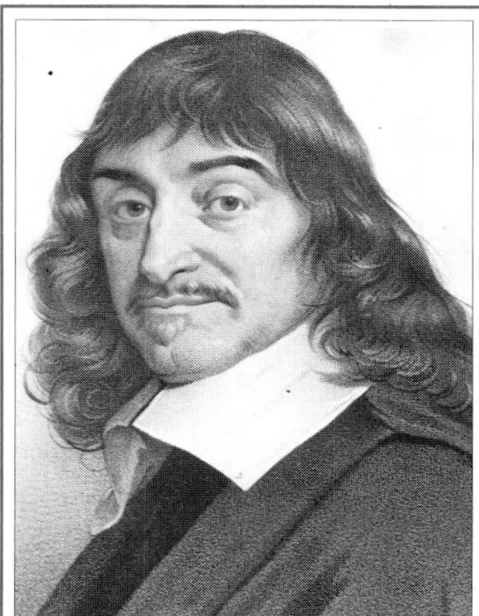

HISTORICAL NOTE

The time was ripe in the early 1600s for the brilliant French mathematician René Descartes (1596–1650) and others to found the subject of *analytical geometry*. The merging of the two great mathematical disciplines of the time, algebra and geometry, into a single unifying body of knowledge was one of the great mathematical developments of all time. Analytical geometry enabled mathematicians to describe curves (geometry), such as the trajectories of the planets, by means of equations (algebra). This new way of looking at the universe was responsible in great part for the "invention" of the calculus, which would come 50 years later.

It is interesting to note here that Descartes was also responsible for popularizing the exponential notation x^n that we studied earlier.

Problems

In Problems 1–5, connect the following points with straight line segments to find the mystery figures.

$A = (0, 0)$	$E = (2, 4)$
$B = (4, 0)$	$F = (4, 3)$
$C = (2, 2)$	$G = (2, 6)$
$D = (0, 3)$	

1. Connect A to C, C to B, C to E, D to E, E to F, and E to G.
2. Connect A to D, D to E, E to F, F to B, and B to A.
3. Connect A to F and D to B.
4. Connect A to G, G to B, and B to A.
5. Connect D to A, A to C, C to B, and B to F.

Find the mystery figures in Problems 6–9 by connecting the points in each list (in order) with straight line segments.

6. (3, 5), (6, −2), (0, −2), (3, 5) (You've seen this before.)
7. (0, 0), (0, 4), (5, 4), (5, 0), (0, 0) (You've seen this before.)
8. (3, −1), (−5, −1), (−2, 4), (6, 4), (3, −1) (What is this called?)
9. (−2, 0), (5, −3), (6, 2), (1, 4), (−2, 0) (What is this called?)

10. Hmmmmm. Connect the following points in the order they are given with straight line segments to find the initials of one of the major universities in the United States.

First initial: (0, 4), (0, 0), (4, 0), (4, 4)
Second initial: (6, 0), (6, 4), (8, 2), (10, 4), (10, 0)

In Problems 11–14, locate the following points in the xy-plane and find the distance between them.

11. (0, 0), (1, 1)
12. (2, 3), (3, 5)
13. (−1, −1), (3, −3)
14. (1, 0), (2, −3)

15. What is the total distance around the perimeter of the triangle that has corner points (1, 1), (2, 3), and (4, −1)?

Graphs of Functions

When both the domain and range of a function consist of real numbers, we can draw a "picture" or **graph** of the function in the plane using cartesian coordinates. We define the graph of a function f to be the collection of points $(x, f(x))$ in the cartesian plane where x lies in the domain of f. Several functions important to business and science are shown in Figure 7.

It is generally possible to approximate the graph of a function by simply plotting some representative points $(x, f(x))$ and then joining them by a smooth curve.

Three-Step Procedure for Graphing Functions

To graph a function f, carry out the following three steps:

Step 1. Evaluate $f(x)$ at a few representative values of x in the domain of f.

Step 2. Plot the points $(x, f(x))$ in the plane.

Step 3. Connect the points plotted in Step 2 with a smooth curve.

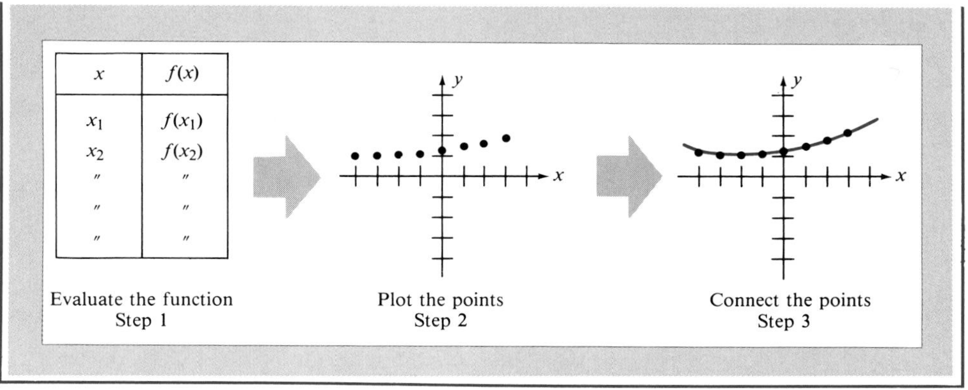

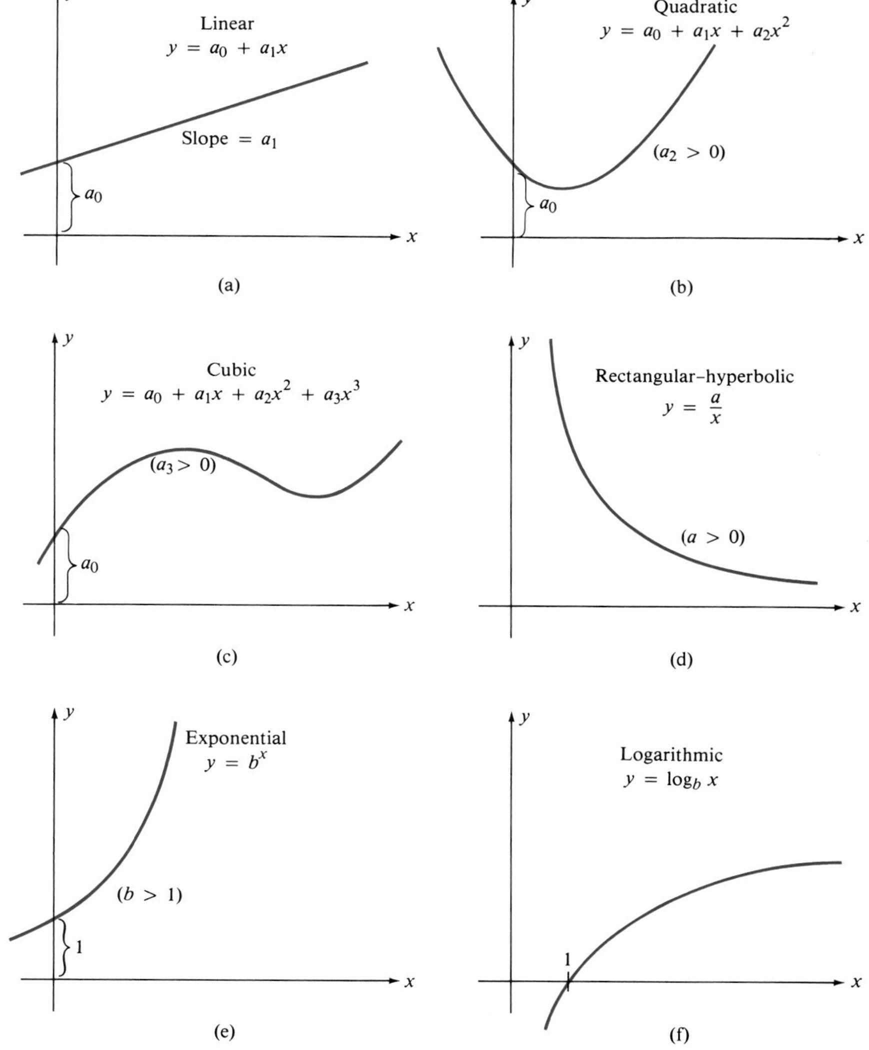

Figure 7
Important graphs in business and science

Example

Graphing a Function Sketch the graph of the function f defined by

$$f(x) = x^2 - 3 \qquad -\infty < x < \infty$$

Solution The domain of the function consists of all real numbers x. The three-step procedure is illustrated in Figure 8.

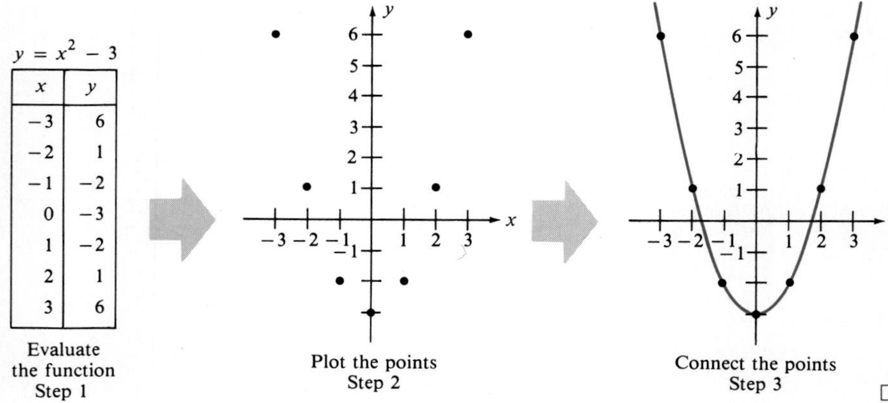

$y = x^2 - 3$

x	y
−3	6
−2	1
−1	−2
0	−3
1	−2
2	1
3	6

Figure 8
Three-step procedure for graphing $f(x) = x^2 - 3$ □

Example

Graphing a Function Draw the graph of the function f defined by

$$f(x) = \sqrt{x} \qquad x \geq 0$$

Solution The domain of the function consists of all nonnegative real numbers $x \geq 0$. The three-step procedure is illustrated in Figure 9.

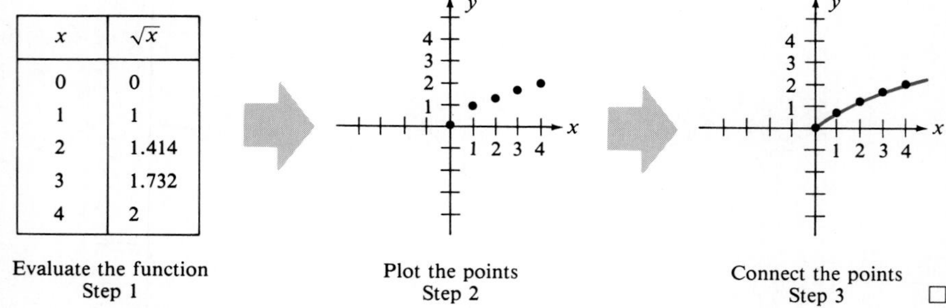

x	$\sqrt{x}$
0	0
1	1
2	1.414
3	1.732
4	2

Figure 9
Three-step procedure for graphing $f(x) = \sqrt{x}$ □

Vertical Line Test for Functions

Inasmuch as a function f assigns to each value x in its domain a single value $f(x)$, this implies that the graph of any function f will touch or cross a vertical line no more than once. Note that the graphs of the functions in the two previous examples intersect each vertical line at most once. The two curves drawn in Figure 10 illustrate the essential difference between the graph of a function and a curve that is not the graph of a function.

Example

Wind Chill Equivalent Temperature Just how cold is it? In cold weather, the air temperature alone does not always provide a reliable indicator of how cold you feel, since it does not take into consideration the wind speed. In 1939,

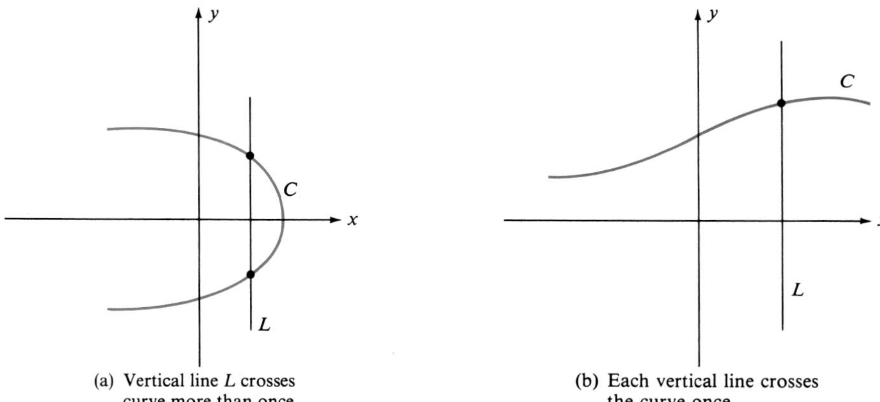

Figure 10
The vertical line test for functions

meteorologists Siple and Passel proposed a function to determine the "equivalent wind chill temperature." For example, on the basis of experiments, Siple and Passel determined that a temperature of 20°F and a 10-mph wind had the same cooling effect as a temperature of 3°F and no wind. From these results, they concluded that a temperature of 20°F and a 10-mph wind would have an equivalent wind chill temperature of 3°F. In the special case in which the air temperature is 0°F, the equivalent wind chill temperature $WC(v)$ for wind velocity v lying between 5 and 50 mph is given by the wind chill function

$$WC(v) = 91 - 91(0.44 + 0.325\sqrt{v} - 0.023v) \qquad 5 \leq v \leq 50$$

Sketch the graph of the equivalent wind chill function $WC(v)$ when the air temperature is 0°F.

Solution For convenience, we have denoted the wind chill function by WC instead of the usual functional notation of f. We first compute the values of $WC(v)$ for wind velocities 5, 10, 15, 20, . . . , 40, 45 mph as shown in Table 4. The points $(v, WC(v))$ listed in Table 4 and a smooth curve connecting them are drawn in Figure 11.

TABLE 4
Equivalent Wind Chill Temperature When the Air Temperature is 0°F

Wind Speed v (mph)	Equivalent Wind Chill Temperature $WC(v)$ (°F) (rounded to nearest integer)
5	−5
10	−22
15	−32
20	−39
25	−45
30	−48
35	−51
40	−52
45	−53

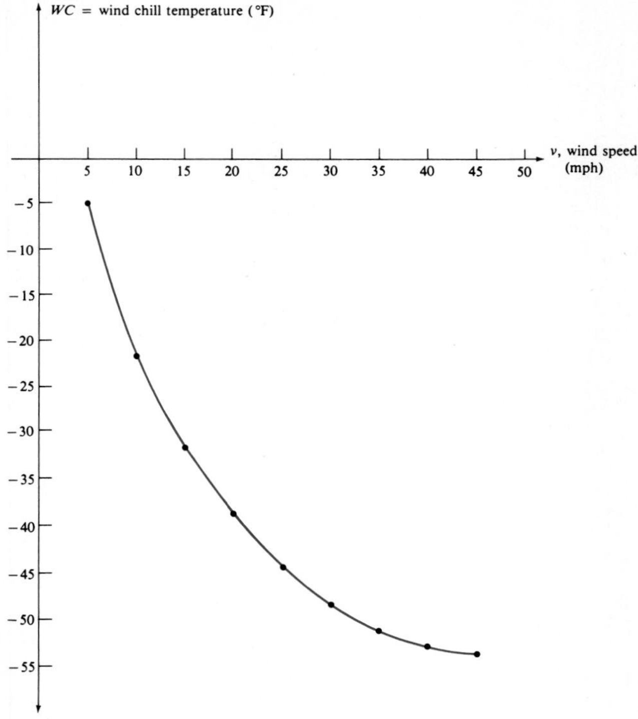

Figure 11
Graph of the equivalent wind chill temperature function when the air temperature is 0°F

□

Problems

For Problems 1–10, draw the graph of the given function using the three-step procedure. Take as the domain of each function the values of x for which the function makes mathematical sense.

1. $f(x) = x$

2. $f(x) = 2x + 1$

3. $f(x) = x^2$

4. $f(x) = x^2 + x + 1$

5. $f(x) = x^3$

6. $f(x) = |x|$

7. $f(x) = |x - 1|$

8. $f(x) = \sqrt{x - 1}$

9. $f(x) = \dfrac{1}{x}$ (Be careful when connecting points.)

10. $f(x) = \dfrac{1}{x^2}$ (Be careful when connecting points.)

Some Interesting Graphs

11. Just How Cold Is It? In International Falls, Minnesota, the temperature is −20°F. At this temperature, the equivalent wind chill temperature function is given by

$$WC(v) = 91 - 111(0.44 + 0.325\sqrt{v} - 0.023v) \quad 5 \le v \le 45$$

Suppose the wind is blowing at 30 mph. What is the equivalent wind chill temperature?

First-Order Polynomials: Straight Lines

Perhaps the simplest function in mathematics is the **first-order polynomial** or linear function

$$f(x) = ax + b$$

where a and b are constants. There are many reasons why this function is so important. First of all, as we shall see in Chapter 1, the first-order polynomial is essential for the study of the differential calculus. Second, and more important from the point of view of applications, linear functions often describe relationships between real-world quantities. For example, a scientific study determined that the number N of deaths in the world each week could be estimated by a linear function depending on the amount of sulfur dioxide produced by burning fossil fuels. In particular, if C is the average concentration of sulfur dioxide (micrograms per cubic meter) in the air, then the estimated number of respiratory deaths N per week can be estimated by the linear function

$$N(C) = 0.031C + 94 \qquad 50 \le C \le 700$$

The graph of this function is shown in Figure 12.

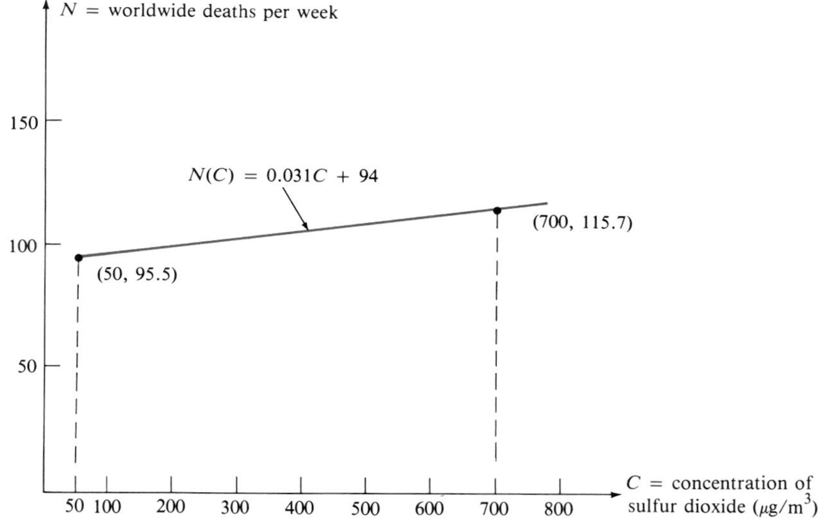

Figure 12
Graph of the number of respiratory deaths per week due to sulfur dioxide

The graph of the linear function $N(C)$ shown in Figure 12 is a straight line. In fact, as we shall see shortly, the graph of any linear function is a straight line. Inasmuch as straight lines are so crucial to the study of calculus and in describing real-world phenomena, we will study them now.

The Straight Line

An equation of the form

$$ax + by = c$$

where a and b are not both zero is called a **linear equation** in the two variables x and y. Examples are

$$\begin{aligned} 2x + 3y &= 3 \\ x - y &= 0 \\ -3x + y &= -2 \\ y &= 5 \end{aligned}$$

A solution of a linear equation in two variables is an **ordered pair** of real numbers (x, y), or point, that satisfies the equation. For example, the pair (1, 3) is a solution of the equation $3x + y = 6$ because $3(1) + 3 = 6$. The **solution set** of a linear equation is the set of all solutions of a linear equation. By the **graph of an equation**, we mean a plot of all its solutions (x, y) in the xy-plane. We will not prove it here, but it can be shown that the graph of a linear equation is a straight line. To graph a linear equation, it is sufficient to plot just two solutions (x, y) in the xy-plane and then draw the straight line that passes through those two points because any straight line is completely determined by any pair of points on it.

Example

Draw the graph of $2x + y = 2$.

Solution It is usually convenient first to set x to zero and solve for y and then set y to zero and solve for x. Doing this, we get

Setting $x = 0$ and Solving for y	Setting $y = 0$ and Solving for x
$2(0) + y = 2$ $y = 2$	$2x + 0 = 2$ $2x = 2$ $x = 1$
So $(0, 2)$ is a point on the graph (the y-intercept).	So $(1, 0)$ is a point on the graph (the x-intercept).

Hence we have

x	y	
0	2	⟵ y-intercept
1	0	⟵ x-intercept

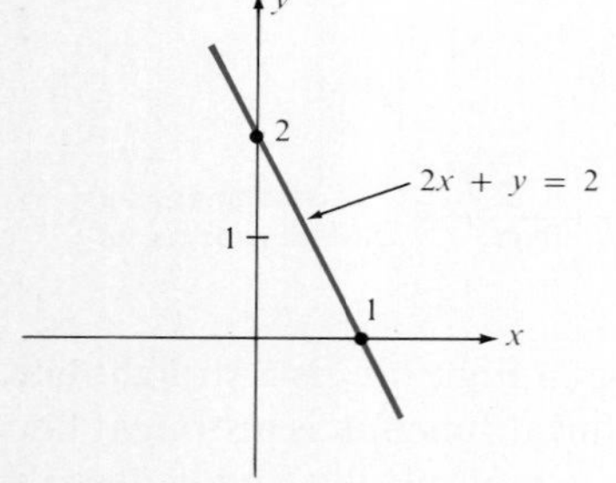

Figure 13
Line passing through (0, 2) and (1, 0)

These values where the graph in Figure 13 crosses the x- and y-axes are called the x- and y-intercepts, respectively. □

Example

Draw the graph of the line $x - 3y = 6$.

Solution After finding the x- and y-intercepts, we can easily graph the line. (See Figure 14.)

x	y	
0	−2	⟵ y-intercept
6	0	⟵ x-intercept

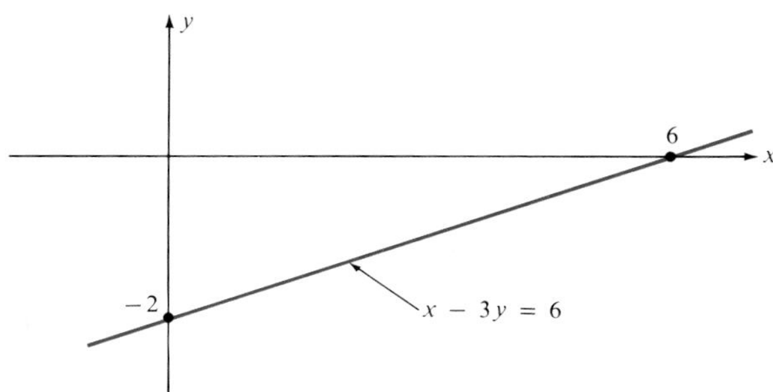

Figure 14
Line passing through (0, −2) and (6, 0)

□

Slope of a Straight Line

An important characteristic of a line is its "steepness." To measure the steepness of a line, we introduce the concept of the **slope** of the straight line that passes through two given points.

Definition of Slope of a Straight Line

The slope of the nonvertical straight line that passes through the points (x_1, y_1) and (x_2, y_2) is given by

$$m = \frac{\text{rise}}{\text{run}} = \frac{y_2 - y_1}{x_2 - x_1} \qquad (x_1 \neq x_2)$$

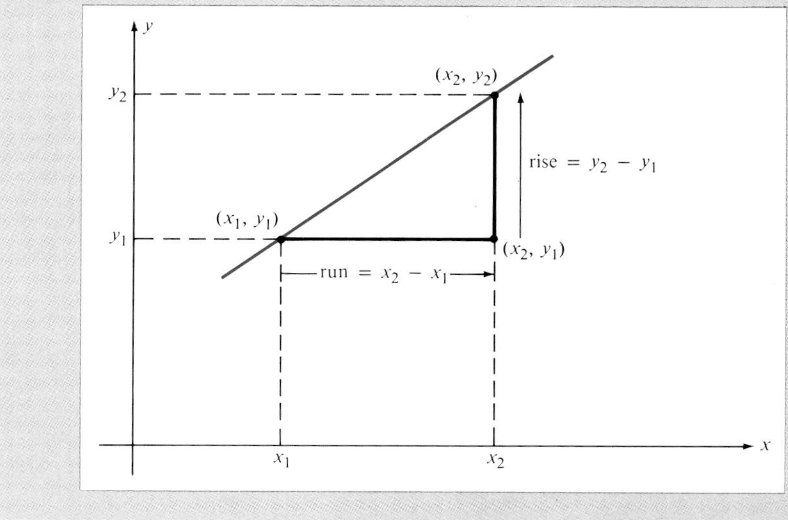

Example

Find the slope of the line that passes through each pair of points

(a) (1, 2) and (3, 5)

(b) (2, −1) and (2, 3)

Solution

(a) If we say that $(x_1, y_1) = (1, 2)$ and $(x_2, y_2) = (3, 5)$, we have

$$m = \frac{y_2 - y_1}{x_2 - x_1} = \frac{5 - 2}{3 - 1} = 1.5$$

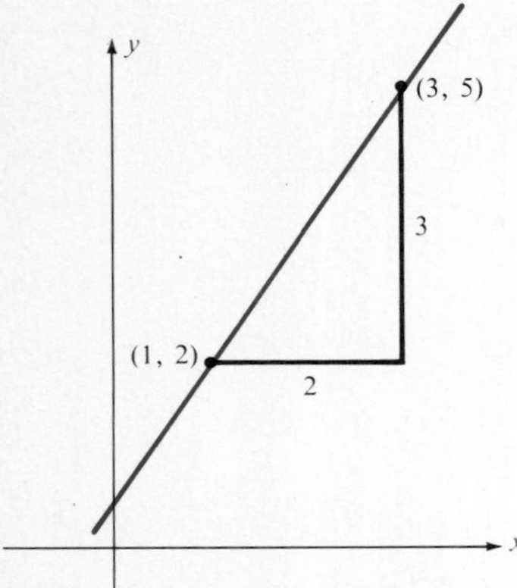

Figure 15
Line passing through (1, 2) and (3, 5)

The reader should know that it does not make any difference how we identify (x_1, y_1) and (x_2, y_2) with the two points. For example if we let $(x_1, y_1) = (3, 5)$ and $(x_2, y_2) = (1, 2)$, we have the same slope

$$m = \frac{2-5}{1-3} = \frac{-3}{-2} = 1.5$$

(See Figure 15.)

(b) If we say that $(x_1, y_1) = (2, -1)$ and $(x_2, y_2) = (2, 3)$, we have

$$m = \frac{y_2 - y_1}{x_2 - x_1} = \frac{3-(-1)}{2-2} = \frac{4}{0} \longleftarrow \textit{Not defined!}$$

(See Figure 16.) □

This last example illustrates the fact that **vertical lines** do not have slopes. Table 5 illustrates the general nature of the slope of a line.

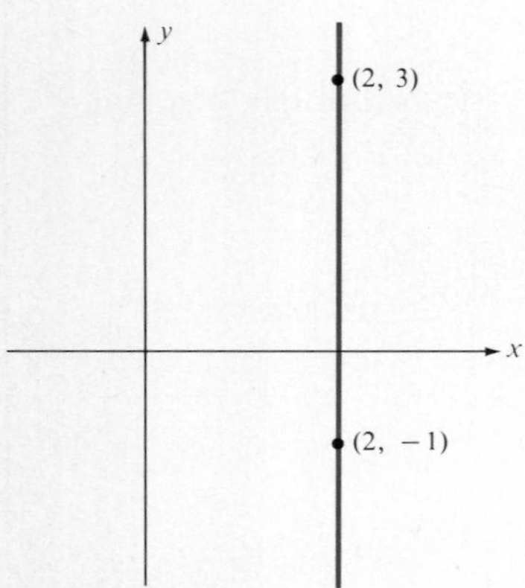

Figure 16
Vertical line x = 2

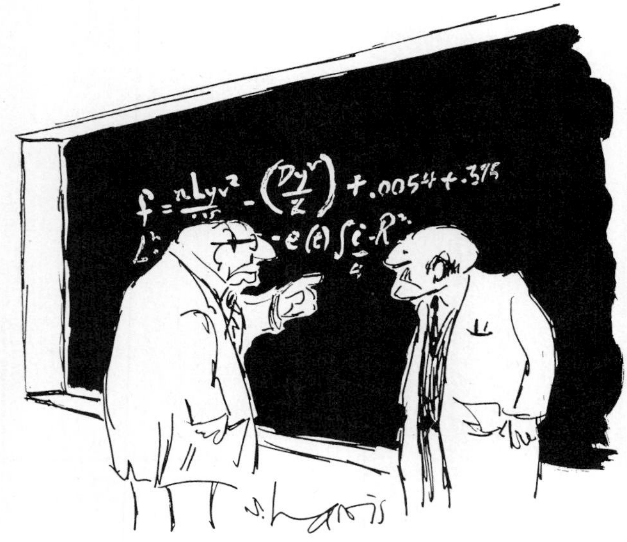

Special Forms of Lines

> **Slope-Intercept Form of a Line**
>
> The graph of the equation
>
> $$y = mx + b$$
>
> where m and b are constants is a nonvertical straight line. This form of a straight line is called the **slope-intercept form** of a line.

TABLE 5
Slope of a Line

Line	Slope	Illustration
Rising	Positive	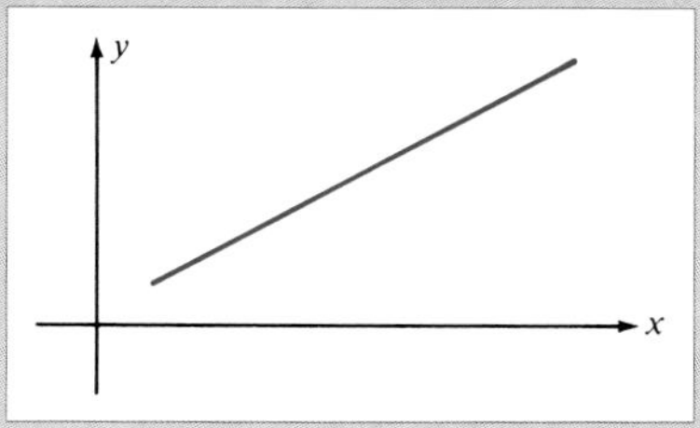
Falling	Negative	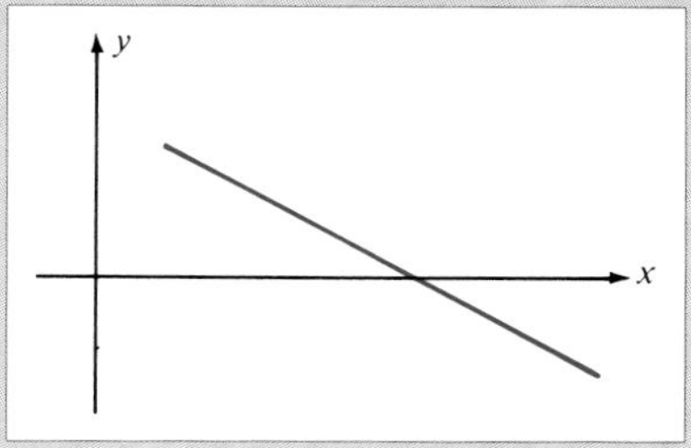
Horizontal	Zero	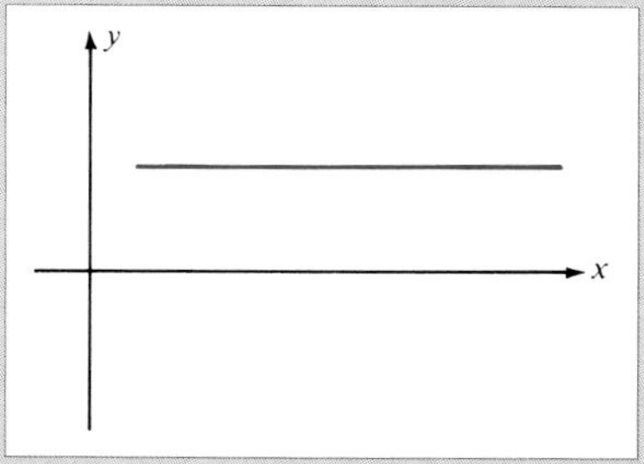
Vertical	Not defined	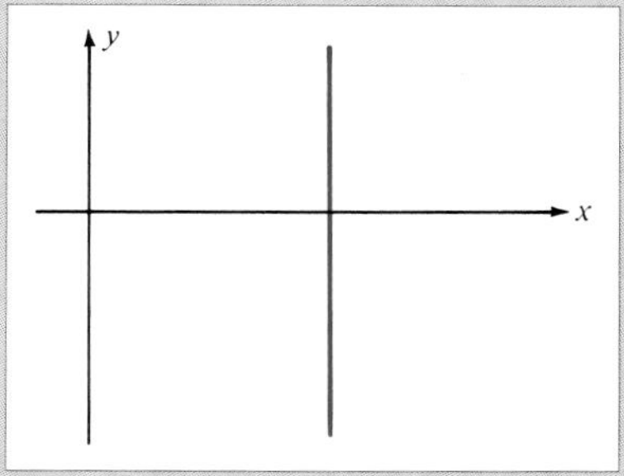

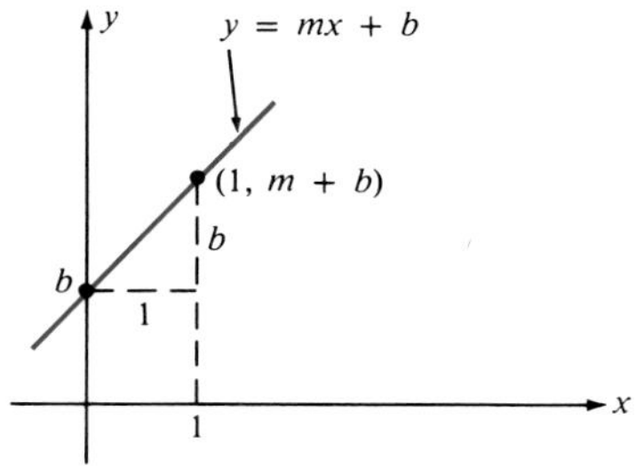

Figure 17
Constructing a line with slope m

Note that the graph of the above equation crosses the y-axis when $x = 0$, or at the point $(0, b)$. The constant b is thus called the **y-intercept** of the line. To determine the significance of m, we consider $x = 0$ and $x = 1$. For these values of x, the line passes through the points $(0, b)$ and $(1, m + b)$. Hence the slope of this line is given by

$$\text{Slope} = \frac{(m + b) - b}{1 - 0} = m$$

In other words, m represents the slope of the line. (See Figure 17.)

Example

Find the slope and y-intercept of the following lines:

(a) $y = 2x + 3$ (b) $y = -x - 2$

(c) $y = 5$

Solution

(a) The slope of the line $y = 2x + 3$ is 2, and the y-intercept is 3. (See Figure 18.)

(b) The slope of the line $y = -x - 2$ is -1, and the y-intercept is -2. (See Figure 19.)

(c) The slope of the line $y = 5$ is 0, and the y-intercept is 5. The line is horizontal. (See Figure 20.)

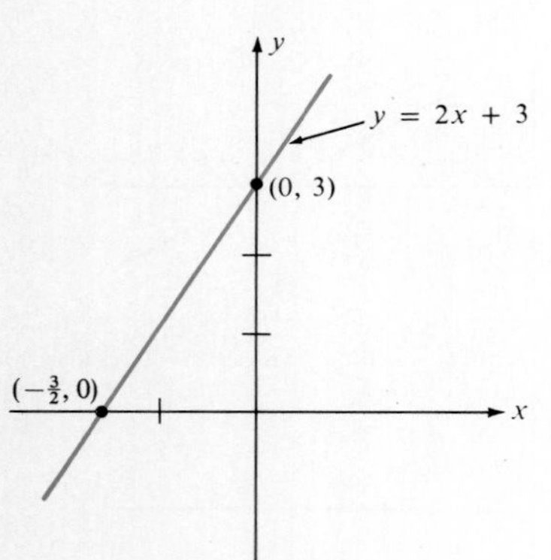

Figure 18
Line with slope 2 and y-intercept 3

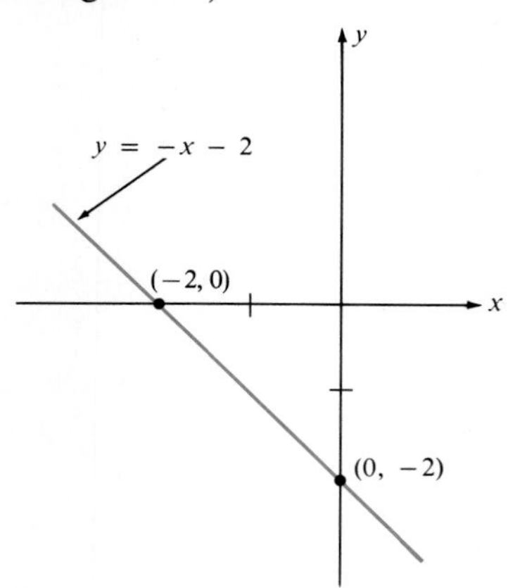

Figure 19
Line with slope −1 and y-intercept −2

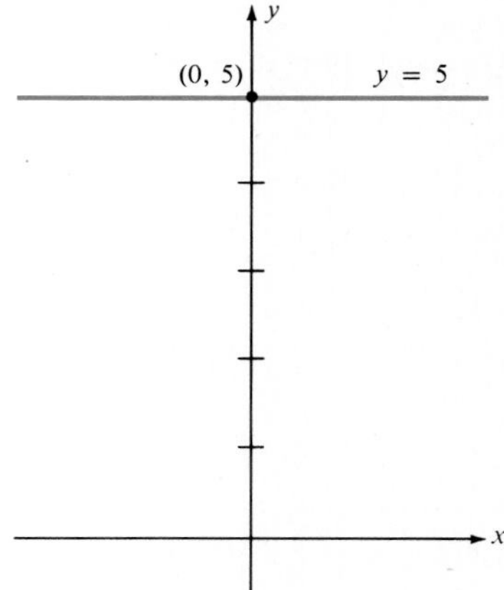

Figure 20
Horizontal line $y = 5$

□

Point-Slope Form of a Line

Imagine a straight line that passes through a fixed point (x_1, y_1) and has a given slope m. (See Figure 21.) The interesting thing about this line is that every *other* point (x, y) on this line satisfies the equation

$$\frac{y - y_1}{x - x_1} = m$$

This gives us the general equation for the **point-slope form** of a straight line.

> **Point-Slope Form of a Straight Line**
>
> The point-slope form of a straight line with slope m that passes through the point (x_1, y_1) is given by the equation
>
> $$y - y_1 = m(x - x_1)$$

The point-slope form of a straight line is useful because it allows us to find the equation of a line when we know the coordinates of a point on the line and the slope.

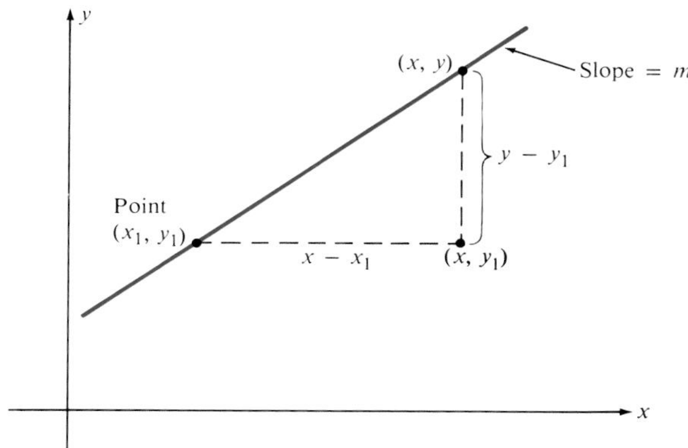

Figure 21
Point-slope form of a line

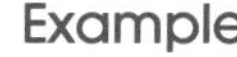

Example

(a) Find an equation of the line that passes through the point (1, 2) and has slope 3.
(b) Find an equation of the line that passes through the two points (1, 3) and (2, 1).

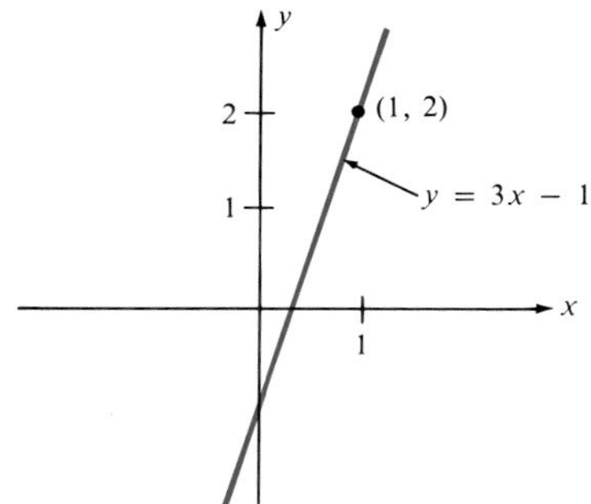

Figure 22
Line passing through (1, 2) with slope 3

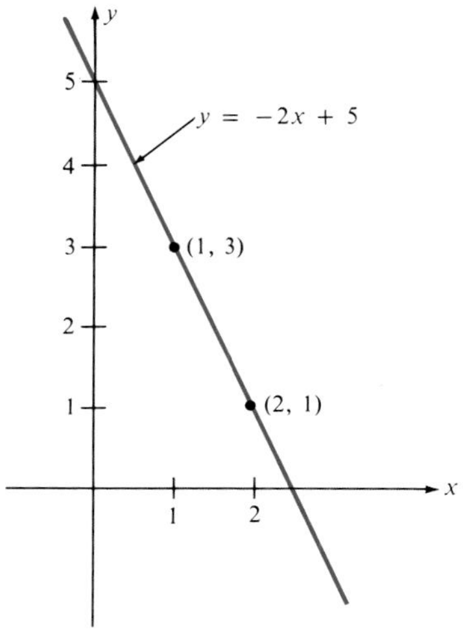

Figure 23
Line passing through (1, 3) and (2, 1)

Solution

(a) If we let $(x_1, y_1) = (1, 2)$ and $m = 3$, we have

$$y - y_1 = m(x - x_1)$$

or

$$y - 2 = 3(x - 1)$$

We can rewrite this equation in slope-intercept form:

$$y = 3x - 1$$

which means that the line has a y-intercept of -1. (See Figure 22.)

(b) If we let $(x_1, y_1) = (1, 3)$ and $(x_2, y_2) = (2, 1)$, we first find the slope $m = (1 - 3)/(2 - 1) = -2$. Using the point-slope formula

$$y - y_1 = m(x - x_1)$$

with $(x_1, y_1) = (1, 3)$, we get

$$y - 3 = -2(x - 1)$$

We rewrite this equation, too, in the slope-intercept form:

$$y = -2x + 5$$

(See Figure 23.)

Note: It is important to observe that in the above point-slope formula, we could have just as well substituted the second point $(x_2, y_2) = (2, 1)$, and we would have gotten the same equation. To convince you of this fact, we make this substitution, getting

$$y - 1 = -2(x - 2)$$

or

$$y = -2x + 5$$

□

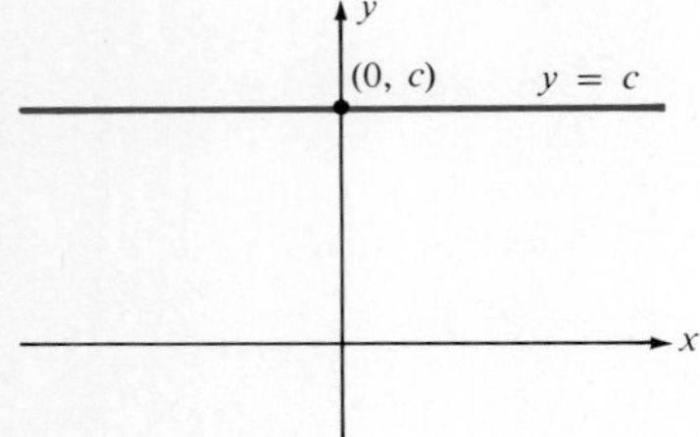

Figure 24
Horizontal line $y = c$

Horizontal and Vertical Lines

The simplest line equations are those for horizontal and vertical lines. Since a horizontal line is satisfied by all points (x, y) that have the same y-coordinate, the equation of the horizontal line whose y-coordinate is always c is given by

$$y = c \qquad \text{(horizontal line)}$$

Note that the slope of a horizontal line is zero and, conversely, that all lines with slope zero are horizontal. (See Figure 24.)

On the other hand, a vertical line consists of points (x, y) whose x-coordinate is a constant. (See Figure 25.) That means an equation of the form

$$x = c$$

As we noted earlier, vertical lines do not have a slope.

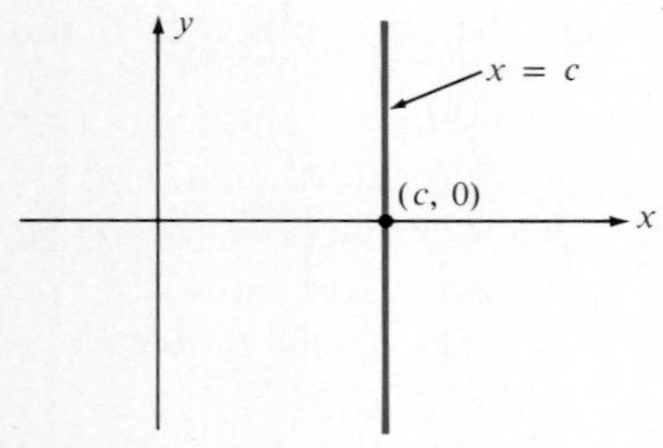

Figure 25
Vertical line $x = c$

Straight Lines in Modern Business (Break-Even Analysis)

Consider a manufacturing plant such as a General Electric plant that produces refrigerators. Suppose the daily cost to operate the plant has been broken into two kinds of costs: **fixed cost** (cost that stays the same no matter how many refrigerators are produced) and **variable cost** (cost that depends on the number of refrigerators produced). Every manufacturing plant has fixed costs, which include such costs as those for building maintenance, electricity, and heating. An important problem in production analysis is the *break-even problem.* Suppose the fixed daily cost at this plant is \$50,000 and the cost to produce a single refrigerator is \$250. If the company sells the refrigerators for \$400 each, how many refrigerators must be produced for the company to break even at this plant for one day?

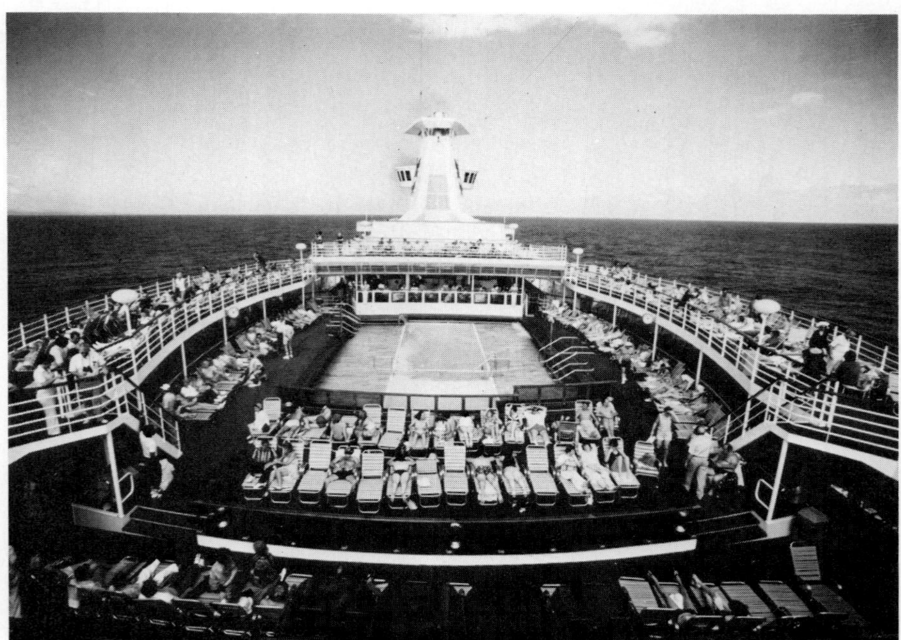

The pool deck on Royal Caribbean Cruise Line's Song of Norway. *The cruise industry is keenly aware of break-even analysis.*

Let

$$x = \text{number of refrigerators produced per day}$$
$$C = \text{daily cost of producing } x \text{ refrigerators}$$
$$R = \text{daily revenue (return) on sales of } x \text{ refrigerators}$$
$$P = \text{daily profit when } x \text{ refrigerators are sold}$$

The company's revenue R and total cost C when x refrigerators are produced (assuming that it sells all it produces) are given by

$$R = \$400x$$
$$C = \text{fixed costs} + \text{variable costs} = \$50{,}000 + \$250x$$

The company's profit P when x refrigerators are produced (we assume that the company sells all that it produces) is simply the revenue minus the cost. That is,

$$P = R - C = 400x - (50{,}000 + 250x) = 150x - 50{,}000$$

Note that when no refrigerators are produced, the daily profit is $-\$50{,}000$, which means that the company suffers a daily loss equal to the fixed costs. As the number of refrigerators produced increases, however, the profit will increase at a rate of \$150 per refrigerator. After a certain number of refrigerators are produced, the company's revenue will finally equal the fixed cost, and the profit will be zero. This gives the number of refrigerators that must be produced in a given day for the company to *break even.* Only when more units are produced is it worthwhile for the company to be in business. In this problem this occurs when

$$150x - 50{,}000 = 0$$

or

$$x = 333.33$$

In other words, the company must produce roughly 333 or 334 refrigerators at this plant each day just to break even. We will pick 334 as the break-even point, since when 333 refrigerators are produced per day, the profit is slightly negative, but when 334 refrigerators are produced, the profit becomes slightly positive.

In other words, when production reaches 334 or more refrigerators per day, the company starts to turn a profit. For instance, if the company produces 750 refrigerators per day, then its daily profit from this plant will be

$$P = 150x - 50{,}000 = 150(750) - 50{,}000 = \$62{,}500$$

The **profit line** $P = 150x - 50{,}000$ is graphed in Figure 26.

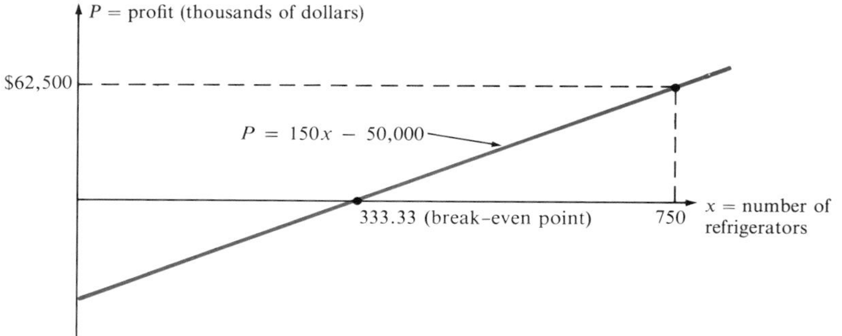

Figure 26
Profit line showing break-even point

Problems

Graph the lines in Problems 1–5 and identify the slopes and y-intercepts (if such exist).

1. $y = 2x + 1$
2. $y = -x + 2$
3. $y - 1 = x + 1$
4. $y = 5$
5. $x = 2$

In Problems 6–10, find the equation of the straight line in slope-intercept form with the given slope that passes through the given point. What is the y-intercept of each line? Sketch the graph of each line.

6. $(x_1, y_1) = (0, 0)$, slope 1
7. $(x_1, y_1) = (1, 2)$, slope 2
8. $(x_1, y_1) = (0, -1)$, slope -2
9. $(x_1, y_1) = (-1, 2)$, slope 3
10. $(x_1, y_1) = (2, 0)$, slope -1

Find the slope-intercept form of the straight line that passes through the points given in Problems 11–15. What are the slope and y-intercepts of each line? Sketch the graph of each line.

11. $(0, 0), (1, 1)$
12. $(0, 1), (1, 0)$
13. $(-1, 1), (1, -1)$
14. $(2, 3), (4, 7)$
15. $(0, 4), (1, 3)$

Mathematics in Business Management

16. Break-Even Analysis. A major publishing company that produces college textbooks generally has large fixed costs but relatively small variable costs. Suppose a publisher has a fixed cost of $200,000 (production costs, artwork, editorial costs, . . .) to produce a mathematics textbook and a variable cost of $8 for each book produced. If the company sells the books for $20 each to college bookstores, how many books must be sold (or produced) for the company to break even? Find the company's loss or profit if it sells
(a) 10,000 books
(b) 15,000 books
(c) 25,000 books

For Problems 17–21, use the following fixed and variable costs in the different industries to determine the break-even point for each. Sketch the graphs of the linear revenue and cost functions.

17. Record company (Warner Brothers, Columbia, . . .)
Fixed costs = $500,000 (one-time cost)
Variable costs = $0.50 per album
Revenue = $5.00 per album

18. Computer company (IBM, Leading Edge, Apple, . . .)
Fixed costs = $100,000 (daily costs)
Variable costs = $250 per computer
Revenue = $450 per computer

19. Food products company (General Foods, Kelloggs, . . .)
Fixed costs = $25,000 (weekly costs)
Variable costs = $0.25 per box of cereal
Revenue = $0.90 per box of cereal

20. Automobile company (Ford, General Motors, . . .)
Fixed costs = $250,000 (weekly costs)
Variable costs = $5000 per car
Revenue = $7000 per car

21. Newspaper publisher (*Boston Globe*, *Denver Post*, . . .)
Fixed costs = $100,000 (daily costs)
Variable costs = $0.15 per newspaper
Revenue = $0.35 per paper

22. Break-Even Analysis in the Airline Industry. Suppose the fixed cost to an airline company to make a particular flight from New York to Los Angeles is $50,000.
(a) If the company's revenue is $200 per passenger, how many passengers must be on this flight for the company to break even?
(b) If the airplane on this flight has a capacity of 400 passengers, what percentage of the plane must be filled for the company to break even?
(c) What expenses would be included in the $50,000 fixed cost?

23. Break-Even Analysis in the Movie Industry. Suppose the fixed cost to a movie theater owner to show a movie is $200.
(a) If the movie theater owner has revenue of $4 per moviegoer, how many tickets must be sold for the owner to break even?
(b) Do the above fixed cost and revenue per moviegoer appear to reflect the true values in the movie industry? How would a theater owner find these values?

Mathematics in the Natural Sciences

24. Celsius to Fahrenheit. Suppose you are in Canada, where the temperature is measured in Celsius instead of Fahrenheit. The relationship between the temperature in Celsius (C) and the temperature in Fahrenheit (F) is the linear function

$$F = \frac{9}{5}C + 32$$

Sketch the graph that relates these two temperatures. Let C vary from -20 to $+40$. (Use C for the x-axis and F for the y-axis.) If tomorrow's weather is predicted to be 25 degrees Celsius, what kind of clothes will you wear outside?

25. Sulfur Dioxide Pollution. A major by-product of burning fossil fuels is the poisonous chemical sulfur dioxide. In an experiment conducted in Oslo, Norway, it was shown that the number N of deaths per week in the world is approximately a linear function of the mean concentration C of sulfur dioxide in the air (measured in parts per million of a gram per cubic meter). The linear function found was

$$N = 94 + 0.031C \qquad 50 \le C \le 700$$

(a) Sketch the graph of this function.
(b) Find the predicted number of deaths per week that will result if the earth's atmosphere contains 100 parts per million of a gram of sulfur dioxide.

Mathematics in the Social Sciences

26. Gasoline Efficiency. An experiment conducted by the Federal Highway Administration showed that (over a given range of speeds) the relationship between the fuel efficiency N of an automobile (in miles per gallon) and the speed S of the automobile (in miles per hour) is a linear one. Suppose that for a certain automobile the relationship is the linear function

$$N = -0.5S + 40$$

(a) Sketch the graph of this function.
(b) What is the predicted mileage for this type of automobile when the speed is 50 miles per hour?
(c) How fast must you drive if you expect to get 20 miles per gallon?

27. Is There an Equation That Predicts World Records? The past world records for the men's mile run are plotted in Figure 27. Statisticians have ways of finding the "best line" that will approximate a given set of observations. A linear approximation to the points in Figure 27 has been found to be the linear function

$$T = -0.00615Y + 16$$

where T is the world record in minutes and Y is the calendar year in which the record was set. Using this linear model as a guide, what will be the world record for the men's mile run in the year 1995? Be sure to convert the time to minutes and seconds.

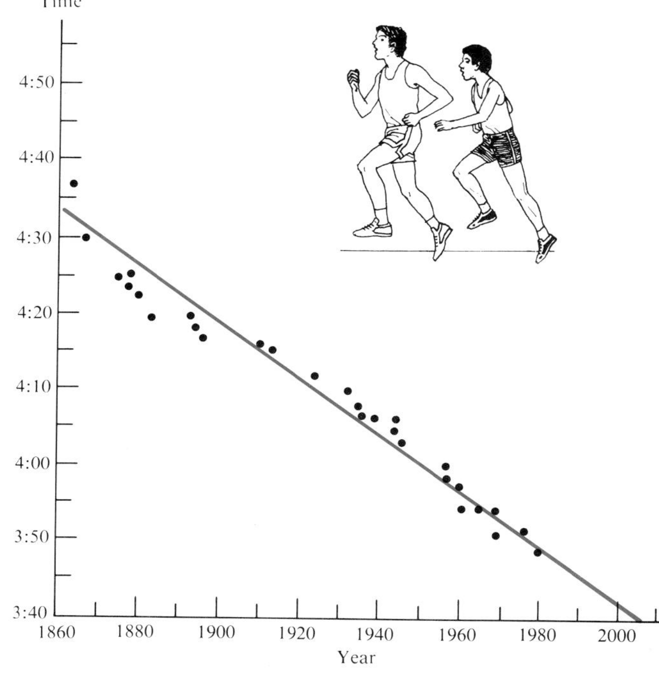

Figure 27
World record times for the mile run (men's)

Interesting Problem

28. How Much Farther Did You Run? The next time you are jogging around a quarter-mile track (or any oval track) and you are running on the outside, with a friend on the inside, just say, "Did you know that the extra distance I'm running does not depend on the length of the track, but is a linear function of the distance we are apart." If you want to be more impressive, tell your friend that the extra distance D the outside runner runs is determined by the linear function

$$D = 2\pi x$$

where $\pi = 3.14159\ldots$ and x is the distance between the runners. For example, if you are 3 feet farther outside than your friend is, you will run

$$D = 2\pi(3)$$
$$\cong 18.8$$

feet farther on each lap than your running partner. Sketch the graph of the distance D as a function of x for $0 < x < 8$. How much farther do you run per lap if you are 5 feet further outside?

The interesting thing about this formula is that it holds for any oval track with circular ends (which is the shape of most tracks).

29. Hmmmmm. The earth is approximately a sphere, and the distance around the equator is roughly 23,000 miles. Suppose you place a rope on the ground at the equator. Now you add an extra 10 feet to the rope and stretch out the slack so that the rope lies above the ground a constant amount. The question is: Is it possible for a mouse to crawl under the rope? *Hint:* Find the linear function that gives the height of the rope above the ground (call it h) in terms of the length of the new rope added (call it R), and evaluate this function at $R = 10$.

Higer-Order Polynomials

The first-order polynomial introduced in the preceding section is a special case of the general **nth-order polynomial**

$$P_n(x) = a_n x^n + a_{n-1}x^{n-1} + \ldots + a_1 x + a_0$$

where $a_0, a_1, \ldots, a_n$ are real numbers, a_n is different from zero, and n is any nonnegative integer. Polynomials are useful mathematical models in both business and science inasmuch as they are easy to manipulate (as we shall see later) and they allow us to describe complex relationships between economic variables. Later, when we study the theory of the firm, we will see that a company's profit, revenue, and cost can often be modeled or described by polynomials of first, second, and third degree.

HISTORICAL NOTE

The letter x in the above polynomial is called the **variable**, while the letters $a_n, a_{n-1}, \ldots, a_0$ are called **coefficients**. The person responsible for the convention of using the last letters of the alphabet (u, v, w, x, y, and z) to represent variables of unknown quantities and the early letters of the alphabet (a, b, c, . . .) to represent constants, or known quantities, was the French mathematician René Descartes (1596–1650).

Quadratic Polynomial

An important polynomial or function in economics is the second-order or **quadratic polynomial**

$$f(x) = ax^2 + bx + c$$

where $a \neq 0$. Whether you know it or not, you have seen the graph of this function, called a **parabola**, many times. In his excellent expository article* on the parabola, Lee Whitt claims that there have been "over one billion sold." He goes on to say that the biggest-selling parabola is the automobile headlight (at least, a slice through the middle of the headlight is a parabola; the entire headlight is called a *paraboloid*). The smallest-selling parabola is the huge 200-inch Hale telescope mirror. Other parabolic designs can be found in bridges and roofs of certain buildings. You can even see parabolas when you go to a basketball, football, or baseball game. Although the path a ball follows is not exactly a parabola (because of air friction), it is often close to being one. From a geometric point of view, a parabola is defined as the set of points in the plane that have the same distance from a given point as they have from a given line.

---

* Lee Whitt, "The Standup Conic Presents: The Parabola and Its Applications," *UMAP Journal*, Vol. 3, No. 3, pp. 285–313, 1982.

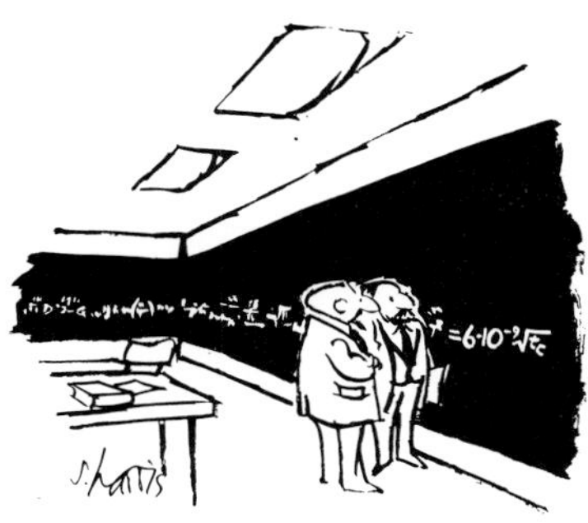

"I TEND TO AGREE WITH YOU — ESPECIALLY SINCE $6 \cdot 10^{-9}\sqrt{F_c}$ IS MY LUCKY NUMBER."

Graph of $y = ax^2 + bx + c$

The graph of a parabola, defined by the quadratic function

$$y = ax^2 + bx + c \qquad (a \neq 0)$$

has its **axis** (line of symmetry) parallel to the y-axis. It opens upward if $a > 0$ and downward if $a < 0$. The point of intersection of the line of symmetry and the parabola is called the **vertex point** of the parabola. The vertex will be the high point of the parabola if the parabola turns downward; it will be the low point of the parabola if the parabola turns upward. The x-coordinate of the vertex point is always given by $x = -b/(2a)$.

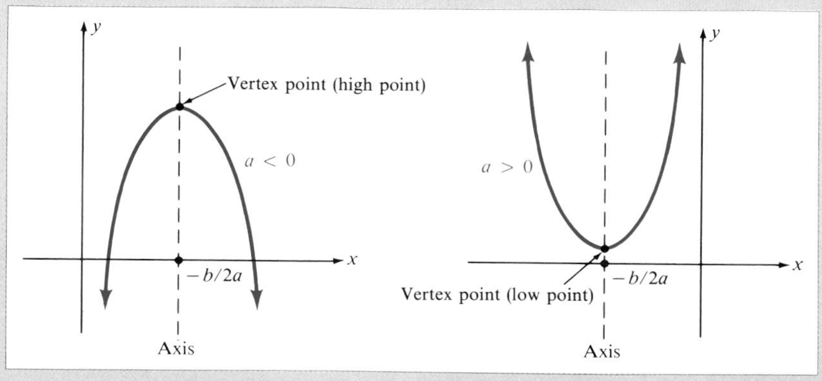

Example

Quadratic Polynomial Cost Function TX Unlimited is a growing firm that produces microcomputers. The total cost per week for producing microcomputers increases as the number of microcomputers produced increases, but not as a first-order polynomial. Because there are setup costs, because the price the company pays to suppliers depends on the quantity ordered, because the company must pay overtime costs, and because of a variety of other reasons, the **average cost** (the total cost divided by the number of computers produced) must be represented by a curve other than a straight line. Suppose in this case that the average cost AC per computer can be approximated by the quadratic polynomial

$$AC(q) = 0.005q^2 - 2q + 1000 \qquad q > 0$$

where q is the number of computers produced each week.

(a) Sketch the graph of this cost function.

(b) From the graph, approximately how many computers should be produced to minimize the average cost per computer?

(c) What is the minimum average cost per computer?

Solution

(a) Of course, we realize that the function $AC(q)$ is defined only when $q = 1, 2, 3, \ldots$. However, since it is generally easier to analyze a curve than a collection of points, economists usually draw the curve for all $q > 0$. We evaluate $AC(q)$ at several values of q and join the points $(q, AC(q))$ with a smooth curve, getting the curve shown in Figure 28.

(b) Observing the graph of $AC(q)$ shown in Figure 28, we see that the average cost attains a minimum value when the number of computers produced per week is 200.

(c) Evaluating the function $AC(q)$ when $q = 200$ gives the minimum average cost:

$$\begin{aligned} AC(200) &= 0.005(200)^2 - 2(200) + 1000 \\ &= \$800 \end{aligned}$$

If the company produces 200 microcomputers per week, then the average cost per computer will be \$800 dollars. Any other number of computers produced will result in a greater average cost. Of course, the company would have to consider whether it could actually sell this many computers.

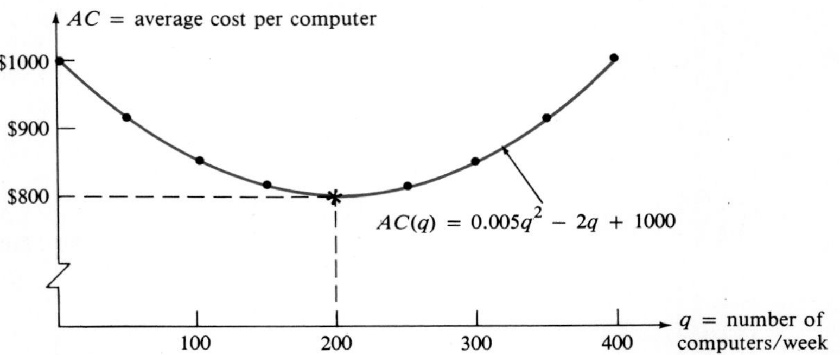

Figure 28
Average cost curve for TX Unlimited

□

Cubic Polynomials

The quadratic polynomial we have just studied can be used to describe many phenomena in business and the real world. Unfortunately, the basic **"U-shaped"** graph of all parabolas (when $a > 0$) and **"inverted U-shaped"** graph (when $a < 0$) is not general enough to describe all the phenomena we wish to study. For example the total cost $C(q)$ (see Figure 29) of producing q items of a given product often obeys the following pattern:

- For small q, the cost $C(q)$ increases rapidly as q increases.
- For larger q, the cost $C(q)$ still increases with increasing q but not as rapidly.
- For still larger q, the cost $C(q)$ increases rapidly again with increasing q.

Fortunately, there are third-order or **cubic polynomials**

$$P(x) = a_3x^3 + a_2x^2 + a_1x + a_0$$

that follow this basic pattern. The following example illustrates this idea.

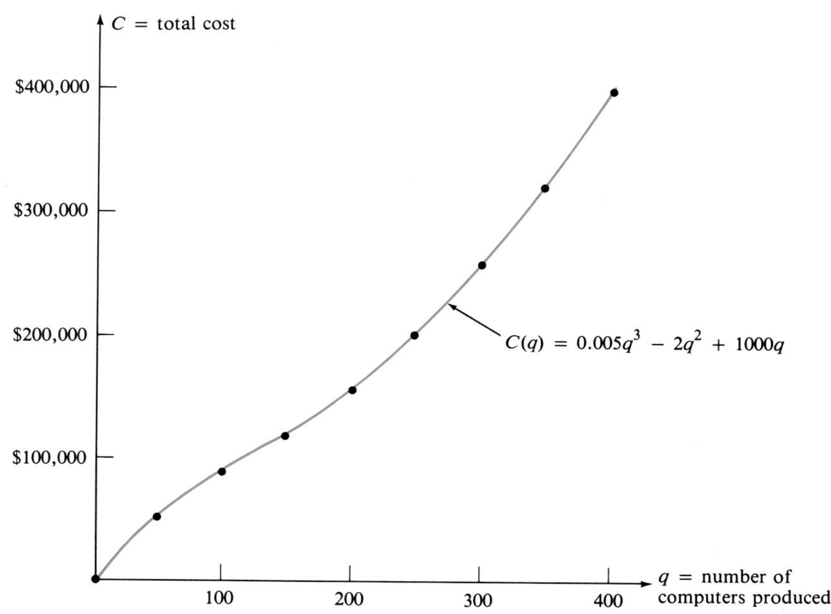

Figure 29
Total cost curve

Example

Total Cost Function We saw in the previous example that for TX Unlimited, the average cost $AC(q)$ of producing q microcomputers is

$$AC(q) = 0.005q^2 - 2q + 1000$$

This means that the **total cost** $C(q)$ of producing q computers is simply the product of the average cost of producing q computers and the number of computers produced. That is, the third-order polynomial

$$\begin{aligned} C(q) &= q \cdot AC(q) \\ &= q(0.005q^2 - 2q + 1000) \\ &= 0.005q^3 - 2q^2 + 1000q \end{aligned}$$

Sketch the graph of $C(q)$.

Solution We evaluate $C(q)$ at several values of q and join the points $(q, C(q))$ with a smooth curve. (See Figure 29.) □

Example

Cubic Profit Function Suppose TX Unlimited sells its computers for $850 per computer. What is the company's profit from the production (and sale) of q computers per week if the weekly cost to produce q computers is

$$C(q) = 0.005q^3 - 2q^2 + 1000q$$

Solution The revenue taken in from producing (and selling) q computers per week is given by the linear function

$$R(q) = 850q$$

Since the profit earned is the revenue minus the cost, the profit is given by the

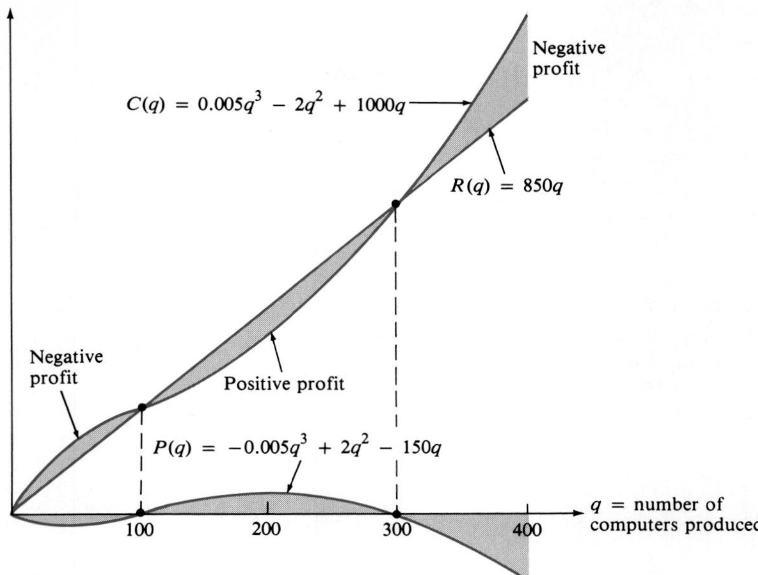

Figure 30
Total cost curve for TX Unlimited

cubic polynomial

$$\begin{aligned} P(q) &= R(q) - C(q) \\ &= 850q - (0.005q^3 - 2q^2 + 1000q) \\ &= -0.005q^3 + 2q^2 - 150q \end{aligned}$$

The graphs of $R(q)$, $C(q)$, and $P(q)$ are shown in Figure 30.

From the graph of the profit curve, we can conclude that TX Unlimited must produce at least 100 computers per week to break even. If the company produces between 100 and 300 computers, it will turn a profit. However, when more than 300 computers are produced, the cost will be larger than the revenue, resulting in a net loss. □

Problems

For Problems 1–10, classify the given function according to whether it is or is not a polynomial. For the polynomials, determine the order of the polynomial.

1. $R(q) = 5q + 1000$ (revenue function)
2. $C(q) = q^3 - 60q + 1400q + 5000$ (cost function)
3. $P(q) = -q^4 + 50q - 500q - 1000$ (profit function)
4. $C(q) = \sqrt{q^2 + 100}$ (cost function)
5. $f(t) = 10e^{-kt}$ $(k > 0)$ (biological decay)
6. $F(t) = 10e^{rt}$ $(r > 0)$ (biological growth)
7. $S(q) = aq + b$ (a, b constants) (supply curve)
8. $D(q) = cq + d$ (c, d constants) (demand curve)
9. $S(q) = \sqrt{q}$ (supply curve)
10. $P(x) = \dfrac{x}{x - 2}$ (rational function)

For Problems 11–18, sketch the graph of the given polynomial over the indicated interval.

11. $f(x) = x^2 - x, 0 \le x$
12. $f(x) = x^2 - x + 1, 1 \le x$
13. $g(x) = x^3 - x, -\infty < x < \infty$
14. $C(q) = 0.01q^2 - 10q + 100, 0 \le q$
15. $C(q) = q^3 - 6q^2 + 10, 0 \le q$
16. $C(q) = 0.1q^3 - q^2 + 2q + 3, 0 \le q$
17. $P(q) = -q^3 + q^2 + q - 3, 0 \le q$
18. $P(q) = 0.01q^3 + 2q^2 - q - 10, 0 \le q$

Some Important Polynomials in Economics

19. Linear Revenue Function. The amount of money R that a company or individual takes in from the sale of q items of a given product is called the *revenue* from the sale of these items. If the amount of money charged for each item is a constant k (and does not change with q), then the revenue taken in from the sale of q items will be given by the linear polynomial

$$R(q) = kq$$

Although in reality q will be an integer 0, 1, 2, . . . , we often draw the curve for all $q > 0$. Sketch the graphs of the following linear revenue curves for $q > 0$:

(a) $R(q) = 0.25q$
(b) $R(q) = 1.5q$
(c) $R(q) = 2.5q$

20. Quadratic Revenue Function. Suppose the number q of items of a given product a company can sell depends on the amount charged for each item according to the linear demand function

$$q = D(p) = 100 - 0.2p \quad p \geq 0$$

Since the revenue the company takes in from the sale of q items of the product is given by

$$R(q) = pq$$

where p is the price charged for each item, we can write the revenue in terms of the price p as

$$R(p) = pq = p\,D(p)$$

Hence in terms of the price p the revenue function $R(p)$ is the quadratic polynomial (or quadratic function)

$$R(p) = p\,D(p) = p(100 - 0.2p)$$
$$= 100p - 0.2p^2 \qquad (p \geq 0)$$

Sketch the graph of this quadratic revenue function.

21. Cubic Cost Function. Quite often, the cost C to a company for the production of q items of a given product can be estimated by a **cubic** polynomial

$$C(q) = aq^3 + bq^2 + cq + d$$

where a, b, c, and d are given constants (a, c, and d will always be positive, and b will always be negative in a cost function). Sketch the graph of the specific cost function

$$C(q) = 0.5q^3 - 0.5q^2 + 100q + 500 \qquad q \geq 0$$

22. Cubic Profit Function. The profit $P(q)$ that a company earns when it produces (and sells) q items of a given product is the revenue $R(q)$ taken in from the sale of these items minus the cost $C(q)$ to produce the items. That is

$$P(q) = R(q) - C(q)$$

(a) What is the profit function $P(q)$ when the revenue and cost functions are

$$R(q) = 5q$$
$$C(q) = 0.5q^3 - 0.3q^2 + 20q + 100$$

(b) Sketch the graph of the profit function.

Absolute Value Function

There are many functions that are important to the study of business and the sciences. Some of these functions, such as rational functions, exponential and logarithmic functions, and the trigonometric functions will be introduced later as we go along. There is one function, however, that is convenient to introduce now. It is the absolute value function. We first define the **absolute value** of a real number a, denoted $|a|$, as

$$|a| = \begin{cases} a & a > 0 \\ 0 & a = 0 \\ -a & a < 0 \end{cases}$$

The definition of the absolute value of a real number determines the **absolute value function** f, which associates with each real number x its absolute value:

$$f(x) = |x|$$

The graph of the absolute value function, which is defined on the entire real line, is shown in Figure 31. Note that the absolute value $|x|$ is never negative, no matter what the value of x may be.

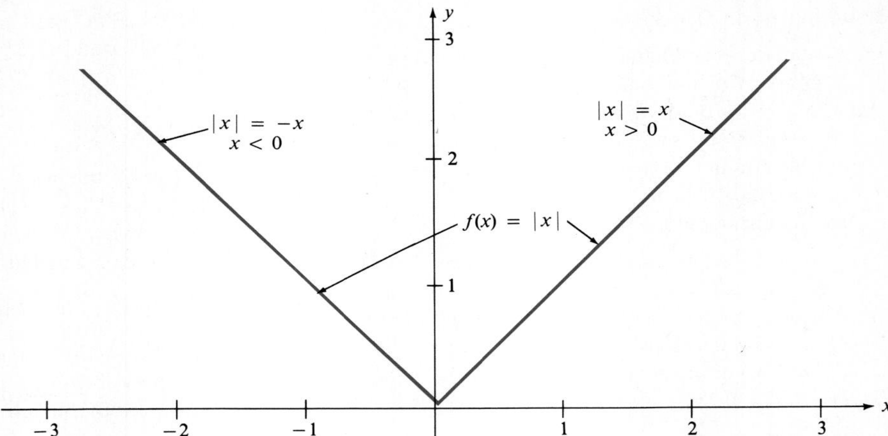

Figure 31
The absolute value function

One of the main reasons for our interest in the absolute value function is the fact that distances between points on the real line can be written in terms of absolute values. For example, the distance between any real number x and 0 on the real number line is simply the absolute value $|x|$. More generally, the distance between any two real numbers x and y on the real line is the absolute value of their difference $|x - y|$. This distance may be written either as $|x - y|$ or $|y - x|$; they are exactly the same.

Example

Distance from 1 The function

$$f(x) = |x - 1|$$

might be named the "distance from 1" function, since the value of $f(x)$ represents the distance of x from the number 1 on the real line. Graph this function.

Solution The graph has the same basic shape as $|x|$, which measures the distance of a number x from 0, only now we are measuring the distance from 1 rather than the distance from 0. Hence we obtain the graph shown in Figure 32. □

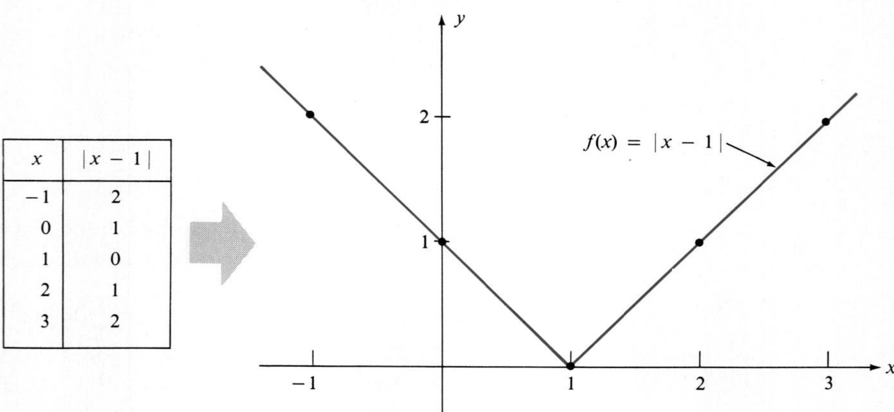

x	$\lvert x - 1\rvert$
−1	2
0	1
1	0
2	1
3	2

Figure 32
The "distance from 1" function

The absolute value function also provides a convenient way to describe intervals of real numbers. For example, if p is a given constant then the function

$$f(x) = |x - p|$$

can be interpreted as the distance from x to p. Hence those numbers x that satisfy

$$|x - p| \leq a$$

for $a \geq 0$ represent the values of x for which the distance from p is less than or equal to a. In other words, the inequalities

$$|x - p| \leq a$$

and

$$p - a \leq x \leq p + a$$

define the same values of x. In general, we can denote other kinds of intervals using the absolute value function. We write these intervals now. □

Writing Intervals with Absolute Values

Let $a \geq 0$ and p be any real number. Then the following pairs of inequalities define the same real numbers:

Absolute Value Form	Interval Form	Interval(s)
$\|x - p\| \leq a$	$p - a \leq x \leq p + a$	$[p - a, p + a]$
$\|x - p\| < a$	$p - a < x < p + a$	$(p - a, p + a)$
$\|x - p\| \geq a$	$x \leq p - a$ or $x \geq p + a$	$(\infty, p - a]$ or $[p + a, \infty)$
$\|x - p\| > a$	$x < p - a$ or $x > p + a$	$(\infty, p - a)$ or $(p + a, \infty)$

Example

Absolute Value Function Defining Intervals

	Absolute Value Form	Interval Form	Interval(s)
(a)	$\|x - 1\| \leq 1$	$0 \leq x \leq 2$	$[0, 2]$
(b)	$\|x - 2\| < 3$	$-1 < x < 5$	$(-1, 5)$
(c)	$\|x + 1\| \leq 1$	$-2 \leq x \leq 0$	$[-2, 0]$
(d)	$\|x - 3\| > 2$	$x < 1$ or $x > 5$	$(-\infty, 1)$ or $(5, \infty)$
(e)	$\|x + 1\| > 3$	$x < -4$ or $x > 2$	$(-\infty, -4)$ or $(2, \infty)$

Problems

For Problems 1–6, is it true that the given equation is true for all values of the given variables? If so, show why. If not, give a number or numbers to show that the equation is not always true.

1. $|x| = |-x|$

2. $|x^2| = |x|^2$

3. $|xy| = |x|\,|y|$

4. $|x^3| = |x|^3$

5. $|2x| = 2|x|$

6. $|x + y| = |x| + |y|$

For Problems 7–15, find the real numbers x, if any, that satisfy the given inequality.

7. $|x| \geq 3$

8. $|x| \leq 3$

9. $|x - 1| < 1$

10. $|x + 1| \geq 1$

11. $|x + 3| < 5$
12. $|x - 9| \geq 1$
13. $|x - 9| \leq -1$
14. $|x + 3| \leq 1$
15. $|x - 1| \geq 0$

For Problems 16–20, which of the numbers is larger?

16. $-|x|$ or $|-x|$
17. $-|x + y|$ or $|x + y|$
18. $-|xy|$ or $|-xy|$
19. $|x + y|$ or $|x| + |y|$
20. $\left|\frac{-x}{y}\right|$ or $-\frac{|x|}{|y|}$
21. **Hmmmmm.** Which is larger, $|-x - y|$ or $|x + y|$?
22. **Double Hmmmmm.** Assume that x is a positive number. Which of the numbers $|x|$, $-|x|$, $|-x|$, and $-|-x|$ is the largest? Which is the smallest?

P.3 Zeros of Linear and Quadratic Functions

Zeros of Linear Functions

A **zero** of a function f is a value of x for which $f(x) = 0$. For example, the graph of the function shown in Figure 33 has zeros at $x = -1$, $x = 2$, and $x = 3$. As we shall see throughout this book, zeros of functions often represent important physical quantities. We show here how zeros of linear functions can be found.

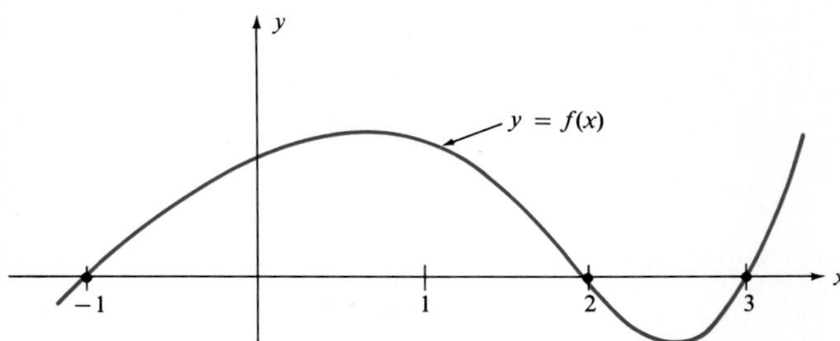

Figure 33
Zeros of a function at $x = -1$, 2, and 3

People find zeros of linear equations every day whether they know it or not. If you see apples advertised at three for 75 cents, you quickly calculate that each apple costs 25 cents. By finding the cost of a single apple, you have essentially solved the linear equation

$$3x = 75$$

Other examples of linear equations are

$$2x + 1 = 0$$
$$-3w + 4 = 7$$
$$2p - 6 = -3$$

The letter in the equation is called the **unknown**, and the convention is that it is denoted by one of the letters in the latter part of the alphabet, such as u, v, w, x, y, and z.

General Linear Equation

The **general linear equation** is an equation of the form

$$ax + b = c$$

where a, b, and c are any real numbers, with the exception that $a \neq 0$.

To solve a linear equation for the unknown variable, we isolate the variable on one side of the equation using various properties of the real numbers. We illustrate these ideas with the example that follows.

Example

Solve the following equation for x:

$$\frac{1}{5}x = 4 - x$$

Solution Multiply each side of the equation by 5 to get

$$x = 20 - 5x$$

Now add $5x$ to each side of the equation, getting

$$x + 5x = 20 - 5x + 5x$$

or

$$6x = 20$$

Finally, if we multiply each side of the equation by $\frac{1}{6}$, we get the value of x:

$$x = \frac{10}{3}$$

The reader should substitute this value back into the equation to see that it is a **solution**. □

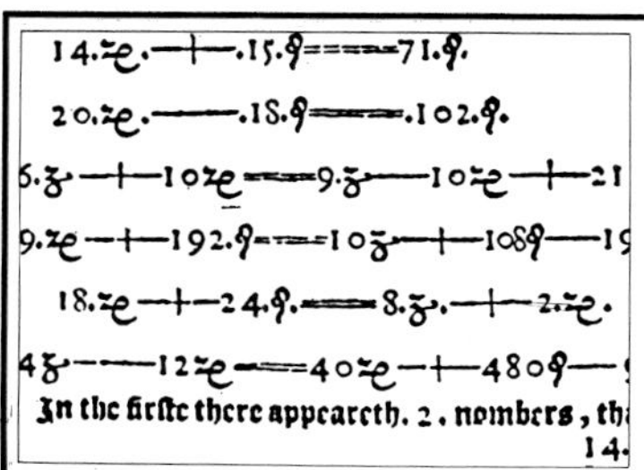
In the firste there appeareth. 2. nombers, th
14.

HISTORICAL NOTE

The English mathematician Robert Recorde (1510–1558) was the first person to use the modern symbolism for the equals sign in an algebra book, *The Whetstone of Witte*, published in 1557. Recorde used the pair of parallel line segments, =, "bicuase noe 2 thynges can be moare equalle."

Problems

Solve the linear equations.

1. $7 - 5x = x - 19$
2. $2(x - 3) = 3(x + 1)$
3. $15x - 10 = 2x + 1$
4. $9x + (1 - x) = -x$
5. $2x + 3(x + 1) = 5$
6. $5x - 5 = 7$
7. $-x + 1 = 5$
8. $5x + 2x = 0$
9. $7x - 2(x - 1) = 3x$
10. $1 - x = x - 1$
11. $2x - 1 = 1 - (2x - 1)$
12. $1 - [1 - (1 - x)] = 0$
13. $1 + [1 + (1 + x)] = 0$
14. $1 - [1 - (1 - x)] = 1 + [1 + (1 + x)]$ (a real good one)

Zeros of Quadratic Functions

The zeros of the general quadratic function

$$f(x) = ax^2 + x + c$$

are simply the solutions of the **quadratic equation**

$$ax^2 + bx + c = 0$$

Sometimes the solutions of this equation can be found by factoring the quadratic expression on the left-hand side of the equation into two linear factors. The following example illustrates this idea.

Example

Factoring Quadratic Equations Solve the following equation for x:

$$x^2 - x - 12 = 0$$

Solution Since the quadratic on the left-hand side of the equation can be factored:

$$x^2 - x - 12 = (x - 4)(x + 3)$$

we have

$$(x - 4)(x + 3) = 0$$

From this we can see that the two values of x that satisfy this equation are

$$x = 4$$
$$x = -3$$

□

Example

An Investor and the Quadratic Equation Suppose you deposit \$100 in a bank that pays interest compounded semiannually. A year later (after two compoundings) the value of your deposit has increased to \$115. What is the annual interest rate paid by the bank?

Solution In general, if an amount P is deposited in a bank that pays an annual interest rate of r compounded semiannually, then after two compoundings (one year) the value F of the account will be

$$F = P\left(1 + \frac{r}{2}\right)^2$$

Hence we set

$$115 = 100\left(1 + \frac{r}{2}\right)^2$$

and solve for r. In this equation it is easiest first to take the square root of each side of the equation, getting

$$10\left(1 + \frac{r}{2}\right) = \sqrt{115}$$

Hence we have

$$1 + \frac{r}{2} = \frac{\sqrt{115}}{10} \cong 1.072$$

or approximately

$$\frac{r}{2} = 0.072$$

$$r = 0.144$$

In other words, the annual interest rate is 14.4%. □

Example

Factoring a Cubic Solve the cubic polynomial equation

$$x^3 - 2x^2 - 11x + 12 = 0$$

Solution The cubic polynomial on the left-hand side of the equation can be written as

$$x^3 - 2x^2 - 11x + 12 = (x - 1)(x + 3)(x - 4)$$

In other words, any of the three numbers $x = 1, -3, 4$ will satisfy the cubic equation. □

Some polynomials of degree two cannot be easily factored and hence are difficult to solve. When a quadratic equation cannot easily be factored, we generally use the quadratic formula to find the solution.

Quadratic Formula

The two solutions of the quadratic equation

$$ax^2 + bx + c = 0 \qquad (a \neq 0)$$

are given by the **quadratic formula**:

$$x = \frac{-b \pm \sqrt{b^2 - 4ac}}{2a}$$

If $b^2 - 4ac < 0$, the solutions are complex numbers. If $b^2 - 4ac = 0$, the quadratic equation is said to have a double root of $-b/2a$.

Example

Quadratic Formula Solve the quadratic equation

$$x^2 + 5x - 2 = 0$$

Solution Since the quadratic polynomial on the left-hand side of this equation is difficult to factor, we use the quadratic formula. Here, we have

$$x = \frac{-5 \pm \sqrt{5^2 - 4(1)(-2)}}{2(1)} = \frac{-5 \pm \sqrt{25 + 8}}{2} = \frac{-5 \pm \sqrt{33}}{2}$$

Evaluating these two numbers, we find

$$x \cong 0.372$$
$$x \cong -5.372$$ □

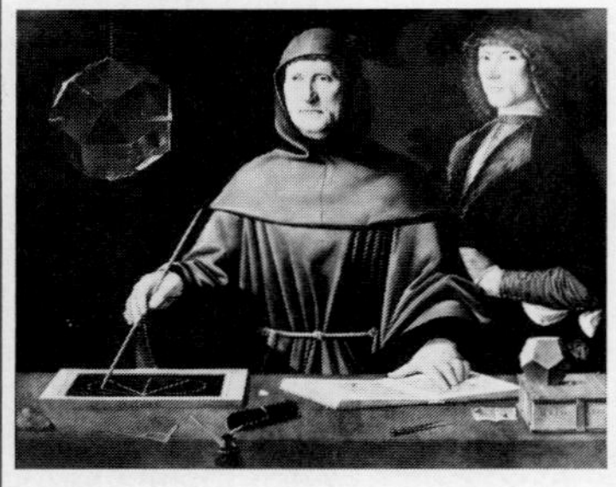

HISTORICAL NOTE

The quadratic equation was solved over 2000 years ago by Babylonian mathematicians (although not in the form we know it today). The cubic equation was solved by the Italian mathematicians Scipione dal Ferro (1465?–1526) and Niccolò Tartaglia (1500?–1557) during the 1500s. The quartic equation (fourth degree) was solved in 1540 by the Italian mathematician Ludovico Ferrari (1522–1565). In 1832 the French mathematician Evariste Galois (1811–1832) proved that there exist fifth-order polynomial equations and higher-order polynomial equations, which cannot be solved in terms of the sums, differences, products, and quotients of the roots of their coefficients.

Problems

For Problems 1–12, solve by factoring.

1. $x^2 + 5x - 14 = 0$
2. $3x^2 + x - 10 = 0$
3. $3x^2 - 27 = 0$
4. $6x^2 - 4x - 10 = 0$
5. $16x^2 - 9 = 0$
6. $3x^2 + 13x = -14$
7. $10x^2 + 4x - 6 = 0$
8. $4x^2 - 12x + 9 = 0$
9. $\dfrac{x}{4} - \dfrac{x}{x+4} = \dfrac{x-1}{6}$
10. $\dfrac{3x-6}{x-1} = \dfrac{2-x}{3+x}$
11. $x^3 - 2x^2 - x + 2 = 0$
12. $x^4 - 6x^3 + 9x^2 = 0$

For Problems 13–22, find real solutions by using the quadratic formula.

13. $3x^2 + 2x - 10 = 0$
14. $5x^2 - 2x - 7 = 0$
15. $12y^2 - 17y + 6 = 0$
16. $4x^2 - 2x - 7 = 0$
17. $x^2 + 8x + 2 = 0$
18. $3x^2 + 2px + q = 0$
19. $x^2 - 4mx + m = 0$
20. $x^2 + x + 1 = 0$
21. $\dfrac{3}{x+1} + \dfrac{2}{x} - \dfrac{1}{1-x} = 0$
22. $\dfrac{4y^2}{y-1} - 5y + 6 = 0$

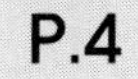

Function Operations

Manipulation of Graphs of Functions

It is surprising how many different ways graphs of functions can be moved around simply by changing the function in a minor manner. By learning a number of little "tricks," you will be able to invert, shrink, expand, shift, and manipulate graphs very easily. Computer graphics systems often use rules such as these to manipulate pictures on a computer screen.

Rules for Manipulating Graphs

The following table lists some common manipulations.

Movement of the Graph	How to Change $f(x)$
Graph moves up or down	$f(x) \longrightarrow f(x) \pm h$
Graph moves to the left or right	$f(x) \longrightarrow f(x \pm h)$
Graph stretches or contracts in the horizontal direction	$f(x) \longrightarrow f(hx)$
Graph stretches or contracts in the vertical direction	$f(x) \longrightarrow hf(x)$
Graph is reflected through the y-axis	$f(x) \longrightarrow f(-x)$
Graph is reflected through the x-axis	$f(x) \longrightarrow -f(x)$
Graph is reflected through the origin, (0, 0)	$f(x) \longrightarrow -f(-x)$

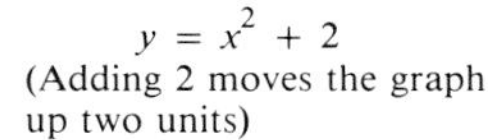

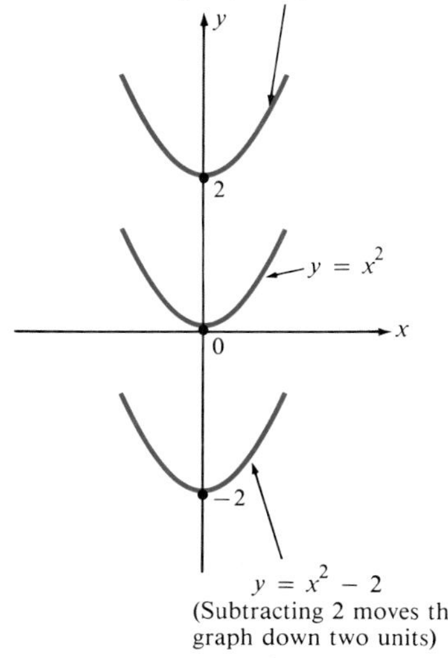

Figure 34
The result of adding or subtracting a constant

We now illustrate the above movements by means of examples.

Moving Graph Up or Down

To move the graph $y = f(x)$ up or down, add or subtract a positive number to or from $f(x)$. (See Figure 34.)

Moving Graph Left or Right

To move the graph $y = f(x)$ to the left or right, replace x by

- $x - h$ for a shift h units to the right ($h > 0$),
- $x + h$ for a shift h units to the left ($h > 0$).

See Figure 35.

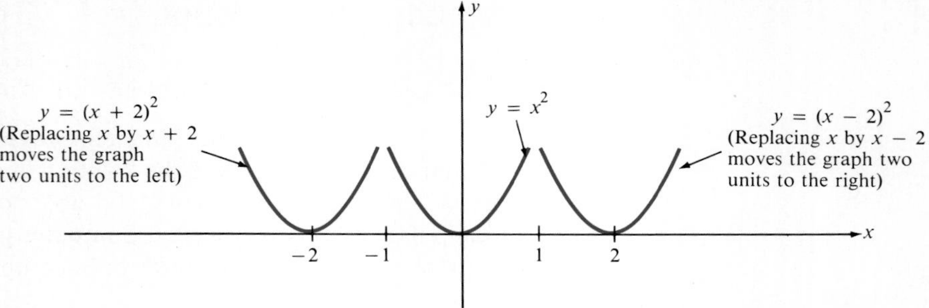

Figure 35
The result of replacing x by x + c or x − c

Horizontal Stretching and Contracting

To stretch or contract the graph $y = f(x)$ in the horizontal direction, replace x in $f(x)$ by hx, where h is a positive number. If $h > 1$, the graph will be contracted toward the y-axis. If $h < 1$, the graph will stretch away from the y-axis. (See Figure 36.)

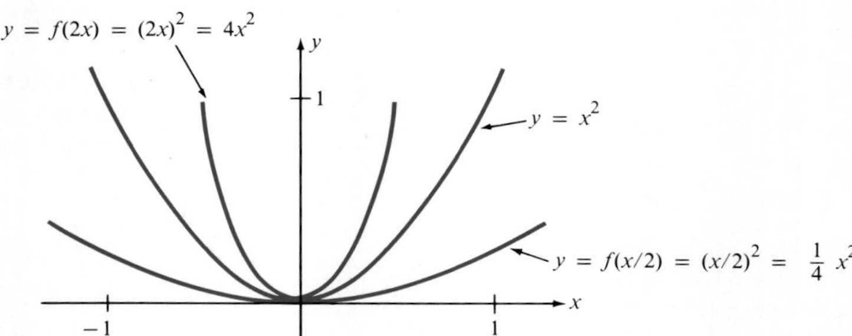

Figure 36
Replacing x by hx in a function stretches or contracts in the x direction, depending on the size of the constant

Vertical Stretching and Contracting

To stretch or contract the graph $y = f(x)$ in the vertical direction, replace $f(x)$ by $hf(x)$, where $h > 0$. (See Figure 37.)

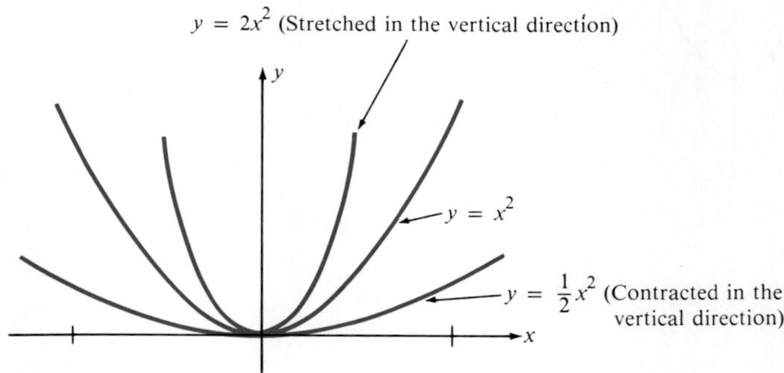

Figure 37
Multiplying a function by a constant stretches or contracts the graph in the y direction, depending on the size of the constant

Reflecting Through the y-Axis

To reflect the graph $y = f(x)$ through the y-axis, replace x by $-x$. (See Figure 38.)

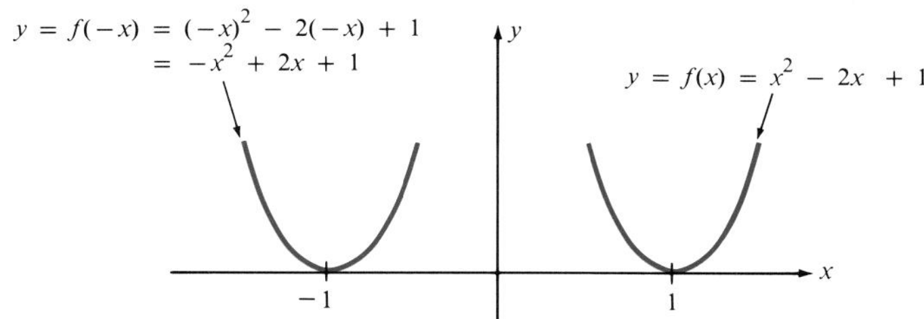

Figure 38
Changing x to $-x$ reflects the graph through the y-axis

Reflecting Through the x-Axis

To reflect the graph $y = f(x)$ through the x-axis, replace $f(x)$ by $-f(x)$. (See Figure 39.)

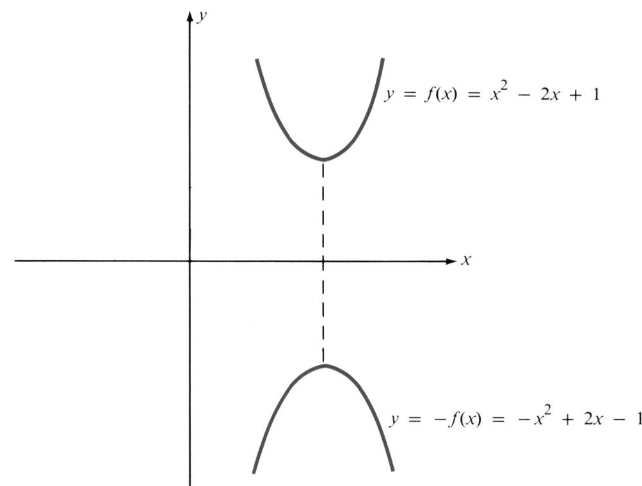

Figure 39
Changing the sign of a function reflects the graph through the x-axis

Reflecting Through the Origin

To reflect the graph $y = f(x)$ through the origin (0, 0), replace $f(x)$ by $-f(-x)$. (See Figure 40.)

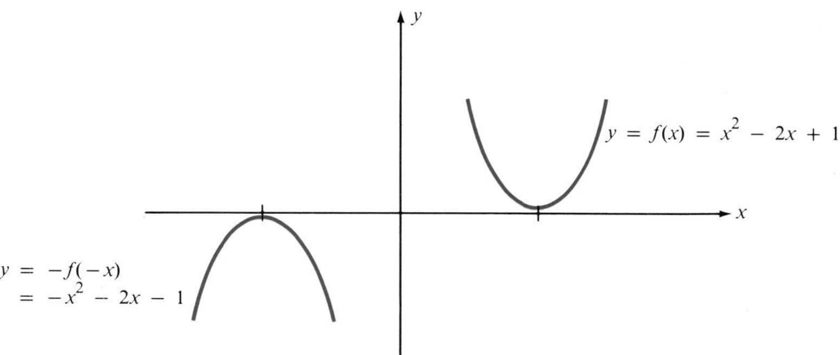

Figure 40
Changing x to $-x$ and then changing the sign of the function reflects the graph through the origin

We now apply the above manipulations to the square root function.

Function Manipulations at Work

The graphs in Figure 41 represent manipulations of the square root function

$$f(x) = \sqrt{x}$$

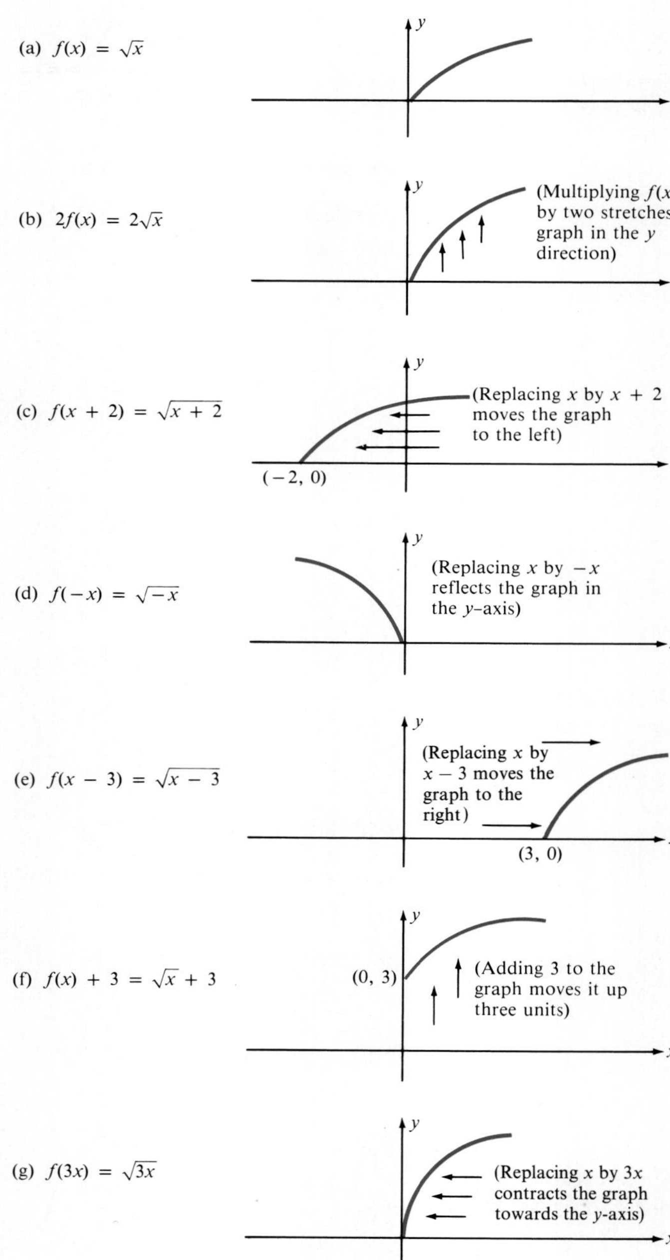

Figure 41
Some manipulations of the square root function

Problems

For each of the operations in Problems 1–11, determine how to change the function $f(x) = x^2$ to bring about the indicated change. Sketch the graphs of both $f(x) = x^2$ and the manipulated function.

1. Move the parabola up three units.
2. Move the parabola down five units.
3. Move the parabola to the left two units.
4. Move the parabola to the right seven units.
5. Stretch the parabola in the vertical direction by a factor of 2.
6. Contract the parabola in the horizontal direction by a factor of 3.
7. Stretch the parabola in the vertical direction by a factor of 5.
8. Shrink the parabola in the vertical direction by a factor of 4.
9. Reflect the parabola through the y-axis.
10. Reflect the parabola through the x-axis.
11. Reflect the parabola through the origin.

Arithmetic Operations of Functions

Just as numbers can be added, subtracted, multiplied, and divided to produce new numbers, it is possible to add, subtract, multiply, and divide functions as well. We define these operations of functions as follows.

> **Arithmetic Operations of Functions**
>
> Given the functions f and g, we define their **sum** $f + g$, **difference** $f - g$, **product** $f \cdot g$, and **quotient** f/g as follows:
>
> - **Sum:** $(f + g)(x) = f(x) + g(x)$
> - **Difference:** $(f - g)(x) = f(x) - g(x)$
> - **Product:** $(f \cdot g)(x) = f(x) \cdot g(x)$
> - **Quotient:** $(f/g)(x) = f(x)/g(x)$
>
> For the functions $f + g$, $f - g$, and $f \cdot g$, the domain is defined to be the real numbers x that lie in *both* the domains of f and g. For the quotient function, f/g, the domain is defined to be the real numbers x that lie in both the domains of f and g with the values of x (if any) for which $g(x) = 0$ excluded.

Example

Arithmetic Operations of Functions Find the sum, difference, product, and quotient of the two functions

$$f(x) = \sqrt{1 - x} \qquad \text{and} \qquad g(x) = x^2 - 4$$

Find the domains of $f + g$, $f - g$, $f \cdot g$, and f/g.

Solution

(a) Sum:
$$\begin{aligned}(f + g)(x) = f(x) + g(x) &= \sqrt{1 - x} + (x^2 - 4)\\ &= \sqrt{1 - x} + x^2 - 4\end{aligned}$$

(b) Difference:
$$\begin{aligned}(f - g)(x) = f(x) - g(x) &= \sqrt{1 - x} - (x^2 - 4)\\ &= \sqrt{1 - x} - x^2 + 4\end{aligned}$$

(c) Product: $(f \cdot g)(x) = f(x) \cdot g(x) = (\sqrt{1-x})(x^2 - 4)$

Since the domain of f is $(-\infty, 1]$ and the domain of g is $(-\infty, \infty)$, the domains of $f + g$, $f - g$, and $f \cdot g$ are $(-\infty, 1]$.

(d) Quotient: $(f/g)(x) = \dfrac{f(x)}{g(x)} = \dfrac{\sqrt{1-x}}{x^2 - 4}$

Since $g(x) = x^2 - 4$ when $x = \pm 2$, we must exclude the point $x = -2$ from the interval $(-\infty, 1]$, so the domain of f/g is all values of x that lie in the interval $(-\infty, -2)$ or in the interval $(-2, 1]$.

Problems

For Problems 1–8, find
(a) $f + g$
(b) $f - g$
(c) $f \cdot g$
(d) f/g
and find the domains of $f + g$, $f - g$, $f \cdot g$, and f/g.

1. $f(x) = 2x$, $g(x) = 1$

2. $f(x) = x^2$, $g(x) = x + 1$

3. $f(x) = |x|$, $g(x) = x - 1$

4. $f(x) = x^3$, $g(x) = x^3 - 2x + 1$

5. $f(x) = \sqrt{1 - x^2}$, $g(x) = \sqrt{x}$

6. $f(x) = \dfrac{1}{x}$, $g(x) = x^2 + 1$

7. $f(x) = \dfrac{x - 1}{x^2 + 1}$, $g(x) = x^2 + 1$

8. $f(x) = \dfrac{x}{1 + x^2}$, $g(x) = \dfrac{1 + x^2}{x}$

Composition of Functions

We often think of complicated things as being made up of several simpler things. In mathematics a "complicated" function can be interpreted as a composition of "simpler" functions. To make this idea more precise, consider the function defined by

$$h(x) = \sqrt{x^2 + 1}$$

where

$$f(x) = \sqrt{x}$$
$$g(x) = x^2 + 1$$

The function h can be interpreted as the **composition** of the functions g and f. That is, the function h does the same thing as g and f together. The first function g takes a real number x and assigns to it the value $x^2 + 1$; the second function f takes this result $x^2 + 1$ and assigns to it the value of the square root $\sqrt{x^2 + 1}$. But this team effort by g and f is exactly what the function h does. (See Figure 42.)

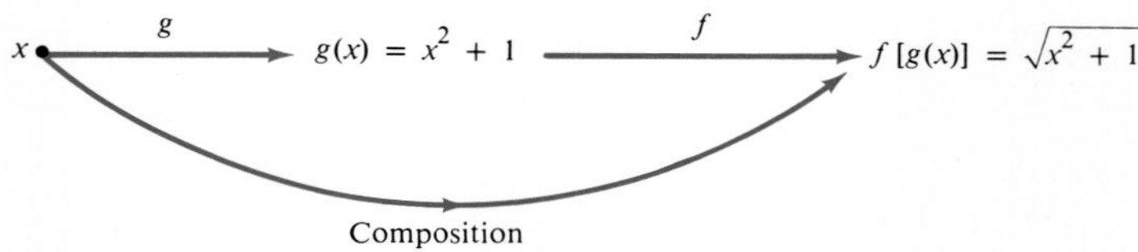

Figure 42
The composition of two functions

Another way of understanding compositions is in terms of the black box idea of a function, as illustrated in Figure 43. Here we consider two machines, working in sequence. We imagine a real number x being fed into the first machine (the "g machine"), which acts on this number and turns out a new number, called $g(x)$. This new number $g(x)$ is then fed into the second machine (the "f machine"), which in turn acts on this number and turns out another number, which we call $f[g(x)]$. These two machines acting in succession would be called the composition of g followed by f.

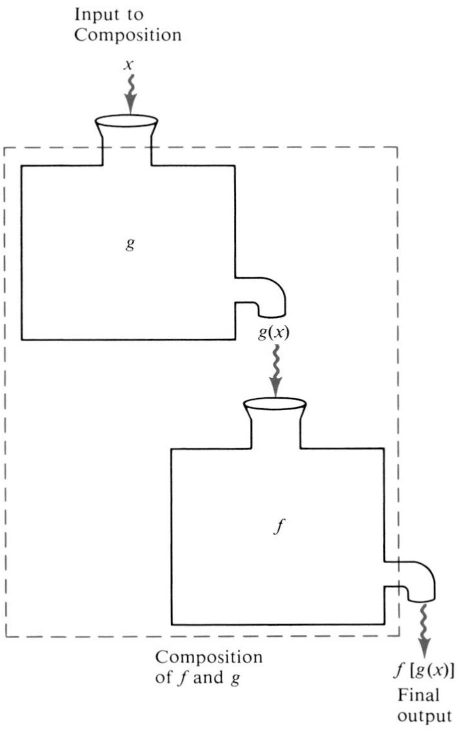

Figure 43
Composition of functions as "machines"

Example

Composition of Functions If the functions f, g, and h are defined by

$$f(x) = x^2 + 1 \qquad g(x) = \sqrt{x} \qquad h(x) = 1 + 2x$$

find the following compositions:

(a) $f[g(x)]$
(b) $h[g(x)]$
(c) $g[f(x)]$

Solution

(a) $$\begin{aligned} f[g(x)] &= [g(x)]^2 + 1 \\ &= [\sqrt{x}]^2 + 1 \\ &= x + 1 \end{aligned}$$

(b) $h[g(x)] = 1 + 2g(x)$
$= 1 + 2\sqrt{x}$

(c) $g[f(x)] = \sqrt{f(x)}$
$= \sqrt{x^2 + 1}$ □

Problems

Find the composition of functions in Problems 1–6 if

$$f(x) = 3x \qquad g(x) = x^2 + 2x + 1 \qquad h(x) = 1 + \frac{1}{x}$$

1. $f[g(x)]$
2. $f[h(x)]$
3. $g[f(x)]$
4. $g[h(x)]$
5. $h[f(x)]$
6. $h[g(x)]$

For Problems 7–15, find the indicated composition and determine the values of x for which the composition is defined if

$$f(x) = \sqrt{x} \qquad g(x) = x^2 + 1 \qquad h(x) = x - 1$$

7. $f[g(x)]$
8. $f[h(x)]$
9. $g[f(x)]$
10. $g[h(x)]$
11. $h[f(x)]$
12. $h[g(x)]$
13. $f[f(x)]$
14. $g[g(x)]$
15. $h[h(x)]$

Practice Test

The following test can be used by students to determine whether they need additional work in the Calculus Preliminaries. Before studying calculus, it is advisable for all students to spend some time and take this test. There are 11 well-chosen questions. Experience has shown that students should use the guidelines in Table 5.

TABLE 5
Guidelines for Calculus Practice Test

Correct Answers	Review Strategy
11	Excellent, no review necessary
10–9	Good, just a little touch-up needed
8–7	Average, review the weak sections
6–5	Advisable to review, quick review
4–0	Necessary to review, detailed review

You should also talk with your professor about your weaknesses.

1. Evaluate the roots (if they are defined) of the following expressions:
   (a) $16^{1/4}$
   (b) $(\frac{1}{64})^{1/5}$
   (c) $(-8)^{2/3}$
   (d) $(-16)^{1/4}$
   (e) $(\frac{1}{27})^{-2/3}$
2. Simplify the following expressions:
   (a) $\sqrt{16x^2}$
   (b) $\sqrt{a^2b^2} + \sqrt{c^2}$
   (c) $\sqrt[3]{8x^3y^6}$
3. Factor the following polynomials as the product of first-order polynomials:
   (a) $x^2 - 9$
   (b) $x^2 - x - 12$
4. Find the roots of the equation
$$x^2 + 5x - 2 = 0$$
5. Rewrite the expression
$$\frac{x-1}{x+1} - \frac{x}{x+3}$$
as a single fraction and simplify as much as possible.
6. Eliminate the square roots from the denominator of
$$\frac{1}{\sqrt{x} - \sqrt{y}}$$
by rationalization.

7. Solve the inequalities
(a) $2x + 3 \leq 7 - x$
(b) $\frac{1}{x} + 2 \geq 0$

8. Graph the line described by the following equation:

$$y = 3x - 1$$

and identify the slope and y-intercept.

9. Find the equation of the straight line that passes through the point (1, 3) with slope 2.

10. Find the equation of the straight line that passes through the points (1, 1) and (2, 0).

11. If $f(x) = x^2$ and $g(x) = 2x + 1$, find
(a) $f[g(x)]$
(b) $g[f(x)]$

Although a stroboscobe can observe the motion of a tennis player several times per second, the derivative can analyze the instantaneous motion of the player.

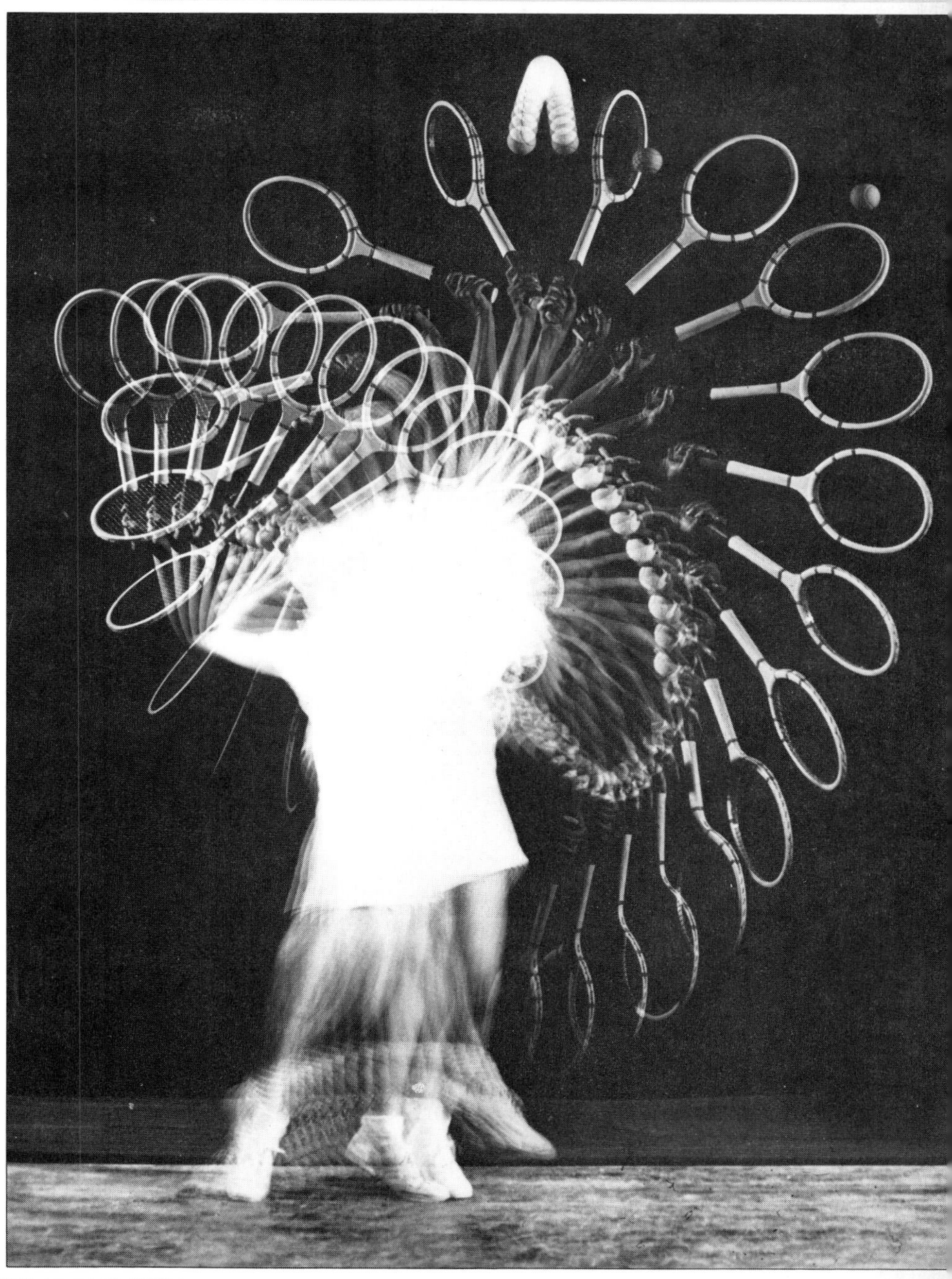

1 The Derivative

Many physical phenomena involve changing quantities. Some examples are the change in economic variables such as interest rates and profit curves, the change in biological populations such as virus and bacteria populations, and the change in physical variables such as the speed of an airplane or automobile. In this chapter we introduce the mathematical tools that are necessary to understand precisely the concept of the rate of change of a quantity.

1.1 An Historical Look at Calculus

PURPOSE

We present an historical overview of the calculus and give a glimpse into the lives of the individuals who were most responsible for making this monumental discovery. We will also introduce the two problems that were partly responsible for motivating the development of the calculus, the tangent problem and the problem of areas. It was the problem of tangents that motivated the study of the derivative (one of the two major areas of the calculus) and the area problem that motivated the study of the integral (the other major area of the calculus).

Introduction

Calculus is many things to many people. Economists often think of calculus in terms of mathematical models for forecasting discount rates, inflation, or the national debt. To an electrical engineer, calculus might represent a body of knowledge that will help to understand the circuitry of a computer. Today, in fact, practically every area of the natural and social sciences uses calculus in some form or another. We will show how calculus is used to describe phenomena in the modern world. Our first goal, however, is to outline its historical development.

Two Major Areas of Calculus

The most basic classification in calculus is the one shown in Figure 1. One of the two major subareas of the calculus is the study of *differential calculus* and the *derivative*. The other major subarea is the study of the *integral calculus* and the *integral*.

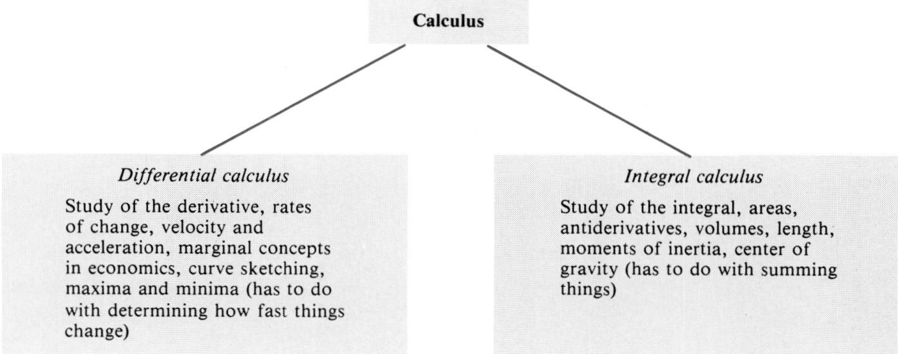

Figure 1
The two major areas of the calculus

The **derivative** is one of the most basic concepts in all of mathematics. It is a mathematical quantity that describes the rate of change of one quantity with respect to another. It is used today to study the motion of objects in space, marginal revenue in economics, the growth of biological populations, and a host of other phenomena.

On the other hand, the **integral** can be interpreted as a process of summing. One use of the integral is to represent the area enclosed by a curve.

Two Historic Problems of Calculus

During the 1600's, two major problems occupied the attention of many leading mathematicians. They were called the **tangent problem** and the **area problem**. We restate them here.

The Tangent Problem

Find the slope of a tangent line to a curve at a point.

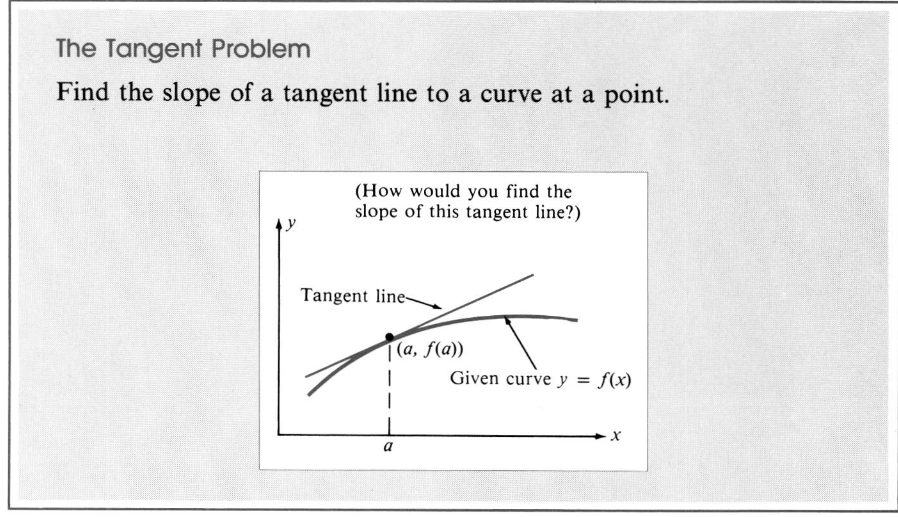

The Area Problem

Find the area enclosed by a curve.

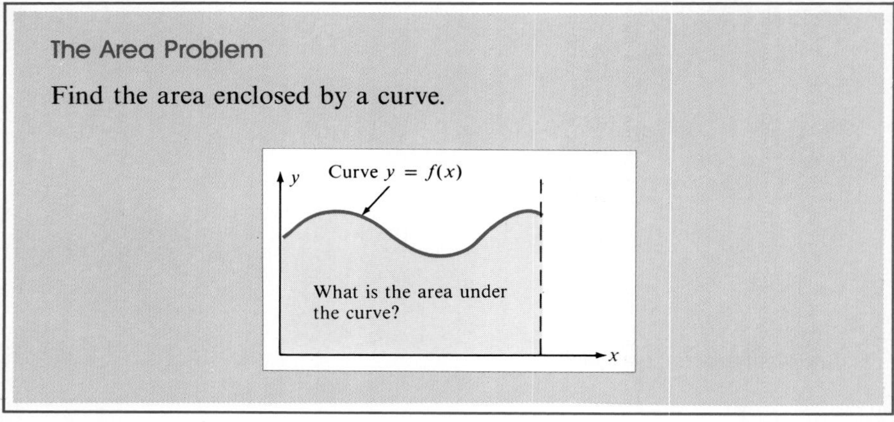

The problems above were solved in the late 1600's by the English mathematician Sir Isaac Newton and the German scholar Gottfried Wilhelm von Leibniz. In addition to solving these problems they developed an extensive body of knowledge that we now call the **calculus**. We now give a glimpse into the lives of these brilliant individuals.

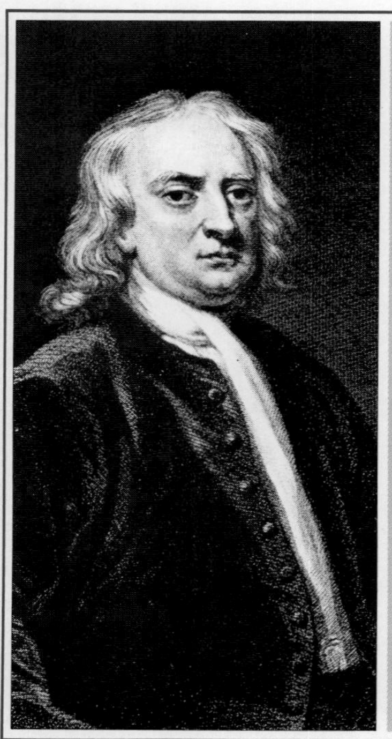

HISTORICAL NOTE

Sir Isaac Newton (1642–1727) was born on Christmas day in 1642 in Woolsthorp, England. As a youth, he showed no exceptional mathematical ability. In 1661 he entered Trinity College at Cambridge University. At Cambridge, Newton was stimulated by a very creative professor, Isaac Barrow (who in fact developed much of the calculus himself). After leaving Cambridge in 1665, Newton returned home and initiated his great works on mechanics, mathematics, and optics. It was in the years 1665–1666, during the great plague of London, that Newton developed his ideas for the calculus. Isaac Barrow, knowing of Newton's towering brilliance, resigned his prestigious position as Lucasian Professor of Mathematics in favor of the young Newton.

Newton was shy about publishing his discoveries, afraid of the criticism that his novel ideas might cause. In fact, when Newton did publish his results on optics in 1672, his theories were criticized by many scientists, including Robert Hooke and Christiaan Huygens. After that experience, Newton decided never to publish again. It is now known that the integral and derivative were developed by Newton during the years 1665–1670 but were not published until the years 1710–1735.

The other mathematician who was responsible for the development of the calculus was Gottfried Wilhelm von Leibniz.

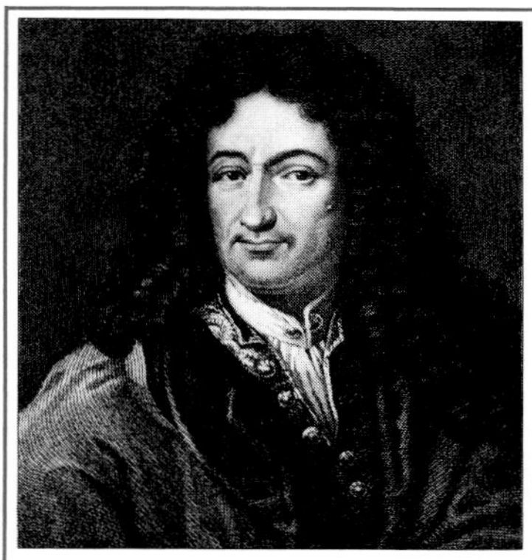

HISTORICAL NOTE

Gottfried Wilhelm von Leibniz (1646–1716) was four years younger than Newton and was born in Leipzig, Germany. Unlike Newton, however, Leibniz was a child prodigy, having mastered Greek and Latin as a young boy. By the time he was twenty, he had mastered mathematics, philosophy, theology, and law. In contrast to Newton, Leibniz never held an academic chair at a university. His life was spent in the diplomatic service, which gave him plenty of time to devote to scholarly work. Most of his creative work in coinventing the calculus was carried out during the years 1682–1692 and appeared in the mathematical journal *Acta Eruditorum*, of which he was the editor. This journal had wide circulation among the leading scholars of Europe, and it was here that the outside world first learned of the calculus.

There is, of course, much more to the story of these two men. It seemed that Newton's followers in England claimed that Leibniz had plagiarized Newton's earlier works. Leibniz too had his own admirers in Europe (Huygens, L'Hôpital, and the Bernoulli brothers), and the fight was on. The controversy grew and grew until many scholars in England and Europe refused to talk to one another.

An interesting point in the development of the calculus was that Newton's approach turned out to be superior to the manner in which Leibniz developed it. Newton introduced a concept known as the *limit*, while Leibniz used another device called the *infinitesimal*. The limit concept won out, and limits are what are used in this book.

It appeared that the infinitesimal concept was dead, but in 1961 the mathematician Abraham Robinson showed how the infinitesimal approach could be used in a much better manner than Leibniz originally imagined. Hence in the last 30 years the infinitesimal has made something of a comeback. In fact there are a few new calculus books that use this "infinitesimals over limits" approach. One is *Infinitesimal Calculus* by James M. Henle and Eugene M. Klienberg (MIT Press, 1979).

1.2 Limits and Continuity

PURPOSE

We introduce the fundamental concept of the calculus, the limit. It is by means of limits that the derivative and integral are defined. Using the limit, we introduce the concept of continuity and continuous functions.

Introduction

If there is one basic concept that might be called the essence of calculus, it is the limit. In later chapters the limit will be used to define the two basic tools of calculus, the derivative and the integral. Indeed, the basic idea of infinity, of which mathematicians are the academic custodians, can be described in terms of limits. Of course, other disciplines are also aware of the infinite. Theologians have been known to say, "Infinity is the hand of God," while one poet has written:

Infinity, it ebbs and flows with the sea
It takes and gives from you and me.
But in the end it's all for naught
The ebbing and flowing of the sea.

When mathematicians speak of infinity and limits, the prose is generally not so lush. Mathematicians do not speak in such superlatives as do poets and theologians. Mathematicians only claim is that they speak of infinity in a precise manner. This is where the limit comes in.

Limits of Functions

One dictionary defines a limit as something that can be "approached but never reached." One wonders exactly what type of thing this would be. It would seem that if something could be approached, it could be reached. For example, the

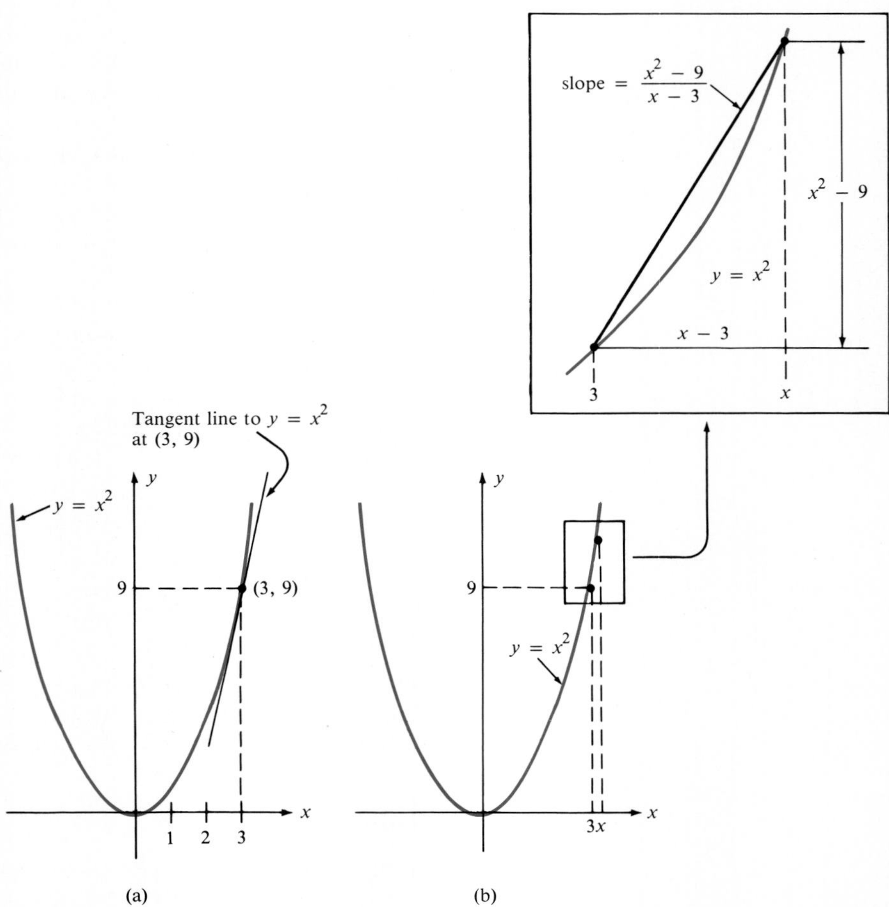

Figure 2
Finding the slope of the secant line

denominator of an algebraic expression may be zero at a point, say a, and hence the expression is not defined at a. The expression may be evaluated at points *approaching* a but not *at* a itself. Hence we might say that the point a can be approached but not reached.

To illustrate this idea, consider the important problem in calculus of finding the slope of a tangent line to a curve. Intuitively, a tangent line to a curve is a straight line that just grazes a curve at a point. The tangent line to the graph of $f(x) = x^2$ at the point (3, 9) is drawn in Figure 2a.

The calculus approach for finding the slope of this tangent line is first to find the slope of the straight line that passes through the two points (3, 9) and some nearby point (x, x^2) on the graph. This straight line is called a **secant line**. Since the slope of a straight line that passes through two points (x_1, y_1) and (x_2, y_2) is

$$m = \frac{y_2 - y_1}{x_2 - x_1} \qquad x_1 \neq x_2$$

the slope of the secant line passing through (3, 9) and (x, x^2) is

$$m = \frac{x^2 - 9}{x - 3}$$

See Figure 2b.

The second step in finding the slope of the tangent line is more difficult. If we let $x = 3$ in the above equation for m, we discover that the expression for m has the form 0/0, which is undefined in mathematics. In other words, the number 3 is the "something" we referred to earlier that can be approached but not reached. Table 1 shows the slopes of the secant lines for values of x close to 3.

TABLE 1
Slopes of Secant Lines Near $x = 3$

	x	Slope of Secant Lines
	2.5	5.5
	2.7	5.7
	2.9	5.9
	2.95	5.95
	2.99	5.99
	2.999	5.999
Can only approach ⟶	**3.000**	**limit**
	3.001	6.001
	3.01	6.01
	3.05	6.05
	3.1	6.1
	3.3	6.3
	3.5	6.5

Note that although we cannot let $x = 3$, the slopes of the secant lines seem to approach 6 as x approaches 3. We say that 6 is the limit of the slope of the secant lines passing through $(3, f(3))$ and $(x, f(x))$ as x approaches 3. We write this as

$$\lim_{x \to 3} \frac{x^2 - 9}{x - 3} = 6$$

In this example the number 6 will represent the slope of the tangent line to the graph $f(x) = x^2$ at the point (3, 9).

The above discussion motivates the following definition of the limit of a function.

Definition of the Limit of a Function

Let f be a function defined at all points near a point a (except possibly at a itself). If the value of the function $f(x)$ approaches a single number L as x approaches a from the *left* ($x < a$) and if the value $f(x)$ also approaches the same number L as x approaches a from the *right* ($x > a$), then we say that L is the **limit** of $f(x)$ at a. We denote this limit by

$$\lim_{x \to a} f(x) = L$$

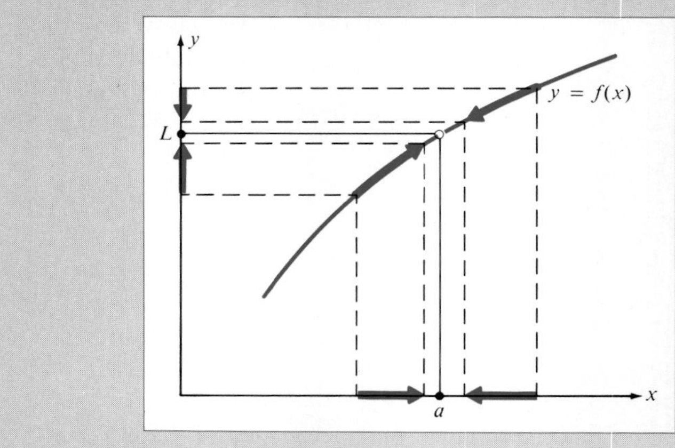

Note that the *limit* of $f(x)$ at $x = a$ is not determined by the *value* of $f(x)$ at $x = a$. In fact, $f(x)$ may not even be defined when $x = a$.

Adversarial Interpretation of the Limit (ε-δ definition)

Another way of thinking about limits is in terms of an adversarial relationship between you and your worst enemy. We say that $f(x)$ has a limit of L at $x = a$ if no matter what positive constant ε (*enemy's constant*) your enemy provides you, you can find a positive *counter number* δ such that for any x ($x \neq a$) closer to a than δ, the value of $f(x)$ will be closer to L than your enemy's ε. Essentially, this says that you can make the value of $f(x)$ closer to L than any preassigned value by picking x sufficiently close to a (without picking $x = a$). This is sometimes called the **epsilon-delta** definition of a limit. It was first introduced into mathematics by the German mathematician Karl Weierstrass (1815–1897). If you translate this statement into mathematical language you will obtain the Weierstrass limit definition of a function.

Weierstrass (ε-δ) Definition of Limit of a Function

Suppose $f(x)$ is defined on an interval $x_0 < x < x_1$ and that a is a point in this interval. Then

$$\lim_{x \to a} f(x) = L$$

if for each $\varepsilon > 0$ there exists a $\delta > 0$ such that for all values of x $(x \neq a)$ that satisfy

$$|x - a| < \delta$$

the functional value $f(x)$ will satisfy

$$|f(x) - L| < \varepsilon$$

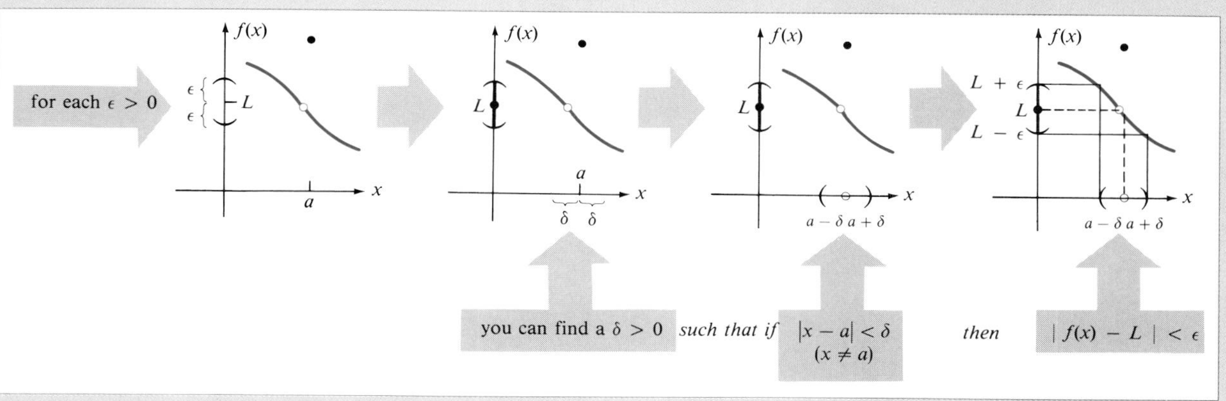

Example 1 Limit of a Function Find the limit

$$\lim_{x \to 2} \frac{x^3 - x^2 + x - 6}{x - 2}$$

Solution First note that this rational function is not defined when $x = 2$, since the denominator is 0. However, we can use a calculator and evaluate the function for values of x approaching 2, as shown in Table 2. From this table we conclude intuitively that the limit is 9. We write this as

$$\lim_{x \to 2} \frac{x^3 - x^2 + x - 6}{x - 2} = 9$$

□

TABLE 2
Values of $f(x)$ with x Close to 2

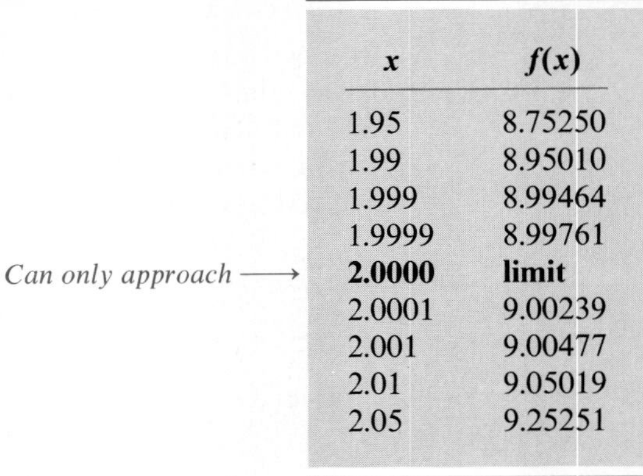

Can only approach ⟶ (row $x = 2.0000$)

x	$f(x)$
1.95	8.75250
1.99	8.95010
1.999	8.99464
1.9999	8.99761
2.0000	**limit**
2.0001	9.00239
2.001	9.00477
2.01	9.05019
2.05	9.25251

Example 2 Limit of a Function Find the limit

$$\lim_{x \to 0} \frac{x}{\sqrt{x+9}-3}$$

Solution The function has no meaning at $x = 0$, since the denominator is 0 when $x = 0$ (again, so is the numerator). Using a calculator, we evaluate the function at points closer and closer to zero. (See Table 3.)

TABLE 3
Values of the Function Close to 0

Can only approach ⟶ (row $x = 0$)

x	$f(x)$
−0.5	5.915476
−0.1	5.983287
−0.01	5.998333
−0.001	5.999833
−0.0001	5.999952
0	**limit**
0.0001	6.000024
0.001	6.000168
0.01	6.001667
0.1	6.016621
0.5	6.082207

We can see that although the function is not defined at 0, the value of $f(x)$ gets closer and closer to 6 as x gets closer and closer to 0. Hence the limit is 6, which we write as

$$\lim_{x \to 0} \frac{x}{\sqrt{x+9}-3} = 6$$

The graph of this function in the neighborhood of 0 is shown in Figure 3. □

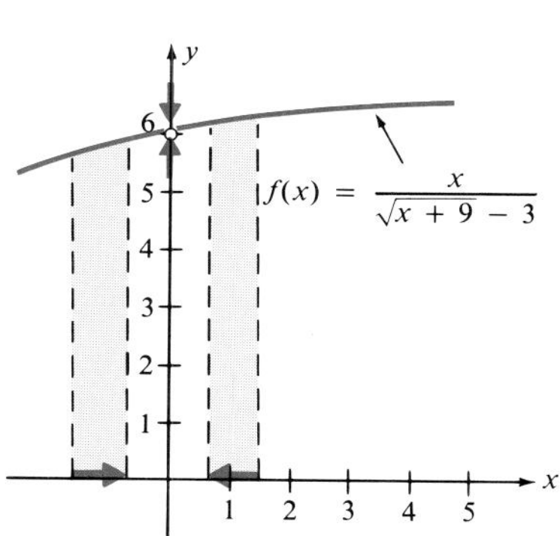

Figure 3

Illustration of $\lim_{x \to 0} \dfrac{x}{\sqrt{x+9} - 3}$

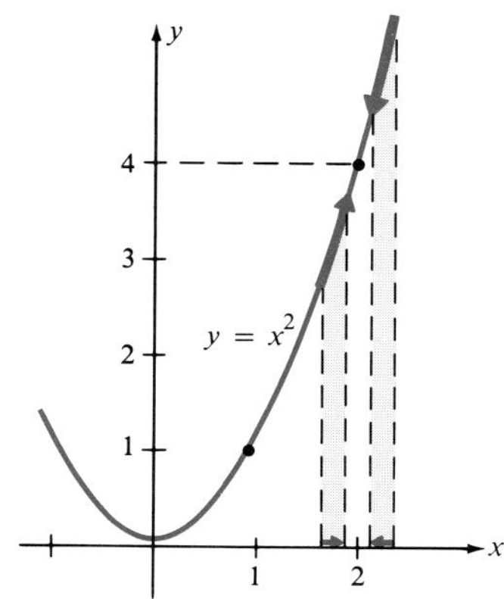

Figure 4

Illustration of $\lim_{x \to 2} x^2$

Example 3

Limit of a Function Find the limit

$$\lim_{x \to 2} x^2$$

Solution If it is easy to graph the function, this should always be done. In this case the graph of $y = x^2$ is shown in Figure 4. We can see that x^2 approaches 4 as x approaches 2. Hence we have

$$\lim_{x \to 2} x^2 = 4$$

In this example the value of the function x^2 at 2 is the same as the limit of x^2 as x approaches 2. This is not always true, but it is true in some cases. Later, we will see that this is true when a function is continuous at a point. □

Example 4

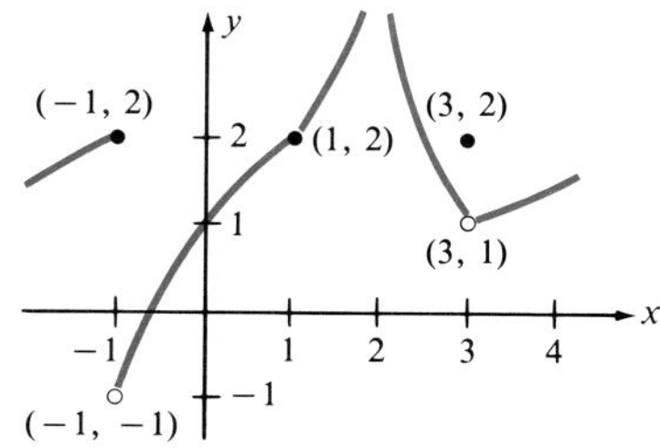

Figure 5
Finding limits

Limits of Functions Find the following limits for the function f graphed in Figure 5.

(a) $\lim_{x \to -1} f(x)$

(b) $\lim_{x \to 1} f(x)$

(c) $\lim_{x \to 2} f(x)$

(d) $\lim_{x \to 3} f(x)$

Solution

(a) The limit

$$\lim_{x \to -1} f(x)$$

does not exist, since $f(x)$ does not approach a unique value as x approaches -1 from different sides. In this case, $f(x)$ approaches 2 as x approaches -1 from the left side and -1 as x approaches -1 from the right side. You should also be aware that $f(-1) = 2$ has nothing to do with the limit at -1.

(b) We have

$$\lim_{x \to 1} f(x) = 2$$

since $f(x)$ approaches 2 as x approaches 1 from both the left and right side of 1.

(c) The limit

$$\lim_{x \to 2} f(x)$$

does not exist, since $f(x)$ does not approach any finite value as x approaches 2 from either side.

(d) As x approaches 3, we have the limit

$$\lim_{x \to 3} f(x) = 1$$

□

Example 5

Limits of Rational Functions Find the limit

$$\lim_{x \to 3} \frac{1}{x - 3}$$

Solution We evaluate the function for x close to 3. (See Table 4.)

TABLE 4
Values of $f(x)$ Close to 3

	x	$f(x)$
	2.900	−10.
	2.990	−100.
	2.999	−1000.
Can only approach ⟶	**3.000**	**limit**
	3.001	1000.
	3.010	100.
	3.100	10.

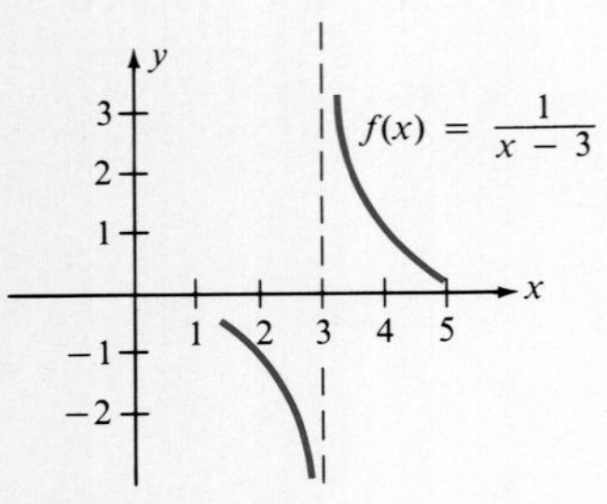

Figure 6
No limit at $x = 3$

It is clear that the values of $f(x)$ do not approach any limiting value as x approaches 3. This can also be seen by looking at the graph of $f(x)$ in Figure 6.

□

The following rules for limits are often helpful in the evaluation of complicated limits.

Rules for Limits

If f and g are functions such that the limits

$$\lim_{x\to a} f(x) \qquad \lim_{x\to a} g(x)$$

exist then the following rules for limits hold:

- The limit of a sum is the sum of the limits:

$$\lim_{x\to a} [f(x) + g(x)] = \lim_{x\to a} f(x) + \lim_{x\to a} g(x)$$

- The limit of a difference is the difference of the limits:

$$\lim_{x\to a} [f(x) - g(x)] = \lim_{x\to a} f(x) - \lim_{x\to a} g(x)$$

- The limit of a product is the product of the limits:

$$\lim_{x\to a} [f(x)g(x)] = \lim_{x\to a} f(x) \cdot \lim_{x\to a} g(x)$$

- The limit of a quotient is the quotient of the limits:

$$\lim_{x\to a} \frac{f(x)}{g(x)} = \frac{\lim_{x\to a} f(x)}{\lim_{x\to a} g(x)} \qquad \text{provided that} \quad \lim_{x\to a} g(x) \neq 0$$

- The limit of a root is the root of the limit:

$$\lim_{x\to a} \sqrt[n]{f(x)} = \sqrt[n]{\lim_{x\to a} f(x)} \qquad \text{provided } \sqrt[n]{\lim_{x\to a} f(x)} \text{ exists}$$

- The limit of a power is the power of the limit:

$$\lim_{x\to a} [f(x)]^n = \left[\lim_{x\to a} f(x)\right]^n$$

Two other useful limits are as follows:

- The limit of a constant is the constant

$$\lim_{x\to a} c = c \qquad \text{for any constant } c$$

- The limit of x at a is a

$$\lim_{x\to a} x = a$$

Example 6 Limit of a Polynomial Find the limit

$$\lim_{x\to 2} (3x^2 - 4x + 1)$$

Solution First, using the rules that the limit of a sum or difference is the sum or difference of the limits, we write

$$\begin{aligned}\lim_{x\to 2}(3x^2-4x+1) &= \lim_{x\to 2}(3x^2)-\lim_{x\to 2}(4x)+\lim_{x\to 2}(1)\\ &= 3\lim_{x\to 2}x^2-4\lim_{x\to 2}(x)+\lim_{x\to 2}(1)\\ &= 3(4)-4(2)+(1)\\ &= 5\end{aligned}$$

□

Example 7 Limit of a Root Find the limit

$$\lim_{x\to 2}\sqrt{x^2-1}$$

Solution Using the rule that the limit of a root is the root of a limit, we have

$$\begin{aligned}\lim_{x\to 2}\sqrt{x^2-1} &= \sqrt{\lim_{x\to 2}(x^2-1)}\\ &= \sqrt{\lim_{x\to 2}(x^2)-\lim_{x\to 2}(1)}\\ &= \sqrt{4-1}\\ &= \sqrt{3}\end{aligned}$$

□

Comment on the Above Limit

Note that in finding the above limit, we used the fact that

$$\lim_{x\to 2}(x^2-1)>0$$

Example 8 Limit of a Product Find the limit of the product

$$\lim_{x\to 2}(x\sqrt{x^2-1})$$

Solution Using the rule that the limit of a product is the product of the limits, we have

$$\begin{aligned}\lim_{x\to 2}(x\sqrt{x^2-1}) &= \lim_{x\to 2}(x)\cdot\lim_{x\to 2}\sqrt{x^2-1}\\ &= 2\sqrt{3}\end{aligned}$$

□

Example 9 Limit of a Quotient Find the limit of the quotient

$$\lim_{x\to 4}\frac{x^2+3x+1}{\sqrt{x}-1}$$

Solution Using the rule that the limit of a quotient is the quotient of the limits, we can write

$$\lim_{x\to 4} \frac{x^2+3x+1}{\sqrt{x}-1} = \frac{\lim_{x\to 4}(x^2+3x+1)}{\lim_{x\to 4}(\sqrt{x}-1)} = \frac{29}{1}$$

□

Comment on the Above Limit

Note that in finding the above limit we used the fact that

$$\lim_{x\to 4}(\sqrt{x}-1) \neq 0$$

Example 10

Limit of a Power Find the limit

$$\lim_{x\to -1}(x+3)^5$$

Solution Using the fact that the limit of a power is the power of a limit, we have

$$\lim_{x\to -1}(x+3)^5 = \left[\lim_{x\to -1}(x+3)\right]^5 = [2]^5 = 32$$

□

Example 11

Factoring out a Common Factor Find the limit

$$\lim_{x\to 2}\frac{x^2-4}{x-2}$$

Solution Note that in the above fraction, both the numerator and denominator approach 0 as x approaches 2. When this happens, we look for a factor of $x-2$ in both the numerator and the denominator. We can write

$$\lim_{x\to 2}\frac{x^2-4}{x-2} = \lim_{x\to 2}\frac{(x-2)(x+2)}{x-2} = \lim_{x\to 2}(x+2) = 4$$

□

Comment on the Above Limit

Although both the numerator and denominator of the above expression get closer and closer to 0 as x gets closer and closer to 2, the value of the numerator will tend to be 4 times the value of the denominator. (See Table 5.)

TABLE 5

x	$\dfrac{x^2 - 4}{x - 2}$
1.9	$\dfrac{-0.39}{-.01} = 3.9$
1.99	$\dfrac{-0.0399}{-0.01} = 3.99$

The Concept of Continuity

Most of the functions graphed thus far could be drawn without lifting the pencil from the paper. Intuitively, a function f is continuous at a point $x = a$ if its graph passes through the point $(a, f(a))$ without a break. Figure 7 shows the graphs of continuous functions from business management and science.

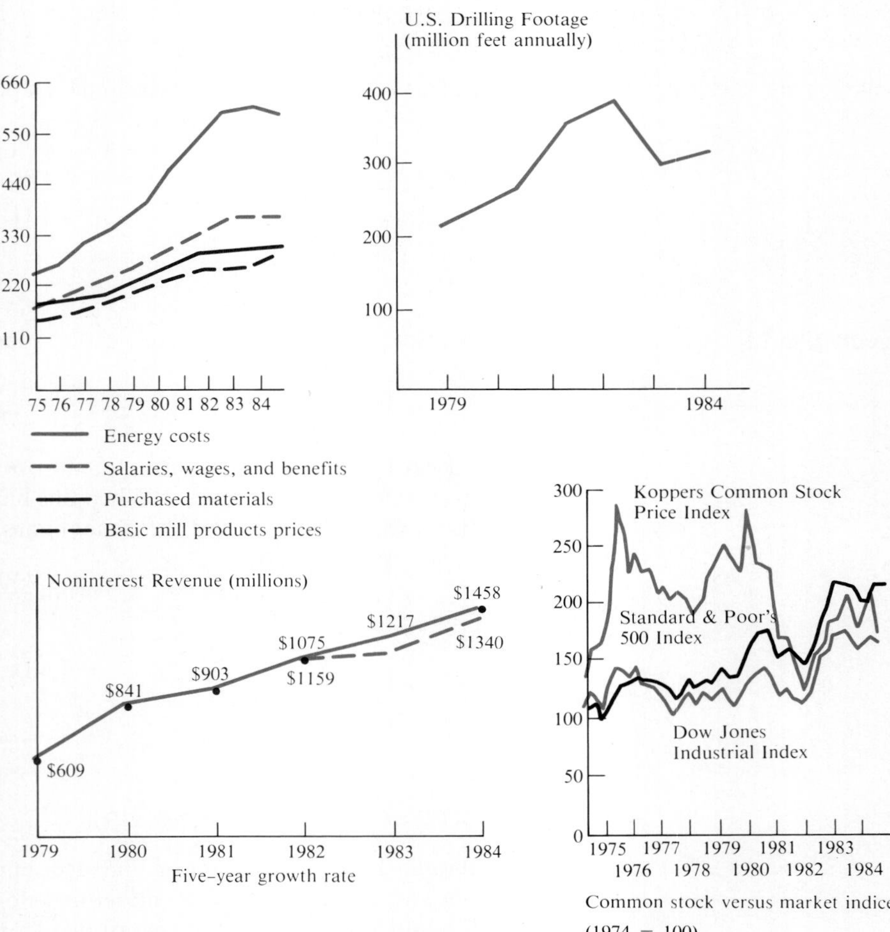

Figure 7
Some continuous functions in the business world

We now define the concept of continuity in terms of the limit.

Definition of Continuity

A function f is continuous at a point $x = a$ if

1. $\lim_{x \to a} f(x)$ exists
2. $f(a)$ exists
3. $\lim_{x \to a} f(x) = f(a)$

If f is not continuous at $x = a$, we say that f is **discontinuous** or has a **discontinuity** at $x = a$.

If a function is continuous at all points on an open interval (a, b), we simply say the function is continuous on that interval.

The above definition of continuity at $x = a$ implies that if a function is continuous at $x = a$, then the function f is defined at $x = a$ and that

$$\lim_{x \to a} f(x)$$

exists.

Figure 8 shows four different ways that a function can fail to be continuous

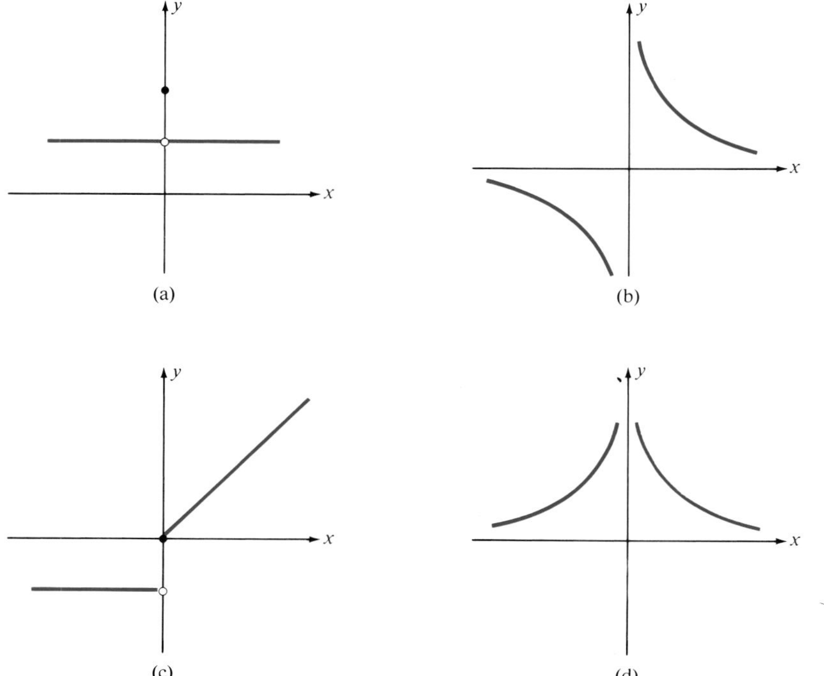

Figure 8
All functions discontinuous at $x = 0$

at a point. All four of these functions are discontinuous at $x = 0$. The functions are, however, continuous at all other points.

Example 12

Continuity on an Interval The graph in Figure 9 of $N(t)$ shows the number of cats that lived in one of the author's homes over the past ten years. Determine whether $N(t)$ is continuous on the following intervals:

(a) (0, 2)
(b) (4, 7)
(c) (7, 9)

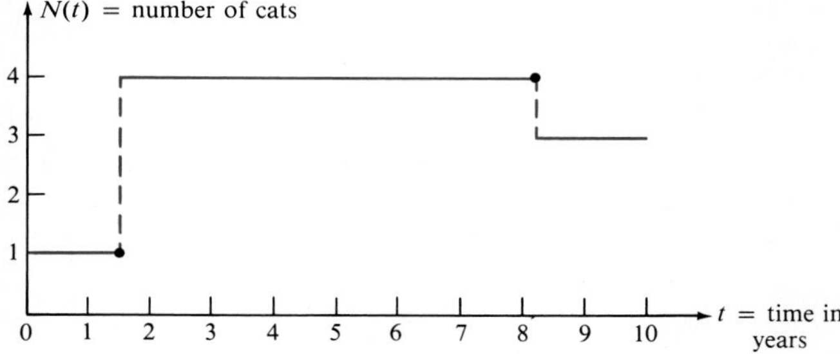

Figure 9
The cat function

Solution

(a) Interval (0, 2): The "cat function" $N(t)$ is not continuous on (0, 2), since the function has a jump discontinuity at $t = 1.5$ years (Daisy had kittens).
(b) Interval (4, 7): The function $N(t)$ is constant and hence continuous on the open interval (4, 7).
(c) Interval (7, 9): The jump discontinuity at $t = 8.2$ means that $N(t)$ is not continuous on the interval (7, 9). □

Constructing New Continuous Functions

Earlier, we said that the limit of a sum of functions was the sum of the limits of the functions. This property can be used to show that the sum of two continuous functions is also continuous. In the same way, the other limit properties can be used to show that the difference, product, and quotient of continuous functions are continuous. We now present an important result stating that polynomials and rational functions (when defined) are continuous functions.

Continuity of Polynomials and Rational Functions

Polynomials of the form

$$p(x) = a_0x^{n+1} + a_1x^n + \cdots + a_nx + a_{n+1}$$

are continuous for all values of x.

Rational functions of the form

$$r(x) = \frac{p(x)}{q(x)}$$

where $p(x)$ and $q(x)$ are polynomials are continuous for all values of x except for those x where $q(x) = 0$.

Example 13 Continuity of Polynomials and Rational Functions Where is each of the following two functions continuous?

(a) $p(x) = x^4 - 3x^3 + 2x^2 + 6x + 7$

(b) $q(x) = \dfrac{x^3 + 3x^2 + 1}{x^2 - 1}$

Solution

(a) The polynomial $p(x)$ is continuous for all values of x.

(b) The rational function $q(x)$ is continuous for all values of x except when x is equal to 1 or -1 where the denominator is equal to 0. □

Continuity in the Real World

The reason for our interest in continuity and continuous functions is that many phenomena in the real world change or move continuously. The height of a ball thrown into the air is a continuous function of time. Temperature, air pressure, electric current, light intensity, and many other physical phenomena change continuously with time. In fact, you might find it difficult to think of a physical phenomenon that does not change continuously with time.

In the business world, although most phenomena such as interest rates and a company's profit change by jumps, it is possible to approximate these changes by continuous models. For instance, although interest rates change by tenths (9.5% and 10.3% are typical interest rates), it is convenient to study continuous interest rate curves. Other curves such as the number of unemployed persons, profit curves, and cost curves also change in jumps, but for simplicity they are often described by such continuous functions as polynomials. In biology, too, population growth changes in discrete jumps but is generally described by continuous models when populations are large.

Discontinuity in the Real World

Although many phenomena are modeled by continuous functions, several types of problems must be described by discontinuous functions. Figure 10 shows some discontinuous phenomena.

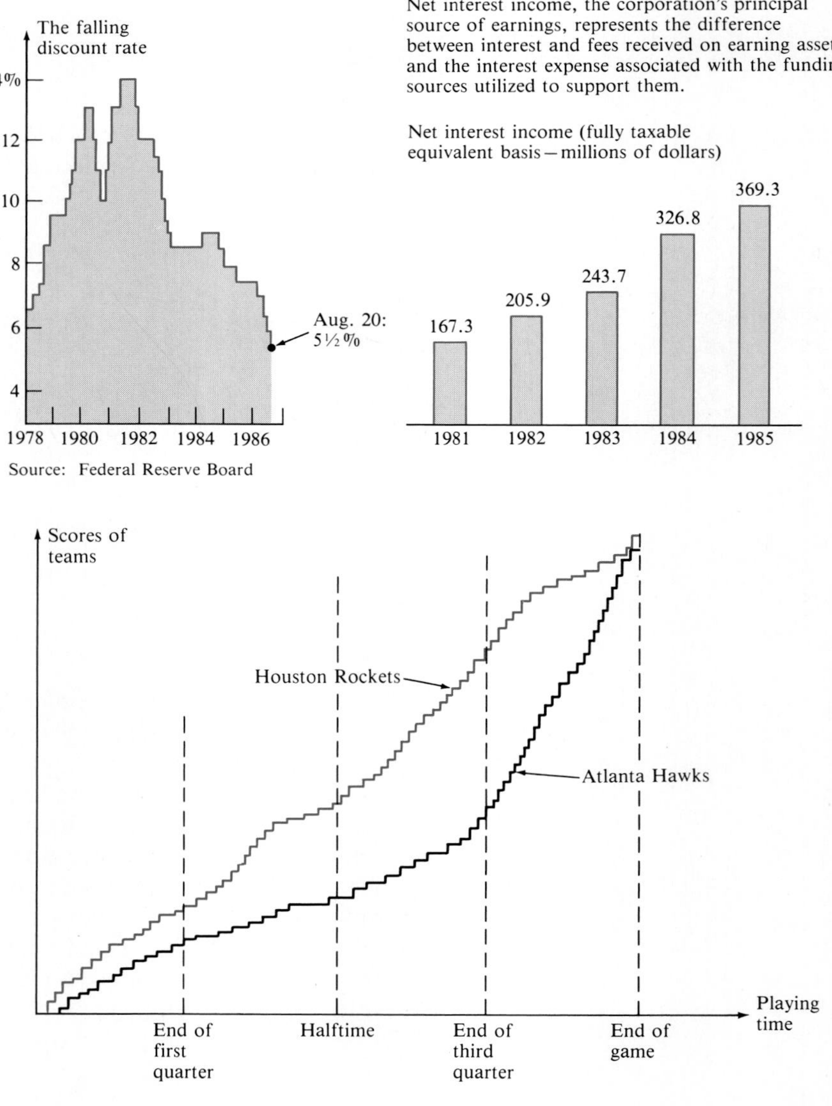

Figure 10
Discontinuous phenomena

Problems

For Problems 1–11, find the limits. If possible, graph the function.

1. $\lim_{x\to 2} 3x$

2. $\lim_{x\to 1} (3x^2 + 1)$

3. $\lim_{x\to 4} \dfrac{x-2}{x+2}$

4. $\lim_{x\to -3} \dfrac{x^2-9}{x^2+9}$

5. $\lim_{x\to 2} \sqrt{9-x^2}$

6. $\lim_{x\to 0} (x^2 + 2x + 1)$

7. $\lim_{x\to 2} \dfrac{x-2}{x^2-4}$

8. $\lim_{x\to 3} \dfrac{x^3-27}{x^2-9}$

9. $\lim_{x\to 3} \dfrac{2}{x+1}$

10. $\lim_{x\to 3} (x^2\sqrt{x^2+7})$

11. $\lim_{x\to 3} \sqrt[3]{x^2-1}$

Limits of Branched Functions

Often a function is defined by different algebraic expressions on different intervals of the real line. Such functions are called *branched functions*. For Problems 12–17, find the limits, if they exist, of the indicated branched functions.

12. $\lim_{x\to 0} f(x),\ f(x) = \begin{cases} x^2 & -\infty < x < 0 \\ 1 & x = 0 \\ -x^2 & 0 < x < \infty \end{cases}$

13. $\lim_{x\to 2} f(x),\ f(x) = \begin{cases} |x-2| & -\infty < x < 2 \\ 1 & x = 2 \\ |x-2| & 2 < x < \infty \end{cases}$

14. $\lim_{x\to 0} f(x),\ f(x) = \begin{cases} 0 & -\infty < x < 0 \\ 1 & x = 0 \\ x & 0 < x < \infty \end{cases}$

15. $\lim_{x\to 0} f(x),\ f(x) = \begin{cases} -1 & -\infty < x < 0 \\ 0 & x = 0 \\ 1 & 0 < x < \infty \end{cases}$

16. $\lim_{x\to 0} f(x),\ f(x) = \begin{cases} x+1 & -\infty < x < 0 \\ 0 & x = 0 \\ x+1 & 0 < x < \infty \end{cases}$

17. $\lim_{x\to 1} f(x),\ f(x) = \begin{cases} \sqrt{1-x^2} & 0 \le x < 1 \\ 1 & 1 \le x < 2 \\ 2 & 2 \le x < \infty \end{cases}$

For Problems 18–23, find the indicated quantities if they exist. Use Figure 11.

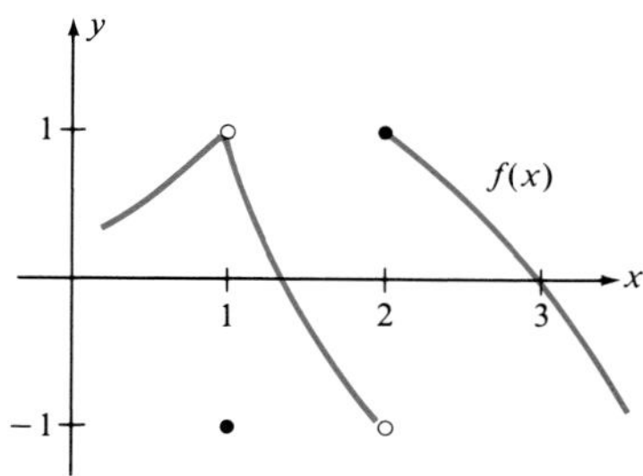

Figure 11
Graph for Problems 18–23

18. $\lim_{x\to 1} f(x)$

19. $\lim_{x\to 2} f(x)$

20. $\lim_{x\to 3} f(x)$

21. $f(1)$

22. $f(2)$

23. $f(3)$

For Problems 24–27, find the limits by evaluating (on a calculator) the function at values of x close to the limiting value of x. For problems in which you can rationalize the denominator, find the limit by the rationalizing technique to check the calculator solution. You can review the process of rationalizing the denominator in the Calculus Preliminaries.

24. $\lim_{x\to 0} \dfrac{x}{\sqrt{x+4}-2}$

25. $\lim_{x\to 0} \dfrac{x}{\sqrt{x+9}-3}$

26. $\lim_{x\to 0} \dfrac{x}{\sqrt{x+16}-4}$

27. $\lim_{x\to 0} \dfrac{x}{\sqrt{x+25}-5}$

For Problems 28–30, find the following limits. Indicate the limit rules used at each step.

28. $\lim_{x\to 3} \left(\dfrac{1}{x+7} - \dfrac{2x}{3x-2}\right)$

29. $\lim_{t\to 4} \dfrac{2t+4}{t-3}$

30. $\lim_{x\to 1} (2x^3 + 4x + 3)$

For Problems 31–37, tell whether the given phenomenon represents a continuous or discontinuous function of time. If the function is discontinuous, tell where the function fails to be continuous.

31. The total score of a basketball game.

32. The number of people infected with a given type of bacteria.
33. The temperature during the day.
34. The amount of inventory of a given product.
35. The daily revenue of a company.
36. Your weight throughout your life.
37. A company's annual profits.

For Problems 38–48, determine the points for which the functions are continuous. Also find any points where the functions are discontinuous.

38. $f(x) = x + 3$
39. $f(x) = x^3 + 3x^2 - 2x + 1$
40. $f(x) = x^5 + x^4 + 3x - 1$
41. $f(x) = \dfrac{x + 1}{x^2 + 1}$
42. $f(x) = \dfrac{2x^2 + 5x + 1}{x^2 - 1}$
43. $f(x) = \dfrac{x^2 + 1}{x + 1}$
44. $f(x) = (x^2 + x + 1)(x^3 - x^2 + 4)$
45. $f(x) = (x^2 + 2)(x^5 - x^3 + x + 1)$
46. $f(x) = (x^3 + 1)\left(\dfrac{x^2 + x + 6}{x^2 + 1}\right)$
47. $f(x) = \dfrac{1}{x + 1} \cdot \dfrac{2x^5 + 1}{x - 3}$
48. $f(x) = \dfrac{1}{x + 5} \cdot \dfrac{x^3 + 3}{x^2 + 5} \cdot \dfrac{5}{2x - 3}$

For Problems 49–51, answer the questions concerning the graph in Figure 12.

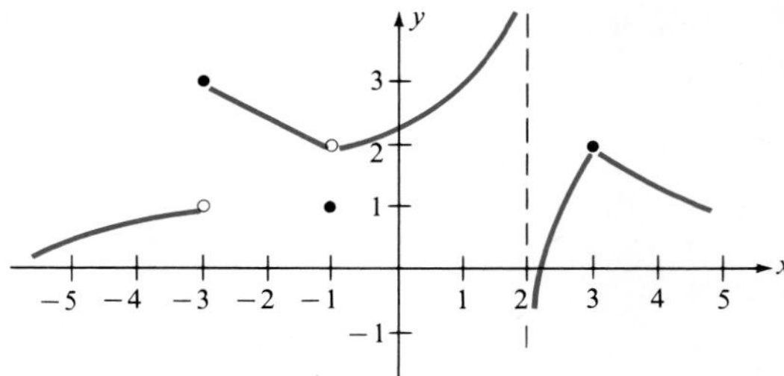

Figure 12
Graph for Problems 49–51

49. At what points (if any) is the function discontinuous? Tell why in terms of limits.
50. Where is the function discontinuous as a result of the limit not existing at a point?
51. Where is the function discontinuous as a result of the limit existing but not being equal to the value of the function at the point?
52. **Population Problem.** Let $S(t)$ be the number of people in a store at time t, where t ranges from 9:00 A.M. to 5:00 P.M. When is such a function continuous? When does this function have a discontinuity?
53. **Postage Problem.** Postage rates in 1989 were 25 cents for a first-class letter weighing no more than one ounce and 20 cents for each additional ounce or fraction thereof. Determine the function that describes the amount of postage required for a first-class letter weighing no more than 12 ounces. At what values is this function continuous? At what values is this function discontinuous?

1.3 An Analysis of Change

PURPOSE

We introduce the three important types of change of a function:

- total change,
- average rate of change, and
- instantaneous rate of change.

We will see that the computation of the total change and the average rate of change of a function involve only simply algebra. However, to introduce the idea of the instantaneous rate of change, we will need to use the concept of the limit of a function. After we introduce the instantaneous rate of change, we will introduce the concept of instantaneous velocity.

Introduction

Throughout the ages, mathematics has been called upon to solve problems that had previously gone unsolved. Four thousand years before Christ, the Sumerians used mathematics in carrying out financial dealings such as computing simple and compound interest, mortgages, and deeds of sale. Later, Egyptian builders used mathematics and geometry to construct the great pyramids of the Pharaohs.

Centuries later, Portuguese and Italian sailors needed mathematics to understand navigational charts and complex navigational equipment. The Renaissance period introduced complex mechanical devices that could be understood and explained by using mathematical principles.

However, the mathematics inherited from previous times was ill-equipped for studying motion. The discoveries by the pioneer Italian astronomer Galileo Galilei, who might be called the "father of dynamics," introduced the study of motion and change into science. It was in this setting that Newton and Leibniz developed the calculus, a mathematical discipline for understanding problems involving changing quantities. It is interesting to note that Newton was born in 1642, the same year that Galileo died.

It has often been said that, with the beginning of the calculus, the modern age of mathematics began. We now show how Newton and Leibniz analyzed change. Since a function is the mathematical device that shows how two quantities are related, we naturally analyze the change in functions.

Total and Average Change of a Function

We illustrate the concept of change by studying the growth of a biological organism. Suppose a medical researcher is monitoring the diameter $D(t)$ of a malignant tumor at day t. Table 6 represents observations recorded at the same time of day over a six-day period (day 20 to day 25).

TABLE 6
Daily Tumor Readings

Day	Diameter of Tumor (mm)	Change in Diameter (mm)
20	150.0	—
21	157.3	7.3
22	166.5	9.2
23	176.4	9.9
24	188.1	11.7
25	200.0	11.9

The total change D in the diameter of the tumor during the period from day 20 to day 25 is given by

$$\begin{aligned}\Delta D &= D(25) - D(20)\\ &= 200 \text{ mm} - 150 \text{ mm}\\ &= 50 \text{ mm}\end{aligned}$$

This change is shown in Figure 13.

A second type of change, the average daily change in the diameter, is found by dividing the total change by the number of days elapsed (five in this case).

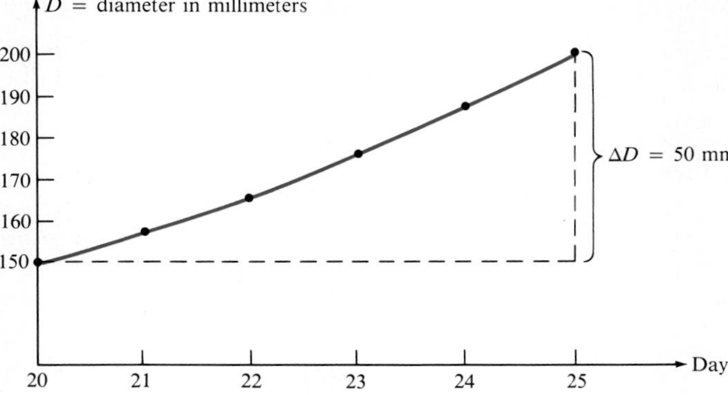

Figure 13
Diameter of tumor

This gives

$$\text{Average daily change} = \frac{D(25) - D(20)}{5}$$

$$= \frac{200 - 150}{5}$$

$$= 10.0 \quad \text{mm per day}$$

In other words, the average daily growth of the tumor during this time period is 10 millimeters per day. Note in Table 6 that during the first two days, growth is less than 10 millimeters per day, while during the last two days the growth is greater than 10 millimeters per day. The average growth, however, is exactly 10 millimeters per day.

The above discussion leads us to the following general definition for the average change in a function.

Definition of the Average Change in a Function

The average change of $f(x)$ on the interval $[a, a + h]$ is given by

$$\text{Average change in } f(x) \text{ on } [a, a + h] = \frac{\text{total change in } f(x)}{\text{total change in } x}$$

$$= \frac{f(a + h) - f(a)}{h}$$

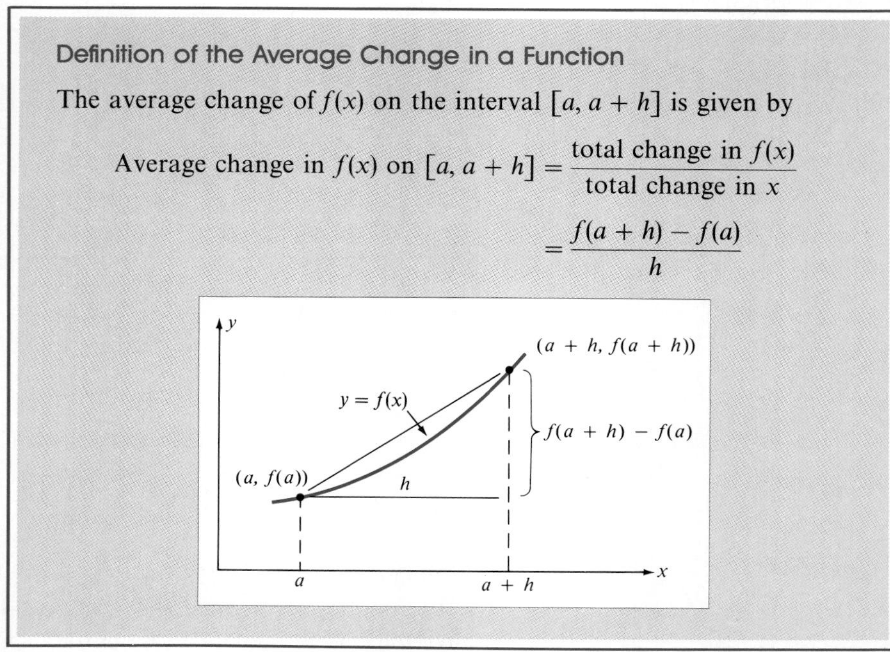

The diagram above shows that the average change in a function of an interval is simply the total change of the value of the function over the interval divided by the length of the interval. Geometrically the average change of a function f over an interval $[a, a + h]$ is the slope of the secant line connecting $(a, f(a))$ and $(a + h, f(a + h))$.

Example 1

Growth of a Tumor Suppose the diameter D of a cancerous tumor grows over a given period of time according to the "power" law

$$D(t) = 0.015t^2 \text{ millimeters}$$

where t is time measured in days and $t = 0$ denotes the time when the tumor begins growth. Find the total change in the diameter during the time period from day 10 to day 60. Use the total change to determine the average daily growth during this time period.

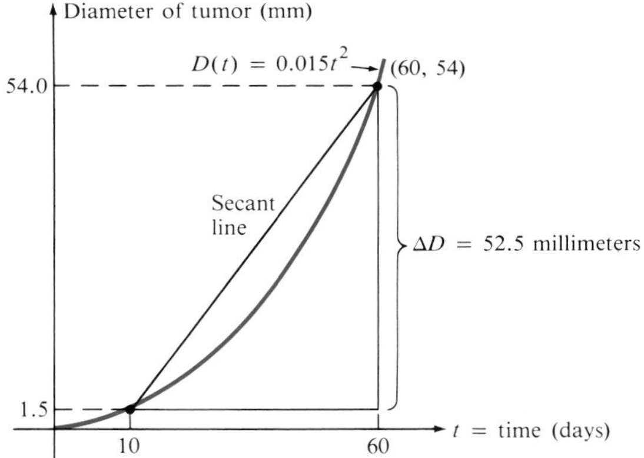

Figure 14
Total and average rate of change in diameter of tumor

Solution The graph of the diameter $D(t)$ is shown in Figure 14. The total change in diameter ΔD during this time period is given by

$$\begin{aligned}\Delta D &= D(60) - D(10)\\ &= 0.015[(60)^2 - (10)^2]\\ &= 52.5 \text{ millimeters}\end{aligned}$$

The average daily change during these days is

$$\begin{aligned}\text{Average daily change} &= \frac{52.5}{50}\\ &= 1.05 \text{ millimeters per day}\end{aligned}$$

□

Instantaneous Rate of Change

Until now, we have used algebra only to define the total and average rate of change in a function. To introduce the concept of the instantaneous rate of change, however, we need to use the idea of the limit.

The **instantaneous rate of change** (or simply the *rate of change*) refers to the rate of change of a function at a point. We have seen that the average change in a function f over an interval $[a, a + h]$ is the slope of the line connecting $(a, f(a))$ and $(a + h, f(a + h))$. This line is called the secant line connecting these two points. If we now let the length h of the interval $[a, a + h]$ approach 0, the secant lines connecting $(a, f(a))$ and $(a + h, f(a + h))$ will approach the tangent line to the graph at $(a, f(a))$. This tangent line is the line that just grazes the graph of $y = f(x)$ at the point $(a, f(a))$. The instantaneous rate of change of a function f at the point $(a, f(a))$ is the slope of the tangent line at this point. We can state this more precisely in terms of limits.

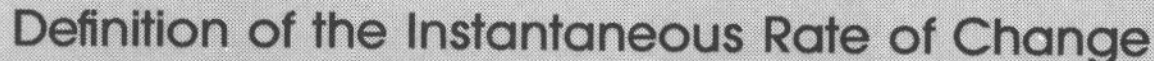

Definition of the Instantaneous Rate of Change

The instantaneous rate of change of $f(x)$ at $x = a$ is given by

$$\text{Instantaneous rate of change} = \lim_{h \to 0} \frac{f(a + h) - f(a)}{h}$$

provided that the limit exists.

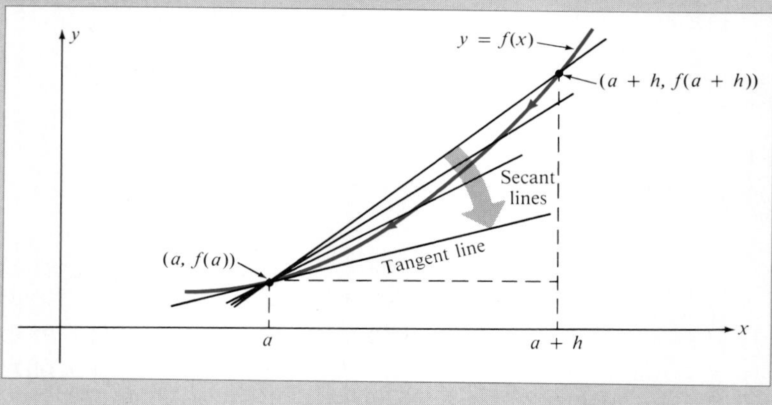

Example 2

Instantaneous Rate of Change Using the same growth function

$$D(t) = 0.015t^2$$

as discussed in Example 1, find the instantaneous rate of change in the diameter D of the tumor on the 20th day.

Solution The instantaneous rate of change in the diameter D when $t = 20$ days is found by computing the limit:

$$\begin{aligned}
\text{Instantaneous rate of change} &= \lim_{h\to 0} \frac{D(20+h) - D(20)}{h} \\
&= \lim_{h\to 0} \frac{0.015(20+h)^2 - 0.015(20)^2}{h} \\
&= 0.015 \lim_{h\to 0} \frac{(400 + 40h + h^2 - 400)}{h} \\
&= 0.015 \lim_{h\to 0} (40 + h) \\
&= 0.6 \quad \text{millimeter per day}
\end{aligned}$$

That is, on day 20 the size of the tumor is increasing at the rate of 0.6 millimeter per day. This instantaneous rate of change is the slope of the tangent line at (20, 6) as shown in Figure 15. □

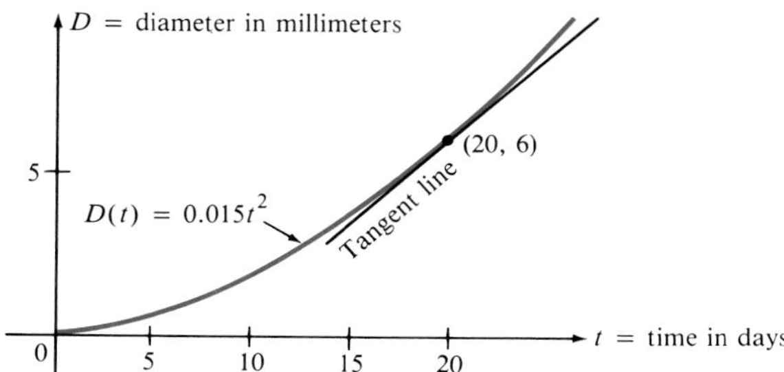

Figure 15
The slope of the tangent line gives the instantaneous growth rate

Instantaneous Velocity

Calculus was introduced originally to study the movement of the earth and the other planets around the sun. This brings us in a natural way to the concept of instantaneous velocity. This book is mostly devoted to the applications of the calculus to business and the life sciences; but since the study of motion is so basic to the calculus, we discuss the basics of motion here.

To illustrate the concept of velocity, imagine driving from Denver to Omaha on Interstate 80. The distance traveled from Denver after t hours is denoted by the position versus time curve $s(t)$ shown in Figure 16.

From Figure 16 we can make the following observations concerning the journey. The total distance traveled from Denver to Omaha during the 10 hours was

$$\begin{aligned}
\text{Distance traveled} &= s(10) - s(0) \\
&= 540 - 0 \\
&= 540 \quad \text{miles}
\end{aligned}$$

Since the car traveled 540 miles during a 10-hour period, we say that the average velocity of the car during the course of the trip was $\frac{540}{10} = 54$ miles per hour.

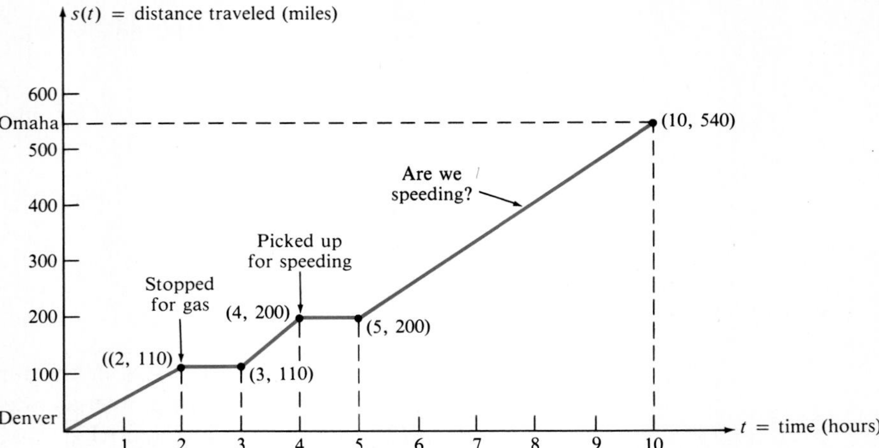

Figure 16
Road trip from Denver to Omaha

We write this as

$$\text{Average velocity} = \frac{s(10) - s(0)}{10}$$

$$= 54 \quad \text{miles per hour}$$

However, just because the average velocity of the car was 54 miles per hour during the 10-hour trip, it does not necessarily follow that the car traveled at exactly that rate of speed during the entire trip. Sometimes the car may have gone faster, and sometimes it may have gone slower.

While the average velocity may be useful for some purposes, it is not always important. If we were to run head-on into a tree, we would no doubt be more concerned with the instantaneous velocity at the exact instant of impact than with the average velocity over the entire trip.

The concept of instantaneous velocity has baffled mathematicians from the very earliest times. It was not until the advent of the calculus that mathematicians gained a clear understanding of the concept. The difficulty of understanding instantaneous velocity lies in the fact that when we use the word "instantaneous," we are referring to something that happens at a certain *instant* of time. This is in contrast to something that happens over an interval—one hour, one minute, one second, and so on. Instantaneous means that something happens so fast that no time elapses. If this is true, then in the case of instantaneous velocity the distance traveled is 0, the elapsed time is 0, and so the average velocity must be $\frac{0}{0}$, which of course is meaningless.

The way we understand instantaneous velocity today, having the power of the calculus at our disposal, is to think in terms of limits. For instance, suppose we wish to find the instantaneous velocity at exactly 25 seconds after leaving Denver for Omaha. Although the velocity of the car may be varying at this instant of time, it is clear that over a short period of time—say, from 25 seconds to 25.1 seconds—the change in velocity will be very small. We can then approximate the instantaneous velocity at 25 seconds by computing the average velocity over the time interval from 25 seconds to 25.1 seconds. This average velocity can be computed by measuring the distance traveled during the time period from 25 seconds to 25.1 seconds and then dividing by the time elapsed, which is 0.1 second. The error that results from approximating the instantaneous velocity by the average velocity will decrease as the length of the time interval over which the average velocity was computed decreases. We would expect that the average velocity between 25 seconds and 25.01 seconds would be a better approximation to the instantaneous velocity at 25 seconds than the average velocity between 25 seconds and 25.1 seconds. Thus if the average velocity is computed for smaller and smaller time intervals, the average velocity should approach the instantaneous velocity.

This discussion leads us to the formal definition of instantaneous velocity.

Definition of Instantaneous Velocity

Let $s(t)$ be a function that gives the location of an object (such as a car) moving along a line (such as a road) as a function of time t. The **instantaneous velocity** of the object at time t_0 is the limiting value of the average velocity of the object during the time from t_0 to $t_0 + h$ as h approaches zero. Since the average velocity of the object during the time from t_0 to $t_0 + h$ is

$$\text{Average velocity on } [t_0, t_0 + h] = \frac{s(t_0 + h) - s(t_0)}{h}$$

the instantaneous velocity at t_0 is the limit

$$v(t_0) = \lim_{h \to 0} \frac{s(t_0 + h) - s(t_0)}{h}$$

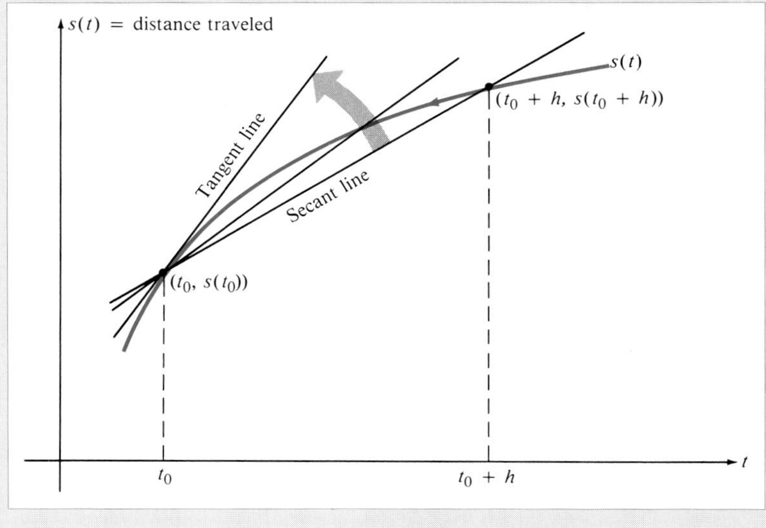

Observe that velocity is the instantaneous rate of change of the position $s(t)$. If $s(t)$ is measured in miles and t in hours, then the instantaneous velocity will have units of miles per hour.

Instantaneous Velocity of a Falling Ball

Suppose you drop a ball from the top of a tall building. Have you ever wondered how far it falls after one second? After two seconds? After three seconds? Galileo discovered that (in the absence of air friction) the exact distance $s(t)$ in feet that the ball will fall in t seconds is given by the quadratic function of time

$$s(t) = 16t^2$$

as illustrated in Figure 17. Table 7 gives the distance the ball falls during given periods of time.

TABLE 7
Object Falling under the Influence of Gravity

Elapsed Time (seconds)	Distance Fallen (feet)
0	0
1	16
2	64
3	144
4	256
5	400
6	576
7	784
8	1024

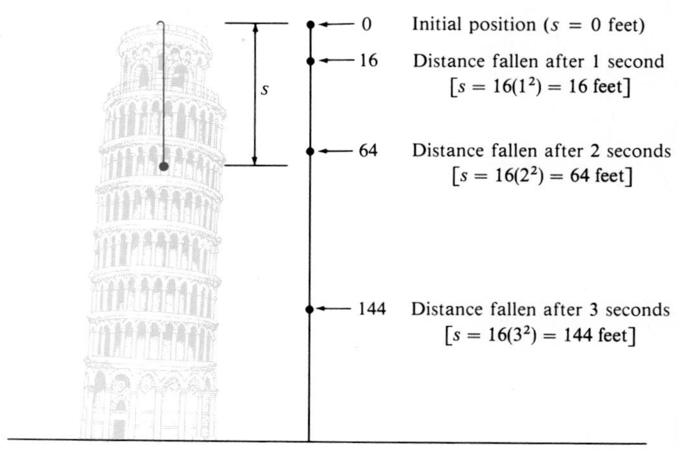

Figure 17
Distance that an object falls in t seconds

To determine the velocity (instantaneous) of the ball after t seconds, we compute the limit of the average velocity during the time interval $[t, t + h]$ as h goes to zero. That is,

$$\begin{aligned} v(t) &= \lim_{h\to 0} \frac{s(t+h) - s(t)}{h} \\ &= \lim_{h\to 0} \frac{16(t+h)^2 - 16t^2}{h} \\ &= \lim_{h\to 0} \frac{16(t^2 + 2ht + h^2) - 16t^2}{h} \\ &= \lim_{h\to 0} 16(2t + h) \\ &= 32t \quad \text{feet per second} \end{aligned}$$

In other words, after t seconds we have

$$\text{Position of the ball} = 16t^2 \text{ feet}$$
$$\text{Velocity of the ball} = 32t \text{ feet per second}$$

Table 8 gives the distance fallen and the velocity of the ball after different periods of elapsed time.

TABLE 8
State of Ball Dropped from Building

Time Elapsed (seconds)	Distance Fallen (feet)	Velocity (feet/seconds)
0	0	0
1	16	32
2	64	64
3	144	96
4	256	128
5	400	160
6	576	192
7	784	224
8	1024	256
9	1296	288
10	1600	320

Problems

For Problems 1–8, graph the function

$$f(x) = 3x + 2$$

and find the following quantities. Interpret the meaning of each quantity.

1. $f(2)$

2. $f(2 + 0.5) - f(2)$

3. $\dfrac{f(2 + 0.5) - f(2)}{0.5}$

4. $f(2 + h) - f(2)$

5. $\dfrac{f(2 + h) - f(2)}{h}$

6. $\lim\limits_{h \to 0} \dfrac{f(2 + h) - f(2)}{h}$

7. $\lim\limits_{h \to 0} \dfrac{f(3 + h) - f(3)}{h}$

8. $\lim\limits_{h \to 0} \dfrac{f(4 + h) - f(4)}{h}$

Problems 9–22 concern themselves with the function $f(x) = x^2$ graphed in Figure 18. For each problem, find the indicated change.

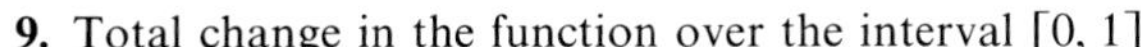

9. Total change in the function over the interval $[0, 1]$.
10. Total change in the function over the interval $[0, 2]$.
11. Total change in the function over the interval $[1, 3]$.
12. Total change in the function over the interval $[-1, 1]$.
13. Total change in the function over the interval $[-2, 0]$.

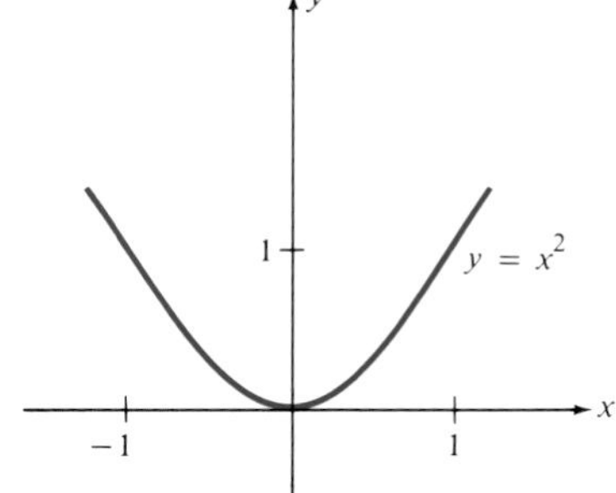

Figure 18
Graph for Problems 9–22

14. Average change in the function over the interval $[0, 1]$.
15. Average change in the function over the interval $[0, 2]$.
16. Average change in the function over the interval $[1, 3]$.
17. Average change in the function over the interval $[-1, 1]$.
18. Average change in the function over the interval $[-2, 0]$.
19. Instantaneous rate of change at $x = 1$.
20. Instantaneous rate of change at $x = 2$.
21. Instantaneous rate of change at $x = -1$.
22. Instantaneous rate of change at $x = -2$.

Falling Ball

For Problems 23–27, the function

$$s(t) = 16t^2$$

represents the distance in feet a ball falls (in the absence of air friction) in t seconds when dropped from a tall building. Assuming no air friction find the indicated quantities.

23. Find the distance fallen during the first 3 seconds.
24. Find the distance fallen during the first 10 seconds.
25. Find the velocity of the ball at time $t = 3$ seconds.
26. Find the velocity of the ball at time $t = 10$ seconds.
27. At what time will the instantaneous velocity be the same as the average velocity over the first 5 seconds?

Instantaneous Velocity

For Problems 28–32, a particle moves along a straight line where $s(t)$ is the distance traveled in feet at time t seconds. Find the velocity of the particle at time t for the given functions.

28. $s(t) = 5$
29. $s(t) = t$
30. $s(t) = 5t + 7$
31. $s(t) = t^2 + 4$
32. $s(t) = 4t^2 + 3t$

Other Rates of Change

Find the instantaneous rate of change of the quantities in Problems 33–34 with respect to the radius r.

33. The circumference C of a circle, where $C = 2\pi r$.
34. The area A of a circle, where $A = \pi r^2$.

Changing Demand for Gasoline

Suppose the daily demand $D(p)$ for automobile gasoline in the United States as a function of price p has been determined to be

$$D(p) = \frac{(p-5)^4}{10} \qquad (0.5 \le p \le 5)$$

where D is measured in millions of gallons and p is measured in dollars. The graph of $D(p)$ is shown in Figure 19.

35. Find the total decrease in demand when the price of gasoline is raised from \$1 to \$5.
36. Find the average decrease in demand in millions of gallons per dollar when the price is raised from \$1 to \$5.
37. Find the total decrease in demand when the price is raised from \$2 to \$5.
38. Find the average decrease in demand when the price is increased from \$2 to \$5.

Seborrheic Lesion

A seborrheic lesion or sore has been treated with a new form of hydrocortisone, and its size is measured over the course of ten days. The observations in Table 9 were taken. Find the quantities in Problems 39–44.

TABLE 9
Observations of Seborrheic Lesion

Day	Lesion Size (cm)
0	5.1
1	4.6
2	3.9
3	3.3
4	2.7
5	2.2
6	1.7
7	1.3
8	0.7
9	0.3
10	0.0

39. The total decrease in lesion size during the ten-day period.
40. The average decrease in lesion size during the ten-day period.
41. The total decrease in lesion size during the first five days.
42. The average decrease in lesion size during the first five days.

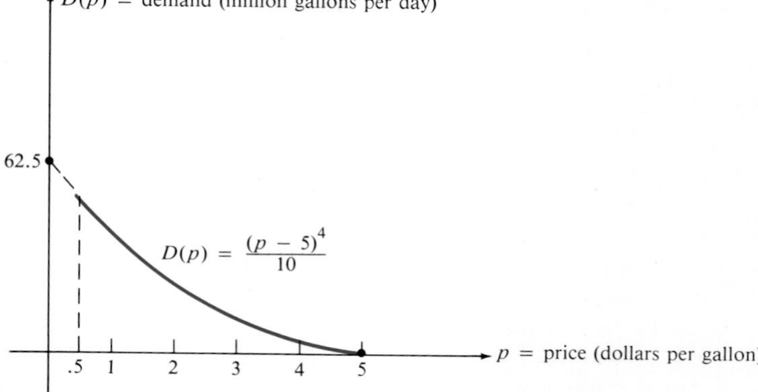

Figure 19
Demand curve for gasoline

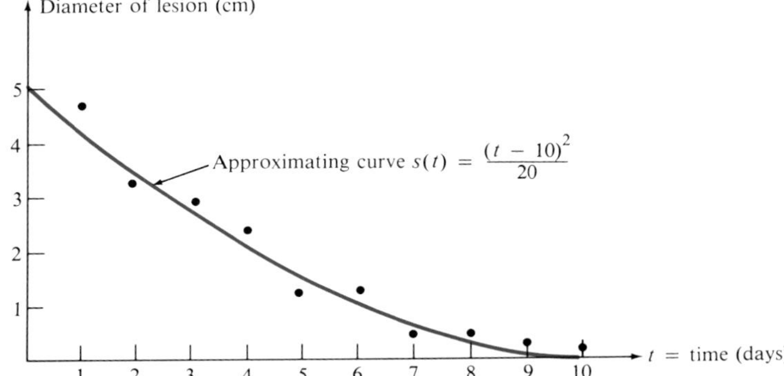

Figure 20
Shrinking of a seborrheic lesion

43. The total decrease in lesion size during the last five days.

44. The average decrease in lesion size during the last five days.

Medical Problem

Suppose a medical researcher constructs a mathematical model or equation describing the size of a lesion. The equation that describes the diameter of a lesion (cm) as a function of time (days) is given by

$$D(t) = \frac{(t-10)^2}{20} \qquad 0 \le t \le 10$$

as illustrated in Figure 20.

45. What is the instantaneous rate of change of the lesion size on day 5?

46. What is the instantaneous rate of change of the lesion size on day 7?

47. What is the instantaneous rate of change of the lesion size on day 1?

Olympic Swimming Times (Are Women Catching Up?)

Table 10 shows the winning Olympic swimming times for the men's and women's 100-meter freestyle event during the time period 1912–1984. The last column shows the percentage dif-

TABLE 10
Winning 100-Meter Freestyle Times (1912–1984 Olympic Games)

Year	Men's 100-Meter Freestyle (min:sec)		Women's 100-Meter Freestyle (min:sec)		Percentage Difference in Times
1912	1:03.4	(U.S.)	1:22.2	(Australia)	29.7%
1920	1:01.4	(U.S.)	1:13.6	(U.S.)	19.9%
1924	0:59.0	(U.S.)	1:12.4	(U.S.)	22.7%
1928	0:58.6	(U.S.)	1:11.0	(U.S.)	21.2%
1932	0:58.2	(Japan)	1:06.8	(U.S.)	14.8%
1936	0:57.6	(Hungary)	1:05.9	(Netherlands)	14.4%
1948	0:57.3	(U.S.)	1:06.3	(Denmark)	15.7%
1952	0:57.4	(U.S.)	1:06.8	(Hungary)	16.0%
1956	0:55.4	(Australia)	1:02.0	(Australia)	11.9%
1960	0:55.2	(Australia)	1:01.2	(Australia)	10.5%
1964	0:53.4	(U.S.)	0:59.5	(Australia)	11.4%
1968	0:52.2	(Australia)	1:00.0	(U.S.)	14.5%
1972	0:51.22	(U.S.)	0:58.59	(U.S.)	14.4%
1976	0:49.99	(U.S.)	0:55.65	(GDR)	11.3%
1980	0:50.40	(GDR)	0:54.79	(GDR)	8.7%
1984	0:49.80	(U.S.)	0:55.92	(U.S.)	12.8%

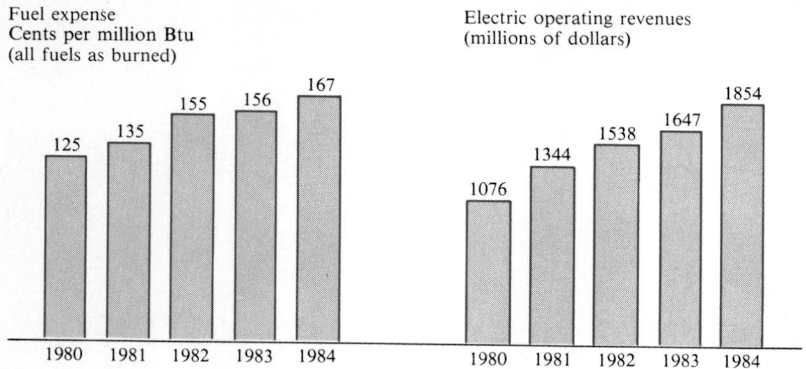

Figure 21
Fuel expense and revenues of a power and light company.

ference between the men's and women's times. That is,

$$\text{Percentage difference} = 100\,\frac{\text{Women's times} - \text{Men's times}}{\text{Men's times}}$$

48. What was the total change in the percentage difference during the years from 1912 to 1984?

49. What was the average change per year in the percentage difference from 1912 to 1984?

50. What was the average change per Olympic Games in the percentage difference during the years from 1912 to 1984? *Hint:* The Olympic Games occurred 28 times in that span of years.

51. What was the average change in the men's times during the period from 1912 to 1984?

52. What was the average change in the women's times during the period from 1912 to 1984?

Annual Report

Figure 21 shows the annual fuel expenses and revenues (what they take in) during the period 1980–1984 for a given power and light company.

53. Find the average yearly increase in cost of fuel during this period.

54. Find the average yearly increase in revenues during this period.

Annual Report

Figure 22, which shows circulation during the period 1976–1985, was taken from the annual report of the Gannett Co., Inc. Gannett has become one of the most innovative media companies in the United States in recent years. For Problems 55–56, find the indicated quantities.

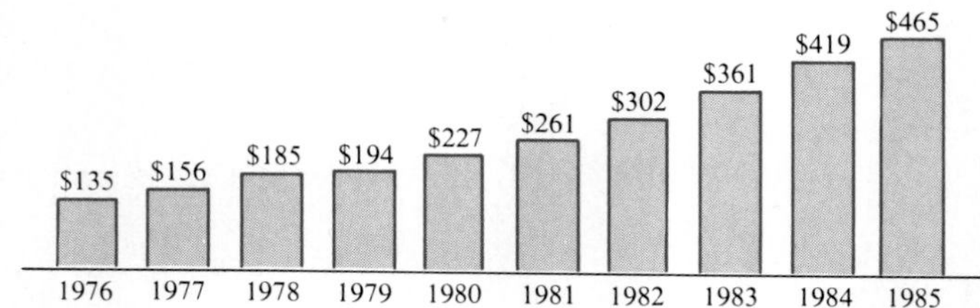

Figure 22
Gannett circulation revenues (in millions of dollars)

55. Find the total change in circulation revenue during the time period from 1976 to 1985.

56. Find the average change in circulation revenue during the time period 1976–1985.

1.4 Introduction to the Derivative

PURPOSE

We define the derivative of a function f at a point x and give

- a geometric interpretation of the derivative and
- a precise definition of the tangent line to a graph.

We will also show how the derivative is used in economics to study the rate of change of supply and demand curves.

What Is and What Is Not a Tangent Line

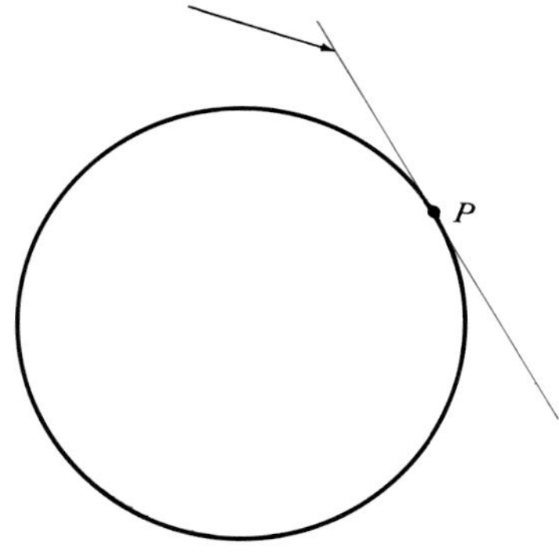

Figure 23
Geometric representation of a tangent line

In plane geometry, we say that a line is **tangent** to a circle if it intersects a circle at exactly one point. (See Figure 23.) However, for more general curves, we need a more general definition. Since the basic idea of a tangent line is so important in the development of differential calculus, it is important that we have an accurate understanding of its meaning.* As is true of other concepts in mathematics, there are many "rough" ideas floating around of what a tangent line is, and they are not only rough, but wrong. Before we tell you what a tangent line is, it is useful for you to know what a tangent line is *not*.

The first misconception of a tangent line is

Misconception 1: "A line is tangent to a curve if it crosses the curve at exactly one point."

This is wrong. The line in Figure 24a crosses the curve at exactly one point, but it is not a tangent line. A second misconception is

Misconception 2: "A tangent line to a curve must cross the curve only once."

This is also wrong. The line in Figure 24b is tangent to the curve at P, but it crosses the curve at three other points. Still another misconception that is often heard is

Misconception 3: "A line is tangent to a curve if it touches the curve at exactly one point but does not cross the curve."

Again, we can find a counterexample to this misconception. (See Figure 24c.) Yet another misconception of a tangent line is

Misconception 4: "A tangent line to a curve is a line that just 'grazes' the curve at a point but does not cross the curve."

* This exposition of the tangent line was motivated by Richard V. Andree, "What Is a Geometric Tangent?" *Mathematics Teacher*, Nov. 1957.

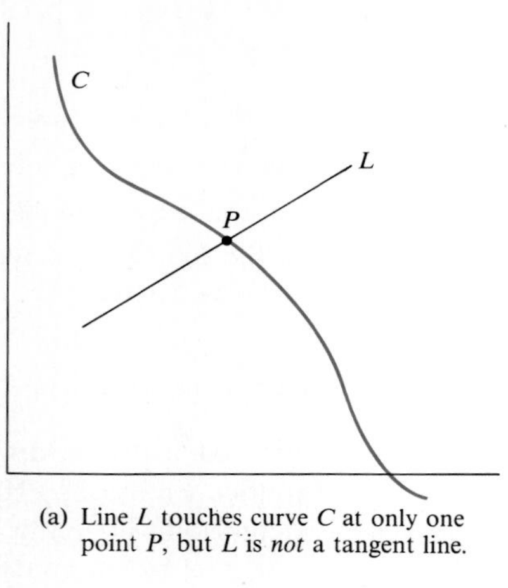

(a) Line L touches curve C at only one point P, but L is *not* a tangent line.

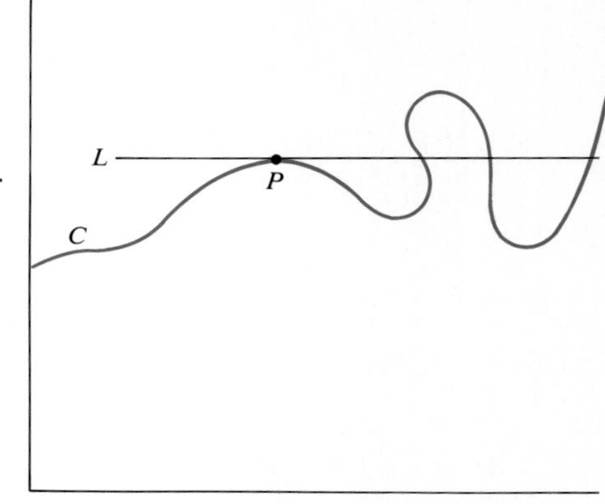

(b) Line L is a tangent to curve C at point P, but it also crosses curve C at three other points.

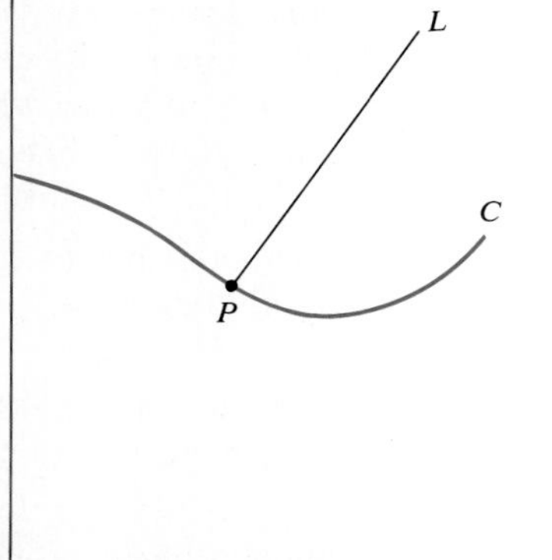

(c) Line segment L touches curve C at point P but does not cross it; however, L is *not* tangent to C at P.

(d) Line L is tangent to curve C at point P, but L also crosses C at P.

Figure 24
What is and what is not a tangent line

This definition would seem to describe our feelings about a tangent line, but it also fails. The line drawn in Figure 24d is tangent to the curve, and it does just "graze" the curve. However, it does cross the curve.

Since we have described some misconceptions that others have made in trying to conceptualize a tangent line, we would like you to spend five minutes writing your own definition.

Now that you have made up your own definition of the tangent line, we will give you the definition mathematicians use today. To this end, we first draw a curve C as shown in Figure 25a on which a fixed point P (the proposed point of tangency) is located. We now select any other point Q on the curve and draw the line, called the **secant line**, passing through P and Q. If we now move Q along the curve toward P, the secant line through P and Q will rotate towards some "limiting" position as shown in Figure 25b. The line occupying this limiting position is called the **tangent line** to the curve at P.

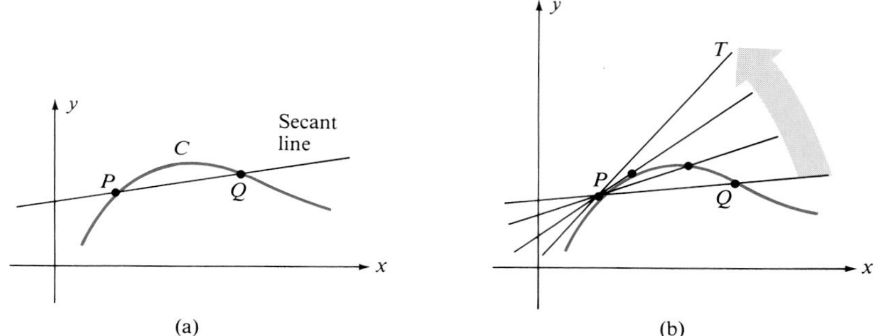

Figure 25
The limiting secant line gives the tangent line

Now that we have a precise meaning of the tangent line, we can introduce the most important concept of this chapter, the derivative.

The Meaning of the Derivative

We select an arbitrary point $P = (a, f(a))$ on the graph of a function $y = f(x)$ and draw the secant line through this point and a neighboring point on the graph $Q = (a + h, f(a + h))$. (See Figure 26.)

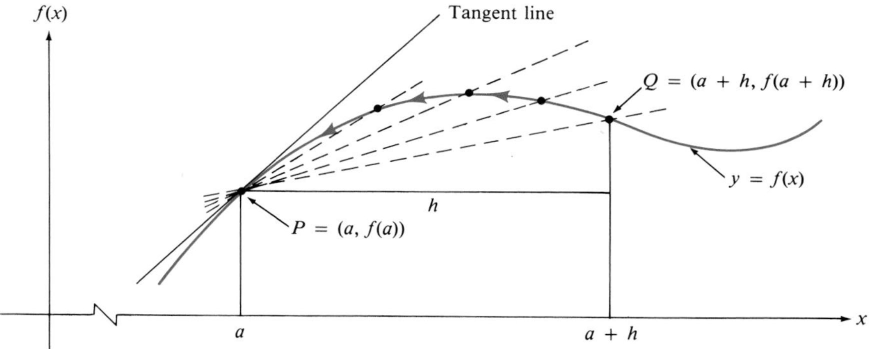

Figure 26
Geometric interpretation of the derivative

The slope of this secant line connecting P and Q is clearly

$$\text{Slope of secant line} = \frac{f(a + h) - f(a)}{h}$$

We now move Q along the graph toward P (or equivalently let h approach 0). As Q approaches P (or $h \to 0$), the secant line connecting P and Q will approach the tangent line at P, and the slopes of the secant lines will approach the slope of the tangent line $m_{\tan}$:

$$m_{\tan} = \lim_{h \to 0} \frac{f(a + h) - f(a)}{h}$$

The above limit is the most important limit in the differential calculus, and it leads to the following definition.

Definition of the Derivative

The derivative of the function f at a point a, denoted $f'(a)$ is defined by

$$f'(a) = \lim_{h\to 0} \frac{f(a+h) - f(a)}{h}$$

provided that the limit exists.

Now that we have defined the derivative as the limiting value of the slopes of the secant lines (provided that this limit exists), we can define the tangent line more formally in terms of the derivative.

Calculus Definition of the Tangent Line

The tangent line to the graph of a function f at the point $(a, f(a))$ is the straight line passing through $(a, f(a))$ with slope

$$f'(a) = \lim_{h\to 0} \frac{f(a+h) - f(a)}{h}$$

provided that the limit exists. If this limit does not exist, the function does not have a tangent line at the point $(a, f(a))$. Using the point-slope formula, we find that the equation of this tangent line is

$$y - f(a) = f'(a)(x - a)$$

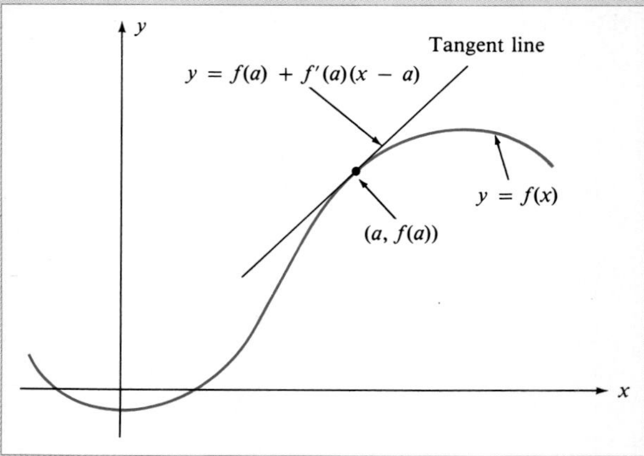

Example 1

Secant and Tangent Line Find the secant line to the graph of $f(x) = x^2$ that passes through the points (1, 1) and (2, 4). Then find the tangent line to the graph at (1, 1).

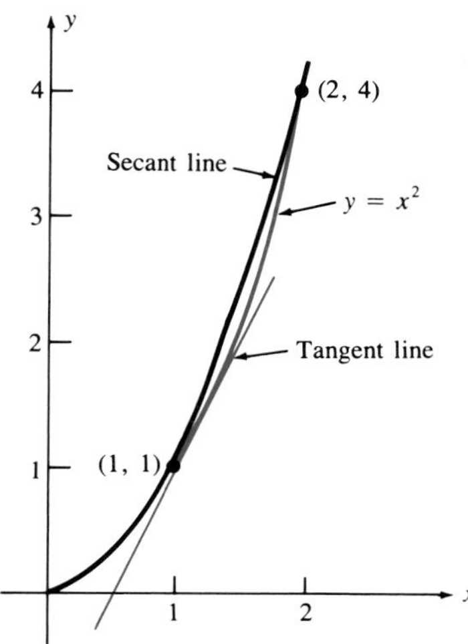

Figure 27
The secant line for $y = x^2$ through (1, 1) and (2, 4) and the tangent line at (1, 1)

Solution The graph of $f(x) = x^2$ along with the secant and tangent lines are draw in Figure 27.

To find the secant line that passes through the points (1, 1) and (2, 4), we first compute its slope:

$$\text{Slope} = \frac{4 - 1}{2 - 1} = 3$$

Hence from the point-slope formula the equation of the secant line is

$$\frac{y - 1}{x - 1} = 3$$

or, written in slope-intercept form

$$y = 3x - 2$$

To find the tangent line to the curve at (1, 1), we first find the derivative of $f(x) = x^2$ when $x = 1$. That is,

$$\begin{aligned} f'(1) &= \lim_{h \to 0} \frac{f(1 + h) - f(1)}{h} \\ &= \lim_{h \to 0} \frac{(1 + h)^2 - 1^2}{h} \\ &= \lim_{h \to 0} \frac{(1 + 2h + h^2) - 1}{h} \\ &= \lim_{h \to 0} (2 + h) \\ &= 2 \end{aligned}$$

In other words, when $x = 1$, the value of x^2 is changing by two units for each unit change in x.

Using this derivative, we find the tangent line to the graph of $f(x) = x^2$ at (1, 1) to be

$$y - f(1) = f'(1)(x - 1)$$
$$y - 1 = 2(x - 1)$$

or

$$y = 2x - 1$$

□

Example 2

Computing the Derivative Find the derivative of $f(x) = x^2$ at an arbitrary point $x = a$.

Solution Using the definition of the derivative, we have

$$\begin{aligned} f'(a) &= \lim_{h\to 0} \frac{f(a+h) - f(a)}{h} \\ &= \lim_{h\to 0} \frac{(a+h)^2 - a^2}{h} \\ &= \lim_{h\to 0} \frac{(a^2 + 2ah + h^2) - a^2}{h} \\ &= \lim_{h\to 0} (2a + h) \\ &= 2a \end{aligned}$$

□

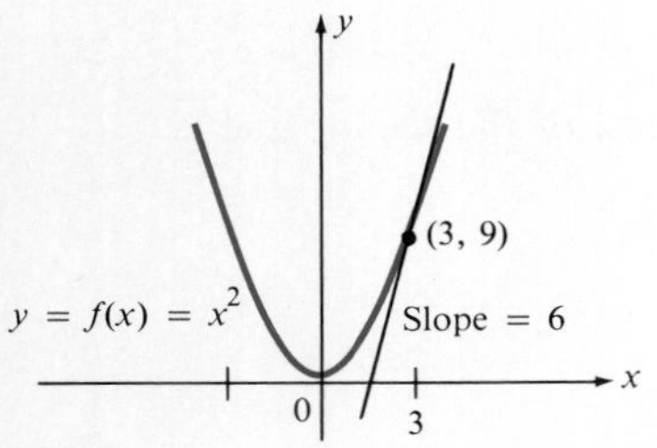

Figure 28
The derivative represents the slope of the tangent line

Since $x = a$ is an arbitrary real number, it is often customary to replace a by x and refer to the derivative at an arbitrary real number x. In this example the derivative of $f(x) = x^2$ at an arbitrary x is

$$f'(x) = 2x$$

This derivative gives the slope of the tangent line to the curve $f(x) = x^2$ at any point $(x, f(x))$. Keep in mind that $f'(x)$ gives the rate of change of the function f at x, whereas $f(x)$ gives the value of the function f at x. Figure 28 illustrates this idea.

HISTORICAL NOTE

Originally, the subject of the limit was a subject for debate. The concept of "infinitely small" quantities, which were the forerunners of the limit, were awfully hard to take by many people. Even the brilliant Johann Bernoulli once said, "A quantity which is increased or decreased by an infinitely small quantity is neither increased nor decreased."

One of the more able critics of the early calculus was the eminent metaphysician Bishop George Berkeley (1685–1753). He once referred to the derivative as "ghosts of departed quantities."

Derivative Notation

The process of finding a derivative is called **differentiation**. If the independent variable is x, then differentiation of some quantity $[*]$ is often denoted by

$$\frac{d}{dx}[*]$$

which is read "the derivative of $*$ with respect to x."

For example, we would write

$$\frac{d}{dx}[x^2] = 2x$$

The d/dx notation can be used to find derivatives of functions involving variables other than x. For example, if the independent variable is t, then we would replace x by t and write

$$\frac{d}{dt}[t^2] = 2t$$

The major failing of the d/dx notation is that it is difficult to express the derivative at a specific point. Here, the **prime notation** is better suited. For example, to represent the value of the derivative of f at the specific point $x = a$, the two notations are

Prime notation: $f'(a)$

d/dx notation: $\left.\frac{df(x)}{dx}\right|_{x=a}$

Clearly, the prime notation is simpler.

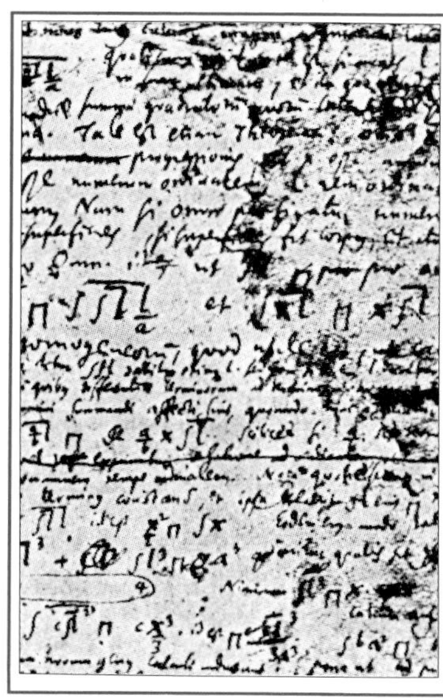

HISTORICAL NOTE

Baron Gottfried Wilhelm von Leibniz was very careful to develop proper mathematical notation. His work in logic had made him aware that symbols should be chosen with great care and should appeal to one's intuition. It was Leibniz who devised the *d/dx* notation for the derivative.

The followers of Newton in England did not use the Leibniz *d/dx* notation; they used Newton's inferior "fluxions." As a result, Newton's followers were unable to solve many problems that Leibniz and his followers found almost trivial, and Newton's followers became helplessly bogged down in a notational quagmire. As a result of these notational difficulties, English mathematics lagged behind the mathematics of Europe during the 1700's. It was not until the 1800's and the arrival of the English school of algebraists, led by Arthur Cayley and James Joseph Sylvester, that English mathematics fully recovered.

Example 3 Finding the Derivative Find the derivative of

$$f(x) = \frac{1}{x}$$

at an arbitrary point $x \neq 0$.

Solution Using the limit definition of the derivative, we can write

$$f'(x) = \lim_{h\to 0} \frac{f(x+h) - f(x)}{h} \qquad \text{(definition of the derivative)}$$

$$= \lim_{h\to 0} \frac{\dfrac{1}{x+h} - \dfrac{1}{x}}{h} \qquad \text{(direct substitution)}$$

$$= \lim_{h\to 0} \frac{x - (x+h)}{x(x+h)h} \qquad \text{(simple algebra)}$$

$$= \lim_{h\to 0} \frac{-1}{x(x+h)} \qquad \text{(more algebra)}$$

$$= \frac{-1}{\lim_{h\to 0} (x^2 + hx)} \qquad \text{(the limit of a quotient is the quotient of the limits)}$$

$$= -\frac{1}{x^2} \qquad \text{(evaluating the above limit)}$$

□

Example 4 Finding Derivatives Find the derivative of $f(x) = \sqrt{x}$.

Solution Using the definition of the derivative, we write

$$f'(x) = \lim_{h\to 0} \frac{\sqrt{x+h} - \sqrt{x}}{h} \qquad \text{(definition of the derivative)}$$

$$= \lim_{h\to 0} \frac{\sqrt{x+h} - \sqrt{x}}{h} \cdot \frac{\sqrt{x+h} + \sqrt{x}}{\sqrt{x+h} + \sqrt{x}} \qquad \text{(multiply the numerator and denominator by the conjugate)}$$

$$= \lim_{h\to 0} \frac{(x+h) - x}{h(\sqrt{x+h} + \sqrt{x})} \qquad \text{(algebra)}$$

$$= \lim_{h\to 0} \frac{1}{\sqrt{x+h} + \sqrt{x}} \qquad \text{(algebra)}$$

$$= \frac{1}{\lim_{h\to 0} (\sqrt{x+h} + \sqrt{x})} \qquad \text{(the limit of a quotient is the quotient of the limits)}$$

$$= \frac{1}{2\sqrt{x}} \qquad \text{(evaluate the above limit)}$$

Figure 29 interprets this derivative by showing some tangent lines to the function $f(x) = \sqrt{x}$. □

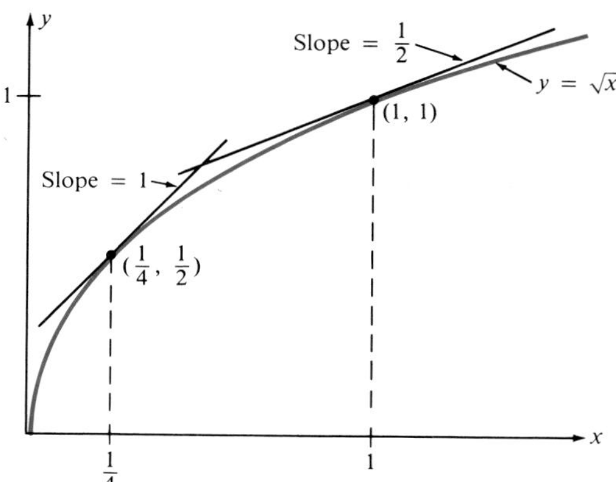

Figure 29
Slopes of tangent lines to $y = \sqrt{x}$ at $x = \frac{1}{4}$ and $x = 1$

Example 5

Derivative at a Point If $y = x^2$, find

$$\left.\frac{dy}{dx}\right|_{x=0} \quad \text{and} \quad \left.\frac{dy}{dx}\right|_{x=3}$$

Solution The derivative of $y = x^2$ at x is

$$\frac{dy}{dx} = 2x$$

Hence simply evaluating this derivative at the points 0 and 3, we have

$$\left.\frac{dy}{dx}\right|_{x=0} = 0 \qquad \left.\frac{dy}{dx}\right|_{x=3} = 6$$

□

Steps for Finding the Derivative

Given $y = f(x)$:

Step 1. Compute the value $f(x + h)$.

Step 2. Compute the difference $f(x + h) - f(x)$.

Step 3. Compute the quotient

$$\frac{f(x + h) - f(x)}{h}$$

Step 4. Compute the limit

$$\frac{df(x)}{dx} = \lim_{h \to 0} \frac{f(x + h) - f(x)}{h}$$

When the Derivative Fails to Exist

There are three common ways in which a function can fail to have a derivative at a point. Roughly, they are

1. The graph of the function has a break.
2. The graph of the function has a corner-point.
3. The graph of the function has a vertical tangent line.

In all of these cases it is impossible to draw a unique, nonvertical tangent line to the graph at the given point. We illustrate in Figure 30 some functions that fail to have derivatives at different points.

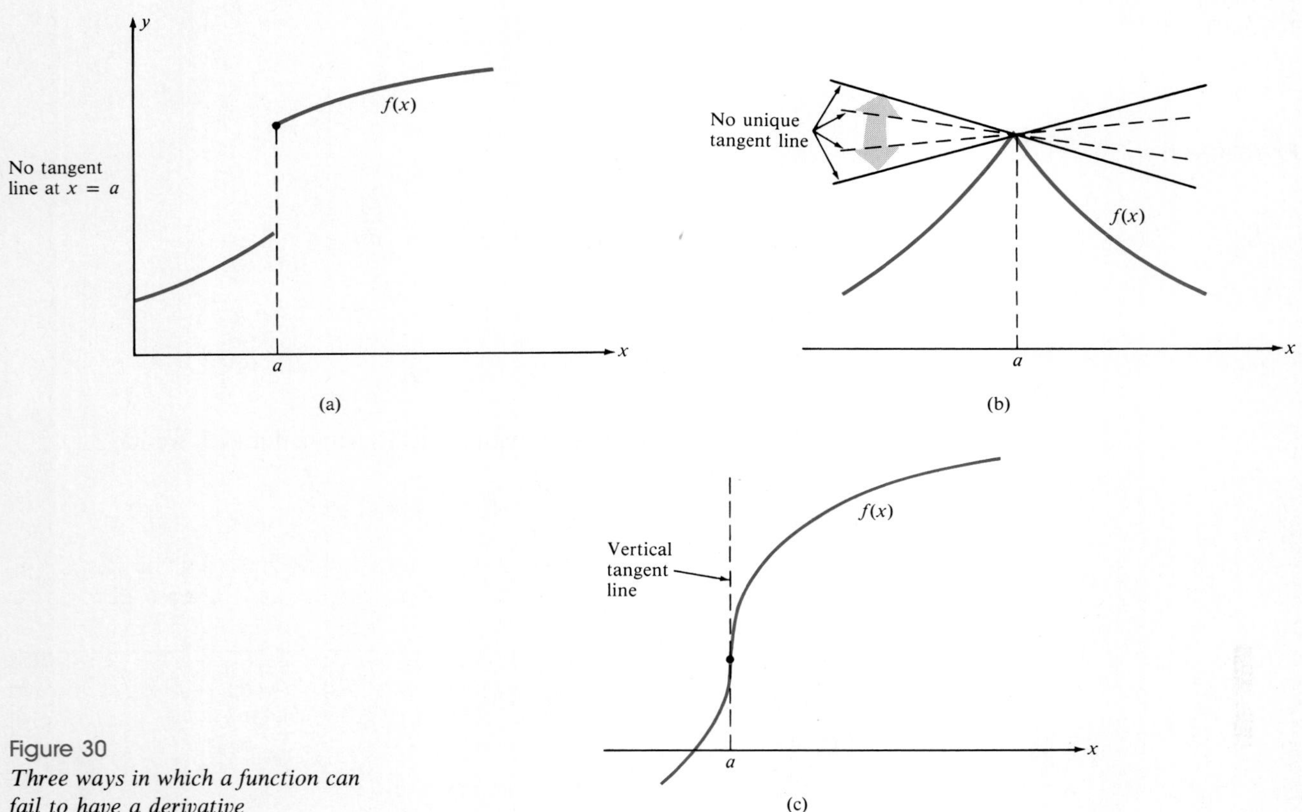

Figure 30
Three ways in which a function can fail to have a derivative

Relationship between Differentiable and Continuous Functions

A differentiable function is generally thought of as an improvement over a continuous function. Whereas a function that is continuous at a point may fail to have a derivative at that point, a function that has a derivative at a point is automatically continuous at that point. We state and verify this basic relationship between the concepts of differentiability and continuity here.

Differentiability Implies Continuity

If f is differentiable at a, then f is continuous at a. To verify this, we write

$$\begin{aligned}\lim_{h\to 0}[f(a+h)-f(a)] &= \lim_{h\to 0}\left[\frac{f(a+h)-f(a)}{h}\right]h \quad &&\text{(divide and multiply by } h\text{)}\\ &= \lim_{h\to 0}\frac{f(a+h)-f(a)}{h}\cdot\lim_{h\to 0}h\\ &= f'(a)\cdot\lim_{h\to 0}h &&\text{(since } f \text{ is differentiable at } a\text{)}\\ &= f'(a)\cdot 0\\ &= 0\end{aligned}$$

Hence

$$\lim_{h\to 0}[f(a+h)-f(a)]=0$$

$$\lim_{h\to 0}f(a+h)-\lim_{h\to 0}f(a)=0$$

Hence

$$\lim_{h\to 0}f(a+h)=\lim_{h\to 0}f(a)=f(a)$$

This verifies that f is continuous at a.

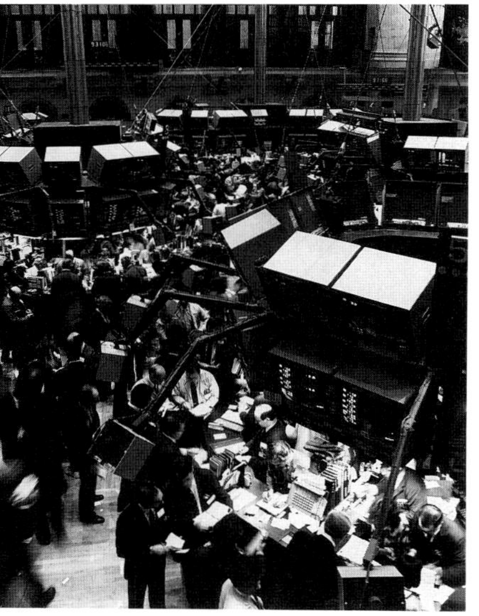

Supply and demand curves play an important role in determining the price of stocks on the New York Stock Exchange.

Derivatives of the Supply and Demand Curves

In recent years, economists have put calculus to good use. Of the past 20 recipients of Nobel prizes in economics, many have used concepts from calculus. For example, the 1978 winner, Herbert Simon, used ideas of calculus to analyze decision-making processes in economic organizations. Two years later, Lawrence Klein from the University of Pennsylvania won the Nobel prize in economics for his studies in economic forecasting. His ideas, too, use concepts of calculus. We now show how differential calculus can be used to analyze the supply and demand curves in economics.

Let us suppose that corn is being sold on the Chicago Board of Trade. The amount of corn offered every day by farmers and other sellers depends on the price offered. Some farmers will be willing to sell their corn at a fairly low price, while others will be willing to sell only at a higher price. The total quantity q of corn that farmers and other sellers will offer for sale at a given price p defines a **supply curve**:

$$q = S(p)$$

On the other hand, from the buyers' point of view the amount q of corn purchased by exporters, traders, and others also depends on the price p of the corn. The higher the price of corn, the smaller the quantity of corn that will be purchased. The lower the price of corn, the greater the quantity of corn that will be purchased by the buyers. The exact relationship between the quantity q that buyers are willing to buy (that they demand) and the price of the corn p defines the **demand curve**:

$$q = D(p)$$

Typical supply and demand curves are graphed in Figure 31.

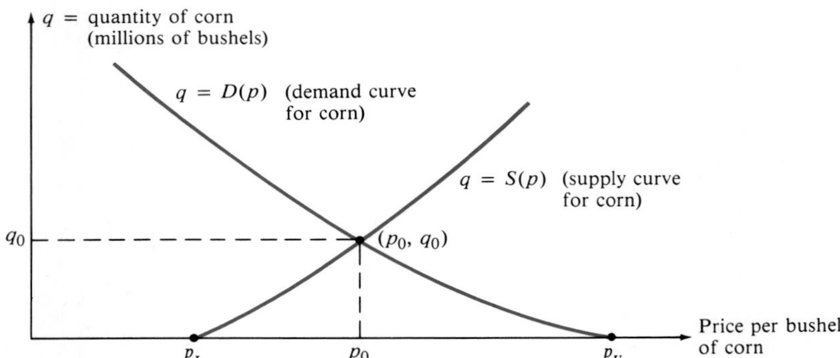

Figure 31
Supply and demand curves for corn

In Figure 31, we see that the supply curve is negative when the price p is less than some value p_L. The number p_L is called the **lower price limit**, and it represents the lowest price at which someone will be willing to sell some corn. If the price is less than p_L, no one will be willing to sell any corn.

Farther up the price scale we have the number p_U, which is called the **upper price limit**. This number represents the highest price at which any buyer will buy corn.

Observe that the supply curve is always increasing with price, while the demand curve is always decreasing with price. (Do you understand why this should be?) The curves will intersect at a point (p_0, q_0). This point of intersection is called the **market equilibrium point**. In a competitive market the price p_0 of the commodity and the amount q_0 of commodity demanded and sold will tend to stabilize at this point. In other words, the price of corn will stabilize at p_0, and the amount of corn demanded and sold will stabilize at q_0.

To see how calculus can be used to analyze the supply and demand curves, first consider the derivative of the supply curve:

$$\frac{dq}{dp} = \frac{dS(p)}{dp}$$

In this problem the derivative represents the rate of change of the corn supplied by sellers as a function of the price of the corn. It can be interpreted as the reaction by the sellers to a given change in price. For example, if

$$\left.\frac{dS}{dp}\right|_{p=\$3.50} = 2 \quad \text{million bushels per dollar}$$

then for every dollar increase (or fraction thereof) in the price of corn up from \$3.50, there will be an increase in the quantity of corn offered of two million bushels. (See Figure 32.)

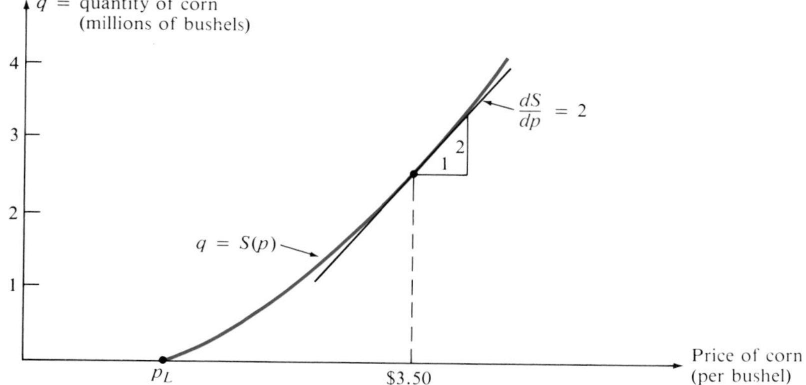

Figure 32
Slope of the supply curve for corn when the price is \$3.50

On the other hand, the derivative of the demand curve

$$\frac{dq}{dp} = \frac{dD(p)}{dq}$$

represents the reaction by the suppliers to a change in the price. Suppose, for example, that corn is selling at \$3.50 per bushel and that the derivative of the demand curve is

$$\left.\frac{dD}{dp}\right|_{p=\$3.50} = -3$$

This means that when the price of corn is \$3.50 per bushel, a one-dollar increase (or some fraction thereof) in price will cause a decrease of three million bushels in the quantity demanded (or some fraction thereof). For example, an increase of \$0.10 in the price for a bushel of corn from \$3.50 to \$3.60 (one-tenth unit) will result in a decrease in demand of 0.3 million bushels (three-tenths unit) of corn by the consumers. (See Figure 33.)

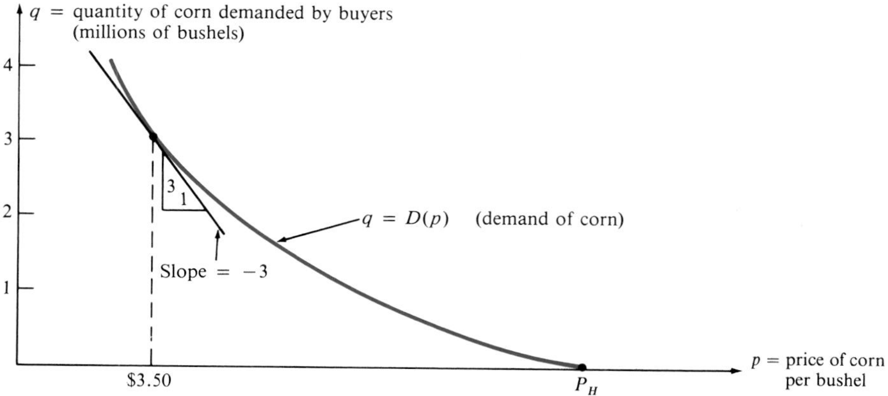

Figure 33
Slope of the demand curve for corn when the price is \$3.50

Example 6

Supply and Demand Suppose the supply and demand curves for corn on the Chicago Board of Trade have been determined by economists to be described by the functions

$$q = S(p) = -1 + 0.10p^2 \qquad \text{(supply curve)}$$
$$q = D(p) = 4 - 0.04p^2 \qquad \text{(demand curve)}$$

Here q is the quantity of corn measured in millions of bushels and p is the price for a bushel of corn measured in dollars.

Suppose corn is currently selling for \$4.00 a bushel. Find and interpret the derivatives of the supply and demand curves at this price.

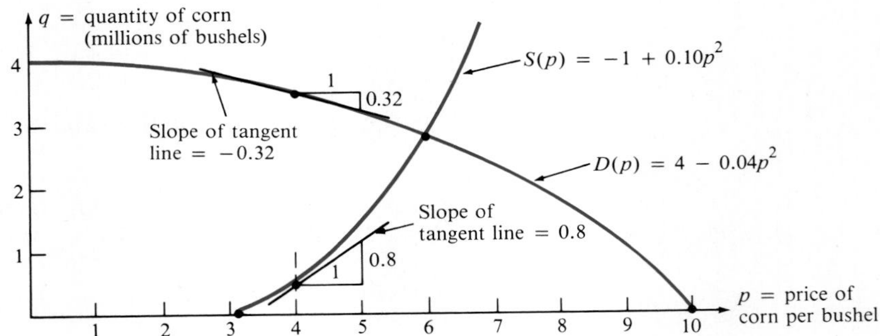

Figure 34
Derivative of supply and demand curves at p = \$4.00

Solution The graphs of the supply and demand curves are shown in Figure 34. The derivative of the supply curve is given by

$$S'(p) = 0.20p$$

When $p = 4.00$, we have

$$\begin{aligned} S'(4.00) &= 0.2(4.00) \\ &= 0.80 \quad \text{million bushels per dollar} \end{aligned}$$

On the other hand, the derivative of the demand curve is

$$D'(p) = -0.08p$$

When $p = \$4.00$, we have

$$\begin{aligned} D'(4.00) &= -0.08(4.00) \\ &= -0.32 \quad \text{million bushels per dollar} \end{aligned}$$

□

Interpretation

Supply derivative: $S'(4.00) = 0.8$

When the price of corn is \$4.00 per bushel, a one-dollar increase in price will result in an increase in supply of 800,000 bushels. If the price of corn increases from \$4.00 to \$4.10 per bushel (one-tenth unit of price), we would expect that sellers (collectively) would increase the supply by 80,000 bushels. On the other hand, if the price falls from \$4.00 to \$3.90, then the supply will decrease by 80,000 bushels.

$$\text{Demand derivative:} \quad D'(4.00) = -0.32$$

When the price of corn is \$4.00 per bushel, a one-dollar increase in price will result in a decrease in demand of 320,000 bushels. If the price of corn increases from \$4.00 to \$4.10 per bushel (one-tenth unit of price), then the demand for corn by the buyers will decrease by 32,000 bushels. On the other hand, if the price falls from \$4.00 to \$3.90, then the demand will increase by 32,000 bushels.

Problems

For Problems 1–4, graph the function

$$f(x) = x^2 + 1$$

and answer the indicated questions. Interpret graphically the quantities computed.

1. What is the equation of the secant line that passes through the points (1, 2) and (2, 5) on the graph of $f(x)$?

2. $f(1 + h) - f(1)$

3. $\dfrac{f(1 + h) - f(1)}{h}$

4. $\lim\limits_{h \to 0} \dfrac{f(1 + h) - f(1)}{h}$

For Problems 5–19, use the definition of the derivative to compute $f'(x)$ for each function. After finding the derivative, compute $f'(0)$ and $f'(1)$.

5. $f(x) = x$

6. $f(x) = 2x$

7. $f(x) = 2x + 3$

8. $f(x) = 5x - 4$

9. $f(x) = x^2$

10. $f(x) = 5x^2$

11. $f(x) = x^2 + x$

12. $f(x) = 3x^2 + 2x$

13. $f(x) = 7x^2 + 5x + 3$

14. $f(x) = 10x^2 - 10x + 20$

15. $f(x) = \dfrac{1}{x}$

16. $f(x) = \dfrac{1}{x + 1}$

17. $f(x) = \dfrac{1}{x^2}$

18. $f(x) = \sqrt{x}$

19. $f(x) = \sqrt{x} + x$

For Problems 20–24, find the slope of the tangent line to the graph at the indicated points. Find the equation of the tangent line.

20. $f(x) = 2x + 3$; (1, 5)

21. $f(x) = x^2$; (2, 4)

22. $f(x) = \dfrac{1}{x + 1}$; (0, 1)

23. $f(x) = \dfrac{1}{x^2}$; (1, 1)

24. $f(x) = \dfrac{1}{x^2}$; (−1, 1)

For Problems 25–30, find the indicated quantities if

$$y = f(x) = x^2$$

25. $f'(0)$

26. $f'(1)$

27. $f'(-1)$

28. $\left.\dfrac{dy}{dx}\right|_{x=3}$

29. $\left.\dfrac{dy}{dx}\right|_{x=4}$

30. $\left.\dfrac{dy}{dx}\right|_{x=-1}$

31. If $y = \sqrt{x} + 1$, find $\left.\dfrac{dy}{dx}\right|_{x=16}$.

32. If $y = \dfrac{1}{x + 1}$, find $\left.\dfrac{dy}{dx}\right|_{x=0}$.

Tangent Lines

For Problems 33–36, find the indicated tangent lines.

33. Find the equation of the tangent line to the graph of

$$f(x) = 3x + 5$$

at the point (0, 5).

34. Find the equation of the tangent line to the graph of

$$f(x) = x^2 + 3$$

at the point (−1, 4).

35. Find the equation of the tangent line to the graph of

$$f(x) = x^2 + 2x$$

at the point (2, 8).

36. Find the equation of the tangent line to the graph of

$$f(x) = \sqrt{x}$$

at the point (1, 1).

Supply and Demand Derivatives

For Problems 37–42, carry out the following steps for the indicated supply and demand curves:

(a) Plot the supply and demand curves.
(b) Find the lower and upper price limits.
(c) Find the equilibrium point.
(d) Find and interpret the derivatives of the supply and demand curves at the indicated prices.

37. $S(p) = 4p - 1$ (linear supply)
$D(p) = 4 - p$ (linear demand)
Price = \$0.50

38. $S(p) = 3p - 5$ (linear supply)
$D(p) = 10 - 2p$ (linear demand)
Price = \$2.50

39. $S(p) = 4p - 1$ (linear supply)
$D(p) = 4 - p^2$ (quadratic demand)
Price = \$1.00

40. $S(p) = p^2 - 16$ (quadratic supply)
$D(p) = -p^2 + 36$ (quadratic demand)
Price = \$4.50

41. $S(p) = p^2 - 2p - 15$ (quadratic supply)
$D(p) = 100 - p^2$ (quadratic demand)
Price = \$7.50

42. $S(p) = p^2 - p - 5$ (quadratic supply)
$D(p) = 50 - p - p^2$ (quadratic demand)
Price = \$4.00

43. Price Elasticity of Demand. Economists refer to the *price elasticity of a demand function* as a measure of the responsiveness between the proportional change in the quantity demanded to the proportional change in the price. That is,

$$E(p) = -\frac{dD/dp}{D/p} \qquad \text{(price elasticity of demand)}$$

(the minus sign is simply to make the sign of the elasticity positive). For the demand function

$$D(p) = 16 - p^2$$

(a) Find the price elasticity $E(p)$ for any price p.
(b) Find and interpret the price elasticity when the price is \$2.00.

44. Price Elasticity of Supply. Economists refer to the *price elasticity of a supply function* as the responsiveness that measures the relationship between the proportional change in the quantity supplied to the proportional change in the price. That is,

$$E(p) = \frac{dS/dp}{S/p} \qquad \text{(price elasticity of supply)}$$

For the supply function

$$S(p) = p^2 - 9$$

(a) Find the price elasticity $E(p)$ for any price p.
(b) Find and interpret the price elasticity when the price is \$5.00.

Points Where Derivatives Do Not Exist

For Problems 45–48, find the points (if any) where the functions do not have derivatives.

45.

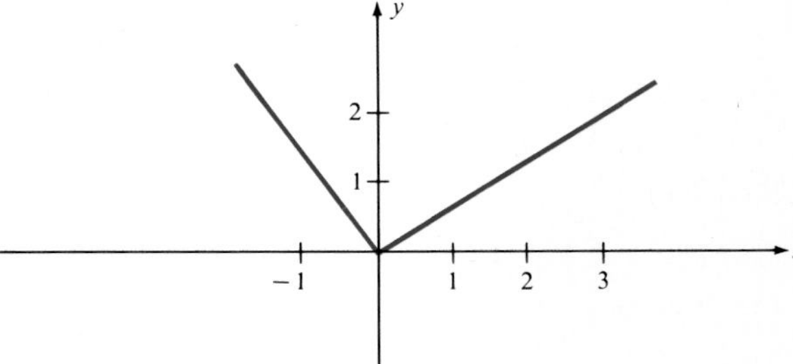

46.

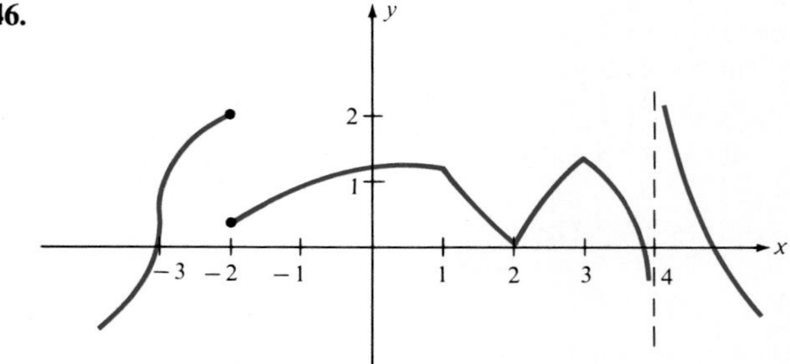

47.

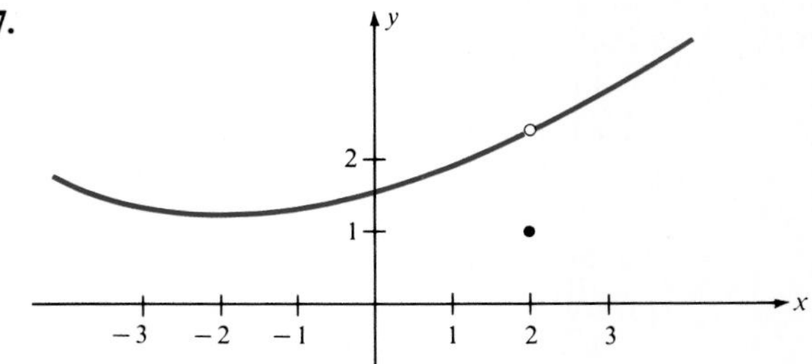

48.

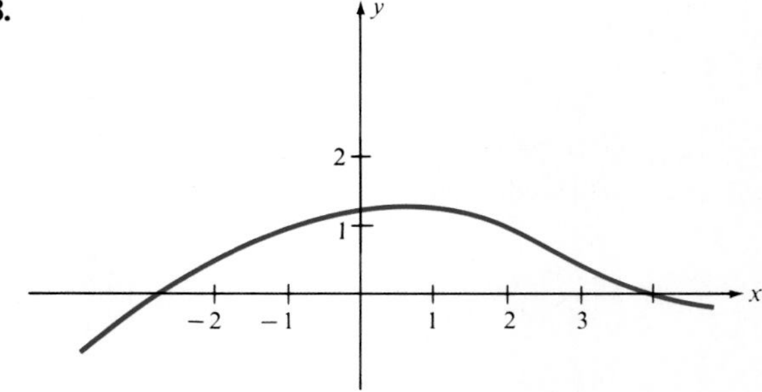

1.5 Derivatives of Polynomials and Sums

PURPOSE

We introduce the general power rule for derivatives and prove some important rules for derivatives. We also continue the analysis of how the derivative is used in economics by introducing the concept of marginal analysis.

Introduction

Until now, we have found the derivative of simple functions at any point x by using the definition of the derivative:

$$f'(x) = \lim_{h \to 0} \frac{f(x + h) - f(x)}{h}$$

We now develop rules that will help simplify the computation of the derivative We start by learning how to differentiate any constant power of x.

Derivative of x^a (a Any Real Number)

In the previous section we differentiated $f(x) = x^2$, using the definition of the derivative. We now show how to find the derivative of any power of x. To do this we begin by drawing **Pascal's triangle** as shown in Table 11. This triangle shows how to expand the binomial expression

$$(a + b)^n$$

for an arbitrary integer n in terms of powers of a and b. The numbers in the Pascal triangle are the coefficients of the individual terms in the expansion.

TABLE 11
Expansions of $(a + b)^n$ by Means of Pascal's Triangle

Binomial Expression		**Binomial Expansion**	
$(a + b)^0$	=	1	
$(a + b)^1$	=	$1a + 1b$	
$(a + b)^2$	=	$1a^2 + 2ab + 1b^2$	*Pascal's*
$(a + b)^3$	=	$1a^3 + 3a^2b + 3ab^2 + 1b^3$	*Triangle*
⋮		⋮ ⋮	
$(a + b)^n$	=	$1a^n + na^{n-1}b + \cdots + nab^{n-1} + 1b^n$	

Using the results of Table 11, we can write

$$\begin{aligned}
\frac{d}{dx}[x^n] &= \lim_{h \to 0} \frac{(x + h)^n - x^n}{h} \\
&= \lim_{h \to 0} \frac{(x^n + nx^{n-1}h + \cdots + h^n) - x^n}{h} \qquad \text{(first and last terms cancel)} \\
&= \lim_{h \to 0} [nx^{n-1} + n(n - 1)x^{n-2}h + \cdots + h^{n-1}] \qquad \text{(cancel } h\text{)} \\
&= nx^{n-1}
\end{aligned}$$

Although we have proven the above power rule only for integer powers of x, it also holds for all real powers. We state the more general result without proof.

> **Power Rule for Derivatives**
>
> If a is any real number, then the power function $f(x) = x^a$ has the derivative
>
> $$\frac{d}{dx} x^a = ax^{a-1}$$

Example 1

Derivatives of Powers of x Table 12 demonstrates the power rule for particular values of a.

TABLE 12
The Power Rule for Some Values of a

a	$f(x) = x^a$	$f'(x) = ax^{a-1}$
0	1	0
1	x	1
2	x^2	$2x$
5	x^5	$5x^4$
-1	x^{-1}	$-x^{-2}$
-2	x^{-2}	$-2x^{-3}$
1.5	$x^{1.5}$	$1.5x^{1/2}$
7.3	$x^{7.3}$	$7.3x^{6.3}$

Factoring Constants Out of the Derivative

We now introduce some useful properties of the derivative. The first property says that we can factor constants outside the derivative. This rule is useful because, although we know the derivative of x^2, we do not know the derivatives of $3x^2$, $2x^2$, and other such constant multiples.

> **Derivative of a Constant Times a Function**
>
> If c is a real number, then for any function $f(x)$, we have
>
> $$\frac{d}{dx}[cf(x)] = c\frac{d}{dx}f(x)$$

Verification of the Above Rule

Since the derivative is a limit, the verification must rely on properties of limits. For a function $f(x)$ and a constant c the function $cf(x)$ has the derivative

$$\frac{d}{dx}[cf(x)] = \lim_{h \to 0} \frac{cf(x+h) - cf(x)}{h}$$

$$= \lim_{h \to 0} c\,\frac{f(x+h) - f(x)}{h}$$

$$= c \lim_{h \to 0} \frac{f(x+h) - f(x)}{h} \qquad \left[\text{by the limit property } \lim_{x \to a} cf(x) = c \lim_{x \to a} f(x)\right]$$

$$= c\,\frac{d}{dx}[f(x)] \qquad \text{(by the definition of the derivative)}$$

Example 2

Factoring Out Constants The following derivatives illustrate the use of the constant rule:

$$\frac{d}{dx}[3x^2] = 3\frac{d}{dx}[x^2] = 6x$$

$$\frac{d}{dx}[5x^{-1}] = 5\frac{d}{dx}[x^{-1}] = -5x^{-2}$$

$$\frac{d}{dx}[8x^{1/2}] = 8\frac{d}{dx}[x^{1/2}] = 4x^{-1/2}$$

$$\frac{d}{dx}[-4x] = -4\frac{d}{dx}[x] = -4$$

Example 3

Derivative of Constants Find the derivative of the constant function

$$f(x) = c \qquad (c \text{ any real number})$$

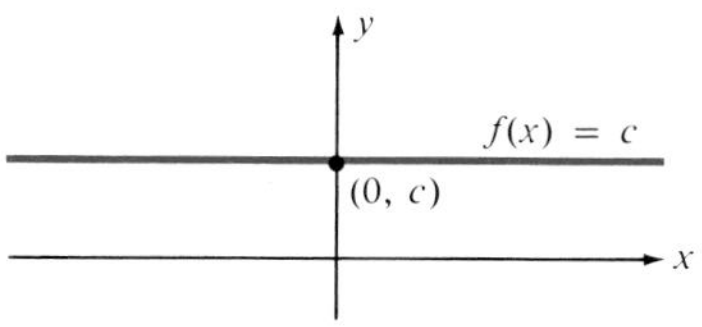

Figure 35
The derivative of a constant function is zero

Solution Using the definition of the derivative, we can write

$$f'(x) = \lim_{h \to 0} \frac{c - c}{h}$$

$$= 0$$

The interpretation of this result is geometrically obvious, since the slope of any tangent line to a horizontal graph is zero. (See Figure 35.) □

Derivatives of Sums and Differences of Functions

The next rules allow us to find the derivatives of sums and differences of functions. For example, we would like to find the derivative of $3x^2 + 2x^4 - 7x^5$ in terms of the derivatives of the individual terms.

Derivative of Sums and Differences

Let f and g be differentiable functions. Then

- The derivative of a sum is the sum of the derivatives:

$$\frac{d}{dx}[f(x) + g(x)] = \frac{d}{dx} f(x) + \frac{d}{dx} g(x)$$

- The derivative of a difference is the difference of the derivatives:

$$\frac{d}{dx}[f(x) - g(x)] = \frac{d}{dx} f(x) - \frac{d}{dx} g(x)$$

Verification of the Sum Rule

The statement that the derivative of a sum is the sum of the derivatives is verified by using the limit rule: The limit of a sum is the sum of the limits. Starting with the definition of the derivative of a sum, we write

$$\begin{aligned}\frac{d}{dx}[f(x) + g(x)] &= \lim_{h\to 0} \frac{[f(x+h) + g(x+h)] - [f(x) + g(x)]}{h}\\ &= \lim_{h\to 0} \frac{[f(x+h) - f(x)] + [g(x+h) - g(x)]}{h}\\ &= \lim_{h\to 0} \frac{f(x+h) - f(x)}{h} + \lim_{h\to 0} \frac{g(x+h) - g(x)}{h}\\ &= \frac{df(x)}{dx} + \frac{dg(x)}{dx}\end{aligned}$$

This completes the verification of the sum rule.

The verification of the difference rule is essentially the same.

Example 4

Derivatives of Sums and Differences Find the derivative of

$$f(x) = 3x^2 + x^{1/2}$$

Solution Using the needed derivative rules, we have

$$\begin{aligned}\frac{d}{dx}(3x^2 + x^{1/2}) &= \frac{d}{dx}(3x^2) + \frac{d}{dx}(x^{1/2})\\ &= 6x + \frac{1}{2}x^{-1/2}\end{aligned}$$

□

Some other functions and their derivatives are shown here:

$$\frac{d}{dx}[\sqrt{x} + 5x^{5/2}] = \frac{1}{2}x^{-1/2} + \frac{25}{2}x^{3/2}$$

$$\frac{d}{dx}[3x^2 + 6x - 5] = 6x + 6$$

$$\frac{d}{dx}[-x^{-1} - x] = x^{-2} - 1$$

$$\frac{d}{dx}\left[8x^3 - \frac{1}{x}\right] = 24x^2 + x^{-2}$$

Using the previous rules for differentiating powers x^n, sums, and differences, along with the rule for factoring out constants, we can now state the general rule for differentiating polynomials.

Derivative of Polynomials

The derivative of a polynomial is given by

$$\frac{d}{dx}[a_0x^n + a_1x^{n-1} + a_2x^{n-2} + \cdots + a_{n-1}x + a_n]$$
$$= a_0nx^{n-1} + a_1(n-1)x^{n-2} + \cdots + a_{n-1}$$

Example 5

Derivative of a Polynomial Differentiate the polynomial

$$\frac{d}{dx}[x^2 - 3x + 5]$$

Solution Using the rule for differentiating polynomials, we have

$$\frac{d}{dx}[x^2 - 3x + 5] = 2x - 3$$ □

Marginal Analysis in Economics

The adjective *marginal* is used in economics to describe the rate of change or derivative of a function describing an economic quantity. For instance, suppose a firm produces q units of a product (computers, candy bars, airplanes, bars of soap, textbooks, or whatever) and we assume that the firm sells all that it produces. Not only is the firm interested in the basic quantities

$C(q) =$ **Cost** to produce q units of the product
$R(q) =$ **Revenue** when q units are produced
$P(q) =$ **Profit** when q units are produced

but also the marginal quantities

$MC = C'(q)$ **(marginal cost)**
$MR = R'(q)$ **(marginal revenue)**
$MP = P'(q)$ **(marginal profit)**

Whereas the *total cost* $C(q)$ represents the cost to produce q units of the product, the *marginal cost* $C'(q)$ represents the rate of change in the cost. By the definition of the derivative the marginal cost is approximately equal to

$$C'(q) \cong \frac{C(q+1) - C(q)}{1} = C(q+1) - C(q)$$

which is simply the increase in cost of producing an additional unit of the product when q units are currently being produced. For instance, if the firm produces computers and if the marginal cost is $C'(10{,}000) = \$250$, then when the production level is 10,000 computers (per week, month, or whatever), it costs the company roughly \$250 to produce each additional computer.

The *total revenue function* $R(q)$ represents the proceeds to the firm when the company sells q units of the product (in other words, the price charged per unit times the number of units sold). The *marginal revenue* $R'(q)$ represents rate of change in revenue. That is, it is the approximate increase in revenue as a result of an additional sale of one more unit of the product when the sales level is q units.

Finally, the *profit* $P(q)$ represents the profit to the firm when it produces (and hence sells) q units of the product. It is simply the revenue minus the cost. That is

$$\text{Profit} = \text{Revenue} - \text{Cost}$$

The *marginal profit* $P'(q)$ is the rate of change in the profit, or approximately the increase in profit as a result of producing one more unit of the product when the current production level is q.

Throughout the remainder of this book we will see how these three important marginal quantities are useful in economics.

Example 6

Revenue, Cost, and Profit For a company that manufactures pocket calculators suppose the revenue and profit from the daily production (and hence sale) of q calculators are given by

$$R(q) = 15q \qquad \text{(revenue function)}$$
$$C(q) = 1000 + 5q + 0.01q^2 \qquad \text{(cost function)}$$

(a) Find the company's daily profit if it produces q calculators.

(b) Find the marginal revenue, marginal cost, and marginal profit.

(c) Find the number q of items produced that makes the marginal cost equal to the marginal revenue.

Solution

(a) The profit $P(q)$ resulting from the sale of q items is given by

$$\begin{aligned} P(q) &= R(q) - C(q) \\ &= 15q - (1000 + 5q + 0.01q^2) \\ &= -0.01q^2 + 10q - 1000 \end{aligned}$$

(b) The marginal functions are

$$MR = R'(q) = 15 \qquad \text{(marginal revenue)}$$
$$MC = C'(q) = 0.02q + 5 \qquad \text{(marginal cost)}$$
$$MP = P'(q) = -0.02q + 10 \qquad \text{(marginal profit)}$$

(c) The marginal revenue is equal to the marginal cost when

$$R'(q) = C'(q)$$

or

$$15 = 0.02q + 5$$
$$0.02q = 10$$
$$q = 500$$

□

Interpretation of Results

The fact that the marginal revenue is always equal to 15 for all q means that the company will always take in an additional \$15 for each additional calculator produced. In other words, \$15 is the selling price of the calculator. Also note that the marginal cost is larger for higher production levels. This could be due to decreased efficiency in the factory at higher production levels. For example, when 100 calculators per day are produced, it costs the company

$$C'(100) = 0.02(100) + 5$$
$$= \$7$$

to produce an additional calculator. However, when 500 calculators per day are produced, the cost to produce an additional calculator has risen to

$$C'(500) = 0.02(500) + 10$$
$$= \$15$$

Note that when 500 calculators are produced, the cost to produce an additional calculator is the same as the selling price of the calculator. Hence there is no reason to produce any more than 500 calculators.

Example 7

Marginal Cost A company that produces microcomputers has determined that the cost $C(q)$ in dollars to produce q computers per week can be approximated by the quadratic polynomial

$$C(q) = 100{,}000 + 400q + 0.06q^2$$

(a) Find the marginal cost when the production level is 1000 computers.

(b) Find the marginal cost when the production level is 2000 computers.

Solution

(a) Since the total cost is

$$C(q) = 100{,}000 + 400q + 0.06q^2$$

the marginal cost, which we denote by MC, is

$$
\begin{aligned}
MC &= \frac{d}{dq} C(q) \\
&= \frac{d}{dq}(100{,}000 + 400q + 0.06q^2) \\
&= 400 + 0.12q \qquad \text{(dollars per computer)}
\end{aligned}
$$

When the production level is 1000 computers per week, the marginal cost is

$$
\begin{aligned}
\left.\frac{dC}{dq}\right|_{q=1000} &= 400 + 0.12(1000) \\
&= \$520 \quad \text{per computer}
\end{aligned}
$$

(b) When the level of production has risen to 2000 computers per week, the marginal cost is

$$
\begin{aligned}
\left.\frac{dC}{dq}\right|_{q=2000} &= 400 + 0.12(2000) \\
&= \$640 \quad \text{per computer}
\end{aligned}
$$

□

Interpretation of Results

When production increases from 1000 to 2000 computers, the marginal cost changes from \$520 to \$640. This means that the production cost per computer has risen by \$120. The reason for this increase might be decreased efficiency caused by insufficient plant facilities, overtime wages, or a combination of these and other factors. It is important that a firm keep track of unit operating expenses for different levels of production. This is where marginal cost analysis plays a key role.

Problems

For Problems 1–10, differentiate the powers of x using the power rule for derivatives.

1. $f(x) = 1$

2. $f(x) = x^5$

3. $f(x) = x^{2.5}$

4. $f(x) = \sqrt{x}$

5. $f(x) = \dfrac{1}{x^2}$

6. $f(x) = \dfrac{1}{\sqrt{x}}$

7. $f(x) = \sqrt{x^3}$

8. $f(x) = x^{7/3}$

9. $f(x) = x^{-3}$

10. $f(x) = x^{-3.5}$

For Problems 11–25, use the rules learned in this section to differentiate the functions. Do not use the definition of the derivative to find the derivatives.

11. $f(x) = 4$
12. $f(x) = c$ (c a constant)
13. $f(x) = 2^{1/2}$
14. $f(x) = 1 - x$
15. $f(x) = 2x + 1$
16. $f(x) = 2x^2$
17. $f(x) = (x + 2)^2$
18. $f(x) = (x - 1)^2$
19. $f(x) = ax^2 + bx + c$ (a, b, and c are constants)
20. $f(x) = x^4 + x^3 + x^2 + x + 1$
21. $f(x) = x^{3/2}$
22. $f(x) = 2x^{-1} + 3x^2 + 3$
23. $f(x) = x^2 + 1/x$
24. $f(x) = 1/x^3 - 7x + 8$
25. $f(x) = 10x^{-4} + 3x^2 + 2x + 7$

Falling Object

A ball dropped from a tall building has fallen a distance of $s(t) = 16t^2$ feet after t seconds.

26. Find the velocity of the ball as a function of time t. What is the velocity after 1 second? After 2 seconds?

27. Find the velocity of the ball after 5 seconds. After 10 seconds.

Biology Problems

28. Fish Population. A new species of fish is introduced into a lake ecosystem. Initially, 100,000 fish are stocked. A marine biologist predicts that the population $P(t)$ of the fish after t years will be

$$P(t) = 100t^2 + 5000t + 100{,}000$$

What is the rate of change in fish per year after year 1? After year 2? After year 5?

29. Flea Jumping. A flea leaping vertically reaches a height of $h(t)$ feet after t seconds where $h(t)$ is given by

$$h(t) = 12t - 16t^2$$

What is the velocity in feet per second of the flea after 1 second? At what time will the velocity of the flea be zero? What is your interpretation of this result?

30. Botany Problem. The proportion of seeds of a certain species of tree that scatter farther than the distance r (measured in feet) is given by

$$p(r) = \frac{2}{r} + \frac{3}{r^{1/2}}$$

Find the rate of change in this proportion as a function of r. What is the value of this rate of change when $r = 100$ feet? What is your interpretation of this result?

31. Protein Synthesis. After t days, protein synthesizing in a cell was found to have a mass (in grams) given by

$$M(t) = 3t^2 + \frac{1}{2t}$$

What is the rate of change (grams per day) at day 1? At day 2?

Bacteria Populations

For Problems 32–35, two types of bacteria (Bacteria 1 and Bacteria 2) grow according to the laws

$$p_1(t) = 50t^2 - 20t + 1000$$
$$p_2(t) = 30t^2 - 80t + 2000$$

where $p_1(t)$ and $p_2(t)$ represent the number of each type of bacteria present at time t (measured in hours).

32. Find the instantaneous rate of growth of Bacteria 1.

33. What is the rate of growth of Bacteria 1 after 4 hours? After 6 hours?

34. Find the instantaneous rate of growth of Bacteria 2.

35. Find the instantaneous rate of growth of the total population.

Finding Tangent Lines to Graphs

36. Tangent Line. Find the points on the graph of

$$y = 2x^3 + 3x^2 - 6x + 1$$

where the curve has a horizontal tangent line.

37. Tangent Line. Find the equation of the tangent line to the graph of

$$y = x^2 + 3x + 3$$

at the point (0, 3).

38. Tangent Line. Find the points on the graph of

$$y = x^2$$

where the slope is equal to its height. Draw a picture to illustrate your conclusions.

Marginal Analysis in Economics

39. Revenue, Cost, and Profit. If the revenue and cost functions are given by

$$R(q) = 10q - 0.01q^2$$
$$C(q) = 5000 + 5q$$

(a) Find the profit function.
(b) Find the marginal revenue, marginal cost, and marginal profit.
(c) For what value of q is the marginal profit equal to zero?

40. Marginal Profit. Why is it true that the marginal profit is equal to the marginal revenue minus the marginal cost? What rule for derivatives do you need to verify this fact?

41. Revenue Found from Demand Curve. The revenue function can always be found by the formula

$$R(q) = (\text{Number of items sold})(\text{Price per item})$$
$$= (q)(\text{Price per item})$$

If the demand function is given by

$$q = D(q) = 4p - 10$$

find the revenue function as a function of q. *Hint:* Solve for the price p in the demand function as a function of q, and substitute this value for the price per item in $R(q)$. This is one way that economists can find the equation for the revenue function.

42. **Finding Profit from Demand Curve and Cost.** The demand function is given by

$$q = D(p) = 2p - 20 \qquad \text{(demand curve)}$$

and the cost function is

$$C(q) = 10{,}000 + 4q \qquad \text{(cost function)}$$

Find the profit function. *Hint:* First find the revenue function by

$$R(q) = (\text{Number of items sold})(\text{Price per item})$$
$$= (q)(\text{Price solved from demand curve})$$

Then compute $P(q) = R(q) - C(q)$.

43. **Marginal Cost.** The cost to produce q units of a product is given by

$$C(q) = 3q^2 - 3q + 12$$

Find the marginal cost of the above cost function. What is the marginal cost when $q = 100$? What is the interpretation of this marginal cost?

44. **Marginal Cost.** The daily cost in dollars to produce q automobiles is found to be given by

$$C(q) = 400{,}000 + 2000q - 10q^2$$

What is the marginal cost when 100 cars are produced in a day? Is the marginal cost increasing or decreasing when more than 100 cars are produced?

45. **Airplane Problem.** An airplane takes off, starting from rest. The distance in feet that it travels during the first few seconds is given by the function

$$s(t) = 2t^2 + 4t + 1$$

How fast is the plane traveling after 10 seconds? After 20 seconds?

46. **Velocity of a Ball.** A ball thrown straight up with an initial velocity of v_0 feet per second will have a height $h(t)$ after t seconds where $h(t)$ is given by the function

$$h(t) = -16t^2 + v_0 t$$

What will be the velocity of the ball after 5 seconds if the initial velocity is $v_0 = 12$?

Velocity

47. **General Law for Falling Object.** The height s in feet reached by a body projected vertically upward with a velocity v feet per second is given by the formula

$$s(t) = -\frac{1}{2}gt^2 + vt$$

where t is time measured in seconds from when the body is projected and g is the acceleration of the body due to gravity, approximately 32 ft/sec^2.
(a) Show that the initial velocity (when $t = 0$) is v.
(b) How long will it take for the object to reach its maximum height?
(c) What is the maximum height attained by the body?

48. **Throwing a Ball.** A ball is thrown upward with an initial velocity of 56 ft/sec. Assuming no air friction, how high will the ball rise and when will it return to the ground?

1.6 Derivatives of Products and Quotients

PURPOSE

We continue the development of the derivative by presenting the product and the quotient rules. These rules allow us to find the derivative of the product or quotient of two functions in terms of the derivatives of the individual functions. We also introduce more marginal concepts of economics.

Introduction

The product and quotient rule introduced in this section will add substantially to the repertoire of functions that we can easily differentiate. For instance, after mastering this section you will be able to differentiate such formidable-looking expressions as

$$f(x) = \frac{\sqrt{x} + x^2}{x^3 + 4x - x^{-2}}$$

We start with the product rule.

Differentiation of Products

In the previous section we learned how to differentiate sums and differences of differentiable functions. We now make the natural progression to differentiating *products* and *quotients*. Although the natural temptation is to think that the derivative of a product is the product of the derivatives, we will see that this is *not* the case. It is also not true that the derivative of a quotient is the quotient of the derivatives. These differentiation rules are more involved.

We begin by presenting a geometric interpretation of the product rule that will help you understand how the derivative should be found.

Geometric Interpretation of the Product Rule

Imagine a rectangle as shown in Figure 36 in which both the width $W(t)$ and the height $H(t)$ of the rectangle change with time. Close your eyes and imagine the rectangle changing in height $H(t)$ and width $W(t)$, maybe getting tall and skinny and then later becoming short and fat. Since the area $A(t)$ of the rectangle is the product $A(t) = W(t)H(t)$, the rate of change of the area is the derivative of the product $W(t)H(t)$. That is,

$$\frac{d}{dt}A(t) = \frac{d}{dt}[W(t)H(t)]$$

To find this rate of change, we allow time to increase by a small amount h from an arbitrary time t to $t + h$. The total change in area of the rectangle will then be

$$\text{Total change in area} = A(t + h) - A(t)$$

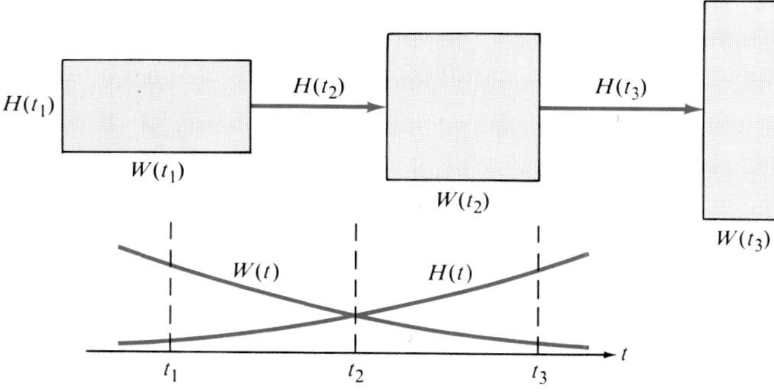

Figure 36
The changing dimensions of a rectangle

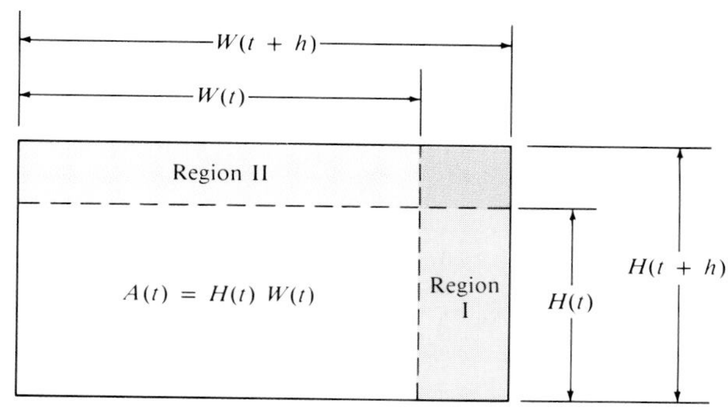

Figure 37
The change in area is essentially the change in Region I and Region II

This change is represented in Figure 37 by the shaded region. If we now ignore the tiny rectangle in the upper right-hand corner of the shaded region, which becomes insignificant when the increase in time h is small, (since the product of two small numbers, i.e., close to zero, is smaller than the numbers themselves) then from Figure 37 we see that the total change in the area is essentially

$$\begin{aligned}\text{Total change in area} &= \text{Region I} + \text{Region II}\\ &= H(t)[W(t + h) - W(t)] + W(t)[H(t + h) - H(t)]\end{aligned}$$

To find the instantaneous rate of change of this area, and hence the derivative of $H(t)W(t)$, we divide this total change by h to get the average change and then take the limit as h approaches zero, getting

$$\frac{d}{dt}[W(t)H(t)] = H(t)\lim_{h\to 0}\frac{W(t+h)-W(t)}{h} + W(t)\lim_{h\to 0}\frac{H(t+h)-H(t)}{h}$$

$$= H(t)W'(t) + W(t)H'(t)$$

The above discussion motivates the general rule for finding the derivative of a product of two functions.

> **Product Rule for Derivatives**
>
> Let f and g be differentiable functions at x. Then
>
> $$\frac{d}{dx}[f(x)g(x)] = f(x)g'(x) + g(x)f'(x)$$
>
> This rule can be stated by saying that the derivative of a product of two factors is the first factor times the derivative of the second factor plus the second factor times the derivative of the first factor.

We now show how the above derivative rule for products can be used to differentiate various functions.

Example 1 Derivative of a Product Find $h'(x)$ where

$$h(x) = 3x^3(3x+4)$$

Solution Calling the two factors

$$f(x) = 3x^3$$
$$g(x) = 3x + 4$$

we first differentiate each factor separately, getting

$$f'(x) = 9x^2$$
$$g'(x) = 3$$

Now, applying the product rule, we have

$$\frac{d}{dx}[f(x)g(x)] = f(x)g'(x) + g(x)f'(x)$$

$$= 3x^3(3) + (3x+4)(9x^2)$$
$$= 36x^2(x+1)$$ □

Example 2 Derivative of a Product Differentiate

$$h(x) = (\sqrt{x} + x)(x^2 + 3)$$

Solution We identify the two factors

$$f(x) = \sqrt{x} + x$$
$$g(x) = x^2 + 3$$

We then differentiate each factor separately, getting

$$f'(x) = \frac{1}{2\sqrt{x}} + 1$$

$$g'(x) = 2x$$

Applying the product rule, we have

$$\frac{d}{dx}[f(x)g(x)] = f(x)g'(x) + g(x)f'(x)$$

$$= (\sqrt{x} + x)(2x) + (x^2 + 3)\left(\frac{1}{2\sqrt{x}} + 1\right)$$ □

Example 3

Differentiation of a Product Find $h'(x)$ where

$$h(x) = (x^3 + 3x)(x + 3)$$

Solution Calling

$$f(x) = x^3 + 3x$$
$$g(x) = x + 3$$

we first differentiate each factor separately, getting

$$f'(x) = 3x^2 + 3$$
$$g'(x) = 1$$

Now, applying the product rule, we have

$$\frac{d}{dx}[f(x)g(x)] = f(x)g'(x) + g(x)f'(x)$$

$$= (x^3 + 3x)(1) + (x + 3)(3x^2 + 3)$$
$$= 4x^3 + 9x^2 + 6x + 9$$ □

The Derivative of a Quotient

Until now, we have found rules for differentiating sums, differences, and products of functions. Another important rule is the **quotient rule**. We state it here without proof.

Quotient Rule for Derivatives

Let f and g be differentiable functions. Then

$$\frac{d}{dx}\frac{f(x)}{g(x)} = \frac{g(x)f'(x) - f(x)g'(x)}{[g(x)]^2}$$

for all points where $g(x) \neq 0$.

This rule can be stated by saying that the derivative of the quotient of two functions is the denominator times the derivative of the numerator minus the numerator times the derivative of the denominator all divided by the denominator squared. (Whew!)

Verification of the Quotient Rule

There is a very clever way to verify the quotient rule once the product rule is known. We begin by writing

$$y(x) = \frac{f(x)}{g(x)}$$

We now write the above equation as

$$f(x) = y(x)g(x)$$

Using the product rule to differentiate this expression, we get

$$f'(x) = y'(x)g(x) + y(x)g'(x)$$

Solving for $y'(x)$, we find

$$y'(x) = \frac{f'(x)}{g(x)} - \frac{y(x)g'(x)}{g(x)}$$

And so if we substitute $f(x)/g(x)$ for $y(x)$ into this equation, we obtain the desired result:

$$\begin{aligned} y'(x) &= \frac{f'(x)}{g(x)} - \frac{f(x)g'(x)}{[g(x)]^2} \\ &= \frac{g(x)f'(x) - f(x)g'(x)}{[g(x)]^2} \end{aligned}$$

Example 4 Derivative of a Quotient

Find dy/dx if

$$y = \frac{1}{x^2 + 1}$$

Solution Calling the numerator and the denominator

$$\begin{aligned} f(x) &= 1 \\ g(x) &= x^2 + 1 \end{aligned}$$

respectively, we have

$$\begin{aligned} f'(x) &= 0 \\ g'(x) &= 2x \end{aligned}$$

Hence using the quotient rule, we get

$$\begin{aligned} \frac{dy}{dx} &= \frac{g(x)f'(x) - f(x)g'(x)}{[g(x)]^2} \\ &= \frac{(x^2 + 1)(0) - (1)(2x)}{(x^2 + 1)^2} \\ &= \frac{-2x}{(x^2 + 1)^2} \end{aligned}$$

□

Example 5

Derivative of a Quotient Find $h'(x)$ where

$$h(x) = \frac{2x + 3}{x^2 + 2x - 3}$$

Solution Calling the numerator and denominator

$$f(x) = 2x + 3$$
$$g(x) = x^2 + 2x - 3$$

respectively, we have

$$f'(x) = 2$$
$$g'(x) = 2x + 2$$

Using the quotient rule, we get

$$\begin{aligned}\frac{d}{dx}\frac{f(x)}{g(x)} &= \frac{g(x)f'(x) - f(x)g'(x)}{[g(x)]^2} \\ &= \frac{(x^2 + 2x - 3)(2) - (2x + 3)(2x + 2)}{(x^2 + 2x - 3)^2} \\ &= \frac{-2(x^2 + 3x + 6)}{(x^2 + 2x - 3)^2}\end{aligned}$$

□

HISTORICAL NOTE

Sir Isaac Newton considered a curve as something that was generated by a continuous motion of a point. The position of the point, which he often denoted by x, was called a "*fluent*" (we would call it a function). Its rate of change, which he denoted by $\dot{x}$, he called the "*fluxion*" (we would call it the derivative). Newton also called the small amount by which a fluent changes over a small interval of time, o, the "*moment*" of the fluent and denoted this moment by $\dot{x}o$ [we would call this the differential $(dx/dt)(dt)$ or dx]. Today we refer to the "dot" notation as the Newtonian notation for the derivative. Today, physics textbooks in mechanics still denote the derivative, dx/dt, by the Newtonian notation $\dot{x}$ in honor of Newton.

Average Cost and Marginal Average Cost

In the previous sections we introduced the idea of marginal analysis in economics and business. Essentially, for every economic quantity that changes over time, there is a corresponding marginal economic quantity that gives the rate of change of this quantity. Suppose, for example, that $C(q)$ is the cost to a firm to manufacture q items. It is clear then that the average cost to produce each item is

$$\text{Average cost per item} = \frac{C(q)}{q}$$

The marginal average cost is the rate of change of this average cost and is found by

$$\text{Marginal average cost} = \frac{d}{dq}\frac{C(q)}{q}$$

To illustrate how the marginal average cost is used in the business world, suppose it has been determined that the monthly cost to a company to manufacture q computers is

$$C(q) = 200\sqrt{q} + 500{,}000$$

From the above cost function it is an easy matter to find the average cost per computer when q computers are produced. It is simply

$$\text{Average cost} = \frac{C(q)}{q} = \frac{200\sqrt{q} + 500{,}000}{q}$$

Knowing the average cost, we can now find the marginal average cost, or the derivative of the average cost. Differentiating the above quotient, we get

$$\frac{d}{dq}\frac{C(q)}{q} = \frac{q(100q^{-1/2}) - (200\sqrt{q} + 500{,}000)(1)}{q^2}$$

$$= \frac{-100(\sqrt{q} + 5000)}{q^2}$$

Graphs of the cost, average cost, and marginal average cost are shown in Figure 38.

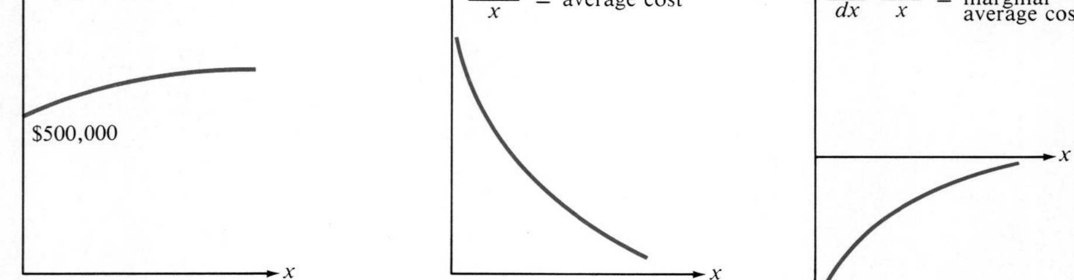

Figure 38
Cost, average cost, and marginal average cost

Interpretation

To interpret the above results, suppose the firm has orders for 10,000 computers for the coming month. The total cost or the cash flow needed to produce these computers will be

$$C(10{,}000) = 200(100) + 500{,}000$$
$$= \$520{,}000$$

As a measure of the efficiency of the firm's production facilities, it is valuable to know the average cost per computer. For this firm it is

$$\frac{C(10{,}000)}{10{,}000} = \frac{520{,}000}{10{,}000}$$
$$= \$52 \quad \text{per computer}$$

This average cost gives a measure of the efficiency to produce all 10,000 computers. On the other hand, the marginal average cost gives a measure of how efficient the firm is at the given production level. For this firm the marginal average cost is

$$\begin{bmatrix}\text{Marginal average cost}\\ \text{when } q = 10{,}000\end{bmatrix} = \frac{(10{,}000)(100/100) - (200 \cdot 100 + 500{,}000)}{(10{,}000)^2}$$

$$= \frac{10{,}000 - 520{,}000}{100{,}000{,}000}$$

$$= -\$0.0051 \text{ per computer}$$

In other words, the average cost to produce a computer (which is \$52 per computer) is coming down at a half cent for each additional computer produced. The reason for this is that at a production rate of 10,000 computers per month it costs much less to make each new computer than it did when the production level was lower. If we compute the marginal cost (rate of change in the cost), we will find

$$C'(x) = \frac{100}{\sqrt{x}}$$

Hence we get the surprising result that

$$C'(10{,}000) = \frac{100}{\sqrt{10{,}000}}$$

$$= \$1$$

which means that it costs the company only \$1 to make a computer when the production level is 10,000 computers. This explains why the average cost per computer is coming down by one-half cent per new computer produced when the production level is 10,000 computers.

Problems

For Problems 1–20, use the product rule or the quotient rule to find the indicated derivatives.

1. $f(x) = x^2(x^2 + x + 3)$
2. $f(x) = (x + 1)(x - 1)$
3. $f(x) = (x^2 + 1)(x^2 - 1)$
4. $f(x) = (x^2 + x + 1)(x^2 - 3x - 4)$
5. $y = (t^2 + 1)(t^2 - 1)$
6. $f(x) = \sqrt{x} \cdot (x^2 - x^{-1})$
7. $g(u) = (u^2 + 1)(u^2 + u - 1)$
8. $f(x) = x^{3/2}(1 - x)$
9. $f(x) = \dfrac{1}{x^2}$
10. $f(x) = \dfrac{1}{x^2 + x + 1}$
11. $f(x) = \dfrac{5}{x^3 + 5}$
12. $g(x) = \dfrac{x}{x - 1}$
13. $h(x) = \dfrac{x^2 - 1}{x + 2}$
14. $f(x) = \dfrac{x(x^2 + 1)}{2x + 3}$
15. $f(x) = x^2 + \dfrac{2}{x + 1}$
16. $f(x) = \dfrac{2x^2 + x + 3}{x^2(x^2 + 1)}$
17. $y = \dfrac{x^2 + 1}{(2x + 1)(x^2 + 3)}$
18. $y = x + \dfrac{1}{x^2 + 1}$
19. $y = \dfrac{1}{\sqrt{x}}$
20. $y = \dfrac{\sqrt{x}}{\sqrt{x} + 1}$

21. **Extended Product Rule.** Show that for functions f, g, and h differentiable at x, the following derivative rule holds:

$$\frac{d}{dx}[f(x)g(x)h(x)] = f'(x)g(x)h(x) + f(x)g'(x)h(x) + f(x)g(x)h'(x)$$

22. **Extended Product Rule.** Use the extended product rule developed in Problem 21 to differentiate

$$\frac{d}{dx}[(x^2 + 1)(x^2 + x + 3)(1 + 2x)]$$

23. **Marginal Revenue.** If $p(x)$ is the price per unit at which x units of a commodity can be sold, then $R = x \cdot p(x)$ is the revenue of the commodity. Show that the marginal revenue is given by

$$\frac{d}{dx}R(x) = p(x) + x\frac{d}{dx}p(x)$$

24. **Marginal Revenue.** Assume that the price per unit is given by

$$p(x) = \frac{50}{x + 5}$$

Find the marginal revenue.

25. **Capital Depreciation.** A firm has determined that a capital investment depreciates according to the rule

$$C(t) = \frac{100{,}000}{t + 2}$$

where $C(t)$ is the value of the investment measured in dollars and t is the age of the investment in years. Find the rate of depreciation of the investment (in dollars per year) after 1 year. After 2 years. After 3 years.

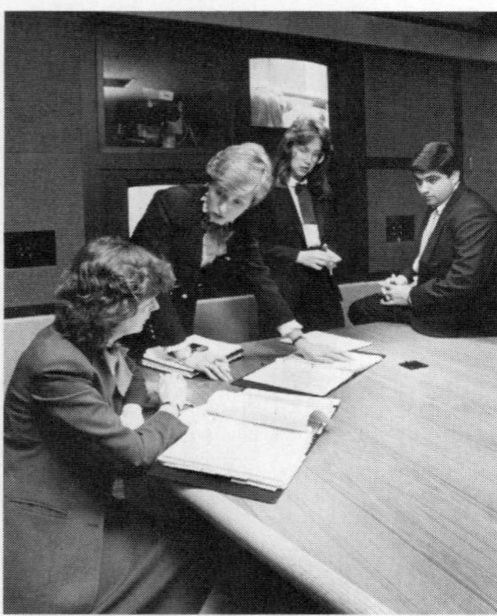

Actuarial scientists at a major insurance company analyze a problem in capital depreciation.

26. **Adrenalin Injection.** Medical data predict that the electrical response y (in millivolts) of a muscle to the amount of adrenalin injected x (in cubic centimeters) is given by the function

$$y(x) = \frac{x}{a + bx}$$

What is the rate of change of y with respect to x? What is your interpretation of this result?

27. **Velocity of a Particle.** The displacement $s(t)$ in feet of a particle from a given reference point is given by

$$s(t) = \frac{100}{t + 1} - 100$$

where t is time measured in seconds. What is the velocity of the particle after 1 second? After 2 seconds? After 3 seconds?

28. **Velocity of a Particle.** The position $s(t)$ of an object on the x-axis is given by

$$s(t) = 10 - \frac{20}{t^2 + 1}$$

where t is measured in seconds. What is the velocity of the object at any time t?

29. **Marginal Revenue.** Find the marginal revenue when x units of a product are sold if the price p charged for each unit is

$$p(x) = 60 - 3x$$

Note that the price charged for each item depends on the number sold. *Hint:* The revenue is given by $R(x) = x \cdot p(x)$.

An Analysis of Costs

A firm has determined that it costs

$$C(x) = 100\sqrt{x} + 100{,}000$$

to produce x units of a given product. For Problems 30–38, determine the types of costs.

30. Find the marginal cost when the firm produces x units.
31. Find the marginal cost when the firm produces 100 units.
32. Find the marginal cost when the firm produces 10,000 units.
33. Find the average cost per unit when the firm produces x units.
34. Find the average cost per unit when the firm produces 100 units.
35. Find the average cost per unit when the firm produces 10,000 units.
36. Find the marginal average cost when the firm produces x units.
37. Find the marginal average cost when the firm produces 100 units.

38. Find the marginal average cost when the production rate is 10,000 units.

39. Blood Flow. According to *Poiseuille's law*, the total resistance R to blood flow in a blood vessel of constant length L and radius r is given by

$$R = \frac{kL}{r^4}$$

where k is a constant of proportionality determined by the viscosity of the blood. How fast is the resistance decreasing when $r = 0.2$ mm?

40. Rate of Change. Assume that the width W and height H of a rectangle depend on time t according to the functions

$$H(t) = 3t^2 + 2t + 1$$
$$W(t) = t - 3$$

What is the area of the rectangle and what is the rate of change of the area after 2 seconds? After 4 seconds?

41. General Derivative Formula. Find y' if

$$y = \frac{xf(x)}{g(x)}$$

Use the result to find the derivative of

$$y = \frac{x(x^2 + 1)}{(x^2 + 3)^2}$$

42. Misconception. A common error for beginners is to differentiate a product of two functions by use of the formula

$$\frac{d}{dx}[f(x)g(x)] = \frac{d}{dx}f(x)\frac{d}{dx}g(x)$$

Are there any pairs of functions from the five functions listed below for which this identity actually holds? Show that this relation does not hold for the other pairs.

(a) $a(x) = 13$

(b) $b(x) = x + 1$

(c) $c(x) = x$

(d) $d(x) = \dfrac{1}{x - 1}$

(e) $e(x) = \dfrac{1}{x}$

43. Fish Population. The total weight W in pounds of a fish population in a certain lake is given by the product

$$W = nw$$

where

n = number of fish in the lake

w = average weight of the fish

Suppose a biologist estimates that n and w will change according to the following functions:

$$n(t) = 0.5t^2 + t + 1000$$
$$w(t) = 0.3t^2 + 2t + 1$$

where t is time measured in years. What is the total weight W of the fish population, and what is the rate of change in the total weight after one year? After two years?

44. Algae Study. The density D of algae in a container is given by the quotient

$$D = \frac{n}{V} \quad \text{(algae per cubic centimeter)}$$

where

n = number of algae

V = volume of the container (cubic centimeters)

Suppose that both the number of algae and the volume of the container change with time according to the functions

$$n(t) = \sqrt{t} + 100 \quad \text{(number of algae)}$$

$$V(t) = \frac{1000}{\sqrt{t}} \quad \text{(cubic centimeters)}$$

where t is time measured in hours. What is the density D and the rate of change D' of the density after 100 hours?

45. Challenge Problem. The following function was mentioned as a complicated function that could be differentiated after learning the material of this section. Can you differentiate this function?

$$f(x) = \frac{\sqrt{x} + x^2}{x^3 + 4x - x^{-2}}$$

1.7 The Chain Rule

PURPOSE

We introduce a rule that shows how to find the derivative of the composition of two differentiable functions

$$y = f[g(x)]$$

in terms of the derivative of $f(x)$ and the derivative of $g(x)$. This rule, called the chain rule, allows us to differentiate a wide variety of functions.

Introduction

We are coming to the end of the line of the rules for differentiation. Although it does not really make sense to say that one rule is more important than any other rule, most people would probably say that the chain rule is the most important. You should understand how this rule works, since it will be used over and over throughout the remainder of this book. In the next chapter, when we study related rates, it will be critical that you understand this rule. To master its use, we must recognize complicated functions as compositions of simpler functions. When the individual components of the composition have been recognized, differentiation by the chain rule is relatively simple. You should review how compositions of functions are formed, as explained in the Calculus Preliminaries.

The Chain Rule

We begin by presenting a geometric interpretation of the chain rule. This will give you an intuitive understanding of this important rule. Let us assume that y depends on u by means of some relationship

$$y = f(u)$$

and that u depends on x by means of a second relationship

$$u = g(x)$$

To find the derivative of y with respect to x, we must determine the relationship between the change in y and the change in x. (See Figure 39.) To find this, suppose a small change in x of $\Delta x = 0.1$ gives rise to a change in u of $\Delta u = 0.4$. Suppose, too, that a small change in u of $\Delta u = 0.1$ gives rise to a change in y of $\Delta y = 0.2$. By knowing how x affects u and how u affects y, we can determine how x affects y. We simply have the ratio of the change in y divided by the change in x as

$$\frac{\Delta y}{\Delta x} = \frac{\Delta y}{\Delta u}\frac{\Delta u}{\Delta x} = \frac{0.2}{0.1}\frac{0.4}{0.1} = (2)(4) = 8$$

In other words, y is changing 8 times faster than x. If we now let Δx tend to zero, we arrive at the following formula:

$$\frac{dy}{dx} = \frac{dy}{du}\frac{du}{dx}$$

This is the **chain rule**. Intuitively, the chain rule says that for small changes in x,

$$\frac{\text{Change in } y}{\text{Change in } x} = \frac{\text{Change in } y}{\text{Change in } u} \cdot \frac{\text{Change in } u}{\text{Change in } x}$$

It is useful to note that in the formula for the chain rule, dy/du is the derivative of $y = f(u)$ with respect to u and du/dx is the derivative of $u = g(x)$ with respect to x.

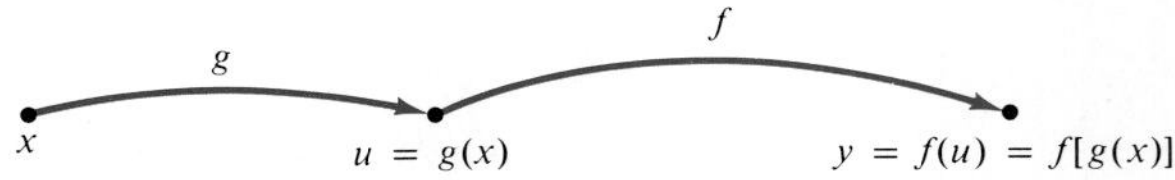

Figure 39
Here y depends on u, and u depends on x

We now give a formal statement of the chain rule.

Chain Rule for Differentiating Compositions

Let

$$y = f(u)$$

be a differentiable function of u, where

$$u = g(x)$$

is a differentiable function of x. Then the composition of these functions

$$y = f(u) = f[g(x)]$$

is also a differentiable function of x whose derivative is

$$\frac{dy}{dx} = \frac{dy}{du}\frac{du}{dx} \qquad \text{(chain rule)}$$

An alternative way of writing the above chain rule is

$$\frac{dy}{dx} = f'[g(x)] \cdot g'(x) \qquad \text{(alternative form)}$$

Example 1

Chain Rule Find dy/dx if

$$y = (x^2 + 2x + 1)^5$$

Solution The above function is a composition, or is "built up" from the two simpler functions

$$y = u^5$$

and

$$u = x^2 + 2x + 1$$

To use the chain rule, first compute the following two derivatives with respect to u and x, respectively:

$$\frac{dy}{du} = 5u^4$$

$$\frac{du}{dx} = 2x + 2$$

The chain rule then gives

$$\begin{aligned} \frac{dy}{dx} &= \frac{dy}{du}\frac{du}{dx} \\ &= 5u^4(2x + 2) \\ &= 5(x^2 + 2x + 1)^4(2x + 2) \end{aligned}$$

The last step above consisted of replacing the value of u by its expression in terms of x so that the final derivative dy/dx is given completely in terms of the variable x. □

Example 2

Find dy/dx if y is given by

$$y = \left(\frac{x-1}{x+1}\right)^3$$

Solution The above function can be interpreted as the composition of

$$y = u^3$$

where u is

$$u = \frac{x-1}{x+1}$$

If we now differentiate y with respect to u and u with respect to x, we have

$$\frac{dy}{du} = 3u^2 \qquad \text{(power rule)}$$

$$\frac{du}{dx} = \frac{(x+1)-(x-1)}{(x+1)^2} \qquad \text{(quotient rule)}$$

$$= \frac{2}{(x+1)^2}$$

Using the chain rule, we get

$$\frac{dy}{dx} = \frac{dy}{du}\frac{du}{dx}$$

$$= 3u^2 \frac{2}{(x+1)^2}$$

$$= 3\frac{(x-1)^2}{(x+1)^2}\frac{2}{(x+1)^2}$$

$$= 6\frac{(x-1)^2}{(x+1)^4}$$

□

Example 3

Chain Rule Find the derivative dy/dx if

$$y = \frac{1}{x^2+1}$$

Solution The above expression is a composition of the two functions

$$y = \frac{1}{u}$$

and

$$u = x^2 + 1$$

If we now differentiate y with respect to u and u with respect to x, we get

$$\frac{dy}{du} = -\frac{1}{u^2} \qquad \text{(power rule)}$$

$$\frac{du}{dx} = 2x \qquad \text{(power rule)}$$

Applying the chain rule, we have

$$\begin{aligned}\frac{dy}{dx} &= \frac{dy}{du}\frac{du}{dx} \\ &= -\frac{1}{u^2}(2x) \\ &= \frac{-2x}{(x^2+1)^2} \qquad \text{(substituting for } u\text{)}\end{aligned}$$

□

Remembering the Chain Rule

The chain rule

$$\frac{dy}{dx} = \frac{dy}{du}\frac{du}{dx}$$

is easy to remember by saying "dee y dee x is equal to dee y dee u times dee u dee x."

Example 4

Alternative Form of the Chain Rule Find the derivative $h'(x)$ of the expression

$$h(x) = \frac{1}{(x^2+1)^2}$$

Solution We use a slightly different notation in this problem so that we can use the alternative form of the chain rule. The above function can be interpreted as the composition

$$h(x) = f[g(x)]$$

of the two simpler functions

$$f(u) = \frac{1}{u^2}$$

where u is

$$g(x) = x^2 + 1$$

First, we differentiate $f(u)$ with respect to u and $g(x)$ with respect to x, getting

$$f'(u) = -\frac{2}{u^3}$$

$$g'(x) = 2x$$

The alternative form of the chain rule gives the derivative of $h'(x)$ as

$$\begin{aligned}h'(x) &= f'[g(x)] \cdot g'(x) \\ &= -\frac{2}{[g(x)]^3}(2x) \\ &= -\frac{4x}{(x^2+1)^3}\end{aligned}$$

□

The chain rule allows us to state the following useful rule.

> **Power Rule for Functions**
>
> Let g be a differentiable function and let a be a real constant. The power rule for differentiating powers of functions states that
>
> $$\frac{d}{dx}[g(x)]^a = a[g(x)]^{a-1}g'(x)$$

Example 5

Power Rule for Functions Find dy/dx if

$$y = (x^3 + 3x + 4)^6$$

Solution Letting

$$g(x) = x^3 + 3x + 4$$

we have

$$g'(x) = 3x^2 + 3$$

Hence the power rule with $a = 6$ states that

$$\frac{d}{dx}(x^3 + 3x + 4)^6 = 6(x^3 + 3x + 4)^5(3x^2 + 3)$$

□

Example 6

Find dy/dx if

$$y = \frac{1}{\sqrt{(x^2 + 1)^3}}$$

Solution Calling

$$g(x) = x^2 + 1$$

we have

$$g'(x) = 2x$$

We now write the above expression as

$$y = \frac{1}{\sqrt{g(x)^3}} = [g(x)]^{-3/2}$$

Using the power rule for functions with $a = -\frac{3}{2}$, we get

$$\frac{dy}{dx} = -\frac{3}{2}[g(x)]^{-5/2}g'(x) = -\frac{3}{2}(x^2 + 1)^{-5/2}(2x) = \frac{-3x}{\sqrt{(x^2 + 1)^5}}$$

□

Example 7 Product and Chain Rule Find the derivative dy/dx if

$$y = 3x^2\sqrt{x^3 + 4}$$

Solution We can interpret y as the product of the two functions

$$f(x) = 3x^2$$
$$g(x) = \sqrt{x^3 + 4}$$

Applying the product and power rule, we have

$$\begin{aligned}
\frac{dy}{dx} &= \frac{d}{dx}[f(x)g(x)] \\
&= f(x)\frac{d}{dx}g(x) + g(x)\frac{d}{dx}f(x) \qquad \text{(product rule)} \\
&= 3x^2\frac{d}{dx}[\sqrt{x^3 + 4}] + \sqrt{x^3 + 4}\frac{d}{dx}[3x^2] \\
&= 3x^2\frac{1}{2}(x^3 + 4)^{-1/2}(3x^2) + \sqrt{x^3 + 4}(6x) \qquad \text{(power rule)} \\
&= \frac{9}{2}x^4(x^3 + 4)^{-1/2} + 6x\sqrt{x^3 + 4}
\end{aligned}$$

□

Example 8 Quotient and Chain Rule Find the derivative of

$$y = \frac{(7x - 4)^5}{x + 1}$$

Solution Calling the numerator and denominator

$$f(x) = (7x - 4)^5$$
$$g(x) = x + 1$$

respectively, we use the quotient rule

$$\begin{aligned}
\frac{dy}{dx} &= \frac{d}{dx}\frac{f(x)}{g(x)} \\
&= \frac{g(x)f'(x) - f(x)g'(x)}{[g(x)]^2} \qquad \text{(quotient rule)} \\
&= \frac{(x + 1)\frac{d}{dx}(7x - 4)^5 - (7x - 4)^5\frac{d}{dx}(x + 1)}{(x + 1)^2} \\
&= \frac{(x + 1)(5)(7x - 4)^4(7) - (7x - 4)^5(1)}{(x + 1)^2} \qquad \text{(chain rule)} \\
&= \frac{(7x - 4)^4(28x + 39)}{(x + 1)^2}
\end{aligned}$$

□

All of the rules that we have learned in this chapter are summarized in Table 13.

TABLE 13
Summary of the Rules of Differentiation

Rule	Function	Derivative
Constant Function	$y = c$	$y' = 0$
Constant Times a Function	$y = cf(x)$	$y' = cf'(x)$
Power Rule	$y = x^a$	$y' = ax^{a-1}$
Derivative of a Sum	$y = f(x) + g(x)$	$y' = f'(x) + g'(x)$
Derivative of a Difference	$y = f(x) - g(x)$	$y' = f'(x) - g'(x)$
Derivative of a Product	$y = f(x)g(x)$	$y' = f(x)g'(x) + g(x)f'(x)$
Derivative of a Quotient	$y = \dfrac{f(x)}{g(x)}$	$y' = \dfrac{g(x)f'(x) - f(x)g'(x)}{[g(x)]^2}$
Chain Rule	$y = f(u)$, $u = g(x)$	$\dfrac{dy}{dx} = \dfrac{dy}{du}\dfrac{du}{dx}$
Power Rule for Functions	$y = [g(x)]^a$	$y' = a[g(x)]^{a-1}g'(x)$

More Theory of the Firm (Profits and Marginal Profits)

The **total profit** $P(q)$ of a firm depends on the number q of items the firm produces if we always assume that the firm sells all that it produces. The derivative $P'(q)$ of the profit is called the **marginal profit** and represents the rate of change of the profit. In practice, it is often interpreted as the additional profit to the firm for making one additional item when the current production level is q.

Example 9

Marginal Profit A firm's weekly profit P (in thousands of dollars) for producing q units of a given product has been determined to be

$$P(q) = \sqrt{500q - q^2} \qquad (0 \le q \le 500)$$

A graph of this profit function is shown in Figure 40. Find the marginal profit when 100 units are produced and when 250 units are produced.

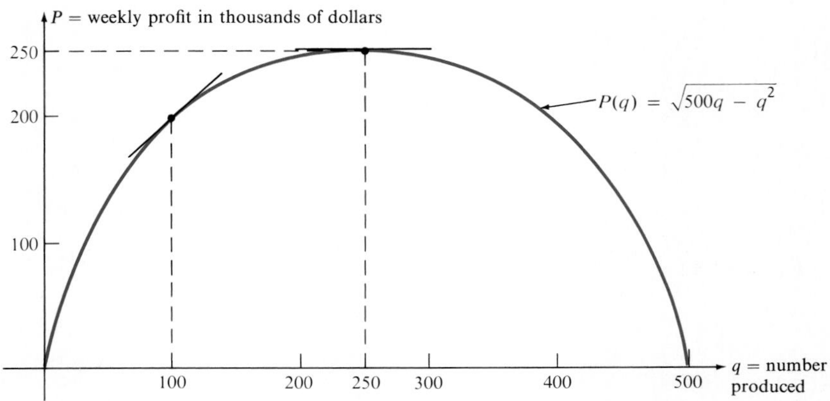

Figure 40
Typical profit function

Solution To find the marginal profit, we differentiate $P(q)$ with respect to q. Using the power rule for functions, we have

$$\frac{d}{dq}\sqrt{500q - q^2} = \frac{d}{dq}(500q - q^2)^{1/2}$$

$$= \frac{1}{2}(500q - q^2)^{-1/2}(500 - 2q)$$

$$= \frac{250 - q}{\sqrt{500q - q^2}} \qquad (0 \le q \le 500)$$

Hence the marginal profit when production levels are 100 and 250 is given by

$$P'(100) = \frac{250 - 100}{\sqrt{50{,}000 - 10{,}000}} = 0.75$$

$$P'(250) = \frac{250 - 250}{\sqrt{125{,}000 - 62{,}500}} = 0$$

□

Interpretation of Results

The interpretation of the above marginal profit calculations is that the firm's profit will increase by an additional 0.75 unit (or $750) when production is raised from 100 units to 101 units per week. On the other hand, when production is at the higher level of 250 items per week, the marginal profit is zero. This means that essentially no additional profit is earned by producing item 251. From Figure 40, we can see that when production is less than 250 items per week, it makes sense to produce more items, since the profit will be increased (provided that the firm can sell the items). When production reaches 250 items per week, however, the marginal profit becomes zero, and no additional profit is earned by increased production. In fact, when production becomes larger than 250 items per week, the marginal profit becomes negative, which means that the firm will lose money on each additional item produced. The reason for this negative return might be decreased efficiency as a result of crowded working conditions, insufficient plant facilities, overtime wages, or a wide variety of other reasons.

Problems

For Problems 1–13, use the chain rule to find the indicated derivatives.

1. $f(x) = (x^2 + 3x + 1)^4$

2. $f(x) = (x^3 + x^2 + 3)^2$

3. $f(x) = \sqrt{x^2 + 3x + 1}$

4. $f(x) = \dfrac{1}{x^2 + 1}$ (Also do this problem using the quotient rule.)

5. $f(x) = \dfrac{1}{\sqrt{(x^2 + x + 1)^3}}$

6. $f(x) = \dfrac{(x^2 + 1)^3}{(x - 2)^2}$

7. $f(x) = \left(x^2 + \dfrac{1}{x}\right)^3$

8. $f(x) = (x^{-1} + x^{-2})^{-3}$

9. $f(x) = [(x + 1)^2 + x]^3$

10. $f(x) = (2x + 1)^{50}$

11. $f(x) = \dfrac{1}{(x^2 + 1)^{10}}$

12. $f(x) = (3x^2 - x)^5(2x + 4)^5$

13. $f(x) = \dfrac{(x + 5)^5}{(x + 4)^3}$

Chain Rule Exercise

For Problems 14–19, let

$$f(x) = (x^2 + 1)^3$$
$$g(x) = 3x - 4$$

Find the indicated quantities.

14. $f[g(x)]$ **15.** $g[f(x)]$

16. $\dfrac{d}{dx} f[g(x)]$ **17.** $\dfrac{d}{dx} g[f(x)]$

18. $\dfrac{d}{dx} f[g(x)]$ when $x = 1$ **19.** $\dfrac{d}{dx} g[f(x)]$ when $x = 1$

20. Find $f'(2)$ if

$$f(z) = \frac{1}{z^2 - 1}$$

For Problems 21–23, find the equation of the tangent line to the graphs of the following functions at the indicated points:

21. $y = (x^2 + 1)^3$; $(1, 8)$ **22.** $y = \dfrac{x + 1}{(x - 1)^{1/2}}$; $(2, 3)$

23. $y = (x^2 + x + 1)^3$; $(1, 27)$

24. General Derivative Rule. Use the derivative rule

$$\frac{d}{dx}\frac{1}{u(x)} = -\frac{u'(x)}{[u(x)]^2}$$

to find the derivative of

$$y = \frac{1}{(x^2 + 1)^2}$$

Alternative Form of Chain Rule

For Problems 25–28, use the alternative form of the chain rule,

$$y' = f'[g(x)] \cdot g'(x)$$

to differentiate the functions. Identify each of the functions $f(x)$, $g(x)$, $f'(x)$, $g'(x)$, $f'[g(x)]$, and dy/dx.

25. $y = (x^2 + 1)^5$ **26.** $y = (x^2 + x + 3)^{-5}$

27. $y = \sqrt{2x + 1}$ **28.** $y = (3x^2 + 1)^3$

Derivatives in the Sciences

For Problems 29–35, the functions have been taken from textbooks in economics, zoology, ecology, sociology, and botany describing phenomena in these areas. Find the rates of change of these functions with respect to the relevant independent variable.

29. $R(q) = 1000\left(2 - \dfrac{q}{500}\right)^2$ (sales revenue)

30. $c(t) = \dfrac{50}{\sqrt{t + 2}}$ (concentration of a hormone)

31. $N(t) = 50\sqrt{t + 4} + 100$ (animal population)

32. $y(t) = 30\sqrt{6t}$ (substrate produced by a hormone)

33. $y(x) = k(x - a)^{1/3}$ (response to visual brightness)

34. $y(x) = k(x - a)^{8/5}$ (response to warmth)

35. $y(x) = k(x - a)^{7/2}$ (response to an electrical stimulus)

36. Tangent Line. Show that there are exactly two tangent lines to the graph of the function

$$y = (x + 1)^3$$

that have x-intercept zero. Find the equation of each of these lines.

37. Related Rates. If Bill is running twice as fast as Mary, and Mary is running three times as fast as Joe, how many times as fast as Joe is Bill running? Set this problem up as a composition and solve it by the chain rule.

38. Related Rates. The radius r of a spherical balloon is expanding according to the function

$$r(t) = 2t^2 + 2t + 3$$

where r is measured in centimeters and t in seconds. What is the rate of change in the radius of the balloon when $t = 2$ seconds? What are the units of this rate of change?

39. Chain Rule. Find dy/dx if

$$y = 2u^2 + 5$$
$$u = 3x^2 - 7$$

40. Chain Rule. Let

$$y = [1 - (2x - 1)^2]^2$$

Identify $f(x)$ and $g(x)$ so that

$$y = f[g(x)]$$

and find dy/dx.

41. Marginal Profit. The daily profit P a company earns from producing q items is given by

$$P(q) = \sqrt{1200q - q^3} \qquad (0 \le q \le 35)$$

What is the marginal profit when the production level is 10 units per day? When the production level is 20 units per day? What are your conclusions?

42. Marginal Revenue. The daily revenue R received from selling q units of a certain product is given by

$$R(q) = \sqrt{400q - q^2} \qquad (0 \le q \le 400)$$

What is the marginal revenue when sales are 50 units a day? When sales are 100 units a day? What can you conclude?

Epilogue: The Snowflake Curve—A Freak or a Beacon?

About 100 years ago, just when mathematicians thought they knew everything there was to know about curves and functions, several strange and exotic curves were discovered that dispelled this myth. Weird curves such as the snowflake or Koch curve, Cantor's stairs, the Weierstrass curve, and the Sierpinski triangle were found by several mathematicians. One of these curves was the snowflake curve named after the mathematician, von Koch, who first studied it in 1904. The curve is fascinating inasmuch as it does not have a tangent line at any point on the curve! In other words, every point on the curve is a corner point. We will not actually draw "the" snowflake curve (since it is impossible) but must imagine it, using other snowflake curves as a guide. To get started, we first picture the four snowflakes shown in Figure 41. The idea now is to imagine the "limiting snowflake" as more and more "spines" are added.

Von Koch proved that this imagined "limiting snowflake" does not have a tangent line at any point on the snowflake. Von Koch also showed that the limiting snowflake has infinite length, and thus we have the weird situation that a curve of infinite length encloses a finite area. (Hmmmmm.)

For roughly 75 years after the time von Koch studied the snowflake curve, mathematicians around the world thought of this curve (and other similar curves) as freaks. Even the great French mathematician Henri Poincaré called these curves the "gallery of monsters." It went so far that the Soviet mathematician, N. Ya. Vilenkin wrote a book in 1965, *Mathematical Art Museum*, which displayed these freaks of mathematics for all to see. Then came Benoit Mandelbrot.

In 1973, Benoit B. Mandelbrot discovered that many of these curves of disrepute, to which he gave the

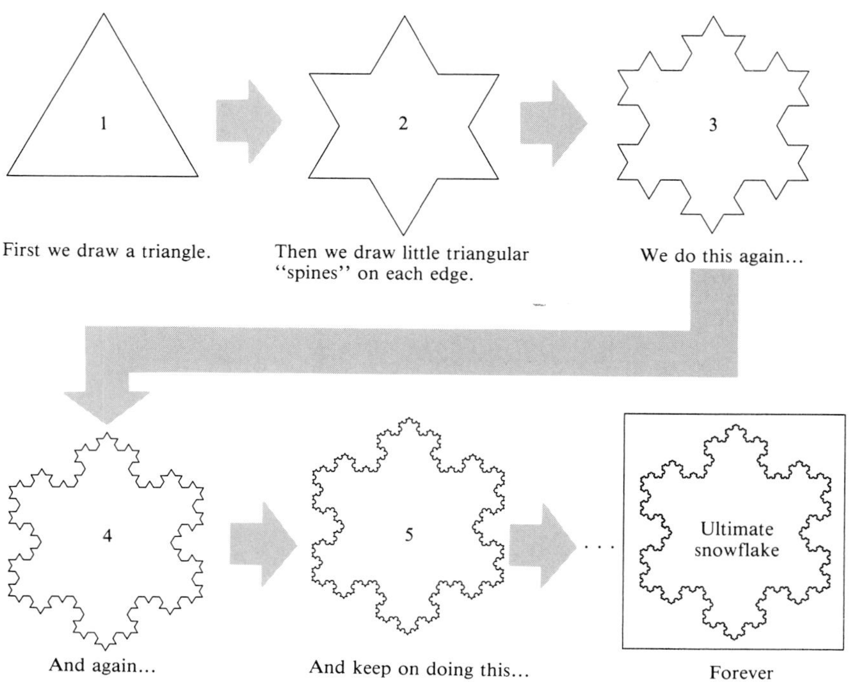

Figure 41
A sequence of snowflakes that look more and more like (converge to) some ultimate limiting snowflake. Can you picture the limiting snowflake?

name **fractals**, could be used to study a wide variety of complex phenomena in a modern complex world. Phenomena such as the distribution of stars and galaxies in the universe, the turbulence of fluids, the study of coastlines of continents, and many others could be studied by using fractals. Just when it seemed that these strange curves should be placed in a mausoleum, Mandelbrot discovered that they led to new theories for the study of chaotic behavior in dynamical systems. Today, the study of fractals and chaotic behavior is considered one of the most active areas of mathematics. The final chapter in this changing area of mathematics has not yet been written.

Interested readers should consult Benoit B. Mandelbrot, *Fractals, Form, Change, and Dimension*, W.H. Freeman and Company, New York, 1977.

Key Ideas for Review

chain rule, 131
continuity
  on an interval, 79
  at a point, 79
derivative
  of a composition, 131
  definition of, 100
  of a difference, 116
  of a polynomial, 117
  of a product, 123
  of a quotient, 125
  of a sum, 116
limit
  of a function, 68
  rules, 75
marginal
  average cost, 128
  cost, 117
  profit, 117
  revenue, 117
secant line, 98
tangent line, 97
tangent problem, 65
velocity, 89

Review Exercises

For Problems 1–10, find the limits.

1. $\lim_{x\to 1} (x^2 + 2x + 1)$

2. $\lim_{x\to -1} \dfrac{x^2 - 1}{x + 1}$

3. $\lim_{x\to 1} (\sqrt{x+1} - \sqrt{x})$

4. $\lim_{x\to 0} (\sqrt{x^2 + x} - \sqrt{x})$

5. $\lim_{x\to 2} \dfrac{2x^2 + 3}{5x^2 + 4}$

6. $\lim_{x\to -1} \dfrac{2x^2 + 3}{5x^2 - 6}$

7. $\lim_{x\to 4} \dfrac{\sqrt{x} - 2}{x^2 - 4}$

8. $\lim_{x\to 2} \sqrt{x^2 + 2x}$

9. $\lim_{x\to 0} \dfrac{\sqrt{x+9} - 3}{x}$

10. $\lim_{x\to 1} \dfrac{x - 1}{|x| - 1}$

For Problems 11–40, differentiate each of the functions.

11. $f(x) = 2x + 1/x$

12. $f(x) = (x + 1)^2$

13. $f(x) = (3x^2 + 4)^3$

14. $f(x) = \sqrt{x} \cdot (2x + 3x^2)$

15. $f(t) = 3\sqrt{t} + t^{-1/2}$

16. $f(z) = \dfrac{z}{1 - z}$

17. $f(z) = (z + \sqrt{z})^{1/2}$

18. $f(z) = (1 + z^2)^{1/3}$

19. $f(r) = 4r^2$

20. $f(x) = (x^2 + 1)(3x^2 + x - 4)$

21. $y = 5^{1/3}$

22. $y = x^{1/2} - x^{-1/2}$

23. $g(t) = 2\sqrt{t} + \dfrac{1}{\sqrt{t}}$

24. $f(x) = \dfrac{x + 1}{x}$

25. $h(t) = 5\sqrt{5} + \dfrac{1}{\sqrt{3}}$

26. $y = (1 + \sqrt{x})^{1/2}$

27. $h(t) = (t^2 - 1)(t^2 + 1)$

28. $y = [x^2 + (x - 1)^2]^5$

29. $f(t) = \dfrac{1}{t^{1/4}}$

30. $f(x) = \dfrac{1}{\sqrt{2x + 3}}$

31. $y = \dfrac{x}{2} + \dfrac{2}{x}$

32. $f(x) = (x^2 + 1)^2$

33. $h(z) = \dfrac{5z}{5z^2 + 1}$

34. $f(x) = \sqrt{2x}(x + 1)^3$

35. $f(t) = (t + 3)\sqrt{t - 2}$

36. $y = [x^3(x + 2)]^4$

37. $y = (5x + 3)(x^2 + 2x - 3)$

38. $f(p) = 5p^{5/4}$

39. $y = \dfrac{1}{\sqrt[3]{x}}$

40. $f(t) = 5 \cdot 3^{0.4} + 2^{-1/4}$

41. If $f(t) = 3t^2$, find $f'(2)$.
42. If $g(x) = x^{-1/2}$, find $g'(1)$.
43. If $f(x) = (x^2 + 1)^2$, find $f'(0)$.

44. If $y = \dfrac{1}{(x+1)^2}$, find $\left.\dfrac{dy}{dx}\right|_{x=3}$.

45. If $h(p) = 3p^{0.5}$, find $h'(1)$.
46. If $f(z) = (1 + z^{1/2})^2$, find $f'(1)$.

For Problems 47–57, find the indicated quantities.

47. $\left.\dfrac{d}{dx}(x^2 + 3x + 1)\right|_{x=1}$

48. $\left.\dfrac{d}{dx}(x^2 + \sqrt{x})\right|_{x=1}$

49. $\left.\dfrac{d}{dx}\left(\dfrac{x+1}{x-1}\right)\right|_{x=-2}$

50. $\left.\dfrac{d}{dz}\sqrt{z^2+1}\right|_{z=0}$

51. Find ds/dt if $s(t) = 16t^2$.
52. Find du/dv if $u = v^4 + v$.

53. Find $\dfrac{d}{dt}(3u^2)$ if $u = 2t + 1$.

54. Find $\dfrac{d}{dx}u(x)$ if $u = 3x^2 + x$.

55. Find $f'(4)$ if $f(x) = \sqrt{x}$.
56. Find $f'(1)$ if $f(z) = 3z^2 + z - 1$.

57. Find $\dfrac{d}{dx}[(x^2+1)(x^2-1)(x^2+2)]$.

Miscellaneous Problems Involving the Derivative

For Problems 58–59, find the equation of the tangent line to the given function at the indicated point.

	Function	Point
58.	$y = x^3 + x + 1$	$(0, 1)$
59.	$y = \dfrac{x}{2} + \dfrac{2}{x}$	$(1, \frac{5}{2})$

For Problems 60–61, determine the point(s) if any at which the graph of the given function has a horizontal tangent line.

60. $y = x^2 - x + 1$

61. $y = x + \dfrac{1}{x}$

62. Moving Water Wave. A circular water wave is moving outward at the rate of 1 foot per second and hence the area of the circle inside this wave is

$$A = \pi t^2$$

How fast is the enclosed area changing after 10 seconds?

63. Related Rates. A right circular cylinder has radius r and height h that are both changing with respect to time according to the functions

$$r(t) = 3t + \frac{1}{t}$$

$$h(t) = 2t^2 + 3t - 1$$

What is the rate of change of the surface area of the cylinder at time $t = 1$ second? *Hint:* The surface area is given by $S = r^2\pi h$.

Marginality

The cost C and revenue R when x units of a product are produced are given by

$$C(x) = x^2 + x + 5$$

$$R(x) = 9x$$

For Problems 64–67, determine the indicated quantities.

64. What is the marginal cost?
65. What is the marginal revenue?
66. What production level makes the marginal revenue equal to the marginal cost? What is your interpretation of this result?
67. What is the profit function $P(x)$? What is the value of the profit when the marginal profit is zero?

68. Marginal Cost. The cost of producing x widgets is given by

$$C(x) = 0.36x^2 - 0.14x + 2$$

What is the marginal cost when the production is 100 widgets?

69. Marginal Profit. If the revenue function for the widgets in Problem 68 is

$$R(x) = 7.06x$$

what is the marginal profit $P(x)$?

70. Hmmmmm. In 1860, the German mathematician Karl Weierstrass (1815–1897) discovered a function that was continuous *everywhere* but differentiable *nowhere* (needless to say, the graph of the function had a lot of corner-points). Although the authors could not convince the art department to draw the graph of this *Weierstrass function* the illustrators objected to drawing an infinite number of corner-points), the four graphs shown in Figure 42 represent better and better approximations to the graph of the Weierstrass function. What argument would you use to convince someone that the Weierstrass curve does not have a derivative anywhere?

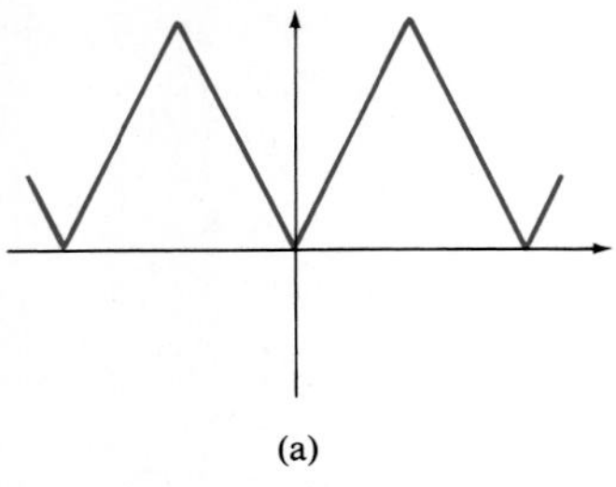

(a)

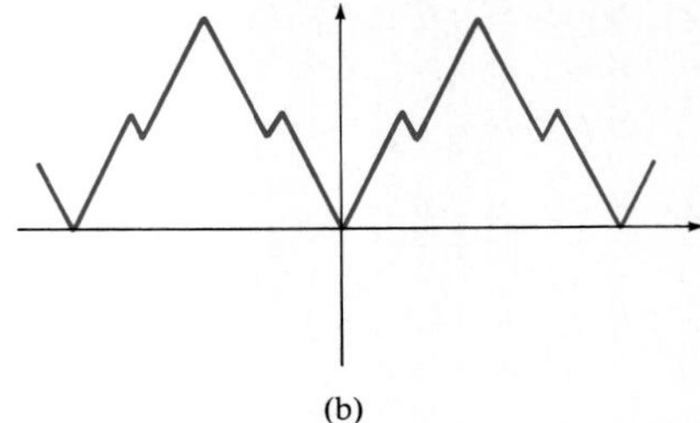

(b)

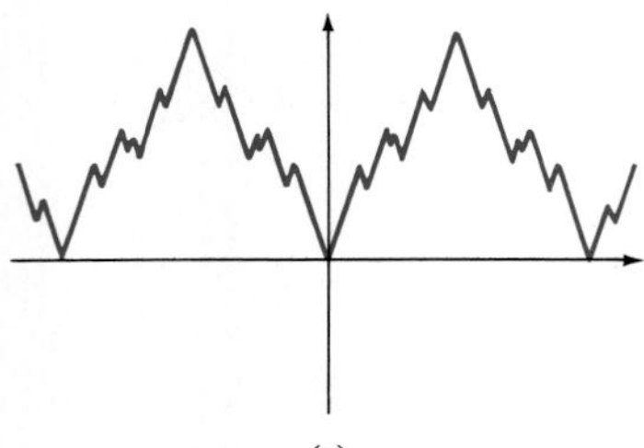

(c)

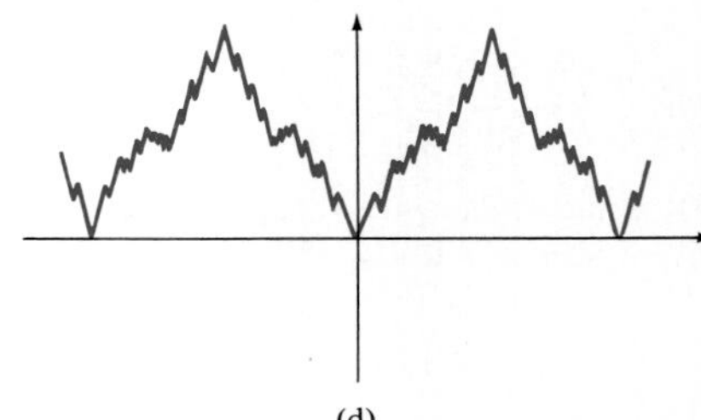

(d)

Figure 42
Approximations to the graph of the Weierstrass function. Can you visualize the limiting curve?

Chapter Test

1. Find the limit

$$\lim_{x \to 36} \frac{6 - \sqrt{x}}{x + 36}$$

2. Find the derivative of

$$f(x) = \frac{1}{x - 3}$$

by using the definition.

3. Find the derivative of

$$f(x) = (\sqrt{x} + 1)^{1/2}$$

4. Find the derivative of

$$f(x) = (x^2 + 1)(5x - 1)$$

using the product rule.

5. Find the derivative of

$$f(x) = x^{4/3} + x^{3/4}$$

6. An object moves along a line so that after t seconds the distance $s(t)$ in feet from a given reference point is

$$s(t) = 50 - 4t - 5t^2$$

Find $s'(1)$ and $s'(2)$. Interpret the results.

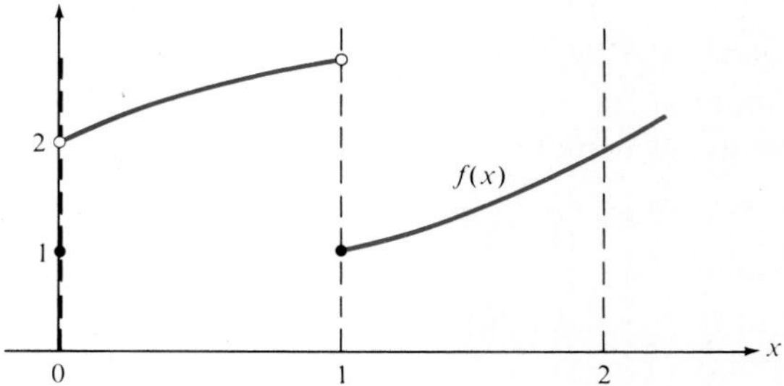

Figure 43
Graph for Problems 7–8

Problems 7–8 refer to the graph in Figure 43.

7. Find the following limit:

$$\lim_{x \to 1} f(x)$$

8. (a) Is f continuous on the interval (0, 1)? Why?
(b) Is f continuous on the interval (1, 2)? Why?
(c) Is f continuous on the interval (0, 2)? Why?

9. How Much Wood Is in a Tree? Foresters know how to approximate the amount of wood in a tree by simply measuring the diameter of the trunk of the tree at a given height. Suppose that it is possible to predict the number B of board feet* of wood in a spruce tree from the tree's diameter d (in inches) at eye level from the equation

$$B = 12 + 0.005(d - 6)^3 \qquad d \geq 6$$

What is the instantaneous rate of change in the volume of the tree when the diameter is 16 inches? Why would this value be useful to a forester?

10. An Experiment You Can Try. A ball thrown straight up into the air has a height of

$$h(t) = 30t - 16t^2$$

feet after t seconds.

(a) What is the initial velocity of the ball?
(b) What is the velocity of the ball after 2 seconds?
(c) When will the ball hit the ground?
(d) What will be the velocity when the ball hits the ground?

11. An Important Equation in Economics: *MR* = *MC*. Suppose that the cost to produce x items of a given product is

$$C(x) = \frac{1}{3}x^3 - 5x^2 + 30x + 100$$

dollars. It is also known that the revenue taken in from the sale of x items is

$$R(x) = 50x - x^2$$

For what value(s) of x will the marginal revenue be equal to the marginal cost? Interpret your results.

---

* One board foot is one square foot, one inch thick.

The concept of instantaneous change of a function as defined by the derivative allows one to study a variety of phenomena otherwise left to speculation.

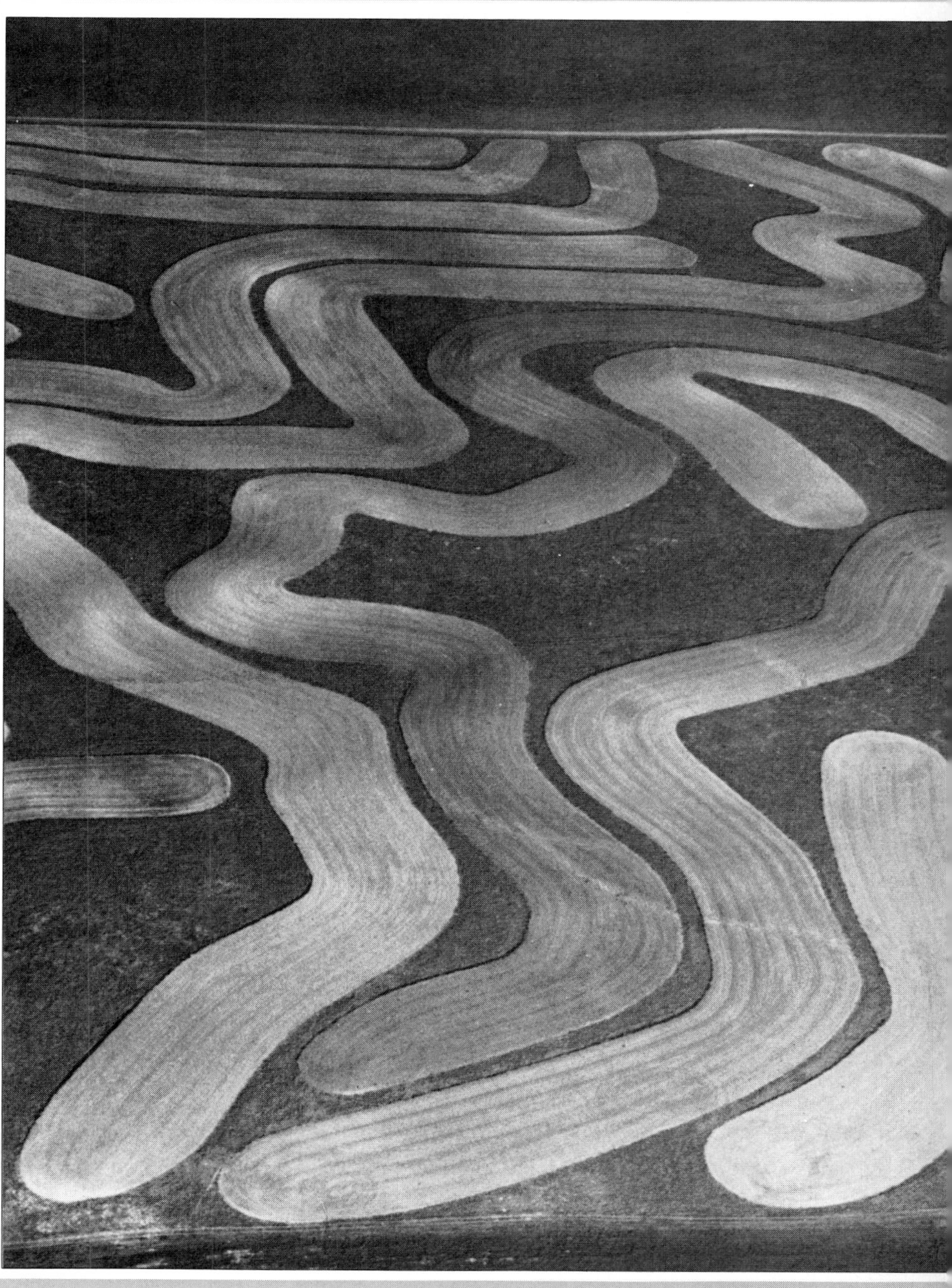

2 Additional Derivative Topics and Applications

The derivative is one of the most useful concepts in all of mathematics. In this chapter we show how it can be used to solve a variety of problems in business and science. In Sections 2.1 and 2.2 we begin by showing how the derivative can be used to analyze in detail the graph of a function. In Sections 2.3 and 2.4 we show how the derivative can be used to find both the maximum and the minimum of a function and to solve an important class of problems known as optimization problems. Finally, in Section 2.5 we introduce what are known as related rates problems, which allow us to find the rate of change of one variable in terms of the rate of change of another variable.

2.1 Use of the Derivative in Graphing

PURPOSE

We introduce several tools used in graphing functions. The major tools are

- the determination of increasing and decreasing regions of a function and
- the determination of critical and stationary points of a function.

Introduction

Beginning students of mathematics usually graph functions by plotting a series of points and then drawing curves of some type connecting the plotted points. Although this point-plotting approach may give a rough shape of the curve, the method does not provide enough detailed information about the function to solve many advanced graphing problems. No matter how many points are plotted, the values of the function between the points can only be surmised. For example, between two successive plotted points, we must guess whether the graph exhibits a downward curvature (Figure 1a), an upward curvature (Figure 1b), or both (Figure 1c).

In this section and the next we will show how the derivative can aid in graphing functions. We begin by determining when a function is increasing and when it is decreasing.

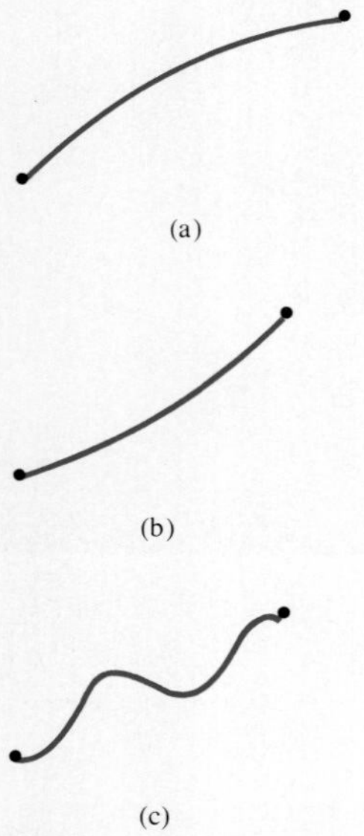

(a)

(b)

(c)

Figure 1
Different shapes of a graph

Increasing and Decreasing Functions

The adjectives *increasing* and *decreasing*, when applied to a function, refer to the behavior of the graph of a function as we move from left to right along the real axis. If the graph is rising as we move from left to right through a point, we say that the function is **increasing** at this point. On the other hand, if the graph is falling at a point as we move from left to right through a point, we say that the function is **decreasing** at this point. The function graphed in Figure 2 is rising or increasing at points in the interval $(-\infty, -2)$, falling or decreasing at points in the interval $(-2, 3)$, and increasing again in the interval $(3, \infty)$.

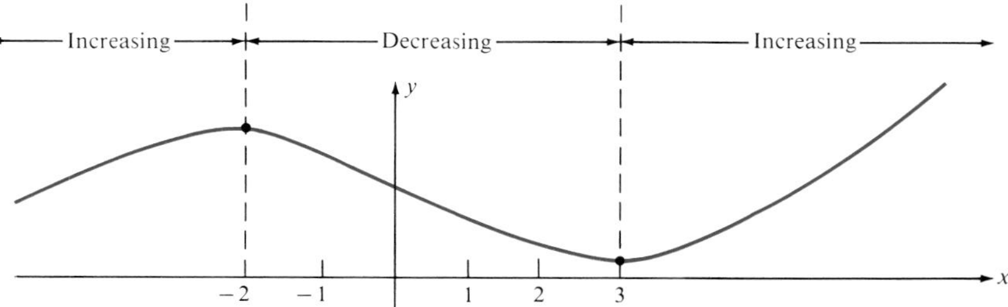

Figure 2
Intervals where a function is increasing and decreasing

It is clear from Figure 2 that on the intervals where the graph is increasing, the derivative $f'(x)$ is positive, and on the intervals where the curve is decreasing, the derivative $f'(x)$ is negative. This leads us to a useful test for determining where the graph of a function is increasing and where it is decreasing.

Finding Increasing and Decreasing Intervals of a Function

Assume that a function f has a derivative at $x = c$. The sign of the derivative $f'(c)$ will determine whether the graph $y = f(x)$ is increasing or decreasing at c. Specifically,

- if $f'(c) > 0$, then f is increasing at c,
- if $f'(c) < 0$, then f is decreasing at c, and
- if $f'(c) = 0$, then f is neither increasing nor decreasing at c.

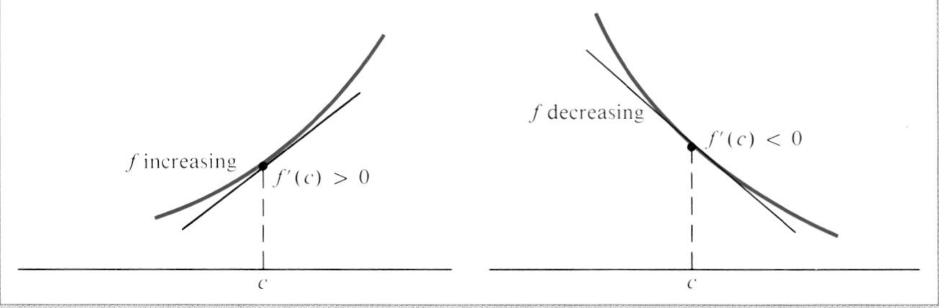

If f is increasing at each point in an interval (a, b), then f is increasing on (a, b).

Example 1 Increasing and Decreasing Functions Given the function

$$f(x) = \frac{1}{3}x^3 - \frac{3}{2}x^2 + 2x + 1$$

find the values of x where the graph $y = f(x)$ is increasing and where it is decreasing. Use this information to graph the function.

Solution We first compute the derivative

$$\begin{aligned} f'(x) &= x^2 - 3x + 2 \\ &= (x-1)(x-2) \end{aligned}$$

To determine where this derivative is positive and where it is negative, it is useful to draw the following diagram showing the intervals where each factor is positive or negative:

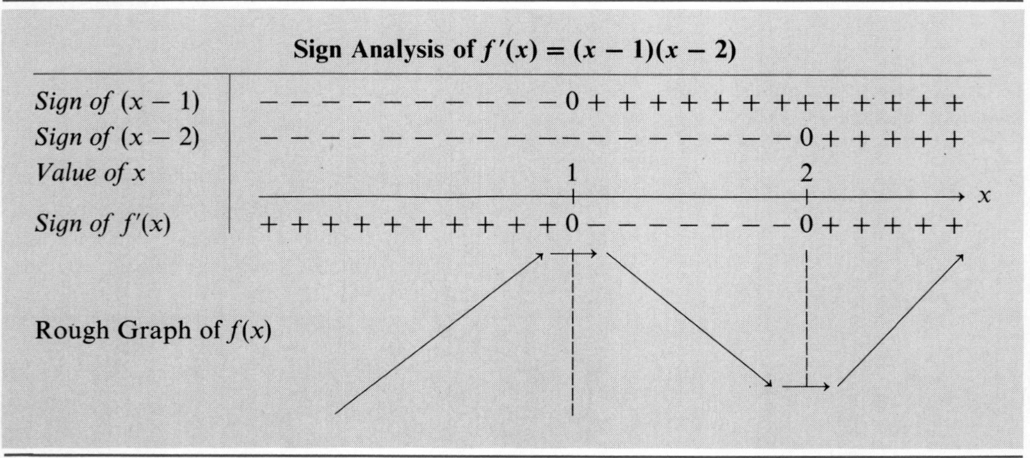

Examining the numerical sign of the derivative (whether it is positive or negative), we see that the graph of f is increasing for x less than 1 or greater than 2 and decreasing for x satisfying $1 < x < 2$. Using this information and plotting a few relevant points (Figure 3), we can draw an accurate graph of the function. □

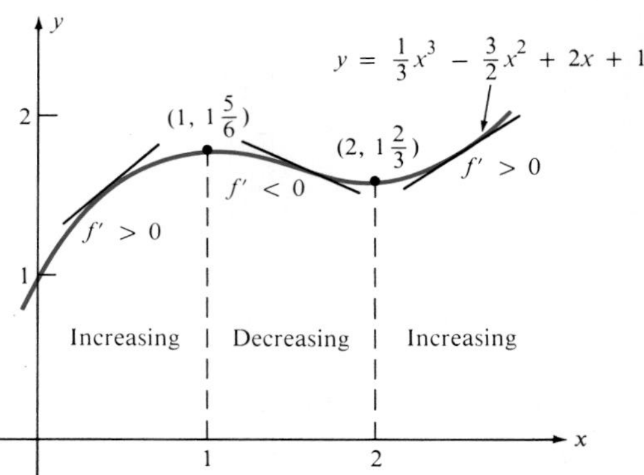

Figure 3
First derivative test

"A Few Relevant Points"

When we drew the graph in Figure 3, we used the fact that we knew where the function was increasing and where it was decreasing. We then selected a few relevant points to draw the graph. By selecting certain points we are using the old point-plotting method, except that now we know much more about what happens between the points. It is a rule of thumb that one of the relevant points is usually chosen by letting $x = 0$ so that we can find the point where the graph crosses the y-axis (the y-intercept). Also, by setting $y = 0$ and solving for x we can find the places where the graph crosses the x-axis. The number of relevant points needed to plot the graph depends on the behavior of the function and how certain we are of the form of the graph.

In the graph in Figure 3 the points $x = 1, 2$ where $f'(x) = 0$ play an important role in the graph of the function. These points are called stationary points. This leads us to the next important tool for graphing.

Definition of Critical and Stationary Points

A **critical point** of a function f is any point where either the derivative f' does not exist or is zero. Critical points where the derivative is zero are called **stationary points**.

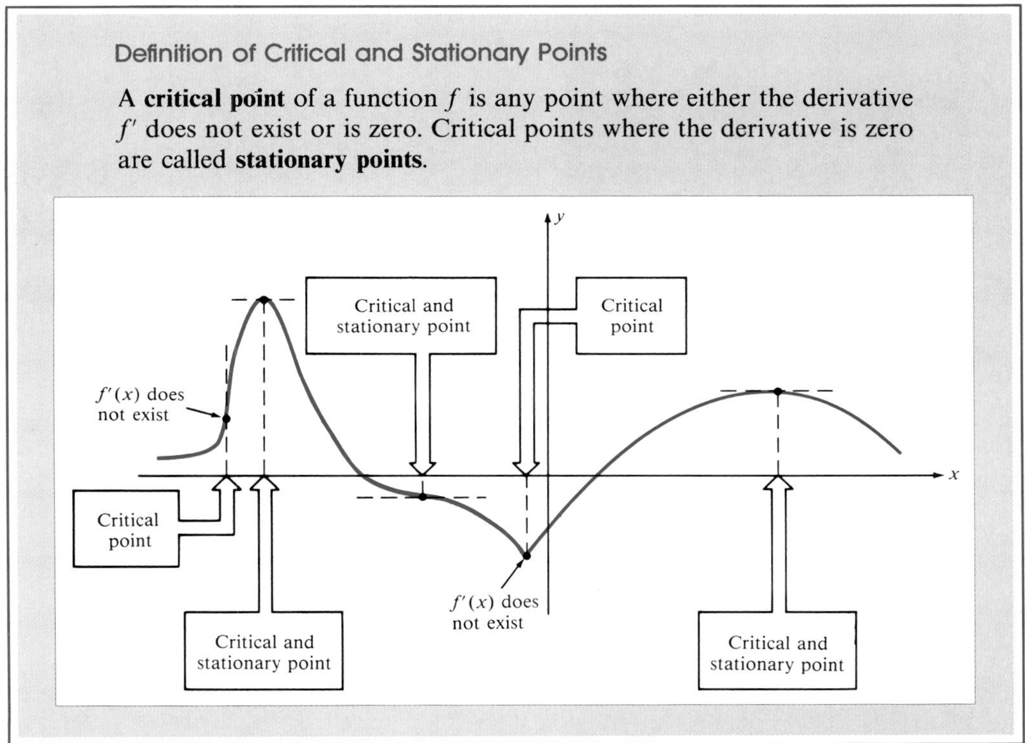

Comments on Critical and Stationary Points

The diagram above illustrates the different ways in which the graph of a function can behave at a critical point. For example, when a function fails to have a derivative at a point, the graph can have a corner-point, it can go straight up, or it can have a discontinuity at such points.

Stationary points are different. They correspond to points on the graph of the function where the function has momentarily stopped increasing or decreasing. The fundamental property that distinguishes a stationary point is the fact that the tangent line to the graph is horizontal at a stationary point. Often the graph of a function reaches its maximum or its minimum values at stationary points. At other times the graph of a function momentarily stops increasing or decreasing at a stationary point. Knowledge about the behavior of a function at its critical points is extremely valuable in graphing functions.

Example 2

Critical and Stationary Points Find both the critical and the stationary points, if any, of the function

$$f(x) = x^2 - 4x + 3$$

Solution Computing the first derivative, we have

$$f'(x) = 2x - 4$$

This derivative exists for all values of x and is zero when x is 2. Hence the function has a critical point (which is also a stationary point) at 2. The graph of the function is shown in Figure 4. □

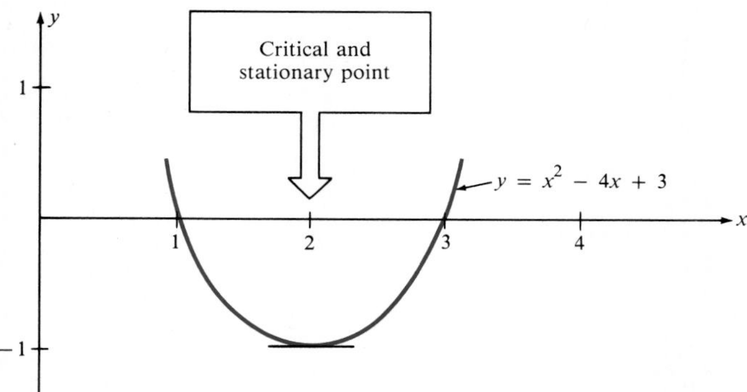

Figure 4
Critical and stationary point at 2

Example 3

Critical and Stationary Points Find both the critical and the stationary points of the absolute value function

$$f(x) = |x|$$

Solution The graph of this function can easily be drawn without resorting to ideas of calculus. It is shown in Figure 5.

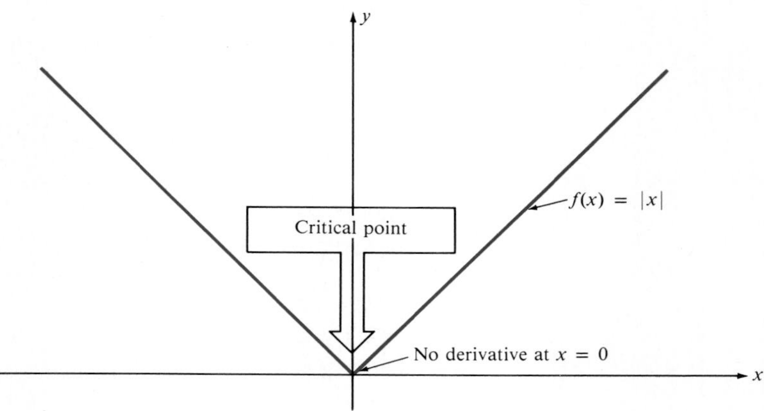

Figure 5
Critical point at 0

The slopes of the tangent lines to the graph of $f(x) = |x|$ are given in Table 1 for different values of x.

TABLE 1
Slope of Tangent Lines for Values of x

Value of x	Slope of Tangent Line to $f(x) = \|x\|$
$x < 0$	-1
$x = 0$	does not exist
$x > 0$	$+1$

Hence the derivative of $f(x) = |x|$ is

$$\frac{d}{dx}|x| = \begin{cases} -1 & (x < 0) \\ \text{does not exist} & (x = 0) \\ +1 & (x > 0) \end{cases}$$

Thus the absolute value function has a critical point at zero. Since the derivative is never zero, the function does not have a stationary point. □

Example 4

Critical and Stationary Points Find both the critical and the stationary points of

$$f(x) = x^{2/3}$$

Also find the regions where the function is increasing and where it is decreasing.

Solution Using the power rule to compute the derivative, we have

$$f'(x) = \frac{2}{3}x^{-1/3}$$

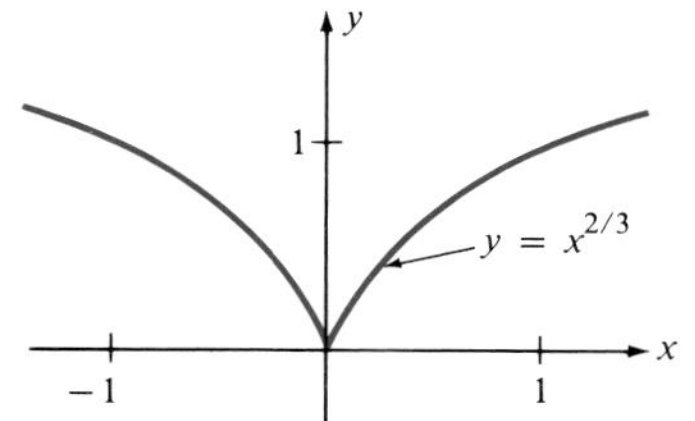

Figure 6
Graph of $y = x^{2/3}$

Since $f'(x)$ does not exist at $x = 0$, we conclude that f has a critical point at zero (observe no stationary points since the derivative is never zero). To find the regions where f is increasing and where it is decreasing, we carry out the following sign analysis:

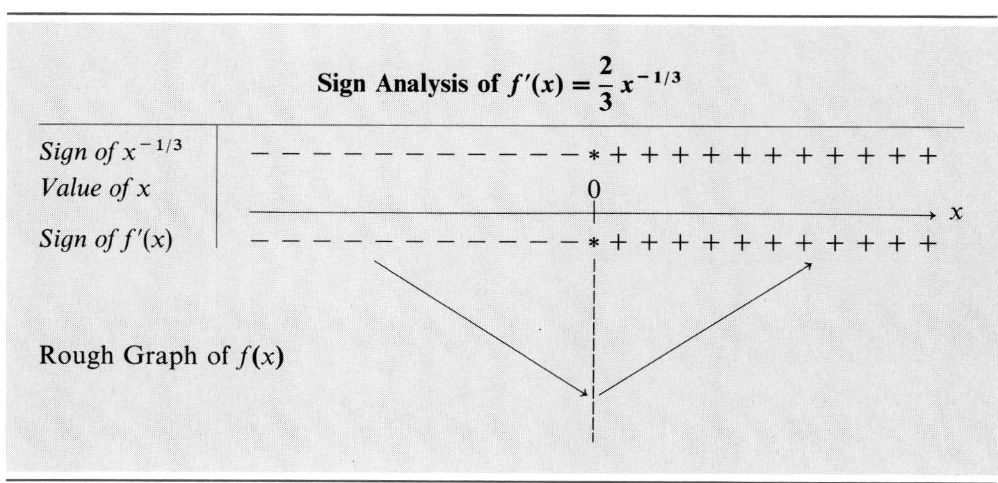

By plotting a few relevant points and using the above information, the graph of $f(x) = x^{2/3}$ can be plotted as shown in Figure 6. □

Finding the Revenue Function from the Demand Curve

The study of a company's revenue, cost, and profit is known as the **theory of the firm** in mathematical economics. We continue our ongoing study of this important topic by showing why the **demand function** $q = D(p)$ is so important in this theory.

Until now we have expressed the revenue $R(q)$ in terms of the number of items q produced. However, revenue can always be computed by the formula

$$R = pq$$

where

$$p = \text{Price of each item}$$
$$q = \text{Number of items produced}$$

If we now substitute the value of q in the demand curve $q = D(p)$ into the above revenue equation, we have

$$R(p) = p\,D(p) \qquad \text{(revenue in terms of price)}$$

This equation is important because it gives the revenue in terms of the price of a product and not the number of items produced. In other words, it gives an alternative way of finding the revenue.

Also, since the profit P from the production of a given product is the revenue R minus the cost C, we can also write the profit in terms of the price. Doing this, we have

$$\begin{aligned} P(p) &= R(p) - C(p) \\ &= p\,D(p) - C(p) \qquad \text{(profit in terms of price)} \end{aligned}$$

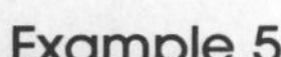

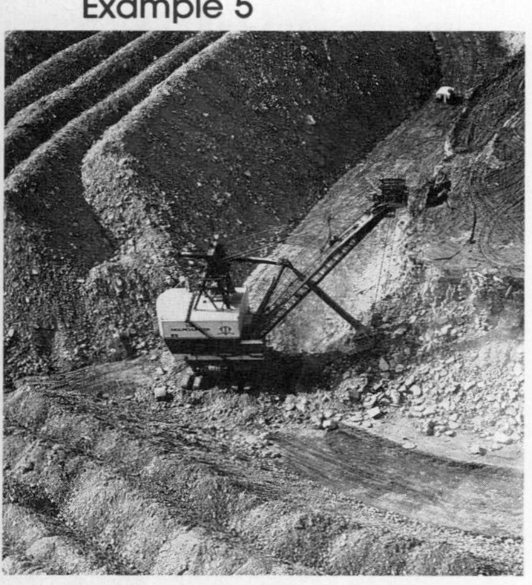

All large mining companies carry out detailed studies to predict revenue, cost, and profit. Failure to determine accurate estimates of these quantities can spell the difference between success and failure.

Theory of the Firm The number q of tons of molybdenum that the Colorado Molybdenum Co. can sell in one day depends on the market price p in dollars for a ton of molybdenum. Suppose the relationship between the daily demand for molybdenum and the market price is

$$q = D(p) = 100 - \frac{p}{10} \qquad (\$100 \le p \le \$1000)$$

(a) Find the company's daily revenue in terms of the price p of molybdenum and evaluate the revenue when the price is \$400 per ton.

(b) Find the company's daily revenue in terms of the number of tons q of molybdenum produced.

Solution

(a) Using the general revenue formula $R = pq$, we can write

$$\begin{aligned} R(p) &= p\,D(p) \\ &= p\left(100 - \frac{p}{10}\right) \\ &= -\frac{p^2}{10} + 100p \qquad (\$100 \le p \le \$1000) \end{aligned}$$

When the price of molybdenum is \$400 per ton, the company's weekly revenue will be

$$R(400) = 400\left(100 - \frac{400}{10}\right)$$
$$= \$24{,}000$$

(b) To find the revenue $R = pq$ in terms of q, we simply solve for p in the demand function

$$q = D(p) = 100 - \frac{p}{10}$$

in terms of q. This gives

$$p = 1000 - 10q$$

Hence we have

$$\begin{aligned} R(q) &= pq \\ &= (1000 - 10q)q \\ &= -10q^2 + 1000q \end{aligned}$$ □

Final Comment

The previous example illustrates one of the reasons why the demand function $q = D(p)$ is useful in the theory of the firm. It allows the revenue, cost, and profit of a firm to be rewritten completely in terms of p.

Problems

Problems 1–6 refer to the graph of $y = f(x)$ in Figure 7.

1. Identify the points where $f(x)$ is increasing.
2. Identify the points where $f(x)$ is decreasing.
3. Identify the critical points.
4. Identify the stationary points.
5. Identify the points where the derivative does not exist.
6. Identify the points where the derivative is zero.

For Problems 7–8, draw a graph $y = f(x)$ that has the given properties.

7. (a) $f'(-1)$ does not exist.
(b) $f(0) = 1$
(c) $f'(1) = 0$
(d) $f'(2) = 1$
(e) $f'(3)$ is negative.
(f) f has a stationary point at $x = 4$.
(g) $f(6) = 0$

8. (a) f has a critical point at $x = 0$.
(b) f has a stationary point at $x = 1$.
(c) $f(1) = 2$
(d) $f'(2) = 1$
(e) $f'(3) = -1$
(f) $f'(4) = 0$

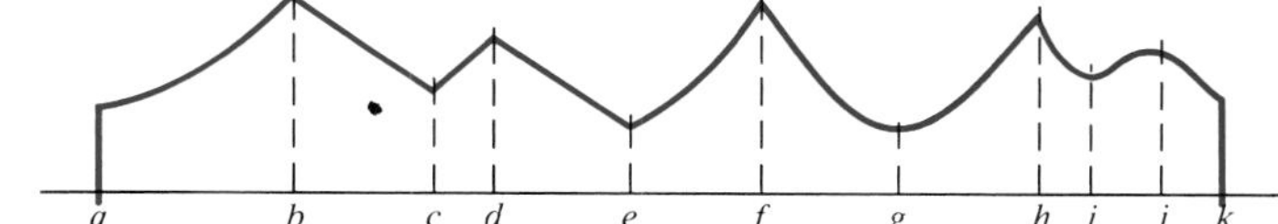

Figure 7
Graph for Problems 1–6

For Problems 9–10, use the information given to make a rough sketch of a plausible graph $y = f(x)$.

9.

x: 0 at the first mark, 1 at the second mark

$f'(x)$ — — — — — — 0 + + + + + + + + 0 — — — — — —

x	$f(x)$
0	1
1	4

10.

x: 1, 2, 3 at the marks

$f'(x)$ — — — — — — 0 + + + + + + + + 0 — — — — — — — 0 + + + + +

x	$f(x)$
1	0
2	1
3	0

11. Sign of the Derivative. In the graph in Figure 8, give the sign of the derivative in each of the intervals:
(a) $(-2, -1)$
(b) $(-1, 0)$
(c) $(0, 1)$
(d) $(1, 2)$

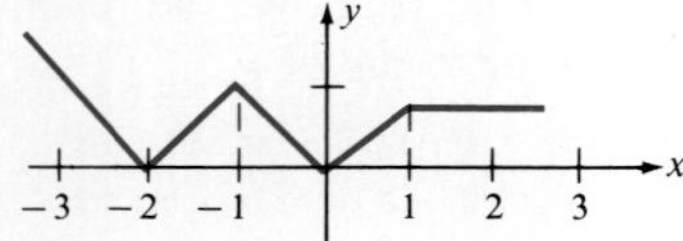

Figure 8
Graph for Problem 11

For Problems 12–36, find the critical and stationary points, and determine the intervals where the functions are increasing and where they are decreasing. Use this information to graph the functions.

12. $f(x) = 5$
13. $f(x) = 3x + 1$
14. $f(x) = x^2$
15. $f(x) = x^2 - 1$
16. $f(x) = x^2 - 2x - 3$
17. $f(x) = (x - 4)^2$
18. $f(x) = x^3$
19. $f(x) = x^3 + 5$
20. $f(x) = x^3 - 4x$
21. $f(x) = (x - 3)^3$
22. $f(x) = 3x^3 - 3x^2 + 1$
23. $f(x) = x + \dfrac{1}{x^2}$
24. $f(x) = x + \dfrac{1}{x}$
25. $f(x) = x^4$
26. $f(x) = (x - 1)^4$
27. $f(x) = (x + 2)^4$
28. $f(x) = \dfrac{x - 1}{x + 1}$
29. $f(x) = x^{1/2}$
30. $f(x) = x^{1/3}$
31. $f(x) = x^{1/5}$
32. $f(x) = x^{4/3}$
33. $f(x) = (x - 4)^{2/3}$
34. $f(x) = 2x - 3x^{2/3}$
35. $f(x) = 1 - x^{2/3}$
36. $f(x) = (x - 1)^{5/3}$

For Problems 37–42, determine the intervals where the functions are increasing and those where the functions are decreasing. Find the critical and stationary points.

37.

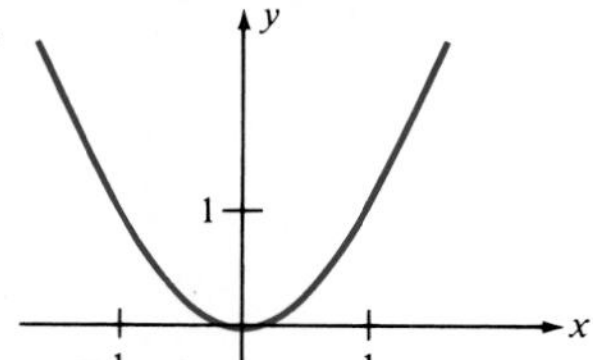

38.

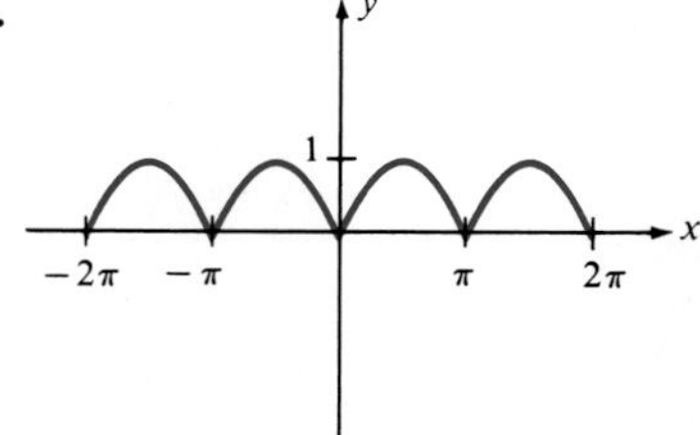

39.

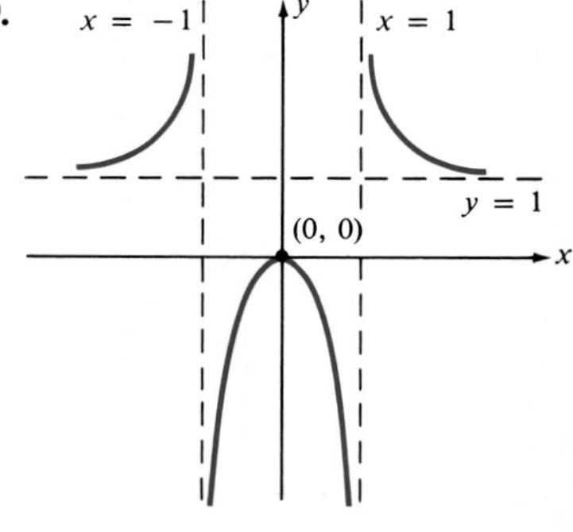

40.

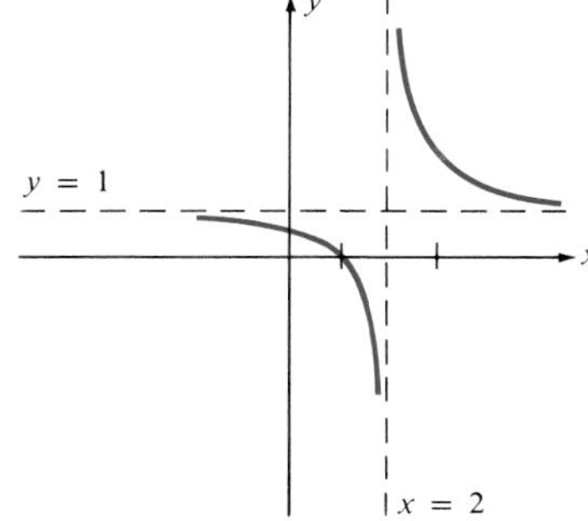

41.

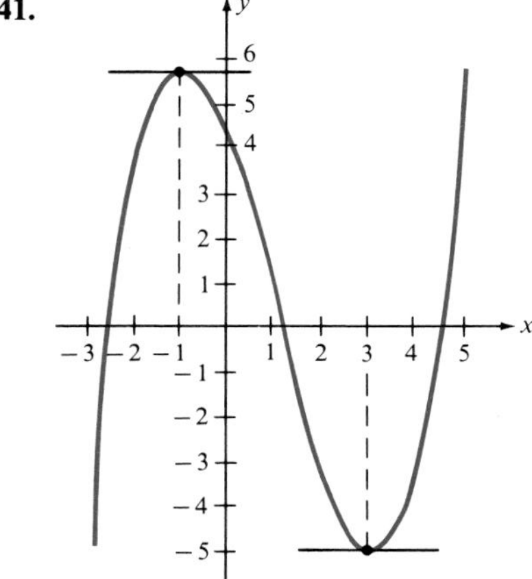

42.

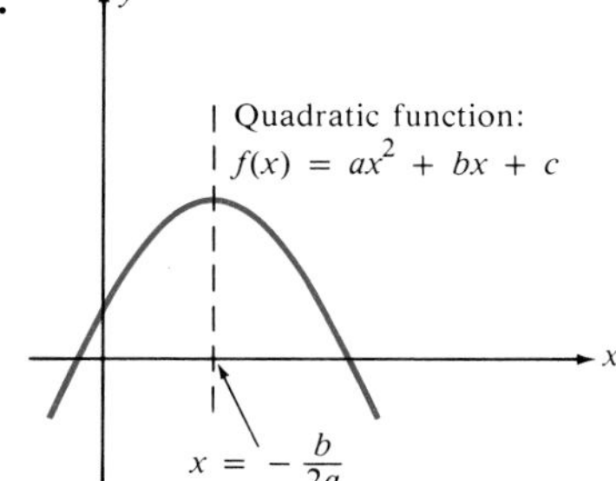

For Problems 43–45, state in common language how the slope of the functions change as one moves from left to right on the real axis.

43.

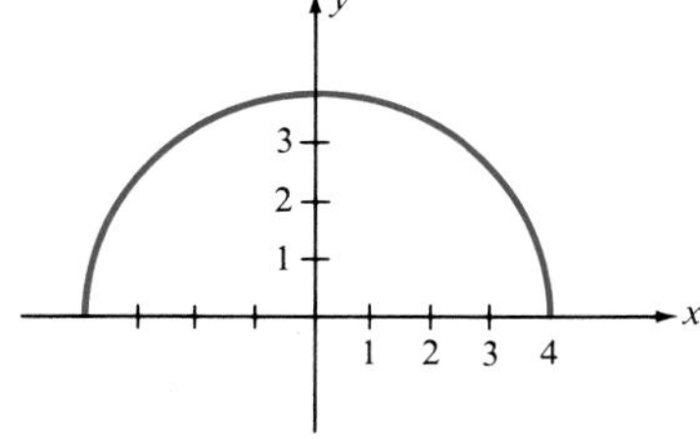

44.

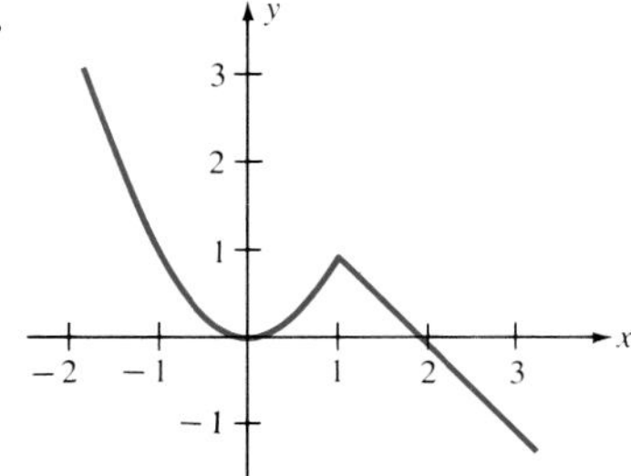

45.

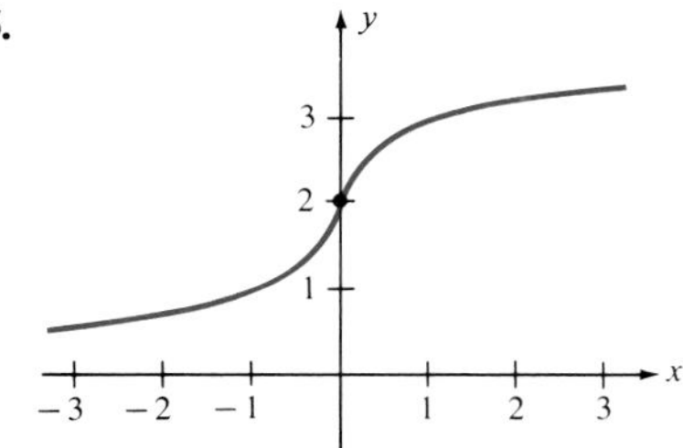

More Theory of the Firm

46. Finding Revenue from the Demand Curve. Find the revenue function $R(p)$ if the demand curve is given by

$$q = D(p) = 20 - 5p$$

47. Finding Revenue from the Demand Curve. Find the revenue function $R(p)$ if the demand curve is given by

$$q = D(p) = 9 - p^2$$

48. Finding Profit from Demand and Cost. Find the profit function $P(q)$ if the demand curve is

$$q = D(p) = 25 - p^2$$

and the cost function is

$$C(q) = 10 + 3q$$

49. Finding Profit from Demand and Cost. Find the profit function $P(q)$ if the demand curve is

$$q = D(p) = 36 - p^2$$

and the cost function is

$$C(q) = 5 + 0.5q$$

50. Finding Marginal Revenue and Marginal Profit. Find the marginal revenue $R'(q)$ and the marginal profit $P'(q)$ if the demand curve is

$$q = D(p) = 25 - p$$

and the cost function is

$$C(q) = 50 + 0.5q$$

51. Finding Marginal Revenue and Marginal Profit. Find the marginal revenue $R'(q)$ and the marginal profit $P'(q)$ if the demand curve is

$$q = D(p) = 64 - p^2$$

and the cost function is

$$C(q) = 100 + 0.5q + 0.001q^2$$

2.2 Use of the Second Derivative in Graphing

PURPOSE

We introduce the concept of higher derivatives and show how the second derivative also gives useful information about the graph of a function. Important topics include

- higher derivatives,
- the concavity and inflection points of a graph, and
- the use of second derivatives for determining concavity.

Introduction

In the previous section we learned how the first derivative can be used to determine when the graph of a function is increasing and when it is decreasing. However, several characteristics of the graph of a function cannot be determined by the first derivative. For instance the two graphs drawn in Figure 9 are both increasing, yet they have a basic qualitative difference in their behavior. Although they both are headed in an "upward" direction, one graph is curved "downward," and the other curved "upward."

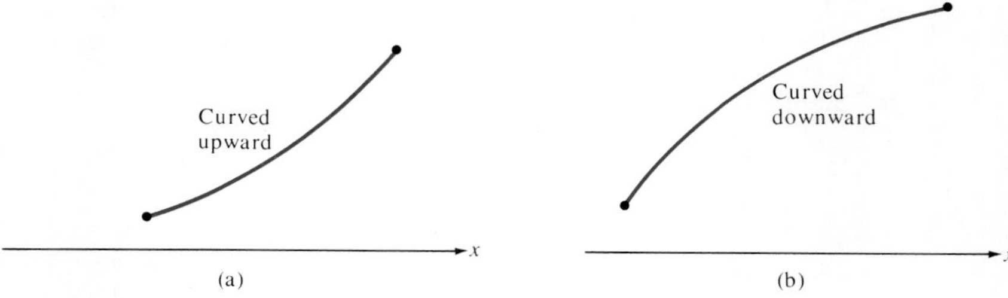

Figure 9
Two increasing functions

To understand some of these additional properties of graphs, we introduce higher derivatives.

Higher Derivatives

The derivative f' is called the **first derivative** or simply the derivative of f. Since this derivative is a new function, we can differentiate it and obtain the derivative of the derivative. This is called the **second derivative** of f. In fact, if we continue this process we can find a third, fourth, and even **higher derivatives**. The general notation for derivatives of all orders are given in Table 2.

TABLE 2
General Notation for Higher Derivatives

Notation	Meaning
f	Function
f'	First derivative
$f'' = (f')'$	Second derivative
$f''' = (f'')'$	Third derivative
$f^{(4)} = (f''')'$	Fourth derivative
$f^{(5)} = (f^{(4)})'$	Fifth derivative
$\vdots \quad \vdots$	$\vdots$
$f^{(n)} = (f^{(n-1)})'$	nth derivative

Example 1

Higher Derivatives Find the first six derivatives of the polynomial

$$f(x) = x^4 + 5x^3 + 3x^2 + 3x + 7$$

Solution Starting with

$$f(x) = x^4 + 5x^3 + 3x^2 + 3x + 7$$

we simply differentiate to get

$$\begin{aligned} f'(x) &= 4x^3 + 15x^2 + 6x + 3 \\ f''(x) &= 12x^2 + 30x + 6 \\ f'''(x) &= 24x + 30 \\ f^{(4)}(x) &= 24 \\ f^{(5)}(x) &= 0 \\ f^{(6)}(x) &= 0 \end{aligned}$$

Note that all derivatives of order five or higher are zero. □

Leibniz "dee" Notation

It is also possible to represent higher-order derivatives by means of the Leibniz "dee" notation. If f is a function of x, then we write

$$\begin{aligned} f'(x) &= \frac{d}{dx}[f(x)] \\ f''(x) &= \frac{d}{dx}\left[\frac{d}{dx}[f(x)]\right] = \frac{d^2}{dx^2}[f(x)] \\ f'''(x) &= \frac{d}{dx}\left[\frac{d}{dx}\left[\frac{d}{dx}[f(x)]\right]\right] = \frac{d^3}{dx^3}[f(x)] \\ &\vdots \qquad \vdots \\ f^{(n)}(x) &= \frac{d^n}{dx^n}[f(x)] \end{aligned}$$

In general, we have two alternative notations for the nth derivative, which are

$$f^{(n)}(x) \quad \text{and} \quad \frac{d^n}{dx^n}[f(x)]$$

Both are read "the nth derivative of f with respect to x."

Example 2

Higher Derivatives Find the first three derivatives of the function

$$y = x^2 + \frac{1}{x} \qquad (x \neq 0)$$

Solution Using the rules of differentiation, we repeatedly differentiate, getting

$$\frac{dy}{dx} = 2x - \frac{1}{x^2}$$

$$\frac{d^2y}{dx^2} = 2 + \frac{2}{x^3}$$

$$\frac{d^3y}{dx^3} = -\frac{6}{x^4}$$

□

Concavity and Inflection Points

Earlier in this chapter we saw that the first derivative provided us with information about when a function is increasing or decreasing. It is natural to wonder whether the second and higher derivatives provide any information about the graph of a function. Although derivatives higher than second order do not provide much information about the graph of a function, the second derivative is very important to the understanding of the graph of a function.

Definition of Concavity and Inflection Points

A function f is **concave up** at a point $x = a$ if in some small region near the point $(a, f(a))$ the graph of f lies above the tangent line to the graph at $(a, f(a))$. On the other hand, a function f is **concave down** at $x = a$ if in some small region near the point $(a, f(a))$ the graph of f lies below the tangent line to the graph at $(a, f(a))$.

An **inflection point** of a graph is a point where the graph changes from concave up to concave down or vice versa.

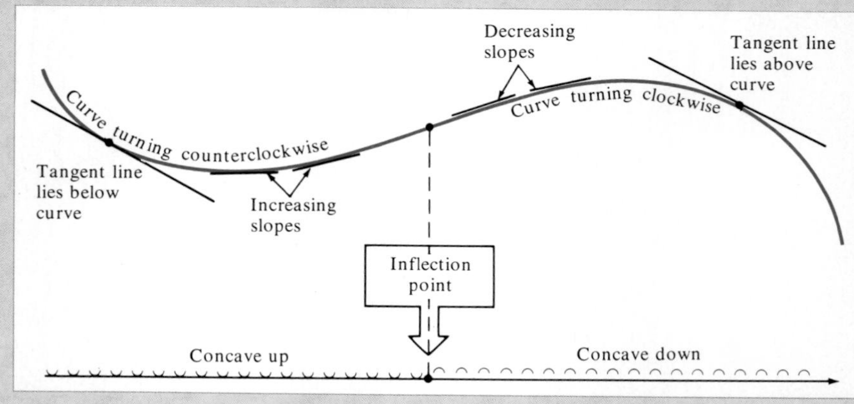

The Calculus Connection to Concavity

It is clear from the definition of concavity that if f is differentiable on an open interval (a, b), then the graph of f is

- *Concave up* on (a, b) if $f'(x)$ is *increasing* as we move from left to right on (a, b), that is, $f''(x) > 0$, for x in (a, b).
- *Concave down* on (a, b) if $f'(x)$ is *decreasing* as we move from left to right on (a, b), that is, $f''(x) < 0$, for x in (a, b).

It turns out that we can use the second derivative of a function to determine where a function is concave up and concave down in much the same way that we used the first derivative to determine when a function was increasing and decreasing.

Use of the Second Derivative

The role of the second derivative in graphing lies in the fact that it can be used to determine where a function is concave up or concave down. We make this clear here.

Second Derivative in Determining Concavity

Let f define a function that has a second derivative $f''(c)$ at $x = c$. Then

- if $f''(c) > 0$, then f is concave up at c,
- if $f''(c) < 0$, then f is concave down at c, and
- if $f''(c) = 0$, then no conclusion can be drawn.

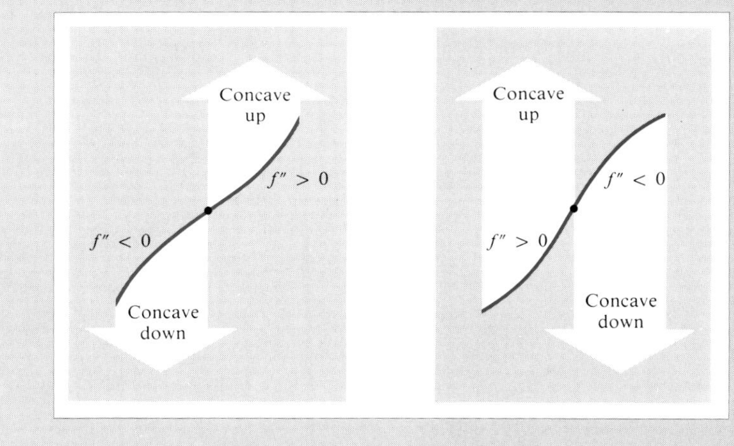

Although no conclusion can be drawn in general when $f''(c) = 0$, it often happens that f has an inflection point at c when $f''(c) = 0$.

Example 3 Determining Concavity Let $f(x)$ be given by

$$f(x) = \frac{1}{3}x^3 - \frac{3}{2}x^2 + 2x + 1$$

Find

(a) The intervals where f is increasing and where it is decreasing
(b) The critical and the stationary points
(c) The intervals on which f is concave up or concave down
(d) The inflection points

Use the above information to graph the function.

Solution

(a) *Increasing and decreasing intervals:* We begin by computing the first derivative. We have

$$\begin{aligned} f'(x) &= x^2 - 3x + 2 \\ &= (x - 1)(x - 2) \end{aligned}$$

To determine where the graph $y = f(x)$ is increasing and where it is decreasing, we determine where the derivative $f'(x)$ is positive and where it is negative.

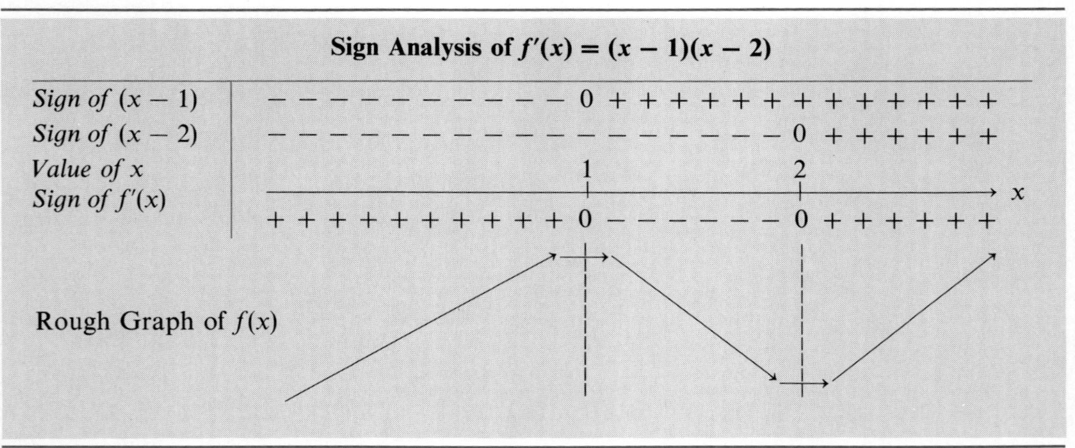

The above sign analysis says that the graph $y = f(x)$ is increasing on the intervals $(\infty, 1)$ and $(2, \infty)$ and decreasing on $(1, 2)$.

(b) *Critical and stationary points:* To find the critical and the stationary points, we observe that the derivative $f'(x)$ always exists and is zero when $x = 1, 2$. Hence these two points are critical points (which are also stationary points).

(c) *Concave up and down:* To determine where the graph is concave up and where it is concave down, we compute the second derivative:

$$f''(x) = 2x - 3 \quad \begin{cases} \text{positive for } x > \frac{3}{2} \\ \text{zero for } x = \frac{3}{2} \\ \text{negative for } x < \frac{3}{2} \end{cases}$$

The second derivative says that the graph is concave up on the interval $(\frac{3}{2}, \infty)$, since $f''(x) > 0$ on that interval. Also the graph is concave down on the interval $(-\infty, \frac{3}{2})$, since $f''(x) < 0$ on that interval.

(d) *Inflection point (changing concavity):* The function has an inflection point at $x = \frac{3}{2}$, since the second derivative $f''(x)$ changes sign at this point. It is often the case that the inflection point occurs when the second derivative is zero.

To graph the function, we first plot the points in Table 3. The graph of f is shown in Figure 10. □

TABLE 3
Relevant Points of the Graph

x	$f(x)$	Why Relevant?
0	1.00	Easy point to plot
1.0	1.83	Stationary point
1.5	1.75	Inflection point
2.0	1.67	Stationary point
4.0	6.33	Typical point

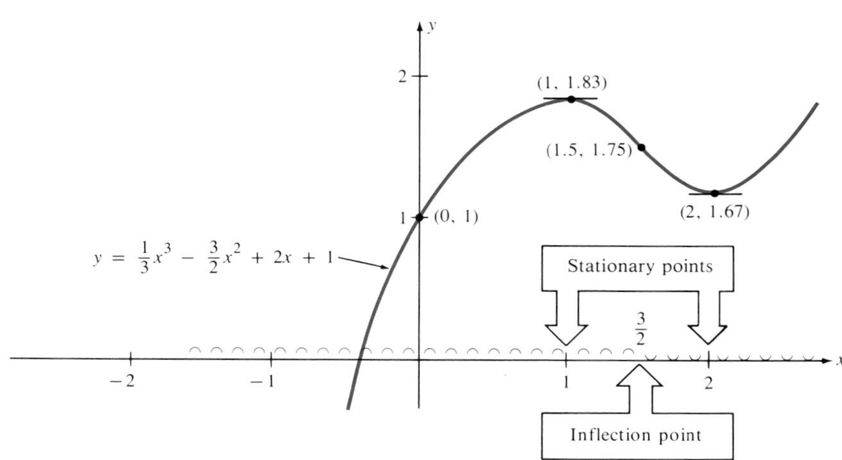

Figure 10
Graph of the cubic equation

Using the first and second derivatives, the following steps can be followed when graphing functions:

Steps in Graphing $y = f(x)$

Step 1. Calculate $f'(x)$ and $f''(x)$.

Step 2. Use $f'(x)$ to determine the critical and the stationary points and to find the intervals where f is increasing and the intervals where f is decreasing.

Step 3. Use $f''(x)$ to determine inflection points and to find the intervals where f is concave up and the intervals where f is concave down.

Step 4. Plot a few strategic points and use the above information to sketch the graph.

Example 4

Advanced Graphing Graph the function

$$f(x) = \frac{1}{3}x^3 - x^2 + 4$$

Solution Using the above four-step process, we have

- **Step 1** [calculate $f'(x)$ and $f''(x)$]. Finding the first and second derivatives, we have

$$f'(x) = x^2 - 2x \quad \begin{cases} \text{Positive} & (x < 0 \text{ or } x > 2) \\ \text{Zero} & (x = 0, 2) \\ \text{Negative} & (0 < x < 2) \end{cases}$$

$$f''(x) = 2x - 2 \quad \begin{cases} \text{Positive} & (x > 1) \\ \text{Zero} & (x = 1) \\ \text{Negative} & (x < 1) \end{cases}$$

- **Step 2** (find intervals where f is increasing and decreasing). The first derivative tells us

  (i) f is increasing on $(-\infty, 0)$ and $(2, \infty)$,
  (ii) f has stationary points at 0 and 2, and
  (iii) f is decreasing on $(0, 2)$.

- **Step 3** (find the intervals of concavity). The second derivative tells us

  (i) f is concave up on $(1, \infty)$,
  (ii) f has an inflection point at 1, and
  (iii) f is concave down on $(-\infty, 1)$.

- **Step 4** (plot some relevant points). We now plot the points given in Table 4. The graph of f is shown in Figure 11. □

TABLE 4
Points Plotted for Example 4

Point Plotted	Why Plotted?
$(0, 4)$	The graph crosses the y-axis at this point. The graph also has a horizontal tangent line at this point.
$(2, \frac{8}{3})$	The graph of the function has a horizontal tangent line at this point (also an inflection point of the curve).
$(3, 4)$	Selected at random.
$(-3, -14)$	Selected at random.

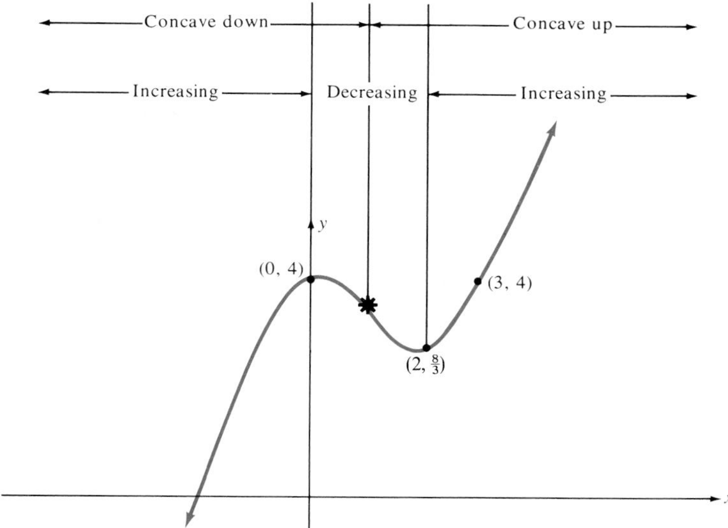

Figure 11
Graph of a cubic polynomial

Asymptotes and Limits at Infinity

We are often interested in how the graph of a function behaves as its argument becomes large positively or large negatively. As an example, consider the rational function defined by

$$f(x) = \frac{5x + 4}{2x} \qquad (x \neq 0)$$

It is interesting to evaluate this function for larger and larger values of x as shown in Table 5.

TABLE 5
Illustration of the Limit at Infinity

x	$f(x)$
1	4.5
10	2.7
100	2.52
1,000	2.502
10,000	2.5002
100,000	2.50002
1,000,000	2.500002
10,000,000	2.5000002

The graph of this function is shown in Figure 12. Note that as x increases, the values of $f(x)$ get closer and closer to the horizontal line $y = 2.5$. This line is called the **horizontal asymptote** of the graph $y = f(x)$ at infinity. We use the

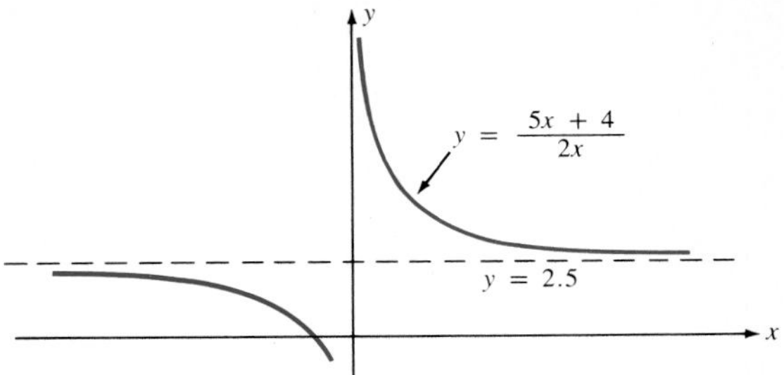

Figure 12
Horizontal asymptote $y = 2.5$

notation $x \to \infty$ (read "x approaches infinity") to indicate that x increases without bound. This discussion leads us to the formal definition of horizontal asymptotes and limits at infinity.

Definitions of Horizontal Asymptotes and Limits at Infinity

A function f has a limit or approaches a **limiting value** of L as $x \to \infty$ if the values of $f(x)$ approach the number L as x increases without bound. We write this limit at infinity as

$$\lim_{x \to \infty} f(x) = L$$

On the other hand, we write the limit of f at minus infinity

$$\lim_{x \to -\infty} f(x) = L$$

to mean that the values of $f(x)$ approach L as x decreases without bound.

If either of these limits exists, we say that the horizontal line $y = L$ approached by the graph $y = f(x)$ is a horizontal asymptote of the graph. It is possible for any graph $y = f(x)$ to have either 0, 1, or 2 horizontal asymptotes.

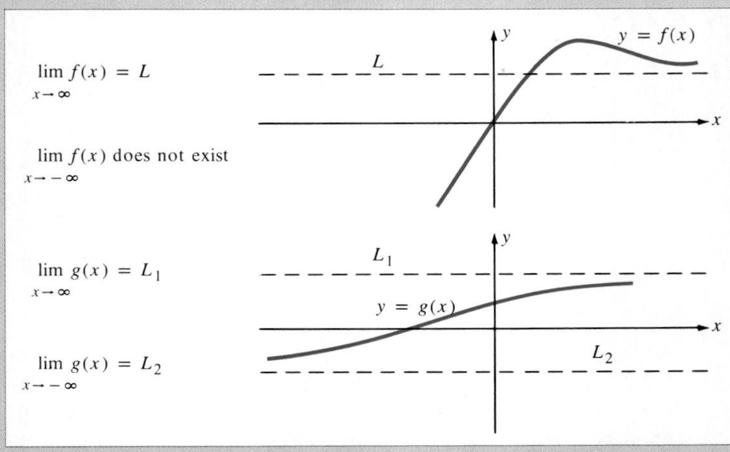

Horizontal Asymptotes of Rational Functions

One class of functions that always has limits at infinity and hence horizontal asymptotes are the **rational functions** (ratios of polynomials) in which the degree of the numerator polynomial is less than or equal to the degree of the denominator polynomial.

Example 5

Horizontal Asymptotes Find the limit at plus infinity (if it exists) of the rational function

$$f(x) = \frac{3x + 5}{4x + 7}$$

and find the horizontal asymptote there.

Solution To calculate the limiting value at infinity of a rational function, a general rule is to divide both the numerator and denominator by the highest power of x in the denominator. This gives

$$f(x) = \frac{3x + 5}{4x + 7} = \frac{3 + \dfrac{5}{x}}{4 + \dfrac{7}{x}}$$

As $x \to \infty$, the two terms with x in the denominator will go to zero. This gives the limiting value at infinity of

$$\lim_{x \to \infty} f(x) = \frac{3 + 0}{4 + 0} = \frac{3}{4}$$

In this case, both the numerator and the denominator polynomials had the same degree. Hence the limit at plus infinity is the ratio of the coefficients of the highest powers of x. Note, too, that the limit of $f(x)$ at minus infinity is also $\frac{3}{4}$. The graph of $f(x)$ is shown in Figure 13. □

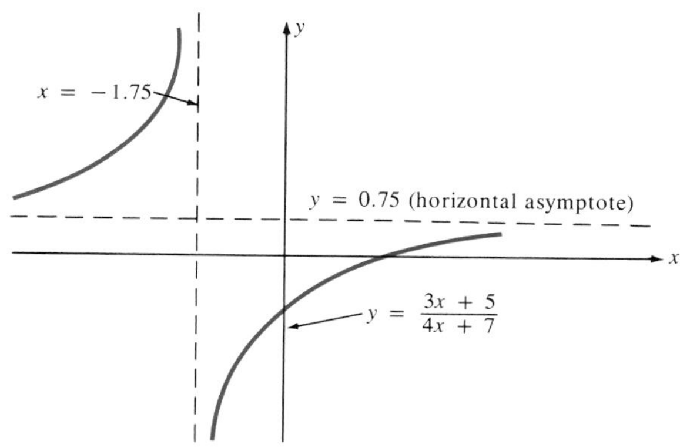

Figure 13
A rational function with a horizontal asymptote

Example 6 Horizontal Asymptotes Find the limit at infinity of the rational function

$$f(x) = \frac{5x^2 + 2x + 3}{2x^2 - x + 9}$$

and find the horizontal asymptote.

Solution Again, the degrees of the numerator and the denominator are the same. Hence we rewrite $f(x)$ as

$$f(x) = \frac{5x^2 + 2x + 3}{2x^2 - x + 9} = \frac{5 + \dfrac{2}{x} + \dfrac{3}{x^2}}{2 - \dfrac{1}{x} + \dfrac{9}{x^2}}$$

Clearly, as $x \to \infty$, we get the limit

$$\lim_{x \to \infty} f(x) = \frac{5 + 0 + 0}{2 - 0 + 0} = \frac{5}{2}$$

Hence the line $y = \frac{5}{2}$ is the horizontal asymptote of $f(x)$ at plus infinity. □

Vertical Asymptotes of Rational Functions

It is often the case that the value of a function $f(x)$ "approaches" plus or minus infinity as x approaches some finite number $x = c$. The graph of the rational function

$$f(x) = \frac{2x}{x - 1}$$

is shown in Figure 14. In this case the vertical line $x = 1$ is called a **vertical asymptote** of the graph of $y = f(x)$. The following is a more formal definition of this concept.

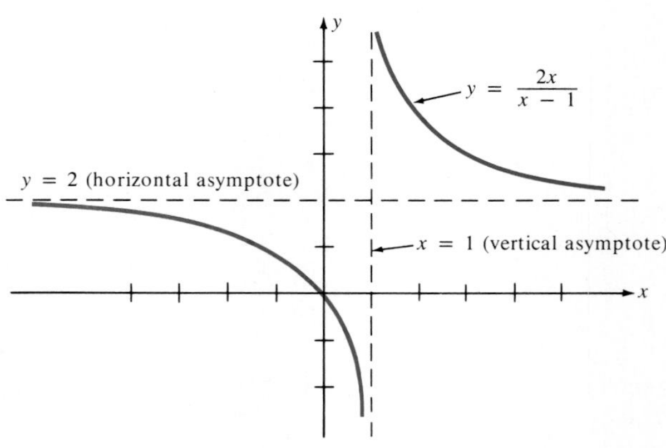

Figure 14
A rational function with both vertical and horizontal asymptotes

Definition of a Vertical Asymptote

If the value of a function $f(x)$ gets large without bound or becomes an arbitrarily large negative number as x approaches a value c from either the left or the right, we say that the vertical line $x = c$ is a vertical asymptote of the graph $y = f(x)$.

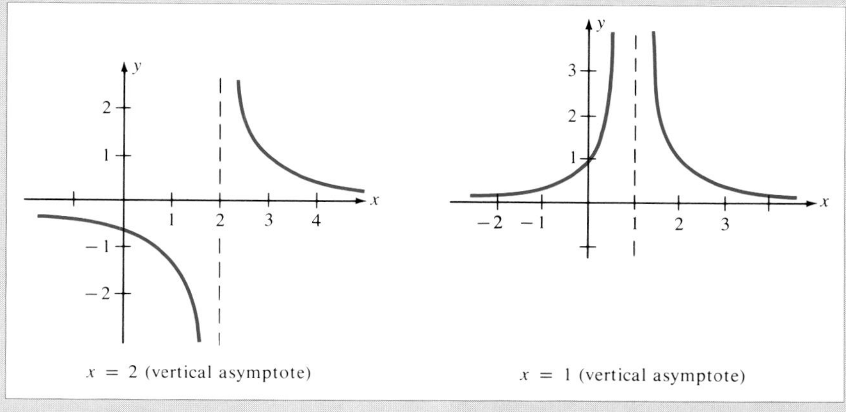

$x = 2$ (vertical asymptote) $x = 1$ (vertical asymptote)

The graph of a function may have either no vertical asymptotes or any number of vertical asymptotes. In fact, there are functions that have an infinite number of vertical asymptotes.

Example 7

Vertical Asymptote Find the vertical asymptotes (if any) of the rational function

$$f(x) = \frac{x + 1}{x - 2}$$

Solution Since the denominator of $f(x)$ is zero at $x = 2$ while the numerator is not zero at $x = 2$, it is clear that the function will approach plus or minus infinity as x approaches 2. To draw the graph of $y = f(x)$ in a small region around $x = 2$, we perform the following sign analysis:

Sign Analysis of $f(x) = \dfrac{x+1}{x-2}$ near the Vertical Asymptote $x = 2$

Sign of $x + 1$	− − − − − − − − 0 + + + + + + + + + + + +
Sign of $x - 2$	− − − − − − − − − − − − − 0 + + + + + + +
Value of x	−1 2 → x
Sign of $f(x)$	+ + + + + + + + 0 − − − − * + + + + + + +

We now use the additional fact that the sign of $f(x)$ is negative in the interval $(-1, 2)$ and positive elsewhere to draw its graph as shown in Figure 15. Note that $f(x)$ has the horizontal asymptote $y = 1$ and the vertical asymptote $x = 2$. □

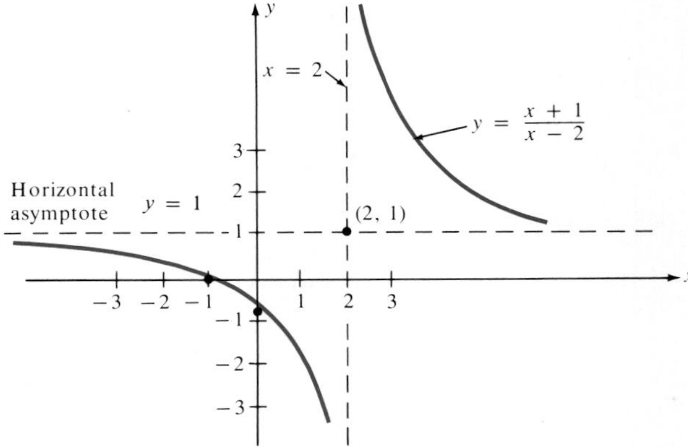

Figure 15
Graph with both a horizontal and a vertical asymptote

In general, if the denominator of a rational function is zero at $x = c$ and the numerator is not zero at c, then $x = c$ will be a vertical asymptote. Hence the rational function

$$f(x) = \frac{x^2 + 1}{(x - 1)(x + 2)}$$

has two vertical asymptotes, $x = 1$ and $x = -2$. It also has one horizontal asymptote, $y = 1$. Table 6 shows the graphs of other rational functions.

Estimating Congressional Seats

After the next presidential election, note the fraction p of the popular vote that the elected president receives. Using this value of p, evaluate the "*House function*"

$$H(p) = \frac{p^3}{p^3 + (1 - p)^3} \qquad 0 \le p \le 1$$

The interesting property of this function, called the *cube law*, is that the value $H(p)$ approximates the proportion of seats in the House of Representatives going to the party of the winning presidential candidate. For example, in 1936 the Democratic candidate, Franklin Delano Roosevelt, won the presidential election with 61% of the popular vote. In that election, the House function would estimate the fraction of Democrats elected to the House of Representatives to be

$$H(0.61) = \frac{(0.61)^3}{(0.61)^3 + (0.39)^3} = 0.79 \quad (79\%)$$

In that election, the Democrats won 333 House seats; and the Republicans won 89 House seats. These values translate to a 78.9% majority for the Democrats.

TABLE 6
Examples of
Rational Functions

Function	Limit at Infinity	Graph of Function
$f(x) = \dfrac{1}{x-1}$	$y = 0$	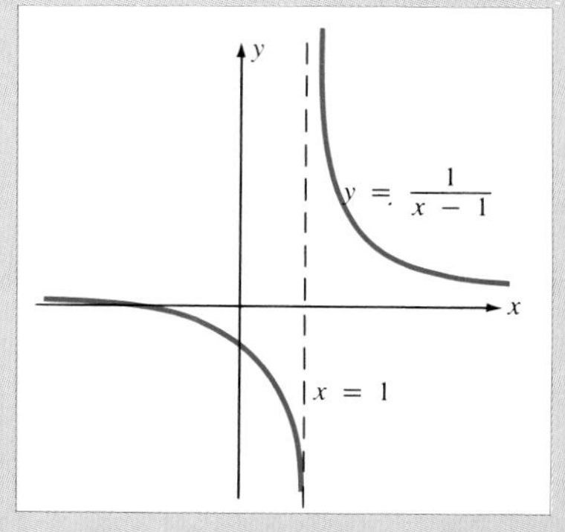
$f(x) = \dfrac{x}{x-2}$	$y = 1$	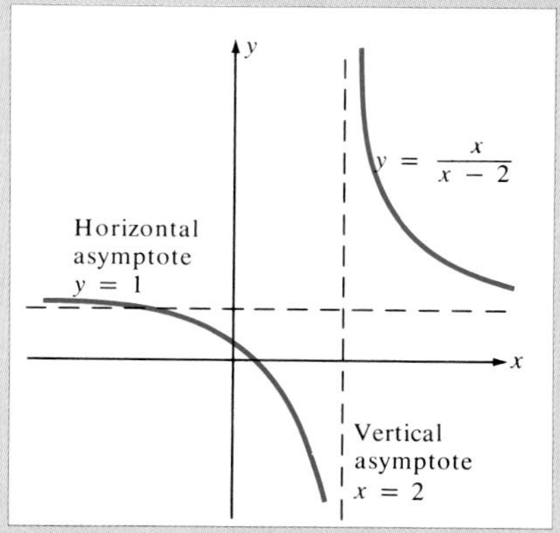
$f(x) = \dfrac{2 + x - x^2}{(x-1)^2}$	$y = -1$	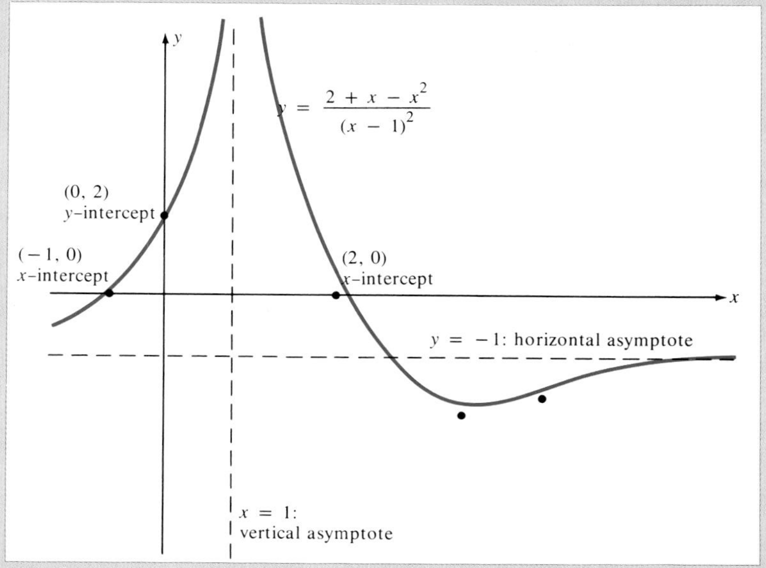

The House function is not always that accurate, but Table 7 shows the results of presidential elections from 1900 to 1988.

TABLE 7
House Function Estimate of the Congressional Seats from the Presidential Results

Year	Elected President, Party, and Percentage of Popular Vote	House Function (estimate of percentage of house members from winning ticket)	Actual Percentage of House Members of Same Party as Elected President (error in estimate)
1900	W. McKinley (R) 54%	62%	58% (4%)
1904	T. Roosevelt (R) 56%	67%	65% (2%)
1908	W. Taft (R) 52%	56%	56% (0%)
1912	W. Wilson (D) 42%	38%	50% (12%)
1916	W. Wilson (D) 50%	50%	49% (1%)
1920	W. Harding (R) 60%	77%	70% (7%)
1924	C. Coolidge (R) 54%	62%	58% (4%)
1928	H. Hoover (R) 58%	72%	62% (10%)
1932	F. Roosevelt (D) 57%	70%	73% (3%)
1936	F. Roosevelt (D) 61%	79%	79% (0%)
1940	F. Roosevelt (D) 54%	62%	62% (0%)
1944	F. Roosevelt (D) 53%	59%	56% (3%)
1948	H. Truman (D) 50%	50%	55% (5%)
1952	D. Eisenhower (R) 55%	65%	65% (0%)
1956	D. Eisenhower (R) 57%	70%	70% (0%)
1960	J. Kennedy (D) 50%	50%	55% (5%)
1964	L. Johnson (D) 61%	79%	72% (7%)
1968	R. Nixon (R) 43%	30%	45% (15%)
1972	R. Nixon (R) 61%	79%	57% (22%)
1976	J. Carter (D) 50%	50%	55% (5%)
1980	R. Reagan (R) 51%	53%	57% (4%)
1984	R. Reagan (R) 59%	75%	48% (27%)
1988	G. Bush (R) 54%	62%	41% (21%)

Figure 16 shows the graph of the House function $H(p)$ and plotted points illustrating the results of presidential and House elections from 1900 to 1988.

Example 8

Derivatives of the House Function Find the first and second derivatives of the House function $H(p)$ and explain why these derivatives are consistent with the graph of $H(p)$ shown in Figure 16.

Solution We first rewrite the House function as

$$H(p) = \frac{p^3}{p^3 + (1-p)^3}$$

$$= \frac{p^3}{3p^2 - 3p + 1}$$

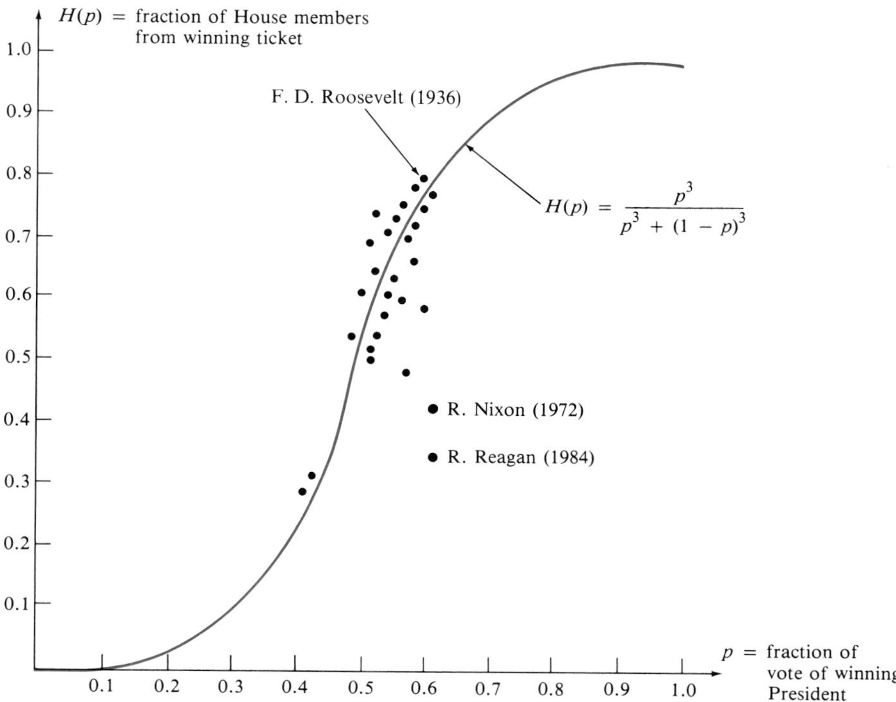

Figure 16
The House function estimates the proportion of elected congressmen from the winning presidential ticket

Hence

$$\begin{aligned}\frac{dH}{dp} &= \frac{(3p^2 - 3p + 1)(3p^2) - p^3(6p - 3)}{(3p^2 - 3p + 1)^2} \\ &= \frac{3p^2(p^2 - 2p + 1)}{(3p^2 - 3p + 1)^2} \\ &= \frac{3p^2(p - 1)^2}{(3p^2 - 3p + 1)^2}\end{aligned}$$

Using the quotient rule one more time, we find

$$\frac{d^2H}{dp^2} = \frac{6p(p - 1)(2p - 1)}{(3p^2 - 3p + 1)^3}$$

From this, we conclude that

$$\frac{dH(p)}{dp} > 0 \qquad 0 < p < 1 \qquad [H(p) \text{ is increasing on } (0, 1)]$$

$$\frac{d^2H(p)}{dp^2} > 0 \qquad 0 < p < \frac{1}{2} \qquad \left[H(p) \text{ is concave up on } \left(1, \frac{1}{2}\right)\right]$$

$$\frac{d^2H(p)}{dp^2} < 0 \qquad \frac{1}{2} < p < 1 \qquad \left[H(p) \text{ is concave down on } \left(\frac{1}{2}, 1\right)\right]$$

Note that the graph of $H(p)$ in Figure 16 has the desired properties of increasing or decreasing and concavity. □

Problems

For Problems 1–12, find $f''(x)$, $f''(0)$, $f''(1)$, and $f''(2)$.

1. $f(x) = x^3 + x^2 + x + 1$
2. $f(x) = 4x^2 + 1$
3. $f(x) = ax^2 + bx + c$
4. $f(x) = \dfrac{1}{x}$
5. $f(x) = \sqrt{x}$
6. $f(x) = \sqrt{x^2 + 1}$
7. $f(x) = \dfrac{x+1}{x-1}$
8. $f(x) = \dfrac{1}{x^2 + 1}$
9. $f(x) = (x + 1)^2$
10. $f(x) = \dfrac{1}{\sqrt{x}}$
11. $f(x) = (x^2 + 1)(x + 2)$
12. $f(x) = (x + 1)(x - 1)$

For Problems 13–17, find $f''(x)$, $f'''(x)$, and $f^{(4)}(x)$.

13. $f(x) = 3x^3 + 4x^2 + x - 5$
14. $f(x) = \dfrac{1}{x}$
15. $f(x) = x^n$ (where $n \geq 5$)
16. $f(x) = \dfrac{x}{x+1}$
17. $f(x) = x^{-3} + x^{1/2}$

For Problems 18–33, find the first and second derivatives of the given functions. Use this information to find
(a) The critical points
(b) The stationary points
(c) The intervals where the functions are increasing
(d) The intervals where the functions are decreasing
(e) The inflection points
(f) Intervals where the functions are concave up
(g) Intervals where the functions are concave down
Use this information to graph the functions.

18. $f(x) = 2x + 1$
19. $f(x) = x^2$
20. $f(x) = x^2 - 1$
21. $f(x) = x^2 - 4x + 3$
22. $f(x) = (x - 1)^2$
23. $f(x) = x^3$
24. $f(x) = x^3 + 1$
25. $f(x) = x^3 - x$
26. $f(x) = 3x^3 + 3x^2 - 2$
27. $f(x) = x + \dfrac{1}{x^2}$
28. $f(x) = x + \dfrac{1}{x}$
29. $f(x) = (x - 2)^3$
30. $f(x) = (x + 5)^3$
31. $f(x) = (x + 2)^4$
32. $f(x) = x^{1/3}$
33. $f(x) = x^{1/5}$

For Problems 34–39, determine the intervals where the graphs are concave up and intervals where the graphs are concave down. Find the inflection points.

34.
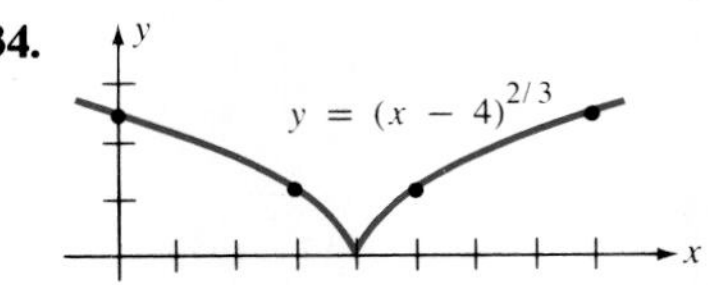

35.
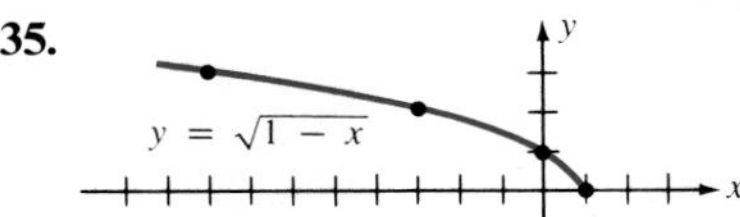

36.
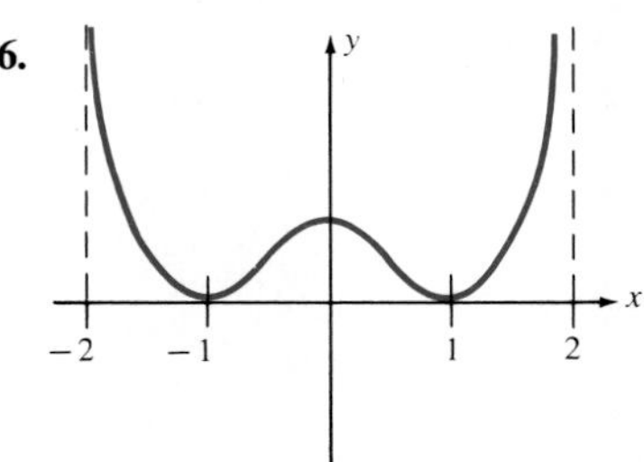

37.
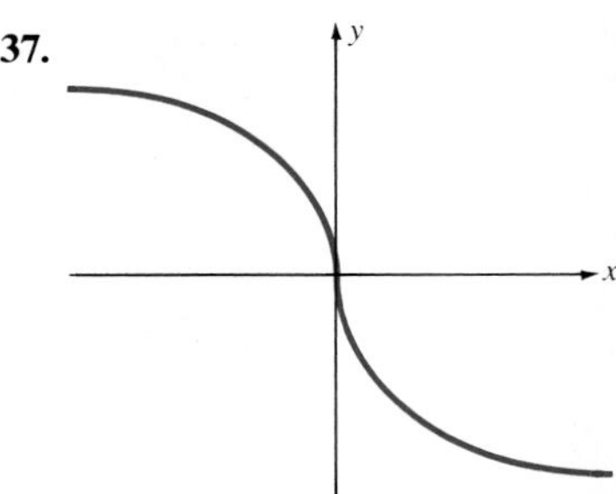

38.
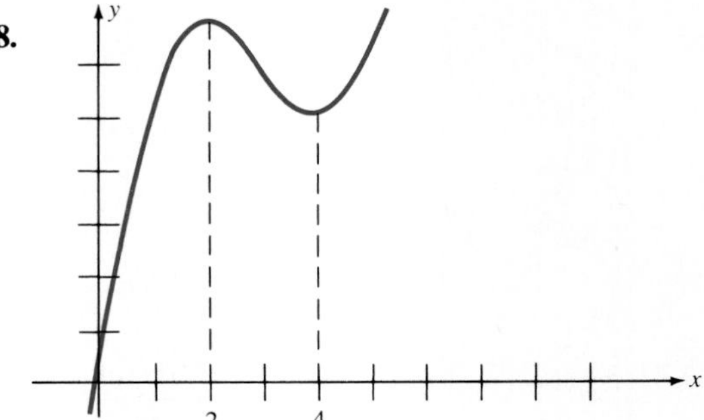

39.
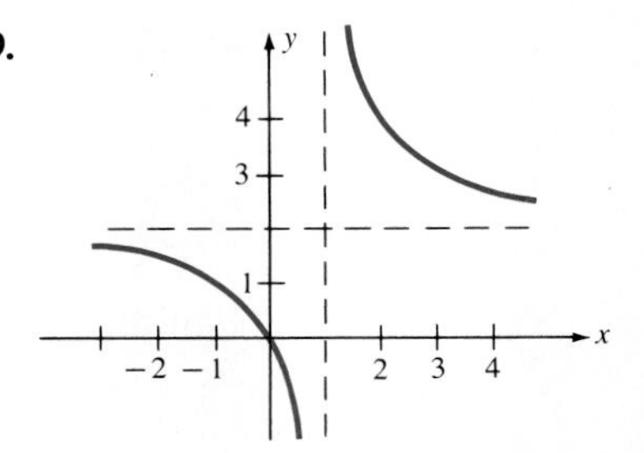

40. First and Second Derivatives. In Figure 17, give the sign of the first and second derivatives in each of the intervals:
(a) $(-2, -1)$
(b) $(-1, 0)$
(c) $(0, 1)$
(d) $(1, 2)$

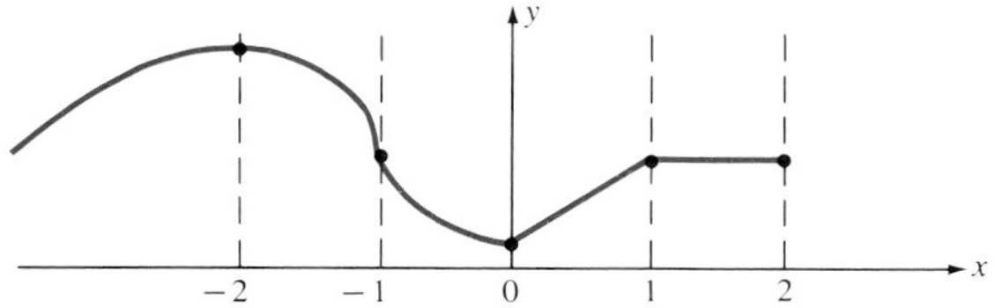

Figure 17
Graph for Problem 40

Limits at Infinity and Horizontal Asymptotes

For Problems 41–50, find the limits both at plus infinity and at minus infinity for the given functions. Find the horizontal asymptotes (if any).

41. $f(x) = 3$

42. $f(x) = \dfrac{1}{x}$

43. $f(x) = 3 + \dfrac{2}{x}$

44. $f(x) = \dfrac{1}{x - 1}$

45. $f(x) = \dfrac{1}{x^2}$

46. $f(x) = \dfrac{2x + 5}{3x - 8}$

47. $f(x) = \dfrac{9x + 10}{x - 4}$

48. $f(x) = \dfrac{x + 1}{x^2 + 1}$

49. $f(x) = \dfrac{3x^2 + 1}{x + 1}$

50. $f(x) = \dfrac{3x^3 + x^2 - 1}{4x^3 - x^2 + x + 5}$

Using Asymptotes to Assist in Graphing

For Problems 51–59, find all vertical and horizontal asymptotes of the graphs determined by the following functions. Use these asymptotes, along with the x- and y-intercepts of the graphs, to plot the graphs of the functions. If necessary, use the first and second derivatives to assist in graphing.

51. $f(x) = \dfrac{1}{x + 1}$

52. $f(x) = \dfrac{x}{x - 1}$

53. $f(x) = \dfrac{x - 1}{x + 1}$

54. $f(x) = \dfrac{x}{x^2 + 1}$

55. $f(x) = \dfrac{1}{x^2 - 1}$

56. $f(x) = \dfrac{x}{x^2 - 1}$

57. $f(x) = \dfrac{x^2 - 1}{x^2 - 3x + 2}$

58. $f(x) = \dfrac{x^2 + 1}{x}$

59. $f(x) = \dfrac{1}{(x - 1)(x - 2)(x - 3)}$

2.3 Maximum and Minimum Values of Functions

PURPOSE

We show how to find both the relative maximum and the relative minimum values of a function and then use these values to find both the absolute maximum and the absolute minimum values. To find the relative maximum and minimum values, we use

- the first derivative test or
- the second derivative test.

We continue our ongoing development of the theory of the firm by determining the optimal pricing strategy of a product.

Introduction

Many problems ultimately reduce to finding the largest and smallest values of a function. In a business environment, profit is always maximized and cost is always minimized. In fact there are very few disciplines in which the concept of optimizing something does not play some role. If the "something" can be described mathematically by a differentiable function, then differential calculus can possibly play an important role in solving such problems. Problems that involve the finding of maximum or minimum points on the graph of a function are called **optimization problems**. To find these points, we first introduce the concept of relative maximum and relative minimum points.

Relative Maximum and Minimum Points of Graphs

The graphs of many functions form hills and valleys. The tops of the hills are called **relative maximum points**, and the low points of the valleys are called **relative minimum points**. (See Figure 18.) The top of any hill need not be the highest point on the entire graph, but it is a high point relative to its neighbors. Likewise, the bottom of a valley need not be the lowest point on the graph, but it is a low point relative to its neighbors. These ideas are formalized in the following definition.

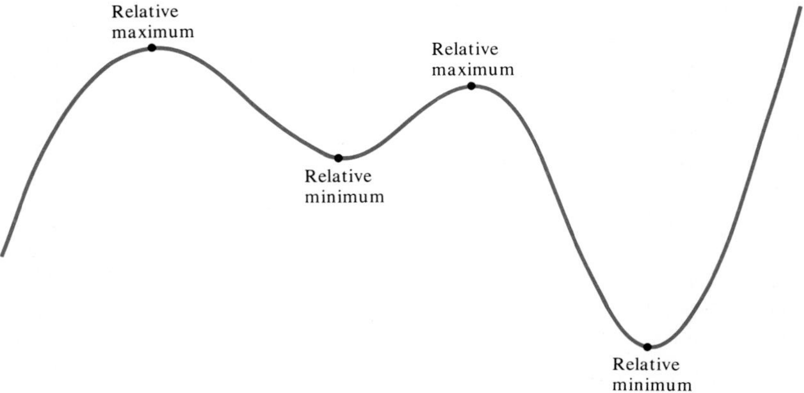

Figure 18
Hills and valleys showing relative maximum and minimum points

Definition of Relative Maximum and Minimum Values

The graph $y = f(x)$ of a function f has a relative maximum value at the point c if there is an open interval (a, b) containing c such that

$$f(c) \geq f(x)$$

for all x in the interval (a, b).

Similarly, the graph $y = f(x)$ has a relative minimum value at the point c if there is an open interval (a, b) containing c such that

$$f(c) \leq f(x)$$

for all x in the interval (a, b).

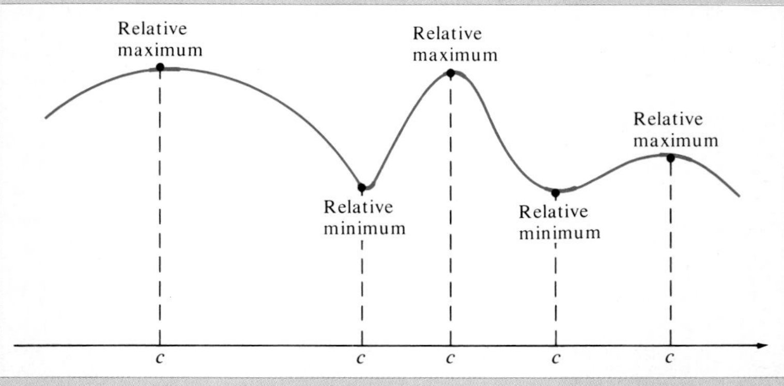

Example 1

Relative Maximum and Minimum Points **Identify the points where the graph in Figure 19 has relative maximum or relative minimum values.**

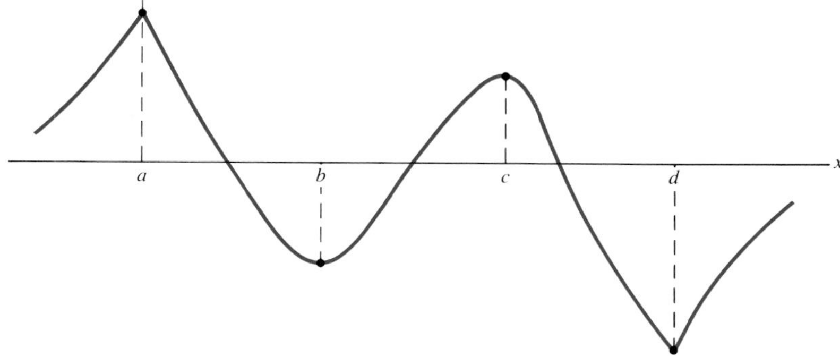

Figure 19
Where are the relative maximum and minimum points?

Solution The graph has relative maximum values at $x = a$ and $x = c$ and relative minimum values at $x = b$ and $x = d$. □

In the previous example we were fortunate to be given a drawing of the graph of a function. Often, however, we may have only an algebraic expression for the function. How is it possible in these situations to find the relative maximum and relative minimum points? This question is answered by the first and second derivative tests. We first study the first derivative test.

The First Derivative Test

The first derivative is used to determine relative maximum and relative minimum points in the following way. If a continuous function is increasing to the left of a point c and decreasing to the right of c, then clearly the graph of f has a relative maximum point at c, as shown in Figure 20. On the other hand, if a function is decreasing to the left of c and increasing to the right of c, then the graph of the function has a relative minimum point at c. These observations are stated more formally below.

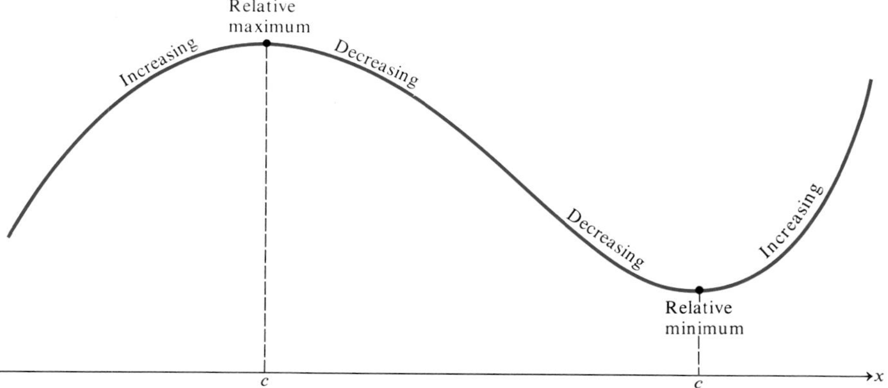

Figure 20
Relative maximum and minimum points occur where the function changes from increasing to decreasing or from decreasing to increasing

First Derivative Test (Relative Maximum and Minimum Points)

Let f be continuous at a real number c where either $f'(c) = 0$ or $f'(c)$ does not exist. The following two conditions can be used to determine whether $f(c)$ is a relative maximum or relative minimum value.

Relative maximum test: If

- $f'(x) > 0$ for all x close to c on the left and
- $f'(x) < 0$ for all x close to c on the right,

then

- $f(x)$ has a relative maximum value at c.

Relative minimum test: If

- $f'(x) < 0$ for all x close to c on the left and
- $f'(x) > 0$ for all x close to c on the right,

then

- $f(x)$ has a relative minimum value at c.

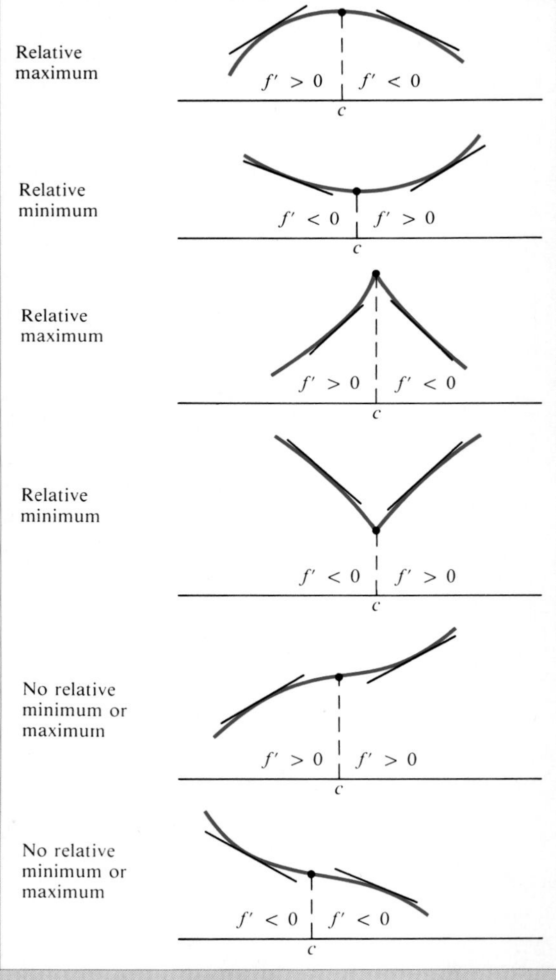

Example 2

Relative Maximum and Minimum Values Find the points on the graph of the function

$$f(x) = \frac{x}{1 + x^2}$$

where the relative maximum and the relative minimum occur.

Solution Computing the first derivative by means of the quotient rule, we have

$$\frac{df(x)}{dx} = \frac{(1 + x^2)\dfrac{dx}{dx} - x\dfrac{d}{dx}(1 + x^2)}{(1 + x^2)^2} = \frac{1 - x^2}{(1 + x^2)^2}$$

The following sign analysis tells where this derivative is positive and where it is negative:

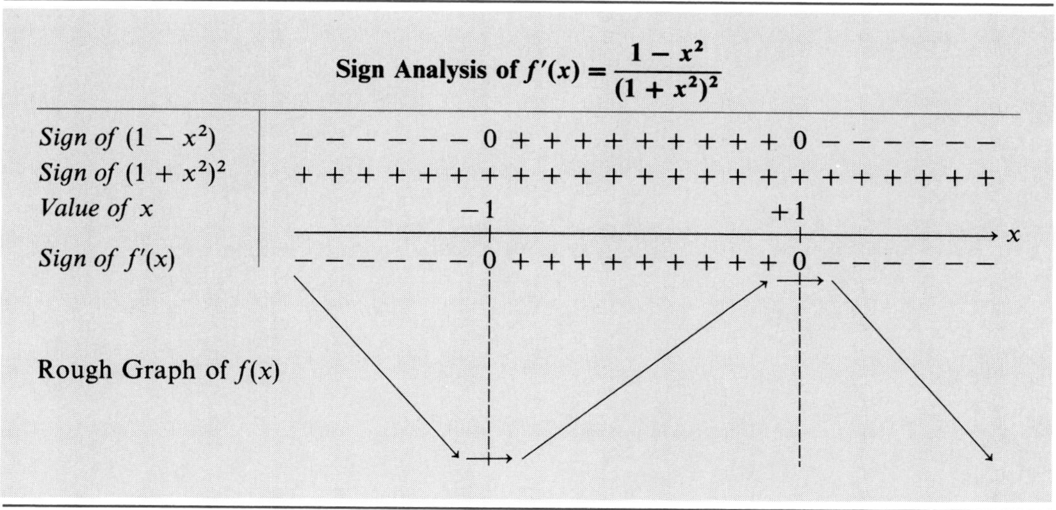

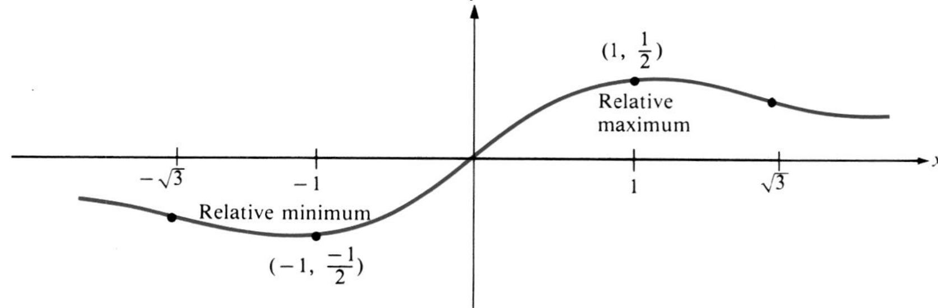

Figure 21
Graph of $f(x) = x/(1 + x^2)$ showing relative minimum and maximum points

Using the first derivative test, we conclude that f has a relative minimum value at -1 [the sign of $f'(x)$ changes from minus to plus there] and a relative maximum value at $+1$ [the sign of $f'(x)$ changes from plus to minus there]. The graph of $y = f(x)$ is shown in Figure 21. □

We have seen that the second derivative of a function contains information about the graph of a function that is not found by the first derivative. Hence it is not surprising that the second derivative can also be used to provide information about both relative maximum and relative minimum points. We now show the role that the second derivative plays in this important problem.

The Second Derivative Test

Since the second derivative of a function determines whether the graph of the function turns up or down, it seems reasonable that it might be used to find either relative maximum or relative minimum points. We see now how the second derivative is used in finding both relative maximum and relative minimum points.

Second Derivative Test (Relative Maximum and Minimum Values)

Assume that a function f has both first and second derivatives at a point c and that $f'(c) = 0$.

Relative maximum test: If $f''(c) < 0$, then the graph of $y = f(x)$ has a relative maximum value at $x = c$.

Relative minimum test: If $f''(c) > 0$, then the graph of $y = f(x)$ has a relative minimum value at $x = c$.

When $f''(c) = 0$ no conclusion can be drawn.

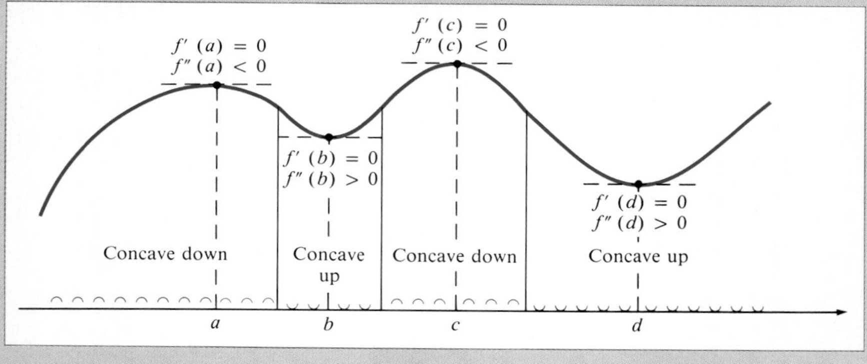

Although the second derivative test requires that we compute the first two derivatives, it is often easier to apply than the first derivative test. The second derivative test is based on the geometrical fact that a relative maximum value occurs at those points where the tangent line to the graph is horizontal and the graph is concave down. Likewise, a graph has a relative minimum value at those points where the tangent line to the graph is horizontal and the graph is concave up.

Example 3

Second Derivative Test Find the relative maximum and minimum points of the function

$$f(x) = x^2 + \frac{1}{x^2} \qquad (x \neq 0)$$

Solution Differentiating, we get

$$f'(x) = 2x - \frac{2}{x^3}$$

We find the stationary points by setting $f'(x)$ to zero and solving for x. This gives

$$f'(x) = 2x - \frac{2}{x^3} = 0$$

Solving for the real roots of this equation, we get the stationary points $x = -1$ and $+1$. Computing the second derivative, we get

$$f''(x) = 2 + \frac{6}{x^4}$$

Evaluating this second derivative at the two stationary points, we have

$$f''(-1) = 8 > 0$$
$$f''(+1) = 8 > 0$$

Since these second derivatives are both positive, we conclude that $y = f(x)$ has relative minimum values at $x = -1$ and $x = +1$. The actual relative minimum values can be found by substituting $x = -1$ and $+1$ into $f(x)$, getting

$$f(-1) = 2$$
$$f(1) = 2$$

To graph the function, we make the following observations:

- The graph has relative minimum points at $(-1, 2)$ and $(1, 2)$.
- The second derivative $f''(x)$ is always positive, and hence the graph $y = f(x)$ is always concave up.
- The graph is not defined at zero.
- The graph is symmetric about the y-axis, since $f(x) = f(-x)$ for all x.

Using these observations, we graph the function as shown in Figure 22. □

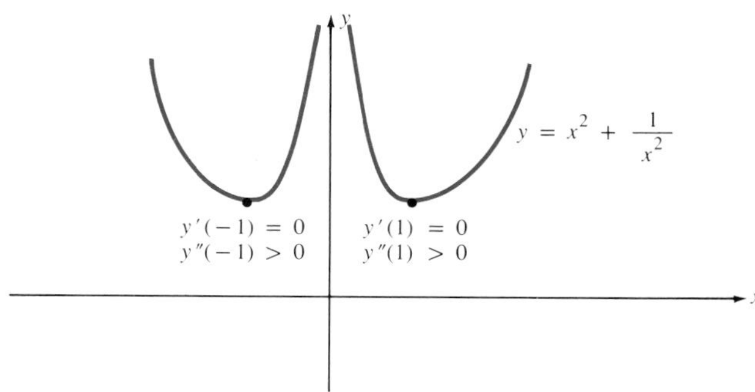

Figure 22
The second derivative test indicates relative minimum values at $x = -1$ and $x = +1$ and a graph that is always concave up

Absolute Maximum and Minimum Values

Many problems in business and science require that we perform a task in an "optimal manner." For example, every firm that sells a product, whether the firm is a manufacturing or a service company, is faced with the problem of determining the best price for its product. If the firm sets the price too low, the volume of sales might be great, but the revenue per item might be so low that the overall revenue will not be maximized. If the price is too high, the revenue per item will be high, but the number of items sold might be so low that again the overall revenue will not be maximized. This is a typical problem in **revenue maximization**. It leads to the mathematical problem of finding the **absolute maximum value** of the revenue function, which in turn leads us to the following definition:

Definition of Absolute Maximum and Minimum Values

A function f has an absolute maximum value at c if

$$f(c) \geq f(x)$$

for all x in the domain of f.

A function f has an absolute minimum value at c if

$$f(c) \leq f(x)$$

for all x in the domain of f.

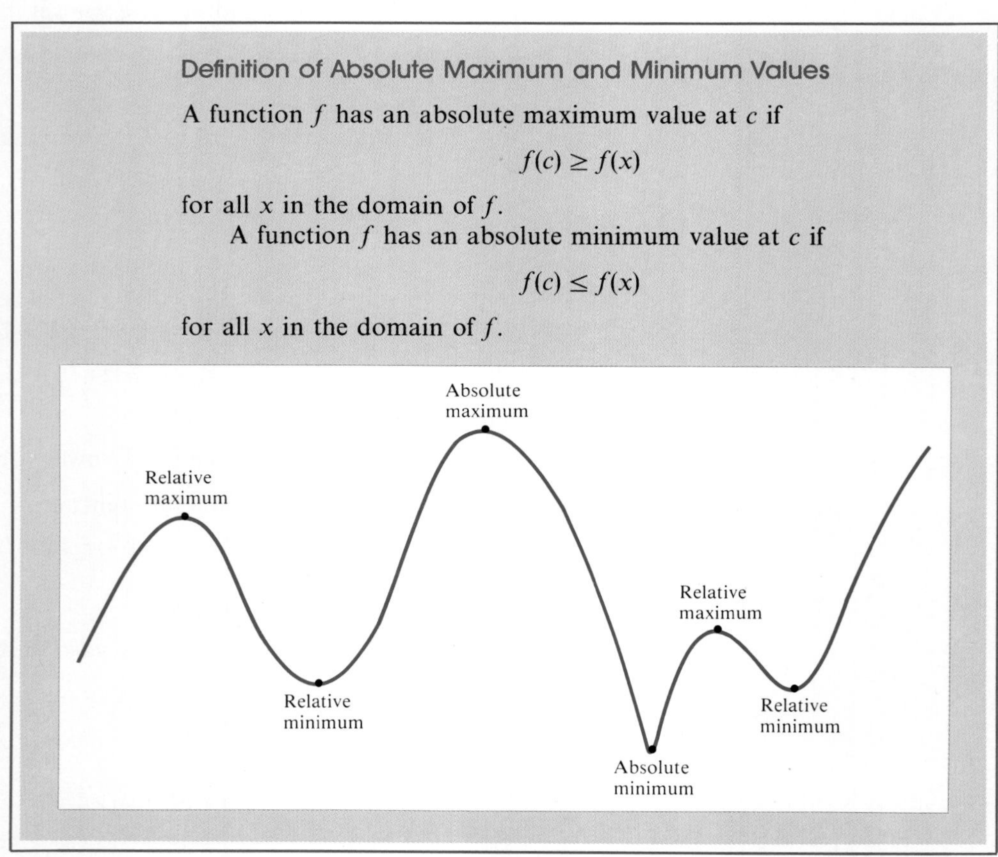

We now give a set of rules that can be used to find the absolute maximum and minimum values of a function. We restrict ourselves to continuous functions defined on closed intervals. It will not be shown here, but it can be proven that for any continuous function defined on a closed interval $[a, b]$ there is always a point in the interval where the function attains its absolute maximum value and a point where it attains its absolute minimum value.

Rules for Finding Absolute Maximum and Minimum Values

To find the points where a continuous function f attains its absolute maximum and minimum values on an interval $[a, b]$ carry out the following steps.

Step 1. Evaluate the function at the endpoints a and b to obtain the values $f(a)$ and $f(b)$.

Step 2. Evaluate $f(x)$ at each critical point in the interval (a, b) [where $f'(x)$ does not exist or where $f'(x) = 0$].

Step 3. Find the largest and smallest of all the values computed puted in Steps 1 and 2. The largest of these values is the absolute minimum of the function on $[a, b]$. The smallest of these values is the absolute minimum of the function on $[a, b]$.

It is useful to note that the absolute maximum and absolute minimum values may occur at points inside the interval $[a, b]$ or at the endpoints a and b.

Example 4

Absolute Maximum and Minimum Values Find the absolute maximum and absolute minimum values of the function

$$f(x) = \frac{1}{3}x^3 - 2x^2 + 3x + 2$$

on the interval $[-1, 4]$.

Solution Using the above three-step process, we have the following:

- **Step 1** (evaluate $f(x)$ at the endpoints). Evaluating $f(x)$ at the endpoints -1 and 4, we have

$$f(-1) = -\tfrac{10}{3}$$
$$f(4) = \tfrac{10}{3}$$

- **Step 2** (evaluate $f(x)$ at the critical points). Computing the derivative of $f(x)$, we get

$$f'(x) = x^2 - 4x + 3$$
$$= (x - 1)(x - 3)$$

Since $f'(x)$ exists at all points in the interval $(-1, 4)$, we find the stationary points of $f(x)$ by solving the equation

$$f'(x) = 0$$

or

$$(x - 1)(x - 3) = 0$$

This gives the two stationary points 1, 3 which both lie in the interval $(-1, 4)$. Evaluating $f(x)$ at these points gives

$$f(1) = \tfrac{10}{3}$$
$$f(3) = 2$$

- **Step 3** (find the largest of the above values). To find the absolute maximum and the absolute minimum values, we find the largest and smallest values among

$$\begin{aligned} f(-1) &= -\tfrac{10}{3} && \text{(left endpoint)} \\ f(4) &= \tfrac{10}{3} && \text{(right endpoint)} \\ f(1) &= \tfrac{10}{3} && \text{(stationary point)} \\ f(3) &= 2 && \text{(stationary point)} \end{aligned}$$

Hence the absolute maximum value of $f(x)$ is $\frac{10}{3}$, which occurs at the two points 1 and 4. The absolute minimum value of $f(x)$ is $-\frac{10}{3}$, which occurs when $x = -1$. The graph of $y = f(x)$ is shown in Figure 23. □

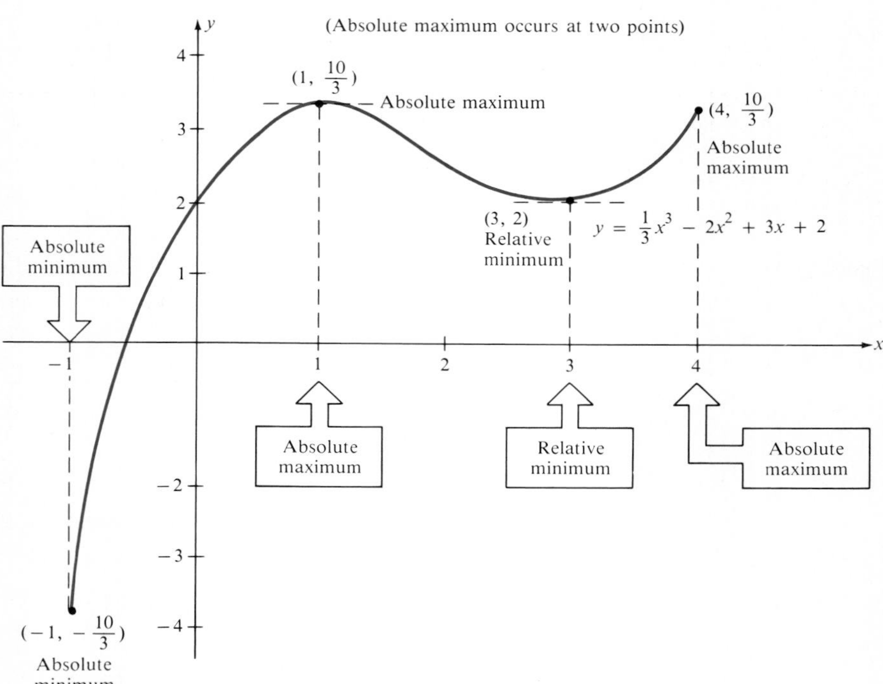

Figure 23
Absolute maximum and minimum values

Determining Price to Maximize Profit

The pricing of a product to maximize profit is a major problem facing companies today. The incorrect pricing of a product can be the difference between success and failure. The overpricing of oil by the OPEC cartel in 1973 resulted in a combination of increased oil exploration and a consumer backlash. The net result was that by the year 1985 there was a worldwide glut of oil, and the price of oil tumbled from \$35 a barrel to \$8 on the spot market. Most economists have felt that if the OPEC cartel had increased the price of oil in a more gradual manner, there would not have been this consumer resistance, and the long-range revenue to OPEC would have been greater.

Although the following example has been simplified from the pricing problems that most companies face, many of the ideas are present in this example.

Example 5

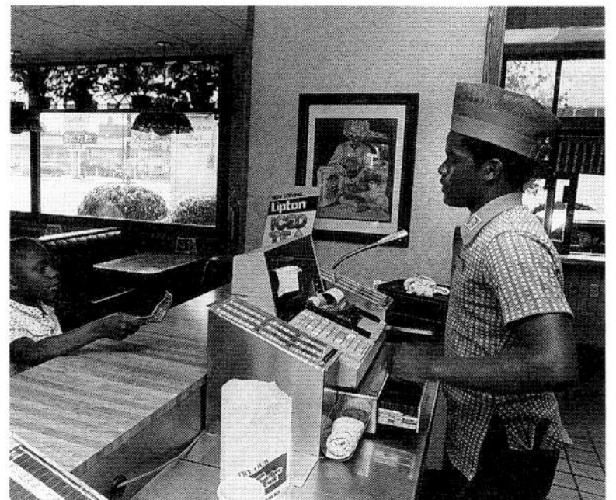

Optimal pricing for many companies is critical for a successful operation. Having good mathematical models to predict profit in terms of the price charged for a product is often worth a million dollars.

Optimal Pricing in the Restaurant Industry Imagine yourself as the operational director for an entire chain of family restaurants (typical chains are Big Boy, Friendly's, and Hot Shoppes). Upon your hiring, you discover that the current price the company charges for their popular Family Platter is \$8.00. Your first job is to determine whether the company is charging too little, too much, or just the right amount to maximize profit. To determine the optimal price, you carry out a market survey and discover that on the average each increase in price of \$0.25 per meal will decrease the company's demand by 20,000 meals per week and that each decrease of \$0.25 per meal will increase demand by 20,000 meals per week. You also know that at the current price of \$8.00 per meal a total of 250,000 meals are sold per week.

It has also been determined that the weekly cost to the company in dollars to serve q Family Platter meals is

$$C(q) = 100{,}000 + 3q$$

What price should be charged for the Family Platter in order that the total revenue be maximized?

Solution The company's weekly profit $P(q)$ when q meals per week are sold is given by

$$P(q) = R(q) - C(q)$$

where

$$\begin{aligned} R(q) &= \text{Revenue from the sale of } q \text{ meals} \\ C(q) &= \text{Cost to produce } q \text{ meals} \end{aligned}$$

With the help of the demand curve $q = D(p)$, the revenue and cost functions can be written as

$$\begin{aligned} R(q) &= pq \\ &= p\,D(p) \\ C(q) &= 100{,}000 + 3q \\ &= 100{,}000 + 3D(p) \end{aligned}$$

where

$$\begin{aligned} p &= \text{Price charged per meal} \\ D(p) &= \text{Number of meals sold when the price per meal is } p \end{aligned}$$

Hence the profit can be written in terms of the price charged per meal as

$$\begin{aligned} P(p) &= R(p) - C(p) \\ &= p\,D(p) - [100{,}000 + 3D(p)] \end{aligned}$$

To maximize the profit $P(p)$, we must first find the equation for the demand $D(p)$. The information given in this problem essentially says that the demand function $D(p)$ is a linear function of p, with slope $-80{,}000$ (the demand goes down by 80,000 for each additional dollar charged). Since the demand function also satisfies $D(8) = 250{,}000$, we can use the point-slope formula for straight lines to write

$$\begin{aligned} D(p) &= 250{,}000 - 80{,}000(p - 8) \\ &= -80{,}000p + 890{,}000 \end{aligned}$$

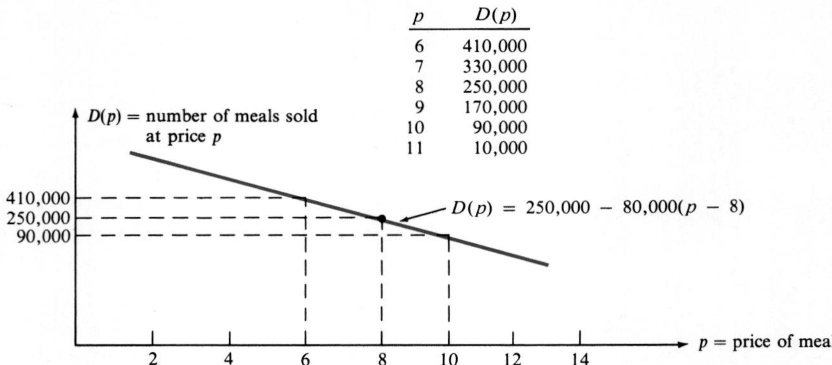

Figure 24
Number-of-meals function

The graph of $D(p)$ is shown in Figure 24. Substituting the expression for $D(p)$ into the equation for $P(p)$ and carrying out a few algebraic steps, we have

$$\begin{aligned} P(p) &= p\,D(p) - [100{,}000 + 3D(p)] \\ &= -80{,}000p^2 + 1{,}130{,}000p - 2{,}770{,}000 \end{aligned}$$

The graph of $P(p)$ is a parabola that, if we set $P(p) = 0$, can be seen to be zero when the price p is (to the nearest penny) \$3.16 or \$10.97. A rough graph of $P(p)$ is shown in Figure 25.

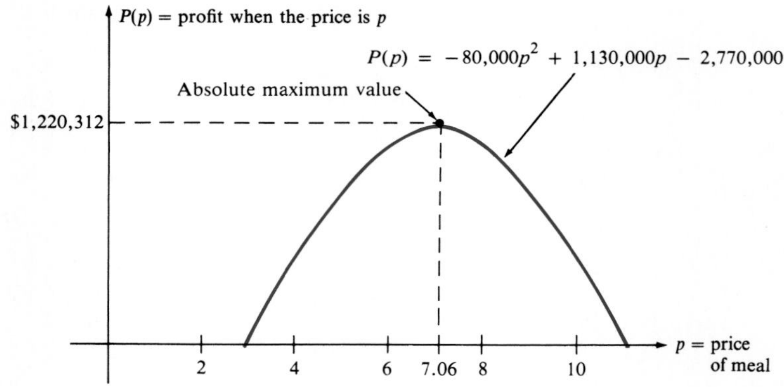

Figure 25
Profit as a function of price p

By an examination of the first and second derivatives,

$$P'(p) = -160{,}000p + 1{,}130{,}000 = \begin{cases} \text{positive for } p < 7.06 \\ \text{negative for } p > 7.06 \end{cases}$$

$$P''(p) = -160{,}000 < 0 \qquad \text{for all } p$$

We conclude that $P(p)$ will be positive only when p is between \$3.16 and \$10.97. Hence we need only find the absolute maximum value of $P(p)$ on the interval [3.16, 10.97]. To do this we carry out the following three-step process:

- **Step 1** (evaluate the function at the endpoints). Evaluating $P(p)$ at the endpoints, we have

$$P(3.16) = 0$$
$$P(10.97) = 0$$

- **Step 2** (evaluate the function at the critical points). Setting the derivative $P'(p)$ equal to zero and solving for p, we have

$$P'(p) = -160{,}000p + 1{,}130{,}000 = 0.$$

This gives

$$p = \$7.06$$

Evaluating $P(p)$ at this stationary point which is in the interval (3.16, 10.97), we have

$$P(7.06) = \$1{,}220{,}312$$

- **Step 3** (find the largest of the above values). The values found in Steps 1 and 2 are

$$\begin{aligned} P(3.16) &= 0 \qquad \text{(not exactly zero but very small)} \\ P(7.06) &= 1{,}220{,}312 \\ P(10.97) &= 0 \qquad \text{(not exactly zero but very small)} \end{aligned}$$

It is clear that the absolute maximum profit is \$1,220,312, which is attained when $p = 7.06$. □

Summary of the Problem

The original price of \$8.00 per meal was too high by \$0.94 per meal. Table 8 gives the weekly profit to the company as a function of the price of a Family Platter.

TABLE 8
Weekly Results for Various Pricing Strategies

	Price per Meal	Meals Sold per Week	Weekly Revenue	Weekly Cost	Weekly Profit
	\$3.16	637,200	\$2,013,552	\$2,011,600	\$1,952
	\$4.00	570,000	\$2,280,000	\$1,810,000	\$470,000
	\$5.00	490,000	\$2,450,000	\$1,570,000	\$880,000
	\$6.00	410,000	\$2,460,000	\$1,330,000	\$1,130,000
	\$7.00	330,000	\$2,310,000	\$1,090,000	\$1,220,000
Optimal →	**\$7.06**	**325,200**	**\$2,295,912**	**\$1,075,600**	**\$1,220,312**
Original →	**\$8.00**	**250,000**	**\$2,000,000**	**\$850,000**	**\$1,150,000**
	\$9.00	170,000	\$1,530,000	\$610,000	\$920,000
	\$10.00	90,000	\$900,000	\$370,000	\$530,000
	\$10.97	12,400	\$136,028	\$137,200	−\$1,172

Note from Table 8 that the company's weekly profit will increase from \$1,150,000 to \$1,220,312 (an increase of \$70,312) when lowering the price from \$8.00 to \$7.06. This example shows the importance of careful mathematical analysis in the pricing of goods and services.

Acceleration

We have seen that the velocity of an object moving along a straight line is given by the derivative of the position function. That is, the velocity describes the rate of change of the position with respect to time. In a similar way, we say that the **acceleration** of an object is the rate of change in the velocity of the object. In other words,

$$s = s(t) \qquad \textit{(position function)}$$

$$v = \frac{ds}{dt} \qquad \textit{(velocity function)}$$

$$a = \frac{dv}{dt} = \frac{d^2s}{st^2} \qquad \textit{(acceleration function)}$$

Example 6

Acceleration of a Falling Ball How many feet straight up can you throw a baseball? Although the authors do not know how strong you are, we do know that if the ball leaves your hand at 64 feet per second, then (neglecting air friction) the height s of the ball in feet will satisfy (fairly accurately) the quadratic function

$$s(t) = -16t^2 + 64t$$

where t is time in seconds measured from when you throw the ball. (See Figure 26.) Suppose you can throw a ball straight up with a velocity of 60 feet per second.

(a) Find the velocity and acceleration of the ball after t seconds.

(b) Find how long it takes for the ball to reach its maximum height.

(c) What is the maximum height the ball will attain?

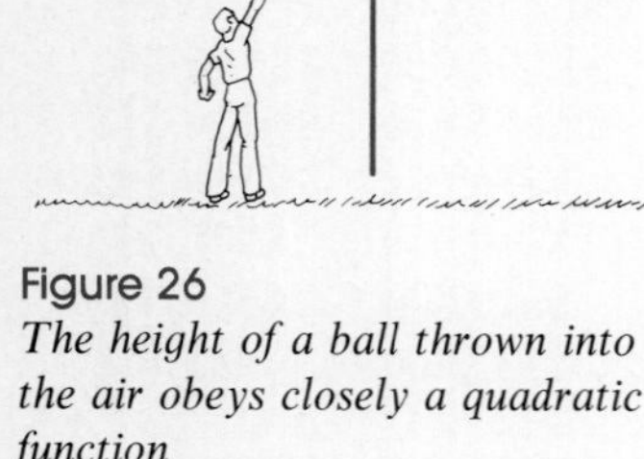

Figure 26
The height of a ball thrown into the air obeys closely a quadratic function

Solution

(a) To find the velocity and acceleration, we differentiate the position function, getting

$$v(t) = \frac{ds}{dt} = \frac{d}{dt}(-16t^2 + 64t)$$
$$= -32t + 64 \text{ ft/sec}$$

$$a(t) = \frac{dv}{dt} = \frac{d}{dt}(-32t + 64)$$
$$= -32 \text{ ft/sec}^2$$

(b) Since the velocity of the ball is zero when the ball attains its maximum height, we set $v(t)$ to 0 and solve for t. This gives

$$-32t + 64 = 0$$

$$t = \frac{64}{32} = 2 \text{ seconds}$$

(c) We find the maximum height of the ball by simply evaluating

$$s(2) = -16(2)^2 + 64(2)$$
$$= 64 \text{ feet}$$

□

Problems

For Problems 1–9, find the intervals or points where the graph in Figure 27 has the indicated properties.

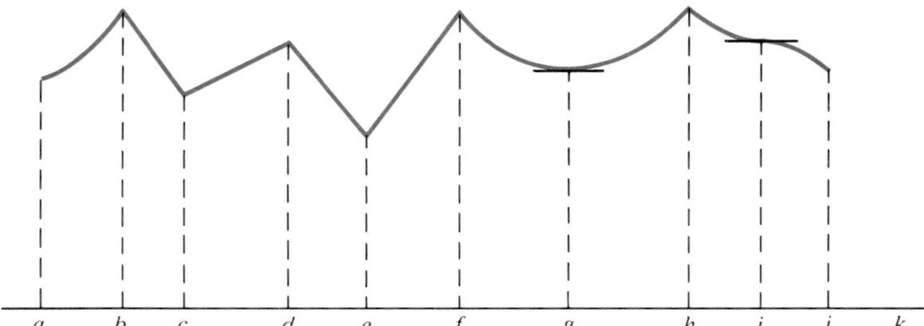

Figure 27
Graph for Problems 1–9

1. $f(x)$ is increasing.
2. $f(x)$ is decreasing.
3. The derivative is zero.
4. The derivative does not exist.
5. $f(x)$ has a relative minimum.
6. $f(x)$ has a relative maximum.
7. $f(x)$ has an absolute minimum.
8. $f(x)$ has an absolute maximum.
9. The second derivative is zero.

For Problems 10–13, use the values of x and $f(x)$ along with the sign of $f'(x)$ on the indicated intervals to give a rough sketch of the graph of f.

10.

Function Information

x	$f(x)$
-1	4
1	0
3	4

Derivative Information

Region	*Sign*
$(-1, 1)$	Negative
1	Zero
$(1, 3)$	Positive

11.

Function Information

x	$f(x)$
-1	-2
$\frac{1}{2}$	$\frac{1}{4}$
2	-2

Derivative Information

Region	*Sign*
$(-1, \frac{1}{2})$	Positive
$\frac{1}{2}$	Zero
$(\frac{1}{2}, 2)$	Negative

12.

Function Information

x	$f(x)$
$\frac{1}{2}$	$\frac{5}{2}$
1	2
$\frac{3}{2}$	$\frac{13}{6}$
2	$\frac{5}{2}$
$\frac{5}{2}$	$\frac{29}{10}$
3	$\frac{10}{3}$

Derivative Information

Region	*Sign*
$(\frac{1}{2}, 1)$	Negative
1	Zero
$(1, 3)$	Positive

13.

Function Information

x	$f(x)$
-2	-8
-1	1
$-\frac{1}{2}$	$\frac{7}{16}$
0	0
$\frac{1}{2}$	$\frac{7}{16}$
1	1
2	-8

Derivative Information

Region	*Sign*
$(-2, -1)$	Positive
-1	Zero
$(-1, 0)$	Negative
0	Zero
$(0, 1)$	Positive
1	Zero
$(1, 2)$	Negative

For Problems 14–30, when possible use the first derivative test to determine the points where $f(x)$ has relative maximum or relative minimum values. If the derivative test does not apply, indicate the reason.

14. $f(x) = 3$

15. $f(x) = 3x - 5$

16. $f(x) = x^2 + 1$

17. $f(x) = 5x^2 - 5x + 3$

18. $f(x) = x^2 + 12x - 10$
19. $f(x) = x^3 - x + 1$
20. $f(x) = x^3 - 18x$
21. $f(x) = 3x^2 - 72x + 15$
22. $f(x) = x^3 + 3x^2 - 24x + 5$

23. $f(x) = x^3 + \frac{9}{4}x^2 - 3x - 6$

24. $f(x) = \frac{x^4}{x^2 - 1}$
25. $f(x) = \sqrt{x}$

26. $f(x) = \sqrt{x^2 - 1}$
27. $f(x) = x^{1/3}$
28. $f(x) = x^{2/3}$
29. $f(x) = x^{4/5}$
30. $f(x) = 6x^{2/3} - 4x$

For Problems 31–43, use the second derivative test to determine whether any of the following functions have relative maximum or relative minimum values at the critical points. If the second derivative test does not apply, explain why.

31. $f(x) = 3x$
32. $f(x) = 3x - 6$
33. $f(x) = x^2$
34. $f(x) = x^2 - 1$
35. $f(x) = x^2 - 2x - 3$
36. $f(x) = x^2 + x + 1$
37. $f(x) = 3x^4 + 8x^3 - 6x^2 - 24x + 10$

38. $f(x) = x^3 - 15x + 4$
39. $f(x) = \frac{x}{x^2 + 2}$

40. $f(x) = x + \frac{1}{x}$
41. $f(x) = 2x^3 - x^6$

42. $f(x) = \frac{x}{\sqrt{x^2 + 4}}$
43. $f(x) = \frac{x^2}{9} + \frac{6}{x}$

For Problems 44–58, find both the absolute maximum and the absolute minimum values of each of the continuous functions on the indicated intervals.

44. $f(x) = 4$ on $[0, 1]$
45. $f(x) = x$ on $[-1, 2]$
46. $f(x) = 3x + 2$ on $[1, 5]$
47. $f(x) = -x + 3$ on $[2, 5]$
48. $f(x) = x^2 - 4x - 3$ on $[-1, 4]$
49. $f(x) = 2x^3 - 15x^2 + 12$ on $[-1, 3]$
50. $f(x) = (x - 1)^3$ on $[-1, 2]$
51. $f(x) = 2x^2 + 2x + 3$ on $[-1, 1]$
52. $f(x) = x^4 - 8x^3 + 22x^2 - 24x + 7$ on $[2, 4]$
53. $f(x) = 2x^3 - 9x^2 + 12x - 5$ on $[2, 4]$

54. $f(x) = x^4 - \frac{4}{3}x^3 - 2$ on $[-1, 1]$

55. $f(x) = \sqrt{x - 1} - \frac{x}{2}$ on $[\frac{3}{2}, 3]$

56. $f(x) = x^{1/3}$ on $[-1, 1]$
57. $f(x) = x^{4/3}$ on $[-1, 1]$
58. $f(x) = 6 - 3x - (x - 1)^{3/2}$ on $[2, 6]$

Theory of the Firm

59. Average Cost. The average production cost per item, when q items are produced, is found by dividing the total cost $C(q)$ by the number of items q. That is,

$$\text{Average cost:} \quad \bar{C}(q) = \frac{C(q)}{q}$$

Assume that the cost to produce q items is given by

$$C(q) = 625 + \frac{q^2}{10}$$

(a) Find the number of items that should be produced to minimize the average cost. Assume that the feasible number of items lies somewhere in the interval $[10, 100]$.
(b) If the value of q that minimizes the average cost is not an integer, how would you find an integer value to use in trying to minimize the average cost?

60. Maximum Revenue. The total revenue $R(p)$ that a company receives depends on the price p the company charges for its product and is given by

$$R(p) = -p^2 + 7p \qquad (0 \le p \le 8)$$

Find the price that will maximize the revenue.

61. Maximum Revenue. The total revenue $R(p)$ that a company receives depends on the price p the company charges for its product and is given by

$$R(p) = -25p^2 + 300p \qquad (0 \le p \le 8)$$

Find the price that will maximize the total revenue.

Maximum Profit

The total profit $P(q)$ that a company earns for producing q units of a product is the total revenue $R(q)$ from the sale of q units of the product minus the total cost $C(q)$ of producing q units of the product. That is,

$$P(q) = R(q) - C(q)$$

Often a firm can determine expressions for $R(q)$ and $C(q)$ as functions of q. For Problems 62–65, find the indicated quantities.

62. Maximum Profit. Suppose $R(q)$ and $P(q)$ can be described by the polynomials

$$R(q) = 100q \qquad (0 \le q \le 10)$$
$$C(q) = q^3 - 3q^2 + 2q \qquad (0 \le q \le 10)$$

Find the number of items that maximizes the total profit. What is the maximum profit for this number of items produced?

63. **Maximum Profit.** For total revenue and cost functions given by

$$R(q) = 500q - q^2 \qquad (0 \le q \le 35)$$
$$C(q) = q^3 - 50q^2 + 500q + 250 \qquad (0 \le q \le 35)$$

find the number of items that maximizes the total profit. What is the maximum profit for this number of items produced?

64. **Maximum Profit.** Suppose $R(q)$ and $C(q)$ are described by the functions

$$R(q) = 50q \qquad (0 \le q \le 100)$$
$$C(q) = 0.5q^2 + 50 \qquad (0 \le q \le 100)$$

Graph these cost and revenue functions. Find the number of items that will maximize the profit. What is the maximum profit?

65. **Maximum Profit.** Suppose $R(q)$ and $C(q)$ are described by the functions

$$R(q) = 5q \qquad (0 \le q \le 5)$$
$$C(q) = 2q^2 \qquad (0 \le q \le 5)$$

Draw graphs of these functions and find the number of items q that will maximize the profit. What is the maximum profit?

66. **Gasoline Mileage.** The Department of Transportation has determined that the number of miles per gallon $M(s)$ that a certain model of automobile will get when it travels s miles per hour is

$$M(s) = -0.025s^2 + 1.40s + 5.5 \qquad (20 \le s \le 55)$$

(a) At what speed will the automobile get the largest number of miles per gallon?
(b) What speed will minimize the miles per gallon?
(c) How many miles per gallon will this model get at these speeds?

Max–Min Puzzlers

67. **Can You Find the Maximum?** What is the absolute maximum value of the function

$$f(x) = x$$

for $0 < x < 1$?

68. **Can You Find the Maximum?** What is the absolute maximum value of the function

$$f(x) = \frac{1}{x}$$

for $-1 < x < 1$?

69. **Mystery Function.** Can you think of a function $f(x)$ defined on some interval that has an absolute maximum value but not an absolute minimum value?

Position, Velocity, and Acceleration

When the position of an object changes, the change is called *velocity*. When the velocity of an object changes, the change is called *acceleration*. The acceleration of an object refers to the change in the velocity of the object. For instance, if you drop a ball from the top of a building, the velocity of the ball will increase (approximately) 32 feet per second *every second*. We say that the acceleration of the ball due to gravity is 32 ft/sec^2. In terms of differential calculus, the acceleration of an object is the first derivative of the velocity of the object and the second derivative of the position. In other words,

$$a(t) = \frac{d}{dt} v(t) = \frac{d^2}{dt^2} s(t)$$

Problems 70–72 are concerned with the concepts of velocity and acceleration.

70. **The Wild Mouse.** Paul has bought a ticket on the Wild Mouse at an amusement park. (See Figure 28.) The ride consists of sitting in a small car (the Wild Mouse) that moves in a straight line on a track. Suppose the position $s(t)$ of the car in feet after t seconds is given by

$$s(t) = -t^3 + 120t^2 \qquad 0 \le t \le 120$$

The position where Paul boards the Mouse is taken as zero. Positive $s(t)$ refers to the position of the Wild Mouse in one direction, while negative $s(t)$ refers to the position in the opposite direction.

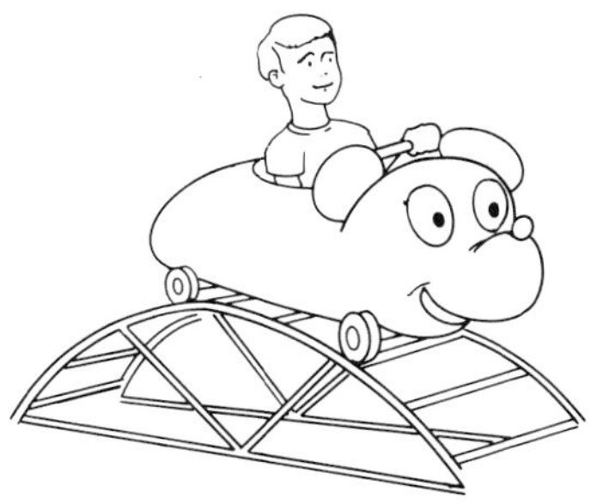

Figure 28
The Wild Mouse

(a) Find the velocity and acceleration of the Wild Mouse after t seconds.
(b) For what values of t does the Wild Mouse come to rest?
(c) Sketch the graphs of the position, velocity, and acceleration curves for the Wild Mouse versus time. Interpret these graphs in terms of Paul's ride. When does the Wild Mouse attain its maximum velocity.

71. Sue's Calculus Book. Sue throws her calculus book out her dormitory window straight up with a velocity of 48 feet per second. (See Figure 29.) Assuming that her dormitory room is 40 feet above the ground, the height of her book after t seconds will be (neglecting air friction)

$$s(t) = -16t^2 + 48t + 40$$

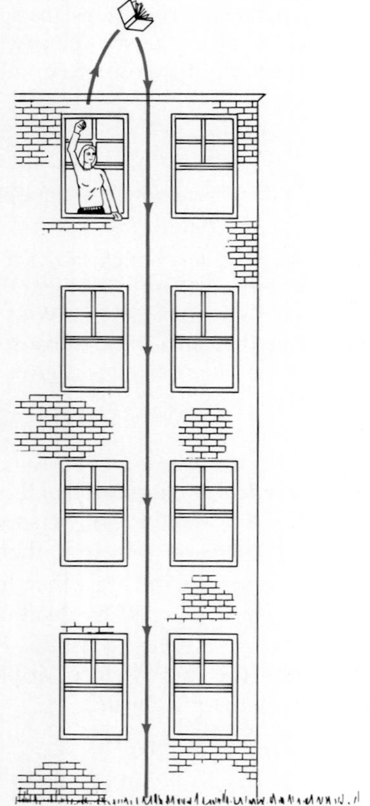

Figure 29
Typical falling object

(a) When will the book reach its maximum height?
(b) What will be the maximum height of the book?
(c) What will be the acceleration of the book after 2 seconds?
(d) When will the book hit the ground?
(e) What will be the velocity of the book when it hits the ground?

72. The Great Zacchini. Back in the 1940's, Emmanuel Zacchini acted regularly as the human cannonball for the Ringling Brothers & Barnum & Bailey Circus. (See Figure 30.) He was fired from a cannon 15 feet above the ground aimed at an angle of 45°, sending him on the parabolic path

$$h(x) = -0.0062x^2 + x + 15 \qquad (0 \le x \le 175)$$

175 feet away into a net (he hoped). What was the maximum height attained by the Great Zacchini?

Social Sciences

73. The Newark Tunnel. Barbara has just accepted a job with the New York City Tunnel Authority. Her first assignment is to determine the speed at which cars should travel through the Newark tunnel so that traffic flow is maximized. She has found a good predictor of the flow f of cars (cars per second) through the tunnel in terms of the average velocity v (miles per hour) of the cars to be the rational function*

$$f(v) = \frac{22v}{v + v^2/22 + 12}$$

(a) What is the average velocity that will maximize the flow of cars through the tunnel?
(b) What is the maximum flow of cars per second that can pass through the tunnel?

* This model was formulated by D. Burghes, I. Huntley, and J. McDonald, *Applying Mathematics*, John Wiley and Sons, New York, 1982.

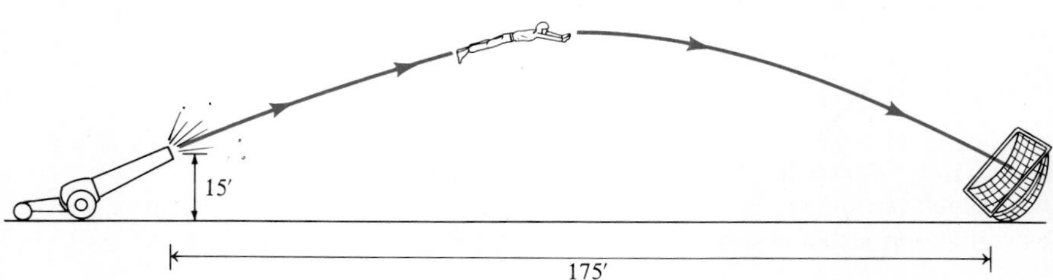

Figure 30
The Great Zacchini

2.4 Optimization Problems (Max–Min Problems)

PURPOSE

We present examples to show how absolute maximum and absolute minimum points of functions are useful in business management and science. These types of problems are called optimization or max–min problems. Some of the optimization problems in this section differ from problems that we have seen so far because they have constraints.

Introduction

One often asks, "What is the best way of doing something?" A business manager might wish to determine how to price a given product in order to maximize the company's profit. A fisheries biologist may wish to determine an optimal feeding program for fish growing in a controlled environment. In many cases the best way of doing something can be reduced to finding the maximum or minimum value of a function. It is here that calculus can come to the rescue. We present some examples of optimization problems that can be solved by using differential calculus.

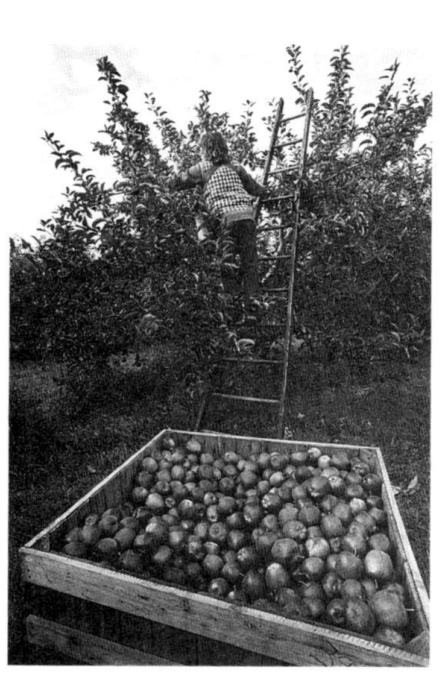

Many companies do not use mathematical modeling, but more and more many successful companies find a way to use mathematical techniques to gain an edge in a competitive world.

The Apple Orchard Problem

An agronomist has been asked to determine the density of apple trees in an orchard that will maximize the total yield of apples. From experiments it is known that if the density of trees is 30 trees or fewer per acre, then each tree will produce 150 bushels of apples on the average. On the other hand, if the density of trees exceeds 30 trees per acre, the yield of each tree will decrease by three bushels per tree for each additional tree planted above 30. How many trees should be planted per acre to maximize the total yield of apples?

From the above information we can plot the graph of

$$N(t) = \text{Number of bushels per tree}$$

as a function of

$$t = \text{Number of trees per acre}$$

This graph is shown in Figure 31.

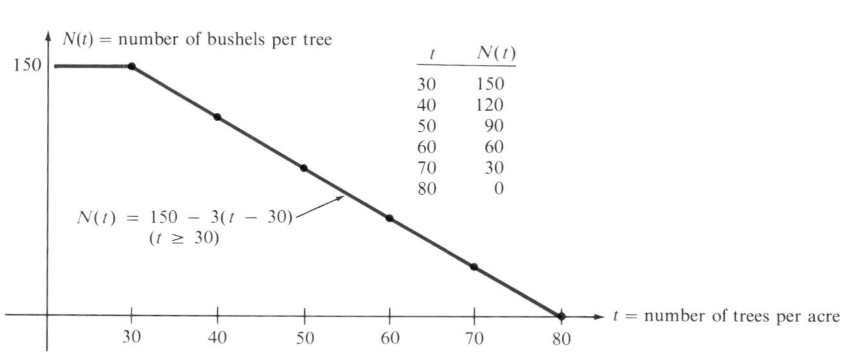

t	$N(t)$
30	150
40	120
50	90
60	60
70	30
80	0

Figure 31
Bushels of apples per tree as a function of the number of trees per acre

Since the yield per tree is always 150 bushels per tree for a tree density less than 30 trees per acre, it makes sense that the number t of trees per acre should be at least 30. However, when the density is greater than 30, the number $N(t)$ of bushels per tree falls by three for each additional tree planted. This information says that $N(t)$ is a linear function with slope -3 that passes through the point $N(30) = 150$. Hence it can be written in point-slope form as

$$\begin{aligned} N(t) &= 150 - 3(t - 30) \\ &= -3t + 240 \qquad (t \geq 30) \end{aligned}$$

If we now call

$$Y(t) = \text{Number of bushels per acre}$$

then we can write

$$\begin{matrix}\text{Number of bushels} \\ \text{per acre}\end{matrix} = \begin{pmatrix}\text{Number of bushels} \\ \text{per tree}\end{pmatrix} \begin{pmatrix}\text{Number of trees} \\ \text{per acre}\end{pmatrix}$$

or

$$\begin{aligned} Y(t) &= N(t)t \\ &= (-3t + 240)t \\ &= -3t(t - 80) \qquad (t \geq 30) \end{aligned}$$

The goal now is to find the value of t where $Y(t)$ has its absolute maximum value. To do this, we first observe that the total yield of apples $Y(t)$ becomes negative when the density t becomes greater than 80 trees per acre. Hence we seek the absolute maximum yield $Y(t)$ of apples when the density t is between 30 and 80 trees per acre (inclusive). Stated mathematically, we wish to find the absolute maximum value of

$$Y(t) = -3t^2 + 240t \qquad (30 \leq t \leq 80)$$

To find this value, we first find the stationary points by solving the equation

$$Y'(t) = -6t + 240 = 0$$

We see that $Y(t)$ has one stationary point when $t = 40$. Evaluating $Y(t)$ at this point, we get

$$\begin{aligned} Y(40) &= -3(40)(40 - 80) \\ &= 4800 \end{aligned}$$

To find the absolute maximum value of $Y(t)$, we pick the largest of the three values

$$\begin{aligned} &Y(30) = 4500 \text{ bushels} && \text{(left endpoint)} \\ &Y(40) = 4800 \text{ bushels} && \text{(stationary point)} \\ &Y(80) = 0 \text{ bushels} && \text{(right endpoint)} \end{aligned}$$

Conclusion

The maximum yield of apples occurs when the tree density is 40 trees per acre. With this density, 4800 bushels will be harvested per acre. Any larger or smaller density of trees per acre will result in a smaller yield of apples per acre. The graph of $Y(t)$ is shown in Figure 32.

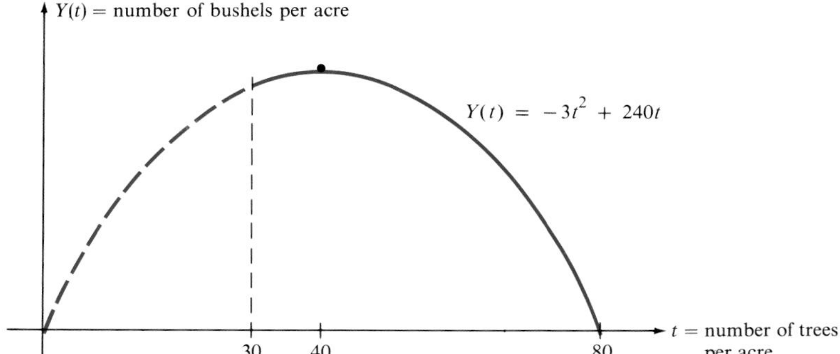

Figure 32
Bushels of apples per acre as a function of the number of trees per acre

Another well-known optimization problem is the maximum-volume box problem. We organize the solution of this problem by subdividing it into small steps.

The Maximum-Volume Box Problem

We start with a square sheet of cardboard for which the length of each side is 12 inches. Next we cut the same size square from each corner of the cardboard and fold the resulting piece of cardboard along the dashed lines as shown in Figure 33 to form a topless box.

The question we ask is, "How many inches should we cut from each corner of the original cardboard square to maximize the volume of the topless box?" How many inches would you guess: 1, 2, 3, 4, or 6 inches?

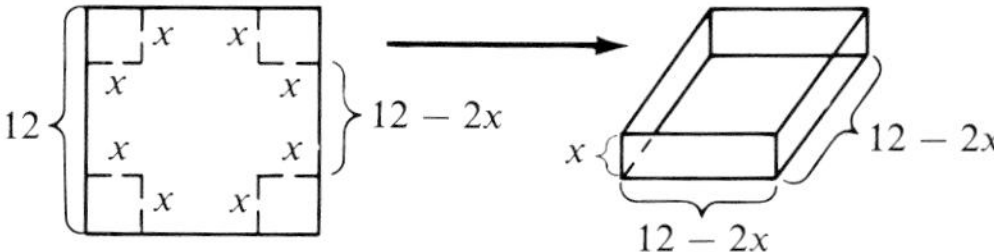

Figure 33
An open box is created by cutting squares of equal size from the corners of a sheet of cardboard

To find the absolute maximum of the volume of the resulting box, we carry out the following steps.

- **Step 1** (draw a picture illustrating the relevant variables). In Figure 33, we have denoted x (in inches) as the length of the sides of the small square cut from each corner.
- **Step 2** (find the equation that relates the relevant variables). The volume $V(x)$ of the topless box is given by

$$\begin{aligned} V(x) &= (\text{length})(\text{width})(\text{height}) \\ &= (12 - 2x)(12 - 2x)(x) \\ &= x(12 - 2x)^2 \qquad (0 \le x \le 6) \end{aligned}$$

Note that we cannot physically cut out squares with sides larger than 6. Hence the restriction on the variable x.

▪ **Step 3** [find the absolute maximum value of $V(x)$]. To find the absolute maximum value of $V(x)$ on the interval $[0, 6]$, we first evaluate it at the endpoints, getting

$$V(0) = 0 \quad \text{cubic inches}$$
$$V(6) = 0 \quad \text{cubic inches}$$

We now find the stationary points by computing the derivative $V'(x)$. We find

$$\begin{aligned} V'(x) &= 12x^2 - 96x + 144 \\ &= 12(x - 6)(x - 2) \end{aligned}$$

Setting this derivative to zero and solving for x, we get the two stationary points $x = 2$ and $x = 6$.

Hence the absolute maximum of $V(x)$ can be found by taking the largest of the quantities

$V(0) = 0$	(left endpoint)
$V(2) = (2)(8)^2 = 128$	(stationary point)
$V(6) = 0$	(right endpoint and stationary point)

Conclusion

To obtain a topless box with a maximum volume, we should cut a square that has 2-inch sides from each corner of the sheet of cardboard. This will result in a topless box with a maximum volume of

$$\begin{aligned} V(2) &= (\text{length})(\text{width})(\text{height}) \\ &= (8)(8)(2) \\ &= 128 \quad \text{cubic inches} \end{aligned}$$

The graph of the volume $V(x)$ of the box as a function of x is drawn in Figure 34.

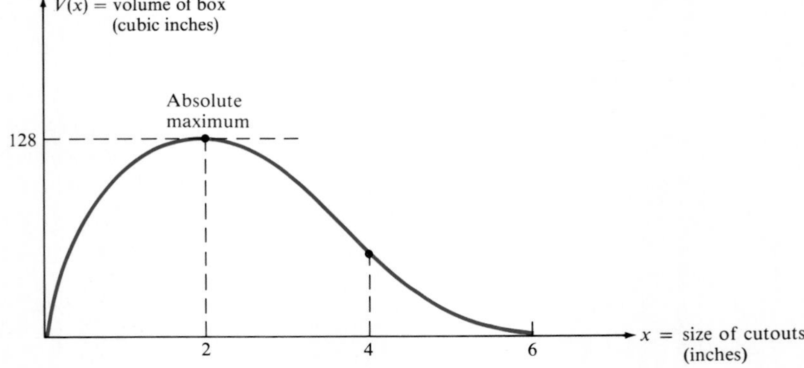

Figure 34
Volume of the box as a function of the cutouts

Max–Min Problems with Constraints

In both the apple orchard problem and the maximum-volume box problem we maximized a function of a single variable. In the remaining problems we will maximize a function of f that depends on two variables x and y which we denote by $f(x, y)$. The method of solution consists of finding a relationship or constraint between the two variables. By substituting this constraint, which we write as $y = g(x)$, into the function $f(x, y)$ we are trying to maximize, we will get an expression $f(x, g(x))$ in one variable. We then find the absolute maximum or minimum value of this function using the methods previously learned. We illustrate these ideas with two fascinating problems.

The Cat Food Can Problem (Minimum Surface Area)

The Carnation Co. of Los Angeles produces and distributes Friskies Buffet cat foods. All flavors come in cylindrical containers, and a 6-ounce can of Friskies Buffet Mixed Grill has a volume of roughly 14.5 cubic inches and dimensions

$$\text{Height} = 1.75 \text{ inches}$$
$$\text{Radius} = 1.62 \text{ inches}$$

The object of our study is to find the radius and the height of the can having a volume of 14.5 cubic inches that has the smallest surface area. In other words, how would we make a can for Friskies Mixed Grill that contains the least amount of metal in its construction? And finally, does the can for Friskies Mixed Grill that the Carnation Co. makes have this smallest surface area?

We begin by drawing typical cans with various diameters and heights as shown in Figure 35. Note that when the can is very tall or very short, the surface area will be large. For instance, when the can is short and fat, although the surface area around the sides is small, the surface area of the top and bottom is large. Also, if the can is tall and skinny, the top and bottom have small surface areas, but the surface area around the sides is large. The can with the smallest surface area lies somewhere between two such extremes.

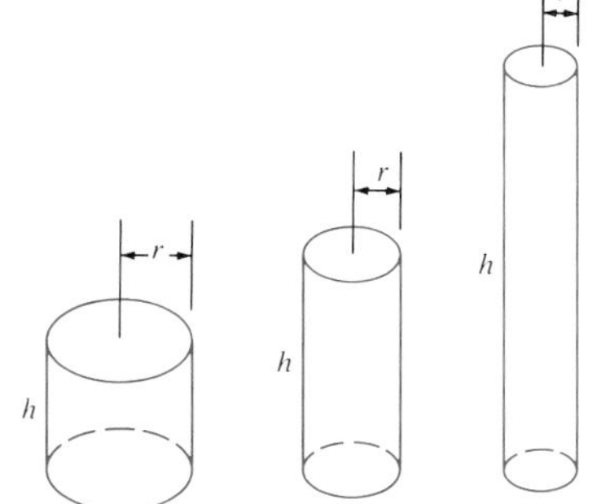

Figure 35
Three cylinders with the same volume but different surface areas

To find the dimensions of the can having volume 14.5 cubic inches with minimum surface area, we begin by writing the surface area S of a cylinder in terms of its radius r and height h. We have

$$S(r, h) = \underbrace{2\pi r^2}_{\text{Area of top and bottom}} + \underbrace{2\pi rh}_{\text{Area of side}} \qquad \text{(surface area of a cylinder)}$$

The goal is to find the values of r and h that minimize $S(r, h)$. Since the surface area S depends on two variables r and h, this maximization problem is different from any we have seen thus far. However, the two variables are not independent of each other, since they are related by the volume constraint:

$$\pi r^2 h = 14.5 \qquad \text{(volume of a cylinder)}$$

Hence we can solve for one of these variables in terms of the other and substitute the solved variable into the equation for S. This will give us $S(r, h)$ as a function of a single variable. Since it is easier in this case to solve for h, we get

$$h = \frac{14.5}{\pi r^2}$$

Substituting this value into the formula for the surface area S, we get

$$\begin{aligned} S(r) &= 2\pi r^2 + \frac{29\pi r}{\pi r^2} \\ &= 2\pi r^2 + \frac{29}{r} \qquad (0 < r < \infty) \end{aligned}$$

Although this function is not defined on a closed interval, it is still possible to find the absolute minimum value of $S(r)$. We begin by computing its first two derivatives:

$$S'(r) = 4\pi r - \frac{29}{r^2}$$

$$S''(r) = 4\pi + \frac{58}{r^3} \qquad \text{(always positive)}$$

Solving the equation $S'(r) = 0$, we find the stationary point

$$\begin{aligned} r &= \sqrt[3]{\frac{29}{4\pi}} \\ &\cong 1.32 \quad \text{inches} \end{aligned}$$

Since the second derivative is always positive, the graph of $S(r)$ is always concave up. It is clear that the surface area $S(r)$ obtains its absolute minimum value at the above stationary point. The graph of the surface area $S(r)$ as a function of the radius r is shown in Figure 36.

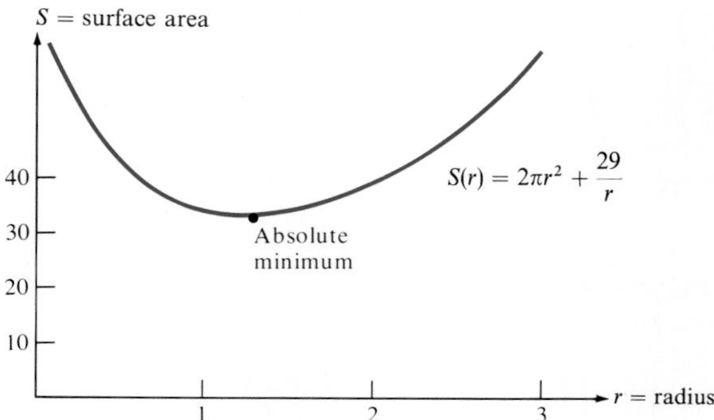

Figure 36
Surface area of a can of Friskies Mixed Grill as a function of its radius

To calculate the corresponding height of the can, we substitute the value $r = 1.32$ inches into the volume constraint, getting

$$\begin{aligned} h &= \frac{14.5}{\pi r^2} = \frac{14.5}{\pi (1.32)^2} \\ &\cong 2.64 \quad \text{inches} \qquad \text{(twice the radius)} \end{aligned}$$

Conclusion

If the volume of a cylindrical can is 14.5 cubic inches, then the dimensions of the can with the minimum surface area will be one for which both the diameter and the height are 2.64 inches. The surface area for such a minimal surface area can was found to be 32.9 square inches.

We conclude that a can of Friskies Buffet Mixed Grill with a diameter of 3.24 inches and a height of 1.75 inches is too short. It is easy to show that the Carnation Co. can save 6.7 square inches of metal for every can of cat food manufactured if they design the cans with height equal to the diameter.

Interested in knowing why the Carnation Co. packaged cat food in such short cans (like many other products such as tuna and canned chicken), we sent a letter to the California office of the Carnation Co. asking the reason why. Here is their reply:

Carnation

Corporate Offices
5045 Wilshire Boulevard
Los Angeles, California 90036
Telephone: (213) 932-6000

April 13, 1987

Jerry Farlow
Professor of Mathematics
Dept. of Mathematics
University of Maine
Orono, ME 04473

Dear Professor Farlow:

We appreciate the interest you expressed in examining the height-to-diameter relationship of containers used in our food products. A 1:1 ratio of height versus diameter is the most efficient use of material, if only the surface area of material is considered. However, there are many other factors which must be considered when designing a can for a particular product. Listed below are some of these other factors:

1) Thermal Processing — There is an inverse relationship between the most efficient design for cans relative to surface area and the amount of processing time required to sterilize the product contained within. In other words, a tall thin can or short wide can will require considerably less processing time and energy to achieve commercial sterility than a can which is nearly equal in height and diameter.

2) Strength Requirements — During thermal processing, considerable internal pressure develops. This pressure can cause the ends of the can to become permanently distorted. Because of this, ends on most cans are made of metal which is substantially thicker than that used in the can cylinder. Therefore, there is not a simple cost-to-surface area relationship relative to metal. As this can becomes taller and the end becomes smaller, thinner metal can be used in both the cylinder and the ends.

3) Can Manufacturing Line Changeover Time — Virtually all can lines run a variety of can sizes. The time required to change over from one can size to another is considerably less if only can height is changed, rather than height and diameter. In addition, since the same ends can be used if only the height is changed, the machinery used to manufacture ends does not have to be changed over to a different diameter. Reduced changeover time translates into reduced downtime and increased line efficiency.

4) Scrap Loss — Generally, more metal scrap is generated as the diameter is increased.

5) Warehouse and Shipping Efficiency — Smaller diameter cans make more efficient use of packaging and shipping space.

As you can see, cost and efficiency of a container are related to factors other than just the amount of material used. These are just a few of the factors which must be taken into consideration when designing a can. We hope that you now better understand that container design is not quite as simple as minimizing surface area.

Once again, thank you for your genuine interest.

Sincerely,

Vince Daukas

Vince Daukas
Assistant Product Manager
Friskies Buffet

The following set of rules can be used for solving optimization problems with constraints. The rules were used in solving the cat food can problem.

Steps in Solving Optimization Problems with Constraints

Step 1 (draw a picture). If possible, draw a picture illustrating the problem and label the relevant variables.

Step 2 (find the objective function). Determine the function to be maximized or minimized, and write it in terms of its variables. This function is called the objective function.

Step 3 (find the constraint). If the objective function depends on two variables, find a relationship or constraint between these variables, and solve for one in terms of the other.

Step 4 (write the objective function in terms of one variable). Substitute the solved variable from Step 3 into the objective function so that the objective function is a function of a single variable.

Step 5 (find the absolute maximum and minimum values). Find the absolute maximum or minimum values of the objective function.

Step 6 (interpretation of results). Interpret the mathematical results obtained in Step 5 in the language of the original problem.

The Salmon Problem (How Fast Should a Salmon Swim?)

The amount of energy $E(v)$ that a salmon expends in swimming upstream with velocity v (relative to the stream) over a period of time T has experimentally been shown to be

$$E(v, T) = cv^3T$$

where c is a constant. Suppose the velocity of the stream is 4 miles per hour and the salmon swims upstream 200 miles. How fast should a fish swim in order to minimize its use of energy?

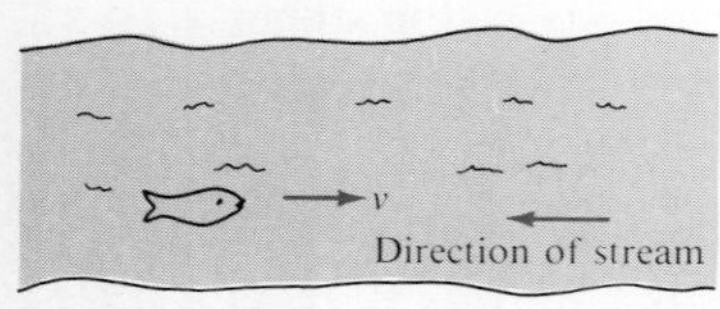

Figure 37
The fish moves with velocity v relative to the velocity of the stream

- **Step 1** (draw a picture). We start by drawing an illustration of the relevant variables, as shown in Figure 37.
- **Step 2** (find the objective function). The quantity or objective function that should be minimized is the energy

$$E(v, T) = cv^3T$$

which depends on the two variables v (velocity) and T (time).

- **Step 3** (find the constraint). The variables v and T are not independent of one another but are related by an equation. To find this equation, observe that the velocity of the fish relative to the ground is 4 miles per hour less than it is relative to the stream. Hence by using the general formula for velocity,

$$\text{Velocity} = \frac{\text{Distance}}{\text{Time}}$$

we can write the constraint equation, which relates v and T:

$$v - 4 = \frac{200}{T} \qquad \text{(constraint equation)}$$

Solving for T in terms of v, we have

$$T = \frac{200}{v - 4}$$

- **Step 4** (write the objective function in terms of one variable). Substituting the above value for T into the objective function $E(v, T)$, we get a function of v alone:

$$\begin{aligned} E(v) &= cv^3T \\ &= 200c\frac{v^3}{v - 4} \qquad (4 < v < \infty) \end{aligned}$$

- **Step 5** (minimize the objective function). To find the absolute minimum value of $E(v)$, we first find its derivative:

$$\frac{dE}{dv} = 400cv^2\frac{v - 6}{(v - 4)^2}$$

Setting dE/dv to zero, we get a single stationary point at $v = 6$. It is also clear that the derivative dE/dv is negative for v less than 6 and positive for v greater than 6. Hence we can conclude that the absolute minimum value of $E(v)$ occurs at $v = 6$.

- **Step 6** (interpret the results). We conclude that for the salmon to minimize its use of energy, it should swim at a rate of $v = 6$ miles per hour or 50% faster than the velocity of the stream (which is 4 miles per hour). Note that the velocity of the fish is 2 miles per hour relative to the bank of the stream. If the fish swims faster than this velocity, it will end up spending more energy. It will, of course, arrive at its destination sooner, but its increased velocity will result in a larger total expended energy. On the other hand, if the fish swims slower than 6 miles per hour, it ends up taking so long that again the total energy expended is not a minimum. It is interesting to note that most salmon do swim at a velocity roughly 50% greater than the velocity of the stream.

The Fence Problem (Minimum Cost)

A nursery wants to add a 1000-square-foot rectangular area to its greenhouse to sell seedlings. For aesthetic reasons they have decided to border the area on three sides by cedar siding at a cost of \$10 per running foot. The remaining side of the enclosure is to be a wall with a brick mosaic that costs \$25 per running foot. What should the dimensions of the sides be so that the cost of the project will be minimized?

- **Step 1** (draw a picture). Calling

$$x = \text{Length of the two cedar fences adjacent to the brick wall}$$
$$y = \text{Length of the brick wall (and the opposite cedar fence)}$$

we draw a diagram and label these variables, as shown in Figure 38.

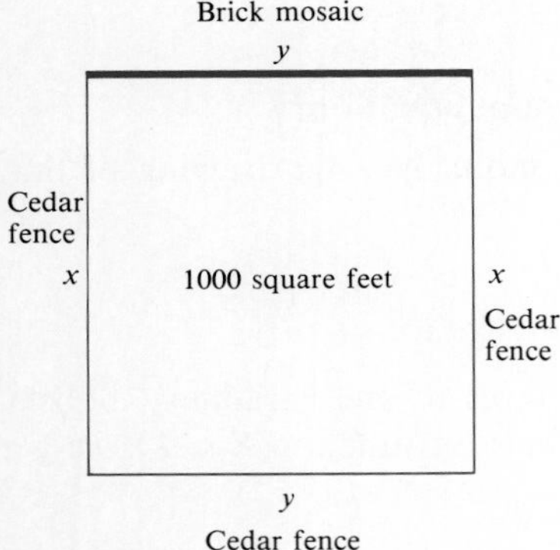

Figure 38
A rectangular area of 1000 square feet is to be enclosed on three sides by cedar fence at a cost of \$10 per running foot and on the fourth side by brick mosaic at a cost of \$25 per running foot

- **Step 2** (find the objective function). The function that we wish to minimize is the total cost of the project. Since the general formula is given by

$$\text{Total cost of fence} = (\text{Cost per foot})(\text{Length in feet})$$

we have

$$\text{Total cost for cedar fence} = (\$10)(2x + y)$$
$$\text{Total cost for brick mosaic} = (\$25)(y)$$

Hence the total cost in dollars of the project will be

$$\begin{aligned} C(x, y) &= 10(2x + y) + 25y \\ &= 20x + 35y \qquad \text{(objective function)} \end{aligned}$$

- **Step 3** (find the constraint). The two variables x and y are not independent but are related by the area constraint

$$xy = 1000 \qquad \text{(constraint equation)}$$

Solving for y in terms of x gives

$$y = \frac{1000}{x}$$

- **Step 4** (write the objective function in terms of one variable). Substituting the above value of y into the objective function $C(x, y)$, we have

$$C(x) = 20x + 35\frac{1000}{x} \qquad (0 < x < \infty)$$

- **Step 5** (minimize the objective function). Computing the derivative of $C(x)$, we have

$$C'(x) = 20 - \frac{35{,}000}{x^2}$$

Setting this derivative to zero, we get

$$20 - \frac{35{,}000}{x^2} = 0$$

or

$$x^2 = \frac{35{,}000}{20}$$

Solving for x, we obtain the stationary point

$$x = 41.83$$

It is clear from the formula for $C'(x)$ that $C'(x)$ is always negative to the left of 41.83 and positive to the right of 41.83. From these observations it is clear that $C(x)$ has an absolute minimum value when $x = 41.83$. Using this value of x, we can find the second dimension y from the constraint equation $xy = 1000$. This gives $y = 23.91$.

▪ **Step 6** (interpret the results). The most economical fence that will enclose an area of 1000 square feet is one 23.91×41.83 feet. The total cost of the fence is

$$\begin{aligned}\text{Total cost} &= 20x + 35y \\ &= 20(41.83) + 35(23.91) \\ &= \$1673.45\end{aligned}$$

Any other rectangular design will cost more. A scale drawing of this optimal design is shown in Figure 39.

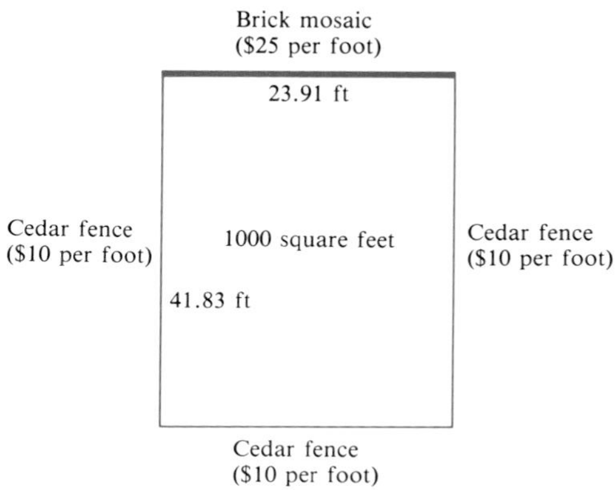

Figure 39
Minimum-cost rectangle

Problems

1. **Maximum Product.** Find two numbers whose sum is 15 and whose product is a maximum.
2. **Minimum Sum of Squares.** Find two numbers whose sum is 10 for which the sum of their squares is a minimum.
3. **Constrained Maximum.** Find nonnegative numbers x and y whose sum is 75 and for which the value of xy^2 is as large as possible.
4. **Constrained Maximum.** Find the maximum value of the function of two variables

$$f(x, y) = x^2y$$

when

$$x + y = 150$$

Theory of the Firm

5. **Minimum Average Cost.** A manufacturer has determined that the total cost C to produce q units of a given product is

$$C(q) = 0.05q^2 + 10q + 250$$

Find the level of production for which the **average cost** per unit is a minimum.

6. **Minimum Operating Costs.** A trucking company has determined that the cost per hour to operate a single truck is given by

$$C(s) = -0.001s^2 + 0.10s + 0.12$$

where s is the speed that the truck travels. At what speed is the total cost per hour a minimum? What is the hourly cost to operate the truck?

7. **Maximum Revenue.** A company has determined that the weekly demand $D(p)$ for its product is a function of the price p that the company charges. The relationship has been determined to be

$$D(p) = -3p + 300$$

How much should the company charge to maximize the revenue? *Hint:* The revenue R is given by $R(p) = p\,D(p)$.

8. **Marginal Revenue.** A company's total revenue is

$$R(q) = 10q - 0.01q^2$$

where q is the number of items produced. Find the number of items produced that will make the marginal revenue zero. What is your interpretation of this value of q?

9. **Maximum Profit.** A manufacturing firm can sell all the items it can produce at a price of \$5 each. The cost in dollars to produce q items per week is given by

$$C(q) = 1000 + 10q - 0.002q^2$$

What value of q should be selected to maximize the total profit? *Hint:* Profit $= 5q - C(q)$.

10. **Maximum Profit.** Suppose the unit sales volume V for a given product depends on the offering price p, according to the equation

$$V(p) = 40{,}000 - 8000p$$

Suppose the cost C to manufacture each item depends on the number V of items produced (same as the number sold) and is given by

$$C(V) = 100{,}000 + 25V$$

Find the price that should be charged for the product that will maximize the profit.
Hint: Profit = (Price)(Volume) − (Cost).

11. **Optimal Pricing.** A real estate company owns 100 apartments in New York City. At \$1000 per month, each apartment can be rented. However, for each \$50 increase, there will be two additional vacancies. How much should the real estate company charge for rent to maximize its revenues?

12. **Optimal Pricing.** A national chain of service stations charges \$28 to replace a muffler. At this rate the company replaces 75,000 mufflers per week. For each additional dollar that the company charges, it tends to lose 1000 customers per week. For each dollar the company subtracts from the \$28, the company gains 1000 customers per week. How much should the company charge to change a muffler to maximize the revenue?

13. **Optimal Density of Pear Trees.** Normally a pear tree will produce 30 bushels of pears per tree when 20 or fewer pear trees are planted per acre. However, for each additional pear tree planted above 20 trees per acre, the yield per tree will fall by one bushel per tree. How many trees should be planted per acre to maximize the total yield?

Minimum-Cost Container Problems

14. **Minimum-Cost Box.** A closed box with a square base is to have a volume of 1600 cubic inches. The material for the top and bottom of the box costs \$3 per square inch, while the material for the sides costs \$1 per square inch. Find the dimensions of the box that will lead to the minimum total cost. What is the minimum total cost?

15. **Minimum Surface Area.** Oversea Containers Inc., builds large wooden containers for secure overseas shipping of goods. Find the dimensions of such a container with a square top, minimal surface area, and a volume of 1000 cubic feet.

16. **Minimum Surface Area.** Find the dimensions of a box with a minimal surface area, a square base, a volume of 100 cubic feet, and no top.

17. **Minimum Surface Area.** Find the dimensions of a carport that is attached to a house, encloses 2000 cubic feet, and has minimal surface area and a height equal to its length. The carport has a flat roof and a side parallel to the house but no front or back wall.

18. **Maximum Volume.** The U.S. Postal Service will accept a package for parcel post only if its length plus girth (shortest distance around the package) does not exceed 108 inches. Mail-It-Secure Co. plans to market a box that will satisfy this condition and have maximum volume. If the box is to have square ends and rectangular sides, what should be the dimensions of the box?

19. **Maximum Volume.** A rectangular sheet of cardboard $3'' \times 5''$ is to be cut as shown in Figure 40 to form a topless box. What dimensions of the box will enclose the maximum volume? What is the maximum volume?

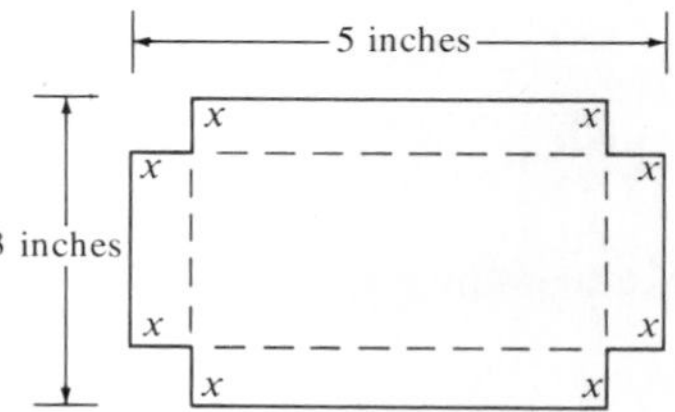

Figure 40
Illustration for Problem 19

20. **Minimum-Cost Box.** A box with a top is three times as long as it is wide and holds a fixed volume V. The material for the sides and bottom costs 20 cents per square foot, while the material for the top costs 30 cents per square foot. What dimensions of the box are most economical?

21. **Wire Problem.** A wire 25 inches long is cut into two pieces. One piece is to be shaped into a square, and the other piece into a circle, as shown in Figure 41. How should the wire be cut to maximize the total area enclosed by the square and the circle?

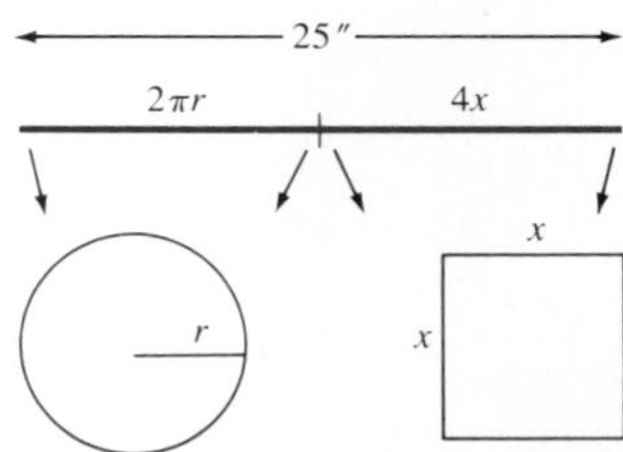

Figure 41
Illustration for Problem 21

22. **Rectangle in a Circle.** What is the rectangle of largest area that can be cut from a circle of radius 20 inches? (See Figure 42.)

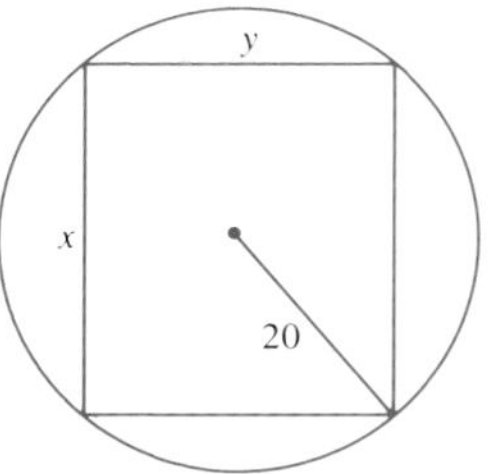

Figure 42
Illustration for Problem 22

23. **Optimal Printing.** Ready Words needs to set up several templates for the printing requirements of its major customers. One type of page should contain 80 square inches of printed matter with 2-inch margins on each side and a 3-inch margin at the top and bottom. Find the dimensions of this type of page that has the minimum total page area.

24. **Norman Window Problem.** A designer of custom windows wishes to build a Norman window with an outside perimeter of 40 feet as shown in Figure 43. How should one design the window to maximize the area of the window? A Norman window consists of a rectangular region bordered above by a semicircle.

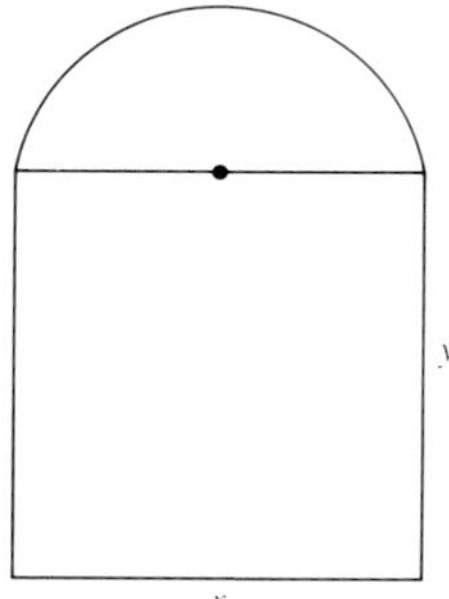

Figure 43
Norman window

25. **Maximum Area.** A strip of metal 12 inches wide is to be formed into an open gutter with a rectangular cross section, as shown in Figure 44. What is the maximum possible area of the cross section?

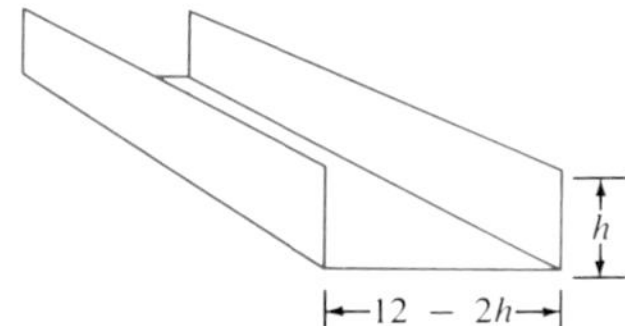

Figure 44
Gutter for Problem 25

26. **Maximum Surface Area.** A tent with a volume of 432 cubic feet is formed with sides shaped as rectangles and ends as equilateral triangles. What should be the dimensions of the tent to minimize its surface area? Does adding a floor to the tent change the answer?

27. **Telephone Lines.** A telephone wire is to be laid to an island seven miles off shore at a cost of \$2000 per mile along the shore and \$3000 per mile under the sea. How should the project be planned to minimize the cost if the distance from A to B is 12 miles? (See Figure 45.)

28. **Maximum Height of a Ball.** A ball is thrown straight up in the air. Its height after t seconds is given by

$$s(t) = -16t^2 + 50t$$

When does the ball reach its maximum height? What is its maximum height?

29. **Maximum Receipts.** A concert promoter knows that 5000 people will attend an event with tickets set at \$10. For each dollar less in ticket price an additional 1000

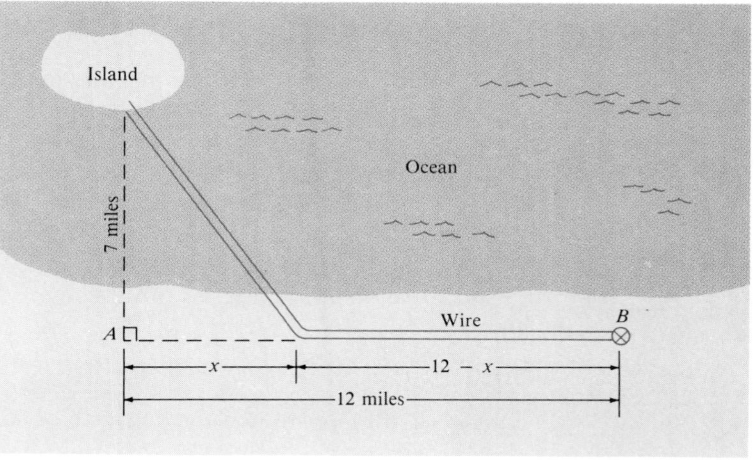

Figure 45
Telephone line to an island

tickets will be sold. What should the ticket price be to maximize total receipts?

30. **Group Travel.** A travel agent is offering charter holidays to Europe for college students. For groups of size up to 100, the fare is \$1000 per person. For larger groups the fare per person decreases by \$5 for each additional person in excess of 100. Find the size of the group that maximizes the travel agent's revenues.

31. **Maximum Area of a Field.** A farmer has 2000 feet of fencing to enclose a pasture area. The field should have the shape of a rectangle with one side bordered by a currently existing rock fence, as shown in Figure 46. What should be the dimensions of the field to enclose the maximum area?

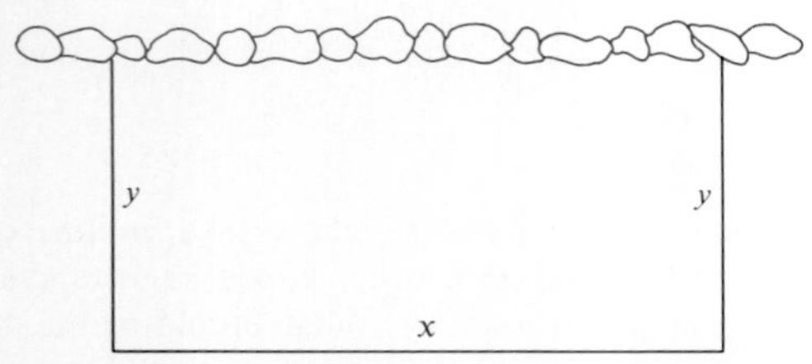

Figure 46
Field bordered by a stone wall

32. **Fish-Stocking Problem.** A fisheries biologist is stocking fish in a lake. She knows that when there are n fish per unit area of water, the average weight $W(n)$ of each fish after one season will be

$$W(n) = 500 - 20n \quad \text{grams}$$

What is the value of n that will maximize the total fish weight after one season? *Hint:* Total weight $= n\,W(n)$.

33. **Bacteria Growth.** The size $N(t)$ of a population of bacteria introduced to a nutrient grows according to the formula

$$N(t) = \frac{5000t}{50 + t^2}$$

where t is measured in weeks. Determine when the bacteria will reach maximum size. What is the maximum size of the population?

34. **Medical Testing.** Blood pressure in a patient will drop by an amount $D(x)$, where

$$D(x) = 0.025x^2(30 - x)$$

and x is the amount of drug injected. Find the dosage that provides the greatest drop in blood pressure. What is the drop in blood pressure?

2.5 Implicit Differentiation and Related Rates

PURPOSE

This section introduces the idea of implicit differentiation and uses it to study the topic of related rates of change. The major ideas introduced are

- implicit differentiation,
- tangent lines to general curves, and
- related rates of change.

Introduction

Until now, we have found the derivative dy/dx when y was related to x by means of an explicit functional relationship $y = f(x)$. We now show how to find the derivative dy/dx when x and y are related *implicitly*, as in a formula such as $x^2 + 3xy^2 + y^2x = 0$. The process used to find dy/dx when x and y are related implicitly is called *implicit differentiation.*

The second portion of this section, which makes use of implicit differentiation, introduces the idea of *related rates.* Here, we find the rate of change of one quantity in terms of the rate of change of other quantities.

Implicit Differentiation

Until now, to find the derivative dy/dx, it was necessary to start with the functional relationship $y = f(x)$. Now, however, we show how to find the derivative

Example 2 **Implicit Differentiation** Find dy/dx given

$$x^3 + y^3 - xy = 0$$

Solution Since it is difficult to solve for y in terms of x, implicit differentiation is the more convenient way to find dy/dx. Keep in mind that since y is a function of x, the chain rule gives the derivative

$$\frac{d}{dx}[y^n] = ny^{n-1}\frac{dy}{dx}$$

Differentiating each side of the above equation with respect to x and remembering that y is a function of x, we get

$$\frac{d}{dx}[x^3 + y^3 - xy] = \frac{d}{dx}[0]$$

$$\frac{d}{dx}[x^3] + \frac{d}{dx}[y^3] - \frac{d}{dx}[xy] = 0$$

$$3x^2 + 3y^2\frac{d}{dx}[y] - x\frac{d}{dx}[y] - y\frac{d}{dx}[x] = 0$$

$$3x^2 + 3y^2\frac{dy}{dx} - x\frac{dy}{dx} - y = 0$$

Other curves where implicit differentiation is useful are shown in Table 10.

TABLE 10
Curves Written in Implicit Form

$f(x, y) = 0$	Type of Curve
$x^2 + y^2 - 1 = 0$	Circle 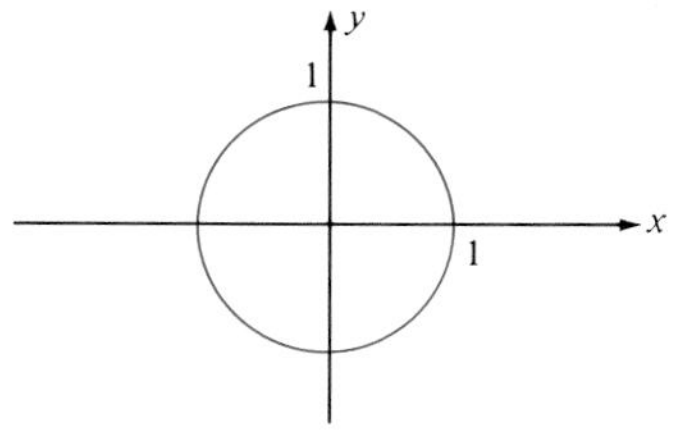
$x^2 - y^2 - 1 = 0$	Hyperbola 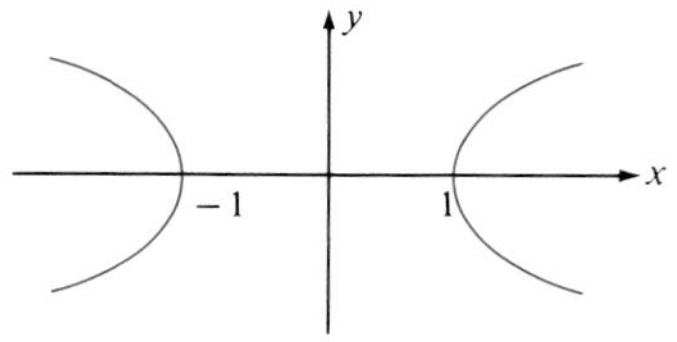
$x^2 + 4y^2 - 16 = 0$	Ellipse 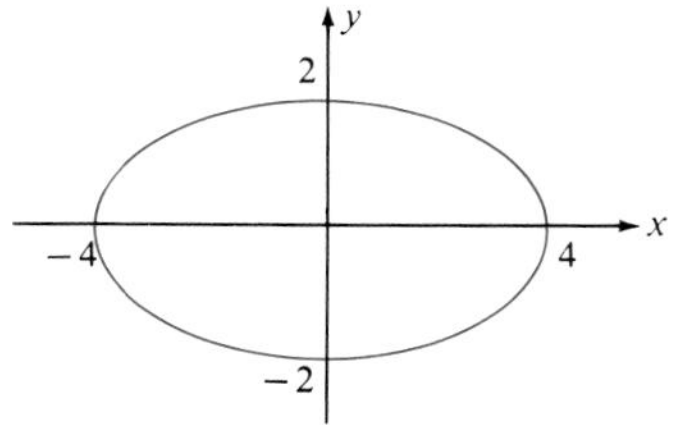

Solving for dy/dx, we have

$$\frac{dy}{dx} = \frac{y - 3x^2}{3y^2 - x}$$

We have found the derivative dy/dx in terms of both x and y. □

In the preceding example, since it was difficult to solve algebraically for y in terms of x in the original equation, we left the result in terms of x and y. Often the derivative is desired at some point (x, y). In those cases there is no disadvantage in having both x and y in the formula for dy/dx.

Tangent Lines to Curves

One of the major applications of implicit differentiation lies in finding tangent lines to curves that are not defined explicitly as $y = f(x)$ but are defined implicitly as $f(x, y) = 0$. If the derivative dy/dx of an implicit function $f(x, y) = 0$ is evaluated at a point (x, y) on the curve $f(x, y) = 0$, then the value of the derivative at the point is the slope of the tangent line to the curve at that point. We illustrate this idea with the following example.

Example 3 Slope of a Tangent Line Let x and y be related by the equation

$$x^2 - y^2 = 1$$

which describes the hyperbola shown in Figure 47. Find the slope of the tangent line to this hyperbola at the point $(2, \sqrt{3})$.

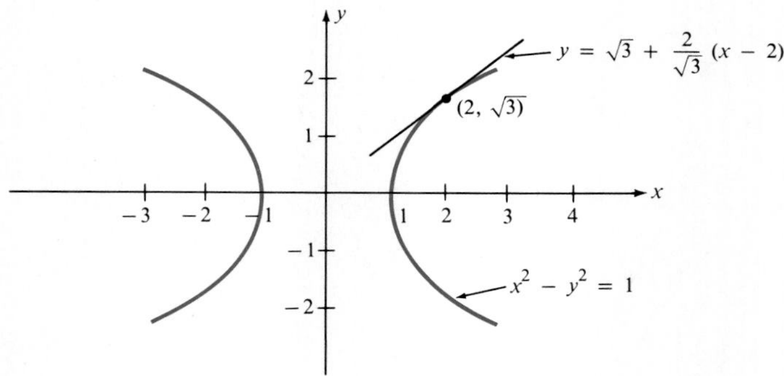

Figure 47
Finding tangent line by implicit differentiation

Solution To find dy/dx at the desired point, we first differentiate implicitly each side of the equation with respect to x. This gives

$$\frac{d}{dx}[x^2 - y^2] = \frac{d}{dx}[1]$$

$$\frac{d}{dx}[x^2] - \frac{d}{dx}[y^2] = 0$$

$$2x - 2y\frac{dy}{dx} = 0$$

Solving for dy/dx gives

$$\frac{dy}{dx} = \frac{x}{y}$$

This derivative says that the slope of the tangent line at any point (x, y) on the hyperbola is given by the ratio x/y. By a simple check we can verify that the point $(2, \sqrt{3})$ lies on the hyperbola $x^2 - y^2 = 1$, and so the slope of the tangent line at this point is $2/\sqrt{3}$. Using the point-slope form of the straight line, we find that the equation of the tangent line at this point is

$$y - \sqrt{3} = \frac{2}{\sqrt{3}}(x - 2)$$

This line is shown in Figure 47. □

We now summarize the technique of implicit differentiation by stating the following rules.

Rules for Implicit Differentiation

To find dy/dx when x and y are related implicitly by $f(x, y) = 0$, use the following three-step procedure:

Step 1. Differentiate $f(x, y) = 0$ with respect to x. Keep in mind that y is a function of x.

Step 2. Solve for dy/dx in terms of x and y.

Step 3. If possible, solve for y in terms of x in the original equation and substitute this value of y into the equation for dy/dx found in Step 2.

Example 4

Tangent Lines to Circles Find the tangent line to the circle

$$x^2 + y^2 = 1$$

at any point (x_0, y_0) on the circle.

Solution Using the above three-step procedure to find dy/dx, we do the following:

- **Step 1** (differentiate the equation with respect to x). Differentiating the given equation with respect to x gives

$$\frac{d}{dx}[x^2 + y^2] = \frac{d}{dx}[1]$$

$$2x + 2y\frac{dy}{dx} = 0$$

- **Step 2** (solve for dy/dx). Solving this equation for dy/dx gives

$$\frac{dy}{dx} = -\frac{x}{y}$$

- **Step 3** (if possible, solve for y in the original equation). Since we cannot solve for a unique value of y in the original equation (we get two values), we leave the derivative dy/dx in terms of both x and y.

Hence the tangent line to any point (x_0, y_0) on the circle

$$x^2 + y^2 = 1$$

will have the slope

$$\frac{dy}{dx} = -\frac{x_0}{y_0}$$

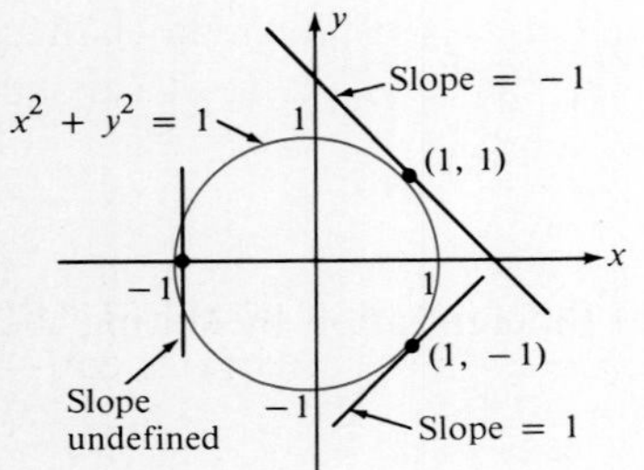

Figure 48
Tangent lines to a circle

Using the point-slope formula for a straight line, this tangent line can be written as

$$y - y_0 = -\frac{x_0}{y_0}(x - x_0)$$

Some of the tangent lines to the circle are shown in Figure 48. □

The remainder of this section will be devoted to the concept of related rates. Implicit differentiation is often required to evaluate many of the derivatives encountered.

Related Rates

If y depends on x, then y will change in some manner when x changes. Suppose now that x changes with time t. Inasmuch as y changes when x changes and x changes when t changes, it follows that y changes when t changes. More specifically, if x and y are related by $y = f(x)$ and x depends on time by means of some function $x = x(t)$, then x and y will be related by the equation $y(t) = f[x(t)]$. From this equation we can find the rate of change in y (dy/dt) in terms of the rate of change in x (dx/dt) by simply using the chain rule and differentiating this equation with respect to t. This gives

$$\frac{dy}{dt} = \frac{d}{dx} f(x) \frac{dx}{dt} \qquad \text{(related rates equation)}$$

Rate of change of y with respect to time — *Rate of change of x with respect to time*

This **related rates equation** gives the relationship between the rate of change in y with respect to time (dy/dt) and the rate of change in x with respect to time (dx/dt). We now present examples to show how this related rates equation can be used to find and solve interesting problems.

Example 5

The Soft Drink Problem Eddie is drinking a soda from a cylindrical can through a straw. The volume of the soda in the can is decreasing at a rate of 0.5 cubic inch per second. If the radius across the top of the can is 1 inch, how fast is the level of soda in the can going down?

Solution We wish to find the rate of change dh/dt of the height h of the soda and are given the rate of change dV/dt of the volume V of the soda. We start by finding the algebraic relationship between V and h. We first write the equation $V = \pi r^2 h$, which expresses the volume V of a cylinder in terms of its radius r and height h. These variables are illustrated in Figure 49.

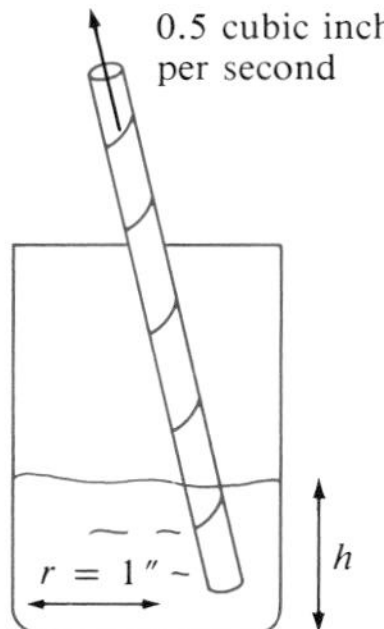

Figure 49
How fast is the soda going down?

As Eddie drinks the soda, the volume V and height h of the soda change with time t. On the other hand, the radius r remains the same, so it can be treated as a constant. If we now differentiate the equation

$$V(t) = \pi r^2 h(t)$$

with respect to time [note that we have denoted the volume and height as $V(t)$ and $h(t)$, since they both change with time], we will get the related rates equation relating dV/dt and dh/dt. Doing this, we get

$$\frac{dV}{dt} = \pi r^2 \frac{dh}{dt} \qquad \text{(related rates equation)}$$

We can now solve for the desired quantity dh/dt in terms of the known quantities r and dV/dt. Since we were given

$$r = 1 \text{ inch}$$

$$\frac{dV}{dt} = -0.5 \quad \text{cubic inch per second}$$

we have

$$\begin{aligned} \frac{dh}{dt} &= \frac{1}{\pi r^2}\frac{dV}{dt} \\ &= \frac{1}{\pi(1)^2}(-0.5) \\ &\cong -0.16 \end{aligned}$$

Note that we let dV/dt be a negative number, since V is decreasing with respect to time as Eddie drinks the soda.

If Eddie drinks the soda at a rate of 0.5 cubic inch per second and if the radius of the can is 1 inch, then the height of the soda will go down (since dh/dt is negative) at a rate of 0.16 inch per second. □

Example 6

The Balloon Problem Imagine yourself blowing up a balloon as in Figure 50, blowing air into a balloon at a rate of 15 cubic inches per second. (That is pretty close to normal for most people.) At the exact moment when the radius of the balloon is 1 inch, how fast will the radius of the balloon be increasing? Make a guess: 1 inch per second? 2 inches per second?

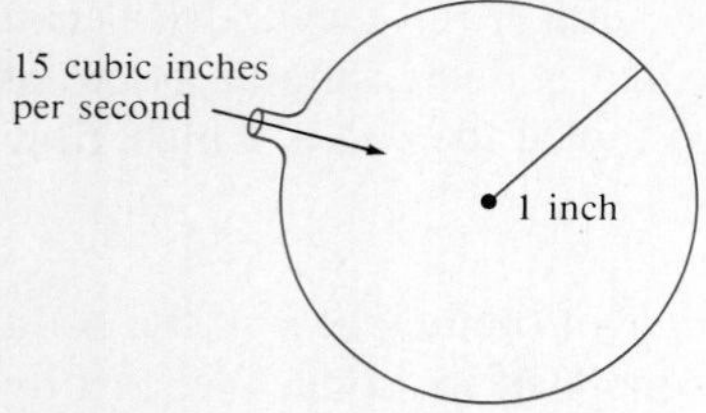

Figure 50
Blowing air into a balloon

Solution The volume and radius of a balloon (sphere) are related by the equation

$$V(t) = \frac{4}{3}\pi r^3(t)$$

To find the relationship between dV/dt and dr/dt, we differentiate with respect to time t, getting the related rates equation

$$\frac{d}{dt}V(t) = \frac{4}{3}\pi\frac{d}{dt}[r^3(t)]$$
$$= 4\pi r^2\frac{dr}{dt}$$

In this problem we are given the two quantities

$$\frac{dV}{dt} = 15 \text{ cubic inches per second}$$
$$r = 1 \text{ inch}$$

Solving for the unknown dr/dt in the related rates equation, we get

$$\frac{dr}{dt} = \frac{1}{4\pi r^2}\frac{dV}{dt}$$
$$= \frac{1}{4\pi(1)^2}(15)$$
$$\cong 1.2 \quad \text{inches per second}$$

□

Conclusion

If you blow air into a balloon at a constant rate of 15 cubic inches per second, then when the radius of the balloon is 1 inch (about the size of a tennis ball), the radius will be increasing at a rate of 1.2 inches per second. As the balloon gets larger, however, the rate at which the radius increases will not be as large. In fact, the graph in Figure 51 shows the relationship between the rate of change dr/dt in the radius and the radius r.

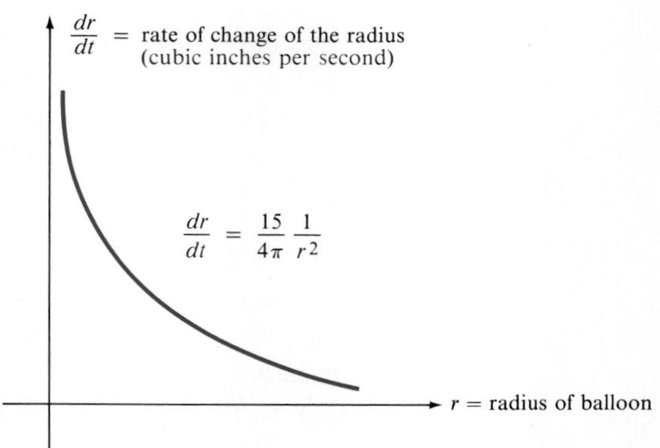

Figure 51
The rate of change in the radius of a balloon as a function of the radius when the air is being blown into it at a rate of 15 cubic inches per second

Steps for Solving Related Rates Problems

Step 1. Draw a picture that describes the problem (if possible) and label all relevant variables (especially the ones that change with time).

Step 2. Find the algebraic equation that relates the variables of the problem.

Step 3. Differentiate the equation from Step 2 with respect to time.

Step 4. Solve for the unknown rate of change (one of the time derivatives).

Example 7

The Ladder Problem Suppose a young man and woman are eloping. The young man has a 20-foot ladder leaning up against the house. However, at the exact moment he is standing at the top of the ladder, the young woman's father starts pulling the ladder away from the house at the rate of 5 feet per second. How fast is the young man coming down the side of the house when the bottom of the ladder is 10 feet from the base of the house?

Solution

Step 1 (draw a picture and label the variables). Figure 52 shows the relevant variables of the problem. The two important variables are

$x(t)$ = Distance from the bottom of the ladder to the house

$y(t)$ = Height of the top of the ladder from the ground

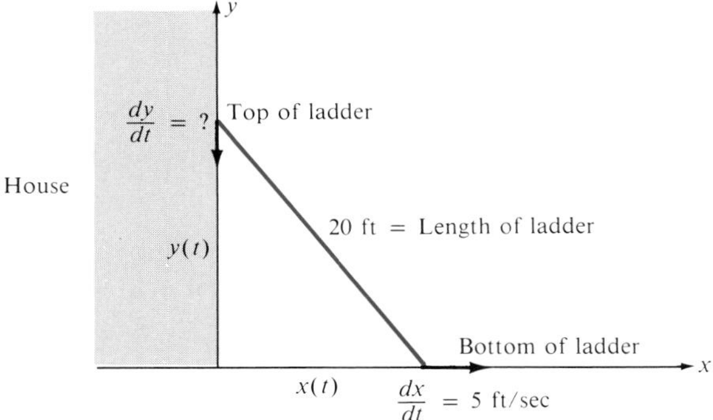

Figure 52
Relevant variables for the ladder problem

Step 2 (find a relationship between the variables). The variables $x(t)$ and $y(t)$ are always related by the Pythagorean theorem:

$$x^2(t) + y^2(t) = 400$$

provided that the ladder is leaning against the house.

- **Step 3** (differentiate with respect to time). We now differentiate this equation implicitly with respect to t to get the related rates equation

$$2x\frac{dx}{dt} + 2y\frac{dy}{dt} = 0$$

- **Step 4** (solve for dy/dt). Solving for dy/dt, which represents the rate at which the young man is coming down the side of the house, we find

$$\frac{dy}{dt} = -\frac{x}{y}\frac{dx}{dt}$$

This equation gives dy/dt in terms of x, y, and dx/dt.

Unfortunately, we are given only dx/dt and x. Hence we must solve for y in terms of x, using the original equation

$$x^2 + y^2 = 400$$

This gives

$$y = \sqrt{400 - x^2}$$

We use the positive root because it represents the height of the ladder above the ground. Substituting this value into the related rates equation, we obtain the unknown rate

$$\frac{dy}{dt} = -\frac{x}{\sqrt{400 - x^2}}\frac{dx}{dt}$$

We now substitute into this equation the given values

$$\frac{dx}{dt} = 5 \text{ ft/sec} \qquad \text{(rate that the ladder is pulled from house)}$$

$$x = 10 \text{ ft} \qquad \text{(distance of ladder from the base of house)}$$

Hence we have

$$\frac{dy}{dt} = -\frac{10}{\sqrt{300}}(5)$$

$$\cong -2.89 \quad \text{feet per second}$$ □

Interesting Conclusion

The value $dy/dt = -2.89$ feet per second means that the function $y(t)$ is decreasing at this rate. This means that when the bottom of the ladder is 10 feet from the house, the top of the ladder is coming down the side of the house at the rate of 2.89 feet per second. We can see in Figure 53 that as the father starts pulling the ladder away from the house, the young man starts falling immediately. Even though the father pulls the ladder at a constant rate of 10 feet per second, the young man falls faster and faster. In fact, the interesting thing is that the speed at which the young man falls approaches infinity immediately before he hits the ground. Is this really true?

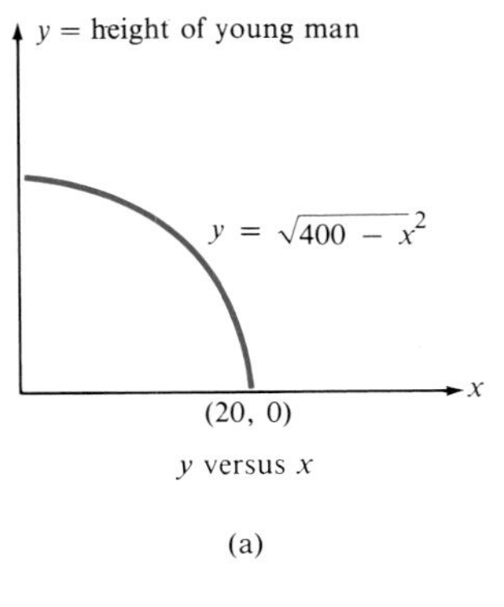

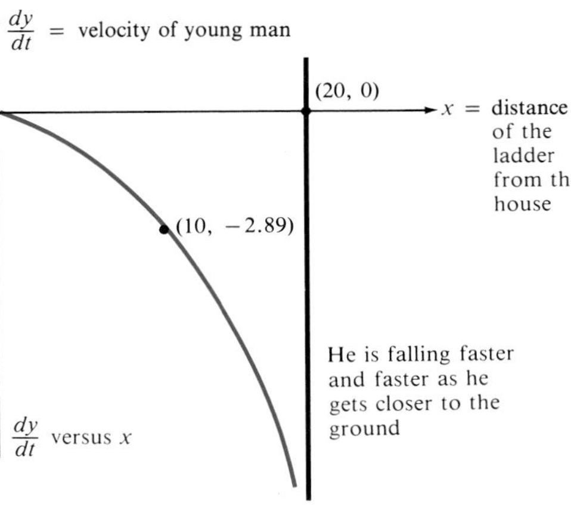

Figure 53
Graphs of y versus x and dy/dx versus x

Problems

In Problems 1–17, find dy/dx using implicit differentiation.

1. $y - x^2 = 0$
2. $y - x^3 = 0$
3. $x^2y = 1$
4. $x^3y = 1$
5. $xy + x = 1$
6. $x^2y + y = 4$
7. $x^3 + xy = x$
8. $xy - 3 + 7x = 0$
9. $xy + y^2 = x$
10. $y^2 + y = x^2(x + 1)$
11. $9x^2 + 16y^2 = 36$
12. $y^5 - 7xy - 18x^3 = 0$
13. $y^2 + xy = x(x - y)$
14. $\dfrac{y + x}{y - x} = x^2$
15. $y^2 = \dfrac{x^2}{x^2 - 1}$
16. $\sqrt{x} + \sqrt{y} = \sqrt{a}$ where a is a positive constant
17. $xy^2 + x^2y = x^3 + 2x^2$

In Problems 18–26, find dy/dx using implicit differentiation and then evaluate dy/dx at the given point.

18. $xy = 4$ at $(1, 4)$
19. $x^2y + y = 1$ at $(0, 1)$
20. $x^3y + x = 0$ at $(1, -1)$
21. $x^2y = 1$ at $(1, 1)$
22. $x^2 - y^2 = 3$ at $(\sqrt{3}, 0)$
23. $x^2 - 3xy = 10$ at $(2, -1)$
24. $x^2y - xy^2 + y - 8 = 0$ at $(-1, 2)$
25. $(\sqrt{x} + 1)(\sqrt{y} + 1) = 6$ at $(1, 4)$
26. $(x - y^2)(x + y) = 15$ at $(4, 1)$

In Problems 27–36, find the equation of the tangent line to the curve at the given point. If possible, draw the curve and the tangent line.

27. $x^2y = 1$ at $(1, 1)$
28. $x^2y + y = 1$ at $(0, 1)$
29. $xy = -1$ at $(1, -1)$
30. $x^3y + xy = 1$ at $(1, 0.5)$
31. $x^2 + y^2 = 9$ at $(0, 3)$
32. $x^2 - y^2 = 9$ at $(3, 0)$
33. $x^2y + xy = 5$ at $(1, \frac{5}{2})$
34. $y^2 - 3x^2 = 1$ at $(-1, 2)$
35. $x^2 - y^2 = 2$ at $(2, \sqrt{2})$
36. $(\sqrt{x} + 1)(\sqrt{y} + 1) = 8$ at $(1, 4)$

Related Rates

37. Particle Moving on a Curve. A particle p is moving along the curve $x^2 = 4y$. Remember that

$$\frac{dx}{dt} = \text{Velocity of the particle in the } x\text{-direction}$$

$$\frac{dy}{dt} = \text{Velocity of the particle in the } y\text{-direction}$$

What is the velocity of the particle in the y-direction when the particle is located at the point $(4, 4)$ and the velocity in the x-direction is 2 units per second?

38. Growing Square. The sides of a square are growing at the rate of 2 ft/min. How fast is the area of the square growing when $x = 3$?

39. Soda Problem. Emma is drinking a soda through a straw. She is drinking at a constant rate of 1 cubic inch per second. If the radius of the can is 1 inch, how fast is the level of soda going down?

40. Price Fluctuations. A certain commodity is priced (in dollars) at the opening of the market each day at

$$p(x) = 5 + \frac{50}{x}$$

where x is the amount (measured in hundreds of pounds) of the commodity available on a given dav. At what rate will the price be changing when there are 75 hundred pounds available and the amount of the commodity is decreasing at a rate of 500 pounds per day?

41. Oil Spill. Hurricane winds have damaged an oil rig and caused a circular oil slick 2 inches thick. Suppose the radius of the slick is currently 100 feet and growing at the rate of 0.5 ft/min. What is the rate at which the oil is spilling? *Hint:* The volume of the oil slick is $V = \pi r^2 h$, where r is the radius and h is the height (or thickness) of the oil slick.

42. Water Waves. Sally throws a rock onto the surface of a lake. A circular pattern of ripples is formed. If the radius of the outermost circle increases at the rate of 10 inches/second, how fast is the area within the outer circle changing after 9 seconds?

43. The Street Lamp Problem. A street light 21 feet off the ground casts a shadow of a pedestrian 6 feet tall who is walking away from the light at a rate of 3 ft/sec. (See Figure 54.) How fast is the shadow lengthening when the pedestrian is 25 feet from the light? How fast is the tip of the shadow moving?

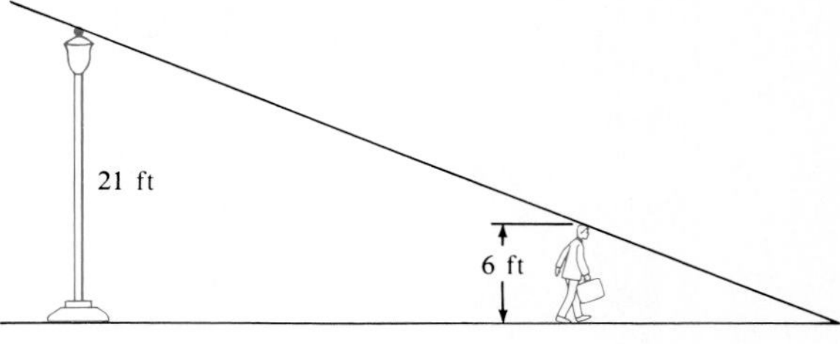

Figure 54
Diagram for Problem 43

2.6 Differentials

PURPOSE

We introduce the concept of the differentials dy and dx. We will show that while a functional relationship relates the size of x to the size of y, the differential relationship shows how a small change in x will give rise to a small change in y.

Introduction

The symbol dy/dx is a bit confusing, since it represents a derivative and not the quotient of two quantities dy and dx. The reason for the dy/dx notation is mostly historical and due to Leibniz. He imagined the derivative dy/dx as the ratio of two infinitely small quantities dy and dx. Nowadays, we interpret dy/dx not as a quotient, but as the limiting value of the quotient

$$\frac{dy}{dx} = \lim_{h \to 0} \frac{f(x+h) - f(x)}{h}$$

It is possible, however, to assign meanings to the quantities dy and dx. We now show how dy and dx can be interpreted in their own right.

Differential Approximation

Consider the function defined by the graph $y = f(x)$ as shown in Figure 55. Pick a point x_0. Let x_0 change by a small amount dx from x_0 to a new value, $x_0 + dx$. The value of $f(x_0)$ will change from the initial value to the new value $f(x_0 + dx)$. The difference between these values is the change f in the function. That is

$$\Delta f = f(x_0 + dx) - f(x_0)$$

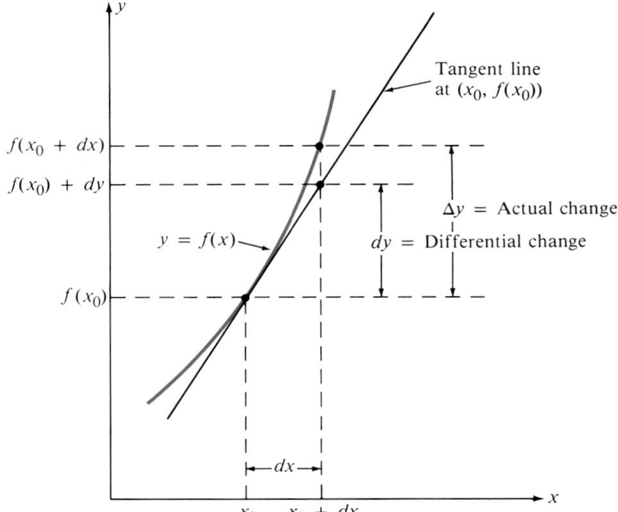

Figure 55
Illustration of the differential $dy = f'(x_0)\,dx$

Now consider the tangent line to the curve $y = f(x)$ at the point $(x_0, f(x_0))$. As we have seen before, the equation of the tangent line is

$$y = f(x_0) + f'(x_0)(x - x_0)$$

Since the tangent line remains close to the graph $y = f(x)$ for values of x close to x_0, the change in y along the tangent line will be approximately the same as the change in y along the graph $y = f(x)$. We see in Figure 55 that as x changes from x_0 to $x_0 + dx$, the change in y along the tangent line will be

$$dy = f'(x_0)\,dx$$

This change is called the **differential change** (or *approximate change*) in $y = f(x)$. When the change dx in x is small, dy approximates the real change in $f(x)$.

Definition of the Differentials *dx* and *dy*

Let $y = f(x)$ have a derivative at the point x_0. The differential change in x, denoted by dx, is simply any change in x (generally taken to be small).

The differential change in y, denoted by dy, which results from a differential change dx from x_0 to $x_0 + dx$, is given by

$$dy = f'(x_0)\,dx$$

Example 1 Differential Change If

$$y = f(x) = x^2$$

find the differential change in y when x changes from 1 to 1.1.

Solution Here we have

$$x_0 = 1 \qquad \text{(starting point)}$$
$$dx = 0.1 \qquad \text{(change in } x\text{)}$$

We first find the derivative

$$f'(x) = 2x$$

The differential dy is found by multiplying the derivative evaluated at $x_0 = 1$ times the differential dx. In other words,

$$\begin{aligned} dy &= f'(x_0)\,dx \\ &= 2x_0\,dx \\ &= 2(1)(0.1) \\ &= 0.2 \end{aligned}$$

The geometric interpretation of the differential dy can be seen in Figure 56. □

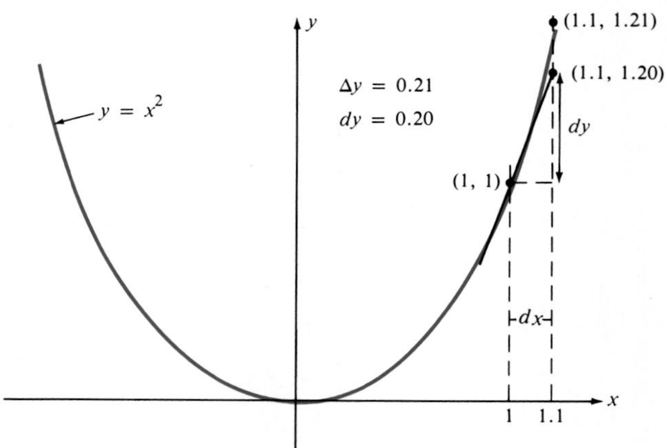

Figure 56
Differential when $x_0 = 1$ and $dx = 0.1$

Reason for an Interest in Differentials

Differentials approximate the exact change in the dependent variable y as a result of a change in the independent variable x. There are a number of reasons why we are satisfied with this approximate change

$$dy = f(x_0)\,dx$$

in contrast to the real change

$$\Delta y = f(x_0 + dx) - f(x_0)$$

The major reason is that it is often impossible to compute the real change, owing to the fact that we cannot evaluate the function at the point $x_0 + dx$. The differential approximation dy uses information only at the point x_0. Also, the differential change dy is generally easier to compute than the real change y, and it is often a good enough approximation for the purpose at hand.

Extrapolation by Differentials

Often, the value of a function and its derivative are known at a point x_0, and from this information we would like to approximate the value of the function at some nearby point $x_0 + dx$. If we draw the tangent line to the graph at $(x_0, f(x_0))$, it is possible to approximate the value $f(x_0 + dx)$ by following along the tangent line, getting the differential approximation

$$\begin{aligned} f(x_0 + dx) &\cong f(x_0) + dy \\ &= f(x_0) + f'(x_0)\,dx \end{aligned}$$

See Figure 57.

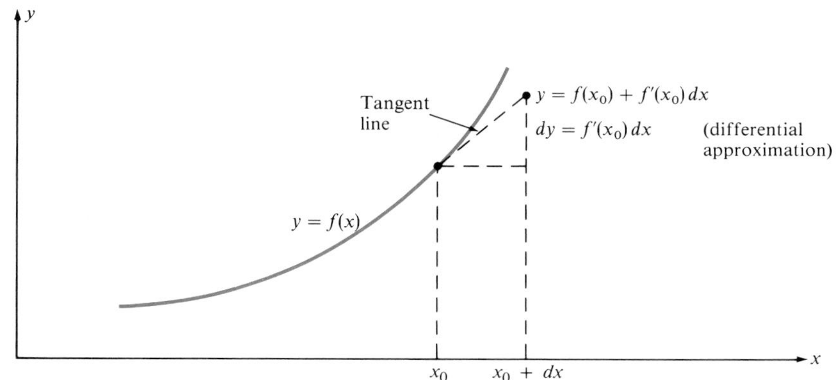

Figure 57
Differential extrapolation is linear extrapolation

Differential Approximation to Extrapolate the World Mile Record

Table 11 lists the previous eight world records in the men's mile run (prior to 1989). These points are plotted in Figure 58.

Statisticians have ways of finding curves that best approximate data points. A quadratic polynomial was found that approximates the data points shown in Table 11. It is given by

$$R(t) = 0.01t^2 - 0.49t + 230.5$$

TABLE 11
World Records in Men's Mile Run, 1975–1985

Runner	Country	Time	Year
Filbert Bayi	Tanzania	3:51.0	1975
John Walker	New Zealand	3:49.4	1975
Sebastian Coe	England	3:49.0	1979
Steve Ovett	England	3:48.8	1980
Sebastian Coe	England	3:48.53	1981
Steve Ovett	England	3:48.40	1981
Sebastian Coe	England	3:47.33	1981
Steve Cram	England	3:46.31	1985

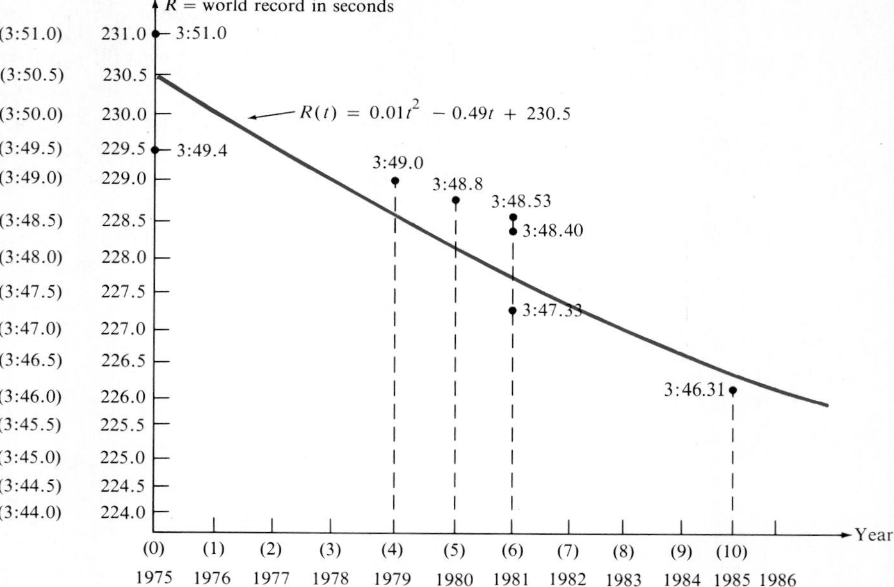

Figure 58
World record times in men's mile run, 1975–1985

In this equation, $R(t)$ is the mile record (in seconds), and t is the year the record was made ($t = 0$ stands for 1975, $t = 1$ stands for 1976, . . . , $t = 10$ stands for 1985). This approximating curve is also drawn in Figure 58. We now differentiate the fitted curve $R(t)$, getting

$$R'(t) = 0.02t - 0.49$$

The value of this derivative at $t = 10$ (which corresponds to 1985) is

$$\begin{aligned} R'(10) &= (0.02)(10) - 0.49 \\ &= -0.29 \end{aligned}$$

To extrapolate the graph $R(t)$ from the year 1985 to the years 1986, 1987, 1988, 1989, and 1990, we compute the different values

$$R(10) + R'(10)\,dt$$

for $dt = 1, 2, 3, 4$, and 5. These values are given in Table 12. You can check the accuracy of these differential approximations by comparing new world records that have occurred since Steve Cram's 1985 record run.

TABLE 12
Differential Extrapolation of World Mile Records

dt	Year	Differential dR $dR = R'(10)\,dt$	Estimated World Mile Record $R(t) = R(10) + dR$
1	1986	$(-0.29)(1) = -0.29$	$226.60 - 0.29 = 226.31$ (3:46.31)
2	1987	$(-0.29)(2) = -0.58$	$226.60 - 0.58 = 226.02$ (3:46.02)
3	1988	$(-0.29)(3) = -0.87$	$226.60 - 0.87 = 225.73$ (3:45.73)
4	1989	$(-0.29)(4) = -1.16$	$226.60 - 1.16 = 225.44$ (3:45.44)
5	1990	$(-0.29)(5) = -1.45$	$226.60 - 1.45 = 225.15$ (3:45.15)

Differentials Used in Error Analysis

Differentials are often used in studying the propagation of errors. For example, suppose that x is a variable that we measure and that y is a variable that is computed by means of a formula

$$y = f(x)$$

If there is an error in the measurement of x, this error will give rise to an error in y. It is important to know how errors in the measured value of x will give rise to errors in y.

To determine these relationships, we introduce some of the language of error analysis. If the **true value** of some quantity is x, but the value determined by some experiment is $x + dx$, then the **error** in the measurement is dx, and the **relative error** in the measurement is

$$\text{Relative error} = \frac{dx}{x}$$

If we multiply the relative error times 100, we get the **percentage error**:

$$\text{Percentage error} = 100\frac{dx}{x}\%$$

Example 2

Relative Error Suppose you approximate the length of the line in Figure 59 using a ruler, and suppose your estimate is 4.06 inches. Suppose that the real length of the line is exactly 4 inches. What are the absolute error, relative error, and percentage error in your measurement?

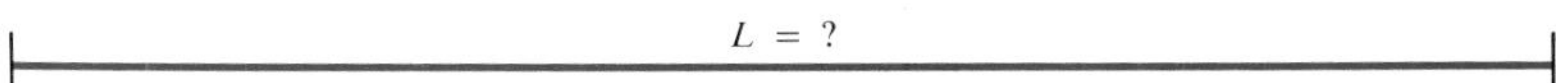

Figure 59
A straight line of unknown length

Solution The error (or absolute error) is simply the difference between the measurement and the real value. Although you can never really determine this value in practice (since you never know the exact real value), in this case it is

$$\text{Absolute error} = 0.06 \text{ inch}$$

The absolute error is always taken to be a positive number. The relative error is the absolute error divided by the real value. In this case it is

$$\text{Relative error} = \frac{0.06}{4} = 0.015$$

If we multiply this quantity times 100, we get the percentage error:

$$\text{Percentage error} = 100(0.015)\% = 1.5\%$$ □

Comment on Relative Error

The relative error is a much more useful measure of the accuracy of a measurement than the absolute error. Someone may tell you that the absolute error in a measurement is 5 pounds but unless you know the size of the measurement, this value is almost meaningless. After all, an error of 5 pounds could be the error in weighing a child or an elephant. If an elephant were being weighed, an error of 5 pounds would not be as startling as an error of 5 pounds in weighing a child.

Example 3

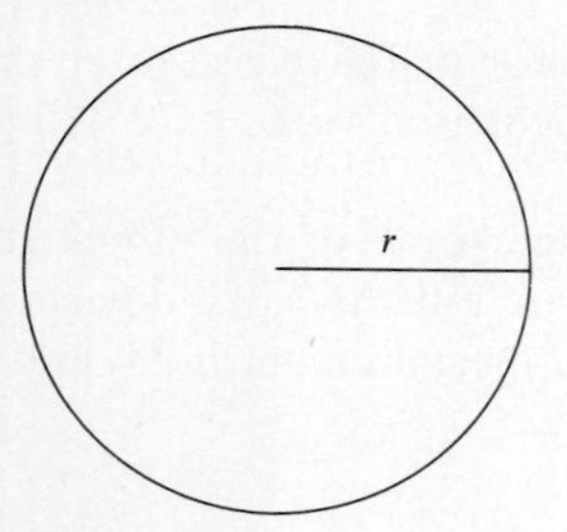

Figure 60
Can you find the area of this circle by measuring the radius?

Propagation of Errors Suppose you approximate the area A of the circle in Figure 60 by estimating the radius r using a ruler and then using the formula $A = \pi r^2$. Suppose you know that your measurement of the radius has an error of less than 0.02 inch. What is the relative error in your estimate in the area?

Solution

- **Step 1** (find the algebraic relationship between the variables). The algebraic relationship between the area of a circle A and its radius r is given by

$$A = \pi r^2$$

- **Step 2** (find the differential relationship between the variables). Finding the derivative of A with respect to r, we compute the differential dA to be

$$\begin{aligned} dA &= \frac{dA}{dr}\,dr \\ &= (2\pi r)\,dr \end{aligned}$$

- **Step 3** (find dA/A in terms of dr/r). Since the goal is to find the relative error dA/A in the area, we divide each side of the above equation by A, getting

$$\frac{dA}{A} = \frac{2\pi r}{A}\,dr$$

Substituting the expression $A = \pi r^2$ for the value of A in the right-hand side of the above equation and rewriting the equation algebraically so that the relative error dr/r appears on the right, we finally have

$$\begin{aligned} \frac{dA}{A} &= \frac{2\pi r}{\pi r^2}\,dr \\ &= 2\,\frac{dr}{r} \\ &= 2(0.02) \\ &= 0.04 \end{aligned}$$

□

Conclusion

If the radius of the circle can be measured with a relative error dr/r less than 0.02, then the area of the circle will have a relative error dA/A less than 0.04. In fact, from the above formula for the relative error dA/A we have the general result that the relative error in the area of the circle is always exactly twice the relative error in the radius.

Example 4

Differentials in Business Suppose you are the sales manager for a business firm and have estimated sales for the coming month to be 2500 items and suppose you are sure that this value is accurate with a maximum percentage error of 2%. If the profit $P(q)$ in dollars from selling q items is given by

$$P(q) = 20q - 0.0003q^2$$

what is the maximum percentage error in your estimation of the monthly profit of

$$\begin{aligned} P(2500) &= 20(2500) - 0.0003(2500)^2 \\ &= \$48,125 \end{aligned}$$

Solution To answer this question, we must find the equation that relates the unknown percentage error of P (which is $100\ dP/P$) to the known percentage error in q (which is $100\ dq/q$). We begin by finding the derivative:

$$\frac{d}{dq} P(q) = 20 - 0.0006q$$

Hence the differential of P is

$$\begin{aligned} dP &= P'(q)\, dq \\ &= (20 - 0.0006q)\, dq \end{aligned}$$

To get $100\, dP/P$ on the left-hand side of the above equation and $100\, dq/q$ on the right-hand side of the equation, we carry out the following steps:

- **Step 1.** Start with

$$dP = (20 - 0.0006q)\, dq$$

- **Step 2.** Divide by P:

$$\frac{dP}{P} = \frac{(20 - 0.0006q)}{P}\, dq$$

- **Step 3.** Multiply and divide the right-hand side by q:

$$\frac{dP}{P} = \frac{(20 - 0.0006q)q}{P} \frac{dq}{q}$$

- **Step 4.** Multiply each side by 100:

$$100 \frac{dP}{P} = \frac{(20 - 0.0006q)q}{P} \left(100 \frac{dq}{q}\right)$$

We now substitute the known values

$$q = 2500$$

$$P(2500) = 48,125$$

$$100 \frac{dq}{q} = 2\%$$

into the right-hand side of the above equation. This gives the percentage error in the cost

$$\begin{aligned} 100 \frac{dP}{P} &= \frac{[20 - 0.0006(2500)](2500)}{48,125} (2) \\ &= 1.9\% \end{aligned}$$

The maximum percentage error in the estimated profit is 1.9%. This means that the real profit will be within 1.9% of the predicted value of $48,125 or between the values of

$$\$48{,}125 - (0.019)(\$48{,}125) = \$47{,}210.62$$

and

$$\$48{,}125 + (0.019)(\$48{,}125) = \$49{,}039.37$$

□

Problems

For Problems 1–10, determine the value of dy at the indicated point x_0 and for the differential in x, dx.

1. $f(x) = 2$, $x_0 = 0, dx = 0.1$
2. $f(x) = 2x + 1$, $x_0 = 2, dx = 0.1$
3. $f(x) = x^2$, $x_0 = 1, dx = 0.01$
4. $f(x) = x^2 + x$, $x_0 = 3, dx = 0.1$
5. $f(x) = 1/x$, $x_0 = 1, dx = 0.1$
6. $f(x) = 1/x^2$, $x_0 = 1, dx = 0.1$
7. $f(x) = 3x^3 - 9x^2 + 5$, $x_0 = 1, dx = 0.01$
8. $f(x) = (2x^2 + x)(x^3 - 2)$, $x_0 = 2, dx = -0.01$
9. $f(x) = \dfrac{x - 1}{x + 2}$, $x_0 = 0, dx = 0.05$
10. $f(x) = \dfrac{1}{x^2 - 2}$, $x_0 = 1, dx = 0.001$

For Problems 11–13, a company had estimated that the next year's net income would be 15 million dollars. Suppose the real net income turned out to be 15.3 million dollars. Determine the following quantities.

11. The absolute error.
12. The relative error.
13. The percentage error.

14. Comparison of Errors. A biologist determines the weight of a rat to be 1 pound. The biologist then determines the weight of an elephant to be 7000 pounds. Suppose the rat actually weighs 1.1 pounds, and the elephant actually weighs 7500 pounds. Determine the following.
(a) Which measurement had the smaller absolute error?
(b) Which measurement had the smaller relative error?
(c) Which measurement had the smaller percentage error?

For Problems 15–19, determine the following errors.

15. Error in the Area of a Square. Find the relative error in the area of a square if the relative error in measuring the side is 2%.

16. Error in the Volume of a Sphere. Find the relative error in the volume of a sphere if the relative error in measuring the radius is 3%.

17. Error in the Volume of a Cube. Find the relative error in the volume of a cube if the relative error in measuring a side is 1%.

18. Error in the Volume of a Cylinder. Find the relative error in the volume of a cylinder with radius equal to one-half the height if the relative error in measuring the radius is 4%.

19. Error in the Surface Area of a Cube. Find the relative error in the surface area of a cube if the relative error in measuring the side is 3%.

Using Differentials to Extrapolate

For Problems 20–26, the value of a function and its derivative are given at a point. Use this information and the differential to extrapolate the value of the function at the indicated point.

20. Given $f(3) = 2$ $f'(3) = 1$, approximate $f(3.1)$.
21. Given $f(2) = 1.3$ $f'(2) = -0.2$, approximate $f(2.05)$.
22. Given $f(10) = 2.4$ $f'(10) = 0.5$, approximate $f(10.3)$.
23. Given $f(-1) = 0$ $f'(-1) = 0$, approximate $f(-0.8)$.
24. Given $f(0) = 35.4$ $f'(0) = 0.25$, approximate $f(0.01)$.
25. Given $f(50) = 2500$ $f'(50) = 0.35$, approximate $f(52)$.
26. Given $f(50) = 2500$ $f'(50) = 0.35$, approximate $f(54)$.

For Problems 27–30, extrapolate the functions at the indicated points, using the differential.

27.

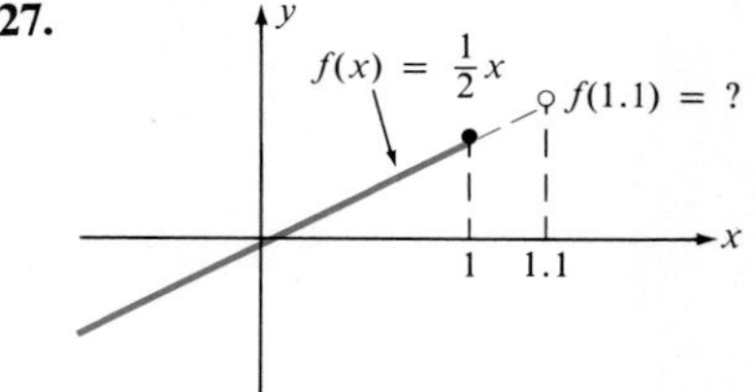

28.

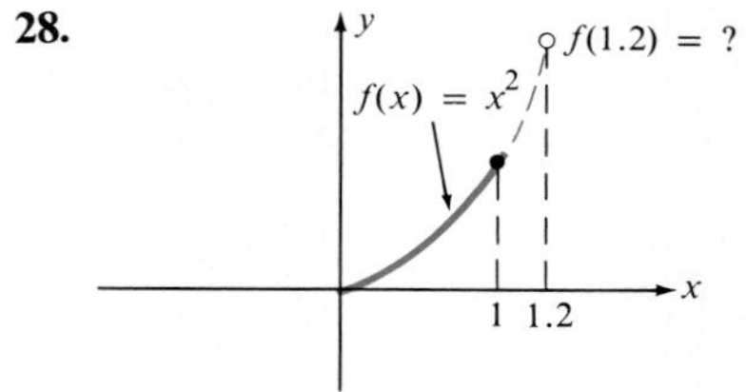

29.

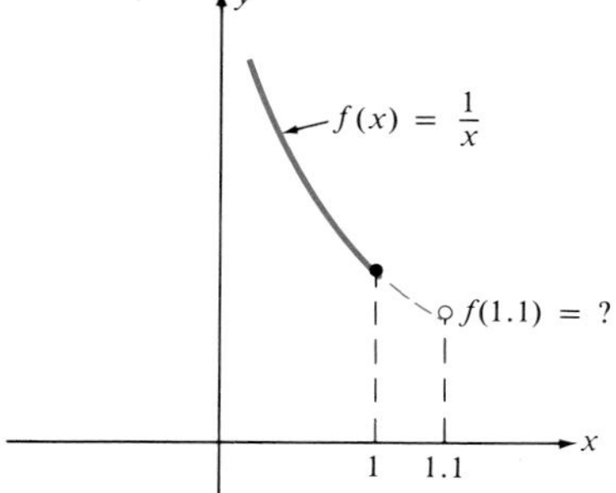

30.

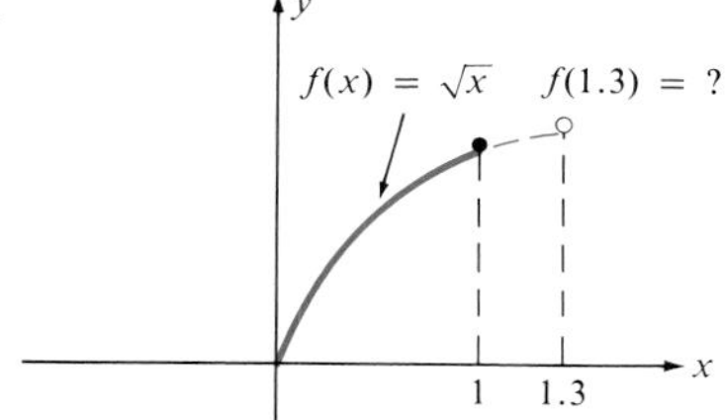

Differentials in Business

31. **Relative Error in the Profit.** The monthly profit of a firm when it produces q items per month is given by

$$P(q) = 3q - 0.001q^2$$

Sales estimates are 1000 items for the coming month with a maximum relative error of 0.02. What is the estimated profit for the next month? What is the relative error in this estimate?

32. **Percentage Error in the Profit.** The monthly profit of a firm when it produces q items per month is given by

$$P(q) = 20q - 0.0005q^3$$

Sales estimates for the coming month are 3000 with a percentage error of 5%. What is the percentage error in the profits?

33. **Relative Error in Revenue.** The monthly revenue $R(q)$ of a firm is given by the formula

$$R(q) = 25q - 0.001q^2$$

where q is the number of items sold during the month. The firm estimates that sales during the coming month will be 5000 items and that this estimate has a maximum relative error of 0.01. What is the estimated revenue for the coming month? What is the relative error in this estimate?

34. **Percentage Error in Revenue.** The monthly revenue $R(q)$ of a firm is given by the formula

$$R(q) = 50q - 0.001q^2$$

where q is the number of items sold during the month. The firm estimates that sales during the coming month will be 3000 items and that this estimate will have a maximum error of 250 items. What is the estimated revenue for the coming month? What is the percentage error in this estimate?

Differentials in Science

35. **Light Intensity.** The intensity of light entering the iris of the eye is given by the function

$$I = cr^2$$

where r is the radius of the pupil and c is a constant depending on the eye. How much does a small change in the radius of the opening of the eye affect the intensity of light entering the iris?

36. **Determination of g.** The acceleration g of an object due to gravity is sometimes determined by measuring the period of the swing of a pendulum. If the length of the pendulum is L and the measured period is T, then g is given by the formula

$$g = \frac{4\pi^2 L}{T^2}$$

Find the relative error in g if
(a) L is measured accurately, but T has an error of 5%.
(b) T is measured accurately, but L has an error of 1%.

37. **Error in Cardiac Output.** A common way to measure cardiac output F (the number of cubic centimeters per minute of blood pumped by the heart) is by using *Fick's formula*:

$$F = \frac{k_1}{x - k_2}$$

The values k_1 and k_2 are constants, and x is the concentration of carbon dioxide in the blood entering the lung. Suppose the measurement of x has a maximum error of 2%. What is the percentage error in the cardiac output?

38. **Thurstone's Learning Curve.** The brilliant psychologist, L. L. Thurstone spent almost all of his professional life developing psychology as a quantitative science. In his Ph.D. thesis (1916), he developed the equation

$$L(x) = \frac{x}{a + bx} \qquad (x \geq 0)$$

$(a \geq 0, b \geq 0)$ as a model to describe the level of attainment L of a given skill (learning to read, shoot a basketball, solve mathematics problems, etc.) in terms of the amount of practice x. Use the first and second derivatives to describe the nature of the graph of this learning curve.

Epilogue: The Stairs Paradox

John is building stairs in a new home connecting a point A on the lower level with a point B on the upper level. (See Figure 61a.) John would like to cover the stairs with one long carpet and would like the total length of the carpet to be as small as possible. Since the carpet is very expensive, the question is: How many steps should he include in the stairs to minimize the total length of the carpet? To answer this question, John first tries a design with only two huge stairs as drawn in Figure 61b). After some thought, however, he decides to double the number of steps to four. (See Figure 61c.) He then thinks that if he keeps doubling the number of steps, the total length of the carpet will get smaller and smaller.

Unfortunately, John has a mathematician friend who tells him that the total length of the carpet is 2 units no matter how many steps he uses. The mathematician also tells John that the various stair designs drawn in Figure 61 illustrate an interesting phenomenon. The mathematician says that there are many things about graphs and curves that we often take for granted but that are not necessarily true. In the case of the stair-steps, we have a series of curves connecting A and B. Calling these curves

$$C_1, C_2, C_3, \ldots, C_n, \ldots$$

we can see that the length of each of these curves is

$$\text{Length } C_1 = \frac{1}{2} + \frac{1}{2} + \frac{1}{2} + \frac{1}{2} = 2$$

$$\text{Length } C_2 = \frac{1}{4} + \frac{1}{4} + \cdots + \frac{1}{4} = 2$$

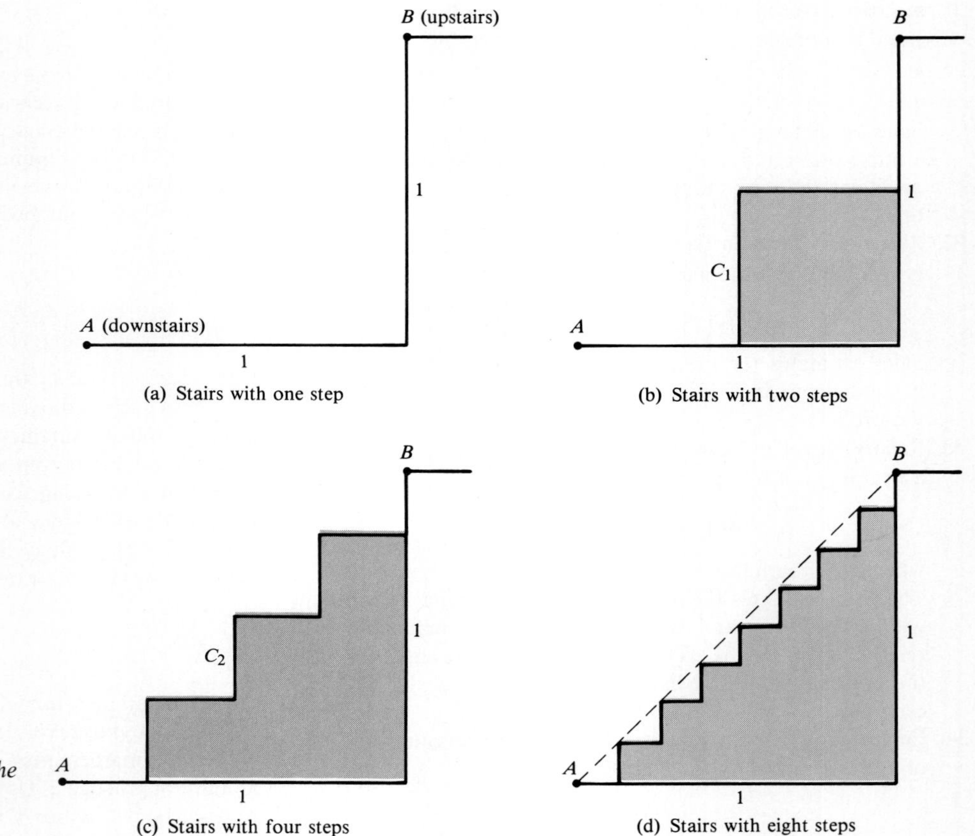

Figure 61

How does the actual length of the stairs change as the number of steps increases?

$$\text{Length } C_3 = \frac{1}{8} + \frac{1}{8} + \cdots + \frac{1}{8} = 2$$

$$\vdots$$

$$\text{Length } C_n = \frac{1}{2^n} + \frac{1}{2^n} + \cdots + \frac{1}{2^n} = 2$$

What is interesting about these curves is that although each of them has a length of 2, they are getting "closer and closer" to the straight line connecting A and B, which has a length of $\sqrt{2} = 1.414\ldots$. In other words, contrary to your intuition, it can happen that two curves are close together but their lengths are not at all close together.

In fact, the mathematician says that if John were really clever, he could construct a series of stairsteps that would get "closer and closer" to the straight line connecting A and B but the lengths of the stairsteps would grow larger and larger without bound.

Purpose of This Epilogue

You might wonder why we included this epilogue. It is kind of clever, but it doesn't have much to do with business management or science. Well, yes and no. A major reason for studying mathematics is not to learn specific facts but to think about and analyze concepts. If you were to spend all your time simply learning facts, your knowledge would quickly become obsolete in a changing world. The modern world needs people who are not afraid to think, and the stairs problem makes you do just that. The stairs problem can be thought of as a series of jagged curves converging to a straight line, yet the lengths of the curves do not converge to the length of the straight line. (Hmmmmm.)

Key Ideas for Review

asymptotes, 165
concavity, 160
critical points, 151
decreasing function, 148
first derivative test, 177
higher derivatives, 158
implicit differentiation, 206
increasing function, 148
inflection points, 161
maximum of a function
  absolute, 182
  relative, 176
minimum of a function
  absolute, 182
  relative, 176
optimization problems, 193
related rates, 212
second derivative test, 180
stationary points, 151

Review Exercises

For Problems 1–10, locate the critical points of the given function. Determine which critical points are relative maximum or relative minimum points using the first derivative test.

1. $f(x) = x^3 - 2x^2 - 4x + 3$
2. $f(x) = x^{2/3}$
3. $f(x) = \dfrac{x}{x^2 + 2}$
4. $f(x) = \dfrac{5x - 6}{3x + 11}$
5. $f(x) = x^2 - x$
6. $f(x) = (x + 1)^3$
7. $f(x) = x^3 - 6x^2 + 9x$
8. $f(x) = x^2 + \dfrac{2}{x}$
9. $f(x) = \dfrac{2x}{x^2 + 4}$
10. $f(x) = 5 + 2(x - 1)^{2/3}$

For Problems 11–20, use the second derivative test to determine whether any of the critical points of the functions are relative minimum or relative maximum points. If the second derivative test does not apply, indicate that nothing is learned.

11. $f(x) = x^3 - 3x^2 - 9x + 5$
12. $f(x) = 3x^4 - 4x^3 - 15$
13. $f(x) = (x - 1)^3$
14. $f(x) = (x - 1)^4$
15. $f(x) = x^{12/5}$
16. $f(x) = 3x^4 - 4x^3$
17. $f(x) = x^3 + 3x - 2$
18. $f(x) = -2x^3 + 3x^2 + 12 + 2$
19. $f(x) = \dfrac{2x}{x^2 + 4}$
20. $f(x) = -\dfrac{4}{3}x^3 - 2x^2 + 3x$

For Problems 21–29, determine both the absolute maximum and the absolute minimum of each function on the indicated interval.

21. $f(x) = 2x^3 - 15x^2 + 12$ on $[-1, 3]$
22. $f(x) = x^4 - 8x^3 + 22x^2 - 24x + 7$ on $[-4, 4]$
23. $f(x) = (x - 2)^4$ on $[0, 4]$
24. $f(x) = (x - 2)^3$ on $[2, 3]$
25. $f(x) = 2x^3 - 15x^2 + 36x$ on $[0, 1]$
26. $f(x) = x$ on $[0, 1]$
27. $f(x) = \sqrt{x - 1}$ on $[1, 4]$
28. $f(x) = \sqrt[3]{x - 1}$ on $[1, 4]$
29. $f(x) = \sqrt{x}$ on $[0, 1]$

Implicit Differentiation

For Problems 30–36, find dy/dx using implicit differentiation.

30. $x^2 + y^2 + 1 = 0$
31. $x^2 + y^2 = 16$
32. $x^3 - y^3 = 1$
33. $x^2y = 1$
34. $x + y = 1$
35. $y - x = 0$
36. $\sqrt{x} + \sqrt{y} = 1$

Differentiation Approximation

For Problems 37–43, use differentials to approximate the given values.

37. $\sqrt{99}$
38. $\sqrt{101}$
39. $\sqrt[3]{1001}$
40. $(0.99)^5$
41. $(1.001)^9$
42. $\dfrac{1}{100.4}$
43. $\dfrac{1}{99.9}$

Applications

44. Related Rates. Let A be the area of a square whose sides have length x. Assume that x changes with time t. How are dA/dt and dx/dt related?

45. Related Rates. Let A be the area of a circle with radius r. Assume that r changes with time t. How are dA/dt and dr/dt related?

46. Ladder Problem Revisited. A 16-foot ladder is leaning against a house. If the bottom of the ladder is being pulled away from the house at a rate of 10 ft/sec, how fast is the top of the ladder coming down when the bottom of the ladder is 5 feet from the house?

47. Street Lamp Problem Revisited. A man who is 6 feet tall is walking at the rate of 4 ft/sec toward a street light that is 20 feet tall. At what rate is the size of his shadow changing?

48. Balloon Tracking Problem. A weather balloon is rising vertically at a rate of 5 ft/sec. An observer is situated 100 feet from a point on the ground directly beneath the balloon. At what rate is the distance between the balloon and the observer changing when the height of the balloon is 300 feet?

49. Maximum Profit. Find the maximum profit and the number of units that should be produced and sold to yield the maximum profit if the revenue and cost from the production of q units of the item are

$$R(q) = 1.5q^2 + 150q + 60 \quad \text{(revenue)}$$
$$C(q) = 1.6q^2 + 60q + 100 \quad \text{(cost)}$$

50. Harry's Problem. Harry is walking at the rate of 5 mph toward the base of a building that is 60 feet high. At what rate is Harry approaching the top of the building when he is 80 feet from the building

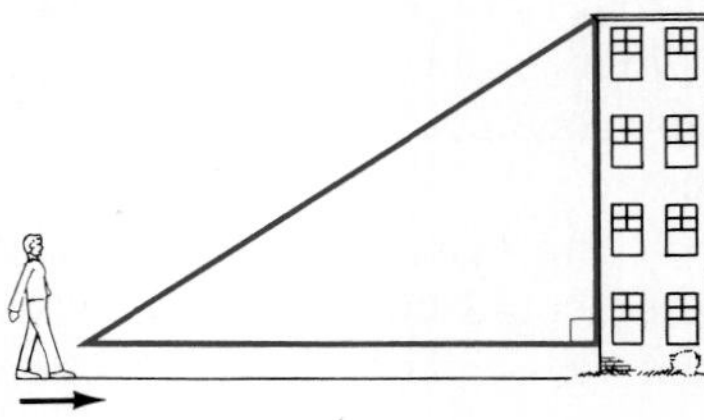

Figure 62
How fast is Harry approaching the top of the building?

51. Moving on a Parabola. A point moves along the parabola

$$y = \frac{1}{6}x^2$$

in such a way that when $x = 6$, the value of x is increasing at a rate of 2 ft/sec. At what rate is the value of y increasing at that instant?

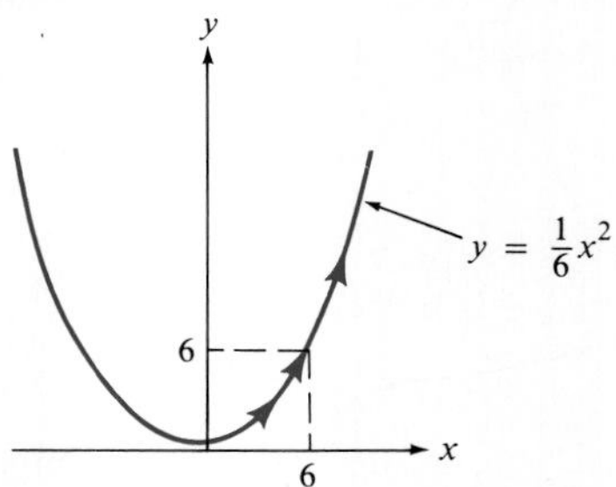

Figure 63
How fast is y changing?

52. More Hot Air. Air is leaking from a spherical balloon at a rate of 1000 in.^{3}/min. At the instant when the radius r is 10 inches, at what rate is the surface S of the sphere decreasing? *Hint:* $S = 4\pi r^2$.

53. Interesting Formula. The surface area S and volume V of a sphere are given in terms of the radius r by the formulas

$$S = 4\pi r^2$$

$$V = \frac{4}{3}\pi r^3$$

Prove and interpret the relation

$$\frac{dV}{dt} = \frac{r}{2}\frac{dS}{dt}$$

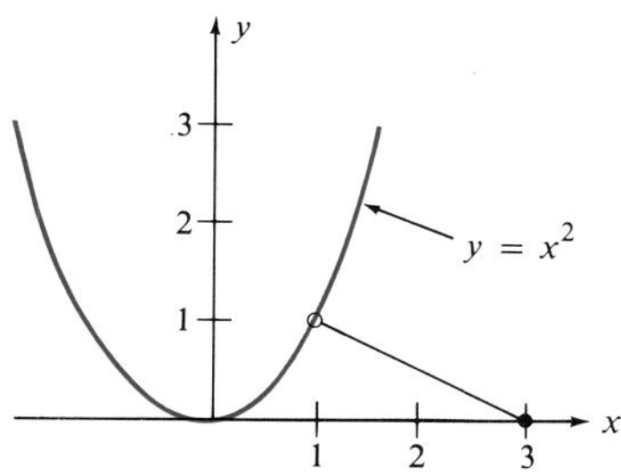

Figure 64
What point on the curve $y = x^2$ is closest to $(3, 0)$?

54. Interesting Distance Problem. Find the point on the graph of

$$y = x^2$$

that is nearest to the point (3, 0).

55. More Apples. An apple orchard now has 30 trees per acre, and the average yield is 400 apples per tree. For each additional tree planted per acre, the average yield per tree is reduced by 10 apples. How many trees per acre will give the largest yield?

56. Marginal Cost. The Express Delivery Co. is planning to add new routes. The added cost of the next expansion phase is given by

$$C(x) = 2x^3 + x^2 - 4x$$

where x is the number of deliveries on the routes added. When is the marginal cost increasing on the interval $[1, 50]$?

57. Inflection Points of a Cubic Equation. Find the inflection point(s) of a function of the form

$$f(x) = ax^3 + bx^2 + cx + d$$

where a, b, c, and d are constants with a different from zero.

58. Error in the Area of a Square. Use differentials to find the approximate relative error in the area of a square. The sides of the square have been measured and found to be 10 inches, with a maximum relative error of 0.05.

59. Error in the Volume of a Cube. Use differentials to find the approximate relative error in the volume of a cube. The sides of the cube have been measured and found to be 10 inches, with a maximum relative error of 0.10.

60. Box Problem Revisited. An open box with a rectangular base is to be constructed from a rectangular piece of cardboard that is 16 inches wide and 25 inches long by cutting out a square from each corner and turning up the sides. Determine the box that will have the largest volume.

61. Number Theory. Find two integers whose difference is 10 and whose product is a minimum.

62. Number Theory. Find two integers whose sum is 10 and whose product is a maximum.

Chapter Test

Problems 1–7 are concerned with the function

$$f(x) = 5x^2 - 5x + 7$$

1. Where is the function increasing and where is it decreasing?

2. What are the critical points?

3. What are the stationary points?

4. What are the relative maximum and the relative minimum points?

5. What are the inflection points?

6. Where is the function concave up and where is it concave down?

7. What is the absolute maximum of this function in the interval $[0, 5]$?

8. Use implicit differentiation to find dy/dx if

$$xy + \sqrt{y} = 1$$

9. If

$$y = x^3$$

and x changes with time t, what is the relationship between dy/dt and dx/dt?

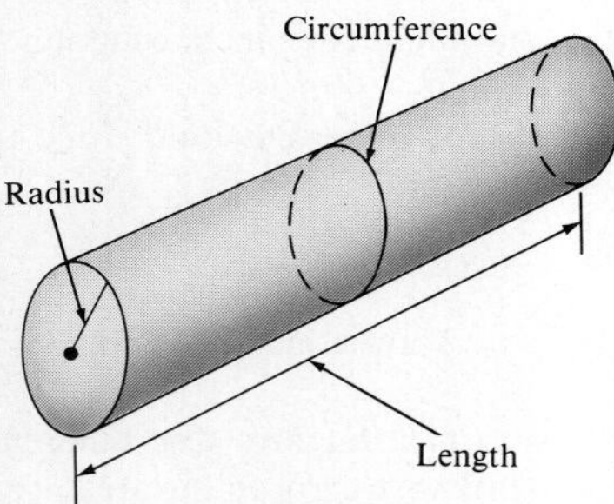

Figure 65
The sum of the length and the circumference of this cylindrical container must not exceed 84 inches

10. What are the two positive real numbers whose sum is 100 that have the largest product?

11. If the sides of a square are measured and found to be 10 inches with a maximum error of 0.05 inch, approximate the relative error in the area of the square.

12. **Hmmmmm.** Peter is sending candy to his girlfriend and is packaging it in a cylindrical container. The U.S. Postal Service requires the length plus circumference of all cylindrical containers to be no more than 84 inches. (See Figure 65.) What are the dimensions of the package (radius and circumference) that will contain the most candy, and how many cubic inches of candy will this cylinder contain?

13. **Yellow Fever Problem.** It is well known that yellow fever is carried by mosquitoes. Suppose a mathematical equation that relates the number N of reported cases of yellow fever to the number of mosquitoes M is given by

$$N = 0.005M^{3/4}$$

If a program is begun that destroys the mosquitoes at a rate of 500,000 per day, then at what rate is the number of reported cases of yellow fever changing when the size of the mosquito population is 10,000,000?

The growth of many phenomena, such as that of a plant or animal, may over a period of time be described by an exponential function. The logarithm function is another useful analytical tool used in the natural and life sciences.

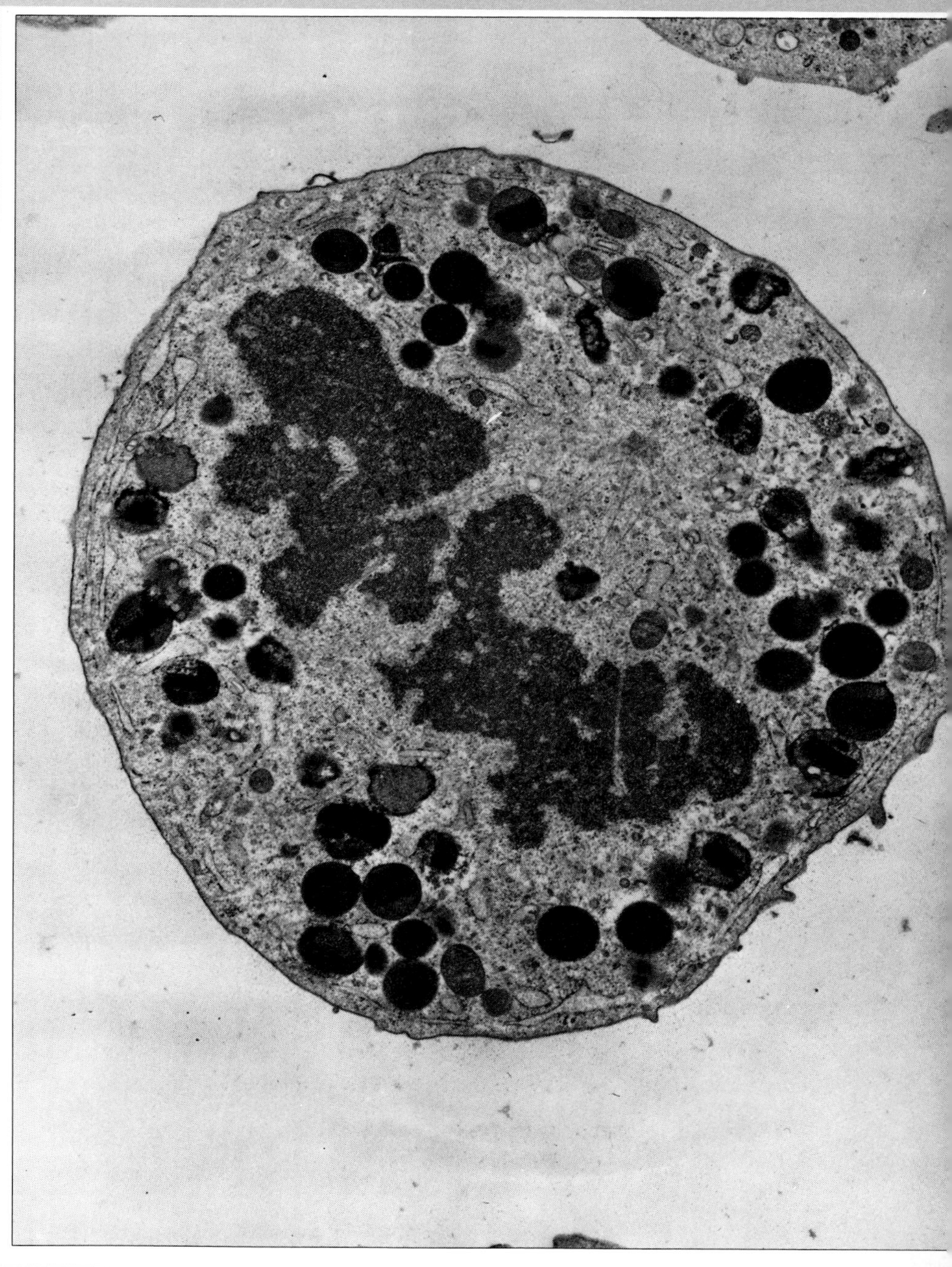

3

Exponential and Logarithmic Functions

In the preceding chapters we saw how polynomials can be used to describe many physical phenomena. However, many natural processes, such as the growth and decay of biological populations, are best described by exponential functions. Also, there are natural phenomena such as earthquake measurements that are best described by logarithmic types of functions. In this chapter we examine these two important types of functions and show how their derivatives can be used to solve a variety of important problems.

3.1 Exponential Growth and Decay

PURPOSE

We introduce the idea of a geometric or exponential sequence and show how it gives rise to the exponential function $f(x) = b^x$. We then introduce the special exponential growth and decay curves and show how these curves are used to describe phenomena such as biological growth and decay and the growth of money due to continuous compounding of interest.

Introduction

Suppose that there are ten fungi spores in a culture and that each spore subdivides into two spores on the average of once every hour. At the end of one hour there will be 20 spores, at the end of two hours 40 spores, at the end of three hours 80 spores, and so on. A related situation occurs when a radioactive substance decays. In the case of the carbon isotope ^{14}C the number of atoms decreases by one-half every 5760 years, which length of time is the **half-life** of the substance. These types of **growth and decay** phenomena are known as **geometric** or **exponential** growth and decay phenomena. They are characterized by the fact that if their population were measured at equally spaced time periods (of any length), then the population at the end of any of these periods would always be some constant b times the population at the end of the previous time period. For example, the population of fungi spores can be found at any time by simply multiplying the size of the population of the spore colony an hour earlier by $b = 2$. Likewise, the number of ^{14}C atoms in a sample can be found at any time by multiplying the number of atoms present 5760 years earlier by $b = 0.5$.

Since the types of physical phenomena in which exponential growth and decay occur are almost endless, it is important that an entire chapter be spent studying the mathematical properties of the functions that describe these phenomena.

Geometric Sequences

A sequence of numbers

$$(1, b, b^2, b^3, b^4, \ldots)$$

where each number in the sequence is found by multiplying the preceding number times a fixed constant is called a **geometric sequence**. The fixed constant used to define the geometric sequence is called the **multiplier** and is denoted by b. A few examples of geometric sequences are

$$\begin{array}{ll} (1, 2, 4, 8, 16, \ldots) & (b = 2) \\ (1, \tfrac{1}{2}, \tfrac{1}{4}, \tfrac{1}{8}, \ldots) & (b = \tfrac{1}{2}) \\ (1, 0.8, 0.64, 0.512, 0.4096, \ldots) & (b = 0.8) \\ (1, -1, 1, -1, \ldots) & (b = -1) \end{array}$$

It is not necessary that a geometric sequence begin with the number 1. If each number in the sequence is multiplied by a constant A, the new numbers

$$(A, Ab, Ab^2, Ab^3, Ab^4, \ldots)$$

still constitute a geometric sequence. More examples of geometric sequences are

$$\begin{array}{ll} (2, 4, 8, 16, 32, \ldots) & (A = 2, b = 2) \\ (8, 4, 2, 1, 0.5, \ldots) & (A = 8, b = \tfrac{1}{2}) \\ (3, -0.6, 0.12, -0.024, \ldots) & (A = 3, b = -0.2) \end{array}$$

Example 1

Population Growth In 1988 the population of the world climbed to 4.9 billion people, and it is currently increasing at an annual rate of 2% per year (every year the population is 1.02 times the population of the year before). If the world's population continues to grow at this rate, what will be its population by the year 2000?

Solution An annual population growth of 2% means that the population at any time can be found by multiplying the population exactly one year earlier times 1.02. This is the same as saying that the population is described by the geometric sequence

$$(P, Pb, Pb^2, Pb^3, \ldots)$$

with $P = 4.9$ and $b = 1.02$. The first few numbers of this sequence, giving the world's population from 1988–2000, are shown in Table 1.

TABLE 1
Geometric Population Growth, 1988–2000

Year	Population (billions)		
1988	P		$= 4.900$
1989	$P(1.02)$		$= 4.998$
1990	$[P(1.02)](1.02)$	$= P(1.02)^2$	$= 5.098$
1991	$[P(1.02)^2](1.02)$	$= P(1.02)^3$	$= 5.200$
1992	$[P(1.02)^3](1.02)$	$= P(1.02)^4$	$= 5.304$
⋮	⋮		⋮
2000	$[P(1.02)^{11}](1.02)$	$= P(1.02)^{12}$	$= 6.214$

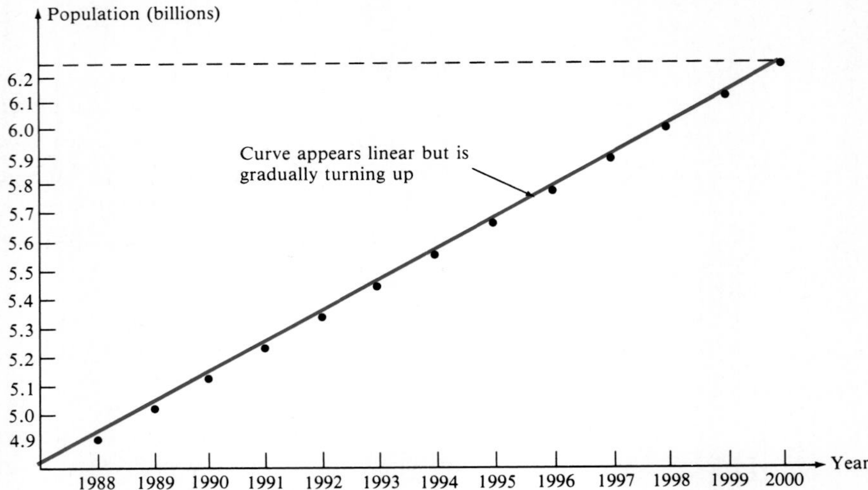

Figure 1
U.S. population, 1988–2000

In other words, if the world's population grows exponentially at the rate of 2% per year until the year 2000, the population of the world will then be 6.214 billion people. A graph of this population curve is shown in Figure 1. □

The Exponential Function b^x

We have seen earlier in the Calculus Preliminaries that the exponential b^n for a positive integer n denotes the product

$$b^n = b \cdot b \cdot b \cdot b \cdot \cdots \cdot b \qquad (n \text{ factors})$$

We have also defined the fractional exponent $b^{m/n}$ by

$$b^{m/n} = (b^{1/n})^m$$

We now find the meaning of b^x when x is not an integer or a fraction. For example, what would be the meaning of 2^π with the irrational number

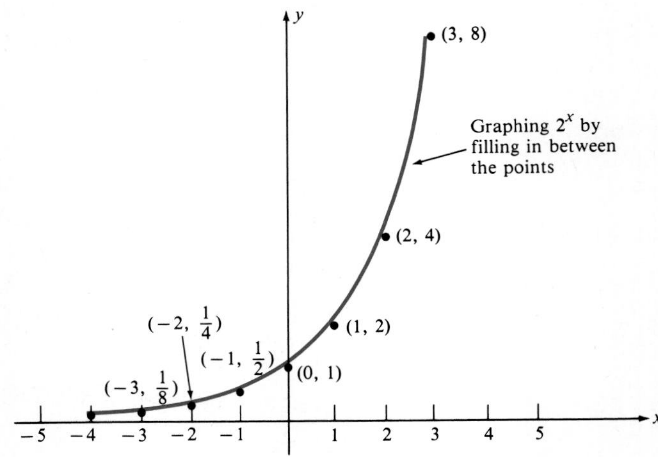

Figure 2
Graph of $y = 2^x$

$\pi = 3.1415927\ldots$ as an exponent? We certainly cannot multiply 2 times itself π times. For the present time we merely interpret the exponential function $y = b^x$ as the smooth curve (called an exponential curve) "filled in" between the points of $y = b^n$ for $n = 1, 2, \ldots$ as shown in Figure 2.

Difference Between Exponential and Power Functions

Students often confuse the **power function**

$$y = x^b$$

and the **exponential function**

$$y = b^x$$

To distinguish the two functions, just remember that for the exponential function b^x the variable x occurs in the exponent, while for the power function x^n the variable x is the *base* of the exponent. Table 2 compares the power function $y = x^2$ with the exponential function $y = 2^x$. Note in Table 2 how fast the exponential function grows. The following example illustrates just how fast.

TABLE 2
Growth of Power and Exponential Functions

x	Power Function x^2	Exponential Function 2^x
0	$0^2 = 0 \cdot 0 = 0$	$2^0 = 1 = 1$
1	$1^2 = 1 \cdot 1 = 1$	$2^1 = 2 = 2$
2	$2^2 = 2 \cdot 2 = 4$	$2^2 = 2 \cdot 2 = 4$
3	$3^2 = 3 \cdot 3 = 9$	$2^3 = 2 \cdot 2 \cdot 2 = 8$
4	$4^2 = 4 \cdot 4 = 16$	$2^4 = 2 \cdot 2 \cdot 2 \cdot 2 = 16$
5	$5^2 = 5 \cdot 5 = 25$	$2^5 = 2 \cdot 2 \cdot 2 \cdot 2 \cdot 2 = 32$
6	$6^2 = 6 \cdot 6 = 36$	$2^6 = 2 \cdot 2 \cdot 2 \cdot 2 \cdot 2 \cdot 2 = 64$
7	$7^2 = 7 \cdot 7 = 49$	$2^7 = 2 \cdot 2 \cdot 2 \cdot 2 \cdot 2 \cdot 2 \cdot 2 = 128$
8	$8^2 = 8 \cdot 8 = 64$	$2^8 = 2 \cdot 2 \cdot 2 \cdot 2 \cdot 2 \cdot 2 \cdot 2 \cdot 2 = 256$
9	$9^2 = 9 \cdot 9 = 81$	$2^9 = 2 \cdot 2 \cdot 2 \cdot 2 \cdot 2 \cdot 2 \cdot 2 \cdot 2 \cdot 2 = 512$
10	$10^2 = 10 \cdot 10 = 100$	$2^{10} = 2 \cdot 2 \cdot 2 \cdot 2 \cdot 2 \cdot 2 \cdot 2 \cdot 2 \cdot 2 \cdot 2 = 1024$

Amazing Exponential Growth

Suppose you tear a page from a newspaper $\frac{1}{250} = 0.004$ inch thick and fold it in half 50 times. How thick will the folded paper be? What is your guess: 2″, 4″, 6″, or even two feet?

To find the thickness is simply an exercise in arithmetic. Each time the paper is folded, the thickness of the folded paper is doubled. Hence the thickness of the paper will grow exponentially according to the geometric sequence

$$(0.004, 0.008, 0.016, 0.032, 0.064, \ldots)$$

Table 3 shows the thickness of the paper as a function of the number of foldings.

TABLE 3
Growth of the Exponential Function $(0.004)2^n$

Number of Foldings	Thickness (inches)	
0	$0.004 \cdot 2^0 = 0.004$	← *Initial thickness*
1	$0.004 \cdot 2^1 = 0.008$	
2	$0.004 \cdot 2^2 = 0.016$	
3	$0.004 \cdot 2^3 = 0.032$	
4	$0.004 \cdot 2^4 = 0.064$	
⋮	⋮	
50	$0.004 \cdot 2^{50} = 4.504 \times 10^{12}$	← *Final thickness*

By using a calculator the thickness of the paper after 50 foldings was found to be approximately 4.504×10^{12} inches. Converting inches to feet and feet to miles, we have

$$\begin{aligned} \text{Thickness} &= 4.504 \times 10^{12} \quad \text{inches} \\ &= (4.504 \times 10^{12})(\tfrac{1}{12}) \quad \text{feet} \\ &= (4.504 \times 10^{12})(\tfrac{1}{12})(\tfrac{1}{5280}) \quad \text{miles} \\ &= 71{,}079{,}540 \quad \text{miles} \end{aligned}$$

In other words, the height of the folded paper is roughly 300 times more than the distance from the earth to the moon. Believe it or not! If you think that this is a rather tall stack of paper, imagine how *wide* the stack of paper will be. After all, the width of the paper will be the width of the original paper *divided* by 2^{50}. It will have a width that is smaller than the diameter of an electron.

We now illustrate how certain populations also satisfy exponential growth over given periods of time.

Example 2

Bacteria Growth A microbiologist has determined that every 12 hours, the size of a colony of *Salmonella* bacteria increases by 15%. Stated another way, as long as the size of the colony obeys this exponential growth, the size of the colony will always be 1.15 times the size of the colony 12 hours earlier. If the initial population of this colony is 200, what will be the population of this colony at any future time t?

Solution Calling P_0 the initial population of the bacteria, the population size $P(t)$ at any time t (and not just at 12-hour intervals) can be described by means of the exponential growth function

$$\begin{aligned} P(t) &= P_0 b^t \\ &= 200(1.15)^t \end{aligned}$$

where t is time measured in 12-hour periods. In other words, $t = 1$ means 12 hours, $t = 2$ means 24 hours, and so on. Using a calculator, we can find the population at any future value of time t, and not just at integer values of t. (See Table 4.) This growth curve is shown in Figure 3. □

TABLE 4
Exponential Growth of Bacteria

Time (hours)	t	Population
0 ← *Present*	0	$200 = 200$
6	0.5	$200(1.15)^{0.5} = 214$
12	1	$200(1.15) = 230$
24	2	$200(1.15)^2 = 264$
36	3	$200(1.15)^3 = 304$
48	4	$200(1.15)^4 = 350$
54	4.5	$200(1.15)^{4.5} = 375$

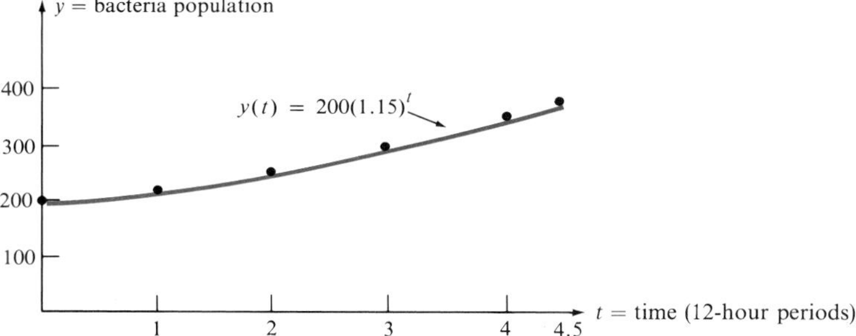

Figure 3
Exponential growth of bacteria

We should point out here that the previous example could just as well have been stated in terms of the growth of a company's revenue. For example, if a company's revenue is 200 million dollars this year and it predicts a 15% annual increase for the next several years, then Table 4 could just as well represent the company's revenue (in millions of dollars) over the next t years.

The Growth and Decay Curves

Although there are many exponential functions such as 2^t, 3^t, $(\frac{1}{2})^t$ that describe exponential growth and decay, there is one class of exponential functions that are special. They are the exponential functions with base e, defined by

$$f(t) = e^{kt}$$

The constant k is an arbitrary constant that describes the rate of growth or decay. In growth problems, k is positive; in decay problems, k is negative. The constant e is a number, sometimes called the **banker's constant*** in financial circles, that has the value $e = 2.71828\ldots$. We will show in the next section (when we can use logarithms) that any exponential function b^x can be rewritten in terms of e^{kt}. Hence all exponential growth and decay phenomena can be studied by using this basic function.

* Although we have called e the banker's constant, mathematicians would probably call it *Euler's constant*. The constant was introduced into mathematics in about 1731 by the Swiss mathematician, Leonhard Euler. The notation was probably chosen as an abbreviation for the word "exponential" and not, as some people think, an abbreviation for Euler's name.

To evaluate $f(t) = e^{kt}$ numerically, it is possible to use either the table of values listed in the Appendix of this book or (probably more conveniently) to use a calculator with an e^t or equivalent key. Graphs of $f(x) = e^{kx}$ for various values of k are shown in Figure 4.

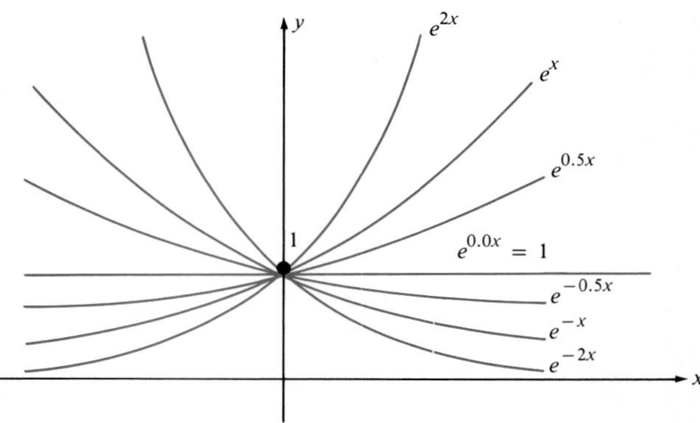

Figure 4
Exponentials e^{kx}

To gain a better understanding of the constant e, use your calculator to verify the computations made to form the second column in Table 5. We see that as k gets larger and larger, the value of

$$\left[1 + \frac{1}{k}\right]^k$$

approaches a limiting value. This limiting value is the constant

$$e = 2.718281828\ldots$$

TABLE 5
Sequence of Numbers Converging to e

k	$\left[1 + \frac{1}{k}\right]^k$
1	2.00000
2	2.25000
5	2.48832
25	2.66584
50	2.69159
100	2.70481
1,000	2.71692
10,000	2.71815
100,000	2.71825

Banker's Constant e

$$e = \lim_{k \to \infty} \left[1 + \frac{1}{k}\right]^k = 2.718281828\ldots$$

The Banker's Constant *e* and the Four Banks

To understand how the number e is used in the calculations of financial matters, consider the following four banks. Each bank pays the same compound interest of 8% per year. However;

- Bank 1 makes interest payments every year (annually).
- Bank 2 makes interest payments every six months (semiannually).
- Bank 3 makes interest payments every month (monthly).
- Bank 4 makes interest payments "continuously" (continuous compounding).

Suppose you deposit $P = \$1000$ in each bank. What will be the value of each of these accounts after five years?

To determine these final amounts, we use the formula for computing the future value F of an initial deposit P. This is given by

$$F = P(1 + i)^n$$

where

$$i = \text{interest rate per compounding period}$$
$$n = \text{number of compoundings}$$

We can now find the amount F in each account from the following formulas:

$$\text{Bank 1:}\quad F_1 = \$1000(1 + 0.08)^5 = \$1469.33$$

$$\text{Bank 2:}\quad F_2 = \$1000\left(1 + \frac{0.08}{2}\right)^{(5)(2)} = \$1480.24$$

$$\text{Bank 3:}\quad F_3 = \$1000\left(1 + \frac{0.08}{12}\right)^{(5)(12)} = \$1489.85$$

$$\text{Bank 4:}\quad F_4 = ?$$

To determine the future value of the account in Bank 4, suppose for a moment that Bank 4 makes k interest payments per year (the interest rate will then be $0.08/k$ per period). After five years the initial \$1000 deposit will be worth

$$\text{Future value for } k \text{ compoundings} = \$1000\left[1 + \frac{0.08}{k}\right]^{5k}$$

For values $k = 1$, 2, and 12 this formula gives the amounts in Banks 1, 2, and 3 at the end of the five years because they compound interest annually, semiannually, and monthly, respectively. If we now let k get larger and larger (interest payments made more often), the above future value will approach the future value F_4 when interest is "compounded continuously." That is, we can perform a little fancy algebra and get

$$F_4 = \lim_{k\to\infty}\left[1000\left(1 + \frac{0.08}{k}\right)^{5k}\right]$$
$$= 100 \lim_{k\to\infty}\left(1 + \frac{1}{k/0.08}\right)^{(k/0.08)(0.08)(5)}$$

However, by looking at the definition of the banker's constant e we see that the expression

$$\left(1 + \frac{1}{k/0.08}\right)^{(k/0.08)}$$

will have a limiting value of e as $k \to \infty$. (The fact that the expression contains $k/0.08$ instead of k only makes the expression approach e more slowly.) Hence we can write the above future value F_4 as

$$\begin{aligned} F_4 &= \$1000e^{(0.08)(5)} \\ &= \$1491.82 \end{aligned}$$

Conclusion of the Four Banks Problem

Although each of the four banks pays the same 8% annual rate of interest, in reality the bank that compounds interest "continuously" pays the most (compare \$1491.82 to the other future values). Of course, no bank can really compound interest continuously. Continuous compounding is simply a mathematical idealization of compounding many, many times with a small time interval between compoundings. Still, the concept is very useful. In reality there is very little difference between the future value of an account when interest is "compounded continuously" and when interest is compounded daily as is done in many banks today. One reason that financial people like to work with continuous compounding is that the exponential function is easy to manipulate mathematically. In general, if interest is compounded continuously at an annual rate of interest r, then after t years an initial deposit of P dollars will have a future value of

$$F = Pe^{rt}$$

Example 3

Compound Interest Sally deposits \$100 in a bank that pays 8% annual interest, compounded continuously. Graph the amount of money in her account after each year for the next ten years.

HISTORICAL NOTE

Three of the most important constants in mathematics are π, i, and e, where π is the ratio of the circumference of a circle to its diameter, i is the unit complex number $i = \sqrt{-1}$, and e is the constant **e**. The symbols π, **i**, and **e** that are used to denote these constants were all introduced into mathematics by the great Swiss mathematician Leonhard Euler (1707–1783). It is fascinating that these three famous constants are related by the celebrated equation $e^{2\pi i} = 1$. This is the reason that students of mathematics often wear tee-shirts with the slogan, "Mathematicians, We're Number $e^{2\pi i}$.

Solution To find this graph, we can use a calculator with an e^x key and construct a table of values for

$$\begin{aligned} F &= Pe^{rt} \\ &= 100e^{(0.08)t} \end{aligned}$$

for $t = 1, 2, \ldots, 10$, as shown in Table 6. Knowing these points, we then connect the points with a smooth curve, as shown in Figure 5.

TABLE 6
Values for Example 3

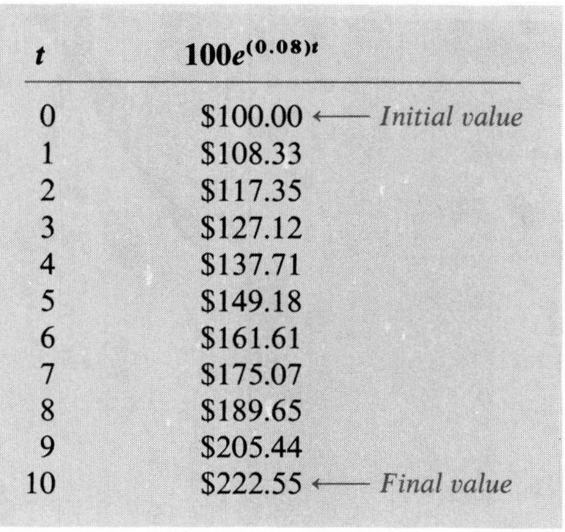

t	$100e^{(0.08)t}$
0	\$100.00 ⟵ *Initial value*
1	\$108.33
2	\$117.35
3	\$127.12
4	\$137.71
5	\$149.18
6	\$161.61
7	\$175.07
8	\$189.65
9	\$205.44
10	\$222.55 ⟵ *Final value*

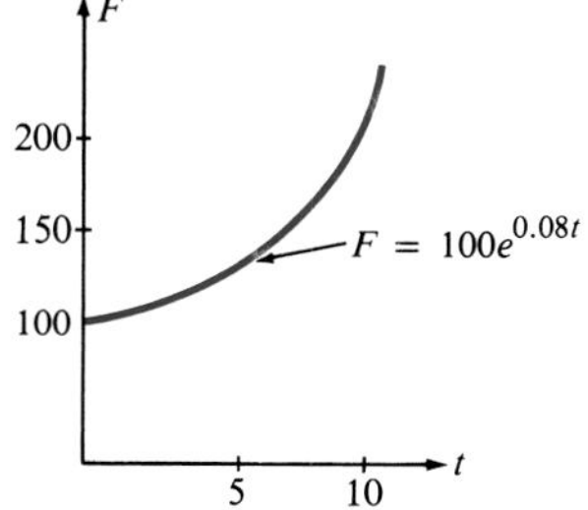

Figure 5
Sally's money growing exponentially over time

The Banker's Constant *e* (an Interpretation)

An interesting interpretation of the banker's constant e is the following. If you were to make an initial deposit of $P = \$1$ in a bank that pays an annual interest r of 10% compounded continuously, then the future value F of the account after ten years would be

$$\begin{aligned} F &= Pe^{rt} \\ &= \$1e^{(0.10)(10)} \\ &= e \qquad \text{(the banker's constant } e\text{)} \end{aligned}$$

In other words, the future value would be \$2.71828 . . . .

Growth and Decay Phenomena

One class of phenomena that can be studied with the help of exponential functions is growth and decay phenomena. We now define this important class of curves.

Definition of Growth and Decay Curves

Let k be any positive constant. For each such k the **exponential growth and decay curves** are defined by

$$y(t) = Pe^{kt} \qquad \text{(exponential growth curves)}$$
$$y(t) = Pe^{-kt} \qquad \text{(exponential decay curves)}$$

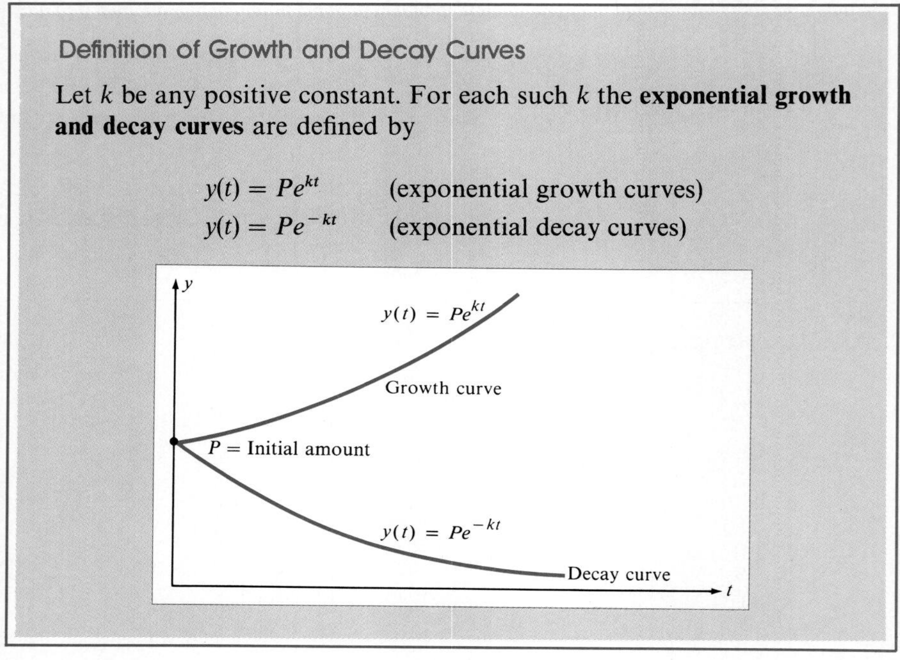

Light Intensity as Exponential Decay

A typical decay phenomenon in science is the decay of sunlight filtering down through water. Anyone who has dived to a depth of 100 feet in most ocean waters will tell you that there is very little light at that depth. Most divers could probably not tell you, however, that the light intensity decays exponentially as a function of depth.

The **Bougour-Lambert law** states that the intensity $I(x)$ of sunlight filtering down through water at a depth x decreases according to the exponential decay function

$$I(x) = I_0 e^{-kx} \qquad (k > 0)$$

Here, I_0 is the intensity of light at the surface, and $k > 0$ is an absorption constant that depends on the murkiness of the water. The murkier the water, the

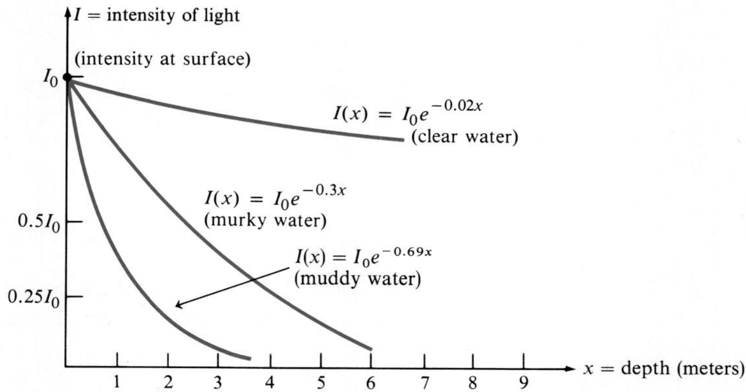

Figure 6
Absorption of light in three typical lakes

larger the value of k. Some examples of light intensity curves for different values of k are shown in Figure 6.

Example 4

Light Intensity in Water Suppose that the light intensity at the surface of a lake is some given value I_0 and that the absorption constant k has been determined experimentally to be $k = 0.69$. How much light has been absorbed by the water at a depth of 2.5 meters?

Solution Using the basic absorption equation

$$I(x) = I_0 e^{-kx}$$

we simply substitute in the given values, getting

$$\begin{aligned} I(2.5) &= I_0 e^{-(0.69)(2.5)} \\ &= 0.178 I_0 \end{aligned}$$

This means that at a depth of 2.5 meters, the light intensity is only 17.8% as intense as on the surface of the water. (See Figure 7.) □

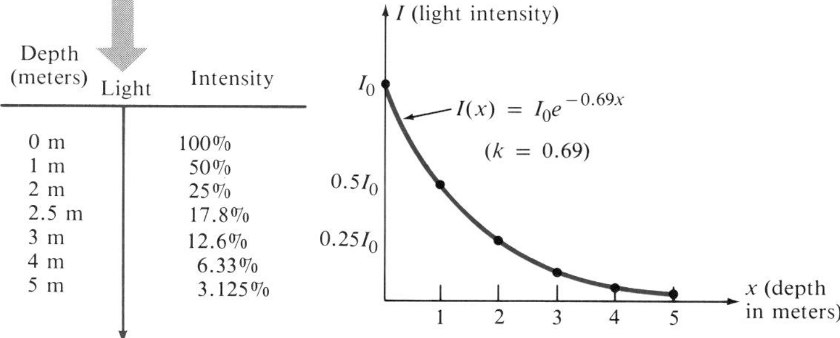

Figure 7
Light intensity decaying exponentially

Example 5

Future Value as a Growth Curve Dorothy has deposited \$1000 in a bank that pays an annual interest rate of 9% compounded continuously. What is the exponential growth function that describes the value of her account after t years?

Solution Here, we are given

$$\begin{aligned} r &= 0.09 \qquad \text{(annual rate of interest)} \\ P &= \$1000 \qquad \text{(initial amount deposited)} \end{aligned}$$

The future value F of her account after t years is given by the exponential growth curve

$$\begin{aligned} F &= Pe^{rt} \\ &= \$1000e^{0.09t} \end{aligned}$$

This growth curve is plotted in Figure 8. □

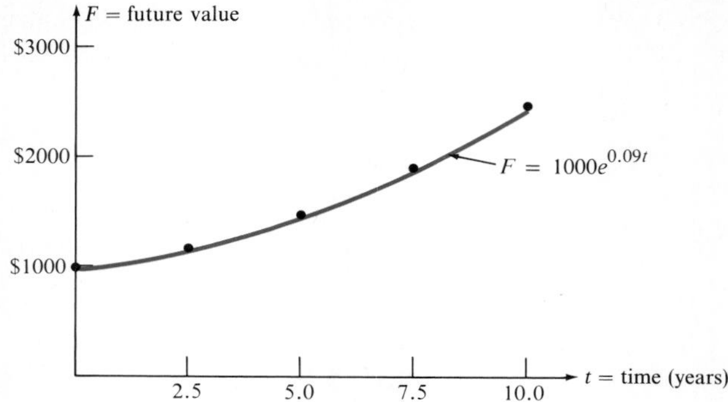

Figure 8
Future value of an account that pays 9% compounded continuously

Problems

For Problems 1–10, find the first six terms of the geometric sequences with given values of A and b.

1. $A = 1, b = 3$
2. $A = 5, b = 2$
3. $A = \frac{1}{2}, b = 4$
4. $A = 1, b = \frac{1}{3}$
5. $A = 2, b = 3$
6. $A = 8, b = \frac{1}{2}$
7. $A = 1, b = 0.1$
8. $A = 4, b = -\frac{1}{2}$
9. $A = 3, b = -3$
10. $A = 6, b = -2$

World Growth

Problems 11–14 refer to Table 7, which gives the world's population (in millions) for different regions of the world for the years 1960–1980.

11. Does the population in North America appear to be increasing exponentially? If so, what would you say is the fractional increase every ten years? In other words, what is the multiplier b in the geometric sequence?

12. Does the population in South America appear to be increasing exponentially? If so, what would you say is the percentage increase every ten years?

13. Assuming the population in North America is increasing exponentially, what would you predict the population to be in 1990? In the year 2000?

14. Which regions of the world have the lowest and highest rate of increase?

TABLE 7
Population Figures for Problems 11–14

Year	North America	South America	Europe	U.S.S.R.	Asia	Africa
1960	199	215	425	214	1683	275
1970	226	283	460	244	2091	354
1980	252	365	484	266	2613	472

For Problems 15–20, graph the given exponential function by plotting the values of the functions at the integers $-2, -1, 0, 1, 2$ and filling in between these points with a smooth curve. Computations can be made by hand or by using a calculator.

15. $y = 2^{-x}$
16. $y = 4^x$
17. $y = 4 \cdot 2^{-x}$
18. $y = 4 \cdot 3^{-2x} + 5$
19. $y = 3 \cdot 2^{-x} + 3$
20. $y = 2^x + 2^{-x}$

For Problems 21–26, solve the exponential equations for x.

21. $(\frac{1}{8})^x = 8$
22. $7^{-x} = 49^{(x+3)}$
23. $5^{-2x} = \frac{1}{25}$
24. $2^{x^2-4x} = 32$
25. $8^{x^2} = 2^{5x}$
26. $3^{(2x+1)} = 3^x$

27. Solving Exponential Equations. Find the points of intersection of the graphs of the functions

$$f(x) = 3^{x^2} \quad \text{and} \quad g(x) = 3^{x+2}$$

28. Solving Exponential Equations. Find the points of intersection of the graphs of the functions

$$f(x) = 5^{x(x^2-3)} \quad \text{and} \quad g(x) = 5^{-2x^2}$$

Annual Growth of Leading Industrial Countries

The Gross National Product (GNP) of a country for a single year is the total value of all goods and services produced by that country for that year. Table 8 lists the 1986 GNP and the average annual growth rate (over the previous ten years) of the GNP for leading industrial countries. For Problems 29–32, assume that the GNPs of the above countries are growing exponentially according to the growth curve

$$\text{GNP}(n) = P(1 + i)^n$$

where

i = average annual growth rate

n = number of years starting from 1986

P = GNP in 1986

TABLE 8
GNP Figures for Problems 29–32

Country	Gross National Product, 1986 (in billions)	Average Annual Growth Rate of GNP, 1977–1986
Canada	420	2.50%
France	569	3.90%
United Kingdom	460	2.75%
Italy	369	2.20%
Japan	1204	4.85%
United States	3662	3.50%
U.S.S.R.	1843	2.20%
West Germany	655	3.10%

29. United States GNP. From the above information, what is the exponential growth function that describes the GNP for the United States? Using this function, what would you expect the GNP of the United States to be in the year 1990?

30. Equation of GNP. From the above information, what would the equation of the GNP be for each of the countries?

31. Leading Economic Country. If economic growth continues as it has during the period 1977–1986, will Japan's GNP surpass the GNP of the United States by the year 2000?

32. Number Two Country. If economic growth continues as it has during the period 1977–1986, will Japan's GNP surpass the Soviet Union's by the year 2000? In the next section, when we study logarithms, we will learn to determine the exact year when these two growth curves intersect.

33. Semiannual Compounding of Money. Sally deposits \$100 in a bank account that pays 10% annual interest, compounded every six months (that is, compounded semiannually). What will be the value of her account after six months, after one year, after 18 months, after two years, and after n compoundings? *Hint:* 10% annual interest compounded semiannually means that every six months the bank pays $\frac{10}{2} = 5\%$ interest on the current value of the account.

34. Quarterly Compounding of Money. Richard deposits \$100 in a bank account that pays 12% annual interest, compounded every three months (quarterly). What will be the value of his account after three months, after six months, after nine months, and after n compoundings? *Hint:* 12% annual interest compounded quarterly means that every three months the bank pays $\frac{12}{4} = 3\%$ interest on the current value of the account.

35. World's Population. Suppose the world's population is falling at the rate of 1% per year. Suppose the current population is 5 billion people. Estimate the world's population for each of the next five years.

36. Bacteria Growth. Find a function that represents the growth of a bacteria population that triples every day if the initial amount of the bacteria is ten cells. Sketch a graph of this function.

37. Bacteria Decay. A bacteria infection is being treated with a new form of hydrocortisone. Suppose that every week the bacteria population falls to 80% of the population of the preceding week. If the initial population is 500, what is the exponential function that describes the population at any time $t > 0$? Sketch a graph of this function.

38. Temperature of Coffee. Suppose that every ten minutes you measure the temperature of your coffee and determine that the temperature is 90% of the temperature ten minutes earlier. If the initial temperature was 180 degrees, what is the exponential function that describes the temperature at any time t? What is the temperature of the coffee after one hour? (Cooling of temperatures is one of many natural phenomena that satisfies an exponential decay law.)

39. Stopping an Oil Tanker. It has been shown that if an oil tanker stops its engines, then its velocity will decrease exponentially. Suppose that the captain shuts off the engines when the speed of the tanker is 20 miles per hour and that every minute the speed of the tanker is only 90% of the speed at the previous minute. What is the exponential decay function that describes the speed of the tanker for any positive time t? What is the speed of the tanker after one hour? Note that the exponential function is never zero, but clearly the tanker will eventually stop. What is the meaning of this discrepancy?

40. Virus Growth. A population of a certain virus grows so that its size $S(t)$ at the end of t days is given by

$$S(t) = S_0 2^{kt}$$

where S_0 is the size of the initial population. For an initial population of 1000 that doubles in 20 days, what is the value of k? What will be the size of the population at the end of 15 and 30 days?

41. Bacteria Population. The size of the population E of a bacteria colony is described by the function

$$E(t) = E_0 2^{t/30}$$

where E_0 is the size of the initial population and t is measured in months. For the initial population size of 500, calculate the population size at times $t = 1, 2, 3, 4,$ and 10 months.

42. The Clever Rat. Psychologists have long held that much about human nature can be learned from rats. Suppose an experimenter places a rat in a maze and that it takes the rat one minute to escape. After that, each time the experimenter places the rat in the maze, it takes only 80% as long for the rat to escape. What is the geometric sequence that describes how long it takes the rat to escape on every trial?

43. Animal Population. The size of an animal population in a given habitat is described by the function

$$P(t) = P_0 2^t$$

where P_0 is the initial population size and t is time measured in years. For an original population size of 400, calculate the population size after 1, 2, 4, 10, and 20 years.

44. Exponential Growth. Would you rather have \$1,000,000 or the value calculated by doubling the amount you have every day for 100 days starting with one cent on the first day? What is the value of each amount at the end of 100 days?

45. Continuous Compounding. Andy deposits \$500 in a bank that pays 9% annual interest compounded continuously. What is the function that describes the value of his account at any time t? What will be the value of the account after one year? After 18 months?

46. Continuous Compounding. Karen deposits \$1000 in a bank that pays 8% annual interest compounded continuously. What is the function that describes the value of her account at any time t? What will be the value of her account after ten years? After 15.5 years?

47. Long-Term Account. Mary inherited the amount contained in a bank account taken out by her grandfather 75 years earlier. The initial deposit in the account was \$10, and the bank paid a constant annual interest rate of 5% compounded continuously. How much did Mary inherit?

48. Which Account Has More Money? Twenty years ago, Harry deposited \$100 in a bank that pays an annual interest rate of 9% compounded continuously. John deposited \$250 in the same bank ten years ago. Which person's account contains more money?

49. Business Learning Curves. Businesses often measure training programs by how fast new employees can learn new skills. Using a given training program, suppose the average number of units L produced by a new employee on the tth week at work can be described by the exponential learning curve

$$L(t) = 100(1 - e^{-0.1t})$$

Use tables or a calculator to find the number of units L that an average employee can produce on week $t =$ 1, 2, 3, 4, and 5. Draw a graph of this learning curve.

50. Sales Decay. Sales of a new product tend to decrease over time. For sales levels described by the function

$$S(t) = 1500 + 750e^{-0.2t}$$

where t is measured in years evaluate the sales level for $t = 0, 1, 2, 3, 4,$ and 10 years.

51. Radioactive Dating of Fossils. Radioactive carbon isotope ^{14}C dating of fossils of plants and animals depends on knowing the amount $C(t)$ of ^{14}C left in the fossil after a given period of time t. The function

$$C(t) = A_0 e^{-t/5760} \qquad (t \geq 0)$$

gives the amount of ^{14}C after t years from the time the plant or animal has died where A_0 is the amount of ^{14}C that was present at the time of death. Find the amount of ^{14}C present $t = 0$, 1000, 2000, 4000, and 8000 years after the plant or animal has died if $A_0 = 1$ gram.

52. Long-Distance Phone calls. Conversations in long-distance telephone calls usually fade out owing to a damping effect on the lines. If I_0 is the initial strength of the signal, then the signal can be measured by

$$I(x) = I_0 e^{-kx}$$

where x is the distance the signal is sent measured in miles and $k > 0$ is the damping constant that depends on the type of wire used in the communication (along with other factors). If $k = 0.002$, what fraction of the signal is lost at 10 miles? After 100 miles? After 500 miles?

53. **Suspension Bridge and the Banker.** The middle span of any suspension bridge is always shaped in the form of a curve called a *catenary*. The equation of this curve is

$$y = \frac{e^x + e^{-x}}{2} \qquad (-1 \le x \le 1)$$

It is interesting that the banker's constant e is the main ingredient of the equation that describes the shape of a suspension bridge. Use a calculator to evaluate this catenary for $x = -1, -0.5, 0, 0.5, 1$. Then fill in between the points with a smooth curve.

Amazing but True Stories (Exponential Growth)

54. **Wise Young Man.** A story is told about a king who offered a young peasant a gold piece for saving the life of the king's daughter. Being humble, however, the young peasant declined and agreed instead to accept one kernel of wheat on the first day, two kernels of wheat on the second day, four kernels of wheat on the third day, eight kernels of wheat on the fourth day, and so on for the next 100 days. How many pieces of grain would the king have to give the young peasant on the 100th day? Assuming there are 1,000,000 kernels of wheat in a bushel, how many bushels of wheat would the king have to give the peasant on the last day?

55. **The Rat's Progeny.** The progeny of a rat numbers about 500 per year. Assume that half of these are females and half are males and that all of them survive. How many progeny will the rat have in 25 years?

56. **A Fast-Growing Function.** We have seen the amazing growth of the exponential function 2^n (remember the paper-folding problem). There is, however, another function that grows much, much faster. That function is the *factorial function*

$$n! = n \cdot (n-1) \cdot (n-2) \cdots 3 \cdot 2 \cdot 1$$

Use a calculator to convince yourself of this fact by computing 2^{25} and $25!$.

3.2 Logarithms and Logarithmic Scales

PURPOSE

We introduce the general logarithmic function with base b and show how it can be used to

- solve algebraic equations and
- describe physical phenomena.

We also introduce the two specific logarithmic functions, the common logarithm and the natural logarithm.

Introduction

Roughly 400 years before you are reading these pages, in around 1590, the Scottish laird John Napier looked at two rows of numbers, similar to the rows of numbers in Table 9, and made a discovery that changed the world.

TABLE 9
Napier's Mystery Numbers

0	1	2	3	4	5	6	7	8	9	10
1	2	4	8	16	32	64	128	256	512	1024

This was a time before computers, calculators, and even slide rules. It was a time when all computations were done by hand with pencil and paper. What

Napier saw in the above rows was an ingenious way to multiply numbers by adding. Since addition is far easier and quicker to perform, he discovered what might be called a sixteenth-century computer.

To understand Napier's discovery, let us suppose we wish to multiply the numbers 16 and 64. If we carry out this multiplication, we will see that the product is 1024. However, there is a far easier way to find this product using the above numbers. (Do you see what it is?) What Napier saw in the above rows of numbers was: If the two numbers directly above 16 and 64 (namely, 4 and 6) are added, then the sum (10) is the number directly above the product of 16 and 64. In fact, this scheme will work for the product of any two numbers in the bottom row (4 times 128 is the number below the sum $2 + 7 = 9$, or 512). Of course, Napier still had a few bugs to work out. Namely, how could he multiply numbers that were not in the bottom row? These problems were all worked out, however, and after 20 years of refinement he published his results in 1614 in a paper entitled "A Description of the Marvelous Rule of Logarithms." We will now learn about these refinements.

The Logarithmic Function

The columns of numbers in Table 10 illustrate the relationship between the exponential function $y = 10^x$ and what is called its **logarithmic inverse**. To understand the logarithmic function, first consider the exponential 10^x. To evaluate 10^x, we start with a value of x—say, $x = 3$—and raise 10 to this power:

$$10^3 = 1000$$

To evaluate the logarithm, we ask the reverse question. That is, given the answer (say 1000), to what power x should we raise 10 in order to get that answer? In other words, find x such that

$$10^x = 1000$$

Clearly, the exponent is 3, and this value is called the logarithm of 1000 to the base 10 and is denoted by

$$\log_{10} 1000 = 3$$

TABLE 10
Relationship Between $y = 10^x$ and $y = \log_{10} x$

Exponential Function		Logarithmic Function	
x	$y = 10^x$	x	$y = \log_{10} x$
-3	$0.001 = 10^{-3}$	0.001	$10^y = 0.001 \longrightarrow y = -3$
-2	$0.01 = 10^{-2}$	0.01	$10^y = 0.01 \longrightarrow y = -2$
-1	$0.1 = 10^{-1}$	0.1	$10^y = 0.1 \longrightarrow y = -1$
0	$1 = 10^0$	1	$10^y = 1 \longrightarrow y = 0$
1	$10 = 10^1$	10	$10^y = 10 \longrightarrow y = 1$
2	$100 = 10^2$	100	$10^y = 100 \longrightarrow y = 2$
3	$1000 = 10^3$	1000	$10^y = 1000 \longrightarrow y = 3$

Table 10 illustrates the relationship between the logarithmic function $\log_{10} x$ and the exponential function 10^x. The relationship between the graphs of exponential and logarithmic functions can be seen in Figure 9.

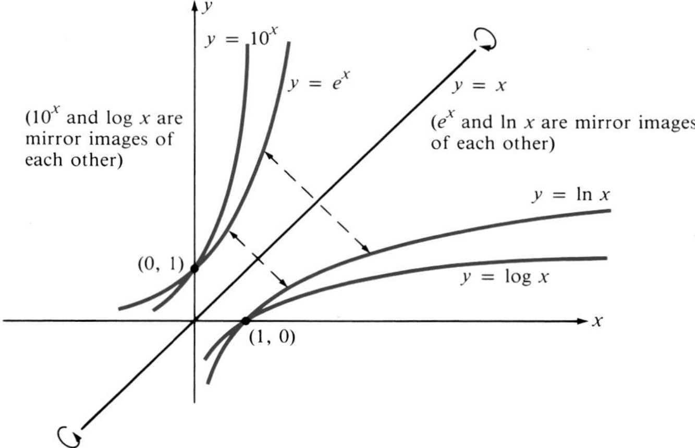

Figure 9
Comparison of log x and ln x

The above discussion leads to the general definition of the logarithm to any base b.

Definition of the Logarithm

The **logarithm** of a positive number x to a base b, denoted $\log_b x$, where b is any positive number different from 1, is the number to which the base b must be raised to equal the number x. If the base is 10, then the logarithm is called the **common logarithm** and is denoted as

$$y = \log x \qquad (x > 0)$$

If the base is the constant $e = 2.718\ldots$, then the logarithm is called the **natural logarithm** and is denoted as

$$y = \ln x \qquad (x > 0)$$

Table 11 illustrates the logarithms with different bases. We can see from Table 11 the general pattern

$$y = \log_b x \quad \text{is the same as} \quad b^y = x$$

TABLE 11
Relationship Between Exponentials and Logarithms

Exponential Form	Logarithmic Form
$10^2 = 100$	$\log 100 = 2$
$4^3 = 64$	$\log_4 64 = 3$
$10^3 = 1000$	$\log 1000 = 3$
$2^{-4} = \frac{1}{16}$	$\log_2(\frac{1}{16}) = -4$
$10^{1.2} = 15.8$	$\log 15.8 = 1.2$
$(\frac{1}{2})^6 = \frac{1}{64}$	$\log_{1/2}(\frac{1}{64}) = 6$
$20^2 = 400$	$\log_{20} 400 = 2$

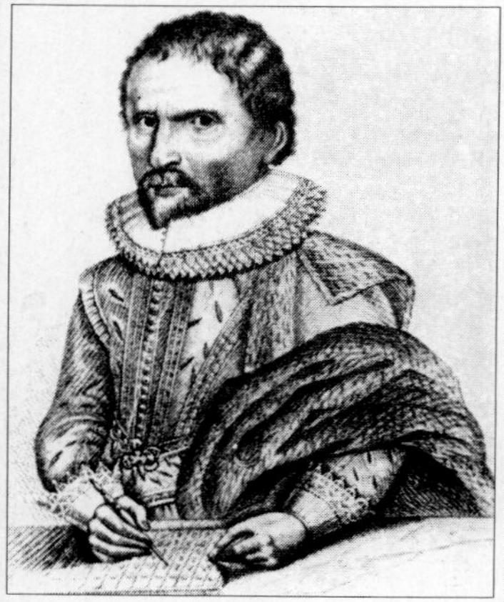

HISTORICAL NOTE

The invention of the logarithm was to the sixteenth century what the computer is to the twentieth century—an evolutionary jump in the speeding up of arithmetic operations. While the logarithm decreased the time that sixteenth century astronomers had to spend on arithmetic computations by more than tenfold, computers have increased the speed of arithmetic operations at least another millionfold.

The inventor of the logarithm, John Napier (1550–1617), was born in Scotland and spent most of his life at the family estate of Merchiston Castle. He was violently anti-Catholic and published a bitter and widely read tirade against the Church of Rome. Napier was very creative and novel in all of his endeavors and thought of mathematics as a diversion from his activities in religion and politics.

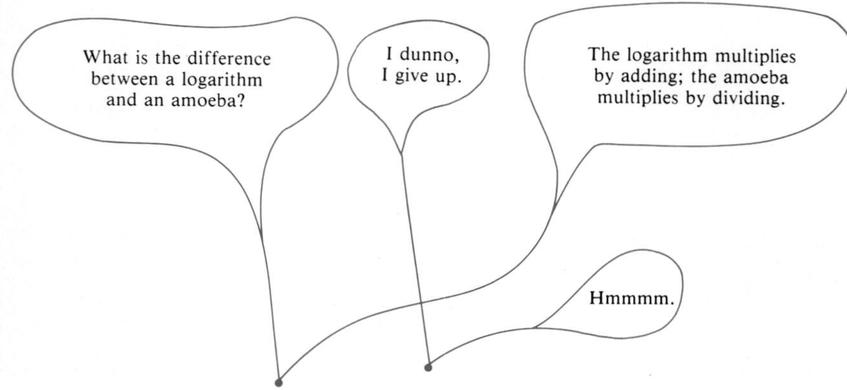

Useful Properties of Logarithms

Logarithms are a valuable tool that are used in many areas of science. They can aid in the solution of algebraic equations when the unknown is in the exponent. They are also useful in the description of physical phenomena. Many applications come about as a result of the following properties of the logarithm.

Six Properties of Logarithms

The following properties of logarithms hold provided that u, v, and b are positive with $b \neq 1$. Some of the examples use the logarithms $\log 2 = 0.301$, $\log 3 = 0.477$, and $\log 17 = 1.230$.

- **Property 1:** $\log_b uv = \log_b u + \log_b v$
  Examples:
$$\begin{aligned} \log 200 &= \log 2 + \log 100 = 0.301 + 2 = 2.301 \\ \log 6000 &= \log 6 + \log 1000 \\ &= \log 2 + \log 3 + 3 \\ &= 0.301 + 0.477 + 3 = 3.778 \end{aligned}$$

- **Property 2:** $\log_b \frac{u}{v} = \log_b u - \log_b v$
  Examples:
$$\log \frac{17}{3} = \log 17 - \log 3 = 1.230 - 0.477 = 0.753$$
$$\log \frac{1}{10} = \log 1 - \log 10 = -\log 10 = -1$$

- **Property 3:** $\log_b u^a = a \log_b u$
  Examples:
$$\begin{aligned} \log 3^2 &= 2 \log 3 = 0.954 \\ \log 2^{14} &= 14 \log 2 = 4.214 \end{aligned}$$

- **Property 4:** $\log_b b = 1$
  Examples:
$$\begin{aligned} \log 10 &= 1 \\ \ln e &= 1 \\ \log_2 2 &= 1 \end{aligned}$$

- **Property 5:** $\log_b 1 = 0$
  Examples:
$$\begin{aligned} \log 1 &= 0 \\ \ln 1 &= 0 \end{aligned}$$

- **Property 6:** $b^{\log_b x} = x$
  Examples:
$$\begin{aligned} 10^{\log_{10} 5} &= 5 \\ 2^{\log_2 3} &= 3 \end{aligned}$$

- **Property 7:** $\log_b b^x = x$
  Examples:
$$\begin{aligned} \log 10^4 &= 4 \\ \ln e^3 &= 3 \end{aligned}$$

Verification of Logarithm Rules

We illustrate the general idea of why the above rules hold by proving Property 1:

$$\log_b uv = \log_b u + \log_b v$$

The proofs of the other rules follow similar lines.

To simplify matters, we let

$$x = \log_b u$$
$$y = \log_b v$$

We rewrite these equations in equivalent exponential form so that we can use properties of exponentials. This gives

$$u = b^x \qquad \text{(exponential form)}$$
$$v = b^y \qquad \text{(exponential form)}$$

We now multiply these quantities, getting

$$uv = b^x b^y$$

However, the product on the right can be written as

$$b^x b^y = b^{x+y} \qquad \text{(basic step in proof)}$$

and hence

$$uv = b^{x+y}$$

Finally, rewriting this equation back in logarithmic form, we have

$$\log_b uv = x + y$$

which is nothing more than

$$\log_b uv = \log_b u + \log_b v$$

Example 1

Uses of Logarithm Properties Provided that the following expressions in x represent positive numbers, we can write the following relationships:

(a) $\log_b x + \log_b(x^2 + 1) = \log_b x(x^2 + 1)$

(b) $\log_b \dfrac{x^2 + 4}{x} = \log_b(x^2 + 4) - \log_b x$

(c) $\log_b(5x^4) = \log_b 5 + \log_b x^4$
$\qquad = \log_b 5 + 4 \log_b x$

Solving Equations Involving Logarithms and Exponentials

Using the properties of logarithms, we can solve many types of equations that would otherwise be extremely difficult to handle. The following examples illustrate how logarithms are used to solve a variety of problems.

Example 2 Equation Involving Logarithms Solve for x:

$$\log x^2 + \log x = 3$$

Solution Using Property 1, we write the left-hand side of this equation as

$$\begin{aligned}\log x^2 + \log x &= \log x^2 \cdot x \\ &= \log x^3\end{aligned}$$

Hence the original equation becomes

$$\log x^3 = 3$$

By the definition of the common logarithm, we get

$$x^3 = 10^3$$

or

$$x = 10$$

□

Example 3 Equation Involving Logarithms Solve for x:

$$\ln(x + 1) - \ln(x - 1) = 1$$

Solution Using Property 2, we can write

$$\ln\left(\frac{x+1}{x-1}\right) = 1$$

By the definition of the natural logarithm we have

$$\frac{x+1}{x-1} = e$$

Multiplying by $x - 1$ and solving for x gives

$$\begin{aligned}x + 1 &= e(x - 1) \\ x(1 - e) &= -1 - e \\ x &= \frac{e+1}{e-1} \\ &\cong 2.16\end{aligned}$$

□

When the unknown variable x is located in an exponent, the general strategy is to take the logarithm of each side of the equation. While it is possible to use a logarithm with any base, the specific problem will generally dictate which logarithm is the most convenient.

Example 4 Unknown in Exponent Solve for x:

$$10^{x^2} = 73$$

Solution Taking the common logarithm of each side of the equation, we have

$$\log 10^{x^2} = \log 73$$

Property 7 says that the left-hand side of this equation is x^2. Hence we have

$$x^2 = \log 73$$

Solving for x, we get

$$\begin{aligned} x &= \pm\sqrt{\log 73} \\ &\cong \pm 1.365 \end{aligned}$$

□

Example 5 Unknown in Exponent Solve for x:

$$2^{2x-1} = 10^x$$

Solution Taking the common logarithm of each side of the equation, we have

$$\log 2^{2x-1} = \log 10^x$$

Using Property 3, we can bring down the exponents, getting

$$\begin{aligned} (2x - 1) \log 2 &= x \log 10 \\ &= x \end{aligned}$$

Finally, solving for x gives

$$\begin{aligned} x &= \frac{\log 2}{2 \log 2 - 1} \\ &\cong -0.756 \end{aligned}$$

□

In the above problem we could have used a logarithm with a different base. However, the final value of x would have been written in terms of this new logarithm. Since common and natural logarithm tables are generally the only ones published, it is best to use these logarithms. Also, most calculators have common and natural logarithm keys.

Logarithm Functions in Growth and Decay Phenomena

In the previous section we introduced exponential growth and decay curves. The main emphasis of the study was to find the exponential functions that described various growth and decay phenomena and to evaluate these functions at different times. We now study what could be called the inverse problem. That is, given an exponential function, such as

$$y = Ae^{kt}$$

what is the value of time t that will make the value of the function y a given amount? In other words, y is the known quantity, and t is the unknown quantity.

For example, suppose Eddie has deposited \$4000 in a bank account that pays 8% annual interest compounded continuously. He hopes that in four years, when he graduates from college, the value of the account will be \$10,000 and he can buy a new car. The question is: When will Eddie's account be worth \$10,000?

To solve this problem, we set the future value of Eddie's account

$$F(t) = \$4000e^{0.08t}$$

equal to \$10,000 and solve for t where t is time in years. In other words, we solve for t in the equation

$$4000e^{0.08t} = 10{,}000$$

Hence

$$e^{0.08t} = 2.5$$

Take the natural logarithm of each side of this equation (remember $\ln e^x = x$) and then solve for t. We get

$$\begin{aligned} 0.08t &= \ln 2.5 \\ t &= \frac{\ln 2.5}{0.08} \\ &\cong \frac{0.916}{0.08} \\ &= 11.45 \quad \text{years} \end{aligned}$$

□

In other words, it will take about 11.45 years for a \$4000 deposit to grow to \$10,000 if interest is paid at an annual rate of 8% compounded continuously. Hopefully, Eddie will not be in college that long.

Example 6

Doubling Time of Money How long will it take money to double in value if invested in a bank that pays 12% compounded continuously?

Solution An initial amount P_0, deposited at 12% annual interest compounded continuously will have a future value F of

$$F(t) = P_0e^{0.12t} \qquad \text{(future value)}$$

after t years. The rate that this future value increases can be seen in Figure 10.

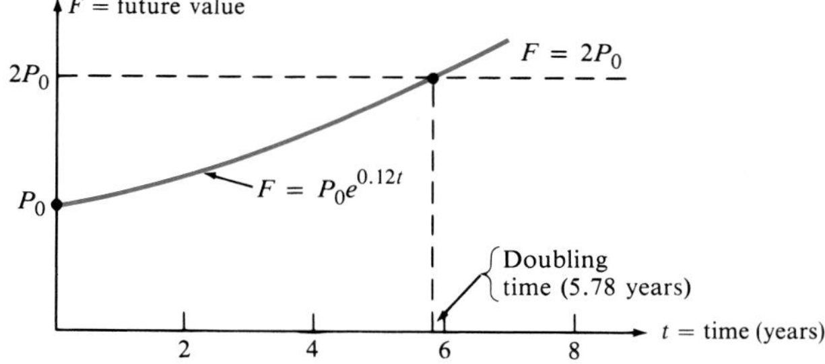

Figure 10
Computation of doubling times

To find the time t where this graph intersects the doubling line

$$F(t) = 2P_0 \qquad \text{(twice the initial amount)}$$

we set the future value equal to this amount and solve for t. That is, we solve for t in the equation

$$P_0e^{0.12t} = 2P_0$$

Dividing each side of this equation by P_0 gives

$$e^{0.12t} = 2$$

Taking the natural logarithm of each side of the equation, we get

$$\ln e^{0.12t} = \ln 2$$

Finally, using the property $\ln e^x = x$ and solving for x, we can write

$$0.12t = \ln 2$$
$$t \cong 5.78 \quad \text{years}$$

In other words, every 5.78 years, money will double in value if invested at 12% compounded continuously. This means that if a student graduates from high school at the age of 18 and deposits a \$1000 graduation gift in a bank that pays 12% annual interest compounded continuously, then by the time the student reaches the age of 65 (roughly eight doubling times), the value of the account will be

$$\begin{aligned}\text{Future value at age 65} &= \$1000 \cdot 2^8 \\ &= \$1000(256) \\ &= \$256{,}000\end{aligned}$$

This gives real meaning to Ben Franklin's adage that "Time Is Money." □

Example 7

Japan Number Two? The 1986 Gross National Product (GNP) of Japan was 1.204 trillion dollars, with an average annual rate of increase over the previous ten years of 4.85%. On the other hand, the GNP of the Soviet Union in 1986 was 1.843 trillion dollars, with an average annual rate of increase over the previous ten years of 2.2%. Assuming that both GNPs will continue to grow at these rates of growth, when will Japan's GNP surpass the GNP of the Soviet Union?

Solution The GNPs of the two countries are described by the following exponential functions:

Japan:	$J(n) = 1.204(1.0485)^n$	(trillions of dollars)
Soviet Union:	$S(n) = 1.843(1.0220)^n$	(trillions of dollars)

where n is the number of years measured from 1986 ($n = 0$ means 1986, $n = 1$ means 1987, and so on). Although n is generally thought to be 0, 1, 2, . . . , we will allow it to be any nonnegative real number. In this way we will be able to interpret a GNP after a fractional number of years (0.5 year, 4.7 years, and so on). These curves are shown in Figure 11.

It is clear that if the present growth rates continue, Japan's GNP will eventually surpass the GNP of the Soviet Union. By examining the curves in Figure 11 it appears that this will happen after roughly 16 or 17 years. To find a better estimate of when the two GNPs intersect, we can solve for n in the equation $J(n) = S(n)$. Doing this, we have

$$1.204(1.0485)^n = 1.843(1.022)^n$$

Moving the quantities involving n to the left-hand side of the equation, we have

$$\frac{(1.0485)^n}{(1.022)^n} = \frac{1.843}{1.204} = 1.531$$

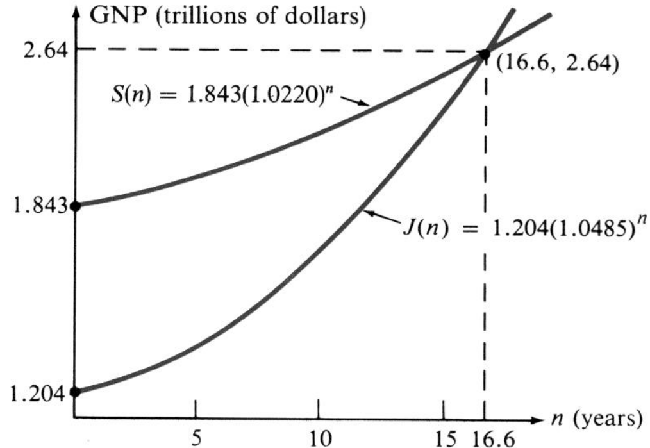

Figure 11
Forecasts of GNPs of Japan and the Soviet Union

Using the property $a^n/b^n = (a/b)^n$ and simplifying, we see

$$(1.026)^n = 1.531$$

Finally, taking the common logarithm of each side of this equation, we have

$$n \log 1.026 = \log 1.531$$

or

$$n = \frac{\log 1.531}{\log 1.026}$$

$$\cong 16.6 \text{ years}$$

If the GNPs of Japan and the Soviet Union continue to grow exponentially at the current rate, then sometime between January 1, 2002, and January 1, 2003, Japan will have the second largest GNP, behind the United States. □

Logarithmic Scales (the Richter Scale)

One of the important uses of the logarithm is in describing phenomena whose measurements are very large, are very small, or range over large intervals. Since logarithms are essentially exponents, their values do not become as large or as small as quickly as other quantities. Observe how the logarithms in the column back in Table 11 do not vary as much as their arguments.

To understand how logarithms are applied in science, we show how the logarithm is used to define the **Richter scale** in seismology. We will see that adding one unit on the Richter (logarithm) scale corresponds to multiplying the seismic activity by ten units. Hence a change of 3 on the Richter scale corresponds to a factor of 1000 in seismic activity.

The energy released by an earthquake at the epicenter is generally measured in units called ergs. In a good-sized quake the energy released might be somewhere around

$$100{,}000{,}000{,}000{,}000{,}000{,}000 \text{ ergs}$$

Since it is difficult to work with numbers of this tremendous size, seismologists use the Richter scale. Imagine the headline

Earthquake Measuring 34,468,346,012,438,547,983 Ergs
Hits Los Angeles!

For this reason, earthquakes are always reported in units R "on the Richter scale" with R defined as

$$R = 0.67 \log E - 7.9 \qquad \text{(Richter scale)}$$

where E is the energy in ergs released by the quake. We illustrate the Richter scale with a few examples.

Example 8

Richter Scale The devastating Mexico City earthquake of 1985 released roughly 4×10^{24} ergs of energy. What was the magnitude of this quake on the Richter scale?

Solution

$$\begin{aligned} R &= 0.67 \log (4 \times 10^{24}) - 7.9 \\ &= 0.67(\log 4 + 24 \log 10) - 7.9 \\ &\cong 0.67(0.60 + 24) - 7.9 \\ &= 8.6 \end{aligned}$$

□

Table 12 shows the effects of various size quakes. Since the Richter scale is a logarithmic scale with base 10, an increase of 1 on the Richter scale represents a tenfold increase in energy released by the quake. Hence an earthquake that measures 8.6 on the Richter scale is 1000 times more powerful than one that measures 5.6 on the Richter scale.

TABLE 12
Types of Earthquakes on the Richter Scale

Magnitude (Richter Scale)	Result at Epicenter	Number per Year
1.0–1.9	Detectable only on a seismograph	Many
2.0–2.9	Noticeable by a few people	800,000
3.0–3.9	Felt by most people, no cause for alarm	20,000
4.0–4.9	Felt by all, some glass broken	2,800
5.0–5.9	Some furniture turned over	1,000
6.0–6.9	Ground cracks, some buildings fall	185
7.0–7.9	Bridges and dams fall	14
8.0+	Disaster on a massive scale, the worst	0.2

Example 9

Energy Released by an Earthquake In 1976 a devastating earthquake measuring 8.9 on the Richter scale struck Guatemala, killing 23,000 people. How much energy was released by that earthquake?

Solution Setting

$$0.67 \log E - 7.9 = 8.9$$

we solve for E. We get

$$\log E = 25.07$$

or

$$E = 10^{25.07} \cong 1.175 \times 10^{25} \text{ ergs}$$

□

Problems

For Problems 1–14, use $\log 5 = 0.70$ and $\log 7 = 0.85$ to determine the numerical value of the expressions.

1. $\log 35$
2. $\log\left(\frac{5}{7}\right)$
3. $\log \sqrt[8]{35}$
4. $\log \sqrt[3]{5}$
5. $\log(0.2)$
6. $\log\left(\frac{125}{49}\right)$
7. $\log(5^4 \cdot 7^5)$
8. $\log \sqrt[5]{7 \cdot 25}$
9. $\log 125$
10. $\log\left(\frac{625}{49}\right)^{10}$
11. $\log \sqrt{5^8 \cdot 7^3}$
12. $\log(1/\sqrt{5^8 \cdot 7^3})$
13. $\log\left(\frac{49}{5}\right)$
14. $\log \sqrt[5]{7^{10}/5^6}$

For Problems 15–20, simplify and/or expand the expressions.

15. $e^{\ln 3 - \ln 4}$
16. $e^{4 \ln 2}$
17. $4^{\log_2 3}$
18. $\log(rt/5)$
19. $\log(e^3/a)$
20. $\log\left[\dfrac{x^2(x+3)}{x+1}\right]$

For Problems 21–36, solve for x.

21. $\log x = 3 \log 2 + 2 \log 3$
22. $\log x = \log 2 - \log 3 + \log 5 - \log 7$
23. $\log \sqrt{x} = 4 \log 2 - 3 \log\left(\frac{1}{2}\right)$
24. $x = \log_2 4$
25. $x = \log_6 36 \log_{25}\left(\frac{1}{5}\right)$
26. $\log x + \log x^2 = 3$
27. $\ln x^2 - \ln x = \ln 18 - \ln 6$
28. $\ln x^2 = 2$
29. $\log_x \dfrac{9}{4} = 2$
30. $\log_3 x^2 - \log_3 x = \log_3 18 - \log_3 6$
31. $\log_4(3x + 5) = \log_4 72 - 3 \log_4 2$
32. $10^{x^2} = 150$
33. $2^{x+1} = 10^{2x}$
34. $3^{4x} = 5^{x+1}$
35. $5^{3x} = 6^{x-1}$
36. $10^x - 2 \cdot 10^{-x} = 1$

Exponential Functions in Finance

37. **Doubling Time for Annual Compounding.** Henry's father and mother have deposited \$1000 in a bank account in his name. The bank pays interest at a rate of 10.5% compounded annually. How long will it take for this account to double in value?
38. **General Doubling Time for Annual Compounding.** How long will it take for a bank account to double in value if the bank pays an annual interest rate of r, compounded annually? How long will it take for this account to triple in value?
39. **Doubling Time for Continuous Compounding.** Sally's father and mother have deposited \$1000 in a bank account in her name. The bank pays an annual interest rate of 10.5% compounded continuously. How long will it take for this account to double in value? Note the difference between this answer and the answer to Problem 37.
40. **General Doubling Time for Continuous Compounding.** How long will it take for a bank account to double in value if the bank pays an annual interest rate of r compounded continuously? How long will it take for this account to triple in value?
41. **Business Growth.** A franchised car repair outlet has $N(t)$ outlets and is expanding this number at the rate of 15% per year compounded continuously. The function that describes this number is

$$N(t) = N_0 e^{0.15t}$$

where t is time measured in years and N_0 is the initial number of franchises. How long will it take for the number of franchises to double? To triple?

42. **How Much Interest Does the Bank Pay?** Suppose you deposited \$100 in a bank that compounds interest continuously, but you forgot to ask the annual interest rate. All you know is that your deposit of \$100 today will be worth \$150 in five years. What is the annual rate of interest that this bank pays?
43. **How Much Interest Does the Bank Pay?** Another bank down the street from the one in Problem 42 also pays compound interest, but this bank compounds interest only every year. Suppose this banker tells you that if you deposit \$100 in the bank today, the deposit will be worth \$175 in six years. How much annual interest does this bank pay?

Brother Can You Spare a Dollar?

What could you buy with a dollar 15 years ago, and what can you buy today for the same dollar? Table 13 compares the value of the dollar in 1988 with the value of the dollar in 1973. For Problems 44–52, find the annual rate of increase r of each product. Assume that the price of each product has increased exponentially according to

$$F = Pe^{rt}$$

where

F = 1988 price

P = 1973 price

r = annual rate of increase

t = time elapsed (years)

44. New house
45. Zenith color TV
46. Texas Instruments calculator
47. Top model new car
48. Round-trip airfare from New York to Los Angeles
49. David Bowie concert
50. Iowa-Illinois football game
51. Big Mac/shake/fries
52. Calculus textbook

TABLE 13
Comparing Prices 1973–1988

Product	**1973**	**1988**	**Percent Change**
The Home and What's Inside			
New house, median price	\$27,500	\$110,000	294%
Zenith color TV	\$499	\$480	−8%
Texas Instruments calculator	\$150	\$10	−93%
Getting Around			
Car (top model)	\$3,700	\$11,800	219%
Round-trip airfare from New York to Los Angeles	\$236	\$1,090	231%
Things to Do			
David Bowie concert	\$6.50	\$21	223%
Iowa-Illinois football game	\$7.00	\$20	185%
Let's Eat			
McDonald's Big Mac/shake/fries	\$1.50	\$2.89	175%
Coca-Cola (6-pack/12-ounce)	\$0.79	\$1.69	114%
Textbooks			
Calculus textbook	\$15	\$40	167%

Social Sciences

53. Is Your Brain Linear, Exponential, or Logarithmic? Curves that describe some kind of learning process over time are called learning curves. Study a photograph of some kind for 30 seconds. Then put it aside and list as many items as you can from the photograph. Wait 5 minutes and repeat the process. Repeat the process a total of five times. Plot the number of items you remembered on each turn versus time. Does your learning curve appear to be linear, exponential, or logarithmic (or none)?

54. Population Growth. In 1988 the population of a certain city was one million people and was increasing at the rate of 4% per year. When will the population of this city reach 1.5 million people?

55. How Fast Do They Walk in Boston? In 1976, Marc and Helen Bornstein systematically observed the time it took pedestrians to walk 50 ft on the main streets of various cities and towns.* They found that in a city with a population of p the average velocity v (in feet per second) that a

* This problem is based on the UMAP Unit 551 module, *The Pace of Life: An Introduction to Empirical Model Fitting* by Bruce King.

person walks can be estimated by the logarithmic function

$$v(p) = 0.86\log p + 0.04$$

(a) Sketch the graph of this "velocity function" $v(p)$ for cities and towns having populations between 100 and 8,000,000.
(b) What is the estimated average walking speed for pedestrians in Boston (population 570,000)
(c) What is the estimated average walking speed for pedestrians in Ayrshire, Iowa (population 315)?

56. **Predicting City Size from Walking Speed.** The equation in Problem 55 can be turned around and solved for the population p in terms of v, giving

$$p(v) = 0.9(14.5)^v$$

(a) Verify this equation for $p(v)$.
(b) The average walking speed for pedestrians in a certain Illinois city is 5.6 ft/sec. What is the size of the city? What is the city? *Hint:* It starts with the letter C.
(c) In a certain town the average pedestrian walks at 2.62 ft/sec. What is the estimated size of this town?

57. **Drinking and Driving.** After a person drinks an alcoholic beverage, the alcohol level $L(t)$ in the person's blood rises to a level of 0.3 mg of alcohol per milliliter of blood. After that time, the amount of alcohol decreases exponentially according to the law

$$L(t) = 0.3(0.5)^t$$

where t is time measured in hours from the time when the peak level was reached. Sketch a graph of the function $L(t)$. If the legal driving limit of alcohol is 0.1 mg of alcohol per milliliter of blood, how long will it be until a person will be able to legally drive?

58. **Surface Area of the Body.** Biologists have found an equation that approximates the surface area S in square feet of the human body in terms of the height h and weight w of the body. The equation is

$$S = 0.1w^{0.425}h^{0.725}$$

where w is a person's weight in pounds and h is a person's height in inches. Approximate the surface area of your own body by substituting your height and weight in the above equation. Rewrite this equation in terms of log S.

59. **Exponential Learning Curve.** Rita is in charge of employee development at a shoe factory. Using her new training methods, she has discovered that the number of shoes that an average new employee can stitch in a day is given by the learning curve

$$L(t) = 25(1 - e^{-0.125t})$$

where t is number of days the employee has been on the job. How many days will it take before the average new employee can stitch 20 shoes per day? Graph the learning curve.

60. **Biological Growth.** The mass in grams of a given bacteria culture grows according to the logistic growth model of the type

$$y(t) = \frac{8}{1 + 7(2^{-t})}$$

where t is time measured in days. (See Figure 12.) When will the mass of the culture reach 7 grams?

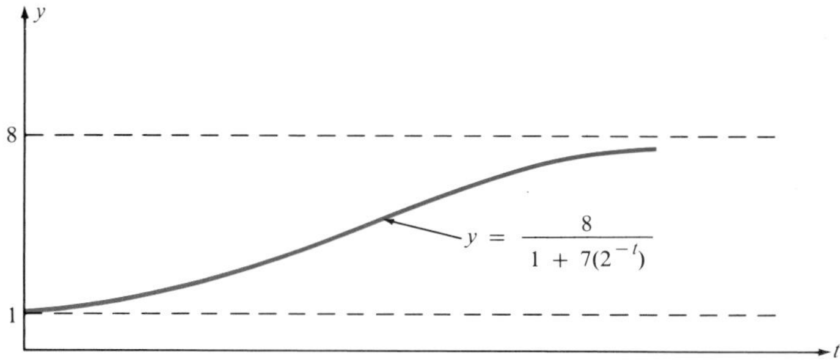

Figure 12
Graph for Problem 60

61. **Logarithmic Production Curve.** The price $P(x)$ of an item depends on the number of units x produced. For the price function

$$P(x) = \log\left(10 + \frac{x}{4}\right)$$

how many units will be produced at a price of \$3?

62. **Hydrogen Ion Concentration.** The acidity of a substance is measured by the concentration (measured in moles per liter) of hydrogen ions (H^+) in the substance. The standard way to describe this concentration is to define the pH of a substance as the negative logarithm of the hydrogen ion concentration. That is,

$$\text{pH} = -\log[H^+]$$

What is the pH of distilled water if its hydrogen ion concentration is 10^{-7} mole/liter?

63. **Hydrogen Ion Concentration.** A substance with pH smaller than 7 is termed an acid, and a substance with pH greater than 7 is called a base. Using the formula in Problem 62, determine the pH for the substances whose hydrogen ion concentrations are given below, and indicate whether they are acids or bases.
    (a) 4.2×10^{-6}
    (b) 8×10^{-6}
    (c) 0.6×10^{-7}
    (d) 6.3×10^{-4} (grapefruit juice)

Decibels

A decibel is a unit of relative loudness. One decibel is the smallest unit of sound detected by the human ear. If x denotes the intensity of a sound wave (measured in watts per square centimeter), then the noise level $L(x)$ in decibels of the wave is given by

$$L(x) = 10 \log\left(\frac{x}{I_0}\right)$$

where I_0 is the intensity of the sound wave at the threshold of audibility (approximately 10^{-16} watt of energy per square centimeter). Use this formula to solve Problems 64–67.

64. What are the noise levels $L(x)$ in decibels for the following intensities x:
    (a) 1000 watts per square centimeter
    (b) 5000 watts per square centimeter
    (c) 10,000 watts per square centimeter
65. The noise level of a whisper is about 20 decibels, and that of ordinary conversation about 65 decibels. Determine the ratio of the intensity of a conversation to the intensity of a whisper.
66. How many decibels are the following phenomena, if they have the following energy levels:
    (a) A motor with an intensity of 10^{-11} watt/square cm
    (b) A typewriter with an intensity of 10^{-4} watt/square cm
    (c) A jet engine with an intensity of 10^{-2} watt/square cm
    (d) A jet with afterburner with an intensity of 10^{-1} watt/square cm
67. What is the difference in the noise levels of two sounds, one of which is 1000 times the intensity of the other?

3.3 Differentiation of Exponential Functions

PURPOSE

We show the role that exponential functions play in the calculus. The major topics introduced are

- how to write b^x in terms of e^{kx},
- how to differentiate e^{kx},
- how to differentiate $e^{g(x)}$, and
- how to differentiate $b^{g(x)}$.

We then introduce the economic concept of discounting and determine the optimal time for a timber company to harvest trees.

Introduction

We have seen that the exponential growth curve

$$G(t) = Ae^{kt} \qquad (k > 0)$$

describes numerous growth phenomena in economics, biology, botany, physics, and other areas. In this section we will learn a remarkable fact about this curve, namely, that the rate of change dG/dt is proportional to the value G. That is,

$$\frac{dG(t)}{dt} = kG(t)$$

The reason that many phenomena obey such a law is that it is the way populations grow. In many insect populations, for example, the population size increases as a result of random mating between insects. That is, the larger the population, the larger the growth becomes (more insects, more mating). Hence we have the phenomenon that the rate of growth is proportional to the size of the population.

Since we will learn how to differentiate the exponential function e^{kx}, we first learn how to rewrite other exponential functions b^x in terms of e^{kx}. In that way we will be able to differentiate them as well.

Rewriting All Exponential Functions b^x in Terms of e^{kx}

Earlier, when we studied exponential growth and decay phenomena, we introduced various exponential functions such as 2^x, $(1.03)^n$, and $(\frac{1}{2})^x$. The interesting thing about these functions is that they can be rewritten in terms of e^{kx}. In this way, all exponential growth and decay phenomena can be restated in terms of the one basic function e^{kx}. Since the independent variable in the following discussion does not necessarily stand for time, we use x instead of t to represent the independent variable.

Rewriting b^x in Terms of e^{kx}

If b is a positive real number and $k = \ln b$, then for any real number x we have

$$b^x = e^{kx}$$

Verification: Using properties of the logarithm, we have

$$\begin{aligned} b^x &= e^{\ln b^x} && \text{(Property 6 of logarithms)} \\ &= e^{x \ln b} && \text{(Property 3 of logarithms)} \\ &= e^{kx} && \text{(definition of } k) \end{aligned}$$

Example 1

Rewriting Exponentials Rewrite the exponential functions 2^x, 3^x, $(0.5)^x$, $(0.8)^x$ in terms of e^{kx}.

Solution Using the basic equation $b^x = e^{(\ln b)x}$, we have

$$\begin{aligned} 2^x &= e^{(\ln 2)x} \cong e^{0.69x} && (b = 2,\ k = 0.69) \\ 3^x &= e^{(\ln 3)x} \cong e^{1.1x} && (b = 3,\ k = 1.1) \\ (0.5)^x &= e^{x \ln 0.5} \cong e^{-0.69x} && (b = 0.5,\ k = -0.69) \\ (0.8)^x &= e^{x \ln 0.8} \cong e^{-0.22x} && (b = 0.8,\ k = -0.22) \end{aligned}$$

The graphs of these exponential functions are shown in Figure 13. □

The Derivative of e^{kx}

Since we have seen how the exponential function b^x can be expressed in terms of e^{kx}, it is important we know how to differentiate e^{kx}. In this way we will be able to differentiate the exponential function b^x as well. We begin by stating the derivative of e^x.

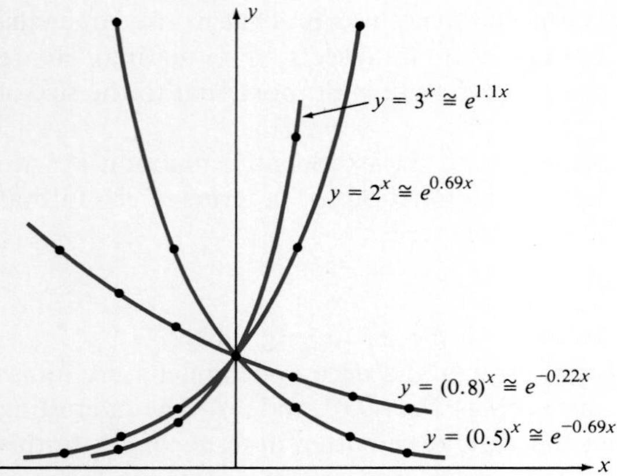

Figure 13
Rewriting exponential functions

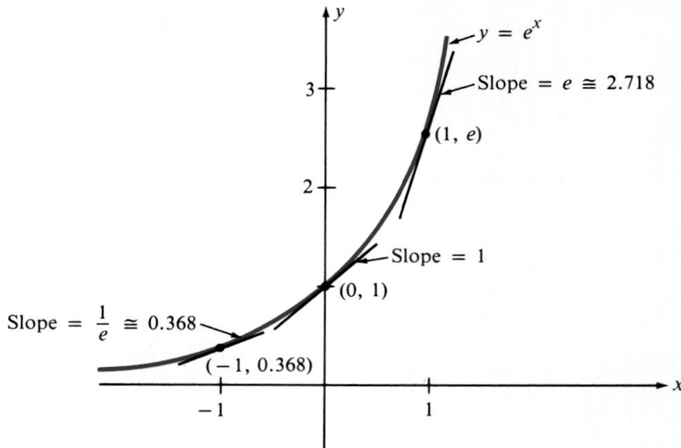

Figure 14
The slope of the tangent line is equal to the height of the graph for $y = e^x$

A Function Whose Derivative Is the Same as the Function

The exponential function e^x has a property that no other function possesses (except for constant multiples Ce^x): The derivative is equal to the function itself. That is,

$$\frac{d}{dx} e^x = e^x$$

Although we will not prove this fact here, the graph shown in Figure 14 illustrates the basic idea. Note that the slope of the tangent line to the graph of $y = e^x$ is always the same as the height of the graph of $y = e^x$.

We now state a number of useful derivatives involving exponential functions.

Summary of Useful Exponential Derivatives

By use of the basic derivative formula $de^x/dx = e^x$ along with the chain rule, we can find the derivative of several other exponential functions. We have the following rules:

$$\frac{d}{dx} e^{g(x)} = e^{g(x)}g'(x) \qquad \text{(general exponential)}$$

$$\frac{d}{dt} e^{kt} = ke^{kt} \qquad \text{(derivative of growth curve)}$$

$$\frac{d}{dt} e^{-kt} = -ke^{-kt} \qquad \text{(derivative of decay curve)}$$

The first rule above for differentiating the general exponential function can easily be remembered by simply realizing that it says

$$\frac{d}{dx}e^{(\text{exponent})} = e^{(\text{exponent})}\frac{d}{dx}(\text{exponent})$$

Example 2

Differentiating Exponentials Find y' if

$$y = e^{(x^2 + 2x)}$$

Solution Here

$$g(x) = x^2 + 2x$$
$$g'(x) = 2x + 2$$

Using the rule for differentiating general exponents, we have

$$\begin{aligned} y' &= e^{g(x)}g'(x) \\ &= (2x + 2)e^{x^2 + 2x} \end{aligned}$$

□

Example 3

Differentiating Exponentials Find y' if

$$y = e^{1/x}$$

Solution Here

$$g(x) = \frac{1}{x}$$

$$g'(x) = -\frac{1}{x^2}$$

Using the rule for differentiating general exponents, we have

$$\begin{aligned} y' &= e^{g(x)}g'(x) \\ &= -\frac{1}{x^2}e^{1/x} \end{aligned}$$

□

Example 4

Differentiating a Growth Curve Find the derivative of the growth curve

$$y(t) = 30e^{0.05t}$$

Solution Using the rule for exponential derivatives, we have

$$\begin{aligned} \frac{dy}{dt} &= 30\frac{d}{dt}e^{0.05t} \\ &= (30)(0.05)e^{0.05t} \\ &= 1.5e^{0.05t} \end{aligned}$$

See Figure 15.

□

Example 5

Differentiating a Decay Curve Find the derivative of the decay curve

$$y(t) = 100e^{-0.25t}$$

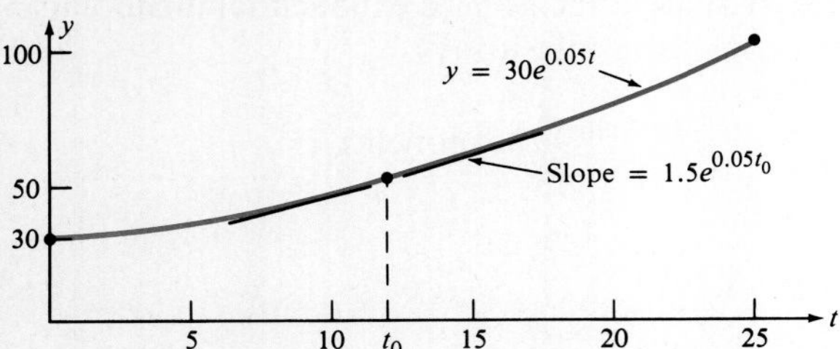

Figure 15
Derivative of an exponential curve

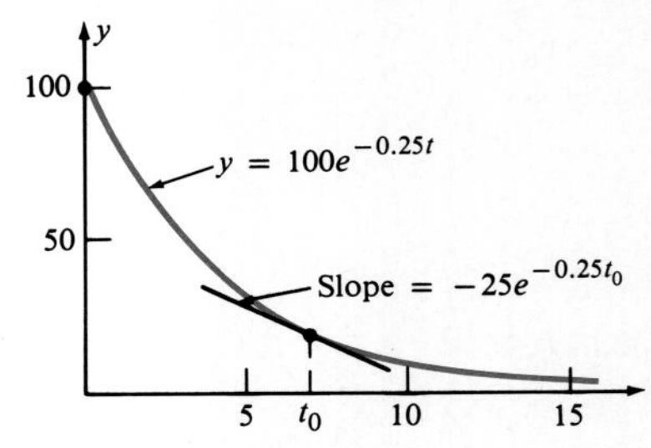

Figure 16
Derivative of a negative exponential curve

Solution Using the rule for exponential derivatives, we have

$$\begin{aligned}\frac{dy}{dt} &= 100\frac{d}{dt}e^{-0.25t}\\ &= (100)(-0.25)e^{-0.25t}\\ &= -25e^{-0.25t}\end{aligned}$$

See Figure 16. □

The Derivative of b^x

Since we now know how to write the exponential b^x for any base b in terms of e^{kx} by means of the formula

$$b^x = e^{(\ln b)x}$$

we can also differentiate b^x.

The Derivative of b^x

If b is any positive number, then the derivative of b^x is

$$\frac{d}{dx}b^x = (\ln b)b^x$$

Verification

Since b^x can be written

$$b^x = e^{(\ln b)x}$$

we have that

$$\begin{aligned}\frac{d}{dx}b^x &= \frac{d}{dx}e^{(\ln b)x}\\ &= (\ln b)e^{(\ln b)x}\\ &= (\ln b)b^x\end{aligned}$$

This completes the verification.

The derivative we have just derived leads naturally to the following more general formula.

General Derivative for Exponential Function with Base b

Using the above derivative and the chain rule, we can state the more general rule

$$\frac{d}{dx} b^{g(x)} = b^{g(x)} \cdot g'(x) \cdot \ln b$$

Example 6

Differentiating Exponentials with Base 2 Find y' if

$$y = 2^x$$

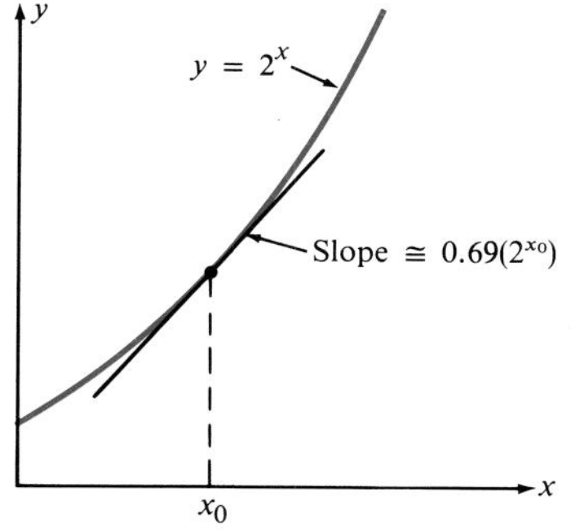

Figure 17
Derivative of 2^x

Solution We have

$$b = 2$$
$$g(x) = x$$
$$g'(x) = 1$$

Using the rule for finding the derivative of $b^{g(x)}$ gives

$$\frac{d}{dx} 2^x = b^{g(x)} \cdot g'(x) \cdot \ln b$$
$$= 2^x \cdot \ln 2$$
$$\cong 0.69(2^x)$$

See Figure 17. □

Example 7

Differentiating Exponentials Find y' if

$$y = 2^{(x^2+1)}$$

Solution We have

$$b = 2$$
$$g(x) = x^2 + 1$$
$$g'(x) = 2x$$

Using the rule for finding the derivative of $b^{g(x)}$ gives

$$\frac{d}{dx} 2^{(x^2+1)} = 2^{(x^2+1)} \cdot 2x \cdot \ln 2$$ □

Example 8

Derivative of Exponentials Find y' if

$$y = 3^{4x}$$

Solution Here

$$b = 3$$
$$g(x) = 4x$$
$$g'(x) = 4$$

Using the rule for finding the derivative of $b^{g(x)}$ gives

$$\frac{d}{dx} 3^{4x} = 3^{4x} \cdot 4 \cdot \ln 3$$
$$\cong 4.39(3^{4x})$$ □

Example 9

Tangent Line to the Exponential Curve Find the tangent line to the curve

$$y = e^x$$

at the point $(1, e)$.

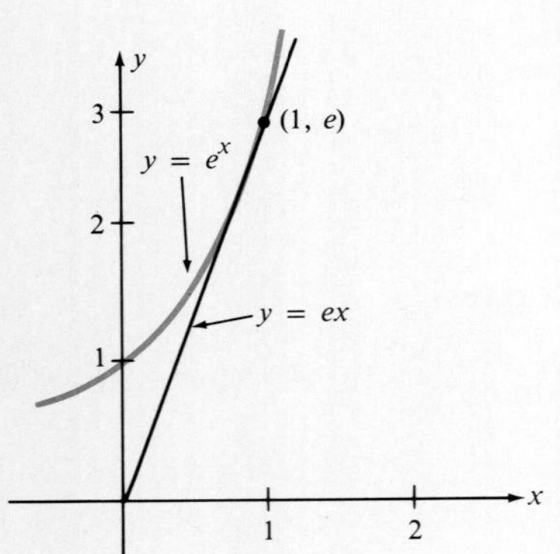

Figure 18
Tangent line to e^x at $(1, e)$

Solution The tangent line to a curve $y = f(x)$ at a point $(a, f(a))$ is given by

$$y - f(a) = f'(a)(x - a)$$

Since

$$\frac{d}{dx} e^x = e^x$$

we have $f(1) = e$, and $f'(1) = e$. Hence the tangent line will be

$$y - e = e(x - 1)$$

or

$$y = ex$$
$$\cong 2.718x$$

See Figure 18. □

Discounting in Economics

In the problem of continuous compounding of interest the goal is to find the future value F from a given present value P. The problem of discounting is the opposite one. In such cases we seek to find the present value P of a given amount F that will be available t years from now. In the case of continuous compounding, an initial principal P will grow to a future value F of

$$F = Pe^{rt}$$

where r is the annual rate of interest. We can also find the corresponding **discount formula** simply by solving for the present value P in terms of the future value F

$$P = Fe^{-rt}$$

The above value of P is called the **discounted value** (or present value) of F; and in this new context, r is often called the **discount rate**. This negative exponential illustrates the fact that if someone were to give you F dollars t years from now, then the value of this money today is only Fe^{-rt} (assuming that money can earn interest at a rate r, compounded continuously). Figure 19 gives the discounted value (or present value) of \$1000 over a 100-year period for various interest rates. The moral of this table is that the value of \$1000 today is not the same as the value of \$1000 in 100 years.

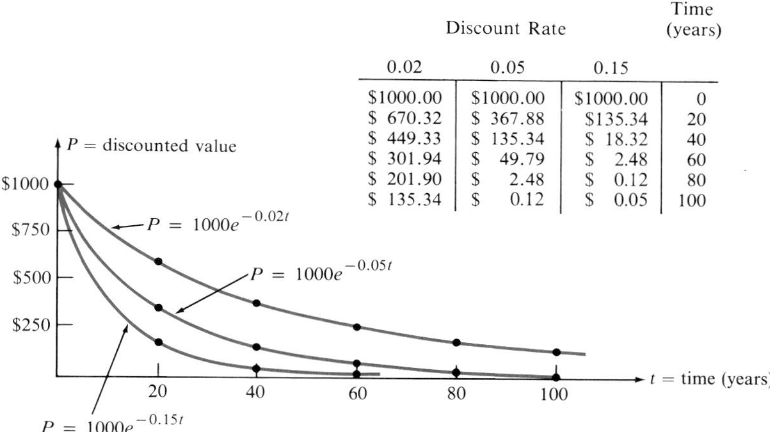

Discount Rate 0.02	0.05	0.15	Time (years)
\$1000.00	\$1000.00	\$1000.00	0
\$ 670.32	\$ 367.88	\$135.34	20
\$ 449.33	\$ 135.34	\$ 18.32	40
\$ 301.94	\$ 49.79	\$ 2.48	60
\$ 201.90	\$ 2.48	\$ 0.12	80
\$ 135.34	\$ 0.12	\$ 0.05	100

Figure 19
Discounted value of \$1000 over 100 years

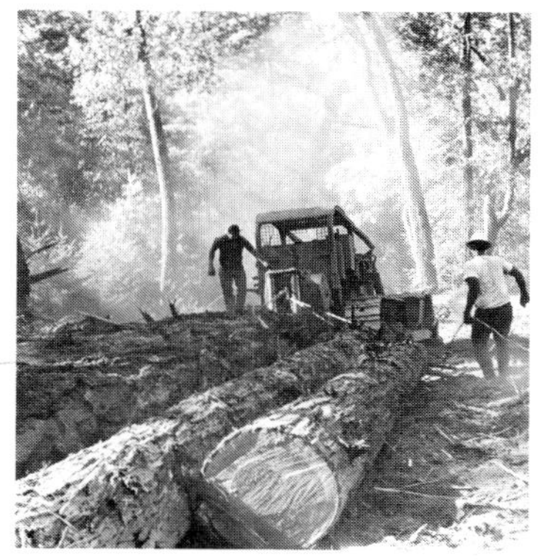

To determine the future value of a product in today's money, economists use a concept known as discounting

Discounting in the Wood Products Industry

To understand the importance of discounting in business management, consider the problem facing a large wood products company in the state of Washington. The company has just planted hybrid tree seedlings on several tracts of land and has determined that the value $V(t)$ of this timber (in millions of dollars) is increasing over time according to the exponential function

$$V(t) = e^{\sqrt{t}}$$

where t is time in years measured from the date the trees were planted. Assuming the world's financial situation to be such that money is discounted at a rate of 8% per year (\$1 today will be worth $\$1e^{0.08t}$ in t years), when should the company cut the timber for maximum revenue? We assume the cost to maintain the trees is negligible in comparison to the value of the trees, and so to maximize the revenue is actually the same as to maximize the profit.

To solve this problem, we proceed as follows. At each future point in time the value of the timber is given by

$$V(t) = e^{\sqrt{t}}$$

However, we must keep in mind that the value $V(t)$ is measured in tomorrow's dollars (the company is paid when the timber is harvested). Hence the present or discounted value P of the timber in today's dollars if the timber is harvested after t years is

$$\begin{aligned} P(t) &= V(t)e^{-0.08t} \qquad \text{(present value)} \\ &= e^{\sqrt{t}}e^{-0.08t} \\ &= e^{\sqrt{t}-0.08t} \end{aligned}$$

The problem now is to find the maximum value of $P(t)$. To do this, we begin by finding the derivative $P'(t)$. Calling

$$g(t) = \sqrt{t} - 0.08t$$

$$g'(t) = \frac{1}{2\sqrt{t}} - 0.08$$

we have

$$\begin{aligned}\frac{d}{dt}P(t) &= \frac{d}{dt}e^{g(t)}\\ &= e^{g(t)}g'(t)\\ &= e^{(\sqrt{t}-0.08t)}\left(\frac{1}{2\sqrt{t}} - 0.08\right)\end{aligned}$$

Setting the derivative to zero to find the critical points, we have

$$e^{(\sqrt{t}-0.08t)}\left(\frac{1}{2\sqrt{t}} - 0.08\right) = 0$$

Since the exponential function on the left is never zero, we have that

$$\frac{1}{2\sqrt{t}} - 0.08 = 0$$

Solving this equation for t gives

$$\sqrt{t} = \frac{1}{(2)(0.08)}$$

$$t = \frac{1}{(4)(0.08)^2} \cong 39 \quad \text{years}$$

Although we have not formally shown that $P(t)$ attains a relative maximum or even its absolute maximum value at this critical point, it is not hard to do so.

Interpretation of the Tree-Harvesting Problem

The company should harvest the trees 39 years after planting to maximize the profit. If this strategy is followed, then the value of the trees in today's dollars, immediately after planting, will be

$$\begin{aligned}P(39) &= e^{\sqrt{39}-(0.08)(39)}\\ &\cong 22.76 \quad \text{million dollars}\end{aligned}$$

Of course, when the trees are harvested in 39 years, the value of the timber will be much more. In fact the value received at that time will be

$$\begin{aligned}V(39) &= e^{\sqrt{39}}\\ &\cong 515.43 \quad \text{million dollars}\end{aligned}$$

This value is the same amount of money the company would have after 39 years if it sold the newly planted timber today for 22.76 million and invested the money in a bank that paid 8% annual interest, compounded continuously.

It is also interesting to note from the above equation for $P(t)$ that if the annual discount rate were r instead of 0.08, then the time the company should harvest their trees would be given by

$$t = \frac{1}{4r^2} \text{ years}$$

Table 14 gives the time when the company should harvest their trees as a function of the discount rate r. The discount rate is often reasonably close to the annual inflation rate.

TABLE 14
When to Harvest Timber Given the Discount Rate

Annual Discount Rate, r	Time to Harvest (years)
0.06	69
0.07	51
0.08	39
0.09	31
0.10	25
0.11	21
0.12	17

Problems

For Problems 1–10, write the exponential functions in the form e^{kx}.

1. 2^x **2.** 3^x
3. 4^x **4.** 8^x
5. $(1.5)^x$ **6.** $(0.7)^x$
7. $(0.9)^x$ **8.** 10^x
9. 100^x **10.** 500^x

For Problems 11–26, find the derivative of the expressions.

11. $y = 2e^{3x}$ **12.** $y = e^{-x}$
13. $y = e^{5x}$ **14.** $y = e^{-9x}$
15. $y = e^{x^2}$ **16.** $y = e^{x+2}$
17. $y = e^{\sqrt{x}}$ **18.** $y = xe^{2x}$
19. $y = \dfrac{e^x}{x}$ **20.** $y = x^2e^{3x}$
21. $y = e^{x^2+x}$ **22.** $y = x^2e^{-x^2}$
23. $y = e^x + e^{-x}$ **24.** $y = \sqrt{e^x + 1}$
25. $y = 2x - e^{4x} + 3e^{x^2}$ **26.** $y = \dfrac{1 + e^x}{x}$

For Problems 27–34, find the derivative of the functions.

27. $y = 5^x$ **28.** $y = 9^x$
29. $y = 2^x$ **30.** $y = 10^x$
31. $y = 2^{x^2}$ **32.** $y = 3^{x^2+1}$
33. $y = 9^{(2x+5)}$ **34.** $y = 10^{-x^2}$

Graphing Problems

35. Shape of e^x. Show that the graph of $y = e^x$ is concave up for all x.

36. Shape of e^{-x}. Is e^{-x} an increasing or decreasing function? Is the graph of e^{-x} concave up or concave down? Sketch the graph of e^{-x}.

37. Shape of 2^x. Show that the graph of $y = 2^x$ is always increasing. What is the concavity of the graph of $y = 2^x$?

38. Tangent Line. Find the equation of the tangent line to

$$y = 2e^{-3x}$$

at $x = 0$. Sketch the graph of the exponential curve and the tangent line at $x = 0$.

39. Tangent Line. Find the equation of the tangent line to

$$y = xe^x$$

at $x = 0$.

Business Management Problems

40. Marginal Revenue. The revenue R in dollars a manufacturer receives when q units of a product are sold is given by

$$R(q) = 0.75qe^{-0.002q}$$

What is the marginal revenue when $q = 100$?

41. **When to Sell Coins.** A coin and stamp dealer calculates that the value $V(t)$ in dollars that a collection will appreciate after t years is given by the formula

$$V(t) = \$1000e^{\sqrt{t/4}}$$

If the annual discount rate is 8%, when should the collection be sold to maximize the return?

42. **Sell No Wine Before Its Time.** A vintner can either sell wine at the present time or age it further for future sales. Suppose the value $V(t)$ of the wine in thousands of dollars is increasing according to the function

$$V(t) = e^{0.2\sqrt{t}}$$

where t is time in years. If the discount rate is 9% per year, when should the vintner sell the wine to maximize profit? We assume that it does not cost anything to store the wine and so profit and revenue are the same thing. What is the value of the wine in today's dollars if this strategy is used?

43. **Wine Problem.** Solve Problem 42 if the value of the wine grows according to the function

$$V(t) = 2^{\sqrt{t}}$$

44. **When to Sell Land.** A landowner owns a piece of property that is increasing in value according to the function

$$V(t) = 100{,}000e^{0.08t}$$

where V is measured in dollars and t is time measured in years. If the discount rate of money is 7% per year, when should the owner sell the land?

45. **Land Speculating.** Another landowner who lives next to the owner mentioned in Problem 44 knows the value of his land is increasing according to the function

$$V(t) = 50{,}000e^{0.06t}$$

where V is measured in dollars and t in years. Assuming the same discount rate of 7% per year, when should this owner sell the land?

46. **Learning Model.** The number of units $P(t)$ produced per day after t days of training is given by

$$P(t) = 150(1 - e^{-kt})$$

where k varies with the individual. Estimate k for an individual who produces 75 units per day after one day of training. Find the derivative $dP(t)/dt$ using this value for k. Find the rate at which $P(t)$ is increasing after five days of training for this individual.

Other Growth Models in Biology

47. **Logistic Growth Curve.** A biologist observes that the weight $w(t)$ of a colony of bacteria is growing according to the logistic growth curve

$$w(t) = \frac{500}{1 + 49e^{-kt}}$$

where t is time measured in days. Here the population starts to grow rapidly; but after some time, certain influences begin to restrict the rate of growth. Figure 20 shows the above logistic curve. Find the rate of change dw/dt of the size of this population of bacteria.

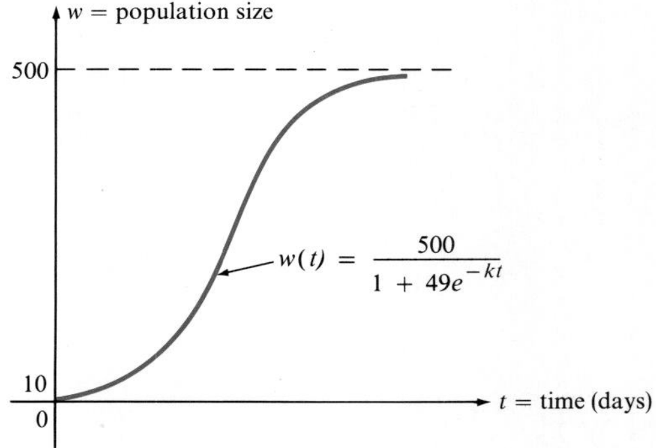

Figure 20
Graph for Problem 47

48. **Gompertz Growth Curve.** A biologist observes that the size of a population of yeast cells is growing according to the Gompertz growth curve

$$N(t) = 500e^{-e^{-0.05t}}$$

where t is time measured in days. (See Figure 21.) Find the rate of change dN/dt of the size of this population.

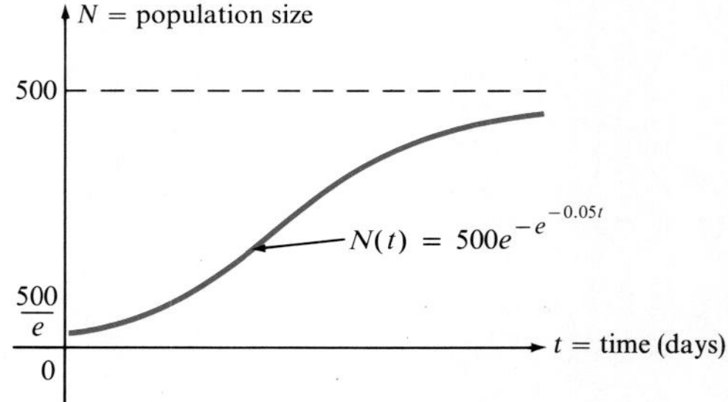

Figure 21
Graph for Problem 48

49. Von Bertalanffy Growth Curve. A biologist observes that the size of a certain virus culture is growing according to the Von Bertalanffy growth curve

$$N(t) = N_0(1 - be^{-kt})^3$$

where t is time measured in hours. (See Figure 22.) Find the rate of change dN/dt of this population.

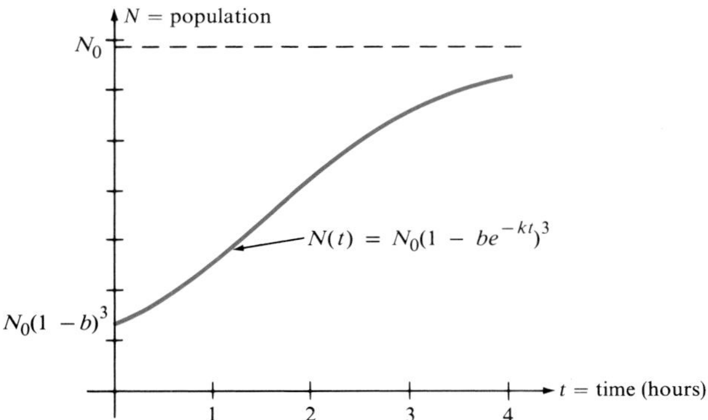

Figure 22
Graph for Problem 49

50. Drug Injection Physiology. The concentration of a drug in the blood that has been injected intramuscularly has been studied theoretically by E. Heinz. He has shown that the concentration y first increases for a given length of time and then decreases to zero. The equation that describes this phenomenon is

$$y = c(e^{-k_2 t} - e^{-k_1 t})$$

where c, k_2, and k_1 are positive constants with $k_2 > k_1$.
(a) Find the value of time when the drug will reach a maximum concentration in the blood?
(b) Graph the concentration curve when $c = 1$ and $k_2 = 2$, $k_1 = 1$. Do not worry about the units for the concentration y and time t.

51. Response of the Body to a Drug. A model used by medical researchers to predict the reaction of the body to a dose of a drug is

$$R(d) = d^2(A - Bd) \qquad 0 \le d \le \frac{A}{B}$$

where $A > 0$ and $B > 0$ are constants whose values depend on the individual and

R = strength of the reaction (such as blood pressure, pulse)
d = amount of drug injected into the body

(a) Find the dosage of the drug for which the reaction is a maximum.
(b) Find the dosage of the drug that maximizes the sensitivity. In other words, find d where $R'(d)$ is a maximum.
(c) Use the first and second derivatives of $R(d)$ to draw its graph when $A = B = 1$.

52. The Monomolecular Curve. The curve

$$W = \frac{W_0}{1 - b}(1 - be^{-kt})$$

is called the **monomolecular curve** in biochemistry because it describes monomolecular reactions.
(a) Find dW/dt.
(b) Find d^2W/dt^2.
(c) Use the information found in parts (a) and (b) to graph the monomolecular curve.

53. Holding Your Breath. When you hold your breath, carbon dioxide (CO_2) diffuses from the blood into the lungs. The curve that describes the pressure p of carbon dioxide in the lungs is given by

$$p(t) = a + be^{-kt}$$

where a, b, and k are positive constants whose values depend on the individual.
(a) Find dp/dt.
(b) Find d^2p/dt^2.
(c) Use the results of parts (a) and (b) to graph $p(t)$ when $a = b = 1$.

An Exponential Curve in Psychology

54. Smart Rat. One of the main uses of calculus in psychology lies in the area of learning theory. In an experiment measuring the intelligence of rats, Estes* designed an experiment in which he put a large rat in a so-called Skinner box. The rat was motivated by a 24-hour thirst, and the experiment was designed in such a way that the more times the rat pushed the "water" lever, the smarter the rat was. Estes was able to estimate the rat's "learning curve" (correct number of selections per minute over a given time period) by the equation

$$r(t) = \frac{13}{1 + 25e^{-0.24t}}$$

where

r = predicted number of correct selections per minute
t = time (min) that the experiment has elapsed.

(See Figure 23.)

* W. Estes, "Toward a Statistical Theory of Learning," *Psychological Review*, Vol. 87, pp. 94–107.

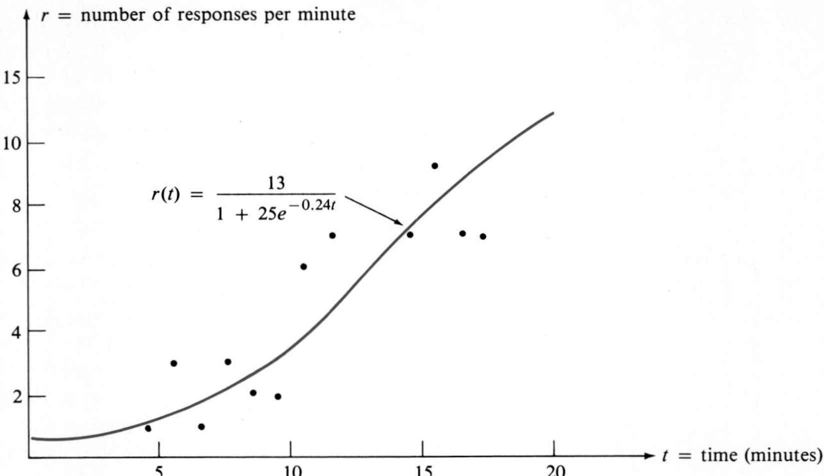

Figure 23
Graph of the theoretical learning curve approximating the observed data points

(a) Show that the learning curve $r(t)$ is always increasing.
(b) At what value of t is $r(t)$ increasing the fastest?
(c) What is the limiting value of $r(t)$ as t approaches infinity? What is the interpretation of this value?

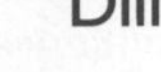

3.4 Differentiation of Logarithmic Functions

PURPOSE

We begin by learning how to differentiate the natural logarithm $\ln x$. After differentiating this basic logarithmic function, we then use the chain rule to differentiate other logarithmic functions, such as $\ln [g(x)]$. We also show how differential calculus is used to introduce the elasticity of the demand function.

Introduction

We have seen that the exponential function 2^x increases very rapidly (remember the paper-folding problem). In fact, all of the exponential functions e^x, 2^x, $3^x, \ldots$ are extremely fast-growing functions. On the other hand, the logarithmic functions $\log x$, $\ln x, \ldots$ are extremely slow-growing functions. They do approach infinity as the argument x gets large, but they do it very slowly. For example, the value of the common logarithm $y = \log x$ has reached only $y = 10$ by the time x has reached 10,000,000,000. We now investigate more than the size of the logarithmic functions. We study the rate of growth and the concavity of these functions.

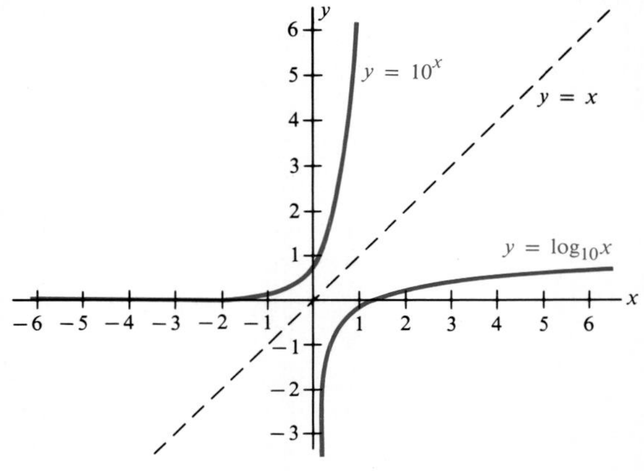

Figure 24
The common logarithm and its inverse function 10^x

Differentiation of the Natural Logarithm

One property of the logarithmic functions (provided that the base b is greater than 1) that can be seen in Figure 24 is that the graphs of the functions are always increasing and are always concave down. These observations lead us to believe that the first derivative is always positive and that the second derivative is always negative.

We begin by stating and verifying the derivative formula for the natural logarithm.

Derivative of ln x

The derivative of the natural logarithm is

$$\frac{d}{dx}\ln x = \frac{1}{x} \qquad (x > 0)$$

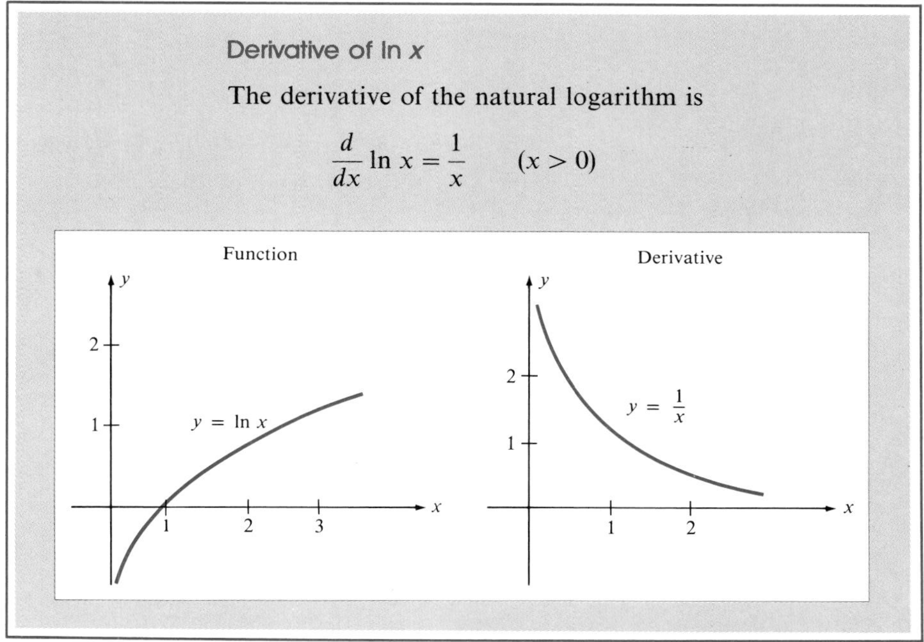

Verification of the Derivative of ln x

We start with the property of logarithms that states

$$e^{\ln x} = x \qquad (x > 0)$$

We now differentiate implicitly each side of this equation with respect to x. Doing this, we get

$$\frac{d}{dx}e^{\ln x} = \frac{dx}{dx}$$

By using the chain rule to find the derivative on the left, the above equation becomes

$$e^{\ln x}\frac{d}{dx}\ln x = 1$$

$$x\frac{d}{dx}\ln x = 1$$

Solving for the derivative

$$\frac{d}{dx} \ln x$$

gives

$$\frac{d}{dx} \ln x = \frac{1}{x}$$

This completes the verification.

Example 1

Differentiating Logarithms If

$$y = \ln x$$

(a) Find y' and y''.
(b) Determine the regions where $\ln x$ is increasing and where it is decreasing.
(c) Determine the regions where $\ln x$ is concave up and where it is concave down.

Solution

(a) Using the formula for the derivative of the natural logarithm, we have

$$y' = \frac{d}{dx} \ln x = \frac{1}{x} \qquad (x > 0)$$

$$y'' = \frac{d^2}{dx^2} \ln x = -\frac{1}{x^2} \qquad (x > 0)$$

(b) Since y' is always positive, we conclude that $\ln x$ is always increasing.
(c) Since y'' is always negative, we conclude that $\ln x$ is always concave down.

Figure 25 shows the derivative of the logarithm at various points. □

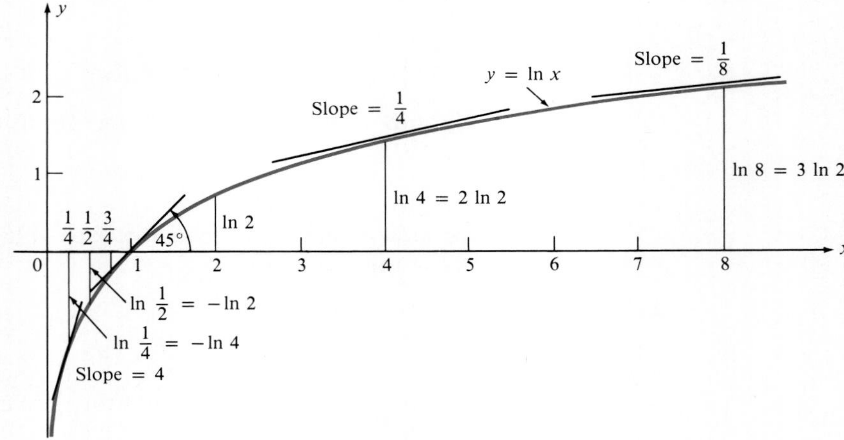

Figure 25
Slopes of the logarithm

Example 2

Differentiating Logarithms Find y' if

$$y = x \ln x \qquad (x > 0)$$

Solution Using the product rule, we have

$$\begin{aligned} y' &= x \frac{d}{dx} \ln x + \ln x \\ &= 1 + \ln x \end{aligned}$$

□

Example 3

Differentiating Logarithms Find y' if

$$y = (\ln x)^3 \qquad (x > 0)$$

Solution Let

$$g(x) = \ln x$$

and apply the generalized power rule

$$\frac{d}{dx} g(x)^n = ng(x)^{n-1} g'(x)$$

In this case we have

$$\begin{aligned} \frac{d}{dx} (\ln x)^3 &= 3(\ln x)^2 \frac{d}{dx} \ln x \\ &= \frac{3(\ln x)^2}{x} \end{aligned}$$

□

Example 4

Differentiating Logarithms Differentiate

$$y = \ln (x^2 + 3x + 5)$$

Solution Letting

$$u = x^2 + 3x + 5$$

we have

$$y = \ln u$$

Using the chain rule

$$\frac{dy}{dx} = \frac{dy}{du}\frac{du}{dx}$$

we can write

$$\frac{dy}{dx} = \frac{1}{u} \cdot (2x + 3)$$

Finally, substituting for u gives

$$\frac{d}{dx} \ln (x^2 + 3x + 5) = \frac{2x + 3}{x^2 + 3x + 5}$$

□

The Derivative of $y = \ln [g(x)]$

Example 4 suggests that we can differentiate the logarithmic function with a more general argument such as $g(x)$. Inasmuch as $\ln [g(x)]$ is the composition of the two functions $g(x)$ and $\ln x$, we can apply the chain rule and obtain the following derivative formula.

Formula for the Derivative of $y = \ln [g(x)]$

If $g(x)$ is differentiable and positive at the value x, then

$$\frac{d}{dx} \ln [g(x)] = \frac{g'(x)}{g(x)}$$

The above derivative formula can be stated verbally as

$$\frac{d}{dx} \ln [\text{argument}] = \frac{1}{(\text{argument})} \frac{d}{dx} (\text{argument})$$

If we select $g(x)$ as the absolute value function $g(x) = |x|$, then we get the formula

$$\frac{d}{dx} \ln |x| = \frac{\frac{d}{dx} |x|}{|x|} = \frac{1}{x} \qquad (x \neq 0)$$

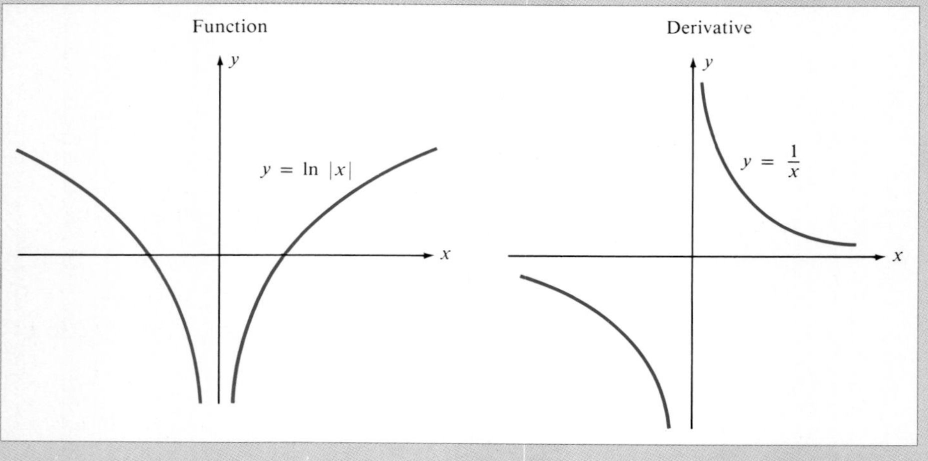

Example 5 Differentiation of Logarithms Find y' if

$$y = \ln x^2$$

Solution Here

$$g(x) = x^2$$
$$g'(x) = 2x$$

By use of the formula for the derivative of $\ln [g(x)]$ we get

$$\frac{dy}{dx} = \frac{g'(x)}{g(x)}$$
$$= \frac{2x}{x^2}$$
$$= \frac{2}{x}$$

□

Example 6 Differentiation of Logarithms Find y' if

$$y = \ln (e^x + x^2)$$

Solution Here

$$g(x) = e^x + x^2$$
$$g'(x) = e^x + 2x$$

Using the formula for the derivative of $\ln [g(x)]$, we have

$$\frac{dy}{dx} = \frac{g'(x)}{g(x)} = \frac{e^x + 2x}{e^x + x^2}$$

□

We now present a useful formula to show how other logarithms, in particular the common logarithm $\log x$, can be written in terms of the natural logarithm $\ln x$.

Change of Base Formula for Logarithms

The logarithms $\log_a x$ and $\log_b x$ with bases a and b are related by the **change of base formula**:

$$\log_b x = \frac{\log_a x}{\log_a b}$$

When the base a is the constant e and $b = 10$, then the change of base formula acts as a conversion formula from the natural to common logarithm

$$\log x = \frac{\ln x}{\ln 10} \cong 0.434 \ln x$$

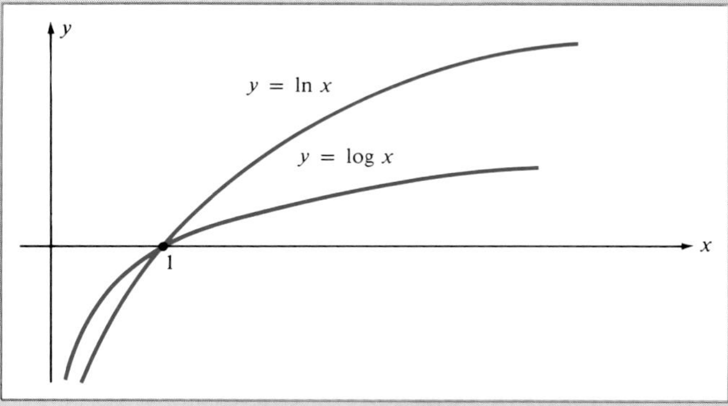

Example 7 Differentiation of the Common Logarithm Find y' if

$$y = \log (x^2 + 1)$$

Solution Rewriting the above common logarithm in terms of a natural logarithm, we have

$$\log(x^2 + 1) \cong 0.434 \ln(x^2 + 1)$$

Hence

$$\frac{d}{dx} \log(x^2 + 1) \cong 0.434 \frac{d}{dx} \ln(x^2 + 1)$$

$$= 0.434 \frac{2x}{x^2 + 1} \qquad \square$$

Elasticity of the Demand Function

Earlier, we studied the economic function known as the demand curve:

$$q = D(p) \qquad \text{(demand curve)}$$

This function gives the number of items q that consumers will buy at a given price p. As everyone knows, q will normally decrease as p increases. A typical demand function is shown in Figure 26.

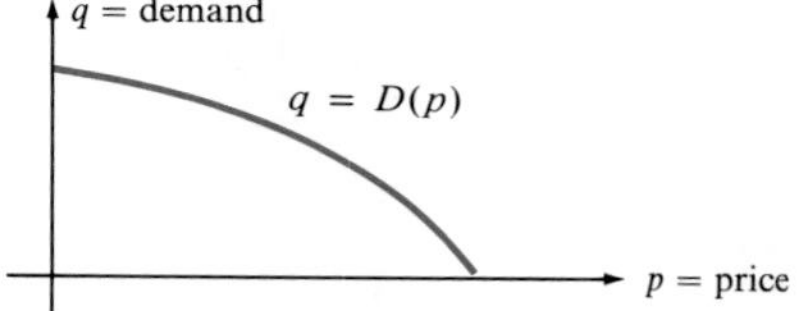

Figure 26
A typical demand function; the demand decreases as the price increases

We also learned that the derivative dD/dp of the demand curve represents the rate of change in the quantity demanded as a function of the price of the goods. For example, if $dD/dp = -2$ when $p = \$5$, then an increase in price of one dollar from \$5 to \$6 would result in a decrease in demand of two units.

The concept of the elasticity of the demand function is closely related to the derivative of the demand function. The difference is that whereas the derivative represents the total change in the demand, the elasticity represents the relative change in the demand. The elasticity is often a more useful measure of change. For example, a change in price of \$2 for a movie ticket would be large, but a change of \$2 would be insignificant in talking about the price of an automobile. For this reason the total change in itself is not too useful, and it is often better to find the relative change in demand. This introduces us to the economic concept of elasticity.

We first define the **relative rate of change** in the demand function. We say that

$$\text{Relative rate of change in demand} = \frac{D'(p)}{D(p)}$$

We can then write the ratio of the relative rate of change in demand to the relative rate of change in the price as

$$\frac{\text{Relative rate of change in quantity}}{\text{Relative rate of change in price}} = \frac{D'(p)/D(p)}{1/p}$$

$$= \frac{pD'(p)}{D(p)}$$

Students are often bothered by the above expression of $1/p$ representing the relative rate of change in the price. Just remember that the derivative of the price p (with respect to p) is 1. Hence the relative rate of change in the price (the derivative of the price divided by the price) is $1/p$. Note, too, that since the demand function $D(p)$ is always decreasing, the above ratio will always be negative. Since economists dislike working with negative numbers, the elasticity of demand is taken to be the above ratio multiplied by -1. This leads us to the definition of the elasticity of the demand function.

Definition of Elasticity of Demand

Let $q = D(p)$ be a demand function. The **elasticity** $E(p)$ of the demand function at a given price p is defined to be

$$E(p) = -\frac{pD'(p)}{D(p)}$$

The elasticity $E(p)$ will always be a nonnegative real number.

Example 8

Elasticity of Demand Suppose the weekly demand for a certain high grade steel is

$$q = 250 - 25p$$

where p is the price per pound and q is the quantity of steel demanded in millions of pounds.

(a) How much steel will be sold per week at \$3 a pound?

(b) Evaluate the derivative $dD(p)/dp$.

(c) Find the elasticity of the demand function.

(d) Evaluate the elasticity of the demand function when $p = \$3$.

Solution For convenience we have graphed the demand function in Figure 27.

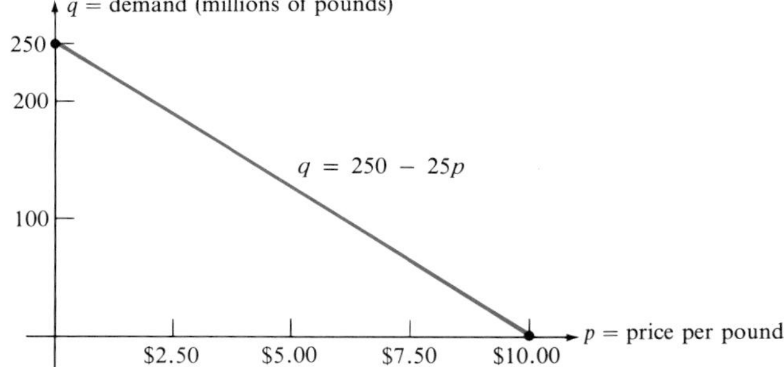

Figure 27
Demand for steel in millions of pounds

(a) *Demand at \$3:* When the price is \$3 per pound, the weekly demand will be

$$\begin{aligned} D(3) &= 250 - (25)(3) \\ &= 175 \quad \text{million pounds} \end{aligned}$$

(b) *Derivative of the demand function:* Given the demand function

$$D(p) = 250 - 25p$$

we have

$$D'(p) = -25$$

(c) *Elasticity of the demand function:* The elasticity of the demand function is given by

$$\begin{aligned} E(p) &= -\frac{pD'(p)}{D(p)} \\ &= \frac{-p(-25)}{250 - 25p} \\ &= \frac{p}{10 - p} \end{aligned}$$

The graph of the elasticity is shown in Figure 28.

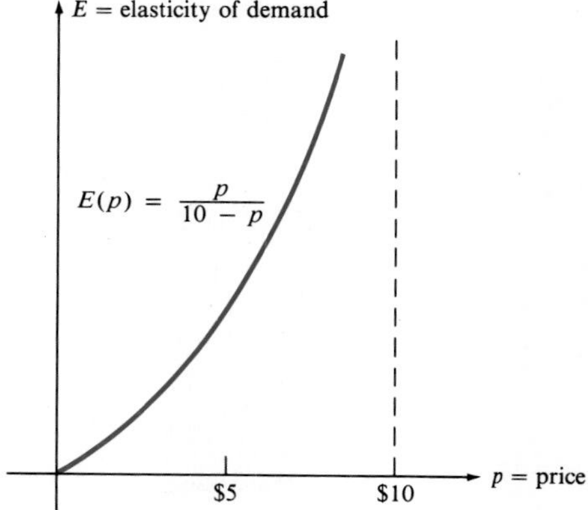

Figure 28
Elasticity of the demand function

(d) *Evaluate elasticity:* When the price of steel is \$3 per pound, the elasticity $E(p)$ is

$$\begin{aligned} E(3) &= \frac{3}{10 - 3} \\ &= \frac{3}{7} \\ &= 0.43 \end{aligned}$$

□

Conclusion

When the price of steel is \$3 per pound a small percentage increase in price will result in a percentage decrease in the demand of 0.43 times the percentage increase in the price. For example, if the price is increased by 5% (from \$3 to \$3.15 per pound), then the weekly demand for steel will fall by $0.43 \cdot (5\%) = 2.15\%$ (or from 175 million tons to 171.24 million tons).

Also, when the price of steel is \$8 then the elasticity is

$$E(8) = \frac{8}{10 - 8}$$
$$= 4$$

This means that when steel is priced at \$8 per pound, a 1% increase (or 8 cents) in the price of steel will result in a corresponding drop in the demand of (4)(1%) = 4%. Of course, it also means that a 1% drop in price would result in a 4% increase in the demand.

Elasticity and Inelasticity

The elasticity of a demand function is a valuable tool for studying the dynamics of consumer behavior. Are there certain prices at which consumers will resist price increases more than others? Why are many consumer goods often priced at \$0.99 or \$1.99? For a company to price its goods effectively, it is useful to study the concepts of elasticity and inelasticity.

Definition of Elasticity and Inelasticity

At a given price p_0 the demand function

$$q = D(p)$$

is called

- **inelastic** if $E(p_0) < 1$,
- of **unit elasticity** if $E(p_0) = 1$,
- **elastic** if $E(p_0) > 1$.

Example 9

Elastic and Inelastic Suppose the daily demand for airline tickets from New York to Los Angeles is given by

$$q = 5000\sqrt{900 - p} \qquad (0 \le p \le 900)$$

where p is the number of dollars charged for a ticket. This demand function is shown in Figure 29.

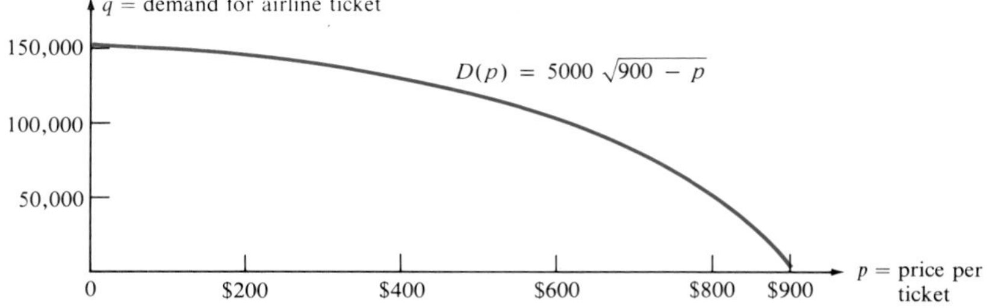

Figure 29
Demand for airline tickets

(a) How many tickets could be sold at \$500 a ticket?

(b) What is the elasticity of the demand function?

(c) At what prices is the demand function elastic and at what prices is it inelastic?

Solution

(a) *Demand:* When the price of a ticket is \$500, the daily demand is

$$\begin{aligned} D(500) &= 5000\sqrt{900 - 500} \\ &= 5000(20) \\ &= 100{,}000 \quad \text{tickets} \end{aligned}$$

(b) *Elasticity:* The elasticity of the demand function can be found to be

$$\begin{aligned} E(p) &= -\frac{pD'(p)}{D(p)} \\ &= \frac{p}{2(900 - p)} \qquad (0 \le p < 900) \end{aligned}$$

The graph of this function is shown in Figure 30.

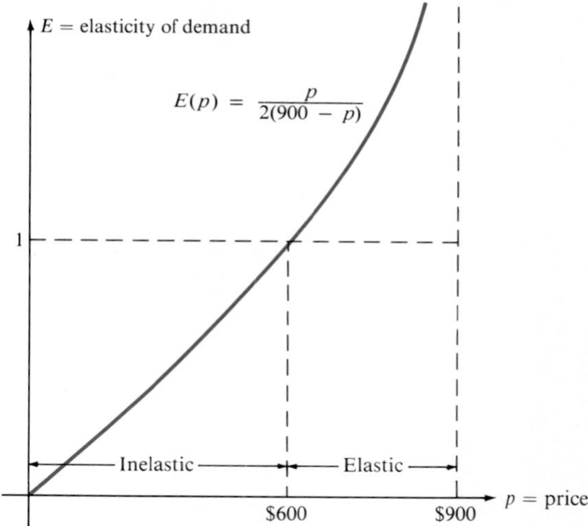

Figure 30
Elasticity of the demand function for airline tickets

(c) *Elastic and inelastic demand:* We begin by finding the prices for which the demand is elastic. That is, find the prices for which

$$E(p) = \frac{p}{2(900 - p)} > 1 \qquad (0 \le p < 900)$$

Subtracting 1 from each side of the inequality, we get

$$\frac{p}{2(900 - p)} - 1 > 0$$

Hence

$$\frac{p - 2(900 - p)}{2(900 - p)} > 0$$

or

$$\frac{3p - 1800}{2(900 - p)} > 0$$

Since the denominator is always positive for p in the interval $[0, 900)$, we seek those prices p in this region for which the numerator is also positive. Hence we write

$$3p - 1800 > 0$$

or

$$p > \$600$$

It is also a simple matter to determine those prices for which the demand function is inelastic ($E < 1$) and those prices for which it has unit elasticity ($E = 1$). We arrive at the following conclusion:

- Demand is inelastic for $0 \le p < \$600$ ($E < 1$).
- Demand has unit elasticity for $p = \$600$ ($E = 1$).
- Demand is elastic for $\$600 < p < \$900$ ($E > 1$). □

Interpretation

If the price of an airline ticket is under \$600, the demand is inelastic, and a percentage increase in price is met with a percentage decrease in demand that is not as great as the percentage increase in price. Hence the airlines will take in more money for each increase in price. However, when the price of a ticket is greater than \$600, the demand is elastic, and a percentage increase in price is met with a larger percentage decrease in demand. Hence an airline company will lose revenue by increasing the price higher than \$600. Therefore, the ideal price is \$600.

Relationship Between Revenue and Elasticity

The elasticity of demand also has a useful relationship to the marginal revenue $R'(p)$. Consider the previous example of selling airline tickets from New York to Los Angeles. If we write the revenue function as

$$\begin{aligned} R(p) &= (\text{Price per ticket})(\text{Tickets sold}) \\ &= p \cdot D(p) \end{aligned}$$

we can differentiate to get the marginal revenue

$$\begin{aligned} R'(p) &= \frac{d}{dp}[D(p) \cdot p] \\ &= D(p) \cdot 1 + D'(p) \cdot p \\ &= D(p)\left[1 + \frac{pD'(p)}{D(p)}\right] \\ &= D(p)[1 - E(p)] \end{aligned}$$

Hence we have the interesting economic law that revenue increases $[R'(p) > 0]$ with increasing prices when the demand for a product is inelastic $[E(p) < 1]$ and revenue decreases $[R'(p) < 0]$ with increasing prices when the demand for a product is elastic $[E(p) > 1]$.

Problems

For Problems 1–15, find dy/dx.

1. $y = \ln(3x + 5)$
2. $y = \ln(x^2 + 4x)$
3. $y = \ln\sqrt{4 - x^2}$
4. $y = \ln(1/x)$
5. $y = \ln(x + 1)$
6. $y = \ln\left(\dfrac{x+1}{x^2+1}\right)$
7. $y = \ln(e^x + e^{-x})$
8. $y = \ln(1 + e^x)$
9. $y = \ln(1/x^2)$
10. $y = \dfrac{\ln x}{x^3}$
11. $y = \dfrac{\ln x^2}{x^2}$
12. $y = \dfrac{\ln(x^2 + 1)}{x^2}$
13. $y = x\ln x - x$ (interesting derivative)
14. $y = \ln x + \ln 2x$
15. $y = e^x \ln(2x)$

Rewriting Logarithms in Terms of Natural Logarithms

For Problems 16–25, write the given logarithms in terms of the natural logarithm.

16. $\log_2 x$
17. $\log_5 x$
18. $\log_{20} x$
19. $\log 10^x$
20. $\log(x + 1)$
21. $\log(x^2 + 3x + 5)$
22. $\log(e^x + 1)$
23. $\log_2(e^x + 1)$
24. $\log_2(2^x)$
25. $\log_2(\log x + 1)$

Differentiating Logarithms with Any Base

For Problems 26–35, find the derivatives of the indicated function. *Hint:* First rewrite the logarithm in terms of the natural logarithm.

26. $\log(9x)$
27. $\log(x + 1)$
28. $\log(3x + 5)$
29. $\log(x^2 + 1)$
30. $\log e^x$
31. $\log(1/x)$
32. $\log x^2$
33. $\log(x^2 + 3x + 1)$
34. $\log_2(x + 1)$
35. $\log_2(1/x)$

Related Mathematical Problems

36. Implicit Differentiation Involving Logarithms. Find dy/dx by implicit differentiation if

$$y + \ln xy = 1$$

37. Implicit Differentiation Involving Logarithms. Find dy/dx by implicit differentiation if

$$\ln y = x$$

Does this agree with the derivative found by solving for y first and then finding dy/dx?

38. Slope of Tangent Line. Find the slope of the tangent line to the graph

$$y = e^x \ln(x + 1)$$

at the point (0, 0).

39. Maximum Value. Find the maximum value of the function

$$f(x) = \frac{\ln x}{\sqrt{x}} \qquad (x > 0)$$

40. Maximum Value. Find the maximum value of the function

$$f(x) = \frac{\ln(x + 1)}{x} \qquad (x > 0)$$

41. Logarithmic Derivative on Entire Real Line. Find the derivative $f'(x)$ where

$$f(x) = \ln|x| \qquad (x \neq 0)$$

Sketch the graph of $f(x)$. *Hint:* Find the derivative for $x < 0$ and then find it for $x > 0$.

Elasticity of the Demand Function

For Problems 42–47, find the elasticity $E(p)$ of the demand functions. Find the prices where the demand functions are elastic and when they are inelastic.

42. $q = 100 - 2p$
43. $q = 10{,}000 - 50p$
44. $q = \dfrac{100}{p^2}$
45. $q = \dfrac{1000}{p^3}$
46. $q = 10{,}000\sqrt{100 - p}$
47. $q = 50{,}000\sqrt{1600 - 2p}$

48. Movie Theater Tickets. A movie theater has a seating capacity of 1000 people. The number of tickets q that can be sold at p dollars is given by

$$q = D(p) = \frac{5000}{p} - 250 \qquad (p > 0)$$

(a) How many tickets could be sold at $3?
(b) Find $D'(p)$.

(c) Find $E(p)$.
(d) Is the demand elastic or inelastic when the price of a ticket is \$5?
(e) What is the marginal revenue $R'(p)$ when the price is \$5? From the value of the marginal revenue, would you increase or decrease the price per ticket to increase revenues?

49. Balance of Trade. To improve its balance of trade position with Korea, the United States has decided to lower the price for some heavy machinery equipment. The demand function is

$$q = \frac{5000}{p^2}$$

(a) Find $E(p)$.
(b) Find $R'(p)$.
(c) Will the United States succeed in raising its revenue by decreasing prices? What is the reason?

50. Regions of Elasticity and Inelasticity. Consider the demand function

$$q = \frac{A}{p^m}$$

where A and m are constants with m a positive integer.
(a) Find $E(p)$.
(b) Find those prices for which the demand function is elastic.
(c) Find the marginal revenue $R'(p)$.

51. Mathematics in the Cruise Ship Industry. The Stella Solaris cruise ship is sailing from Miami on an Amazon cruise. The number of cabins that can be filled is determined by the demand function

$$q = 20\sqrt{1600 - 0.2p} \qquad (0 \le p \le 8000)$$

(a) Find $E(p)$.
(b) Is the demand elastic or inelastic when the price of a cabin is \$2000?
(c) Is the demand elastic or inelastic when the price of a cabin is \$5000?
(d) When the price of a cabin is \$2000, should the price be raised or lowered to increase the total revenue?
(e) When the price of a cabin is \$5000, should the price be raised or lowered to increase the total revenue?

Relative Rates of Change

52. Relative Rate of Change. Suppose the value of a business investment is given by the function

$$I(t) = 100{,}000e^{0.5\sqrt{t}} \qquad (t > 0)$$

Determine the relative rate of increase in this investment after 10 years. *Hint:* It is easiest simply to take the natural logarithm of each side of the equation and then differentiate. This will give the desired value

$$\frac{d}{dt}\ln I(t) = \frac{I'(t)}{I(t)}$$

53. Constant Relative Rate of Change. Show that if the value of an investment increases according to the function

$$y(t) = Pe^{rt}$$

then the relative rate of increase is a constant. What is this relative rate of increase?

54. Changing Interest Rates. Suppose the Federal Reserve Board forecasts that interest rates will increase over the next several months according to the function

$$I(t) = 0.05 + 0.05t + 0.10e^{-0.5t}$$

where t is time measured in months. What is the relative change in interest rates over the next six months?

55. Bacteria Growth. The size of a population of bacteria growing in a liquid medium is given by the function

$$p(t) = 100e^{0.04t}$$

where t is time measured in months. Draw a graph of the relative rate of increase $p'(t)/p(t)$ in the population over the next ten months.

Interesting Derivatives of Logarithms

56. Rate of Change in Doubling Time. We have seen before that if money is deposited in a bank that pays interest at an annual rate of r compounded continuously, then the time T it takes a deposit to double in value is

$$T = \frac{\ln 2}{\ln(1 + r)}$$

Find dT/dr.

57. The Logarithmic Derivative. Find the derivative of the function

$$y = \frac{x^3}{(x^2 + 1)(3x - 4)}$$

Hint: One of the virtues of the logarithm is its ability to turn products into sums and quotients into differences. Take the natural logarithm of each side of this equation and write

$$\begin{aligned}\ln y &= \ln\frac{x^3}{(x^2 + 1)(3x - 4)}\\ &= \ln(x^3) - \ln(x^2 + 1) - \ln(3x - 4)\end{aligned}$$

Now differentiate implicitly with respect to x, and then solve for dy/dx.

Epilogue: History of Mathematical Economics

Only in the past 40 years has mathematics gained widespread acceptance among economic theorists. At one time many people thought that mathematics was used in economics only to confuse outsiders or to add some dignity to an otherwise vacuous subject.

Originally, only the values of graphs and symbols were acknowledged as being important tools to speak the language of economics. Today, the entire subject of economics has been embodied into an axiomatic framework. To gain a perspective on the importance of mathematics in modern economic theory, you should be aware that the work of most of the recent Nobel Prize winning economists has been formulated in the language of mathematics.

Some of the important early developments in mathematical economics, such as marginal revenue and cost, supply and demand curves, and discounting, which are the basis for much of economic development in this book, are listed below. All of the references that follow, with the exception of the first two, rely heavily on differential calculus.

- *1711 (Early Rumblings)*. First book dealing with the applications of mathematics to economics was written by an Italian engineer, Giovanni Ceva.
- *1760 (Early Rumblings)*. An Italian, Cesare Beccaria, used algebra to show the hazards of "profits and smuggling" in the book *Tentativo Analytico Sui Contrabbandi.*
- *1776 (The Wealth of Nations)*. In 1776 the Scottish economist Adam Smith wrote the first genuine analytical work in economics with the two-volume work, *The Wealth of Nations*. His work formed the foundations for the work of later mathematical economists such as David Ricardo.
- *1817 (Mathematical Rigor Raised to a New Level)*. The British economist David Ricardo published the book *Principles*, in which he established a theory of value. Ricardo raised the mathematical level of economics from intuition and common sense to a higher mathematical level.
- *1838 (Supply and Demand Introduced)*. Antoine Augustin Cournot wrote the first major economic treatise, *Researches into the Mathematical Principles of the Theory of Wealth*. Many people believe that this book initiated the study of mathematical economics. Cournot (1801–1877) was a French mathematician who first defined the concepts of supply and demand as mathematical functions. Unfortunately, the book was too advanced and was not appreciated by economists of the time.
- *1871 (Marginality Introduced)*. William Stanley Jevons published the treatise *Theory of Political Economy*. In this book, Jevons introduced the idea of marginality, which is familiar to every modern-day student of economic theory. The book was a major influence on researchers of the time. Jevons once stated, "If economics is to be a science at all, it must be a *mathematical science*."
- *1874 (Utility Theory and Equilibrium Theory Introduced)*. *Elements of Pure Economics* was published by Leon Walras and introduced the concept of marginal utility theory and general equilibrium theory. Walras, Austrian Carl Menger, and Englishman William Stanley Jevons are often given credit for bringing the "marginal revolution" into economics.
- *1884 (Theory of Interest)*. The Austrian economist Eugan Bohm-Bawerk introduced many of the ideas that ultimately led to the theory of interest.
- *1907 (Present and Future Value of Money Introduced)*. *The Rate of Interest* was published by Irving Fisher. In this book, Fisher introduces the ideas of present value, future value, and discounting.
- *1909 (Theory of Equilibrium)*. The most famous untranslated book in the history of economics, *Manuel d'économie Politique*, was published by the Swiss economist Vilfredo Pareto. It covers much of the theory of equilibrium in economics. The book uses calculus extensively.
- *1920 (Price Elasticity Introduced)*. One of the epic contributions to mathematical economics was the book *Principles of Economics* by English economist Alfred Marshall. Marshall made major contributions to utility theory and de-

mand curves. Marshall was the first economist to define mathematically the concept of price elasticity.

- *1928 (Theory of Savings Introduced by Ramsey).* A research paper, "A Mathematical Theory of Savings," was published by F. P. Ramsey. In this paper a mathematical theory based on calculus is developed to determine how much capital to place in savings.
- *1928 (Cobb-Douglas Production Function Introduced).* The now famous Cobb-Douglas production function was introduced by Charles Cobb and Paul Douglas in a research paper, "A Theory of Production," in the *American Economic Review.* This function shows the relationship between the amount of a product produced as a function of the amounts of labor and capital used.
- *1936 (Keynesian Economics).* John Maynard Keynes has dominated twentieth century economics more than any other economist. Although it is hard to pinpoint any single accomplishment, his 1936 book *The General Theory of Employment, Interest, and Money* is a well-known classic. This is the work on which all the Keynesian models are based. Although this specific work contains little mathematics, much of Keynes's work is highly mathematical.

We have presented here a listing of some of the major contributions to the history of mathematical economics. However, the list is in no way complete. Other important names come to mind in such a review. Names like Edgeworth, Wicksell, Wicksteed, Pigou, and Carey are important.

In more recent years, areas of mathematics other than calculus have played an important role in economics. We mention the introduction of game theory into economics by Oskar Morgenstern and John von Neumann in 1931.

Key Ideas for Review

Review Exercises

For Problems 1–5, solve the equations for x.

1. $3^{-x} = \frac{1}{9}$

2. $8^x = 2^{x^2}$

3. $7^x = 49^{(x+1)}$

4. $2^{x+1} = \frac{1}{16}$

5. $7^x = 49$

For Problems 6–11, solve for x.

6. $\log x^2 = 3 \log 2 - 4 \log 5$

7. $\log_2 x = 2$

8. $\ln x^2 + \ln x = \ln 8$

9. $\ln x - \ln x^2 = 1$

10. $\ln (x + 1) = 1$

11. $\ln (x + 1) = 0$

For Problems 12–40, find the derivative of the given function.

12. $f(x) = xe^x$

13. $f(x) = e^{(2x+1)}$

14. $f(x) = e^x \ln x$

15. $f(x) = e^x \log x$

16. $f(x) = (\log x)^2$

17. $f(x) = \ln \sqrt{x}$

18. $f(x) = x \ln x$

19. $f(x) = \ln (e^x)$

20. $f(x) = e^{\ln x}$

21. $f(x) = \dfrac{e^x + e^{-x}}{2}$

22. $f(x) = e^{x^2} \ln x^2$

23. $f(x) = \log_2 x$

24. $f(x) = (\ln x^2)^3$

25. $f(x) = \ln \left(\dfrac{x^2 + 1}{x^2 - 1}\right)$

26. $f(x) = \ln [(x^2 + 1)(x^2 - 1)]$

27. $y = \ln (ax^n)$

28. $y = \ln (ax + b)$

29. $f(t) = \ln (x + \sqrt{1 + x^2})$

30. $f(x) = 10^{nx}$

31. $y = e^{\sqrt{x}}$

32. $f(x) = x^2 \ln (x^2)$

33. $y = \log \frac{2}{x}$

34. $y = \frac{e^x - 1}{e^x + 1}$

35. $y = \ln (x^2 e^x)$

36. $f(x) = x^n(a + bx)^m$

37. $y = 1^x$

38. $y = b^{2x}$

39. $y = \frac{\ln x^2}{x^2}$

40. $y = e^{\ln x}$

Logarithmic Differentiation

It is possible to find the derivative of an expression like

$$y = x^x \qquad (x > 0)$$

by first taking the logarithm of each side of the equation, getting

$$\ln y = \ln x^x = x \ln x$$

If we then differentiate this equation implicitly with respect to x, we get

$$\frac{y'}{y} = \ln x + 1$$

and solving for y', we get

$$y' = y(\ln x + 1) = x^x(\ln x + 1)$$

This general process of finding a derivative is called **logarithmic differentiation**. For Problems 41–47, find the derivative of the given function by using logarithmic differentiation.

41. $y = 2^x$

42. $y = x^{\sqrt{x}}$

43. $y = (x + 1)^3(3x - 1)$

44. $y = x^{\ln x}$

45. $y = (2x + 1)^x$

46. $y = e^x\sqrt{x^2 + 1}$

47. $y = \frac{\sqrt{x + 1}(x - 3)}{x^2 + 1}$

Economics and Financial Problems

48. **Tripling Time.** An amount P_0 is deposited in a bank that pays interest at an annual interest rate of r, compounded continuously. How long will it take this deposit to triple in value?

49. **Marginal Revenue.** The revenue R in dollars that a manufacturer receives when q units of a product are sold is given by

$$R(q) = 0.5qe^{-0.01q}$$

What is the marginal revenue when $q = 100$?

50. **Discounted Investments.** A speculator in precious stones has purchased a ruby that is increasing in value according to the function

$$V(t) = V_0e^{\sqrt{t}}$$

where t is time measured in years. If the discount rate is 8% per year, when should the speculator sell the ruby to maximize profits?

51. **Emerald Speculator.** The same speculator as in Problem 50 has now invested in an emerald that will increase in value according to the function

$$V(t) = V_0e^{0.2\sqrt{t}}$$

When should the emerald be sold to maximize profits?

52. **Which Is Increasing Faster?** The price for a new car is \$12,000. This price is increasing at the rate of \$800 per year. The cost of silver is \$6.00 per ounce and is increasing at the rate of 25 cents per year. What is the relative change in each item per year? Which relative change is larger?

53. **When to Sell.** An investment is valued approximately by the function

$$f(t) = 50{,}000e^{0.2\sqrt{t}}$$

What will be the relative change in the value of this investment in ten years?

54. **Art Investment.** A painting has its value given approximately by

$$v(t) = 5000e^{\sqrt[3]{t}/2}$$

What is the relative rate of change in the investment after five years? After 15 years? What is the percentage rate of change after this length of time?

55. **Changing Annual Compounding to Continuous Compounding.** If interest is paid by a bank at an annual interest rate of i, compounded annually, then an initial amount P will have a future value of

$$F = P(1 + i)^n$$

after n years. Rewrite the above equation in the form

$$F = Pe^{rn}$$

to determine the effective rate r that this bank pays if it compounded interest continuously.

56. **Elasticity of the Demand Function.** Given the demand function

$$q = 5000 - 5p^2$$

(a) Find $E(p)$.
(b) Determine the values of p for which the demand is inelastic and those for which it is elastic.
(c) Find $R(p)$.
(d) Find $R'(p)$.

57. **Elasticity of the Demand Function.** Suppose that the demand q is 100 when the price p is 5 and that the demand is 90 when the price is 10. Assuming the demand function

is a straight line, find the demand function

$$q = a + bp$$

Use this demand function to find:

(a) $E(p)$

(b) The regions where the demand function is inelastic and where the demand function is elastic

(c) $R(p)$

(d) $R'(p)$

Biology and Scientific Problems

58. Finding the Growth Equation. Every day the size of a bacteria population grows by 10%. If the initial size of the population is 100, write the size of this population in the form

$$P(t) = P_0e^{kt}$$

59. Finding the Decay Equation. Every day the size of a bacteria population declines by 15%. If the initial size of the population is 65, write the size of this population in the form

$$P(t) = P_0e^{-kt}$$

60. Finding the Proper Dosage. A virus has been exposed to X-rays. The number of surviving virus cells N depends on the number of roentgens r applied and is given by

$$N(r) = N_0e^{-0.2r}$$

How many roentgens must be applied for 95% of the virus cells to be destroyed?

61. Radioactive Decay. The radioactive carbon isotope ^{14}C decays according to the exponential decay

$$C(t) = C_0e^{-t/5760}$$

where C_0 is the initial amount and t is time measured in years. How long will it take for the substance to decrease to $\frac{1}{10}$ of the original amount?

62. Richter Scale. The Richter scale is given by

$$R = 0.67 \log E - 7.9$$

where E is the energy in ergs released by an earthquake. If the Richter scale measures 4.5, how many ergs of energy are released?

63. Richter Scale. Two earthquakes are reported. One earthquake is in Colombia and measures 4.5 on the Richter scale; the other is in Indonesia and measures 5.3. How many times more energy is released by the Indonesia earthquake?

Chapter Test

1. Find y' if

$$y = x^2 \ln(x^2 + 1)$$

2. Use properties of logarithms to find y' if

$$y = \log \frac{\sqrt{x^2 + 2x + 1}}{\sqrt{x}}$$

3. If the population of a bacteria is increasing exponentially at the rate of 5% every 12 hours, what is the population at any time t? Write the growth function in the form

$$P(t) = P_0e^{kt}$$

4. Suppose the population of bacteria is increasing according to the function

$$P(t) = P_0e^{0.05t}$$

where t is time measured in months. How long will it take the bacteria population to quadruple in size?

5. Find the maximum value of the function

$$f(x) = \frac{\ln x^2}{x} \qquad (x \neq 0)$$

6. Suppose you deposit \$500 in a bank that compounds interest annually. Suppose that in ten years your account will be worth \$1500. What is the annual rate of interest paid by this bank?

7. Hmmmmm. Find the derivative of $y = x^{x/2}$. *Hint:* Take the natural logarithm of each side of the equation before differentiating.

8. Finding the Rate Constant. Suppose a colony of bacteria is growing according to an exponential law

$$P(t) = P_0e^{kt}$$

and suppose the colony doubles in size every 25 days. What is the rate constant k?

9. **Timber Cutting.** Suppose the value of timber (in thousands of dollars) on a given tract of land is given by

$$V = 2^{\sqrt{t}}$$

where t is time measured in years from the present time. Assuming an annual discount rate of 8%, when would be the optimal time to cut the timber for sale?

10. **An Important Function.** The exponential function

$$y = e^{-x^2}$$

plays an important role in probability and statistics. Show that

(a) $y > 0$ for all x.

(b) y approaches 0 both as x approaches plus infinity or minus infinity.

(c) The function attains its maximum value when $x = 0$.

(d) The inflection points occur when $x = \pm 1/\sqrt{2}$.

Projects and Problems (Chapters 1–3)

Cumulative Exercises

For Problems 1–10 compute the derivative of the given quantity.

1. $y = e^{x^2} + e^{-x^2}$

2. $y = \ln(x^2) + \ln^2 x$

3. $y = 5x^4 \ln x$

4. $y = (\ln x)^{-1}$

5. $y = \ln(\ln x)$

6. $y = \sqrt{1 + e^x}$

7. $y = e^{\ln x}$

8. $y = 3x^3 + 2x - 6$

9. $y = x^{1/2} + x^{-1/2}$

10. $y = \dfrac{1}{1 - x^2}$

For Problems 11–14, find the equation of the tangent line at the given point.

11. $y = x^2 - 3x + 4$ at $(0, 4)$

12. $y = e^{2x}$ at $(1, e^2)$

13. $y = \dfrac{x}{x + 1}$ at $(1, \frac{1}{2})$

14. $y = x \ln x$ at $(1, 0)$

For Problems 15–18, determine where each function is increasing and where it is decreasing.

15. $y = x^2 + 3x - 2$

16. $y = x\, e^x$

17. $y = x^2 \ln x \quad (x > 0)$

18. $y = \dfrac{1}{1 + x} \quad (x \neq -1)$

Calculators and Computers

Calculators and computers are so prevalent in the real world that anyone who is ignorant of them is working with a handicap. The following problems allow you to sharpen your computing skills and illustrate how computing can be useful in the study of calculus. For all the problems in this section, use either a calculator or a computer.

19. Graphing with the Computer. Evaluate the function

$$f(x) = x^3 - 2x + 3$$

for $x = -5, -4.5, -4, \ldots, 4, 4.5, 5$. Use these computed values to sketch a rough graph of the function.

20. Limits with a Computer. To estimate the limit

$$\lim_{x \to 1} \frac{x - 1}{\sqrt{x} - 1}$$

complete the following table:

x	$x - 1$	$\sqrt{x} - 1$	$\dfrac{x - 1}{\sqrt{x} - 1}$
0.9			
0.99			
0.999			
0.9999			
1.0			limit
1.0001			
1.001			
1.01			
1.1			

Observe that while the numerator and denominator both approach 0 as x approaches 1 (and in fact are zero at 1), their ratio approaches a nonzero value at 1. The question is: What is this value?

21. Limits with a Computer. To estimate the limit

$$\lim_{x \to 4} \frac{x - 4}{\sqrt{x} - 2}$$

complete the following table:

x	$x - 4$	$\sqrt{x} - 2$	$\dfrac{x - 4}{\sqrt{x} - 2}$
3.9			
3.99			
3.999			
3.9999			
4			limit
4.0001			
4.001			
4.01			
4.1			

Note that although both $x - 4$ and $\sqrt{x} - 2$ approach 0 as x approaches 4 (and in fact are 0 at 4), their ratio approaches a nonzero value. The question is: What is this value?

For Problems 22–24 use a calculator or computer to estimate the following limits. For each problem, compute the value of the numerator, denominator, and quotient at several points near the limiting point. Note that although the numerator and denominator both approach zero, their ratio approaches a nonzero value.

22. $\lim_{x \to 0} \frac{\sqrt{x+1}-1}{x}$

23. $\lim_{x \to 3} \frac{x-3}{\sqrt{3x}-3}$

24. $\lim_{t \to 0} \frac{\sqrt{t+9}-3}{t}$

25. Finding a Derivative. Estimate the derivative of the function $f(x) = x^4$ at $x = 1$ by completing the following table. What is the interpretation of the values in the rightmost two columns?

h	$(1+h)^4 - 1^4$	$\frac{(1+h)^4 - 1^4}{h}$
0.1		
0.01		
0.001		
0.0001		
0.0		derivative

26. Finding the Derivative. Estimate the derivative of

$$f(x) = 2^x$$

at $x = 1$ by computing the values in the following table. What is the interpretation of the values in the two rightmost columns?

h	$f(1+h) - f(1)$	$\frac{f(1+h) - f(1)}{h}$
0.1		
0.01		
0.001		
0.0001		
0.0		derivative

27. Finding the Second Derivative. The second derivative of a function f at a point a can be written as the limit

$$f''(a) = \lim_{h \to 0} \left[\frac{f(a+2h) - 2f(a+h) + f(a)}{h^2} \right]$$

Use this formula to estimate the derivative of $f(x) = x^3$ at $x = 1$ by completing the following table:

h	$f(1)$	$f(1+h)$	$f(1+2h)$	$\frac{f(1+2h) - 2f(1+h) + f(1)}{h^2}$
0.1				
0.01				
0.001				
0.0001				
0.0				second derivative

28. Finding e. The value of e can be defined as the limit

$$e = \lim_{n \to \infty} \left(1 + \frac{1}{n}\right)^n$$

The value of e to 7 places is 2.718281. How large must you choose n in order that

$$f(n) = \left(1 + \frac{1}{n}\right)^n$$

approximates e to 7 places?

Interesting Problems and Applications

29. Interesting Function. The function $y = x^x$ $(x > 0)$ where the base and the exponent are both variables is interesting inasmuch as it is not a power function x^a (a a constant) nor is it an exponential function a^x (a a constant). Hence the derivative rules for power functions and exponential functions do not apply. However, it is possible to find the derivative of this function by first taking the natural logarithm of each side of the equation before differentiating implicitly with respect to x. Use this hint to find the derivative of $y = x^x$.

30. Very Interesting Function. Similar to the function x^x discussed in Problem 29, the function $y = x^{x^x}$ $(x > 0)$ is also neither a power function nor an exponential function. Use the hint given in Problem 29 to find the derivative of $y = x^{x^x}$.

For each of Problems 31–35, find a function that satisfies the indicated property.

31. A continuous function defined on an interval that has no maximum value.

32. A continuous function defined on an interval that has no minimum value.

33. A continuous function defined on an interval that has a maximum value but no minimum value.

34. A function that is continuous at $x = 1$ but has no derivative at $x = 1$.

35. A function whose first derivative is positive but whose second derivative is negative at zero.

36. Do You Know the Rules? Which of the following rules are true? For the rules that are not true, give an example to which the rule does not apply (a counterexample) and replace the rule by the correct rule.

(a) $\lim_{x \to a} f(x)g(x) = \lim_{x \to a} f(x) \lim_{x \to a} g(x)$

(b) $(fg)' = f'g'$ (c) $(f/g)' = f'/g'$

(d) $\frac{d}{dx} f[g(x)] = f'(x)g'(x)$

(e) $\log(A - B) = \log(A) - \log(B)$

(f) $\log(A/B) = \log(A) - \log(B)$

(g) $e^{x+y} = e^x + e^y$

37. Hmmmmm—An Algebra Puzzler. Pick any three-digit number, form a second number by reversing the digits, and then subtract the smaller of the two numbers from the larger. To the resulting difference, add the number formed by reversing the digits of this difference. The final number will be 1089. For example, if you picked the number 521, then you would think: 521, 125, 521 − 125 = 396, 396 + 693 = 1089. Explain why this puzzle works.

38. Making Your Own Puzzle. How would you go about making up your own puzzle similar to the one in Problem 37? Make up such a puzzle and explain why it works.

39. Hmmmmm—A Derivative Puzzler. Watch carefully. We start with the obvious identity

$$x^2 = x \cdot x = x + x + x + \cdots + x \qquad (x\ x\text{'s})$$

If we now differentiate each side of this equation with respect to x, we get

$$\frac{d}{dx} x^2 = \frac{d}{dx}(x + x + \cdots + x)$$

or

$$2x = 1 + 1 + \cdots + 1 \qquad (x\ 1\text{'s})$$

Hence we have

$$2x = x$$

or

$$2 = 1$$

What did we do wrong?

40. Spread of AIDS. At the beginning of 1987 the Surgeon General estimated that there were 50,000 cases of AIDS in the United States and that this number was doubling every 10 months. Assume that the Surgeon General's estimates are accurate.

(a) What is the growth equation of the form

$$N(t) = N_0 b^t$$

for the number of cases of AIDS where t is time measured in 10-month periods starting from the beginning of 1987?

(b) What is the continuous growth equation of the form

$$N(t) = N_0 e^{kt}$$

where t is still measured in 10-month periods.

41. Alcohol Absorption. The percent P of alcohol in a person's blood often decays exponentially according to the decay law

$$P(t) = P_0 e^{-kt}$$

where

P_0 = percent of alcohol in the blood at the time the last drink was consumed

t = time measured from the time the last drink was consumed

(See Figure 1.) The decay constant $k > 0$ depends on the individual. Suppose Sally drinks a gallon of her grandmother's apple cider. Immediately after she drinks the cider, the percent of alcohol in her blood is 0.25%. One hour later the percent of alcohol in her blood has fallen to 0.18%. How long will it be before Sally will legally be able to drive? (Assume that Sally lives in Maine, where the legal alcohol limit is 0.08%.)

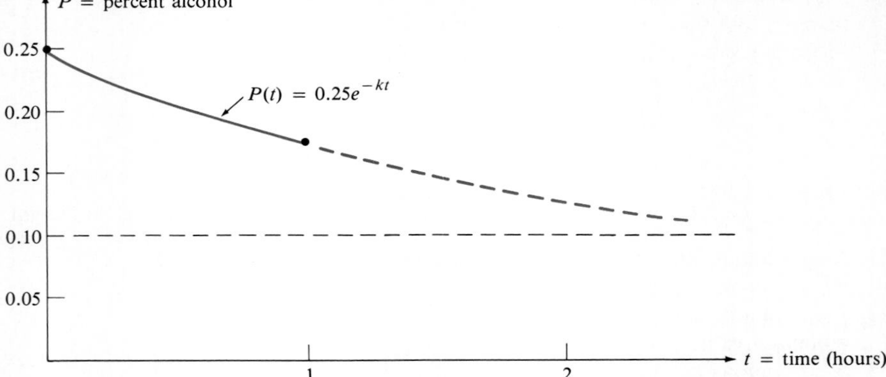

Figure 1
Decay in the percentage of alcohol in the bloodstream

42. The Rule of 70. On the television program "Wall Street Week" a financial expert suggested that people start taking their money out of the stock market and buying long-term bonds. She then said that since bonds pay interest at a rate of 7% compounded continuously, by the **Rule of 70** your money will double every 10 years. It was not clear that the expert understood the mathematics behind this useful rule, but in general the Rule of 70 states that the time it takes money to double is $70/r$, where r is the annual rate of return. What is the reasoning behind the Rule of 70?

43. Is This Page Optimal? The publisher of the book you are now reading wanted each page to have a printed area of approximately 58 square inches (which it does). It was also desired that the margins at the top and bottom of each page be roughly 1″ (which they are). Finally, the margins at the left and right of each page were to be 1.25″ and 0.75″, respectively (which they also are). (See Figure 2.)

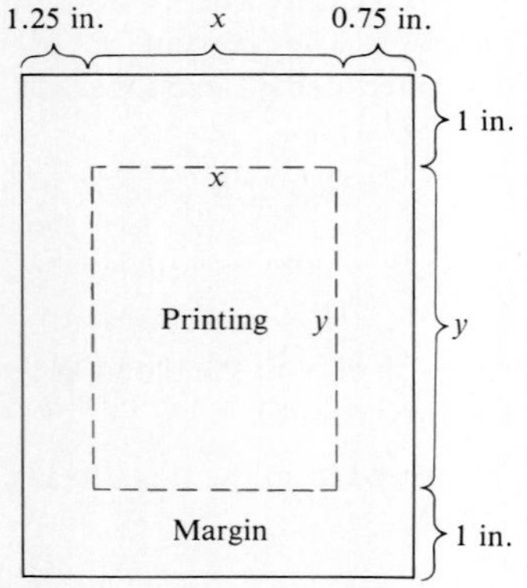

Figure 2
The optimal page problem

(a) What should be the dimensions x and y (width and height) of the printed material of each page in order that the above criteria are met but at the same time the total area of the page is minimized?

(b) Does the page you are now reading have the minimum area?

44. Think Before You Leap. Mary dives from a diving board 32 feet above the water (Figure 3). The distance $s(t)$ in feet that she falls in t seconds is given by

$$s(t) = 16t^2$$

(a) How long will it take for Mary to hit the water?

(b) What is her velocity when she hits the water?

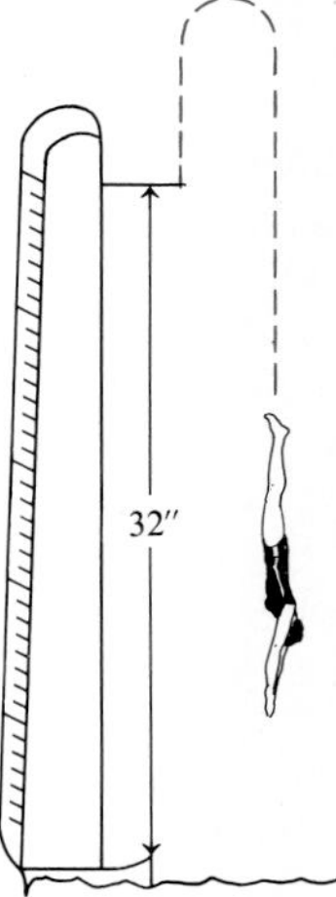

Figure 3
How long will it take for Mary to hit the water?

45. Free Falling on the Moon. Mary has become an astronaut and has gone to the moon. She knows that on the surface of the moon she weighs only $\frac{1}{6}$ as much as she does on earth. Knowing this, she decides to jump off a 1000-foot cliff. The number of feet she falls in t seconds is given by

$$s(t) = \frac{8}{3}t^2$$

(a) How long will it take before Mary hits the ground?
(b) How fast will she be traveling when she lands?

46. Free Falling on Jupiter. After surviving her jump in Problem 45, Mary next voyages to Jupiter, where her weight is 2.5 times her weight on earth. Under these conditions, if she jumps off a cliff, the number of feet she will fall in t seconds will be given by

$$s(t) = 40t^2$$

Since she has survived her moon jump, suppose she decides to jump off a 100-foot cliff.
(a) How long will it take before she hits the ground?
(b) How fast will she be traveling when she lands?

47. World Series Time. This problem is being written one hour after the Minnesota Twins beat the St Louis Cardinals in the seventh game of the 1987 World Series. The game of baseball involves all sorts of related rates problems. Suppose Willie McGee is attempting to steal third base and is 40 feet from third base running at a speed of 30 ft/sec. How fast is he approaching home plate?

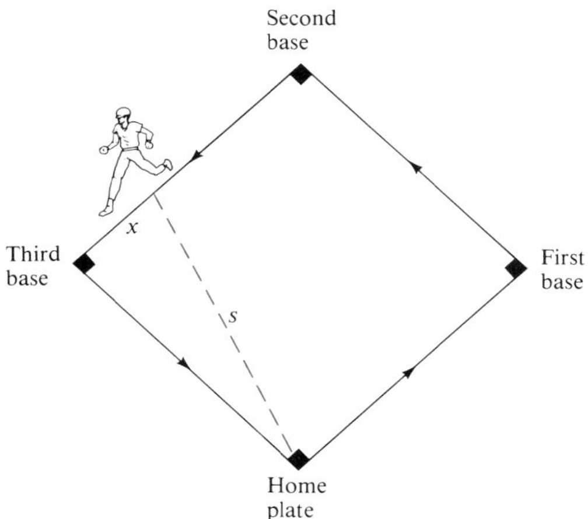

Figure 4
How fast is the runner approaching home plate?

48. Sunflower Problem. Suppose the rate of change in the height H of a sunflower plant follows the logistic growth law

$$\frac{dH}{dt} = H(125 - H)$$

where the height of the sunflower is measured in inches and t is time measured in weeks. At what height will the rate of growth be a maximum? (See Figure 5.)

49. Radioactive Tracer. It is well known that if radioactive iodine is injected into the bloodstream, the concentration I of iodine in the blood will decrease according to the exponential law

$$I(t) = I_0 e^{-kt}$$

where I_0 is the initial concentration of iodine and $k > 0$ is the decay constant. Medical people often say that this exponential law implies that the rate of decrease in iodine is proportional to the amount of iodine present, the decay constant k being the constant of proportionality. Symbolically, this says

$$\frac{dI}{dt} = -kI$$

Show that if $I(t)$ satisfies the exponential law, it also satisfies the "rate proportional to the amount law."

Learning Through Writing

50. Discussion of the Derivative. Write your own definition of the derivative using language that allows the general "derivative concept" to be intuitively understood by a person who has not studied calculus.

51. You Can Be the Author. Compose a word problem that illustrates an important topic studied in Chapters 1–3. The problem should have a title and should illustrate an important idea. What important mathematical idea is illustrated in your problem?

52. You Make Up the Problem. Using a different situation, perhaps one relevant to your own academic discipline, write a problem that illustrates the same mathematical principle as Example 5 in Chapter 2. Solve the problem.

53. Biology Project. In an excellent article ("The Calculus of Leaves: A Modeling Project for a Calculus Class," *UMAP Journal*, Vol. 4, No. 1, 1983), Professor Svoboda from Indiana/Purdue University at Fort Wayne designed a project to model leaf growth. Carry out Professor

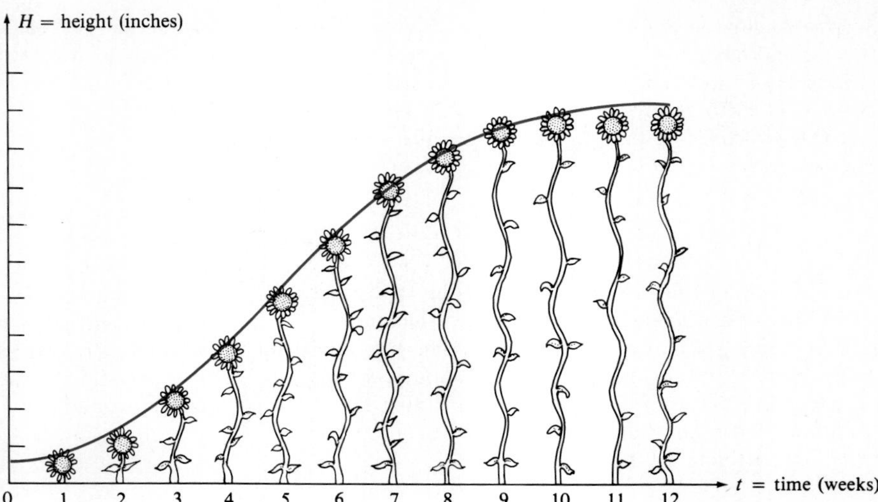

Figure 5
Typical logistic growth curve for many plants and animals

Svoboda's project and write a term paper summarizing your results.

54. Social Science Project. In a fascinating article ("Glottochronology: An Application of Calculus to Linguistics," *UMAP Journal*, Vol 3, No. 1, 1983), Professor Lo Bello from Allegheny College shows how calculus can be used to determine how languages change over time. Summarize Professor Lo Bello's article in a written paper.

The integral calculus is the second major area of the calculus, the differential calculus being the first. The basic idea that characterizes the integral calculus is that it is the inverse of the differential calculus; namely, instead of finding the derivative of a function, one finds the function from the derivative.

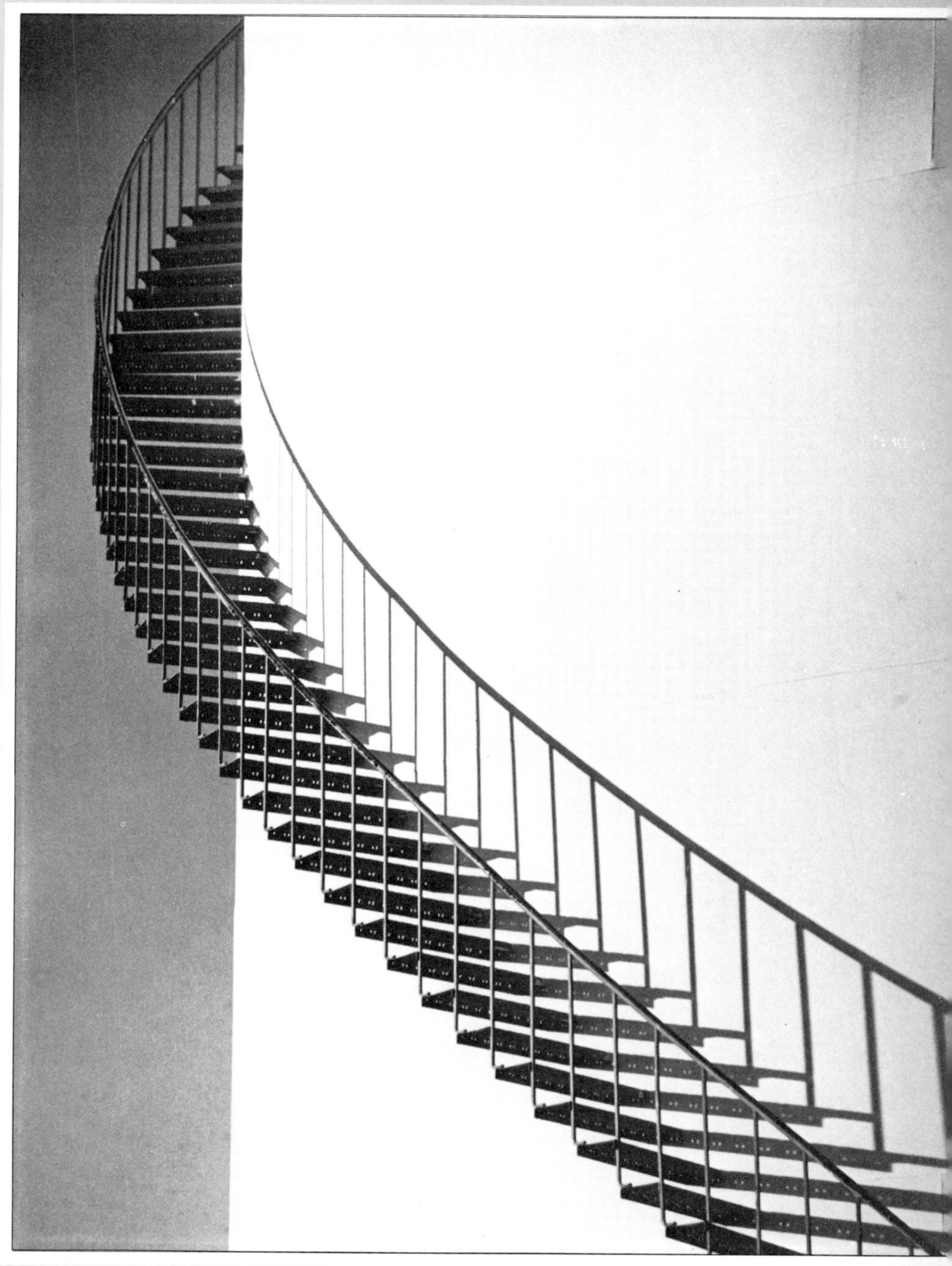

4 Integration

In this chapter we introduce the second of the two major processes of the calculus, integration. We begin in Section 4.1 by introducing the concept of the antiderivative, which may be thought of as the reverse or inverse of the derivative. In Section 4.2 we then define the definite integral of a continuous function and show how it can be used to find areas of regions in the plane. In Section 4.3 we link Sections 4.1 and 4.2 together by means of the fundamental theorem of calculus, which shows how an antiderivative of a function can be used to evaluate the definite integral of a function. Finally, in Section 4.4 we introduce the method of substitution, which is an aid in finding antiderivatives and hence the definite integral of a function.

4.1 The Antiderivative (Indefinite Integral)

PURPOSE

We begin the study of integral calculus by introducing the concept of the antiderivative. In particular, we introduce

- the meaning of an antiderivative and
- the way to find antiderivatives.

We finish by showing how the antiderivative can be used in mathematical economics and science.

Introduction

You can open a door, and then you can close it. You can square a positive number, and then you can take the positive square root of the answer. These pairs of operations have the property that the second operation undoes the first. The door is returned to its original position, and the number that we squared was refound by taking the positive square root.

Operations like these are **inverse operations**. In mathematics, operations like the operations of squaring and taking the positive square root are inverses, as are addition and subtraction. It is now time to study the inverse operation of the derivative, the antiderivative.

Doing the "Inverse" of Differentiation (the Antiderivative)

For demonstration purposes, consider the function defined by $f(x) = x^2$. So far, we have learned that its derivative is $f'(x) = 2x$. However, we can perform another operation on $f(x) = x^2$ called **antidifferentiation**. Instead of "going forward" and finding the derivative

$$x^2 \longrightarrow 2x \qquad \text{(differentiation)}$$

we can "go backward" and find the function whose derivative is x^2.

$$\frac{1}{3}x^3 \longleftarrow x^2 \qquad \text{(antidifferentiation)}$$

That is, we find the antiderivative of x^2.

We are now ready for the formal definition of the antiderivative.

Definition of an Antiderivative of f

A function F is an **antiderivative** of f on the interval (a, b) if

$$\frac{d}{dx}F(x) = f(x)$$

for all x in (a, b).

The word "an" in this definition indicates that there is more than one antiderivative of a function. We now see from an example why we always expect a function to have more than one antiderivative.

Example 1 Finding Antiderivatives Find the antiderivative(s) of

$$f(x) = x^3$$

Solution Using the power rule for the derivative, we know that

$$\frac{d}{dx}\frac{1}{4}x^4 = x^3$$

Hence an antiderivative of $f(x) = x^3$ is

$$F(x) = \frac{1}{4}x^4$$

But the two functions

$$F_1(x) = \frac{1}{4}x^4 + 2 \qquad \text{and} \qquad F_2(x) = \frac{1}{4}x^4 - 100$$

are also antiderivatives. In fact, any function of the form

$$F(x) = \frac{1}{4}x^4 + C$$

where C is any constant is an antiderivative of f. (See Figure 1.)

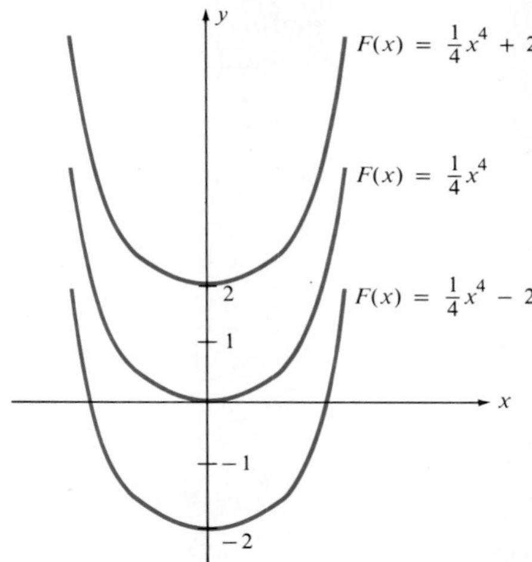

Figure 1
A few antiderivatives of $f(x) = x^3$

In other words, if $F(x)$ is an antiderivative of $f(x)$, then so is each of the functions

$$F(x) + C$$

where C is any real number. □

Notation for Antiderivatives

In differential calculus we denote the derivative of $f(x)$ as $f'(x)$ or $df(x)/dx$. In integral calculus the antiderivative or **indefinite integral** of $f(x)$ is denoted by

$$\int f(x)\,dx = F(x) + C$$

The elongated S, or $\int$, is called the **integral sign**, and $f(x)$ is called the **integrand** of the indefinite integral. The symbol dx indicates the variable in which the antiderivative is taken and is called the **variable of integration**. Later in this chapter, when we study the integration technique of the method of substitution, we will learn why it is convenient to use this differential notation.

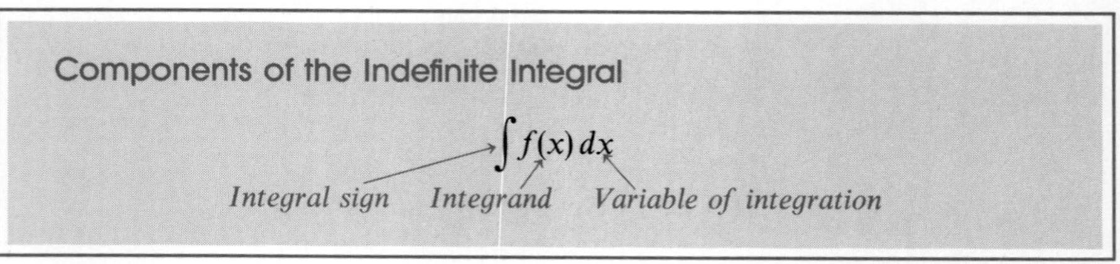

Antiderivatives of Power of x

In differential calculus we learned the power rule

$$\frac{d}{dx}\frac{x^{a+1}}{a+1} = x^a \qquad \text{(power rule for differentiation)}$$

This derivative formula leads to the following antiderivative formula.

Power Rule for Antiderivatives

Let a be any real number such that $a \neq -1$. The **power rule for antiderivatives** says that

$$\int x^a\,dx = \frac{x^{a+1}}{a+1} + C$$

Verification of the Power Rule for Antiderivatives

It is easy to see that this antiderivative formula is correct. All we need to do is observe that the derivative of the antiderivative is the integrand. That is,

$$\frac{d}{dx}\left[\frac{x^{a+1}}{a+1} + C\right] = x^a.$$

Example 2 Power Rule for Antiderivatives Find the antiderivatives of

$$f(x) = \sqrt{x}$$

Solution Using the power rule for antiderivatives with $a = \frac{1}{2}$, we have

$$F(x) = \int x^{1/2}\,dx = \frac{x^{3/2}}{\frac{3}{2}} + C$$

$$= \frac{2}{3}x^{3/2} + C$$

Check:

$$\frac{d}{dx}\left[\frac{2}{3}x^{3/2} + C\right] = x^{1/2}$$

□

Just as there are many general rules for finding derivatives, there are general rules for antiderivatives. These rules will allow us to find the antiderivatives of more complex expressions.

Rules for Antiderivatives

Let f and g both have antiderivatives, and let c be a constant. Then

Constant rule: $\int cf(x)\,dx = c\int f(x)\,dx$

Sum rule: $\int [f(x) + g(x)]\,dx = \int f(x)\,dx + \int g(x)\,dx$

Difference rule: $\int [f(x) - g(x)]\,dx = \int f(x)\,dx - \int g(x)\,dx$

Verification of the Rules for Antiderivatives

To convince yourself of the correctness of the above rules, try restating the meaning of each rule in words. For example, to convince yourself that the sum rule is reasonable, ask yourself whether it is true that a function whose derivative is $f(x) + g(x)$ is equal to the sum of two functions, one whose derivative is $f(x)$ and another whose derivative is $g(x)$. From your knowledge of the properties of the derivative, you know that this is correct. You should also restate in words the other two antiderivatives.

Example 3

Using Rules for Antiderivatives Find

$$\int (3x^2 + 2x + 1)\,dx$$

Solution Using the sum followed by the constant rule, we can write

$$\begin{aligned}\int (3x^2 + 2x + 1)\,dx &= \int 3x^2\,dx + \int 2x\,dx + \int dx\\ &= 3\int x^2\,dx + 2\int x\,dx + \int dx\\ &= 3\left[\frac{x^3}{3} + C_1\right] + 2\left[\frac{x^2}{2} + C_2\right] + [x + C_3]\\ &= x^3 + x^2 + x + (3C_1 + 2C_2 + C_3)\\ &= x^3 + x^2 + x + C\end{aligned}$$

Since the three constants C_1, C_2, and C_3 represent arbitrary real numbers, the sum $3C_1 + 2C_2 + C_3$ is also an arbitrary real number. Hence we denote it simply by C and usually call it the **constant of integration**.

Check:

$$\frac{d}{dx}[x^3 + x^2 + x + C] = 3x^2 + 2x + 1$$ □

How do we pick out a specific one of these antiderivatives? Is there one antiderivative that is the "desirable" one? For example, a few members of the entire "family" of antiderivatives

$$F(x) = \frac{1}{3}x^3 + C$$

of the function $f(x) = x^2$ are indicated in Figure 2.

Many problems dictate that we should find the specific antiderivative that satisfies an additional side or initial condition of the form $F(x_0) = y_0$. Figure 2 illustrates that in the above example we seek the specific antiderivative that passes through the point (0, 1). In other words, we seek the antiderivative that satisfies the side condition $F(0) = 1$. Since this condition says that

$$F(0) = \frac{1}{3}0^3 + C = 1$$

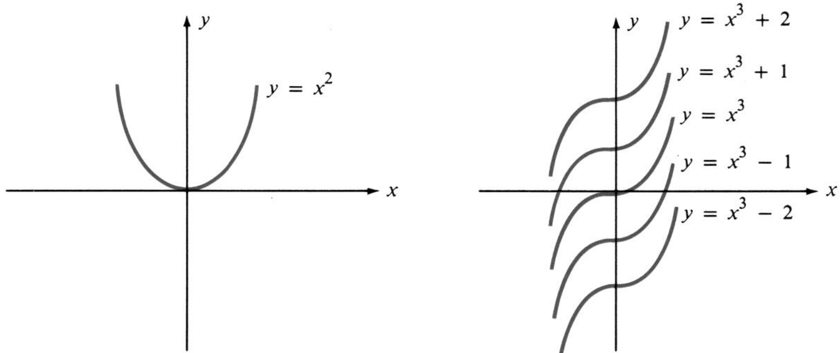

Figure 2
A function and a few of its antiderivatives

it implies that the constant of integration C is 1 and hence the desired antiderivative is

$$F(x) = \frac{1}{3}x^3 + 1$$

Example 4

Finding a Particular Antiderivative Find the specific function $F(x)$ whose derivative is

$$f(x) = 3x^2 + 4x + 5$$

that also satisfies the condition $F(1) = 2$.

Solution Using the rules for antiderivatives, we obtain

$$F(x) = x^3 + 2x^2 + 5x + C$$

Using the condition $F(1) = 2$, we get the equation

$$F(1) = 1^3 + 2(1^2) + 5(1) + C = 2$$

Solving for C, we find

$$C = -6$$

Hence the desired function is

$$F(x) = x^3 + 2x^2 + 5x - 6$$

Check:

$$\frac{d}{dx}(x^3 + 2x^2 + 5x - 6) = 3x^2 + 4x + 5$$

$$F(1) = 1^3 + 2(1^2) + 5(1) - 6 = 2$$

□

General Power Rule for Antiderivatives

In Section 1.7, when we studied the chain rule, we learned the general power rule for derivatives

$$\frac{d}{dx}[g(x)]^{a+1} = (a + 1)[g(x)]^a g'(x)$$

This equation also says that the antiderivative of the expression on the right-hand side is equal to $[g(x)]^{a+1}$. This fact leads to the following rule (stated slightly differently).

Rule for Finding the Antiderivative of General Powers

Let g be a differentiable function and a be any real number such that $a \neq -1$. Then

$$\int [g(x)]^a g'(x)\,dx = \frac{1}{a+1}[g(x)]^{a+1} + C$$

Verification of the General Power Rule

Antiderivative formulas are generally easy to verify. To verify such a rule, all we have to do is differentiate the antiderivative to see that we get the integrand of the indefinite integral. In the above rule we need to verify

$$\frac{d}{dx}\left\{\frac{1}{a+1}[g(x)]^{a+1} + C\right\} = [g(x)]^a g'(x)$$

By using the chain rule and the properties of the derivative we see that this statement is true.

Example 5 Indefinite Integral Find the indefinite integral

$$\int (x^2 + 1)^3 2x\,dx$$

Solution For this integral we interpret the integrand as $[g(x)]^a g'(x)$ where

$$g(x) = x^2 + 1$$
$$g'(x) = 2x$$
$$a = 3$$

Using the generalized power rule, we get

$$\begin{aligned}\int (x^2 + 1)^3 2x\,dx &= \int g(x)^3 g'(x)\,dx \\ &= \frac{1}{4}[g(x)]^4 + C \\ &= \frac{1}{4}(x^2 + 1)^4 + C\end{aligned}$$

Check:

$$\frac{d}{dx}\left[\frac{1}{4}(x^2 + 1)^4 + C\right] = (x^2 + 1)^3 2x$$

□

A New Look at Marginal Analysis

In the theory of the firm we have seen that the revenue, cost, and profit functions (called **total functions** by economists) have derivatives which are called the marginal revenue, marginal cost, and marginal profit functions, respectively. We can now "go backward" and find the antiderivatives of the marginal functions to get the total functions. Since it is often easy for economists to empirically find the marginal functions from economic data, it is possible to find the total functions by finding antiderivatives. For instance, the marginal cost $C'(q)$ represents approximately the added cost of producing one more item of a product when the production level is q units. A company may be able to determine this information much more readily than finding the total cost $C(q)$ of producing q items. Often the total cost $C(q)$ is difficult to determine, since it depends on the fixed cost (the cost when no items are produced), whereas the marginal cost does not depend on the fixed cost.

Example 6

Finding Total Cost from Marginal Cost Suppose the marginal cost of producing q units of a given product is

$$C'(q) = 3q^2 - 2q$$

with a fixed cost of \$10,000. Find the total cost function $C(q)$. What is the cost of producing 25 items?

Solution The problem is to find $C(q)$, given

$$C'(q) = 3q^2 - 2q$$
$$C(0) = 10{,}000$$

We begin by finding the indefinite integral or antiderivative of $C'(q)$. This is given by

$$\begin{aligned} C(q) &= \int C'(q)\,dq \\ &= \int (3q^2 - 2q)\,dq \\ &= q^3 - q^2 + K \end{aligned}$$

We use K instead of C to denote the constant of integration so as not to confuse it with the cost $C(q)$. To find K, we evaluate $C(q)$ at the point $q = 0$, knowing that at this point the cost function satisfies the condition $C(0) = 10{,}000$. This gives

$$C(0) = (0)^3 - (0)^2 + K = 10{,}000$$

Solving for K gives

$$K = 10{,}000$$

Hence the total cost is

$$C(q) = q^3 - q^2 + 10{,}000$$

The cost to the firm to produce 25 items will be

$$\begin{aligned} C(25) &= (25)^3 - (25)^2 + 10{,}000 \\ &= \$25{,}000 \end{aligned}$$

□

Example 7

Finding Total Revenue from Marginal Revenue A wholesaler charges its retailers \$250 for a television set. To encourage retailers to buy in volume, the wholesaler deducts \$2 from the price of each additional set sold up to 50 sets. In other words, the price of the second set is \$248, that of the third set is \$246, and so on, until the 50th set and thereafter, each of which costs \$150. For this wholesaling scheme:

(a) What is the marginal revenue?

(b) What is the total revenue?

(c) What is the total revenue when 30 sets are sold?

Solution

(a) *Marginal revenue.* Since the marginal revenue $R'(q)$ is approximately the amount of money taken in on the sale of the next television set when q sets have been sold, we can write $R'(q)$ mathematically as

$$R'(q) = 250 - 2q \qquad (0 \le q \le 50)$$

(b) *Total revenue.* The total revenue R is the antiderivative of the marginal revenue function. Hence

$$\begin{aligned} R(q) &= \int R'(q)\,dq \\ &= \int (250 - 2q)\,dq \\ &= 250q - q^2 + K \end{aligned}$$

To find the constant K, we use the fact that the revenue is zero when the number of sets sold is zero. That is,

$$R(0) = 0$$

Using the condition that $R(0) = 0$, we get

$$R(0) = 250(0) - 0^2 + K = 0$$

Finally, solving for K, we find

$$K = 0$$

Substituting this value into $R(q)$, we have the total revenue function

$$R(q) = 250q - q^2$$

(c) *Finding* $R(30)$. When 30 television sets are sold, the revenue will be

$$\begin{aligned} R(30) &= (250)(30) - (30)^2 \\ &= \$6600 \end{aligned}$$

□

Comparison Between the Calculus and the Exact Solution

You should realize that the revenue function $R(q)$ found in the previous example approximates the real revenue only when q television sets have been sold. The reason for this discrepancy is that the marginal revenue function $R'(q)$ is only an approximation of

$$R(q + 1) - R(q)$$

which is the true amount of money taken in on the sale of a new television when q sets have been sold. Using calculus, however, makes the analysis much easier.

The revenue problem discussed in Example 7 shows how we can effectively use calculus to approximate the real revenue. It is useful to compare the calculus solution with the exact solution. For example, if the previous wholesaler were to sell three television sets, the revenue function $R(q)$ found by computing the antiderivative of $R'(q)$ would say that the revenue (amount taken in) is

$$\begin{aligned} R(3) &= 250(3) - (3)^2 \\ &= \$741 \end{aligned}$$

On the other hand, without using calculus the company accountant could simply add up the receipts from the sale of the three sets, getting

$$\begin{aligned} \text{Revenue from the sale of three sets} &= \$250 + \$248 + \$246 \\ &= \$744 \end{aligned}$$

In other words, there is an error of \$3 (or 0.4% percentage error) in the calculus solution.

Table 1 shows the difference between the exact revenue from the sale of q television sets and the value of the revenue function $R(q)$ found from the marginal revenue function.

TABLE 1
Error in Treating the Number Sold q as a Continuous Variable

Number of Sets Sold, q	Exact Revenue from the Sale of q Sets	Value of $R(q)$	Absolute and Percentage Error
0	0	0	0
1	\$250	\$249	\$1 (0.4%)
2	\$498	\$496	\$2 (0.4%)
3	\$744	\$741	\$3 (0.4%)
4	\$988	\$984	\$4 (0.4%)
5	\$1,230	\$1,225	\$5 (0.4%)
10	\$2,410	\$2,400	\$10 (0.4%)
20	\$4,620	\$4,600	\$20 (0.4%)
30	\$6,630	\$6,600	\$30 (0.5%)
40	\$8,440	\$8,400	\$40 (0.5%)
50	\$10,050	\$10,000	\$50 (0.5%)

Indefinite Integral of the Exponential Function

In the previous chapter we learned the derivatives

$$\frac{d}{dx} e^{kx} = ke^{kx}$$

$$\frac{d}{dx} \ln x = \frac{1}{x} \qquad (x > 0)$$

It is possible to restate these two equations in terms of antiderivative equations by saying that the antiderivatives of the expressions on the right-hand side are equal to the expressions being differentiated on the left-hand side. These antiderivative forms of the above equations are stated now.

Antiderivatives of Exponential and Logarithm Functions

Exponential: $\int e^{kx}\,dx = \frac{1}{k}e^{kx} + C \qquad (k \neq 0)$

Special Exponential: $\int e^{x}\,dx = e^{x} + C$

Logarithm: $\int \frac{dx}{x} = \ln|x| + C \qquad (x \neq 0)$

Special Logarithm: $\int \frac{dx}{x} = \ln x + C \qquad (x > 0)$

Example 8

Antiderivatives of Exponentials Find the antiderivative of

$$f(x) = e^{0.08x}$$

Solution Using the rule for antiderivatives of exponential functions with $k = 0.08$, we have

$$F(x) = \int e^{0.08x}\,dx$$

$$= \frac{1}{0.08}e^{0.08x} + C$$

Check:

$$\frac{d}{dx}\left[\frac{1}{0.08}e^{0.08x} + C\right] = e^{0.08x}$$

□

Example 9

Antiderivatives of Exponentials Find the antiderivative of

$$f(t) = e^{-t}$$

Solution Using the rule for the antiderivative of exponentials with $k = -1$, we have

$$F(t) = \int e^{-t}\,dt$$

$$= -e^{-t} + C$$

Check:

$$\frac{d}{dt}[-e^{-t} + C] = e^{-t}$$

□

More Uses for Antiderivatives (Finding Totals from Rates)

Indefinite integrals have many applications. In many areas of science we are often able to measure by an experiment the rate of change at which something occurs. For instance, we can often determine the rate of change in the size of a population of bacteria. The problem then is to find the size of the population after a given period of time.

A typical experience that is familiar to most people is driving a car. Suppose you drive your car for a given period of time at varying rates of speed but your odometer is broken, so you cannot determine how far you have traveled. However, you have kept a record of your velocity $v(t)$ during the trip. Knowing the velocity, how can you determine the distance you have traveled? The answer to this question is obtained by finding the antiderivative of the velocity function. If $v(t)$ represents the velocity (miles per hour) at time t (hours), then the antiderivative

$$s(t) = \int v(t)\,dt$$

represents the distance traveled. We illustrate this idea with an example.

Example 10

Finding Distance from Velocity You are driving along an interstate and your velocity is initially 40 miles per hour. Over the next hour you gradually increase your velocity $v(t)$ to 55 miles per hour according to the function

$$v(t) = 40 + 15t^2 \qquad (0 \le t \le 1)$$

How far did you travel during this hour?

Solution By finding the antiderivative of a velocity function $v(t)$ we can find the distance $s(t)$ that an object has traveled. In the case of the car we have

$$\begin{aligned} s(t) &= \int v(t)\,dt \\ &= \int (40 + 15t^2)\,dt \\ &= 40t + 5t^3 + C \end{aligned}$$

To find the constant C, we simply use the fact that $s(0) = 0$. This gives

$$s(0) = 40(0) + 5(0)^3 + C = 0$$

or

$$C = 0$$

Hence the position of your car at any time t (between 0 and 1) is given by

$$s(t) = 40t + 5t^3$$

After one hour you would have traveled

$$\begin{aligned} s(1) &= 40(1) + 5(1)^2 \\ &= 45 \quad \text{miles} \end{aligned}$$

Table 2 shows the velocity and distance traveled during this one-hour period.

□

TABLE 2
Relationship Between Velocity and Distance

Time, t (hours)	Velocity, $v(t) = 40 + 15t^2$ (miles/hr)	Distance Traveled, $s(t) = 40t + 5t^3$ (miles)
0 (0 min)	40.0	0
0.2 (12 min)	40.6	8.04
0.4 (24 min)	42.4	16.32
0.6 (36 min)	45.4	25.08
0.8 (48 min)	49.6	34.56
1.0 (60 min)	55.0	45.00

Problems

For Problems 1–16, find the antiderivatives for each derivative.

1. $\frac{dy}{dx} = x + 3$

2. $\frac{ds}{dt} = t^2 - 2t + 3$

3. $\frac{dy}{dx} = \frac{1}{2}x^3 - \frac{2}{3}x^2 + \frac{1}{5}$

4. $\frac{dy}{dt} = t^3 + \frac{2}{t}$

5. $\frac{dy}{dx} = 4x^3 - 3x^{-2} + x - 3$

6. $\frac{dx}{dt} = t^{5/2} + 3t^{3/2} - t^{1/2} + 3t^{-1/2}$

7. $\frac{dx}{dt} = e^{2t} + 3e^{-3t}$

8. $\frac{dx}{dt} = \frac{2}{3}t + \frac{3}{t^3} + e^{4t} - \frac{6}{t}$

9. $\frac{dy}{dx} = 7\sqrt{x} + \frac{2}{e^{2x}}$

10. $\frac{dy}{dx} = e^x + \frac{5}{x^2} + x^3$

11. $\frac{dy}{dt} = e^{-3t}$

12. $\frac{dy}{dx} = e^x + e^{-x}$

13. $\frac{dy}{dt} = e^{-0.5t}$

14. $\frac{dy}{dx} = (x^2 + 1)^3(2x)$

15. $\frac{dy}{dx} = \sqrt{x^3 + 2x + 3}\,(3x^2 + 2)$

16. $\frac{dy}{dx} = (5x^3 - 1)^{50}\,(15x^2)$

For Problems 17–30, find the general antiderivative.

17. $\int (2x^2 + 5x^3 + x^4)\,dx$

18. $\int \left(\frac{y-1}{y^2} + y^2\right) dy$ (*Hint*: First perform division.)

19. $\int (2t + 3)^2\,dt$ (*Hint:* Expand the integrand.)

20. $\int (2x + 1)(x - 3)\,dx$ (*Hint:* First perform multiplication.)

21. $\int \frac{6x^5}{(x^6 - 3)^3}\,dx$

22. $\int 3x^2(x^3 + 1)^{1/2}\,dx$

23. $\int e^{5x}\,dx$

24. $\int (e^{2x} + e^{-2x})\,dx$

25. $\int e^{-0.04t}\,dt$

26. $\int \left(x^2 + \frac{1}{x^2}\right) dx$

27. $\int 3\sqrt{3x + 2}\,dx$

28. $\int 4(1 + 4x)\sqrt{1 + 2x + 4x^2}\,dx$

29. $\int (x^2 + 1)^3\,(2x)\,dx$

30. $\int (x^3 + 2x + 10)^5\,(3x^2 + 2)\,dx$

For Problems 31–50, find the particular antiderivative of the given derivative determined by the value of the function.

31. $f'(x) = 0,\ f(0) = 1$

32. $f'(t) = 1,\ f(0) = 0$

33. $f'(s) = -1,\ f(0) = 1$

34. $f'(t) = t + 3,\ f(2) = 9$

35. $f'(x) = 3x + 4,\ f(6) = 70$

36. $f'(x) = \frac{x^3}{2} + 2x,\ f(0) = 100$

37. $f'(u) = (u - 2)^2,\ f(4) = 2$

38. $f'(x) = x^3 - \frac{2}{3}x^2 - x - 3,\ f(6) = 200$

39. $f'(u) = 2u + u^{-2},\ f(1) = -1$

40. $f'(t) = \frac{(t + 2)(t - 5)}{t^3},\ f(1) = 4$

41. $f'(x) = x^{-2/3}(x + 16)$, $f(8) = 11.4$

42. $f'(u) = \dfrac{1 - u}{u^2}$, $f(e) = e$

43. $f'(t) = t + \sqrt{t}$, $f(4) = 2$

44. $f'(x) = e^{2x}$, $f(0) = 0$

45. $f'(t) = e^{-0.01t}$, $f(0) = 1$

46. $f'(t) = e^t + e^{-t}$, $f(0) = 1$

47. $f'(x) = 2x\sqrt{x^2 - 9}$, $f(5) = 5$

48. $f'(t) = \dfrac{1}{t}$ $(t > 0)$, $f(1) = 2$

49. $f'(x) = (x^2 + 1)^3(2x)$, $f(0) = 0$

50. $f'(x) = (x^3 + 2x + 5)^2(3x^2 + 2)$, $f(0) = -1$

Marginal Analysis

For Problems 51–59, find the total cost, revenue, and profit given the marginal cost, revenue, and profit.

51. $C'(q) = 40q - 0.01q^2 + 100$ $\quad C(0) = 100$
52. $C'(q) = 3 + 5q - 0.05q^2$ $\quad C(0) = 250$
53. $C'(q) = 2q - 0.02q^2$ $\quad C(0) = 500$
54. $C'(q) = 0.5q^3 - 2q^2 + 6q + 3$ $\quad C(0) = 1000$
55. $C'(q) = 7.5e^{0.15q}$ $\quad C(0) = 80$
56. $P'(q) = 5 - 0.2q$ $\quad P(0) = 0$
57. $P'(q) = 10 - 0.5q$ $\quad P(0) = 0$
58. $R'(q) = 15 - 0.05q - 0.05q^2$ $\quad R(0) = 0$
59. $R'(q) = 10 - 0.08q - 0.10q^2$ $\quad R(0) = 0$

60. **Finding Total Cost from Marginal Cost.** The marginal cost MC of producing the qth unit is given by

$$MC(q) = 8 + 0.03q^2$$

Find the total cost of producing q units if the fixed cost is \$20.

61. **Finding Total Cost from Marginal Cost.** The Acme Hardware Co. has determined its marginal cost is

$$MC(q) = \frac{q^2}{50} - q + 75$$

where q is the number of items produced per day. Find the total cost of producing 100, 200, and 500 units per day. Assume that the fixed cost is zero.

62. **Finding Total Revenue from Marginal Revenue.** A marginal revenue function MR is given by

$$MR(q) = 75 + 0.4q + 0.2q^2$$

where q is the number of units sold. Find the total revenue from selling q units.

Finding Total Size from Growth Rates

63. **Spread of Contagious Diseases.** There have been many studies about the spread of diseases. Assume that the rate at which a certain disease spreads has been determined to be

$$p'(t) = e^{-0.02t}$$

where $p(t)$ is the percentage of the general population that has contracted the disease in year t. If no one has the disease initially (negligible number), how many people will have the disease after t years?

64. **Fruit Flies.** A biologist has determined that the rate of growth in the size of a colony of fruit flies on day t is given by

$$P'(t) = 100\left(2 + \frac{1}{t^2}\right) \qquad (t \ge 1)$$

where the population on day one is $P(1) = 100$. Find the population for any day $t \ge 1$.

65. **How Far Have You Traveled?** Suppose you are initially driving your car at 40 miles per hour, and during a one-hour period you gradually increase your velocity $v(t)$ to 60 miles per hour according to the function

$$v(t) = 40 + 20t$$

where t is time in hours. How far have you traveled after one hour?

66. **How Far Have You Traveled?** Suppose you drive your car for two hours at the constant velocity of

$$v(t) = 50$$

miles per hour. It is clear that you have traveled 100 miles. Find this answer using calculus.

67. **How Far Has the Ball Fallen?** If a ball is dropped from the top of a tall building, the velocity at which the ball falls is given by

$$v(t) = 32t$$

feet per second, where t is time measured from the time that the ball is dropped. How far has the ball fallen after five seconds?

Reverse Problem to Finding the Tangent Line

68. **Finding the Curve from the Tangent Line.** Suppose the slope of the tangent line to a curve is given by

$$f'(x) = 2x$$

If the curve passes through the point (0, 0), what is the curve?

69. **Finding the Curve from the Tangent Line.** Suppose the slope of the tangent line to a curve is given by

$$f'(x) = e^x$$

If the curve passes through the point (0, 2), what is the curve?

4.2 Area and the Definite Integral

PURPOSE

We introduce the definite integral and show how this integral solves one of the two original problems of calculus, the problem of areas. Major topics are

- the calculation of an area using the concept of the limit and
- the definite integral.

Introduction

Mathematicians have struggled with the problem of finding the area of a region in the plane for over 3000 years. Until the invention of the integral calculus, however, the regions considered were mostly those regions bounded by straight lines, called polygons, with a few exceptions such as the circle and the ellipse. For example, it is not necessary to use integral calculus to find the area of a polygon. Figure 3 illustrates how the Greek mathematicians found the area of a polygon by

1. First finding the area of a rectangle
2. Using the area of a rectangle to find the area of a parallelogram
3. Using the area of a parallelogram to find the area of a triangle
4. Using the area of a triangle to find the area of a polygon

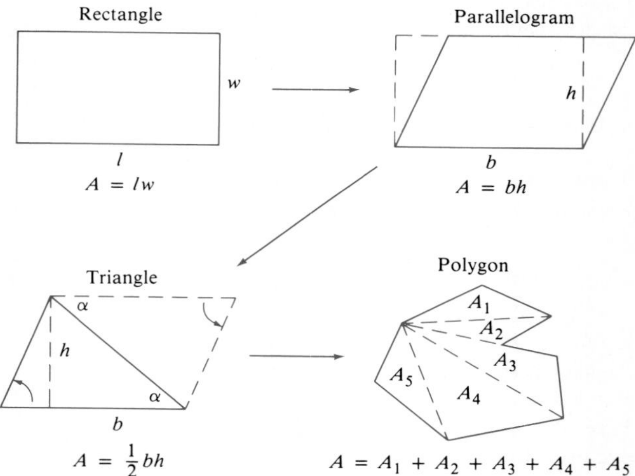

Figure 3
Steps in finding the area of a polygon

Continuing Where the Greeks Left Off (General Areas)

If we know how to find the area of a polygon, we can use this information to approximate, and sometimes even find exactly, the area of a region bordered by curved boundaries. Consider finding the area of a circle. Over 2000 years ago the brilliant Greek mathematician Archimedes (287(?)–212 B.C.) found the area of a circle by drawing a sequence of **inscribed polygons** $P_3, P_4, P_5, \ldots$ that

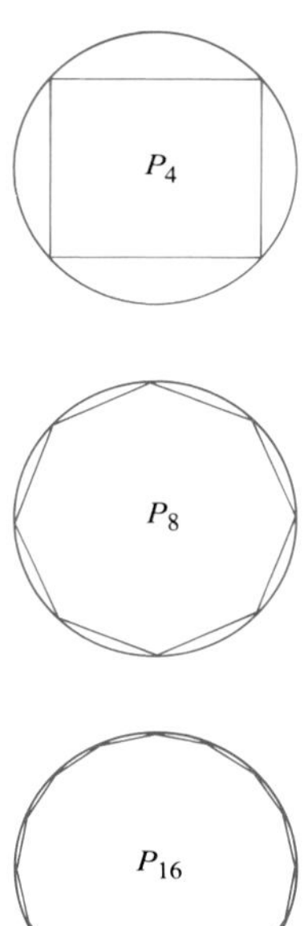

approximate the circle more and more accurately. Figure 4 shows a few representative polygons.

Although mathematicians have studied the concept of area throughout the ages, it was the discovery of the integral calculus by Newton and Leibniz that allowed for the more general determination of areas. For that reason it would certainly be reasonable to give much of the credit for solving the problem of areas (discussed earlier) to Newton and Leibniz. However, the mathematical determination of areas understood by Newton and Leibniz is quite primitive in comparison to the ideas that we will learn in this book. The common mathematical tool for determining area that is learned by students today, the definite integral, was discovered much later, in the mid-1800's, by the French mathematician Augustin Louis Cauchy (1789–1857) and the German mathematician Georg Friedrich Bernhard Riemann (1826–1866).

The way in which we find areas today using integral calculus is to find a formula for the area $A(P_n)$ of n inscribed polygons (in other words treat n as a variable). Then by taking the limit of $A(P_n)$ as n grows without bound ("goes to infinity") this expression will approach the exact area of the circle. That is,

$$\text{Area of circle} = \lim_{n \to \infty} A(P_n)$$

We illustrate how this process works by finding the exact area under the curve $y = x^2$. It is not critical that the approximating polygons be inscribed polygons but merely approximate the area of the region in question more closely as the number of polygons increases.

Figure 4
Three typical polygons whose areas are getting closer to the area of a circle

Example 1

Approximating an Area by Rectangles Approximate the area under the graph of the function

$$f(x) = x^2 \qquad (0 \le x \le 1)$$

as shown in Figure 5, using four rectangles as the approximating polygons.

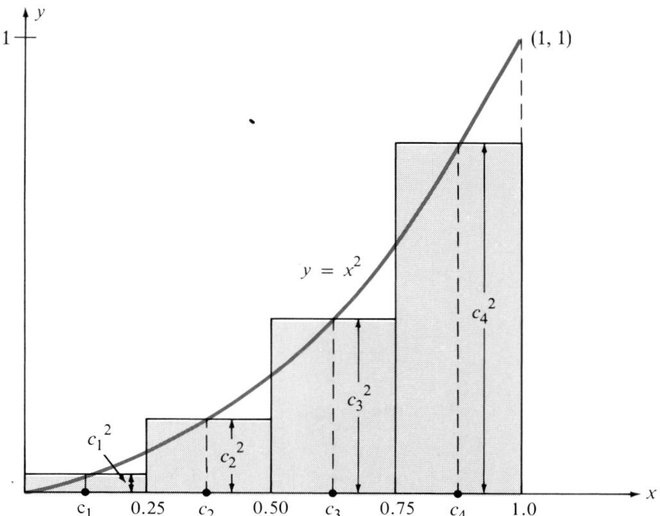

Figure 5
Approximation of the area under a curve by four rectangles

Solution

- **Step 1** (find the length of the subintervals). Subdivide the interval [0, 1] into four subintervals of equal length and compute the length h of each subinterval from the formula

$$h = \frac{\text{Length of interval}}{\text{Number of subintervals}} = \frac{1-0}{4} = \frac{1}{4}$$

- **Step 2** (find midpoints and heights of rectangles). Find the midpoint of each subinterval:

$$c_1 = \frac{h}{2} = \frac{0.25}{2} = 0.125$$

$$c_2 = c_1 + h = 0.125 + 0.250 = 0.375$$
$$c_3 = c_2 + h = 0.375 + 0.250 = 0.625$$
$$c_4 = c_3 + h = 0.625 + 0.250 = 0.875$$

Next draw the four rectangles; the width of each is $h = 0.25$, and the heights are given by

$$f(c_1) = {c_1}^2 = (0.125)^2 = 0.0156$$
$$f(c_2) = {c_2}^2 = (0.375)^2 = 0.1406$$
$$f(c_3) = {c_3}^2 = (0.625)^2 = 0.3906$$
$$f(c_4) = {c_4}^2 = (0.875)^2 = 0.7656$$

Note that the resulting rectangles (polygons) are not entirely beneath the graph of $y = x^2$. It is generally convenient to select the midpoint of each subinterval as the location where we determine the height of each rectangle. In other problems we may decide to choose other points in the subintervals as dictated by computational convenience.

- **Step 3.** Compute the total area of the four rectangles:

$$\begin{aligned}\text{Area of rectangles} &= f(c_1)\cdot h + f(c_2)\cdot h + f(c_3)\cdot h + f(c_4)\cdot h \\ &= 0.25[f(0.125) + f(0.375) + f(0.625) + f(0.875)] \\ &= 0.25[(0.125)^2 + (0.375)^2 + (0.625)^2 + (0.875)^2] \\ &= 0.25[0.0156 + 0.1406 + 0.3906 + 0.7656] \\ &= 0.3281 \qquad \text{(the exact area is } \tfrac{1}{3}\text{)}\end{aligned}$$

□

Example 2

Better Approximation Approximate the area under the graph of the function

$$f(x) = x^2 \qquad (0 \le x \le 1)$$

using $n = 8$ rectangles.

Solution Using the same steps as in Example 1 but now using eight subintervals, we find the midpoints, heights, and areas of the eight rectangles. Table 3 shows the results of these computations.

TABLE 3
Eight Rectangles Used to Approximate the Area Under $f(x) = x^2$

Subintervals	Midpoints, c_i	Heights of Rectangles, $f(c_i)$	Areas of Rectangles, $nf(c_i)$
[0.000, 0.125]	0.0625	0.0039	0.0005
[0.125, 0.250]	0.1875	0.0352	0.0044
[0.250, 0.375]	0.3125	0.0977	0.0122
[0.375, 0.500]	0.4375	0.1903	0.0238
[0.500, 0.625]	0.5625	0.3164	0.0396
[0.625, 0.750]	0.6875	0.4727	0.0591
[0.750, 0.875]	0.8125	0.6602	0.0825
[0.875, 1.00]	0.9375	0.8789	0.1099
		Total:	0.3320

Note in Table 3 that the length of each subinterval, which is the width of each rectangle, is $\frac{1}{8} = 0.125$. Note too that the areas of the eight rectangles are computed by multiplying the heights of the rectangles by their common width of 0.125. The rectangles are shown in Figure 6.

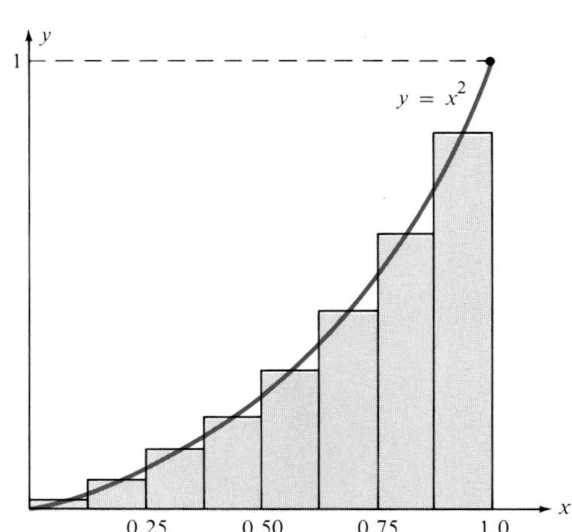

Figure 6
Approximation of the area under a curve by eight rectangles

When the number of rectangles is doubled from $n = 4$ to $n = 8$, the total area of the rectangles changes from 0.3281 to 0.3320, which is closer to the exact area of $\frac{1}{3}$. □

Table 4 gives the approximation of the area under the curve $y = x^2$ using n rectangles for different values of n. It seems clear that the area of n rectangles is approaching $\frac{1}{3}$ as n gets larger and larger.

TABLE 4
Approximating the Area Under $y = x^2$ $(0 \le x \le 1)$ by n Rectangles

Number of Rectangles, n	Area of Rectangles
1	0.2500
2	0.3125
3	0.3241
4	0.3281
5	0.3300
6	0.3310
7	0.3316
8	0.3320
9	0.3323
10	0.3325
15	0.3330
20	0.3331
30	0.3332
40	0.3333
50	0.3333

The Definite Integral

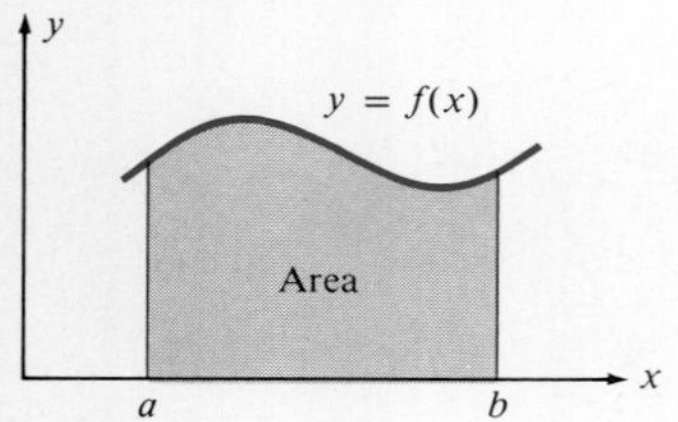

Figure 7
Finding the area under the graph of a function by the definite integral

We have seen that it is easy to find the area of squares, triangles, and other polygons by simple methods. However, finding the areas of regions with curved boundaries, such as the area under a portion of the curve $y = x^2$, requires the use of the limiting process. For the most part we will concentrate on finding areas between the graphs of functions and the x-axis. (See Figure 7.)

Geometrically, the definite integral can be interpreted as finding the area between the graph of a function and the x-axis by finding an algebraic expression for the area of n "approximating rectangles" and then letting n approach infinity. If this limit exists, it can often be shown to approach the exact area under the graph and above the x-axis. (See Figure 8.)

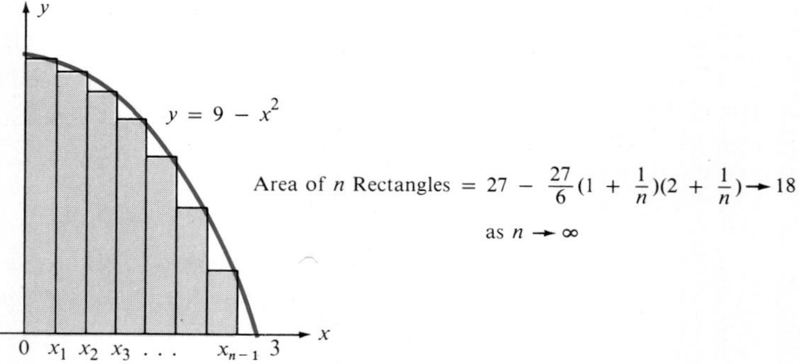

Figure 8
Area under n rectangles approaches 18 as n gets big

Intuitive Comments About the Definite Integral

When the graph of a function $y = f(x)$ lies above the x-axis, the limiting value of the area of n rectangles as n approaches infinity represents the area under the curve. When all of these rectangles have the same width h, height $f(c_i)$, and area $hf(c_i)$, the general expression for these n approximating rectangles is

$$A(R_n) = hf(c_1) + hf(c_2) + \cdots + hf(c_n)$$

As n gets larger and larger, the "shape" of these n rectangles will look more and more like the region between the graph of $y = f(x)$ and the x-axis. This limit

$$\lim_{n \to \infty} A(R_n)$$

is called the definite integral regardless of whether the graph of $y = f(x)$ is always above the x-axis.

If the graph of the function does not lie completely above the x-axis, the definite integral does not represent the area between the graph and the x-axis but can be modified so that the area between the graph and the x-axis can be found.

We now give the formal definition of the definite integral.

Definition of the Definite Integral

Let f be a continuous function on the interval $[a, b]$. The **definite integral** of f is defined as the limiting value of the sum

$$\int_a^b f(x)\,dx = \lim_{n \to \infty} [f(c_1)h + f(c_2)h + \cdots + f(c_n)h]$$

provided that the limit exists (note that n represents the number of terms in the series). The constant h is given by

$$h = \frac{b - a}{n}$$

and the constant c_i for $i = 1, \ldots, n$ is an arbitary number in the ith subinterval

$$x_{i-1} \leq c_i \leq x_i$$

The function f is called the **integrand** of the definite integral, and the numbers b and a are the **upper limit** and **lower limit** of integration, respectively. The following diagram illustrates the relevant variables:

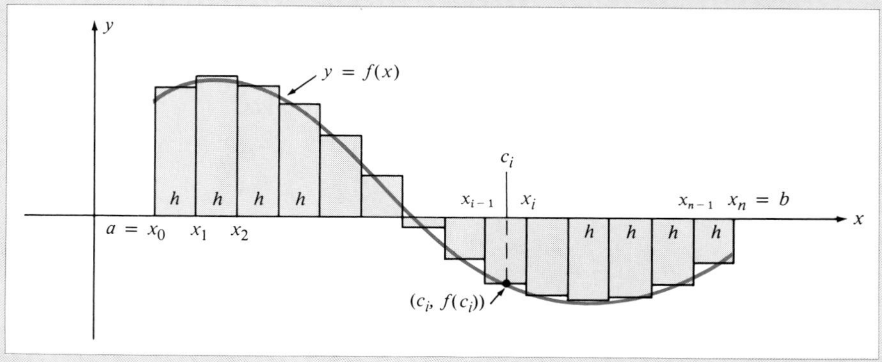

Note that a major difference between the definite integral of this section and the indefinite integral of the previous section is that the definite integral is a number, whereas the indefinite integral is a function.

Example 3 **Definite Integral** Evaluate the definite integral

$$\int_0^2 3x\,dx$$

Since the graph of $y = 3x$ is always above the x-axis over the interval $[0, 2]$, the value of its definite integral will be equal to the area between its graph and the x-axis. (See Figure 9.)

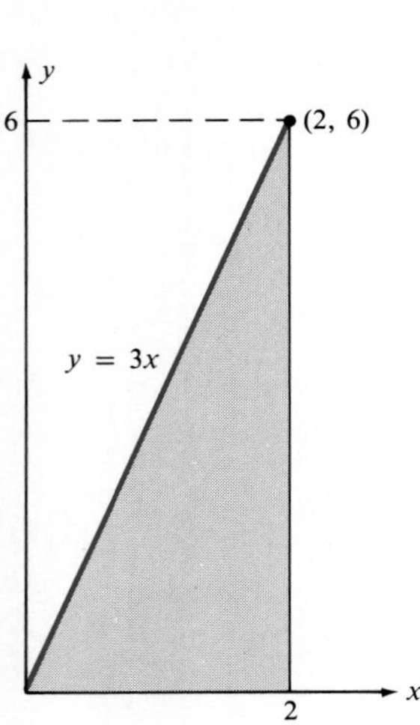

Figure 9
Find the shaded area

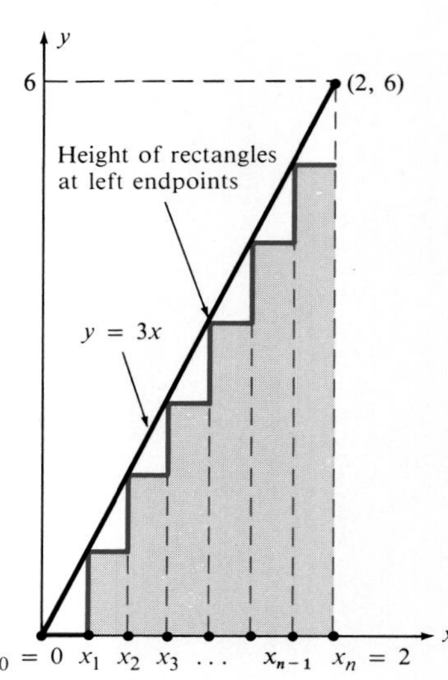

Figure 10
An approximation by n rectangles

Solution Note that the upper and lower limits of integration are

$$b = 2 \quad \text{(upper limit of integration)}$$
$$a = 0 \quad \text{(lower limit of integration)}$$

We begin by finding an algebraic formula A_n for the area under n rectangles. We then compute the limit of A_n as n increases without bound. (See Figure 10.) For convenience we have chosen the heights of the rectangles to be the values of $y = 3x$ at the left endpoints of the subintervals (instead of at the midpoints). If we choose n rectangles, then the widths and heights of these rectangles will be given by the formulas:

$$h = \frac{b-a}{n} = \frac{2-0}{n} = \frac{2}{n} \quad \text{(width of the rectangles)}$$

$$c_i = 0 + (i-1)\left(\frac{2}{n}\right) = (i-1)\left(\frac{2}{n}\right) \quad \text{(left endpoint of } i\text{th subinterval)}$$

$$f(c_i) = 3c_i = 3(i-1)\left(\frac{2}{n}\right) \quad \text{(height of } i\text{th rectangle)}$$

for $i = 1, 2, \ldots, n$.

Hence the formula for the total area of these n rectangles is simply the sum of the areas of each individual rectangle. That is,

$$\begin{aligned}
A_n &= f(c_1)h + f(c_2)h + \cdots + f(c_n)h \\
&= (3c_1)\frac{2}{n} + (3c_2)\frac{2}{n} + \cdots + (3c_n)\frac{2}{n} \\
&= \frac{6}{n}(c_1 + c_2 + \cdots + c_n) \\
&= \frac{6}{n}\left[0 + \frac{2}{n} + \frac{4}{n} + \frac{6}{n} + \cdots + \frac{2(n-1)}{n}\right] \\
&= \frac{12}{n^2}[1 + 2 + 3 + \cdots + (n-1)] \\
&= \frac{12}{n^2}\frac{n(n-1)}{2} \quad * \\
&= \frac{6n^2 - 6n}{n^2} \\
&= 6 - \frac{6}{n} \qquad \text{(area under } n \text{ rectangles)}
\end{aligned}$$

This expression gives the area for those n inscribed rectangles under the curve $y = 3x$. For example, if the number of rectangles is 10,000,000, the area would be

$$6 - \frac{6}{10{,}000{,}000} = 5.9999994$$

The beauty of this formula lies in the fact that it gives the area for any number of rectangles. It is easy to see that as more and more rectangles are included, the total area gets closer and closer to the value 6. In other words, the limiting value and hence the definite integral are given by

$$\begin{aligned}
\int_0^2 3x\,dx &= \lim_{n\to\infty} [f(c_1)h + f(c_2)h + \cdots + f(c_n)h] \\
&= \lim_{n\to\infty}\left(6 - \frac{6}{n}\right) = 6
\end{aligned}$$

□

Comment on the Choice of c_i

In the above example we chose the left endpoints of the subintervals as the locations c_i at which to determine the heights of the rectangles. This decision was for convenience more than anything else. We can choose these locations c_i at any

---

* This step is the result of the following formula which gives the sum of the sequence of $n - 1$ consecutive integers beginning with 1:

$$1 + 2 + 3 + \cdots + (n-1) = \frac{n(n-1)}{2}$$

You can check this result by substituting different values of n.

place in the ith subinterval and the limiting value of the total area of the rectangles will approach the same limit. Of course, for a given finite number of rectangles n the areas of the rectangles will be different from the value of the definite integral, but for larger and larger n this difference will go to zero.

Problems

For Problems 1–9, approximate the areas under the curves, using rectangles with the indicated number of subintervals. For each problem, calculate the approximate area by using the following three ways to determine the height of the rectangles:

- Left endpoint: Pick the left endpoint of each subinterval.
- Right endpoint: Pick the right endpoint of each subinterval.
- Midpoint: Pick the midpoint of each subinterval.

1. One rectangle.

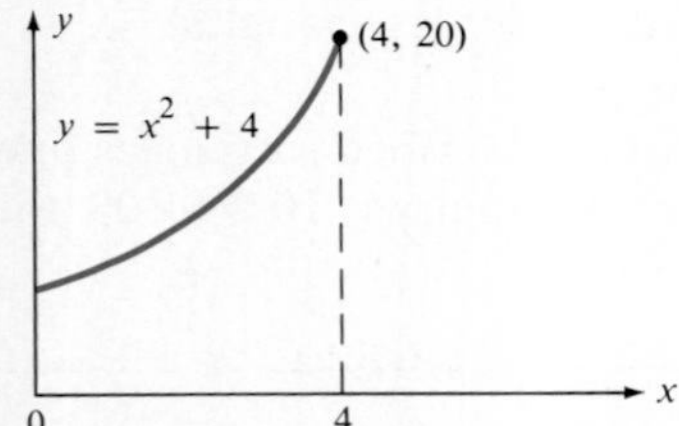

2. Two rectangles.

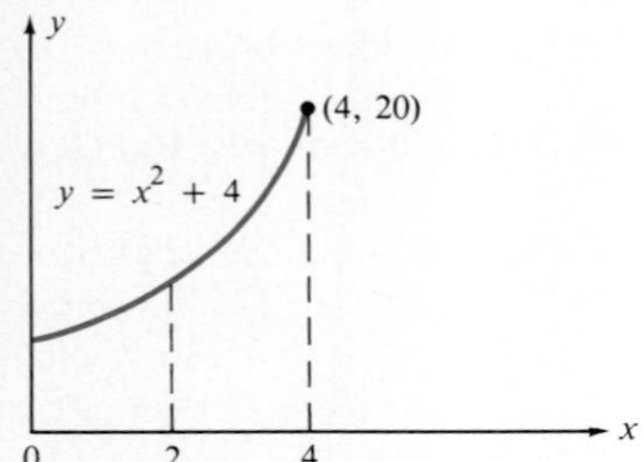

3. Four rectangles.

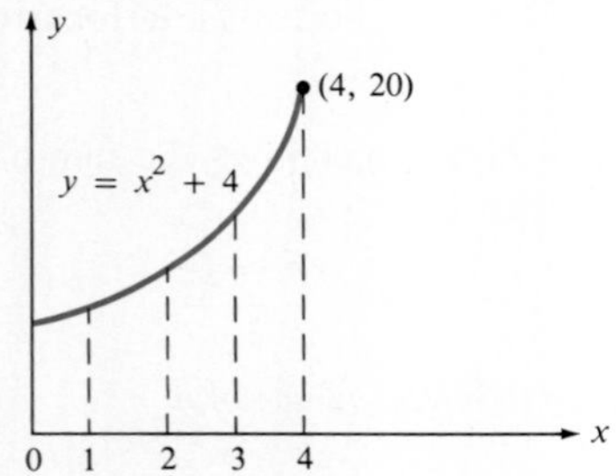

4. One subinterval.

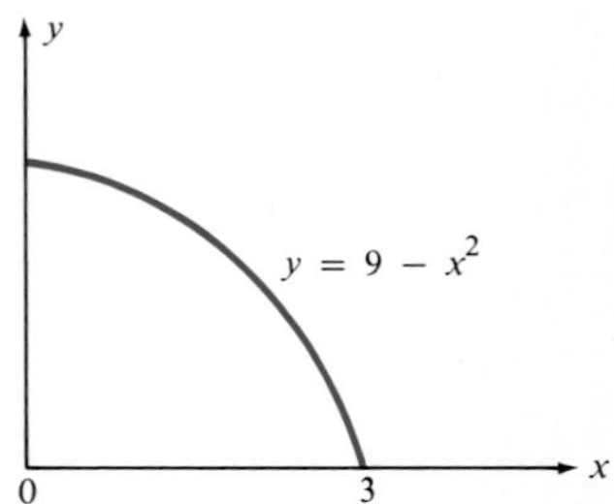

5. Two subintervals.

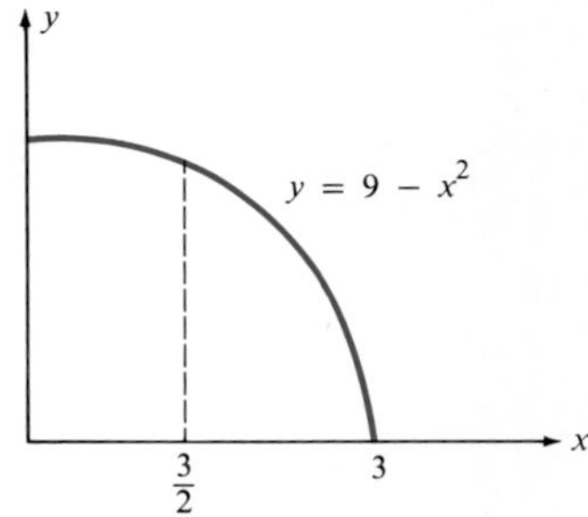

6. Three subintervals.

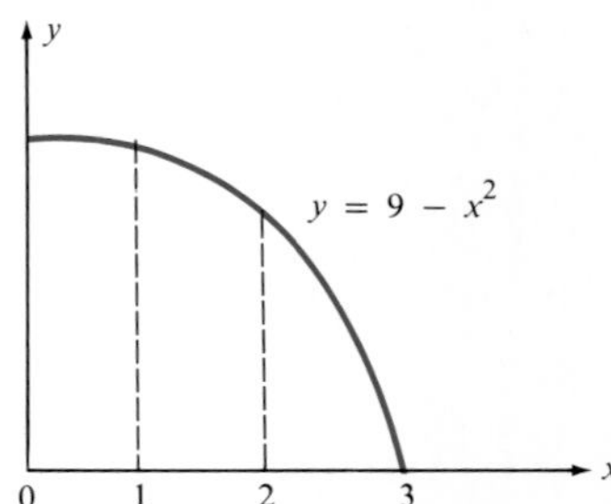

7. One subinterval.

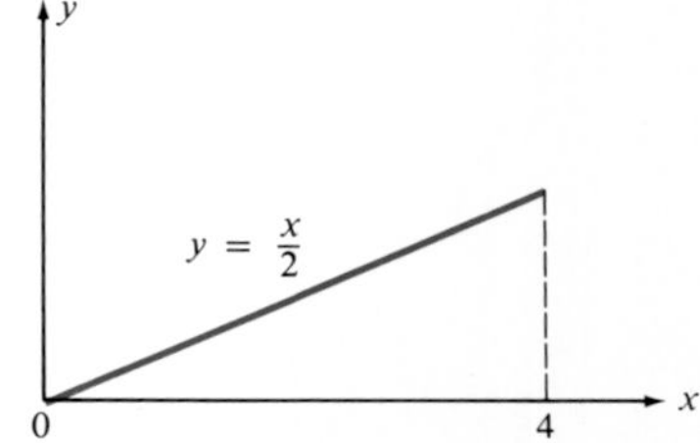

8. Two rectangles.

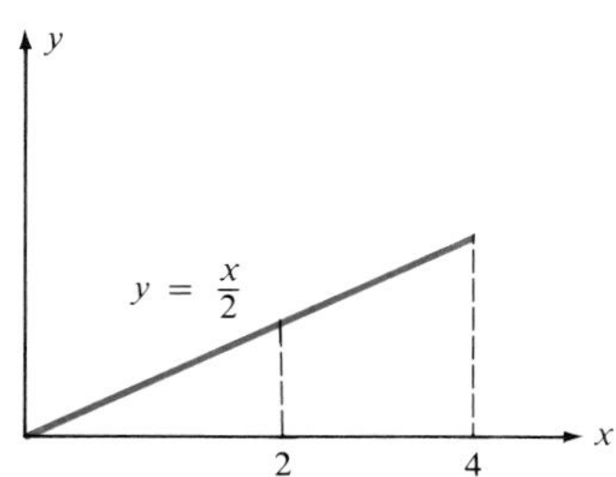

9. Four rectangles.

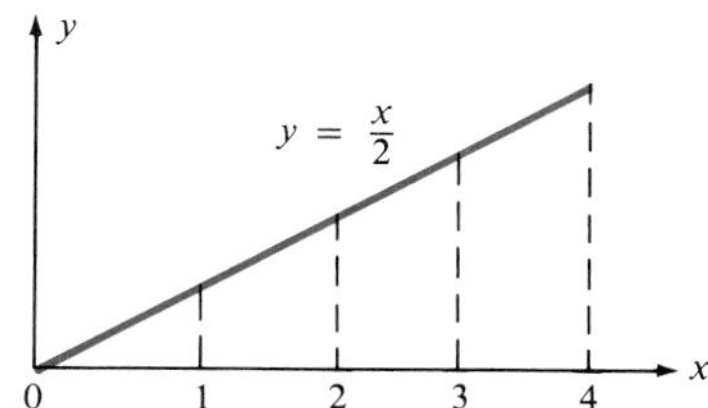

For Problems 10–18, approximate the area under the curves over the indicated intervals. Find approximations for both two and four subintervals, and let the height of the rectangles be the value of the function at the midpoint of each subinterval.

10. $f(x) = 6$ $[0, 1]$ **11.** $f(x) = x$ $[0, 2]$
12. $f(x) = 3x - 2$ $[1, 5]$ **13.** $f(x) = x + 1$ $[1, 5]$
14. $f(x) = x^2$ $[-1, 1]$ **15.** $f(x) = x^2 + 3$ $[4, 6]$
16. $f(x) = x^3$ $[1, 3]$ **17.** $f(x) = \frac{1}{x}$ $[1, 2]$
18. $f(x) = \frac{1}{x^2}$ $[1, 2]$

For Problems 19–22, find the exact area under the curves over the indicated intervals using the definition of the definite integral. Use the value of the function at the right endpoint of each subinterval to calculate the height of a rectangle.

19. $\int_2^5 5\,dx$

20. $\int_1^3 (x + 4)\,dx$ $\left[\textit{Hint: } 1 + 2 + \cdots + n = \frac{n(n+1)}{2}\right]$

21. $\int_0^1 x^2\,dx$

$\left[\textit{Hint: } 1^2 + 2^2 + 3^2 + \cdots + n^2 = \frac{n(n+1)(2n+1)}{6}\right]$

22. $\int_0^1 x^3\,dx$ $\left[\textit{Hint: } 1^3 + 2^3 + 3^3 + \cdots + n^3 = \frac{n^2(n+1)^2}{4}\right]$

Areas in Business

23. Total Sales. Find the total sales for the last four years by finding the area under the curve described in Figure 11. The units for the y-axis are in \$100,000 of sales. Only formulas from geometry are needed.

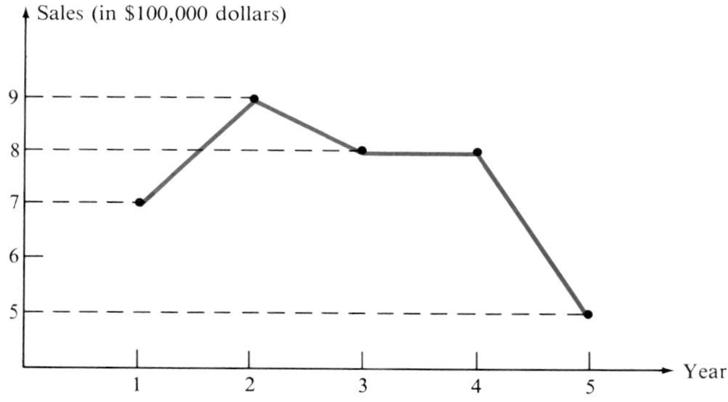

Figure 11
Graph for Problem 23

24. Total Cost. Estimate the total advertising cost for the past six months by finding the area under the curve in Figure 12. The graph below gives the advertising costs by day. The vertical axis has units of \$100. Use any convenient point to determine the heights of the rectangles over each of the six subintervals. The location of the point need not be the same for each subinterval.

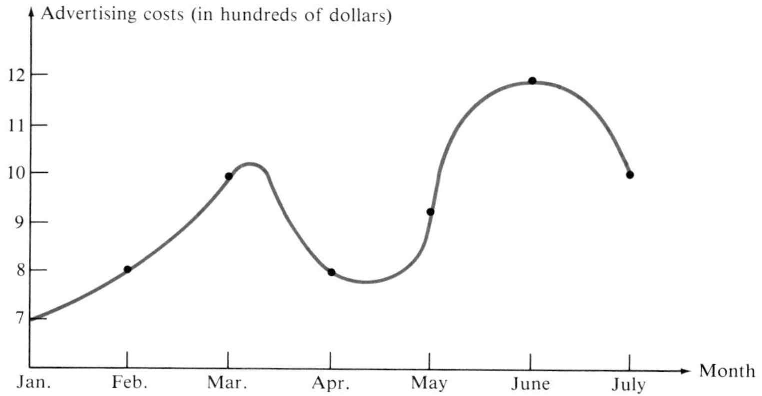

Figure 12
Graph for Problem 24

4.3 The Fundamental Theorem of Calculus

PURPOSE

We introduce the fundamental theorem of calculus. This theorem tells us how to evaluate the definite integral of a function using the antiderivative of the integrand without having to evaluate the limit found in the definition. Using the fundamental theorem, we then evaluate definite integrals used in economics and science.

Fundamental Theorem

In the previous section we evaluated the definite integral of a function f defined on a given interval $[a, b]$ by evaluating the limit

$$\int_a^b f(x)\,dx = \lim_{n \to \infty} [f(c_1)h + f(c_2)h + \cdots + f(c_n)h]$$

This definition is hardly an operational one. It does not provide a practical method for integrating functions and giving answers. Trying to find the definite integral of a function such as

$$f(x) = x^5 - e^x + \ln x$$

using the definition would be almost impossible. There is an important theorem in calculus that allows us to bypass the complicated limit in the definition of the definite integral and evaluate definite integrals by using the antiderivative. This theorem is the **fundamental theorem of calculus**.

Statement of the Fundamental Theorem of Calculus

Let f be a continuous function defined on the interval $[a, b]$ and let F be any antiderivative of f. The definite integral of f can be evaluated from the formula

$$\int_a^b f(x)\,dx = F(b) - F(a)$$

The difference $F(b) - F(a)$ is often denoted in shorthand by the expression

$$F(b) - F(a) = F(x)\Big|_a^b$$

Comments on the Fundamental Theorem

Many students wonder what is so significant about this theorem that it warrants the special name, the fundamental theorem of calculus. What is there about it that gives it this central place in the theory of calculus? Of course, from a practical point of view it is obviously an extremely useful tool for evaluating definite integrals. By applying this theorem, all we have to do to evaluate the definite integral

$$\int_a^b f(x)\,dx$$

is carry out the following steps.

> **Evaluating Definite Integrals Using the Fundamental Theorem**
>
> **Step 1.** Find any antiderivative $F(x)$ of the integrand $f(x)$.
>
> **Step 2.** Evaluate the antiderivative found in Step 1 at the upper and lower limits b and a, getting $F(b)$ and $F(a)$.
>
> **Step 3.** Calculate $F(b) - F(a)$ to obtain the value of the definite integral.

Although the above steps for evaluating definite integrals are extremely useful, they are still not the reason for the name "fundamental theorem." The reason can be seen if we rewrite the theorem in a slightly different manner. Since an integrand $f(x)$ and its antiderivative $F(x)$ are related by

$$F'(x) = f(x)$$

we can rewrite the fundamental theorem in the alternative form

$$\int_a^x F'(x)\,dx = F(x) - F(a)$$

where we have decided to replace the upper limit b by the variable x. (We can do this because b was arbitrary.) If the lower limit of integration a is chosen so that $F(a) = 0$, then we have

$$\int_a^x F'(x)\,dx = F(x)$$

In other words, the fundamental theorem relates the two basic operations of the calculus, differentiation and integration. It says that differential calculus is not a completely unrelated subject from integral calculus. But it even says more. It says that the operation of integration "undoes" the operation of differentiation. In other words, the two basic operations of the calculus are inverse operations.

We now apply the fundamental theorem of calculus to evaluate some definite integrals.

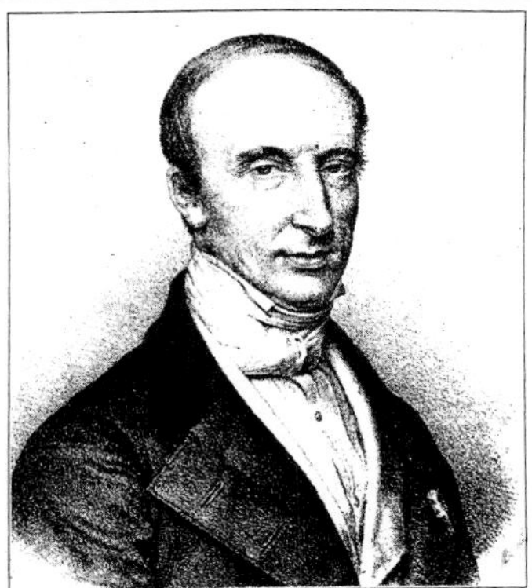

HISTORICAL NOTE

Historically, the definite integral evolved from an attempt to find the area of some region of the plane. Regions were thought to be subdivided into an "infinite number" of rectangles having a height y and an "infinitely small" width dx. The area was then found by "summing" the areas of these rectangles. The sum of the areas of these rectangles was denoted by Leibniz by an elongated S, or $\int$ (now called the integral sign) taken from the Latin word "*summa*." Hence Leibniz denoted the area in question as

$$\int f(x)\,dx$$

The actual word "integral" was first used by the Swiss mathematician Jakob Bernoulli in 1690 to denote "a putting together of component parts."

The modern development of the integral was begun in the 1820's by Augustin Louis Cauchy, who first defined the integral as the limiting value of sums of areas of rectangles.

Example 1 Evaluating Definite Integrals Evaluate the definite integral

$$\int_0^1 x^3\,dx$$

Solution

- **Step 1** (find an antiderivative). Finding an antiderivative of $f(x) = x^3$, we get

$$F(x) = \frac{1}{4}x^4 + C$$

- **Step 2** (evaluate $F(b)$ and $F(a)$). Evaluating the antiderivative at the upper and lower limits, we have

$$F(1) = \frac{(1)^4}{4} + C = \frac{1}{4} + C$$

$$F(0) = \frac{(0)^4}{4} + C = C$$

- **Step 3** (calculate $F(b) - F(a)$). Finding the difference between the antiderivative at the upper and lower limits, we have

$$\begin{aligned}\int_0^1 x^3\,dx &= F(1) - F(0)\\ &= \left(\frac{1}{4} + C\right) - C\\ &= \frac{1}{4}\end{aligned}$$

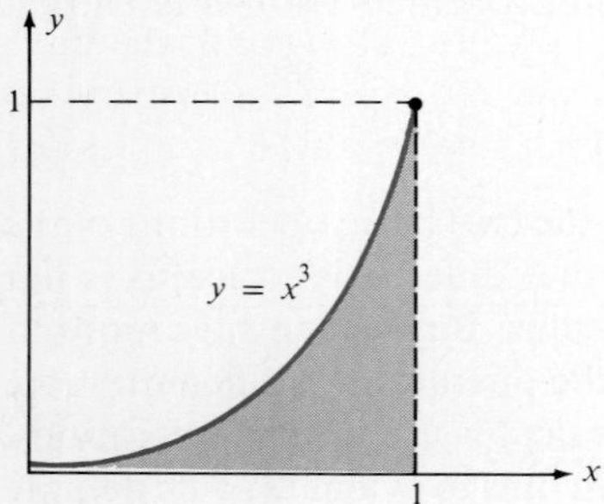

Figure 13
Area under $y = x^3$

Note that the constant C in the antiderivative has canceled and hence does not affect the value of the definite integral. For this reason we will always pick an antiderivative $F(x)$ with $C = 0$ when evaluating definite integrals.

The definite integral represents the area under the curve $y = x^3$ over the interval $[0, 1]$ as shown in Figure 13. □

Example 2 Finding Areas Find the area under the curve

$$y = 1 + e^x$$

over the interval $[0, 2]$ as shown in Figure 14.

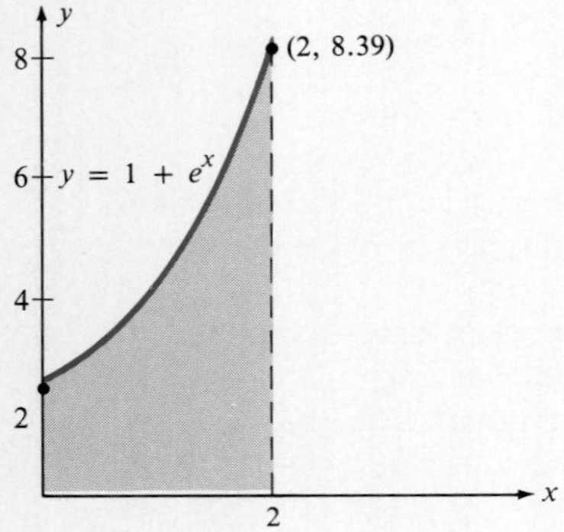

Figure 14
Area under an exponential curve

Solution Since the given function is positive, the area is the value of the definite integral

$$\int_0^2 (1 + e^x)\,dx$$

Now that we have seen the three-step process carried out in Example 1, we will streamline our operation and simply write

$$\begin{aligned}\int_0^2 (1 + e^x)\,dx &= F(x)\Big|_0^2\\ &= (x + e^x)\Big|_0^2\\ &= (2 + e^2) - (0 + e^0)\\ &= e^2 + 1\end{aligned}$$

□

Example 3 Finding a Definite Integral Evaluate the definite integral

$$\int_{-1}^{1} (t^2 + 1)\, dt$$

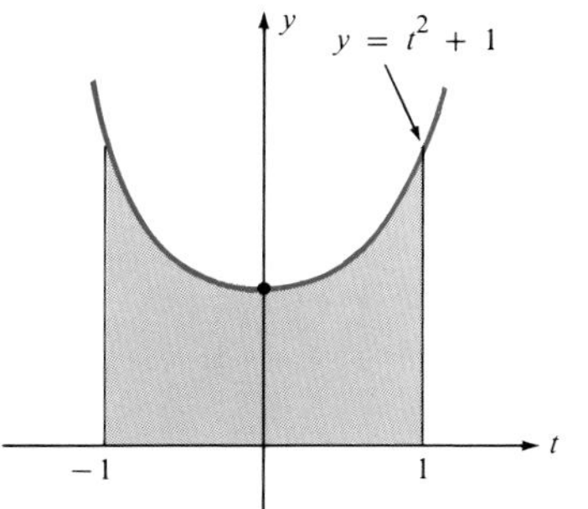

Figure 15
Finding the area under a parabola

Solution Using the fundamental theorem of calculus, we have

$$\begin{aligned}\int_{-1}^{1} (t^2 + 1)\, dt &= \left[\frac{1}{3}t^3 + t\right]\Bigg|_{-1}^{1} \\ &= \left[\frac{1}{3}(1)^3 + 1\right] - \left[\frac{1}{3}(-1)^3 + (-1)\right] \\ &= \frac{4}{3} + \frac{4}{3} \\ &= \frac{8}{3}\end{aligned}$$

This value represents the value of the area shown in Figure 15. □

Rules of Integration

Just as we have rules for evaluating derivatives of sums, differences, products, quotients, and compositions of functions, we can also develop rules for the integration of such combinations of functions. These rules, along with the fundamental theorem of calculus, will allow us to evaluate a wide assortment of definite integrals. If we interpret the integral of a positive function as an area, then for such functions these rules can be intuitively verified.

Rules for Evaluating Definite Integrals

Let f and g be functions such that the following integrals exist and let a, b, and c be constants. Then

- Constants can be factored outside the integral.

$$\int_a^b cf(x)\, dx = c\int_a^b f(x)\, dx$$

- The integral of a sum is the sum of the integrals.

$$\int_a^b [f(x) + g(x)]\, dx = \int_a^b f(x)\, dx + \int_a^b g(x)\, dx$$

- The integral of a difference is the difference of the integrals.

$$\int_a^b [f(x) - g(x)]\, dx = \int_a^b f(x)\, dx - \int_a^b g(x)\, dx$$

Verification of the Integration Rules

The previous rules can be verified intuitively for positive functions by interpreting the definite integral as an area. For instance, the second rule stating that the integral of a sum is the sum of the integrals has a visual interpretation as shown in Figure 16. Essentially, the rule says that the area under the graph of the sum of two functions is the sum of the areas under each individual graph.

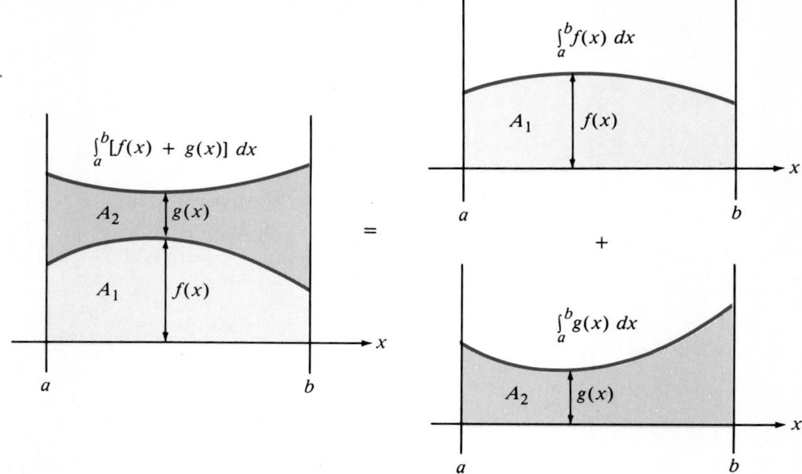

Figure 16
Geometric interpretation of the sum rule for integrals

Example 4

Using the Rules of Integration Evaluate the definite integral

$$\int_0^1 5x\,dx$$

Solution Bringing the constant 5 outside the integral, we have

$$\begin{aligned}\int_0^1 5x\,dx &= 5\int_0^1 x\,dx\\ &= 5\left[\frac{1}{2}x^2\Big|_0^1\right]\\ &= 5\left[\frac{1}{2}(1)^2 - \frac{1}{2}(0)^2\right]\\ &= \frac{5}{2}\end{aligned}$$

□

Example 5

Using the Rules of Integration Evaluate the definite integral

$$\int_0^1 (3x^2 + 2x + 4)\,dx$$

Solution Using the rules of integration, we can write

$$\begin{aligned}\int_0^1 (3x^2 + 2x + 4)\,dx &= \int_0^1 3x^2\,dx + \int_0^1 2x\,dx + \int_0^1 4\,dx \quad \text{(sum rule)}\\ &= 3\int_0^1 x^2\,dx + 2\int_0^1 x\,dx + 4\int_0^1 dx \quad \text{(constant rule)}\\ &= 3\left[\frac{1}{3}x^3\Big|_0^1\right] + 2\left[\frac{1}{2}x^2\Big|_0^1\right] + 4\left[x\Big|_0^1\right]\\ &= 3\left(\frac{1}{3}\right) + 2\left(\frac{1}{2}\right) + 4(1)\\ &= 6\end{aligned}$$

□

The Use of the Definite Integral in Economics

If $C(q)$ denotes the total cost of producing q units of a given commodity, then $C'(q)$ represents the marginal cost. Applying the fundamental theorem of calculus, we can write

$$\int_a^b C'(q)\,dq = C(b) - C(a)$$

The value of this formula lies in the fact that the quantity $C(b) - C(a)$ simply represents the change in cost when the production level is raised from a items to b items. Hence we have the useful rules.

Integral Rules in Economics

Let MR, MP, and MC denote marginal revenue, marginal profit, and marginal cost, respectively. The changes in the total revenue R, total profit P, and total cost C, when the level of production q is changed from a units to b units are given by the following definite integrals:

$$\text{Change in revenue} = \int_a^b MR(q)\,dq$$

$$\text{Change in profit} = \int_a^b MP(q)\,dq$$

$$\text{Change in cost} = \int_a^b MC(q)\,dq$$

Example 6

Finding Increased Costs Suppose you have just been hired as production manager for a large firm that makes stuffed bears. When the production of bears is q bears per hour, your analysis of various costs has determined that the cost (in dollars) of making one more bear is

$$MC(q) = 22 - 0.02q$$

In other words, the first bear costs \$22 to produce, while the cost of making each succeeding bear goes down by two cents. Find the increase in the company's cost when the hourly production level of bears is raised from 100 to 200 bears.

Solution The increase in total cost C, which is $C(200) - C(100)$, can be found by using the fundamental theorem of calculus:

$$\begin{aligned}\text{Increase in cost} &= \int_{100}^{200} MC(q)\,dq \\ &= \int_{100}^{200} (22 - 0.02q)\,dq \\ &= (22q - 0.01q^2)\Big|_{100}^{200} \\ &= (4400 - 400) - (2200 - 100) \\ &= 1900\end{aligned}$$

In other words, the hourly increase in cost necessary to increase production from 100 units to 200 units is \$1900. It is important to note that we did not need to know the value of the fixed costs to find this answer. This is important, since it is often difficult to find this value. □

Determination of Cardiac Output (Dye Dilution Method)

Sally is a member of the university swimming team. To determine her potential as a long-distance swimmer, her coach decides to measure Sally's cardiac output. By cardiac output we simply mean the number of liters of blood that Sally's heart pumps every minute. The technique for measuring cardiac output is known as the dye dilution method. The procedure is quite simple. A dye (Evans blue) is injected into a vein (vena cubiti) near her heart. The dye then goes to the right heart, then through the vascular bed of the lungs, back to the left heart and thence into the aorta and systemic arteries. (See Figure 17a.)

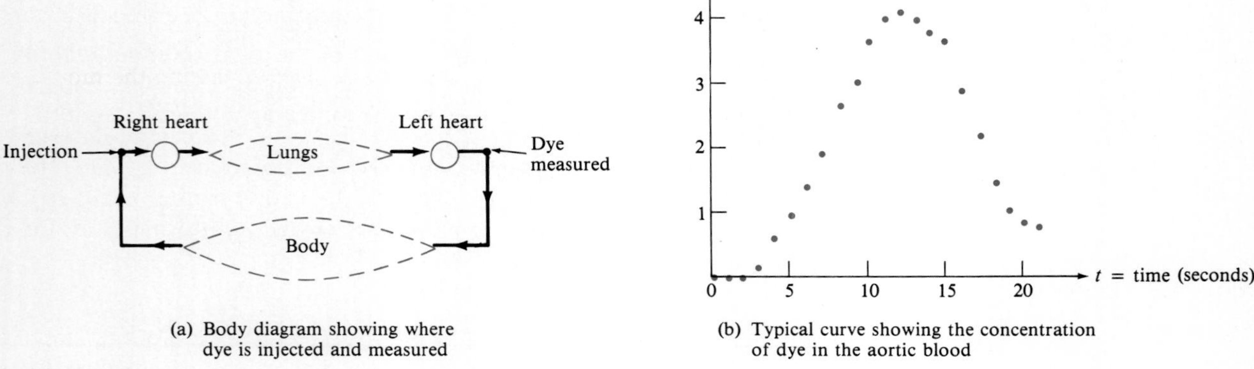

(a) Body diagram showing where dye is injected and measured

(b) Typical curve showing the concentration of dye in the aortic blood

Figure 17
To determine cardiac output, dye is injected into a vein near the heart and then measured in the aortic artery

Samples of blood are then taken at frequent time intervals (1 second, for example) from the aortic artery where the dye first appears a few seconds after injection. Since the injected particles of dye will traverse different pathways through the pulmonary vessels of the lung, they will take varying amounts of time to travel from the injection site to the sampling site. These circumstances lead to the particular shape of the concentration curve shown in Figure 17b.

To develop the mathematics required to determine Sally's cardiac output, we let

$$D = \text{amount of dye injected into the blood (mg)}$$
$$R = \text{cardiac output (liters/min)}$$
$$c(t) = \text{concentration of dye in the blood (mg/liter)}$$

To understand the dye dilution principle, you must understand that the amount of dye that passes the monitoring point in a small time interval of dt minutes from t to $t + dt$ is equal to (approximately) the observed concentration $c(t)$ times the cardiac output R times the length of the time interval dt; that is,

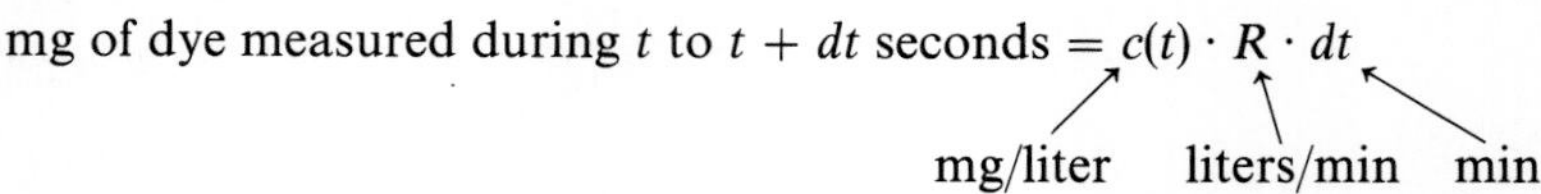

Since all of the injected dye will eventually pass the monitoring point, the total amount of injected dye (mg) will be equal to the sum of the amounts passing

the monitoring point during subsequent intervals. This gives rise to the integral

$$D = \int_0^{T_0} c(t)R\,dt$$
$$= R\int_0^{T_0} c(t)\,dt$$

where t is time measured in minutes and T_0 is the total time it takes for the dye to pass the monitoring point. Hence Sally's cardiac output R is given by

$$R = \frac{D}{\int_0^{T_0} c(t)\,dt}$$

Interpretation

This equation allows us to compute Sally's cardiac output R from a knowledge of the amount D of injected dye and the area under the concentration curve. The concentration curve $c(t)$ is meant to reflect the dye passing the monitoring point on the "first pass." Since the dye will circulate through the body and return back to the heart and thence to the monitoring point in about every 20 seconds, we must in fact integrate the concentration curve over a finite interval, such as [0, 20]. We would have to observe the concentration curve $c(t)$ and determine how long it takes until the dye passes the monitoring point for the first time.

Example 7

Sally's Cardiac Output Sally's physician injects 5.0 mg of Evans blue dye into her vena cubiti. A monitoring device inserted into the aortic artery measures the concentration of dye in the blood every second for 20 seconds, and the results are recorded. (See Figure 18.)

There are techniques (such as the method of least squares, which we will study later) for finding a curve that approximates the data points. Suppose the

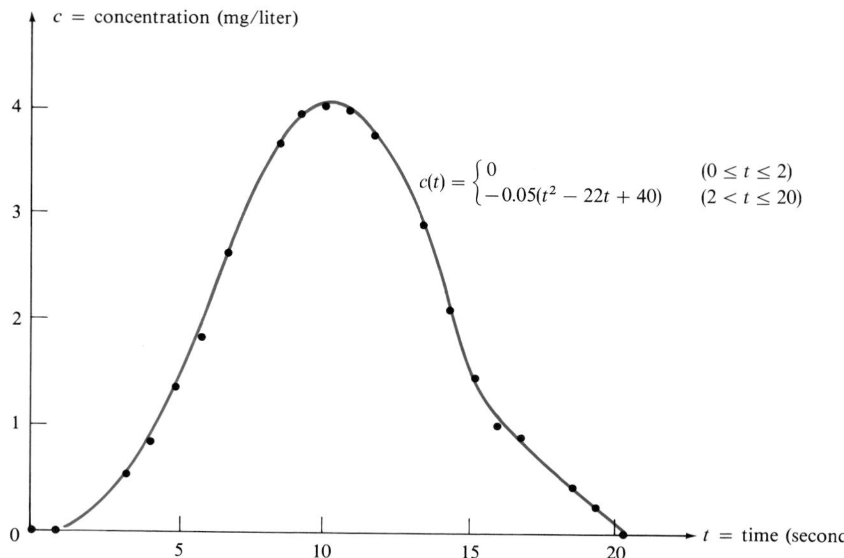

Figure 18
Concentration of dye at the monitoring point as a function of time

best least squares curve that "fits" the observed values of $c(t)$ has been found and is

$$c(t) = \begin{cases} 0 & (0 \le t \le 2) \\ -0.05(t^2 - 22t + 40) & (2 < t \le 20) \end{cases}$$

Integrating this curve, we find

$$\int_0^{20} c(t)\,dt = -0.05 \int_2^{20} (t^2 - 22t + 40)\,dt$$
$$= 48.6$$

Since we have been measuring time in seconds, we can compute Sally's cardiac output R_{sec} in liters per second from the equation

$$R_{sec} = \frac{D}{\int_0^{20} c(t)dt} = \frac{5}{48.6}$$
$$= 0.102 \text{ liters/sec}$$

To find Sally's cardiac output in liters per minute, we multiply the above result by 60 giving

$$R = 60(0.102)$$
$$= 6.12 \text{ liters/min}$$

Hence Sally has a cardiac output of 6.12 liters per minute, which places her in the top 10 percentile for women of her age. □

Problems

For Problems 1–25, evaluate the definite integrals using the fundamental theorem of calculus.

1. $\int_{-3}^{2} 2\,dx$
2. $\int_0^4 5x\,dx$
3. $\int_2^5 (x + 3)\,dx$
4. $\int_1^5 (7t - 3)\,dt$
5. $\int_1^8 (y^3 - 1)\,dy$
6. $\int_1^4 (x^2 - 2x + 2)\,dx$
7. $\int_0^2 (x^3 + x + 3)\,dx$
8. $\int_{-1}^{2} (9x^2 + 2)\,dx$
9. $\int_{-2}^{4} (5 - 3x + 2x^2)\,dx$
10. $\int_1^3 (x - 1)(x + 2)\,dx$ (*Hint:* Do the multiplication first.)
11. $\int_1^4 (9 - x)\sqrt{x}\,dx$
12. $\int_3^4 (x + 1)^2\,dx$
13. $\int_1^5 2x(x^2 + 3)\,dx$
14. $\int_0^1 (8x^2 + 4)(x^2 + 2)\,dx$
15. $\int_1^e \left(x + \frac{1}{x^2}\right)dx$
16. $\int_0^1 \left(\frac{3}{2}e^x - \frac{1}{2}e^{-x}\right)dx$
17. $\int_1^4 \left(\sqrt{x} + \frac{1}{x^2}\right)dx$
18. $\int_0^1 (e^{-x} + x^2)^3(2x - e^{-x})\,dx$
19. $\int_2^5 \frac{x^2 + 1}{x^2}\,dx$
20. $\int_1^3 20x(x^2 + 7)^3\,dx$
21. $\int_2^3 \frac{6x^2 + 4}{\sqrt{x^3 + 2x}}\,dx$
22. $\int_1^4 \frac{x^2 + 3x + 4}{\sqrt{x}}\,dx$
23. $\int_0^1 \frac{2x}{(3 + x^2)^2}\,dx$
24. $\int_5^{10} \frac{8}{\sqrt{4u + 3}}\,du$
25. $\int_0^1 (ax^2 + bx + c)(2ax + b)\,dx$
(*a*, *b*, *c* are positive constants)

For Problems 26–45, find the area between the nonnegative functions and the x-axis over the indicated interval.

26. $f(x) = 2x - 5$, $[3, 6]$
27. $f(t) = 9 - t^2$, $[-2, 1]$
28. $f(x) = x^3$, $[0, 2]$
29. $f(u) = 1 + 2u$, $[0, 3]$

30. $f(x) = x^2 + x^3$, [0, 2]

31. $f(x) = x^3 - 3x^2 + 5$, [0, 2]

32. $f(t) = 4t + t^3$, [1, 2]

33. $f(x) = 2x + x^2$, [0, 5]

34. $f(x) = \sqrt[3]{x}$, [1, 8]

35. $f(w) = \sqrt{w} + \frac{1}{w^2}$, [2, 4]

36. $f(x) = 5 + 2x\sqrt{x^2 + 1}$, [1, 2]

37. $f(x) = e^x$, [0, 1]

38. $f(x) = 4e^{-4x}$, [1, 3]

39. $f(t) = 3e^{-t/5}$, [0, ln 2]

40. $f(u) = 2e^{4u}$, [−1, 1]

41. $f(t) = e^{-t} + 1$, [0, 2]

42. $f(x) = xe^{-x^2}$, [0, 1]

43. $f(x) = xe^{x^2}$, [0, 1]

44. $f(t) = e^{-t}$, [0, 5]

45. $f(t) = 3e^t + 1$, [1, 2]

Finding the Change in Functions

46. Increase in Revenue. The marginal revenue for a firm when sales are q is given by

$$MR(q) = 10 - 0.05q$$

Find the increase in revenue when the sales level increases from 100 to 200 units.

47. Increase in Revenue. The marginal revenue when sales are q items is given by

$$MR(q) = 2 - 0.05q + 0.006q^2$$

What is the revenue increase resulting from a sales increase from 50 to 100 units?

48. Increase in Cost. The marginal cost for Gadgets Inc. is given by

$$MC(q) = 2 - 0.03q + 0.005q^2$$

where q is the number of units produced. What is the total cost to raise production from 100 to 200 units?

49. Increase in Profits. The marginal cost of a certain firm is given by

$$MC(q) = 15 - 0.002q$$

whereas the marginal revenue is

$$MR(q) = 20 - 0.003q$$

where q is the number of units produced. Find the increase in profits when sales are increased from 500 to 700 units.

50. Increased Population. A population of bacteria adds $2000/\sqrt{t}$ new bacteria to its colony each week. How many bacteria are added to the population from week 3 to week 5?

51. Total Revenue. Find the total revenue for 540 units given the marginal revenue

$$MR(q) = 3000 - 4q$$

Hint: Use $R(0) = 0$ to evaluate the constant of integration.

52. Total Cost. Find the total cost of producing 100 items if the marginal cost is

$$MC(q) = 3q^2 - 4q + 5$$

and the fixed cost is zero.

53. Distance Traveled. If a ball is dropped from a tall building, the velocity of the ball in feet per second will be

$$v(t) = 32t$$

where t is time in seconds measured from the time that the ball is dropped. How far will the ball fall between the third second and the fifth second?

54. Lifting Weights. A weight lifter is exercising by repeatedly stretching a spring to its full extension of 2 feet. The amount of work W done in foot-pounds to stretch this spring L feet is given by

$$W = \int_0^L 50x\,dx$$

How much work does the weight lifter perform on each stretch of the spring?

4.4 Evaluating Integrals by the Method of Substitution

PURPOSE

We introduce the method of substitution, which is a method that is helpful in finding an antiderivative $F(x)$ of a function $f(x)$. Knowing an antiderivative, we can then use the fundamental theorem of calculus to evaluate the definite integral. We also present a new economic application of the definite integral, the coefficient of inequality for income distributions.

Introduction

The evaluation of the definite integral

$$\int_a^b f(x)\,dx$$

by the use of the fundamental theorem of calculus is dependent on finding an antiderivative $F(x)$ of the integrand $f(x)$. However, finding an antiderivative of a function is generally much more difficult than finding the derivative. When we find the derivative, we can always use one of the useful rules such as the sum, difference, product, quotient, or chain rule. However, when we seek to find an antiderivative, there are no clear guidelines to follow, and we can often try several different approaches.

The diagram in Figure 19 illustrates our predicament. When we go to the right to find the derivative, there is always a clear path to follow. However, when we go to the left, choices must be made. Here is where the method of substitution is useful. It helps us to make these choices.

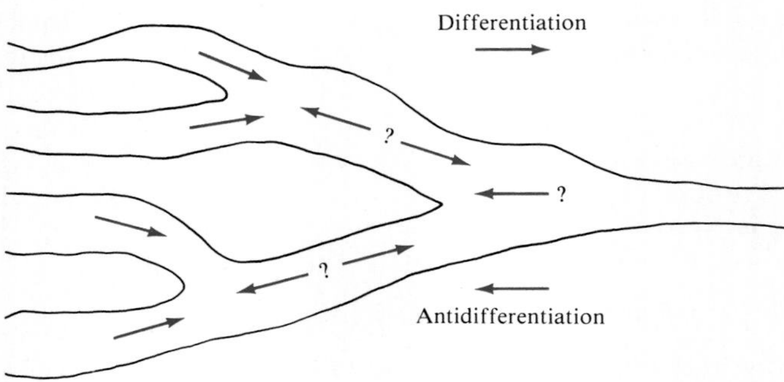

Figure 19
There are specific rules for differentiation but not for antidifferentiation

The Method of Substitution

To understand the method of substitution, it is useful that we review the concept of the differential. For example, if

$$y = (x^2 + 1)^3$$

then the differential is

$$\begin{aligned} dy &= f'(x)\,dx \\ &= 3(x^2 + 1)^2(2x)\,dx \end{aligned}$$

Suppose now that we wish to find the antiderivative

$$\int (x^2 + 1)^2(2x)\,dx$$

Here is where the method of substitution comes into play. To find the above antiderivative, we make a substitution by letting

$$u = x^2 + 1$$

which has the differential

$$du = 2x\,dx$$

Substituting these values into the above indefinite integral, we get

$$\int (x^2 + 1)^2(2x)\,dx = \int u^2\,du$$

We can now find the antiderivative on the right-hand side of this equation by using the power rule. It is simply

$$\int u^2\,du = \frac{1}{3}u^3 + C$$

Finally, substituting $u = x^2 + 1$ for u in the above antiderivative, we get the desired antiderivative in terms of x:

$$\int (x^2 + 1)^2(2x)\,dx = \frac{1}{3}(x^2 + 1)^3 + C$$

The hardest part of the method of substitution is knowing how to define the substitution variable (what should u be). Expertise comes with practice, and one often ends up making a few trial substitutions to find one that actually works.

Example 1

Method of Substitution Find the antiderivative

$$\int \sqrt{2x + 3}\,dx$$

Solution It is often unclear how to make the proper substitution; in fact, sometimes no substitution will work. A good rule of thumb when solving problems involving square roots is to set u equal to the expression under the radical. We carry out the following steps:

- **Step 1.** Introduce the new variable $u = 2x + 3$ and find the differential $du = 2\,dx$.
- **Step 2.** Solve for dx and $2x + 3$ in terms of u and du so that it is possible to transform the original indefinite integral in x to an indefinite integral in u. Doing this, we have

$$2x + 3 = u$$

$$dx = \frac{1}{2}du$$

and hence

$$\int \sqrt{2x + 3}\,dx = \int \frac{\sqrt{u}}{2}\,du$$

- **Step 3.** Find the antiderivative of the new integral in u. Doing this, we get

$$\frac{1}{2}\int \sqrt{u}\,du = \frac{1}{3}u^{3/2} + C$$

- **Step 4.** Substitute back in terms of the original variable. Doing this, we find

$$\int \sqrt{2x + 3}\,dx = \frac{1}{3}(2x + 3)^{3/2} + C$$

Check:

$$\frac{d}{dx}\left[\frac{1}{3}(2x + 3)^{3/2} + C\right] = \sqrt{2x + 3}$$ □

In Example 1 we found the antiderivative in four steps. We list these steps now.

Steps in the Method of Substitution

To find the integral

$$\int f(x)\,dx$$

carry out the following steps:

Step 1 (find u and du). Introduce a new variable u that will be some function of the original variable x and compute the differential du.

Step 2 (find the new integral). Substitute u and du found in Step 1 into the original integral. This gives the new indefinite integral in u:

$$\int f(x)\,dx = \int g(u)\,du$$

where $g(u)$ is the new integrand.

Step 3 (find the new indefinite integral). Find the antiderivative $G(u)$ of $g(u)$:

$$\int g(u)\,du = G(u) + C$$

Hopefully, this step will be easy.

Step 4 (substitute back). Substitute the expression that defined u in terms of x in Step 1 into the antiderivative $G(u)$ to get the final answer in terms of x.

Example 2

Method of Substitution Evaluate the indefinite integral

$$\int \frac{3x^2 + 4}{(x^3 + 4x)^2}\,dx$$

Solution Here we recognize that the numerator is the derivative of the expression being squared in the denominator. This suggests the following substitution:

- **Step 1** (find u and du). We let

$$u = x^3 + 4x$$
$$du = (3x^2 + 4)\,dx$$

- **Step 2** (find the new integral). Substituting these expressions into the above integral gives the new integral in u:

$$\int \frac{3x^2 + 4}{(x^3 + 4x)^2}\,dx = \int \frac{1}{u^2}\,du$$

- **Step 3** (integrate the new integral). Finding the antiderivative of the new integral, we have

$$\int \frac{1}{u^2}\, du = -\frac{1}{u} + C$$

- **Step 4** (substitute back). Finally, the last step is to substitute back $u = x^3 + 4x$ to get the desired antiderivative in terms of x. This gives

$$\int \frac{3x^2 + 4}{(x^3 + 4x)^2}\, dx = \frac{-1}{x^3 + 4x} + C \qquad \square$$

We illustrate the method once again with another example.

Example 3

Method of Substitution Find the indefinite integral

$$\int \frac{x}{\sqrt{x^2 + 2}}\, dx$$

Solution Here we note that the derivative of the quantity inside the radical sign is $2x$, or twice the numerator. This suggests the following substitution:

- **Step 1** (find u and du). We let

$$u = x^2 + 2$$
$$du = 2x\, dx$$

- **Step 2** (find the new integral). We now manipulate these quantities so that we can rewrite the original integral in terms of u and du. We write

$$\sqrt{x^2 + 2} = \sqrt{u}$$
$$x\, dx = \frac{1}{2}\, du$$

This will result in the new integral in u and du:

$$\int \frac{x}{\sqrt{x^2 + 2}}\, dx = \frac{1}{2}\int \frac{du}{\sqrt{u}}$$

- **Step 3** (integrate the new integral). Finding the above indefinite integral in u, we get

$$\frac{1}{2}\int \frac{du}{\sqrt{u}} = \sqrt{u} + C$$

- **Step 4** (substitute back). Replacing the u in the above equation by $u = x^2 + 2$, we get the desired result:

$$\int \frac{x}{\sqrt{x^2 + 2}}\, dx = \sqrt{x^2 + 2} + C$$

Check:

$$\frac{d}{dx}\left(\sqrt{x^2 + 2} + C\right) = \frac{x}{\sqrt{x^2 + 2}} \qquad \square$$

Comment on the Method of Substitution

At this point you should note that it would have been possible (although maybe difficult) to find the previous antiderivatives by a purely trial-and-error approach. In other words, simply asking yourself what is the function whose derivative is the integrand in the original integral. If one's differentiation skills are sharp, one can sometimes use this approach. In fact, students with a great deal of experience may try to find antiderivatives directly and, if that fails, *then* use the method of substitution.

Method of Substitution and Definite Integrals

Until now we have seen how the method of substitution can be used to find antiderivatives. We now use this method to find definite integrals. Here, the strategy is to find the antiderivative of the integrand by the method of substitution and then use the fundamental theorem of calculus. The following example illustrates this idea.

Example 4

Method of Substitution Evaluate the definite integral

$$\int_0^1 x^2 e^{x^3}\,dx$$

Solution

- **Step 1** (find u and du). Observe that the integral is of the form

$$\int f'(x)e^{f(x)}\,dx$$

where

$$f(x) = x^3$$

except for a constant factor of 3. This suggests the substitution

$$u = x^3$$
$$du = 3x^2\,dx$$

- **Step 2** (find the new integral). The expressions found in Step 1 can be rewritten as

$$x^3 = u$$

$$x^2\,dx = \frac{1}{3}\,du$$

Hence we have the new integral

$$\int x^2 e^{x^3}\,dx = \int \frac{1}{3}e^u\,du$$

- **Step 3** (integrate the new integral).

$$\int \frac{1}{3}e^u\,du = \frac{1}{3}e^u + C$$

- **Step 4** (substitute back). Letting $u = x^3$, we have

$$\int x^2 e^{x^3}\,dx = \frac{1}{3}e^{x^3}$$

where we have let the constant of integration be zero, since it always cancels in applying the fundamental theorem. Now that we know the antiderivative, we can apply the fundamental theorem of calculus:

$$\int_0^1 x^2 e^{x^3}\,dx = \frac{1}{3} e^{x^3}\Big|_0^1$$

$$= \frac{1}{3}(e - 1) \qquad \square$$

Example 5 Method of Substitution Find the area under the curve

$$y = x\sqrt{1-x}$$

for x between 0 and 1. (See Figure 20.)

Solution The above area is represented by the definite integral

$$\int_0^1 x\sqrt{1-x}\,dx$$

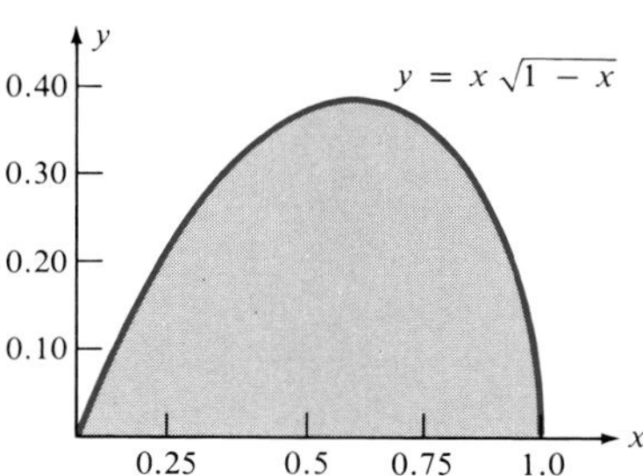

Figure 20
Area under $y = x\sqrt{1-x}$

We first must find the indefinite integral

$$\int x\sqrt{1-x}\,dx$$

Here we let

$$u = 1 - x$$
$$du = -dx$$

These expressions can be rewritten as

$$x = 1 - u$$
$$dx = -du$$

Hence we have the new integral in u:

$$\int x\sqrt{1-x}\,dx = \int (1-u)\sqrt{u}(-du)$$

$$= \int (u-1)u^{1/2}\,du$$

$$= \int (u^{3/2} - u^{1/2})\,du$$

$$= \frac{2}{5}u^{5/2} - \frac{2}{3}u^{3/2}$$

Substituting back in terms of x gives

$$\int x\sqrt{1-x}\,dx = \frac{2}{5}(1-x)^{5/2} - \frac{2}{3}(1-x)^{3/2}$$

Calling the above antiderivative $F(x)$ and applying the fundamental theorem of calculus, we have

$$\begin{aligned}\int_0^1 x\sqrt{1-x}\,dx &= F(1) - F(0)\\ &= \left[\frac{2}{5}(1-1)^{5/2} - \frac{2}{3}(1-1)^{3/2}\right] - \left[\frac{2}{5}(1-0)^{5/2} - \frac{2}{3}(1-0)^{3/2}\right]\\ &= \frac{4}{15}\end{aligned}$$

□

The following rules should be kept in mind when using the method of substitution.

Common Forms for Using the Method of Substitution

Power of function:	$\int [u(x)]^n u'(x)\,dx = \frac{[u(x)]^{n+1}}{n+1} + C$
Function in exponent:	$\int e^{u(x)} u'(x)\,dx = e^{u(x)} + C$
Numerator is derivative of denominator:	$\int \frac{u'(x)}{u(x)}\,dx = \ln\lvert u(x)\rvert + C$

Example 6

Recognizing Special Forms Find the antiderivative

$$\int \frac{x}{x^2+1}\,dx$$

Solution Except for a constant factor, this integral has the form

$$\int \frac{f'(x)}{f(x)}\,dx$$

We let

$$u = x^2 + 1$$
$$du = 2x\,dx$$

Transforming the original integral to the new integral, we get

$$\begin{aligned}\int \frac{x}{x^2+1}\,dx &= \frac{1}{2}\int \frac{1}{u}\,du\\ &= \frac{1}{2}\ln\lvert u\rvert + C\\ &= \frac{1}{2}\ln(x^2+1) + C\end{aligned}$$

Note that we do not need the absolute value sign, since $x^2 + 1$ is always positive.

Check:

$$\frac{d}{dx}\left[\frac{1}{2}\ln(x^2+1)+C\right]=\frac{x}{x^2+1} \qquad \square$$

Example 7 Algebraic Manipulation Before Integration Find the antiderivative

$$\int \frac{t}{t+1}\,dt \qquad (t > 0)$$

Solution This integrand does not fall within any of the standard forms that can be solved by the method of substitution. However, whenever integrating a rational function in which the degree of the numerator is greater than or equal to the degree of the denominator, the first step is to divide the numerator by the denominator. In this instance we get

$$\frac{t}{t+1}=1-\frac{1}{t+1}$$

Hence we can write

$$\begin{aligned}\int \frac{t}{t+1}\,dt &= \int\left(1-\frac{1}{t+1}\right)dt\\ &= \int 1\,dt-\int\frac{1}{t+1}\,dt\end{aligned}$$

The first indefinite integral is clearly t. The second indefinite integral

$$\int \frac{1}{t+1}\,dt$$

can be found by letting

$$\begin{aligned}u &= t+1\\ du &= dt\end{aligned}$$

Thus we have

$$\begin{aligned}\int\frac{1}{t+1}\,dt &= \int\frac{du}{u}\\ &= \ln|u|+C\\ &= \ln(t+1)+C\end{aligned}$$

Note that we do not need the absolute value sign in the above expression, since we have restricted t to be positive. Finally, putting the above two antiderivatives together, we have

$$\int\frac{t}{t+1}\,dt = t-\ln(t+1)+C$$

Note too that the algebraic sign in front of the constant C is immaterial, since C represents an arbitrary constant. Hence the convention is to always place a plus before the C.

Check:

$$\frac{d}{dt}[t - \ln(t+1) + C] = 1 - \frac{1}{t+1}$$

$$= \frac{t}{t+1} \qquad \square$$

The Lorentz Curve (Calculus in the Social Sciences)

Social philosophers have always tried to find measures of social and economic injustices in the world. Injustices might mean that certain people or groups of people have unfair privileges over others. In other words, certain people might have an inordinate amount of power, wealth, honor (social respect), and so on. What does it mean to say that one person is "privileged," and how is it possible for mathematics to measure these social ills and injustices? In recent years, social scientists and economists have found several mathematical measures of social and economic inequities. One of the most useful of these measures is the **Lorentz curve**, which measures the fraction of society's value possessed by a given fraction of society's people.

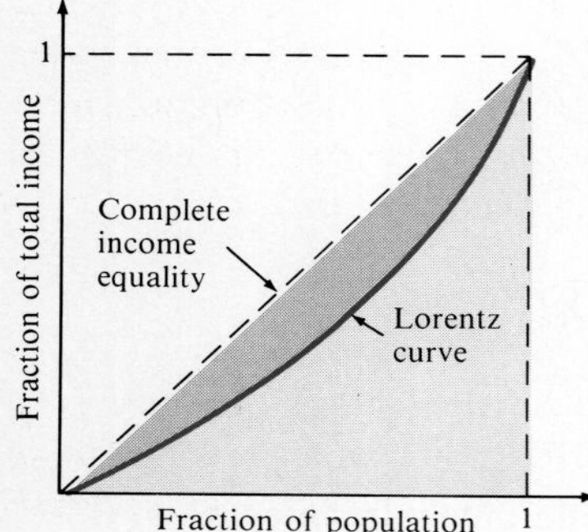

Figure 21
A typical Lorentz curve

To introduce the Lorentz curve, consider a study of wage earners in the United States in 1985. According to studies carried out by the U.S. Department of Labor, the lowest-paid 25% of all wage earners earned only about 10% of the total wages paid in the country during that year. The bottom 50% of all wage earners earned 26% of the total wages paid. The lower 75% of all wage earners earned roughly 50% of the total wages. Table 5 gives in more detail the fraction of the total wages earned by wage earners in various income categories.

The information in Table 5 can also be displayed by drawing the Lorentz curve as shown in Figure 21. The **Lorentz curve** $y = L(x)$ is defined as

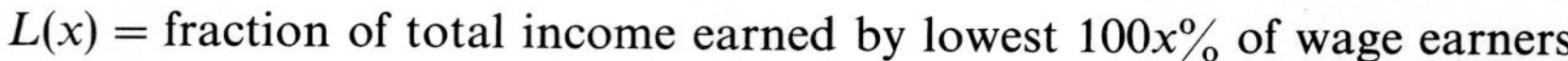

$L(x)$ = fraction of total income earned by lowest $100x\%$ of wage earners

TABLE 5
Points on a Lorentz Curve

Fraction of Lowest-Paid Wage Earners, x	Fraction of Total Wages Earned, $y = L(x)$
0	0
0.10 (10%)	0.02 (2%)
0.20 (20%)	0.06 (6%)
0.30 (30%)	0.12 (12%)
0.40 (40%)	0.17 (17%)
0.50 (50%)	0.26 (26%)
0.60 (60%)	0.32 (32%)
0.70 (70%)	0.46 (46%)
0.80 (80%)	0.58 (58%)
0.90 (90%)	0.72 (72%)
1.00 (100%)	1.00 (100%)

For example, the fact that $L(0.40) = 0.17$ in Figure 21 means that 17% of the total income is earned by the lowest 40% of wage earners.

Every economic society has its own Lorentz curve, which will change over time. The usefulness of the Lorentz curve lies in its ability to be an effective tool for comparing different economic societies and for comparing a single economic environment over time. All Lorentz curves $L(x)$ are defined for $0 \leq x \leq 1$, and all lie below the 45 degree line $y = x$. They also all satisfy the two conditions

$$L(0) = 0 \qquad \text{("nobody earns nothing")}$$
$$L(1) = 1 \qquad \text{("everybody earns everything")}$$

We say that the line $y = x$ represents complete equality of income because when $L(x) = x$, the lowest $100x\%$ of all wage earners earn $100x\%$ of the total income. In other words, the bottom 25% of the workers earn 25% of the wages, the bottom 50% of the workers earn 50% of the total wages, and so on. The farther the Lorentz curve lies below the line $y = x$, the more inequity in the wages of the workers. We can measure this inequity by computing the area under the curve $x - L(x)$, which is the same as the area between the Lorentz curve $L(x)$ and the line $y = x$. This area multiplied times 2 is called the **coefficient of inequality** (CI) and is defined by the definite integral

$$CI = 2 \int_0^1 [x - L(x)]\, dx$$

The factor of 2 is included simply for convenience to make this quantity vary from 0 to 1 (instead of from 0 to 0.5). When CI is 0, the Lorentz curve is $L(x) = x$, and there is complete uniform distribution of income. As CI gets closer and closer to 1, the inequity in the distribution of income is greater. Table 6 lists some coefficients of inequalities for countries in 1980.

TABLE 6
Coefficient of Inequality for Different Countries

Country	Coefficient of Inequality
Brazil	0.34
United Kingdom	0.31
Italy	0.28
United States	0.26
France	0.24
Canada	0.22
U.S.S.R.	0.19
Sweden	0.18

Example 8

Coefficient of Inequality The following Lorentz curves describe the distribution of wages in Squareland and Cubeland:

$$\text{Squareland:} \quad L_s(x) = x^2$$
$$\text{Cubeland:} \quad L_c(x) = x^3$$

Graphs of these curves are shown in Figure 22. Which country has the fairer income distribution among its workers?

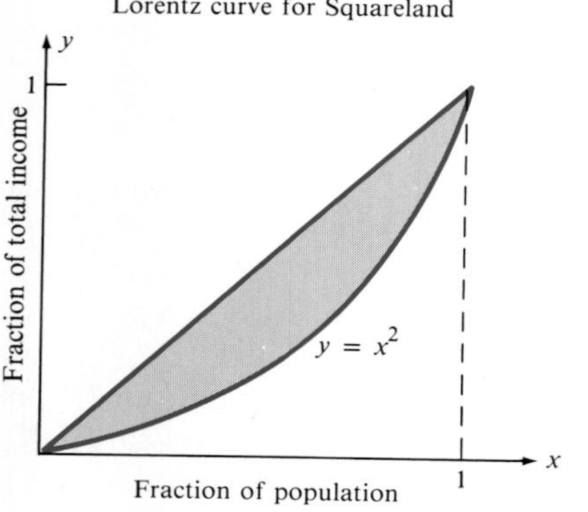

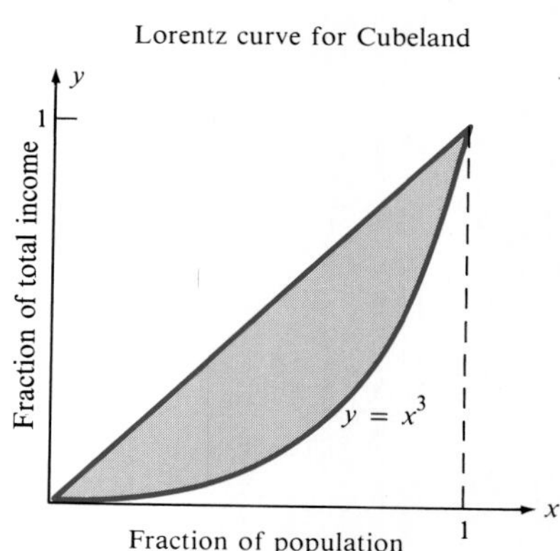

Figure 22
Comparing Lorentz curves

Solution The two coefficients of inequality are found in Table 7. Since Squareland has a smaller coefficient of inequality, there is more equity in its wage distribution. □

TABLE 7
Coefficients of Inequality for Squareland and Cubeland

Squareland	Cubeland
$CE_s = 2\int_0^1 [x - L_s(x)]\,dx$	$CE_c = 2\int_0^1 [x - L_c(x)]\,dx$
$= 2\int_0^1 (x - x^2)\,dx$	$= 2\int_0^1 (x - x^3)\,dx$
$= 2\left[\left(\frac{x^2}{2} - \frac{x^3}{3}\right)\Big\vert_0^1\right]$	$= 2\left[\left(\frac{x^2}{2} - \frac{x^4}{4}\right)\Big\vert_0^1\right]$
$= \frac{1}{3}$	$= \frac{1}{2}$

Legislative Equality and the Lorentz Curve

In the epic 1964 Supreme Court decision on legislative apportionment (*Reynolds* v. *Sims*) the Court declared that "the fundamental principle of representative government in this country is one of equal representation for equal number of people, without regard to race, sex, economic status, or place of residence within a state." As a result of this decision the state apportionments of Alabama, New York, Maryland, Virginia, Delaware, and Colorado were held to be unconstitutional. Although Justice Stewart argued for the minority when he said, "Nobody's right to vote has been denied," Justice Warren argued for the majority by saying that "diluting the weight of votes because of place of residence impairs basic rights under the 14th Amendment. . . . " The majority of the Supreme Court used several measures of inequality to support their decision, and one of those measures was the Lorentz curve (and the coefficient of inequality). As a representative Lorentz curve for a state legislature the Lorentz curve for the 1960 New York State Assembly is shown in Figure 23. Without going into the details of how the curve was constructed, the curve illustrates that certain people in the State of New York (within certain voting districts) have (or had before reapportionment) more voting power than others.* The coefficient of inequality for this curve was found to be 0.22, which indicates that the New York State Assembly is $\frac{22}{100}$ toward complete inequality.

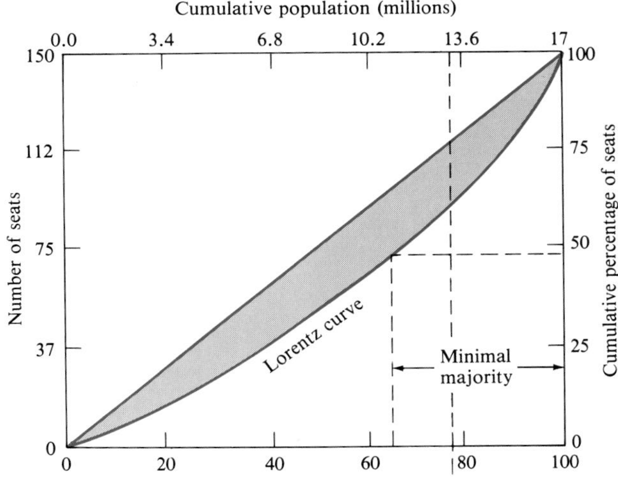

Figure 23
The Lorentz curve used to study "fairness" in the New York State election

Problems

For Problems 1–25, use the method of substitution to find the antiderivatives.

1. $\int x(3x^2 - 5)^3\,dx$

2. $\int (t^3 - 2)(t^4 - 8t + 6)^3\,dt$

3. $\int 2w(w^2 + 3)^2\,dw$

4. $\int \frac{x+1}{x^2 + 2x + 1}\,dx$

5. $\int 6(2x - 5)^{3/2}\,dx$

6. $\int (7t - 11)^{5/6}\,dt$

7. $\int \frac{1}{t+3}\,dt$

8. $\int \frac{3}{1+2y}\,dy$

9. $\int \frac{2}{x-3}\,dx$

10. $\int \frac{5x^2}{(x^3 - 7)^2}\,dx$

11. $\int \frac{(\sqrt{x} + 2)^5}{\sqrt{x}}\,dx$

12. $\int 6u^4\sqrt{1 - u^5}\,du$

13. $\int \sqrt{x^3 + 12x^2 + 3}(3x^2 + 24x)\,dx$

14. $\int \frac{e^x}{e^x + 1}\,dx$

15. $\int e^x\sqrt{e^x + 1}\,dx$

16. $\int 7x^3 e^{x^4}\,dx$

17. $\int \frac{e^{2u} - e^{-2u}}{e^{2u} + e^{-2u}}\,du$

* Details of how this Lorentz curve was constructed can be found in Ruth Silva, "Apportionment of the New York State Legislature," *American Political Science Review*, Dec. 1961.

18. $\int \frac{\ln 5x}{3x}\,dx$

19. $\int \frac{2x \ln (x^2+4)}{x^2+4}\,dx$

20. $\int (1+e^{-2t})(2t-e^{-2t})^3\,dt$

21. $\int xe^{-x^2}\,dx$

22. $\int x\sqrt{x-3}\,dx$

23. $\int \frac{x}{x+2}\,dx$ (*Hint*: Do the division first.)

24. $\int \frac{t}{t-3}\,dt$ (*Hint*: Do the division first.)

25. $\int (u-2)\sqrt{u-1}\,du$

For Problems 26–45, use the method of substitution to evaluate the definite integrals.

26. $\int_{-3}^{1} x^2(1+x^3)^2\,dx$

27. $\int_{2}^{3} (3w-2)^3\,dw$

28. $\int_{2}^{4} \frac{2x-1}{(x^2-x+3)^2}\,dx$

29. $\int_{1}^{3} \frac{t+\frac{3}{2}}{t^2+3t-2}\,dt$

30. $\int_{1}^{2} \frac{3u}{u^2+1}\,du$

31. $\int_{1}^{4} \frac{1}{2u+3}\,du$

32. $\int_{0}^{7} \sqrt{t+2}\,dt$

33. $\int_{0}^{1} \frac{1}{\sqrt{3w+1}}\,dw$

34. $\int_{-2}^{1} \frac{x}{\sqrt{x^2+16}}\,dx$

35. $\int_{0}^{3} s\sqrt{9-s^2}\,ds$

36. $\int_{0}^{3} \frac{r}{\sqrt{4-r}}\,dr$

37. $\int_{2}^{6} \sqrt{10+3x}\,dx$

38. $\int_{0}^{1} (s^5+3)\sqrt{s^6+18s}\,ds$

39. $\int_{1}^{4} 2x^3\sqrt{1+5x^4}\,dx$

40. $\int_{-1/3}^{2/3} \frac{1}{\sqrt{2+3t}}\,dt$

41. $\int_{2}^{4} \frac{2+2x^3}{\sqrt[4]{4x+x^4}}\,dx$

42. $\int_{1}^{3} \sqrt{4s+5}\,ds$

43. $\int_{0}^{1} \frac{3u}{\sqrt{4-u^2}}\,du$

44. $\int_{0}^{2} x^2\sqrt{x^3+1}\,dx$

45. $\int_{0}^{\sqrt{3}} \frac{t}{(4-t^2)^{3/2}}\,dt$

Antiderivative in Business

46. **Finding Total Cost.** Marginal cost is given by

$$C'(q) = \frac{6}{\sqrt{q+5}}$$

where q is the number of units produced. What is the cost in increasing production from 50 to 100 units? From 100 to 200 units?

Coefficient of Inequality

47. **Coefficient of Inequality.** Let the Lorentz curve be

$$L(x) = \frac{7}{8}x^2 + \frac{1}{8}x$$

Find the coefficient of inequality.

48. **Coefficient of Inequality.** The Lorentz curves for two countries are given below:

$$\text{Country A:}\quad L_A(x) = \frac{15}{16}x^2 + \frac{1}{16}x$$

$$\text{Country B:}\quad L_B(x) = \frac{7}{8}x^2 + \frac{1}{8}x$$

What are the coefficients of inequality for each of the countries? Can you say anything about the economic environment in these two countries?

A common mathematical model that is often used to describe the Lorentz curve is

$$L(x) = \frac{k-1}{k}x^2 + \frac{1}{k}x$$

for $k = 1, 2, \ldots$ and $0 \le x \le 1$. In other words, a given country may be described by some constant k.

49. Show that $L(x)$ satisfies the two boundary conditions $L(0) = 0$ and $L(1) = 1$.
50. Find the coefficient of inequality as a function of k.
51. Sketch the graphs of $L(x)$ for $k = 1, 2, 3$, and 10.
52. Verify that for any k the above Lorentz curve lies below the line $y = x$.

Other Measures of Social Inequality

53. **The Ratio of Advantage.** The Lorentz curve (Figure 23) describing inequities in electing the 1960 New York State Assembly is described roughly by

$$L(x) = 0.75x^2 + 0.25x \qquad (0 \le x \le 1)$$

The derivative of the Lorentz curve is called the **ratio of advantage curve**.

(a) What is the ratio of advantage curve for voters in New York? Plot this curve.

(b) The derivative $L'(x_0)$ provides a measure of privilege or discrimination [depending on whether $L'(x_0) < 1$ or $L'(x_0) > 1$, respectively] for people ranked in the x_0th percentile from the bottom of the social scale. What is the ratio of advantage for people ranked 20% from the bottom on the voting power scale?

54. **Comparison of Voting Power.** Compare the ratio of advantage (defined in Problem 53) of voters in New York ranked 75% from the bottom of the voting power scale with the ratio of advantage of voters ranked 20% from the bottom of the scale.

55. Equal Share Coefficient. Where are the voters ranked in the voting power scale that have a ratio of advantage equal to 1? In other words, what is the solution of $L'(x_0) = 1$? This value of x_0 is called the **equal share coefficient**. Why is it called by this name?

56. Elite Minority. What is the value of x_0 that satisfies $L'(x_0) = 0.50$? Voters "to the right" of this value are called the **elite minority**. What percent of the voters in the State of New York belong to this elite minority? What is the reason for this name?

Epilogue: Typical Lorentz Curves

The following Lorentz curves and their coefficients of inequality illustrate how economists compare incomes between different groups and classes of people.*

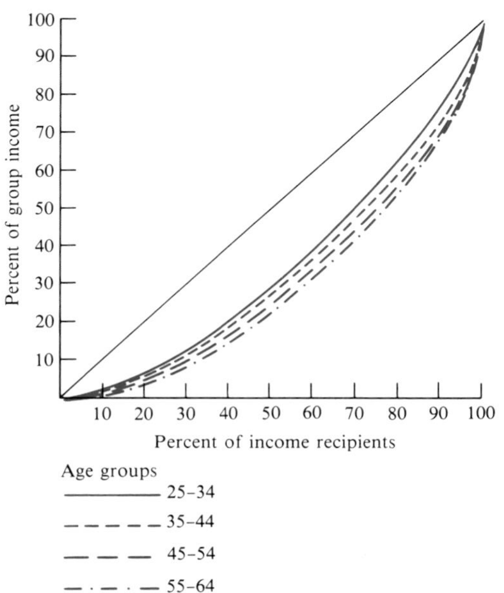

Figure 24

TABLE 8

Age Group	Coefficient of Inequality
25–34	0.25
35–44	0.27
45–54	0.29
55–64	0.31

Coefficient of inequality as a function of age. See Figure 24 and Table 8.

Coefficient of inequality as a function of education. See Figure 25 and Table 9.

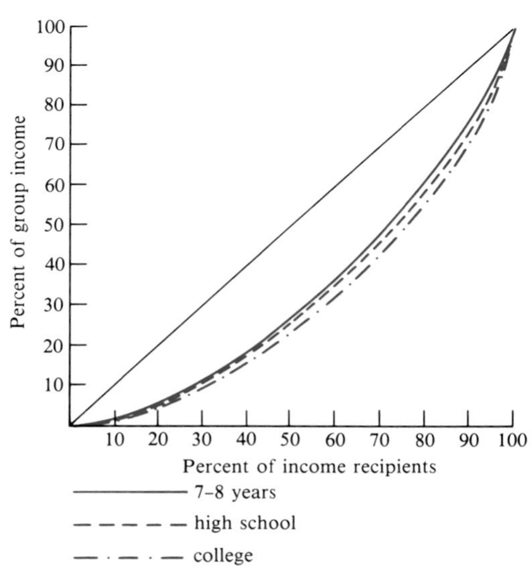

Figure 25

TABLE 9

Education	Coefficient of Inequality
7–8 years	0.31
High school	0.32
College	0.34

Coefficient of inequality as a function of occupation. See Figure 26 and Table 10.

* These Lorentz curves were taken from the Ph.D thesis of Jacob Mincer, "A Study of Personal Income Distribution," Columbia University, 1957.

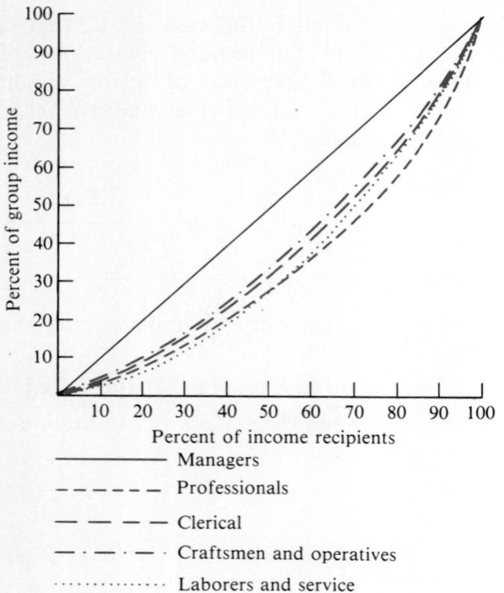

Figure 26

Coefficient of inequality as a function of sex. See Figure 27 and Table 11.

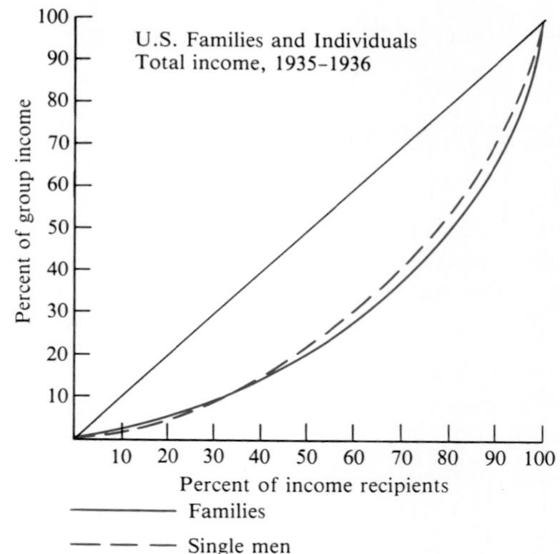

Figure 27

TABLE 10

Occupation	Coefficient of Inequality
Managers	0.25
Professionals	0.27
Clerical	0.29
Craftsmen	0.31
Laborers and service	0.34

TABLE 11

Sex	Coefficient of Inequality
Families	0.23
Single men	0.26

Key Ideas for Review

Review Exercises

For Problems 1–10, find the indefinite integrals.

1. $\int 7\,dx$
2. $\int (x^4 + 3x^2 + 1)\,dx$
3. $\int \sqrt{u}(u^2 + 1)\,du$
4. $\int \sqrt{x}(x + 1)(x - 1)\,dx$
5. $\int (e^x + e^{-x})\,dx$
6. $\int \frac{t + t^2}{t}\,dt$
7. $\int \frac{dx}{\sqrt[3]{x}}\,dx$
8. $\int \sqrt{ax}\,dx$
9. $\int \sqrt{x}(3x - 2)\,dx$
10. $\int \frac{4x^2 - 2\sqrt{x}}{x}\,dx$

For Problems 11–16, find the particular antiderivative of the given derivative determined by the value of the function.

11. $f'(t) = 2t + 5$ $\quad f(0) = 0$
12. $f'(t) = t^2$ $\quad f(1) = 0$
13. $f'(x) = e^x$ $\quad f(0) = 1$
14. $g'(x) = 2x + e^x$ $\quad g(0) = 5$
15. $h'(u) = u\sqrt{u^2 - 9}$ $\quad h(5) = 0$
16. $f'(x) = 0$ $\quad f(0) = 0$

For Problems 17–19, find the total cost given the marginal cost.

17. $C'(q) = 45q - 2q^2$, $C(0) = 10{,}000$
18. $C'(q) = 100q - q^2$, $C(0) = 1000$
19. $C'(q) = 10 - 2e^{-0.5q}$, $C(0) = 1000$

For Problems 20–30, evaluate the definite integrals.

20. $\int_0^1 (x + 1)\,dx$
21. $\int_{-1}^1 (1 - x^2)\,dx$
22. $\int_5^{10} 5\,dx$
23. $\int_0^1 (x + e^{-x})\,dx$
24. $\int_1^3 2x(x^2 + 3)\,dx$
25. $\int_1^e \left(1 + \frac{1}{x}\right)dx$
26. $\int_0^1 \frac{1}{\sqrt{4u + 3}}\,du$
27. $\int_0^a (a^2 z - z^3)\,dz$
28. $\int_0^1 \frac{1}{\sqrt{3 - 2y}}\,dy$
29. $\int_0^4 (2 - \sqrt{x})^2\,dx$
30. $\int_0^2 \frac{z^3}{z + 1}\,dz$

For Problems 31–38, sketch the graph of the function over the indicated interval. Evaluate the integral that gives the area between the curve and the x-axis over the indicated interval.

31. $f(x) = x + 1$ $\quad [0, 5]$
32. $f(x) = 4 - x$ $\quad [0, 4]$
33. $f(x) = 4 - x^2$ $\quad [0, 2]$
34. $f(x) = 1 + e^x$ $\quad [0, 1]$
35. $f(x) = e^x + e^{-x}$ $\quad [-1, 1]$
36. $f(x) = x^n$ $\quad [0, 1]$ for $n \geq 0$
37. $f(x) = \frac{1}{x^n}$ over $[1, 2]$ for $n \geq 2$
38. $f(x) = \sqrt{x} + 1$ over $[0, 1]$

For Problems 39–49, use the method of substitution to find the indefinite integral.

39. $\int x(x^2 - 1)^3\,dx$
40. $\int (x + 1)(x - 1)^4\,dx$
41. $\int u(u + 1)^5\,du$
42. $\int u(u^2 + 4)^2\,du$
43. $\int 5(x + 1)^{10}\,dx$
44. $\int \frac{1}{1 + 2x}\,dx$
45. $\int \frac{5}{x - 1}\,dx$
46. $\int \frac{x^2}{(x - 1)^2}\,dx$
47. $\int \frac{1}{t + 1}\,dt$
48. $\int \frac{e^{2r}}{e^{2r} + 1}\,dr$
49. $\int \frac{x + 4}{2x + 3}\,dx$

For Problems 50–58, use the method of substitution to evaluate the definite integrals.

50. $\int_0^1 x^2(1 + x^2)^3\,dx$
51. $\int_0^4 s\sqrt{s^2 + 1}\,ds$
52. $\int_0^1 \frac{r}{\sqrt{1 + r}}\,dr$
53. $\int_1^6 \sqrt{10 + x}\,dx$
54. $\int_0^2 \frac{s}{(4 - s)^{5/2}}\,ds$
55. $\int_0^3 \sqrt{x + 1}\,dx$
56. $\int_{-1}^1 \frac{2x}{(4 + x^2)^2}\,dx$
57. $\int_{-2}^2 \frac{x}{\sqrt{1 + 8x^2}}\,dx$
58. $\int_{-1}^1 z(1 - z^2)^5\,dz$

Business Management Problems

59. **Total Revenue.** The marginal revenue of a firm is given by

$$MR(q) = 100 - 5q$$

Find the total revenue.

60. Change in Revenue. If the marginal revenue is given by

$$MR(q) = 250 - 10q$$

determine the increase in revenue if the number of items produced q is increased from 100 to 150.

61. Change in Cost. If the marginal cost is given by

$$MC(q) = 10$$

find the increase in cost if the number of items produced q is increased from 1000 to 1500.

62. Change in Profit. If the marginal profit is

$$MP(q) = 10 - q$$

find the increase in profit if the number of items produced q is increased from 50 to 75.

63. Lorentz Curve. The wages in a given country are described by the Lorentz curve

$$L(x) = 0.9x^2 + 0.1x$$

(a) What percent of the total wages of the country are earned by the lowest-paid 10% of the work force?
(b) What percent of the total wages of the country are earned by the lowest-paid 50% of the work force?
(c) Show that $L(x)$ is an increasing function.
(d) Show that $L(x)$ is concave up.
(e) What is the coefficient of inequality?

64. Puzzle. You have inherited 50 annual payments from a rich uncle. You can receive the payments in one of two ways: in increasing order or decreasing order as shown in Table 12. Which order should you choose if banks pay an interest of 8% annually compounded continuously? What is the present value of each continuous cash flow? *Hint:* The decreasing payments can be approximated by the continuous revenue function

$$R_1(t) = \$1000(0.9)^t = \$1000e^{-0.105t}$$

TABLE 12
Payments for Problem 64

Decreasing Payments		Increasing Payments	
$1000	= $1000.00	$1000(0.9)^{49}$ =	$5.73
$1000(0.9)	= $900.00	$1000(0.9)^{48}$ =	$6.36
$1000(0.9)^2$	= $810.00	⋮	
$1000(0.9)^3$	= $729.00		
⋮		$1000(0.9)^3$	= $729.00
		$1000(0.9)^2$	= $810.00
$1000(0.9)^{48}$ =	$6.36	$1000(0.9)	= $900.00
$1000(0.9)^{49}$ =	$5.73	$1000	= $1000.00

and the increasing payments can be approximated by the continuous revenue function

$$R_D(t) = \$1000(0.9)^{49-t} = \$5.73e^{0.105t}$$

Integrals in Science

65. Hitting the Brakes. Mary is driving her car at 60 miles per hour when she suddenly hits the brakes. The car decelerates linearly until coming to rest 8 seconds later.
(a) What is the equation for the velocity of the car (calling time zero the moment when Mary hits the brakes)?
(b) How far will the car travel during the first three seconds after Mary hits the brakes?
(c) How far will the car travel before coming to rest?

66. Length of a Curve. The length L of the graph $y = f(x)$ for $a \le x \le b$ is given by

$$L = \int_a^b \sqrt{1 + [f'(x)]^2}\, dx$$

Use this formula to determine the length of the curve $y = x^{3/2}$ for $0 \le x \le 1$.

67. Falling on the Moon. For a falling body near the surface of the moon the velocity of the object in meters per second is

$$v = 1.62t$$

where t is time in seconds measured from when the object begins falling. Suppose you drop an object from a height of 100 meters above the surface of the moon. How far will the object fall during the first second?

68. Drug Measurements. A patient is given an oral dose of a drug that is assimilated in the body and then excreted through the urine. By measuring the amount of drug in a few specimens, the researcher determines the rate R of the drug being excreted by the patient after t hours can be approximated by the continuous function

$$R(t) = te^{-0.3t} \qquad \text{(mg/hr)}$$

Find the total amount of drug in milligrams that will be excreted during the first 10 hours after the drug is taken.

69. Life Table Function. In population studies the **life table function** $L(x)$ represents the number of individuals who are at least x years old. For example, in 1988 in the United States the life table function had the value $L(50) =$ 80 million, which means that there were 80 million citizens at least 50 years of age. Suppose in a population of whales the life function has been estimated by ecologists to be

$$L(x) = 10{,}000(1 - e^{-0.05x})$$

Estimate the number of whales that are between 2 and 5 years old inclusively. *Hint:* Integrate the life table function from 2 to 5.

Chapter Test

1. Find the following antiderivative:

$$\int \frac{t^2 + t + 1}{t}\, dt$$

2. Evaluate the definite integral

$$\int_0^1 \frac{x}{(x^2 + 1)^3}\, dx$$

3. Use the method of substitution to find the antiderivative of

$$\int u^2\sqrt{1 - u^3}\, du$$

4. The marginal cost of a product is given by

$$C'(q) = 10 + 2e^{-0.10q}$$

Find the increase in cost if the number of items produced q is increased from 10 to 20.

5. If the marginal profit is

$$MP(q) = 5 - 2q$$

find the increase in profit if the number of items produced q is increased from 100 to 200.

6. **Predicting Oil Consumption.** An economist assumes that the annual rate of consumption of oil in the United States (in billions of barrels per year) is given by

$$c(t) = 175e^{0.03t}$$

where t is time in years measured from January 1, 1988. If this trend continues, how much oil will the United States consume during the period from January 1, 1989, to January 1, 1998?

7. **How Far Has the Ball Fallen?** Suppose you throw a ball straight down from the top of the World Trade Center with an initial velocity of 20 ft/sec. The velocity (neglecting air friction) in feet per second at which the ball falls is given by the linear function

$$v(t) = 20 + 32t$$

where t is time in seconds measured from the time the ball was thrown. How far will the ball fall during the first 3 seconds?

8. **A Learning Curve.** The number of words per minute Q the average student can type after spending t weeks in a beginning typing class is given by

$$Q(t) = 75(1 - e^{-0.02t})$$

How many words per minute will the average student type after 10 weeks?

9. **Flooding on the Mississippi.** After heavy melting of snow the Army Corp of Engineers predicts flooding along the Mississippi River. They predict that water will flow into the Mississippi from the Missouri River at a rate of

$$R(t) = 100 - 0.5t^2 \qquad (0 \le t \le 10)$$

million cubic feet of water per day where t measures time in days with $t = 0$ corresponding to March 1. (The interval $[0, 1]$ would correspond to the entire day of March 1.) How many cubic feet of water will flow into the Mississippi River from the Missouri River during the three days of March 2, March 3, and March 4?

Just as the derivative is used to study many phenomena in the natural and life sciences, so is the integral also an important tool used by these sciences.

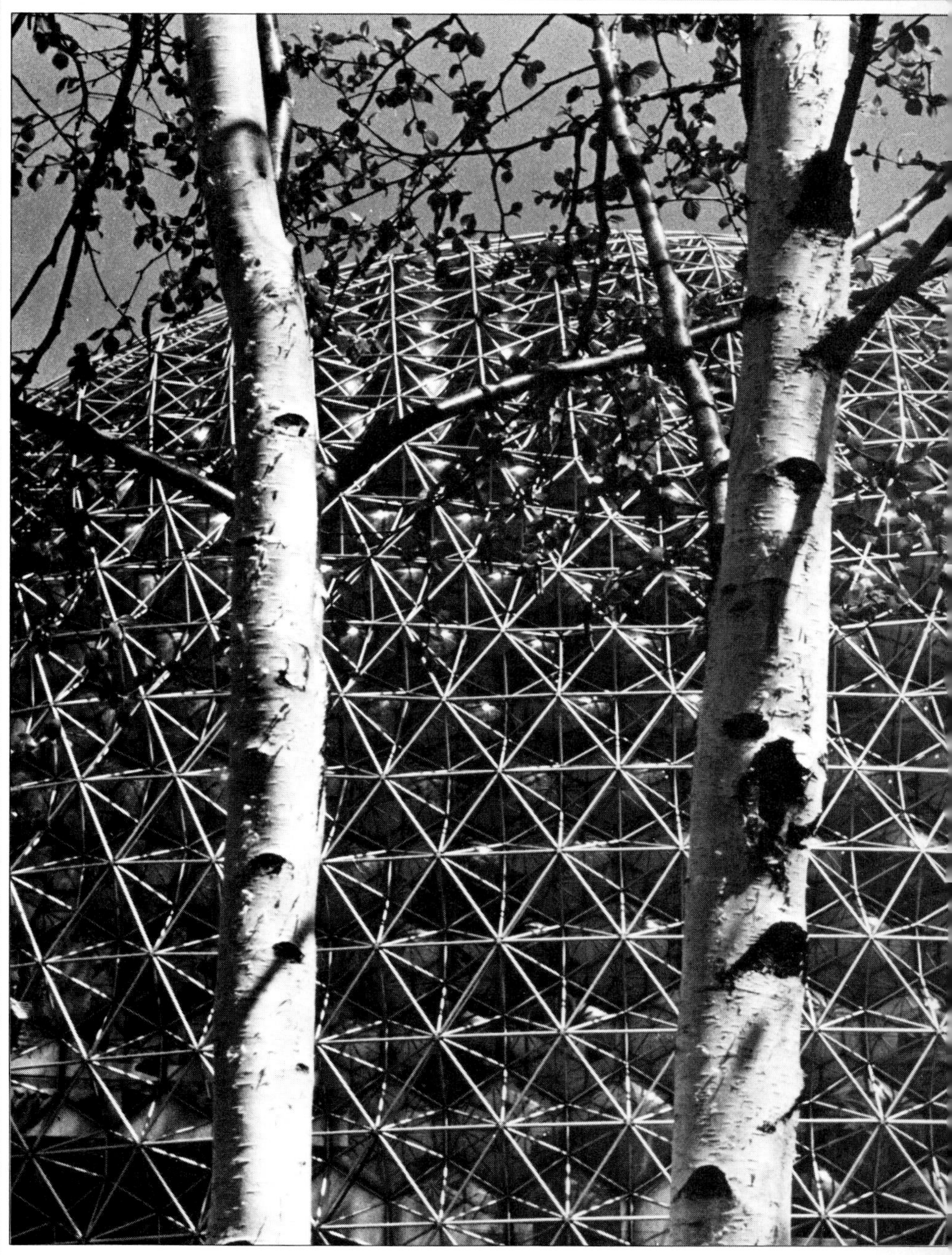

5 Integration Techniques and Applications

In this chapter we introduce a number of important ideas that are related to the integral. We begin in Section 5.1 by showing how to find the area of an unbounded region in the plane using the concept of the improper integral. Next, in Section 5.2 we introduce a technique known as integration by parts, which helps to find the antiderivative of a function and thus to evaluate its definite integral. Then in Section 5.3 we show how the definite integral can be used to find the area between two graphs as well as to find the volume of certain solids in three dimensions. In Section 5.4 we show how to approximate the integral of functions that cannot be integrated by the usual methods using numerical methods. Finally, in Section 5.5 we introduce differential equations and show they can be used to describe growth and decay phenomena.

5.1 Improper Integrals

PURPOSE

We show how it is possible to find the area of an unbounded region of the plane by taking the limit of a sequence of integrals, each defined over a finite interval. This introduces the idea of the improper integral. The concept of the improper integral is then used to find the present value of a continuous cash flow.

Introduction

Consider for a moment a region in the plane that is unbounded. That is, it goes off in some direction to infinity as illustrated by the regions in Figure 1. One is tempted to say that the area of such an unbounded region is infinite. It is often true that the area of an unbounded region is infinite. Certainly, we would say that the area of the entire plane is infinite. However, there are unbounded regions for which it is perfectly reasonable to assign finite areas. A region of the plane may be unbounded, but if the portion of the region that goes off to infinity becomes narrower and narrower, it might be the case that the total area is finite. (See Figure 2.)

In fact, there are unbounded regions in the plane that may reach to the moon from where you are now sitting but have an area equal to the area of the page you are now reading. The problem is to find these areas, and the tool for doing this is the improper integral.

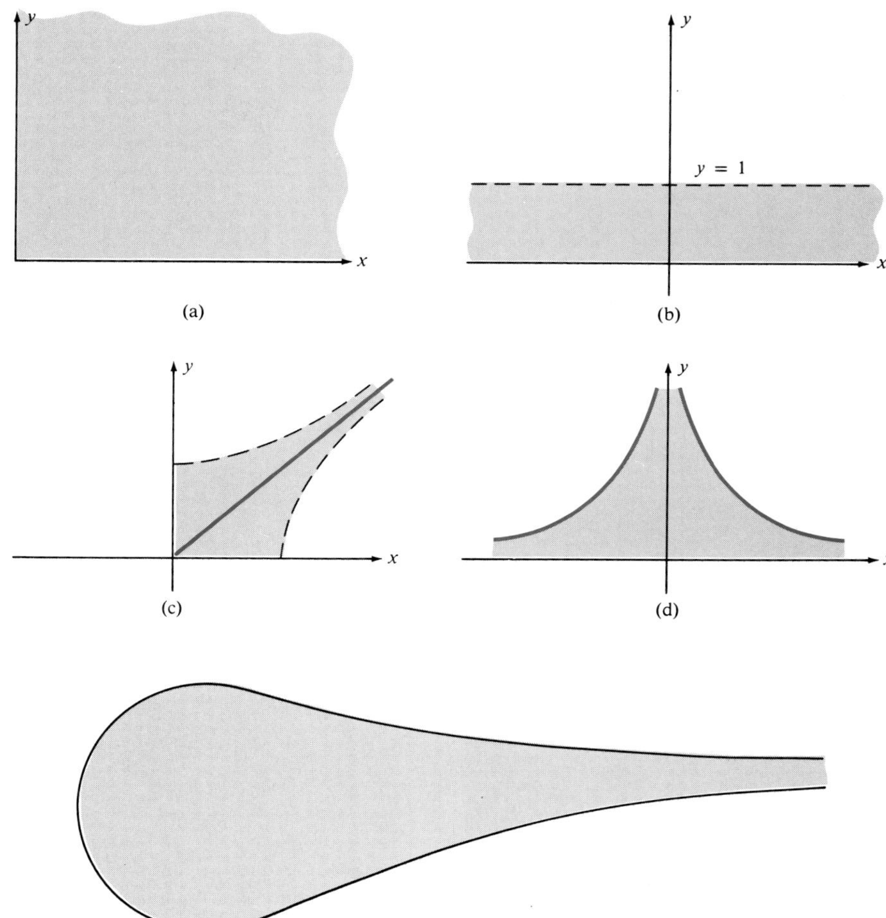

Figure 1
Four unbounded regions in the plane

Figure 2
Is this area finite?

Improper Integrals

We begin with a simple unbounded region. We consider the region that lies between the graph of the function

$$f(x) = \frac{1}{x^2} \qquad (1 \leq x < \infty)$$

and the x-axis for x greater than or equal to 1. (See Figure 3.) We ask if it is possible to assign a finite area to this region. The problem is fascinating because, although the region is unbounded, its height becomes shorter and shorter as we move farther and farther to the right. Clearly, as we enclose more and more of the region by moving to the right, the area of the enclosed region will become larger and larger. The important question is, "Does the enclosed area grow without bound, or does it approach some finite limit?" If it approaches a finite limit, we call this limit the **area** of the region. If the limit does not exist, we say that the area of the region is infinite or that the area is **diverging**.

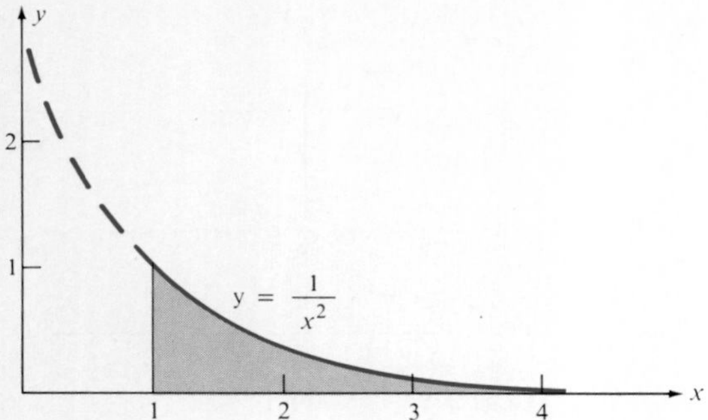

Figure 3
Finding the area of an unbounded region

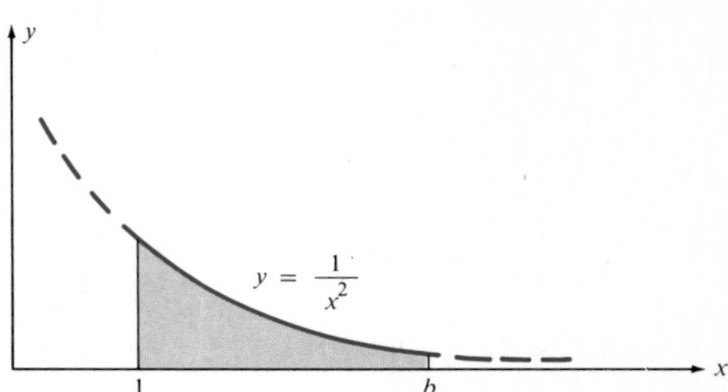

Figure 4
Finding the area over a finite interval

To determine whether the area exists, we begin by selecting an arbitrary number $b > 1$ and evaluate the integral

$$\int_1^b \frac{dx}{x^2}$$

(See Figure 4.) Evaluating this integral, we have

$$\begin{aligned}\int_1^b \frac{dx}{x^2} &= \int_1^b x^{-2}\,dx \\ &= -x^{-1}\Big|_1^b \\ &= -\left(\frac{1}{b} - 1\right) \\ &= 1 - \frac{1}{b}\end{aligned}$$

This expression in b gives the area of the shaded region between 1 and b as shown in Figure 4. For example, when $b = 1000$, we see that the area under the graph between 1 and 1000 is

$$\text{Area between 1 and 1000} = 1 - \frac{1}{1000} = 0.999$$

To find the area under the entire curve for $x \geq 1$, we take the limit as $b \to \infty$. This gives

$$\text{Area of unbounded region} = \lim_{b\to\infty}\left(1 - \frac{1}{b}\right) = 1$$

In other words, although the region is unbounded, the area is only one square unit. This limiting value (1 in this case) is called the value of the improper integral and is denoted by

$$\int_1^\infty \frac{dx}{x^2}$$

The above discussion suggests the following definition of improper integrals.

Definition of Improper Integrals

Let f be a continuous function defined over the indicated intervals and assume the following limits exist. We define the **improper integrals** as follows:

- Right infinite integral:

$$\int_a^{\infty} f(x)\,dx = \lim_{b\to\infty} \int_a^b f(x)\,dx$$

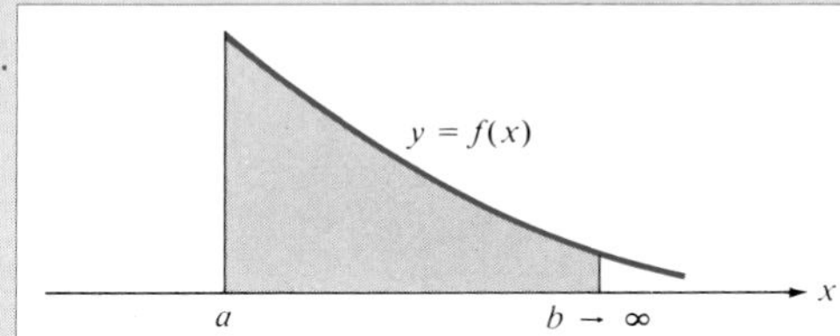

- Left infinite integral:

$$\int_{-\infty}^{b} f(x)\,dx = \lim_{a\to-\infty} \int_a^b f(x)\,dx$$

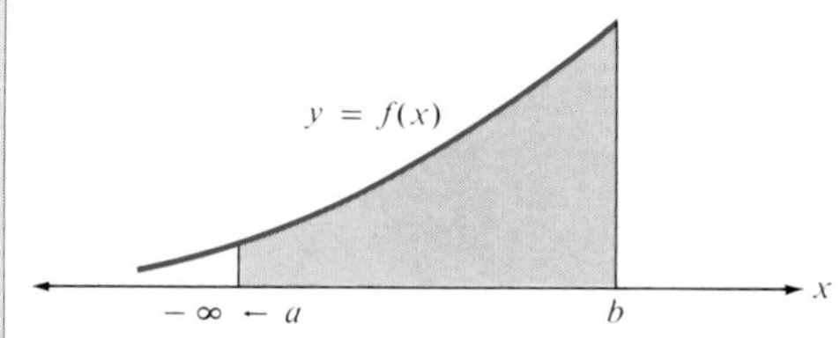

- Doubly infinite integral:

$$\int_{-\infty}^{\infty} f(x)\,dx = \int_{-\infty}^{c} f(x)\,dx + \int_c^{\infty} f(x)\,dx$$

$$= \lim_{a\to-\infty} \int_a^c f(x)\,dx + \lim_{b\to\infty} \int_c^b f(x)\,dx$$

The value of c can be chosen in any way one likes. It will not affect the result. It is often convenient to pick zero for the value of c.

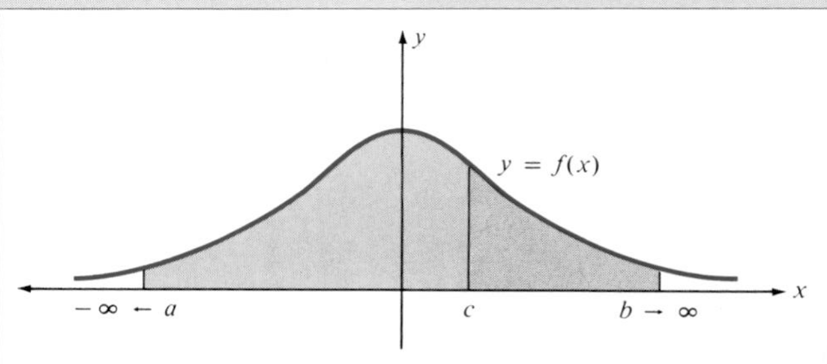

Example 1

Improper Integral Determine whether the area between the graph of $y = 1/x$ and the x-axis for $x \geq 1$ is finite or infinite. (See Figure 5.)

Solution The area is given by the improper integral

$$\int_1^\infty \frac{dx}{x}$$

Using the definition of the improper integral, we have

$$\begin{aligned}\int_1^\infty \frac{dx}{x} &= \lim_{b\to\infty} \int_1^b \frac{dx}{x} \\ &= \lim_{b\to\infty} \ln x \Big|_1^b \\ &= \lim_{b\to\infty} (\ln b - \ln 1) \\ &= \lim_{b\to\infty} \ln b\end{aligned}$$

Since $\ln b \to \infty$ as $b \to \infty$, we say that the improper integral diverges or that the area is infinite. □

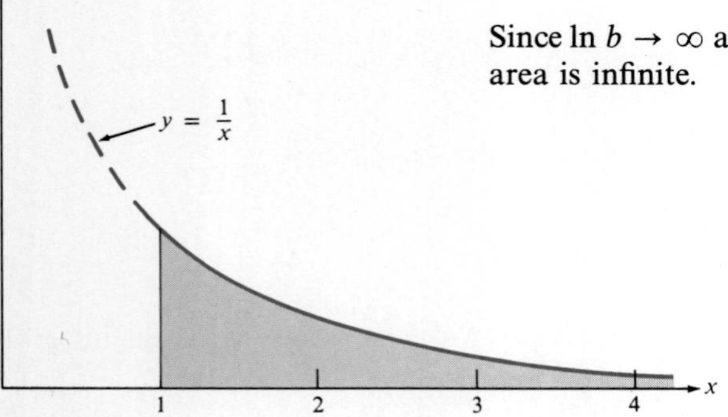

Figure 5
Is the area between the graph of $y = 1/x$ and the x-axis for $x \geq 1$ finite or infinite?

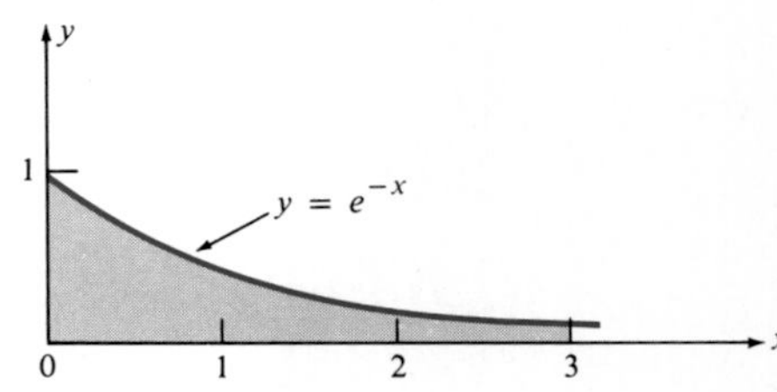

Figure 6
The area between the graph of $y = e^{-x}$ and the x-axis for $x \geq 0$ is described by an improper integral

Example 2

Improper Integral Find the area between the graph of $y = e^{-x}$ and the x-axis for $x \geq 0$. (See Figure 6.)

Solution The area is described by the improper integral

$$\int_0^\infty e^{-x}\,dx$$

Using the definition of the improper integral, we have

$$\begin{aligned}\int_0^\infty e^{-x}\,dx &= \lim_{b\to\infty} \int_0^b e^{-x}\,dx \\ &= \lim_{b\to\infty} (-e^{-x})\Big|_0^b \\ &= \lim_{b\to\infty} (-e^{-b} + 1) \\ &= \lim_{b\to\infty} \left(1 - \frac{1}{e^b}\right) \\ &= 1\end{aligned}$$

In other words, although the region has a "width" that is wider than the length of the United States (much, much wider), the area shown in Figure 6 is only one square unit. □

Example 3

Improper Integral Evaluate the improper integral

$$\int_{-\infty}^{\infty} xe^{-x^2}\,dx$$

See Figure 7.

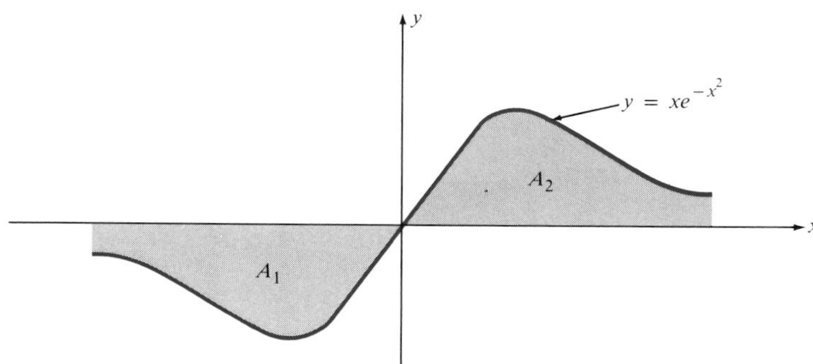

Figure 7
Area under the curve $y = xe^{-x^2}$

Solution The area of this region is given by the value of the improper integral

$$\int_{-\infty}^{\infty} xe^{-x^2}\,dx$$

By definition we can write

$$\begin{aligned}
\int_{-\infty}^{\infty} xe^{-x^2}\,dx &= \int_{-\infty}^{0} xe^{-x^2}\,dx + \int_{0}^{\infty} xe^{-x^2}\,dx \\
&= \lim_{a\to-\infty}\int_{a}^{0} xe^{-x^2}\,dx + \lim_{b\to\infty}\int_{0}^{b} xe^{-x^2}\,dx \\
&= \lim_{a\to-\infty}\left(-\frac{1}{2}e^{-x^2}\right)\Bigg|_{a}^{0} + \lim_{b\to\infty}\left(-\frac{1}{2}e^{-x^2}\right)\Bigg|_{0}^{b} \\
&= -\frac{1}{2}\lim_{a\to-\infty}(e^{-0^2} - e^{-a^2}) - \frac{1}{2}\lim_{b\to\infty}(e^{-b^2} - e^{-0^2}) \\
&= -\frac{1}{2}(1-0) - \frac{1}{2}(0-1) \\
&= -\frac{1}{2} + \frac{1}{2} \\
&= 0
\end{aligned}$$

The improper integral has a value of 0. Since the graph of the function is not always positive, the integral will not represent any area. Notice, however, in Figure 7 by the symmetric nature of the graph that the area A_1 that lies below the x-axis is the same as the area A_2 that lies above the x-axis. When this is true, we expect the value of the improper integral to be 0. □

Present Value of a Continuous Cash Flow

It often happens in financial transactions that an individual or firm will receive a continuous cash flow or revenue stream over a period of time. For example, an oil well might yield a company continuous revenue over a period of time. A pension fund might be paid to a retiree in varying amounts for a number of years.

Suppose a baseball player has just signed a five-year contract that calls for annual payments to the player (or to his estate in event of death) over the next 50 years according to Table 1. The first payment consists of \$75,000, and each succeeding payment is 2% less than the previous payment.

TABLE 1
Revenue Stream of Fifty Annual Payments

Year	Annual Payment	
1988	\$75,000	= \$75,000.00
1989	\$75,000(0.98)	= \$73,500.00
1990	$\$75{,}000(0.98)^2$	= \$72,030.00
1991	$\$75{,}000(0.98)^3$	= \$70,598.40
1992	$\$75{,}000(0.98)^4$	= \$69,177.61
⋮	⋮	⋮
2035	$\$75{,}000(0.98)^{47}$	= \$29,019.29
2036	$\$75{,}000(0.98)^{48}$	= \$28,438.91
2037	$\$75{,}000(0.98)^{49}$	= \$27,870.13

Although the revenue flow described in Table 1 is not paid to the player continuously (it is paid in 50 discrete payments), it can fairly accurately be described as a continuous cash flow and approximated by the continuous revenue function

$$R(t) = \$75{,}000e^{-0.02t}$$

where t is time in years measured from when the payments are begun. The graph of this function is shown in Figure 8.

The value of the continuous revenue function for $t = 0, 1, \ldots, 50$ gives almost the same payments as those listed in Table 1. Also, the area between the revenue function and the t-axis for t between 0 and 50 is very close to the sum of the 50 payments made to the player. Since it is easier to analyze $R(t)$

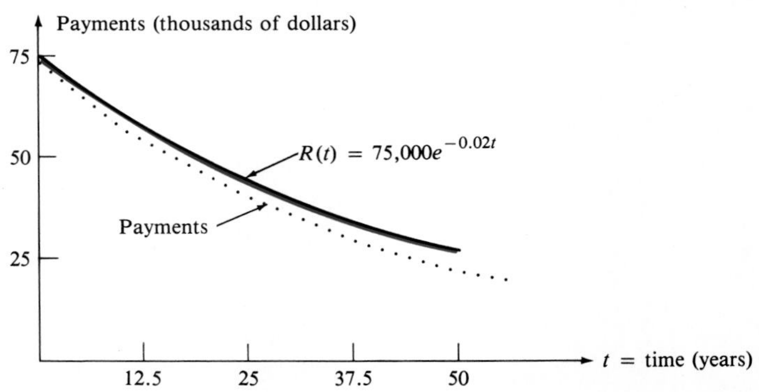

Comparison of continuous revenue and actual payments

than an entire table of numbers, it is easy to see the usefulness of approximating the table of payments by a continuous function $R(t)$.

In the mathematics of finance, one learns that if a present amount P is deposited in a bank that pays an annual interest of r percent compounded continuously, then the future value F of that account after t years will be given by

$$F = Pe^{rt}$$

Turning this equation around and solving for P, we see that if an account will be worth F dollars t years from now, then it has a present value P today of

$$P = Fe^{-rt}$$

However, if a steady cash flow $R(t)$ is deposited into this account during these t years, then the present value of the account is given by the following **present value integral**.

> **Present Value of a Continuous Cash Flow**
>
> If $R(t)$ is the rate at which money flows into an account (dollars per year) over the next T years, and if the account pays an annual interest of r percent compounded continuously, then the present value of this account in today's dollars is
>
> $$P = \int_0^T R(t)e^{-rt}\,dt$$
>
> In the special case of perpetual cash flow (goes on forever), the present value of the account is given by the improper integral
>
> $$P = \int_0^\infty R(t)e^{-rt}\,dt$$

Example 4

Perpetual Cash Flow An opera singer signs a contract that calls for her and her heirs to receive constant payments of \$100,000 per year forever. What is the value of this contract in today's dollars? Assume that money will always earn an annual interest of $r = 10\%$, compounded continuously.

Solution If the annual interest rate paid for borrowing money is 10%, then the current value of a constant perpetual cash flow of $R = \$100{,}000$ per year is

$$\begin{aligned}
P &= \int_0^\infty Re^{-rt}\,dt \\
&= \$100{,}000 \lim_{b\to\infty} \int_0^b e^{-0.10t}\,dt \\
&= \$100{,}000 \lim_{b\to\infty} \left(-\frac{1}{0.10}e^{-0.10t}\right)\Bigg|_0^b \\
&= \frac{\$100{,}000}{0.10} \lim_{b\to\infty} (1 - e^{-0.10b}) \\
&= \frac{\$100{,}000}{0.10} \\
&= \$1{,}000{,}000
\end{aligned}$$

In other words, the contract is worth \$1,000,000 today. This is the same as saying that the owner of the opera company can make the annual \$100,000 payments out of a special \$1,000,000 bank account that pays 10% annual interest compounded continuously. These payments would not draw on the principal of the account but would represent interest paid by the bank. Of course, the owner will pay a much larger sum than \$1,000,000 over the infinite period of time (in fact the total sum of annual \$100,000 payments in perpetuity is infinite). Fortunately for the owner, this number is meaningless. A payment of \$100,000 has no meaning unless one says *when* it is made. One should realize that a payment of \$100,000 today is not the same as this same payment in 100 years. If one assumes that inflation increases at the same 10% rate that the bank pays for borrowed money, then \$100,000 in 100 years will be worth (in today's dollars) roughly the price of a movie ticket (\$4.54). □

Example 5

Present Value of a Perpetual Fund You have inherited an old gold mine that generates a cash flow given by

$$R(t) = \$50{,}000e^{-0.2t}$$

where t is time measured in years. In other words, the mine is dwindling out at the rate given by the values in Table 2. If the annual interest rate paid by banks is 8% compounded continuously, what is the present value of this mine?

TABLE 2
Cash Flow of a Mine

Year, t	Yearly Earnings
0 (present)	\$50,000
1 (next year)	$\$50{,}000e^{-0.2} = \$40{,}936.54$
2	$\$50{,}000e^{-0.4} = \$33{,}516.00$
3	$\$50{,}000e^{-0.6} = \$27{,}440.58$
4	$\$50{,}000e^{-0.8} = \$22{,}466.45$
5	$\$50{,}000e^{-1} = \$18{,}393.97$
⋮	⋮ ⋮

Solution The current value of this mine is given by the present value integral

$$\begin{aligned} P &= \int_0^\infty R(t)e^{-0.08t}\,dt \\ &= \$50{,}000 \int_0^\infty e^{-0.2t}e^{-0.08t}\,dt \\ &= \$50{,}000 \int_0^\infty e^{-0.28t}\,dt \\ &= \$178{,}571.43 \end{aligned}$$

In other words, your inheritance is worth \$178,571.43, which is the present value of the mine. □

Problems

For Problems 1–25, evaluate (if the integrals exist) the following integrals:

1. $\int_0^\infty dx$

2. $\int_1^\infty \frac{1}{x^2}\,dx$

3. $\int_1^\infty \frac{1}{x^{3/4}}\,dx$

4. $\int_1^\infty \frac{1}{(x+1)^3}\,dx$

5. $\int_0^\infty t\,dt$

6. $\int_1^\infty \frac{t}{1+t^2}\,dt$

7. $\int_0^\infty \sqrt{t}\,dt$

8. $\int_0^\infty \frac{1}{x^{2/3}}\,dx$

9. $\int_{-\infty}^{-1} x^{-3}\,dx$

10. $\int_0^\infty \frac{x}{\sqrt{x^2+5}}\,dx$

11. $\int_{-\infty}^0 \frac{1}{1-x}\,dx$

12. $\int_{-\infty}^0 \frac{1}{(x-3)^2}\,dx$

13. $\int_{-\infty}^0 \frac{dx}{x-3}$

14. $\int_{-\infty}^{-4} \frac{2-3x}{x^2}\,dx$

15. $\int_{-\infty}^0 \frac{x+3}{x-3}\,dx$

16. $\int_{-\infty}^\infty \frac{3t^2}{(1+t^3)^3}\,dt$

17. $\int_{-\infty}^\infty \frac{x^3}{(x^4+1)^3}\,dx$

18. $\int_{-\infty}^\infty \frac{x}{\sqrt{x^2+2}}\,dx$

19. $\int_0^\infty e^{3x}\,dx$

20. $\int_0^\infty e^{-x}\,dx$

21. $\int_0^\infty e^{-kt}\,dt \ (k > 0)$

22. $\int_0^\infty xe^{-x^2}\,dx$

23. $\int_{-\infty}^0 xe^{-x^2}\,dx$

24. $\int_{-\infty}^\infty \frac{e^x - e^{-x}}{e^x + e^{-x}}\,dx$

25. $\int_{-\infty}^\infty f(x)\,dx$ where $f(x) = \begin{cases} e^x & \text{for } -\infty < x \le 0 \\ 1 & \text{for } \quad 0 < x < \infty \end{cases}$

Continuous Cash Flows (over Finite Time)

26. **Value of Graduation Present.** You have been given a graduation present consisting of a continuous cash flow of \$500 per year for the next ten years. What is the present value of the gift if banks pay an annual rate of interest of 10% compounded continuously?

27. **Insurance Policy.** Upon retirement an annuity will pay a retiree \$15,000 for the first year with payments increasing by 3% per year thereafter for 25 years. If banks pay interest at an annual rate of 10%, what is the value of this policy? *Hint:* Approximate this revenue stream by the formula

$$R(t) = \$15{,}000e^{0.03t}$$

where R is the annual payment and t is time measured from the time payments begin.

28. **Basketball Contract.** According to the newspapers, a basketball player has just signed a ten-million-dollar contract that calls for the player to be paid \$250,000 this year, with an increase of 2% per year for the next 25 years. If banks are paying an annual interest of 12%, compounded continuously, how much is this contract really costing the owner?

29. **Company Buyout.** Grandma's Cookies is being bought out by General Cookie Corporation. As payment, General Cookie Corp. has agreed to make annual payments according to the revenue function

$$R(t) = \$100{,}000e^{0.03t}$$

for the next 50 years. If banks pay annual interest at an annual rate of 9%, compounded continuously, how much is General Cookie Corp. actually paying for the new company?

Continuous Cash Flow in Perpetuity

30. **Perpetuity Trust.** What is the value of a trust that pays \$2000 per year in perpetuity (forever) if interest is compounded continuously at a rate of 8% per year?

31. **Perpetuity Trust.** Find the present value of a perpetual income trust that pays a yearly amount given by

$$R(t) = \$10{,}000e^{-0.05t}$$

Assume that interest rates are 8% per year, compounded continuously. What would interest rates have to be for the present value to be infinite?

32. **Perpetuity Trust.** What is the present value of a perpetual income trust that pays a yearly amount given by

$$R(t) = \$10{,}000e^{-0.05t}$$

if interest rates are 6% compounded continuously?

33. **Value of Constant Payments.** Someone offers to set up a trust fund in which you (and your estate) will be given \$10 per year in perpetuity (forever). Assuming that banks pay annual interest of 8% compounded continuously, how much is this person giving you?

34. **Value of Constant Payments.** Someone offers to set up a trust fund in which you (and your estate) will be given R dollars per year in perpetuity. Assuming that banks pay annual interest of r percent compounded continuously, how much is this person actually giving you? This is the general formula for the present value of constant payment in perpetuity funds.

35. **Puzzler.** Would you rather collect \$150 per year for 50 years or \$100 per year in perpetuity? Assume that banks pay an annual interest of 10% compounded continuously.

36. Super Baseball Contract. In their attempt to finally win the Central League pennant, the Toledo Cubs have signed the Puerto Rican sensation, Rico Hernandez. They have agreed to give him almost everything except the clubhouse. The final 20-year contract calls for a yearly salary $R(t)$ of

$$R(t) = \$500{,}000e^{-0.04t}$$

where t is time measured in years. If annual interest rates being paid by banks are 8% compounded continuously, how much is this contract worth?

5.2 Integration by Parts

PURPOSE

We introduce the powerful integration by parts formula, which will allow us to evaluate many integrals that cannot be evaluated by other methods. We will see that the integration by parts formula is "analogous" to the product formula for differentiation.

Introduction

There are many types of integrals that we cannot yet evaluate. For example, the integral

$$\int xe^x \, dx$$

cannot be evaluated by the method of substitution or any other method that we have seen thus far. It would take a clever reader indeed to find this antiderivative by picking and choosing functions by a trial-and-error method. We have already seen how the chain rule for finding derivatives motivated the substitution method for finding antiderivatives. We will see now that the product rule for finding derivatives gives rise to another method for finding antiderivatives, the integration by parts method.

The Integration by Parts Formula

Earlier, we learned the following rule for differentiating products:

$$\frac{d}{dx} f(x)g(x) = f'(x)g(x) + f(x)g'(x)$$

If we set the antiderivative of the left-hand side of this equation (with $C = 0$) equal to the antiderivative of the right-hand side, we get

$$f(x)g(x) = \int f'(x)g(x)\, dx + \int f(x)g'(x)\, dx$$

By simply rewriting this equation as

$$\int f(x)g'(x)\, dx = f(x)g(x) - \int f'(x)g(x)\, dx$$

we get a powerful formula for finding the antiderivative on the left, provided that we can find the antiderivative of the right-hand side of the equation. This equation is the integration by parts equation. To use this equation, it is convenient to let

$$u = f(x)$$
$$v = g(x)$$

and hence

$$du = f'(x)\,dx$$
$$dv = g'(x)\,dx$$

The integration by parts formula can now be rewritten in the following more concise form.

Integration by Parts Formula for Indefinite Integrals

The integration by parts formula for indefinite integrals states that

$$\int u\,dv = uv - \int v\,du$$

The integration by parts method consists of using this formula.

To remember this formula just say, "u dee v equals uv minus v dee u."

The strategy to follow when using the integration by parts formula is to identify part of the integral in question as u and the other part as dv. If we identify u and dv correctly, the integration by parts formula will reduce the problem to evaluating an integral simpler than the original integral. We illustrate the process with a few examples.

Example 1 Integration by Parts Find the antiderivative of

$$\int xe^x\,dx$$

Solution There are two possibilities for u, either $u = x$ or $u = e^x$. Let us try

$$u = x$$
$$dv = e^x\,dx$$

Hence we have

$$du = dx$$
$$v = e^x$$

The integration by parts formula then gives

$$\int \underset{u\,dv}{\underset{\uparrow}{xe^x\,dx}} = \underset{u\,v}{\underset{\uparrow}{xe^x}} - \int \underset{v\,du}{\underset{\uparrow}{e^x\,dx}}$$

The new integral on the right-hand side of the above equation is easy to integrate. Integrating it, we get the antiderivative of the original integral as

$$\int xe^x\,dx = xe^x - e^x + C$$

Check:

$$\frac{d}{dx}(xe^x - e^x + C) = (xe^x + e^x) - e^x = xe^x$$

□

Note that if we made the alternative substitution

$$u = e^x$$
$$dv = x\,dx$$

the integration by parts formula would give us

$$\int xe^x\,dx = \frac{x^2}{2}e^x - \int x^2e^x\,dx$$

Although this formula is mathematically correct, the integral on the right-hand side of the equation is more difficult to integrate than is the original integral.

Example 2

Integration by Parts Find the antiderivative

$$\int \ln x\,dx$$

Solution It is convenient to construct a table in which the substitutions for u and dv along with v and du are displayed. We call this table the Integration by Parts (IBP) table. (See Table 3.)

TABLE 3
IBP Table for Example 2

Original Integral: $\int \ln x\,dx$

Let	*Then*
$u = \ln x$	$du = \frac{dx}{x}$
$dv = dx$	$v = x$

IBP formula: $\int u\,dv = uv - \int v\,du$

$$\int \ln x\,dx = x\ln x - \int dx$$

Rewriting the above IBP formula and evaluating the simple integral on the right-hand side with the integrand 1, we get the desired antiderivative

$$\int \ln x\,dx = x\ln x - \int dx$$
$$= x\ln x - x + C$$

Check:

$$\frac{d}{dx}(x\ln x - x + C) = \ln x + \frac{x}{x} - 1 = \ln x$$ □

It is possible to find antiderivatives by repeated application of the integration by parts formula. In the following example we must use the integration by parts formula two times.

Example 3

Repeated Integration by Parts Find the antiderivative of

$$\int x^2 e^x\,dx$$

Solution Looking at the IBP formula in Table 4, we see that we have reduced the problem to finding a new antiderivative

$$2\int xe^x\,dx$$

TABLE 4
IBP Table for Example 3

Original Integral: $\int x^2 e^x\,dx$

Let	*Then*
$u = x^2$	$du = 2x\,dx$
$dv = e^x\,dx$	$v = e^x$

IBP formula: $\int u\,dv = uv - \int v\,du$

$$\int x^2 e^x\,dx = x^2 e^x - 2\int xe^x\,dx$$

We have already found this antiderivative in Example 1 to be

$$\begin{aligned}\int xe^x\,dx &= xe^x - \int e^x\,dx\\ &= xe^x - e^x + C\end{aligned}$$

Substituting this antiderivative into the IBP formula in Table 4, we get

$$\begin{aligned}\int x^2 e^x\,dx &= x^2 e^x - 2\int xe^x\,dx\\ &= x^2 e^x - 2(xe^x - e^x + C)\\ &= (x^2 - 2x + 2)e^x + C_1\end{aligned}$$

where $C_1 = -2C$. (Do not be bothered by the notation; C_1 is still just an arbitrary constant.)

Check:

$$\begin{aligned}\frac{d}{dx}\left[(x^2 - 2x + 2)e^x + C_1\right] &= (2x - 2)e^x + (x^2 - 2x + 2)e^x\\ &= x^2 e^x\end{aligned}$$ □

We now recap the properties that we look for in an integrand when deciding whether the integration by parts method is an appropriate method for integration.

Tips for Choosing u and dv

- You must be able to integrate dv.
- The IBP formula should produce an integral that is easier to integrate.
- For antiderivatives of the form $\int x^p e^{kx}\,dx$, let $u = x^p$ and $dv = e^{kx}\,dx$.
- For antiderivatives of the form $\int x^p(\ln x)^q\,dx$, let $w = (\ln x)^q$ and $dv = x^p\,dx$.

Evaluating Definite Integrals by Integration by Parts

We can evaluate definite integrals as well as indefinite integrals using the integration by parts formula. By using the fundamental theorem of calculus it is a simple matter to verify the following formula.

Integration by Parts Formula for Definite Integrals

$$\int_a^b u\,dv = uv\Big|_a^b - \int_a^b v\,du$$

Example 4

Integration by Parts Evaluate

$$\int_0^1 x\sqrt{x+1}\,dx$$

Solution We make the substitutions shown in Table 5.

TABLE 5
IBP Table for Example 4

Original Integral: $\int_0^1 x\sqrt{x+1}\,dx$

Let	*Then*
$u = x$	$du = dx$
$dv = \sqrt{x+1}\,dx$	$v = \frac{2}{3}(x+1)^{3/2}$

IBP formula: $\int_a^b u\,dv = uv\Big|_a^b - \int_a^b v\,du$

$$\int_0^1 x\sqrt{x+1}\,dx = \frac{2x}{3}(x+1)^{3/2}\Big|_0^1 - \frac{2}{3}\int_0^1 (x+1)^{3/2}\,dx$$

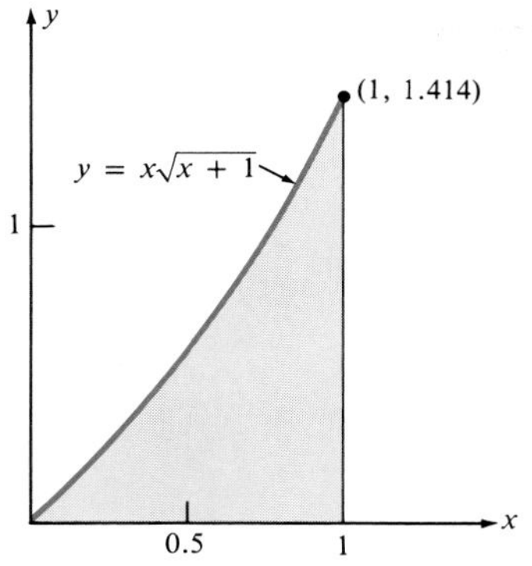

Figure 9
The area under $y = x\sqrt{x+1}$

By evaluating the integral on the right-hand side of the above IBP formula we get

$$\begin{aligned}\int_0^1 x\sqrt{x+1}\,dx &= \frac{2x}{3}(x+1)^{3/2}\Big|_0^1 - \frac{(2)(2)}{(3)(5)}(x+1)^{5/2}\Big|_0^1 \\ &= \frac{2}{3}(2^{3/2}) - (0)(1) - \frac{4}{15}(2^{5/2} - 1) \\ &\cong 0.6438\end{aligned}$$

The numerical value of the definite integral represents the area under the curve shown in Figure 9. □

Phenomena That Start Big and Die Out

Many phenomena initially increase in size or population with a burst of activity but decrease in size or population after a period of time. For instance, a population of bacteria might grow initially but then die out owing to natural factors. Also, the flow of oil from a newly drilled well might increase initially for a number of years but then start to decrease. Phenomena like this are common and can often be described by an equation of the form

$$f(t) = Ate^{-kt}$$

where A and k are positive constants. The general shape of the graph of this function is shown in Figure 10. The exact values of A and k depend on the phenomenon being described.

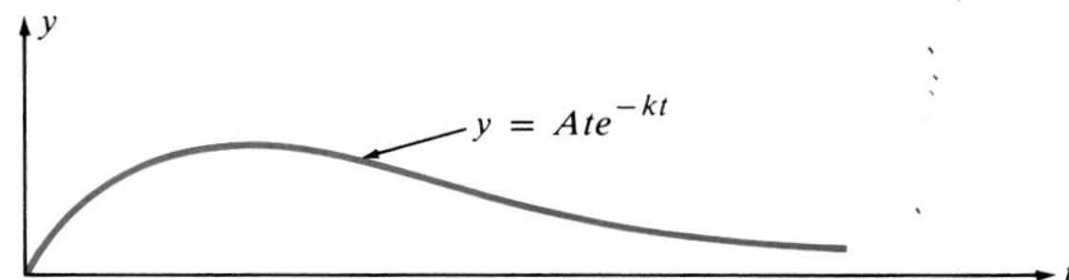

Figure 10
The general curve of $y = Ate^{-kt}$

Example 5

Gas Production Oil engineers have started pumping gas from a new well in the Gulf of Mexico. On the basis of preliminary tests and past experience they predict that the monthly production of gas t months after pumping begins will be given by the function

$$p(t) = 3te^{-0.02t}$$

where $p(t)$ is measured in millions of cubic feet of gas. Estimate the total production in the first 12 months of operation.

Solution The graph of the production curve $p(t)$ is shown in Figure 11. The total production during the first 12 months is found by evaluating the integral

$$\int_0^{12} 3te^{-0.02t}\,dt$$

To evaluate this definite integral, we construct the IBP table in Table 6.

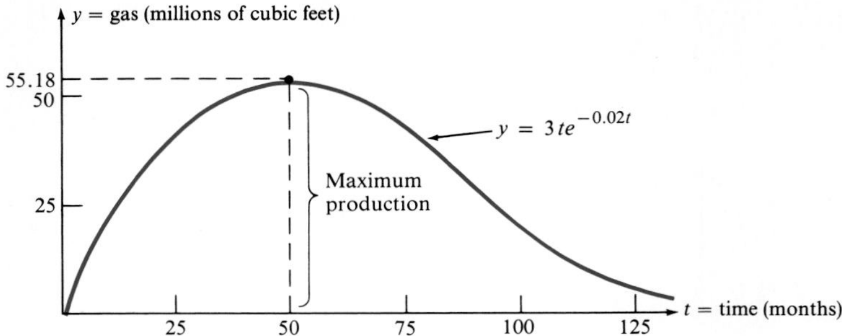

Figure 11
Monthly production of gas

TABLE 6
IBP Table for Example 5

Original Integral: $\int_0^{12} 3te^{-0.02t}\,dt$

Let	*Then*
$u = 3t$	$du = 3\,dt$
$dv = e^{-0.02t}\,dt$	$v = -50e^{-0.02t}$

IBP formula: $\int_a^b u\,dv = uv\Big|_a^b - \int_a^b v\,du$

$$\int_0^{12} 3te^{-0.02t}\,dt = -150te^{-0.02t}\Big|_0^{12} + 150\int_0^{12} e^{-0.02t}\,dt$$

We can now evaluate the new integral on the right-hand side of the IBP formula, getting

$$\begin{aligned} 150\int_0^{12} e^{-0.02t}\,dt &= -(150)(50)e^{-0.02t}\Big|_0^{12} \\ &= -7500(e^{-0.24} - 1) \\ &= 7500(1 - e^{-0.24}) \\ &\cong 1600 \end{aligned}$$

Substituting this back into the IBP formula, we have

$$\begin{aligned} \int_0^{12} 3te^{-0.02t}\,dt &= -150te^{-0.02t}\Big|_0^{12} + 1600 \\ &= -150[(12)e^{-0.24} - 0] + 1600 \\ &\cong 184 \quad \text{million cubic feet} \end{aligned}$$

Interpretation: The engineers can expect to pump 184 million cubic feet of gas during the first 12 months of production. We could also find the total production for any time period by integrating $p(t)$ over the appropriate interval. Table 7 gives the total production of this well for a number of time periods.

It would be interesting to evaluate the improper integral

$$\int_0^{\infty} 3te^{-0.02t}\,dt$$

to determine the total amount of gas in the well as predicted by the model. Without carrying out all the details of the computations we find that the improper

TABLE 7
Gas Pumped Over the First t Years

First t Years	Production (million cubic feet)
1	184
2	631.5
3	1221
4	1871
5	2530
6	3164
7	3754
8	4289
9	4767
10	5187
50	7499
100	7500

integral has the value

$$\begin{aligned}\int_0^{\infty} 3te^{-0.02t}\,dt &= \lim_{b\to\infty}\int_0^b 3te^{-0.02t}\,dt \\ &= \lim_{b\to\infty}\left(-150te^{-0.02t}\Big|_0^b - 7500e^{-0.02t}\Big|_0^b\right) \\ &= 7500 \quad \text{million cubic feet of gas}\end{aligned}$$

In other words, the engineers estimate that the well contains 7.5 billion cubic feet of gas. □

Problems

For Problems 1–10, use integration by parts to evaluate the indefinite integrals.

1. $\int xe^{3x}\,dx;$ $\quad u = x,\quad dv = e^{3x}\,dx$
2. $\int x\ln 2x\,dx$ $\quad u = \ln 2x,\quad dv = x\,dx$
3. $\int (\ln x)^2\,dx$ $\quad u = (\ln x)^2,\quad dv = dx$
4. $\int \sqrt{x}\ln x\,dx$ $\quad u = \ln x,\quad dv = \sqrt{x}\,dx$
5. $\int x^3(x^2+2)^{1/2}\,dx$ $\quad u = x^2,\quad dv = x(x^2+2)^{1/2}\,dx$
6. $\int 3xe^{-(2x+3)}\,dx$ $\quad u = 3x,\quad dv = e^{-(2x+3)}\,dx$
7. $\int x(\ln x)^2\,dx$ $\quad u = (\ln x)^2,\quad dv = x\,dx$
8. $\int \frac{x^3}{\sqrt{x^2-1}}\,dx$ $\quad u = x^2,\quad dv = \frac{x}{\sqrt{x^2-1}}\,dx$
9. $\int \frac{x^3}{\sqrt{1-x^2}}\,dx$ $\quad u = x^2,\quad dv = \frac{x}{\sqrt{1-x^2}}\,dx$
10. $\int x(x+2)^4\,dx$ $\quad u = x,\quad dv = (x+2)^4\,dx$

For Problems 11–14, find a formula for the indefinite integrals using integration by parts.

11. $\int axe^{-bx}\,dx,\ a, b > 0$
12. $\int axe^{bx}\,dx,\ a, b > 0$
13. $\int ax\ln(bx)\,dx,\ a, b > 0$
14. $\int ax\sqrt{bx+c}\,dx,\ a, b, c > 0$

For Problems 15–16, find a formula for the indefinite integrals using integration by parts. The answers should be given in terms of the integrals in Problems 11–12. Let a and b be positive constants.

15. $\int ax^2e^{-bx}\,dx$ **16.** $\int ax^2e^{bx}\,dx$

For Problems 17–20, evaluate the definite integrals using integration by parts.

17. $\int_1^e x\ln x\,dx$ **18.** $\int_0^4 xe^{-2x}\,dx$

19. $\int_1^5 x^2e^{2x}\,dx$ **20.** $\int_0^8 x^2\sqrt{1+x}\,dx$

21. Area Under the Curve. Find the area bounded by the curve $y = xe^x$, the x-axis, and the lines $x = 1$ and $x = e$.

22. Area Under the Curve. Find the area under the curve $y = x\ln x$ for x between 1 and e.

23. Total Revenue. Find the total revenue for a product for the next ten years if the demand is given by

$$D(t) = 100(1 - e^{-t})$$

and the price is given by

$$P(t) = 2t + 3$$

Hint: Revenue at time t is $R(t) = D(t)P(t)$.

24. Total Production. On the basis of preliminary estimates the number of barrels of oil per day (in millions) that a new oil field in Alaska is estimated to produce is given by

$$p(t) = 2te^{-0.10t}$$

where t is time measured in years. How much oil will be pumped in the first ten years?

25. Finding the Robot's Batting Average. On the basis of artificial intelligence principles a computer scientist is building a robot that can learn to hit a baseball. Initially, the robot cannot hit anything, but it learns quickly. A pitching machine is set up to throw 250 pitches every hour to the robot. On the basis of the design of the robot, the number of hits per hour the robot is expected to get satisfies the learning curve

$$H(t) = 250(1 - e^{-0.02t})$$

Sketch a rough graph of the learning curve. What is the total number of hits the robot is expected to get during the first 50 hours? With the total number of hits the robot gets, what will be its batting average after the first 50 hours?

26. Average Life of Carbon Isotope. The amount of radioactive material remaining in a substance at time t is given by the decay curve

$$f(t) = Ae^{-kt} \qquad (k > 0)$$

where A is the amount of radioactive substance present in the material at time zero. The average life M of an atom of the radioactive substance is given by

$$M = \frac{1}{A}\int_0^\infty tkf(t)\,dt$$

Find the average life of a carbon 14 atom if $k = 1.24 \times 10^{-4}$. *Hint:*

$$\lim_{n\to\infty} \frac{n}{e^n} = 0$$

Present Value Problems

27. Present Value of an Oil Well. Suppose a newly discovered oil well is expected to earn income of

$$f(t) = 5t$$

where the income is given in millions of dollars and t is time measured in years. If money is discounted at the rate of 10% per year, then the present value of this oil well in today's dollars is given by

$$V = \int_0^\infty 5te^{-0.10t}\,dt$$

Find the present value of this new oil well. Would you be willing to sell the drilling rights for this well for 25 million dollars?

28. Present Value of an Oil Well. A second oil well, much larger than the one in Problem 27, is found, and geologists predict a steady stream of income from this new well of

$$f(t) = 10t$$

How much is this well worth in today's dollars with money discounted at the rate of 10% per year? *Hint:*

$$\lim_{n\to\infty} \frac{n}{e^{kn}} = 0 \qquad (k > 0)$$

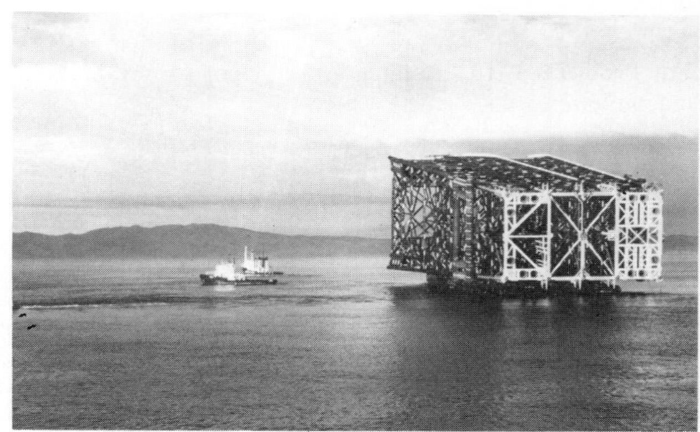

5.3

Areas and Volumes

PURPOSE

We show how the definite integral can be used to find the area between two graphs in the plane. We then move to three dimensions and show how to find the volume of a solid of revolution by the method of disks.

We also introduce the important economic concepts known as the consumers' surplus and the producers' surplus.

Introduction

Today, we sometimes think that without the integral calculus it would be impossible to find areas other than those of simple figures such as rectangles, triangles, and the like. This is not exactly true. Over 2000 years ago, the brilliant Greek mathematician Archimedes of Syracuse [287(?)–212 B.C.] proved that the area of a circle is the same as the area of a right triangle (a triangle with one right angle) with the length of one leg equal to the circumference of the circle and the length of the other leg equal to the radius of the circle. (See Figure 12.)

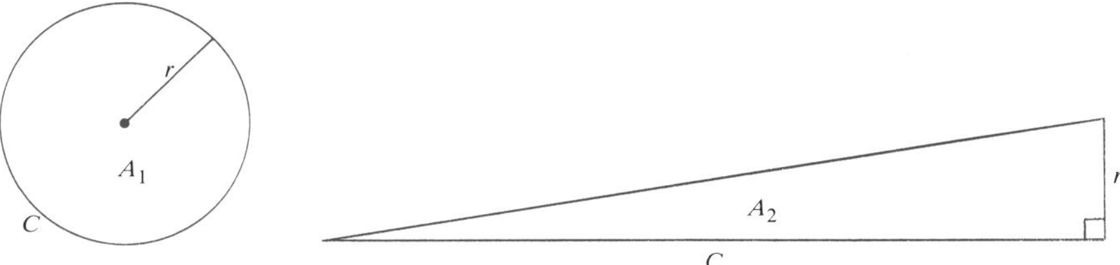

Figure 12
Archimedes' great discovery: $A_1 = A_2$

This fact essentially proves the formula $A = \pi r^2$ for the area A of a circle in terms of its radius. However, to find the area of most regions in the plane, it was necessary to wait another 1900 years until the development of the integral calculus.

Area Between Graphs

We saw earlier how the integral of a nonnegative function f represented the area between the graph of $y = f(x)$ and the x-axis. We can generalize this concept to find the area between two graphs, since the x-axis is merely the graph $y = 0$. Consider finding the area A shown in Figure 13 that lies between the graphs $y = f(x)$ and $y = g(x)$ and the two vertical lines $x = a$ and $x = b$.

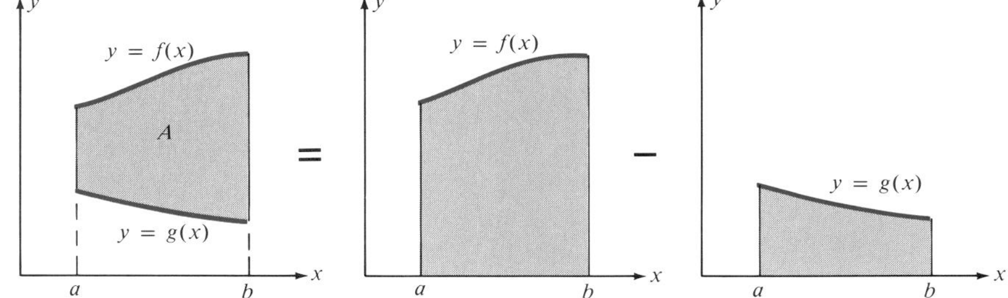

Figure 13
Area expressed as the difference between two areas

Since the area between the two graphs is clearly the area under the top graph $y = f(x)$ minus the area under the bottom graph $y = g(x)$, we can write

$$\begin{aligned}\text{Area between } f(x) \text{ and } g(x) &= \text{Area under } f(x) - \text{Area under } g(x)\\ &= \int_a^b f(x)\,dx - \int_a^b g(x)\,dx\\ &= \int_a^b [f(x) - g(x)]\,dx\end{aligned}$$

This gives rise to the general formula for finding areas between two graphs.

Area Between the Graphs of Two Functions

Let f and g be continuous functions defined on the interval $[a, b]$ with $f(x) \geq g(x)$ for all x in this interval. The area A of the region between the graphs $y = f(x)$ and $y = g(x)$ over the interval $[a, b]$ is given by

$$A = \int_a^b [f(x) - g(x)]\,dx$$

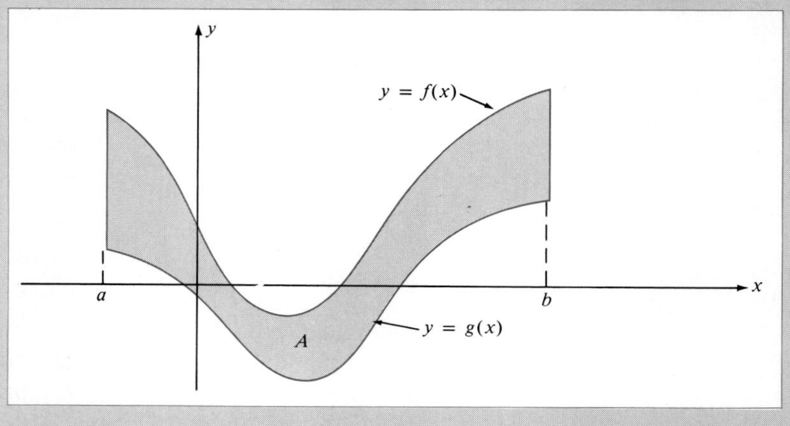

Example 1 **Areas Between Graphs** Find the area between the curves $y = e^{-x}$ and $y = x^2$ on the interval $[1, 2]$.

Solution It is always useful to sketch the graphs of the two functions to determine which graph is the upper boundary and which graph is the lower boundary. (See Figure 14.)

We see that $y = x^2$ is the upper boundary and $y = e^{-x}$ is the lower boundary. Hence we write

$$\begin{aligned} A &= \int_1^2 (x^2 - e^{-x})\,dx \\ &= \left(\frac{x^3}{3} + e^{-x}\right)\Bigg|_1^2 \\ &= \left(\frac{8}{3} + e^{-2}\right) - \left(\frac{1}{3} + e^{-1}\right) \\ &= \frac{7}{3} + e^{-2} - e^{-1} \\ &\cong 2.101 \quad \text{square units} \end{aligned}$$

□

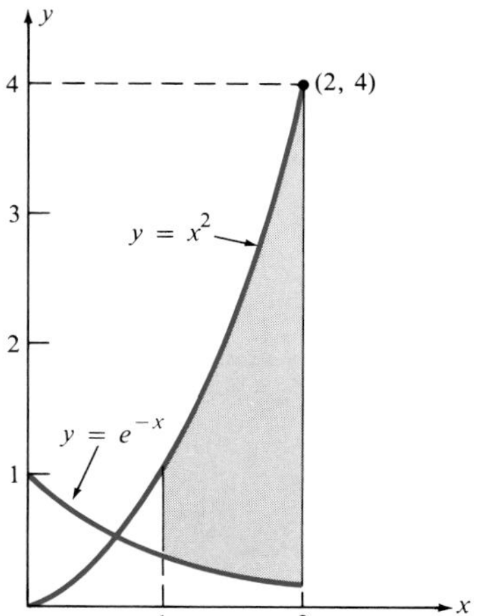

Figure 14
The area between the two curves:
$y = x^2$ and $y = e^{-x}$

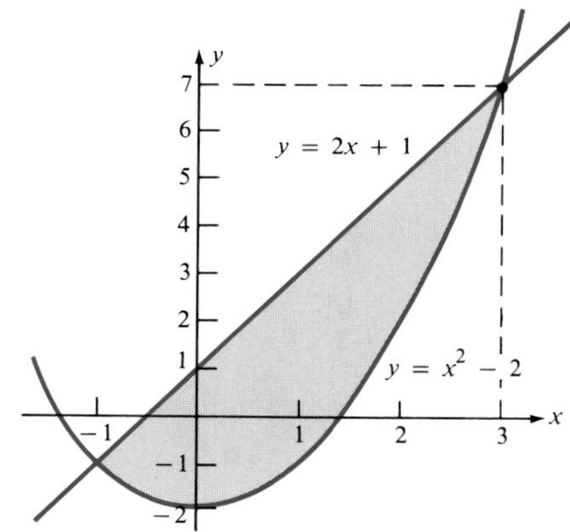

Figure 15
The area bounded by two graphs:
$y = 2x + 1$ and $y = x^2 - 2$

Example 2

Area Between Graphs Find the area between the graphs $f(x) = x^2 - 2$ and $g(x) = 2x + 1$.

Solution The graphs of the functions are shown in Figure 15. To find the area of the region enclosed between the graphs, we must find the values of x where the graphs intersect. We find these values by setting $f(x)$ equal to $g(x)$ and solving for x. This will give us the endpoints of the interval needed as the limits of integration. Doing this, we get

$$\begin{aligned} x^2 - 2 &= 2x + 1 \\ x^2 - 2x - 3 &= 0 \\ (x - 3)(x + 1) &= 0 \end{aligned}$$

Hence the limits of integration are

$$x = -1, 3$$

and the area of the region bounded by the two graphs is found by computing

$$\begin{aligned} A &= \int_{-1}^{3} (\text{Upper boundary} - \text{Lower boundary})\, dx \\ &= \int_{-1}^{3} [(2x + 1) - (x^2 - 2)]\, dx \\ &= \left[(x^2 + x) - \left(\frac{x^3}{3} - 2x \right) \right]_{-1}^{3} \\ &= \frac{32}{3} \text{ square units} \end{aligned}$$

□

We often wish to find the area between two graphs where the graphs cross each other somewhere in the interval of interest. The next example illustrates how to handle such problems.

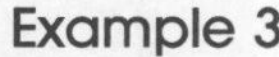

Example 3

Areas Between Intersecting Graphs Find the area A of the region between $f(x) = x^2$ and $g(x) = \sqrt{x}$ over the interval $[0, 4]$.

Solution Again, these functions are easy to graph. (See Figure 16.)

This problem differs from the previous ones, since on the interval $[0, 4]$ neither graph always lies completely above the other. In problems like these, in which the two graphs "switch over" at some intermediate point, we subdivide the interval into subintervals and find the area over each subinterval. We then simply add these areas to find the total area.

From Figure 16 we see that the square root function $\sqrt{x}$ lies above x^2 on the interval from 0 to 1. When x is equal to 1, the two graphs intersect; then for x greater than 1, the graph of x^2 lies above the graph of $\sqrt{x}$. Hence to find the two areas A_1 and A_2 shown in Figure 16, we compute

$$A_1 = \int_0^1 (\sqrt{x} - x^2)\, dx = \left(\frac{2}{3} x^{3/2} - \frac{x^3}{3} \right)\bigg|_0^1 = \frac{1}{3}$$

$$A_1 = \int_1^4 (x^2 - \sqrt{x})\, dx = \left(\frac{x^3}{3} - \frac{2}{3} x^{3/2} \right)\bigg|_1^4 = \frac{49}{3}$$

Adding these two areas, we get the total area

$$\begin{aligned} A &= A_1 + A_2 \\ &= \frac{1}{3} + \frac{49}{3} \\ &= 16\frac{2}{3} \end{aligned}$$

□

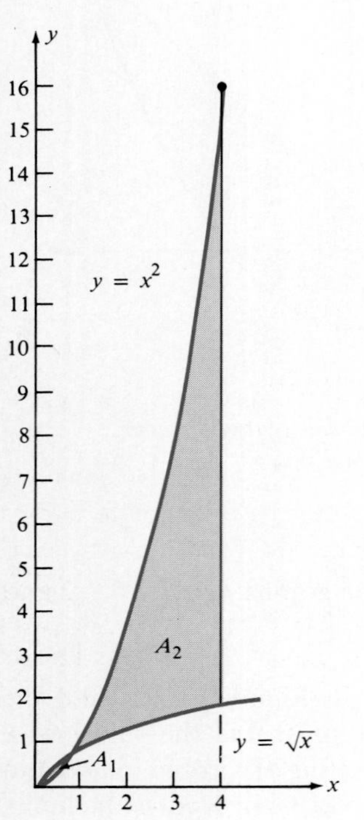

Figure 16
The area between the two curves: $y = x^2$ *and* $y = \sqrt{x}$

The Theory of Consumers' Surplus and Producers' Surplus

In a competitive market the price at which a commodity is sold is determined by the law of supply and demand. Suppose hot dogs are being sold by several vendors on the boardwalk in Atlantic City. From the point of view of the vendors the higher the price, the larger the number of vendors who will be willing to sell hot dogs. When the price is low, fewer vendors will be able to sell hot dogs at a profit, and hence the supply will be lower. The quantity q that producers are willing to supply at a price p defines the **supply curve**

$$q = S(p)$$

On the other hand, from the consumers' point of view the number q of hot dogs purchased depends on the price p of the hot dogs. The higher the price, the fewer hot dogs the consumers will buy. The lower the price, the more hot dogs the consumers will buy. The exact relationship between the quantity q demanded by the consumers and the price p of the hot dogs defines the **demand curve**

$$q = D(p)$$

Typical supply and demand functions are shown in Figure 17. We see that the supply curve is always increasing and the demand curve is always decreasing. Also, these two curves intersect at a point (p_0, q_0). The point at which the supply is equal to the demand is called the **equilibrium point**. In a competitive market the price p and quantity q will tend to stabilize at this point.

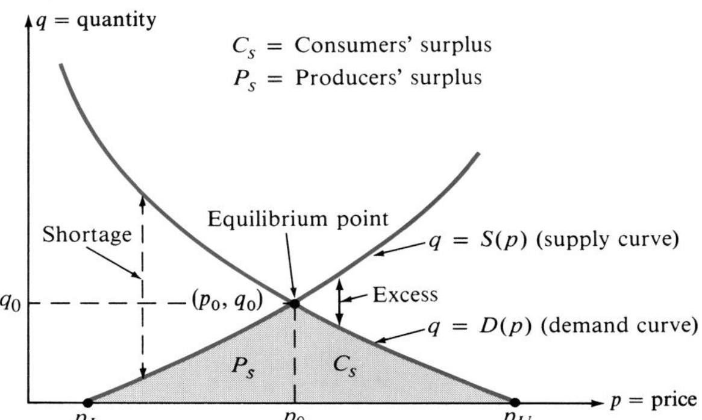

Figure 17
Typical supply and demand curves

There are two economic indicators, known as the producers' surplus and the consumers' surplus, that can be found from the supply and demand curves. To understand their meaning, suppose the going price p_0 (equilibrium price) of a hot dog in Atlantic City is $p_0 = \$0.50$. Of course, some people would be willing to pay more for a hot dog; hence in a certain sense they benefit from the price of $p_0 = \$0.50$. The total amount of money saved by these consumers is known by economists as the **consumers' surplus**. As a very simple example, if eight people were willing to pay \$0.60 for a hot dog and another five were willing to pay \$0.70, then these consumers are collectively saving a total of

$$\begin{aligned}\text{Consumers' surplus} &= 8(\$0.60 - \$0.50) + 5(\$0.70 - \$0.50)\\ &= \$1.80\end{aligned}$$

every time these thirteen people buy a hot dog. The producer (hot dog vendors) would somehow like to get at this money by means of clever market strategies. Can you think of a good market strategy by which the vendors can get some of this money?

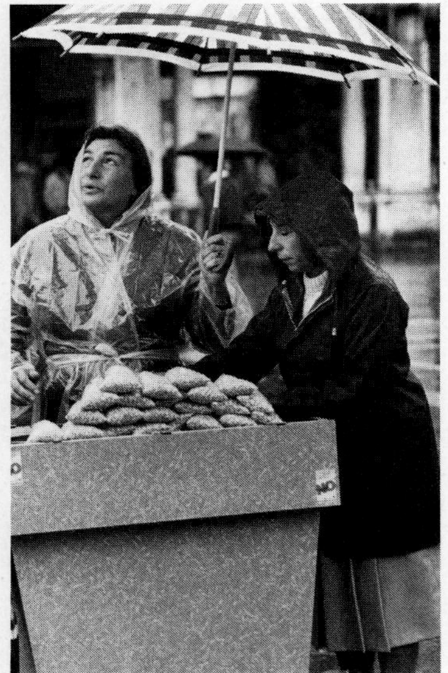

The concepts of producers' and consumers' surplus are fundamental to both large businesses and small.

On the other hand, if the price of a hot dog is $p_0 = \$0.50$, there are probably several vendors who would be willing to sell hot dogs at a cheaper price. In a sense these vendors are earning "extra" money by being able to get the higher price of \$0.50. This extra money earned by these vendors is called the **producers' surplus**. For instance, if ten vendors were willing to sell hot dogs for \$0.40 and another seven were willing to sell hot dogs for \$0.30, then for each hot dog that these vendors sell (for \$0.50 each), they will collectively "earn" an extra

$$\begin{aligned}\text{Producers' surplus} &= 10(\$0.50 - \$0.40) + 7(\$0.50 - \$0.30)\\ &= \$2.40\end{aligned}$$

The consumers would like to get this money by shopping intelligently.

The area C_s in Figure 17 represents the consumers' surplus, while the area P_s is the producers' surplus. They can be found in terms of the supply and demand curves by evaluating the two definite integrals

$$C_s = \int_{p_0}^{p_U} D(p)\,dp \qquad \text{(consumers' surplus)}$$

$$P_s = \int_{p_L}^{p_0} S(p)\,dp \qquad \text{(producers' surplus)}$$

The two numbers p_L and p_U in the above limits of integration are known as the **lower** and **upper price limits**, respectively. The lower price limit p_L is the lowest price at which any producer will be willing to supply the product, and the upper price limit p_U is the highest price at which any consumer is willing to buy the product.

Example 4

Producers' and Consumers' Surpluses Suppose the supply and demand curves for a given commodity are the following:

$$S(p) = 4p - 1 \qquad \text{(supply curve)}$$
$$D(p) = 4 - p^2 \qquad \text{(demand curve)}$$

where $S(p)$ and $D(p)$ are measured in millions of items and the price p is measured in dollars. What is the producers' surplus and what is the consumers' surplus for this commodity?

Solution Graphs of the supply and demand curves are shown in Figure 18. The producers' surplus is given by

$$\begin{aligned}P_s &= \int_{p_L}^{p_0} S(p)\,dp\\ &= \int_{0.25}^{1} (4p - 1)\,dp\\ &= 1.125 \quad \text{million dollars}\end{aligned}$$

The consumers' surplus is given by

$$\begin{aligned}C_s &= \int_{p_0}^{p_U} D(p)\,dp\\ &= \int_{1}^{2} (4 - p^2)\,dp\\ &= 1.667 \quad \text{million dollars}\end{aligned}$$

□

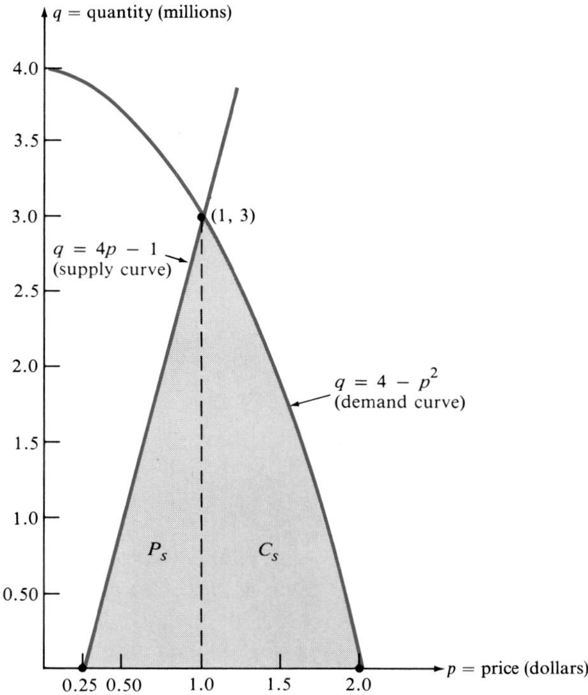

Figure 18
Supply and demand curves

Interpretation

A producers' surplus of 1.125 million dollars means that the producers have collectively "earned" an extra 1.125 million dollars in the sense that certain producers would have produced the product for less than the market price of p_0. It represents the amount of money out there that a smart entrepreneur might earn by buying from producers who are willing to produce at a cheaper price and then reselling the commodity at the going market price of p_0.

A consumers' surplus of 1.667 million dollars means that 1.667 million dollars was collectively "saved" by the consumers in the sense that certain consumers would have paid a higher price for the commodity (if the lower price were not available). If a smart entrepreneur could find these people, it would be possible to earn 1.667 million dollars by buying the commodity at the market price of p_0 and then reselling this commodity to these people at a higher price.

Volumes of Solids of Revolution

Besides finding areas under and between curves, the definite integral can also be used to find volumes of solid regions in three dimensions. The general method of attack is to subdivide the solid region into small subregions, each with known volume (such as cubes or cylinders) in much the same way that we used rectangles when finding areas in the plane. We then use a limiting process that is similar to the way we let the number of rectangles go to infinity in finding areas. The value of the limit will be the exact volume.

This section considers a particular type of solid region in three dimensions known as a **solid of revolution**. There are other solids that are *not* solids of revolution, but we can illustrate the idea of finding volumes by means of this particular type of region. To understand a solid of revolution, consider the graph of the function $y = f(x)$ for x between a and b as shown in Figure 19a. If we revolve the region under the curve, called R, about the x-axis, this action will "sweep out" a three-dimensional solid as shown in Figure 19b. This solid is called the solid of revolution of R about the x-axis.

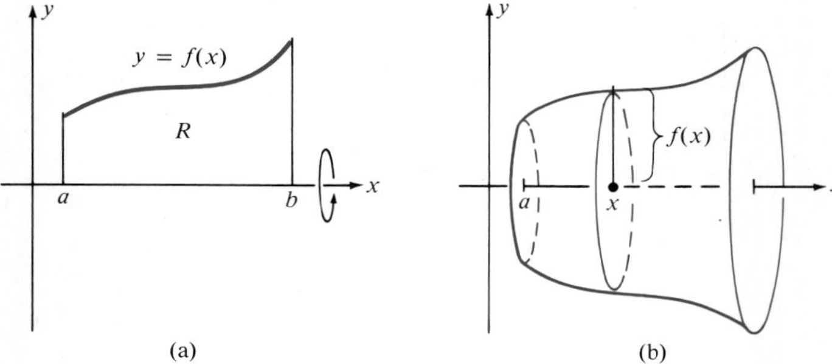

Figure 19
Solid of revolution of R

To find the volume of the solid of revolution, observe in Figure 20a that each small rectangle of width dx in the region R will sweep out a disk (like a penny or nickel) when revolved about the x-axis. Because it is the functional value $f(x)$ that determines the radius of the disk at x, the disk located at x will have a volume of

$$\text{Volume of disk} = \pi[f(x)]^2\, dx$$

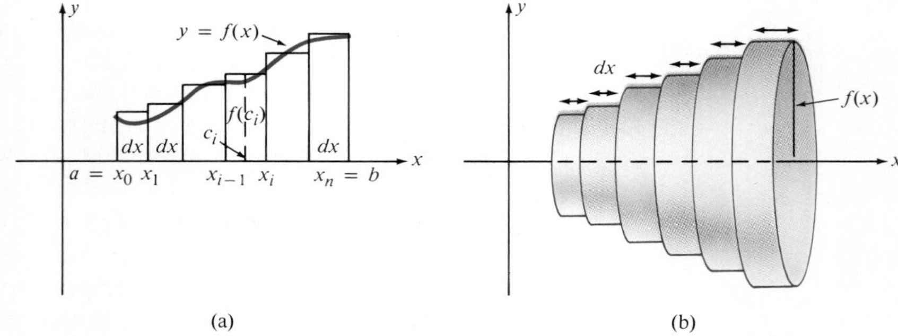

Figure 20
Volume V_n of n disks

We can now approximate the volume of the solid of revolution by summing the volume of n individual disks as demonstrated in Figure 20b.

The sum of the volumes of these n disks is given by

$$V_n = \pi[f(c_1)^2 + f(c_2)^2 + \cdots + f(c_n)^2]\, dx$$

If we now increase the number of disks where the width dx of each individual disk becomes smaller and smaller, the approximation to the volume of the solid of revolution will become better and better. Taking the limiting value of this sum as the number of disks approaches infinity, we get the definite integral

$$\lim_{n\to\infty} V_n = \pi \int_a^b [f(x)]^2\, dx$$

This gives the following result.

Volume of a Solid of Revolution

Let f be a nonnegative and continuous function on the interval $[a, b]$. Let a solid of revolution be defined by revolving the region bounded by $y = f(x)$ and the vertical lines $x = a$ and $x = b$ around the x-axis. The volume of this solid of revolution is given by

$$V = \pi \int_a^b [f(x)]^2\, dx$$

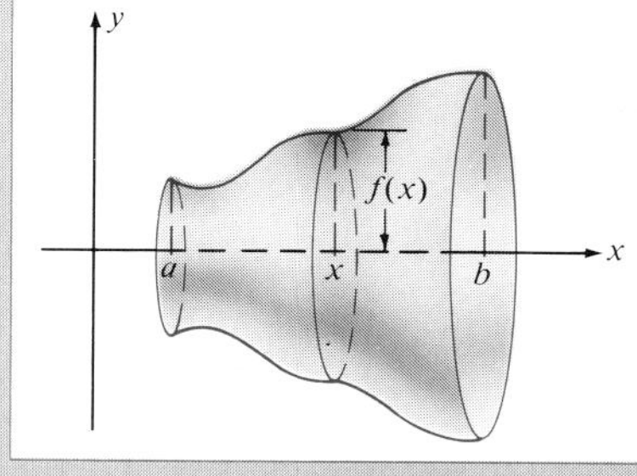

Example 5

Solid of Revolution Find the volume of the solid of revolution generated by revolving $f(x) = \sqrt{x}$ around the x-axis over the interval $[0, 4]$.

Solution The solid of revolution is shown in Figure 21. The volume of the solid of revolution is given by

$$\begin{aligned} V &= \pi \int_0^4 [f(x)]^2\, dx \\ &= \pi \int_0^4 x\, dx \\ &= \pi \left(\frac{x^2}{2} \bigg|_0^4 \right) \\ &= \pi \frac{16 - 0}{2} \\ &= 8\pi \quad \text{cubic units} \end{aligned}$$

□

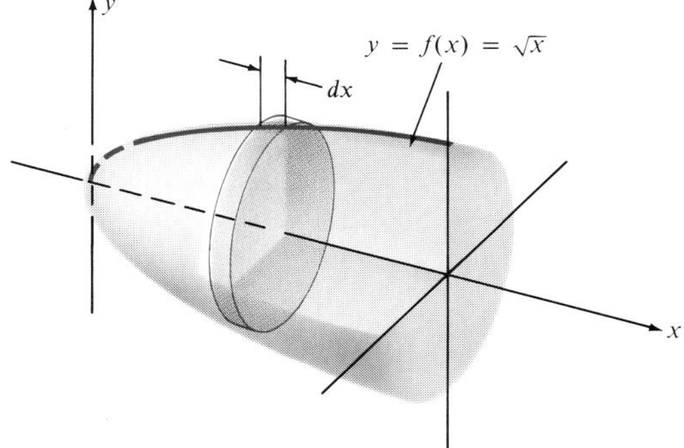

Figure 21
Solid of revolution of $y = \sqrt{x}$

One of the most important solids of revolution is the sphere that is obtained by rotating a semicircle about the x-axis. No calculus book would be complete without finding the volume of this important solid.

Example 6

Volume of a Sphere Find the volume of a sphere of radius a.

Solution The sphere of radius a with center at the origin is the solid of revolution obtained by rotating the region bounded by the graph

$$y = \sqrt{a^2 - x^2} \qquad (-a \le x \le a)$$

about the x-axis. (See Figure 22.)

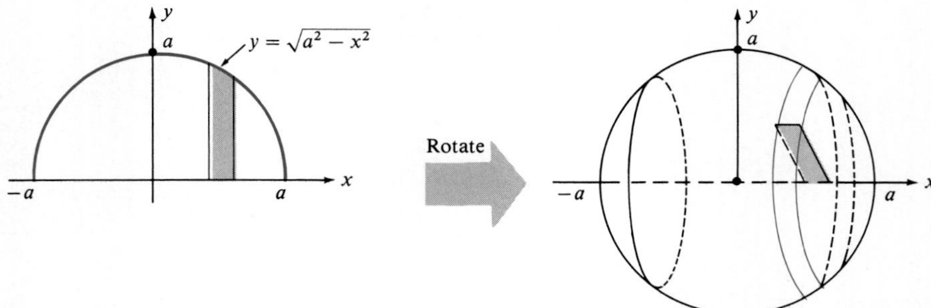

Figure 22
Revolving a hemisphere produces a sphere

Hence the volume of the sphere is

$$\begin{aligned} V &= \pi \int_{-a}^{a} (a^2 - x^2)\,dx \\ &= \pi\left(a^2x - \frac{1}{3}x^3\right)\Big|_{-a}^{a} \\ &= 2\pi\left(a^3 - \frac{1}{3}a^3\right) \\ &= \frac{4}{3}\pi a^3 \end{aligned}$$

□

The Paint Can Paradox

We close this section by presenting a puzzling result known as the **paint can paradox**. The paradox occurs when we revolve the curve $y = 1/x$ about the x-axis for $x \ge 1$. We will let you fall into this paradox by working the following example.

Example 7

The Paint Can Paradox Find

(a) The area under the curve $y = 1/x$ for $x \ge 1$

(b) The volume of the solid of revolution obtained by revolving $y = 1/x$ around the x-axis

Solution Both the curve $y = 1/x$ and its solid of revolution are shown in Figure 23.

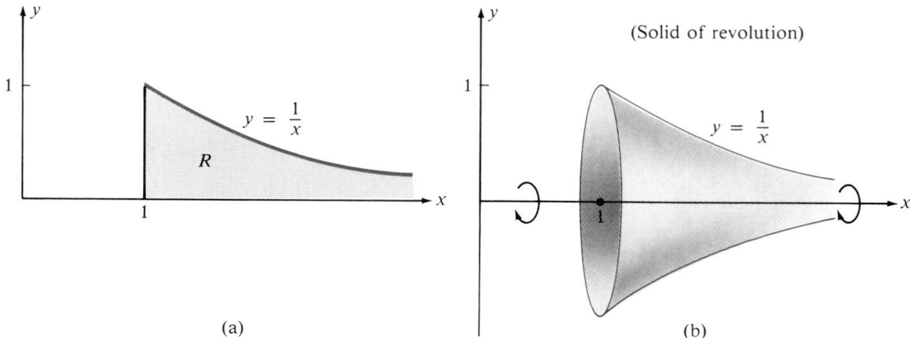

Figure 23
The region under $y = 1/x$ and its solid of revolution

(a) *Area under the curve:* The area A (if it exists) can be found by evaluating the improper integral

$$\begin{aligned} A &= \int_1^\infty \frac{1}{x}\,dx \\ &= \lim_{b\to\infty} \int_1^b \frac{1}{x}\,dx \\ &= \lim_{b\to\infty} (\ln x)\Big|_1^b \\ &= \lim_{b\to\infty} (\ln b - \ln 1)\Big|_1^b \\ &= \lim_{b\to\infty} \ln b = \infty \end{aligned}$$

In other words, the area under the curve will grow without bound as we move farther and farther to the right. We say that the area is infinite.

(b) *Volume of the solid of revolution:* The volume of the solid of revolution can also be found easily and is given by the improper integral

$$\begin{aligned} V &= \pi \int_1^\infty \frac{1}{x^2}\,dx \\ &= \pi \lim_{b\to\infty} \int_1^b \frac{1}{x^2}\,dx \\ &= \pi \lim_{b\to\infty} \left(-x^{-1}\Big|_1^b\right) \\ &= \pi \lim_{b\to\infty} \left(-\frac{1}{b} + 1\right) \\ &= \pi \quad \text{cubic units} \end{aligned}$$

□

The Paradox

We have just seen that the area under the curve $y = 1/x$ is infinite, whereas the volume of the solid of revolution generated by this curve is finite ($\pi \cong 3.14$ cubic units). What this says in effect is that if the units of x and y were chosen as inches, then all the paint in the world couldn't paint the region under the curve $y = 1/x$, whereas the solid of revolution generated by this curve could be filled with roughly 3.14 cubic inches of paint (about a fourth of a cup). Believe it or not!

What is even more disturbing is that the surface area of the solid of revolution obtained by revolving $y = 1/x$ about the x-axis for $x \geq 1$ is also infinite. (We will not work this problem here.) This says in effect that we can fill the solid of revolution but cannot paint its surface. What is more amazing still is that if we filled the solid of revolution with paint, then the inside surface, which naturally has the same area as the outside surface, would appear to be covered with paint, yet the mathematics says that we cannot paint the outside surface. How can this be?

Interpretation of the Paint Can Paradox

Paradoxes in mathematics show that mathematics is relevant to the real world only when models accurately reflect real-world situations. In the paint can paradox the fact that a coat of paint actually has some thickness, and hence volume, has not been included in the discussion. There is a vast difference between painting with a paintbrush and "painting mathematically" in one's head.

Problems

For Problems 1–14, find the area between the given curves over the indicated interval. Sketch the region between the two curves.

	Curve 1	Curve 2	Region
1.	$y = x^2 + 2$	$y = 1$	$[2, 5]$
2.	$y = 3x + 5$	$y = -2x + 4$	$[2, 4]$
3.	$y = 3x + 5$	$y = -2x + 4$	$[-2, -\frac{1}{2}]$
4.	$y = e^x$	$y = \ln x$	$[1, 2]$
5.	$y = \sqrt{x + 1}$	$y = 5x - 2$	$[2, 5]$
6.	$y = 3x^2 - 2$	$y = 3x^2 + 4$	$[-2, \frac{1}{2}]$
7.	$y = xe^x$	$y = x \ln x$	$[1, 2]$
8.	$y = 3x^2 + 2$	$y = -x + 4$	$[2, 5]$
9.	$y = 3x^3$	$y = 3x + 2$	$[-1, 1]$
10.	$y = x^3 - 4$	$y = -5x - 1$	$[1, 3]$
11.	$y = 2x + 3$	$y = -x + 5$	$[1, 4]$
12.	$y = x^3$	$y = x^2$	$[0, 1]$
13.	$y = 2x^2 - 3$	$y = 5 - 2x^2$	$[-1, 1]$
14.	$y = e^x$	$y = e^{-x}$	$[1, \ln 8]$

For Problems 15–21, find the area between the curves. It will be necessary to find where the two curves intersect in order to find the limits of integration. Sketch the region whose area is being calculated.

	Curve 1	Curve 2
15.	$y = 2x^2 + 2$	$y = 18$
16.	$y = 3x^2 - 2$	$y = -2x^2 + 8$
17.	$y = x^3$	$y = x^2$
18.	$y = 3x^2 + 2$	$y = 7x$
19.	$y = 8 + 2x - x^2$	$y = x + 2$
20.	$y = \sqrt{x}\ (x \geq 0)$	$y = -x + 6$ and the y-axis
21.	$y = x^2 + 3$	$y = 12 - x^2$

For Problems 22–28, find the volume of the described solids of revolution about the x-axis. Sketch the volume being described.

22. $y = 3x$ on $[0, 2]$

23. $y = 2x^2 + 3$ on $[0, 3]$

24. $y = 6$ on $[1, 4]$

25. $y = \sqrt{1 - x^2}$ on $[0, 1]$

26. $y = \begin{cases} x & \text{on } [0, 1] \\ 2 - x & \text{on } [1, 2] \end{cases}$

27. $y = e^{-2x}$ on $[1, 4]$

28. $y = \ln x$ on $[e^2, e^4]$ (*Hint:* Use integration by parts.)

For Problems 29–37, find the consumers' and producers' surplus for the supply and demand curves.

	Supply	Demand
29.	$S(p) = p + 2$	$D(p) = -0.5p + 10$
30.	$S(p) = p + 1$	$D(p) = -2p + 5$
31.	$S(p) = 3p - 10$	$D(p) = -0.5p + 25$
32.	$S(p) = 5p - 50$	$D(p) = -p^2 + 100$
33.	$S(p) = p^2 + 2p + 5$	$D(p) = (p - 8)^2$
34.	$S(p) = p^2$	$D(p) = -p + 4$
35.	$S(p) = p^2$	$D(p) = -7p + 30$
36.	$S(p) = 0.01p^2$	$D(p) = -0.99p^2 + 400$
37.	$S(p) = 0.01p^2 - 1$	$D(p) = -0.99p^2 + 99$

Integrals in Business Management

38. Consumers' and Producers' Surpluses. Suppose the supply and demand curves for a commodity are

$$S(p) = 5p - 2$$

$$D(p) = \frac{9}{p} - 1$$

where $S(p)$ and $D(p)$ are measured in millions of items and p is measured in dollars.

(a) Sketch the supply and demand curves.

(b) Find the equilibrium point (p_0, q_0).

(c) Find the consumers' and producers' surpluses, and interpret these values.

39. Consumers' and Producers' Surpluses. An economic study was carried out on a given commodity and the supply and demand tables in Table 8 were constructed.

TABLE 8
Supply and Demand Tables for Problem 39

Supply Table		Demand Table	
Price p (Dollars)	*Supply q (Millions of Items)*	*Price p (Dollars)*	*Demand q (Millions of Items)*
0	0	0	∞
1	0	1	50
2	1	2	30
3	2	3	15
4	4	4	10
5	7	5	7
6	11	6	3
7	16	7	2
8	20	8	1
9	25	9	0
10	31	10	0

Plot the points in the pq-plane and determine the following:

(a) The equilibrium point (p_0, q_0)

(b) The total amount of money that changes hands from the consumers to the producers at this equilibrium point

(c) The surplus (supply minus demand) of the commodity when the price of the commodity is \$9

(d) The shortage (demand minus supply) of the commodity when the price of the commodity is \$3

40. Consumers' and Producers' Surpluses. Supply and demand curves are often approximated by linear curves. The general form for these functions is

$$S(p) = Ap - B \quad \text{(supply curve)}$$
$$D(p) = C - Dp \quad \text{(demand curve)}$$

where A, B, C, and D are nonnegative constants. (See Figure 24.) In terms of the general constants A, B, C, and D, find

(a) The lowest price p_L at which some producer will supply some of the product

(b) The highest price p_U that some consumer will pay for the product

(c) The equilibrium point (p_0, q_0)

(d) The consumers' surplus (leave in integral form)

(e) The producers' surplus (leave in integral form)

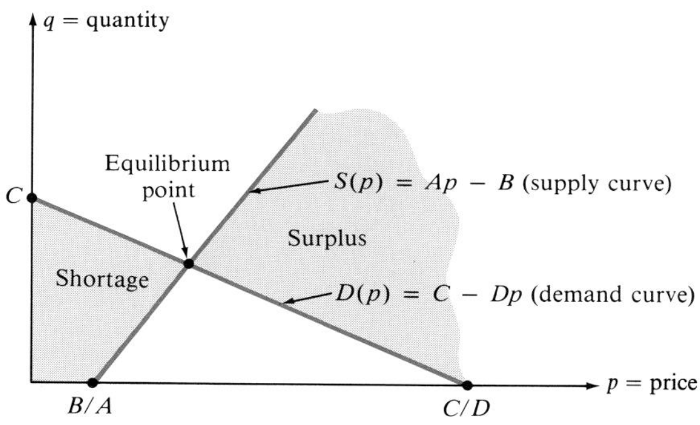

Figure 24
Graph for Problem 40

5.4 Numerical Integration (Calculus and Computers)

PURPOSE

We show how to approximate the value of a definite integral by

- the trapezoid rule and
- Simpson's Rule.

These methods are often used to approximate definite integrals that cannot be found exactly by the fundamental theorem of calculus. Because a great deal of computation is generally involved in carrying out these approximations, these methods are usually carried out on a computer or with the aid of a hand-held calculator.

Introduction

In our studies of the definite integral you may have the misguided impression that all definite integrals can be evaluated quickly and easily, either by a direct application of the fundamental theorem of calculus or by getting help from the method of substitution or by integration by parts. This is far from the truth. There are simple functions, such as

$$f(x) = e^{-x^2}$$

and others for which no elementary antiderivative exists. In such instances (as long as the function is continuous) the definite integral exists, and we may wish to evaluate it. This is where numerical integration is useful. Then too, it often happens in applied problems that the integrand is not provided as an algebraic expression at all but by a collection of data points such as Table 9. The y-values of these data points can often be thought of as the value of a function $y = f(x)$ at the points x_i for $1 \le i \le n$, and we may wish to integrate this function. Hence we again resort to numerical integration.

TABLE 9
Finding "Areas" Under Data Points

x	y
x_1	y_1
x_2	y_2
x_3	y_3
$\vdots$	$\vdots$
x_n	y_n

The Trapezoid Rule

We begin by presenting one of the simplest but most powerful techniques for approximating a definite integral, the trapezoid rule. Consider a function f whose graph $y = f(x)$ is shown in Figure 25a and whose area under the graph is represented by the definite integral

$$\int_a^b f(x)\,dx$$

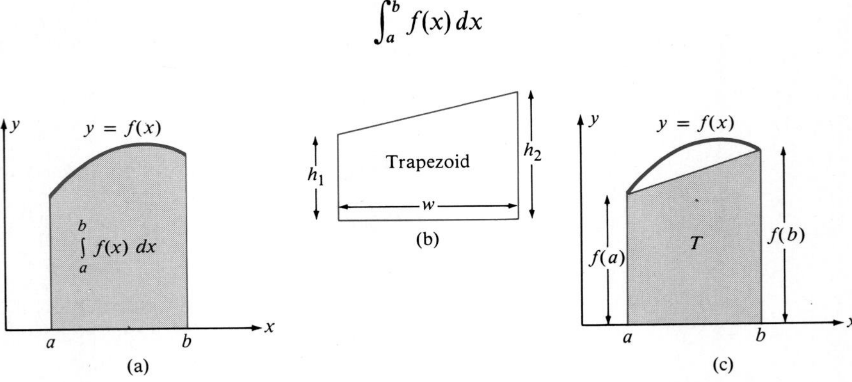

Figure 25
Single trapezoid approximation of a function

When we defined the definite integral we saw that the area under the graph of a function could be approximated by finding the area of approximating rectangles. We now see that the area under the graph can be approximated more accurately by approximating with trapezoids. It can be proven quite easily that the area T of a trapezoid, such as the one drawn in Figure 25b with width w and heights h_1 and h_2, is given by

$$T = w\frac{h_1 + h_2}{2}$$

Hence to approximate the integral

$$\int_a^b f(x)\,dx$$

we first draw the straight line that connects the endpoints $(a, f(a))$ and $(b, f(b))$. If we then compute the area of the resulting trapezoid as shown in Figure 25c, we will get the trapezoid approximation to the integral

$$\int_a^b f(x)\,dx \cong (b - a)\frac{f(a) + f(b)}{2}$$

The power of the trapezoid rule, however, is to approximate the area under the curve not with one trapezoid, but with several. Consider again the integral

$$\int_a^b f(x)\,dx$$

but now subdivide the interval $[a, b]$ into four equal parts. On each subinterval, find the area of the shaded trapezoid as shown in Figure 26. Then add these areas to get an estimate of the integral on the entire interval $[a, b]$.

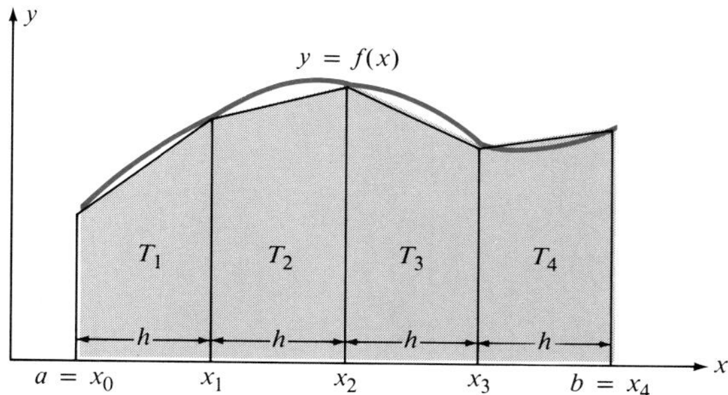

Figure 26
Trapezoid rule with four trapezoids

The length h between two adjacent points is computed by

$$h = \frac{b - a}{4}$$

Hence the approximation of the integral can be found by adding the areas T_1,

T_2, T_3, and T_4 of the four trapezoids shown in Figure 26. That is,

$$\begin{aligned}
\int_a^b f(x)\,dx &= \int_{x_0}^{x_1} f(x)\,dx + \int_{x_1}^{x_2} f(x)\,dx + \int_{x_2}^{x_3} f(x)\,dx + \int_{x_3}^{x_4} f(x)\,dx \\
&\cong T_1 + T_2 + T_3 + T_4 \\
&= (x_1 - x_0)\frac{f(x_0) + f(x_1)}{2} + (x_2 - x_1)\frac{f(x_1) + f(x_2)}{2} \\
&\qquad + (x_3 - x_2)\frac{f(x_2) + f(x_3)}{2} + (x_4 - x_3)\frac{f(x_3) + f(x_4)}{2} \\
&= \frac{h}{2}\{[f(x_0) + f(x_1)] + [f(x_1) + f(x_2)] \\
&\qquad + [f(x_2) + f(x_3)] + [f(x_3) + f(x_4)]\} \\
&= \frac{h}{2}[f(x_0) + 2f(x_1) + 2f(x_2) + 2f(x_3) + f(x_4)]
\end{aligned}$$

This formula motivates the general trapezoid rule.

Trapezoid Rule for Numerical Integration

A definite integral can be approximated by the area of n trapezoids by the formula

$$\int_a^b f(x)\,dx \cong \frac{h}{2}[f(x_0) + 2f(x_1) + 2f(x_2) + \cdots + 2f(x_{n-1}) + f(x_n)]$$

where $h = (b - a)/n$ is the width of each subinterval and $x_j = a + jh$ for $j = 0, 1, 2, \ldots, n$.

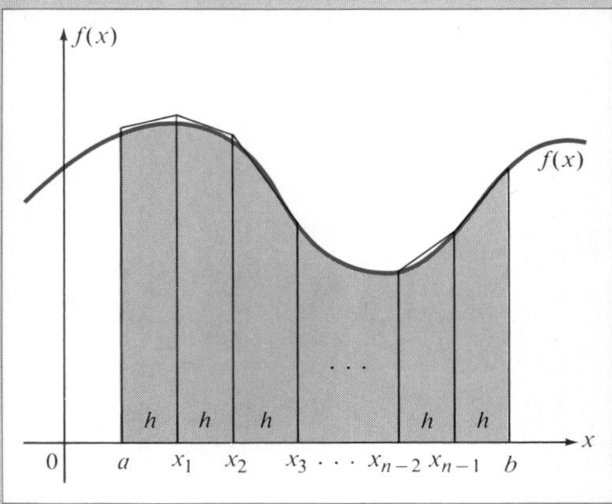

Note that the two endpoints a and b are denoted by x_0 and x_n, respectively, to give more uniformity in the notation.

Example 1

Trapezoid Rule Approximate the definite integral

$$\int_1^3 \frac{dx}{x}$$

by the trapezoid rule using two trapezoids.

Solution Here we are given

$$\begin{aligned} n &= 2 \\ a &= x_0 = 1 \\ b &= x_2 = 3 \end{aligned}$$

We begin by computing the width h of each trapezoid. We have

$$h = \frac{b-a}{n} = \frac{3-1}{2} = 1$$

The endpoints of the interval are $x_0 = 1$, $x_2 = 3$, and there is one intermediate value x_1 given by

$$\begin{aligned} x_1 &= a + jh \qquad (j = 1) \\ &= 1 + 1 \\ &= 2 \end{aligned}$$

The value of $f(x)$ at this point is

$$\begin{aligned} f(x_1) &= \frac{1}{x_1} \\ &= 0.50 \end{aligned}$$

Substituting the above values into the formula for the trapezoid rule, we find

$$\begin{aligned} \int_1^3 \frac{dx}{x} &\cong \frac{h}{2}[f(x_0) + 2f(x_1) + f(x_2)] \\ &= 0.50[f(1) + 2f(2) + f(3)] \\ &= 0.50[1 + 2(0.5) + 0.333] \\ &= 1.167 \end{aligned}$$

Observation: If the above integral were evaluated by using the fundamental theorem of calculus, we would get

$$\begin{aligned} \int_1^3 \frac{dx}{x} &= \ln x \Big|_1^3 \\ &= \ln 3 - \ln 1 \\ &= \ln 3 \\ &= 1.09861\ldots \end{aligned}$$

The trapezoid rule approximation gives a value that is slightly larger than the real value. We can see from the graph of $y = 1/x$ in Figure 27 the reason for the discrepancy. □

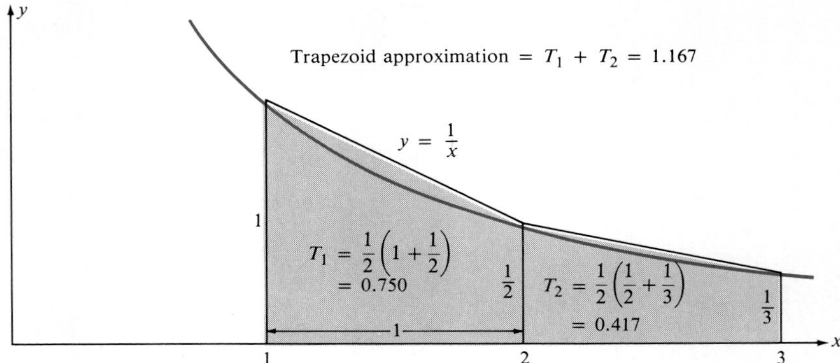

Figure 27
Trapezoid approximation with two trapezoids

We now show how the approximation by the trapezoid rule changes if four subintervals are used instead of two. Intuitively, it is clear that approximating with four trapezoids should be better than with two trapezoids.

Example 2 Trapezoid Rule Approximate the integral

$$\int_1^3 \frac{dx}{x}$$

using the trapezoid rule with four trapezoids.

Solution Here we have

$$n = 4$$
$$a = x_0 = 1$$
$$b = x_4 = 3$$

Again, we first compute the width of the trapezoids. We have

$$h = \frac{b - a}{n} = \frac{3 - 1}{4} = 0.50$$

(See Figure 28.) The endpoints of the interval are $x_0 = 1$, $x_4 = 3$, and there are three intermediate values:

$$\begin{aligned} x_j &= a + jh \\ &= 1 + 0.50j \qquad (j = 1, 2, 3) \end{aligned}$$

The heights of the trapezoids are

$$f(x_j) = \frac{1}{x_j} \qquad (j = 1, 2, 3)$$

These values are displayed in Table 10. We now substitute these values into the trapezoid rule, getting

$$\begin{aligned} \int_1^3 \frac{dx}{x} &\cong \frac{h}{2}[f(x_0) + 2f(x_1) + 2f(x_2) + 2f(x_3) + f(x_4)] \\ &= \frac{0.50}{2}[f(1) + 2f(1.5) + 2f(2) + 2f(2.5) + f(3)] \\ &= 0.25\left[1 + 2\left(\frac{2}{3}\right) + 2\left(\frac{1}{2}\right) + 2\left(\frac{2}{5}\right) + \frac{1}{3}\right] \\ &= 1.1167 \end{aligned}$$

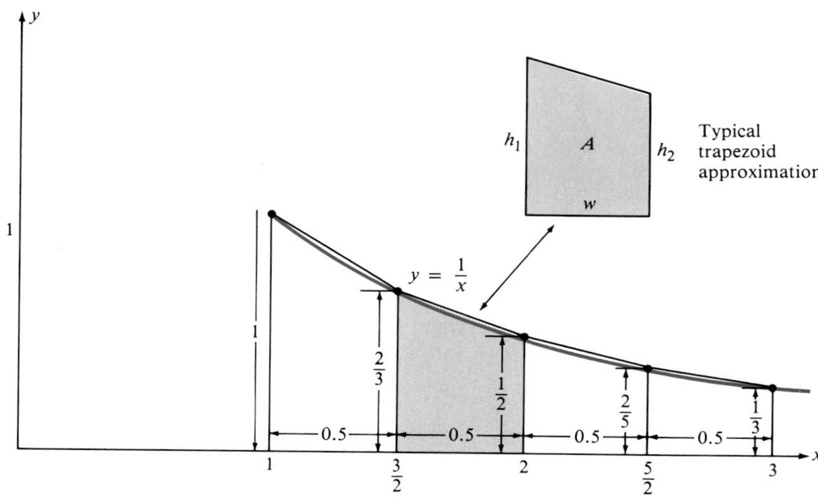

Figure 28
Use of the trapezoid rule

TABLE 10
Endpoints of Subintervals and Heights of Trapezoids

	j	$x_j = 1 + 0.50j$	$f(x_j) = 1/x_j$
Endpoint ⟶	0	$x_0 = 1 + 0 \quad = 1.0$	$f(1.0) = 1/1.0 = 1$
	1	$x_1 = 1 + 0.5 = 1.5$	$f(1.5) = 1/1.5 = \frac{2}{3}$
	2	$x_2 = 1 + 1.0 = 2.0$	$f(2.0) = 1/2.0 = \frac{1}{2}$
	3	$x_3 = 1 + 1.5 = 2.5$	$f(2.5) = 1/2.5 = \frac{2}{5}$
Endpoint ⟶	4	$x_4 = 1 + 2.0 = 3.0$	$f(3.0) = 1/3.0 = \frac{1}{3}$

Table 11 shows how the trapezoid approximation approaches the real value of the integral ln 3 = 1.09861 . . . as the number of trapezoids increases. Note that the error goes to zero as the number of subintervals increases.

TABLE 11
Approximation of $\int_1^3 \frac{dx}{x}$ by the Trapezoid Rule

Number of Trapezoids	Trapezoid Approximation	Error (Approximation − ln 3)	
1	1.3333	0.2347	
2	1.1667	0.0680	⟵ *Example 1*
3	1.1301	0.0315	
4	1.1167	0.0180	⟵ *Example 2*
5	1.1103	0.0144	
6	1.1067	0.0081	
7	1.1046	0.0060	
8	1.1032	0.0046	
9	1.1022	0.0036	
10	1.1016	0.0030	
20	1.0993	0.0007	
30	1.0989	0.0003	
40	1.0988	0.0002	
50	1.0987	0.0001	

A good rule of thumb in estimating the accuracy of the trapezoid rule is to try different numbers of trapezoids and observe whether the approximations are converging to some value as the number of trapezoids increases. Given the values in Table 11, we would be tempted to say that the first three digits of the integral are 1.09. This in fact is correct. □

Figure 29 shows a flow diagram that illustrates the steps required in using the trapezoid rule.

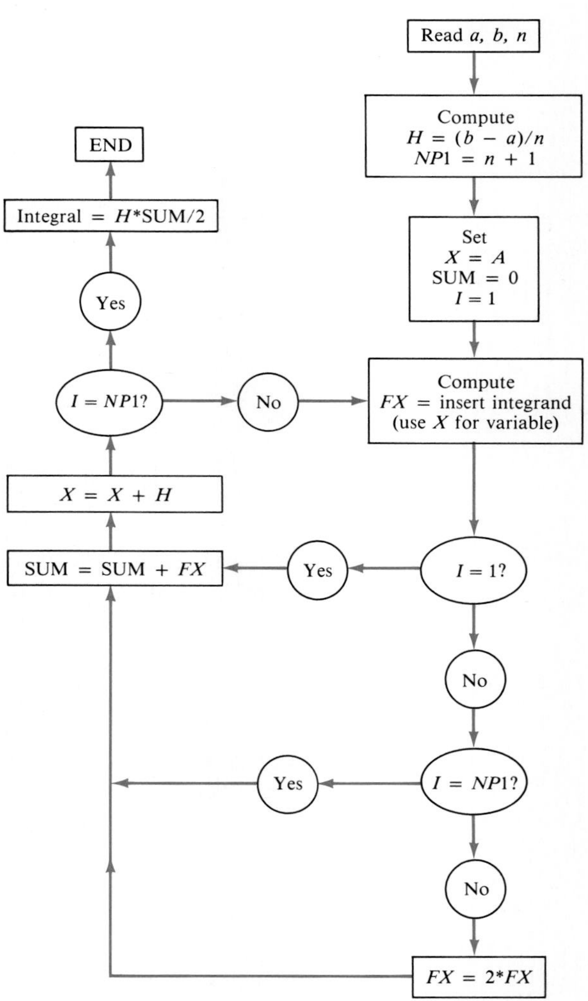

Figure 29
Flow diagram for the trapezoid rule

The following BASIC program carries out the computations described in the flow diagram in Figure 29.

```
10 REM    TRAPEZOID RULE
20 PRINT ''ENTER LEFT AND RIGHT ENDPOINTS''
30 INPUT A,B
```

```
 40  PRINT ''ENTER NUMBER OF SUBINTERVALS''
 50  INPUT N
 60  H = (B - A)/N
 70  SUM = 0
 80  NP1 = N + 1
 90  X = A
100  FOR I = 1 TO NP1
110    REM     INSERT INTEGRAND NEXT
120    FX = 1/X
130    IF I = 1     THEN GO TO 160
140    IF I = NP1   THEN GO TO 160
150    FX = 2*FX
160    SUM = SUM + FX
170    X = X + H
180  NEXT I
190  INTEGRAL = H*SUM/2
200  PRINT ''INTEGRAL IS''; INTEGRAL
210  END
```

BASIC Computer Program for Trapezoid Rule

We mentioned earlier in this section that the function $f(x) = e^{-x^2}$ had no "elementary" antiderivative, and hence a definite integral of this function could not easily be found by using the fundamental theorem of calculus. We now approximate a definite integral of this function using the trapezoid rule.

Example 3

Trapezoid Rule Approximate the definite integral

$$\int_0^1 e^{-x^2}\,dx$$

using the trapezoid rule with four trapezoids.

Solution The graph of $f(x) = e^{-x^2}$ is shown in Figure 30. The basic values used in the trapezoid rule are

$n = 4$ (number of trapezoids)

$a = 0$ (lower limit of integration)

$b = 1$ (upper limit of integration)

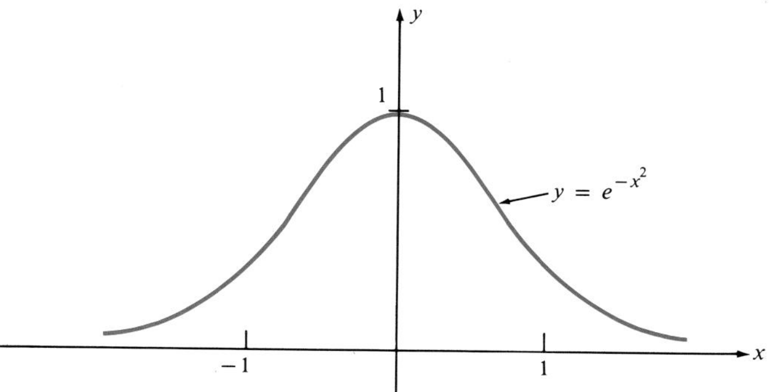

Figure 30
Graph of $f(x) = e^{-x^2}$

Hence we can compute

$$h = \frac{b-a}{n} \qquad \text{(width of trapezoids)}$$
$$= \frac{1-0}{4}$$
$$= 0.25$$

TABLE 12
Intermediate Points and Heights of Trapezoids

	j	$x_j = a + jh$	$f(x_j) = e^{-x_j^2}$
Endpoint ⟶	0	0	$e^{-(0)^2} \cong 1.0000$
	1	0.25	$e^{-(0.25)^2} \cong 0.9394$
	2	0.50	$e^{-(0.50)^2} \cong 0.7788$
	3	0.75	$e^{-(0.75)^2} \cong 0.5698$
Endpoint ⟶	4	1.00	$e^{-(1)^2} \cong 0.3679$

The intermediate points and heights of the trapezoids are found from the formulas in Table 12. Hence the trapezoid rule gives the approximation

$$\int_0^1 e^{-x^2}\,dx \cong \frac{h}{2}[f(x_0) + 2f(x_1) + 2f(x_2) + 2f(x_3) + f(x_4)]$$
$$= 0.125[1 + 2(0.9394) + 2(0.7788) + 2(0.5698) + 0.3679]$$
$$= 0.7430$$

□

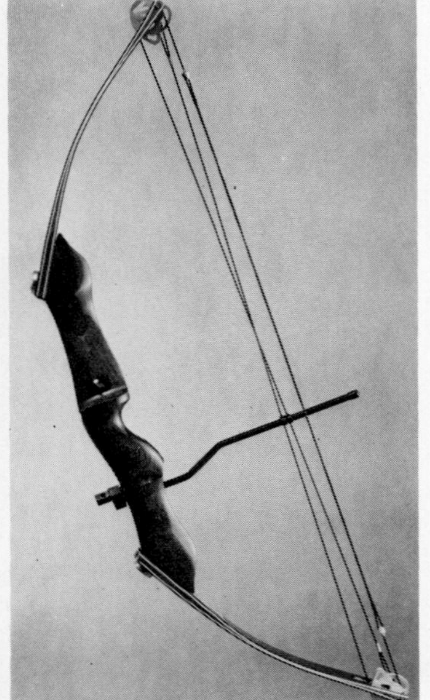

The area under the force curve of a compound bow measures the work performed when the bow is drawn

Using the Trapezoid Rule with Data Points

In the experimental sciences such as biology, psychology, and chemistry an experimenter often obtains observed values of two variables x and y. The values of y can often be interpreted as values of a function at specific values of x. It is often desirable to find the area under the curve defined by this function. The following example illustrates this idea.

Bows and arrows have changed since the good old days of Robin Hood. Today, the serious archer uses a compound bow. The compound bow is designed so that the force required to bend the bow is not directly proportional to the amount that the bow is bent. The force required to hold an arrow steady when the string is completely extended is actually much less than when the string is half-extended. This desirable property allows the archer to hold the arrow in the "cocked" position for long periods of time without tiring.

An experiment is conducted in which the string of a compound bow is slowly pulled until the bow is completely extended. As the string is pulled, the distance x the string is pulled and the force y applied to the string are periodically measured. The resulting observations are shown in Figure 31. A physical principle says that the area under this resulting curve of y versus x represents the energy stored in the bow and hence the energy transferred to the arrow upon release of the string.

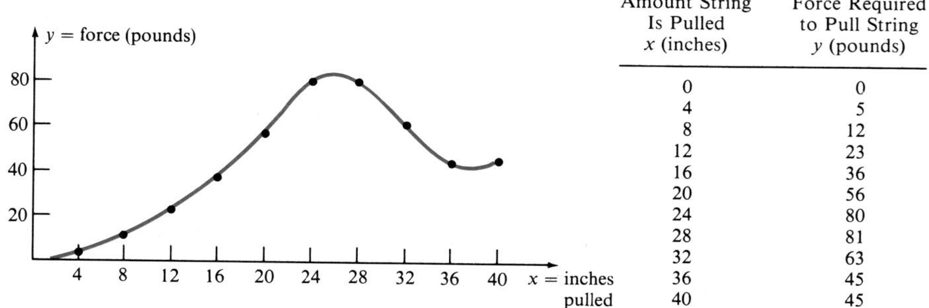

Amount String Is Pulled x (inches)	Force Required to Pull String y (pounds)
0	0
4	5
8	12
12	23
16	36
20	56
24	80
28	81
32	63
36	45
40	45

Figure 31
Force y required to pull a compound bow x inches

Example 4

Energy of a Compound Bow Find the amount of energy stored by the compound bow represented by the observations in Figure 31.

Solution The energy in inch-pounds stored by the bow is the area under the curve that approximates the data points in Figure 31. This force curve is shown in Figure 32.

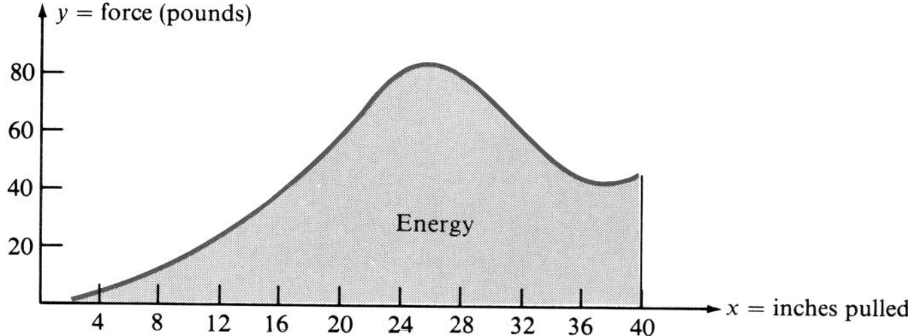

Figure 32
Energy is given by the area under the force curve

Since the observed force y applied to the string can be interpreted as values of a function $y = f(x)$ at 11 equally spaced points, we can use the trapezoid rule with

$$a = 0$$
$$b = 40$$
$$n = 10$$

Computing the width of each trapezoid, we have

$$h = \frac{b - a}{n} = 4$$

and so the trapezoid rule states that

$$\int_0^{40} f(x)\,dx \cong \frac{h}{2}[f(a) + 2f(x_1) + 2f(x_2) + \cdots + 2f(x_9) + f(b)]$$

$$= \frac{4}{2}[0 + 2(5) + 2(12) + \cdots + 2(45) + 45]$$

$$= 1694 \quad \text{inch-pounds}$$

Interpretation: The energy stored by the bow is 1694 inch-pounds or $\frac{1694}{12} = 141$ foot-pounds of energy. To an archer studying compound bows the energy stored by a compound bow is an important statistic. □

Simpson's Rule (Approximating by Parabolas)

Intuition suggests that the trapezoid rule can be improved by replacing trapezoids by parabolas (second-order polynomials). The general idea behind Simpson's Rule is quite simple. Since it is possible to find a unique parabola that will pass through any three points on a graph (other than points on a straight line), we simply replace the integrand of the definite integral by the part of the parabola and integrate the parabola (which is easy to do). The value of the definite integral of the parabola will approximate the definite integral of the original function. We can also extend this idea by replacing the integrand by pieces of several parabolas and integrating each piece separately. (See Figure 33.)

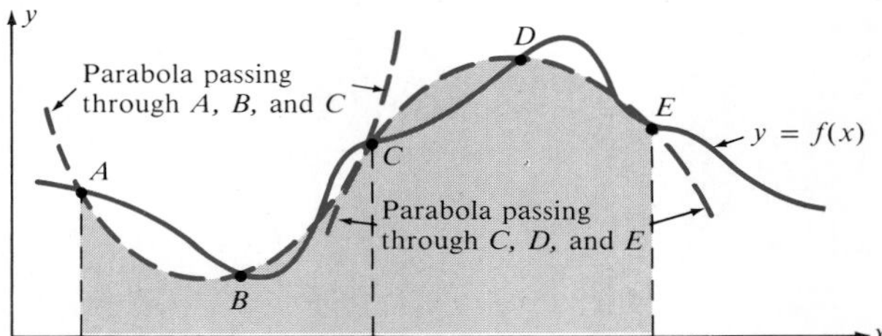

Figure 33
Approximating areas by areas under parabolas

To be more specific, it can be shown that the area under the part of the parabola that passes through the three points $(a, f(a))$, $(a + h, f(a + h))$, and $(a + 2h, f(a + 2h))$ is

$$A = \frac{h}{3}[f(a) + 4f(a + h) + f(a + 2h)]$$

This is illustrated in Figure 34.

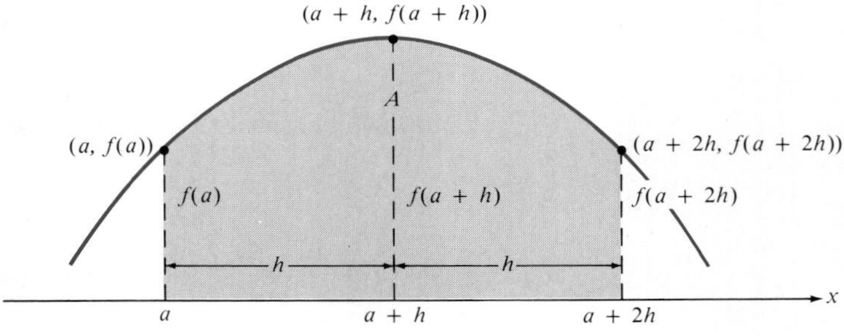

Figure 34
The area under a parabola

We can now approximate the integral

$$\int_a^b f(x)\,dx$$

by subdividing the entire interval $[a, b]$ into an even number (the number of subintervals must be 2, 4, 6, . . .) of subintervals and then applying the above parabola formula to successive pairs of subintervals. This line of reasoning will result in the following approximation.

Simpson's Rule for Approximating Integrals

Let f be a continuous function defined on the interval $[a, b]$ and subdivide the interval into an even number n of subintervals of equal length. An approximation to the integral of f over $[a, b]$ based on replacing the integrand $f(x)$ by a series of parabolas is called **Simpson's Rule** and is given by

$$\int_a^b f(x)\,dx \cong \frac{h}{3}[f(x_0) + 4f(x_1) + 2f(x_2) + 4f(x_3) + \cdots + 2f(x_{n-2}) + 4f(x_{n-1}) + f(x_n)]$$

where

$$h = \frac{b-a}{n}$$

is the width of each subinterval and $x_j = a + jh$ for $j = 0, 1, 2, \ldots, n$.

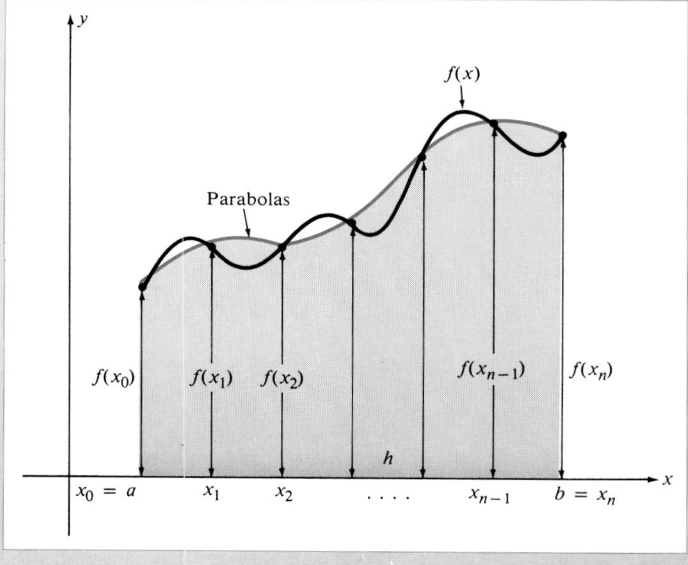

We have denoted the limits of integration as $a = x_0$ and $b = x_n$. Note that the coefficients in the formula for Simpson's Rule have the pattern

$$[1\ 4\ 2\ 4\ 2\ 4\ 2 \cdots 2\ 4\ 2\ 4\ 2\ 4\ 1]$$

Example 5 Simpson's Rule Approximate the definite integral

$$\int_1^3 \frac{dx}{x}$$

using Simpson's Rule with $n = 4$ subintervals.

Solution We are given

$$a = 1$$
$$b = 3$$
$$n = 4$$

and so the length of each subinterval is

$$h = \frac{b-a}{n} = \frac{3-1}{4} = \frac{1}{2}$$

See Figure 35

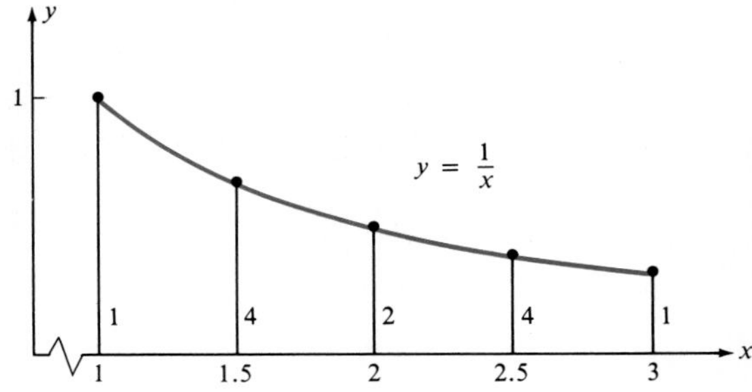

Figure 35
Simpson's Rule must have an even number of subintervals

TABLE 13
Relevant Points Used by Simpson's Rule

	j	$x_j = a + jh$	$f(x_j) = 1/x_j$
Endpoint ⟶	0	$x_0 = 1.0$	$f(1.0) = 1$
	1	$x_1 = 1.5$	$f(1.5) = \frac{2}{3}$
	2	$x_2 = 2.0$	$f(2.0) = \frac{1}{2}$
	3	$x_3 = 2.5$	$f(2.5) = \frac{2}{5}$
Endpoint ⟶	4	$x_4 = 3.0$	$f(3.0) = \frac{1}{3}$

Finding the intermediate points x_j and the values of $f(x_j)$, we compute the values in Table 13. Substituting these values into Simpson's Rule, we have

$$\int_1^3 \frac{dx}{x} \cong \frac{h}{3}[f(1) + 4f(1.5) + 2f(2.0) + 4f(2.5) + f(3.0)]$$
$$= \frac{1}{6}\left(1 + \frac{8}{3} + 1 + \frac{8}{5} + \frac{1}{3}\right)$$
$$= 1.10$$

Interpretation: The exact value of the above integral is ln 3 = 1.09861 . . . , which means that Simpson's Rule with four subintervals has an error of 0.00039. This compares with the trapezoid rule using four subintervals, which has a much larger error of 0.0180. □

HISTORICAL NOTE

Thomas Simpson (1710–1761) was born to the wife of an English weaver and had no formal education. His interest in mathematics was aroused when he received an arithmetic book from a peddler. His first break in life came as a young man when he married his landlady, a marriage that allowed him to be partially financially independent.

In 1736, Simpson moved to London and published his first mathematical work in a periodical called *Ladies Diary*, of which he later became editor. In 1737 he published one of the all-time successful calculus textbooks. After that he concentrated on his textbook writing until one Robert Heath accused him of plagiarism. The publicity was great, and Simpson proceeded to dash off a series of popular textbooks that made him a wealthy man.

It is interesting to note that the rule that made Simpson famous was not discovered by Simpson at all, having been discovered in 1668 by the English mathematician James Gregory.

Problems

In Problems 1–15, calculate the definite integral using both the trapezoid method and Simpson's Rule with $n = 4$ subintervals. Compare the accuracy of these methods when the exact answer can be found by using the fundamental theorem of calculus.

1. $\int_0^4 2\,dx$

2. $\int_0^4 x\,dx$

3. $\int_1^5 (2x+1)\,dx$

4. $\int_{-1}^3 x\,dx$

5. $\int_0^1 x^2\,dx$

6. $\int_1^3 (x^2-1)\,dx$

7. $\int_0^4 x^3\,dx$

8. $\int_{-2}^2 x^3\,dx$

9. $\int_{-2}^2 (x^3+2)\,dx$

10. $\int_0^8 \sqrt{x+1}\,dx$

11. $\int_1^2 \frac{dx}{x}$

12. $\int_0^4 e^{-x}\,dx$

13. $\int_0^1 e^{x^2}\,dx$

14. $\int_0^1 xe^{-x^3}\,dx$

15. $\int_0^1 xe^x\,dx$

In Problems 16–22, approximate the definite integrals using both the trapezoid rule and Simpson's Rule with $n = 6$ subintervals.

16. $\int_0^1 \sqrt{x^3+1}\,dx$

17. $\int_{-1}^1 \sqrt{x^4+1}\,dx$

18. $\int_0^1 \sqrt{1-x^2}\,dx$

19. $\int_0^2 \frac{1}{1+x^2}\,dx$

20. $\int_1^7 \frac{1}{\sqrt{1+x^2}}\,dx$

21. $\int_1^5 \frac{\ln x}{x}\,dx$

22. $\int_1^3 (x\ln x - x)\,dx$

23. Trapezoid Rule. Approximate $\ln 3$ by calculating the integral

$$\int_1^3 \frac{dx}{x}\,dx$$

using the trapezoid rule with $n = 6$ subintervals. Sketch the graph of the integrand showing the trapezoids used in the approximation.

24. Simpson's Rule. Approximate $\ln 5$ by evaluating the integral

$$\int_1^5 \frac{dx}{x}$$

using Simpson's Rule with $n = 8$ subintervals. Sketch the graph of the integrand showing the trapezoids used in the approximation.

25. Simpson's Rule. Using a calculator or tables, approximate the value of the definite integral

$$\int_2^4 e^{-x^2}\,dx$$

using Simpson's Rule with $n = 10$ subintervals.

26. Trapezoid Rule. A well-known identity in mathematics is

$$\int_0^1 \frac{dx}{1+x^2}\,dx = \frac{\pi}{4}$$

Approximate this integral using the trapezoid rule with $n = 10$ subintervals. Use this value to approximate the value of π.

27. Trapezoid Rule with Data Points. The integral

$$S = \int_a^b v(t)\,dt$$

gives the distance traveled by an object moving at the velocity $v(t)$ during the time interval $[a, b]$. Suppose you are driving a car and you record the velocities in Table 14 every 30 minutes (0.5 hour). Use the trapezoid rule to approximate the total distance that you have traveled.

TABLE 14
Velocities for Problem 27

t (hours)	$v(t)$ (miles/hour)
0.0	0
0.5	45
1.0	52
1.5	60
2.0	35
2.5	45
3.0	53
3.5	48
4.0	37
4.5	49
5.0	53

28. Computing the Wood in a Tree. The circumference of a tree trunk is measured at 3-foot intervals from the base of the tree to a height at which the tree is to be cut. Assuming the cross section of the tree to be circular, what is the estimate of the volume of wood in the tree described by the values in Table 15 when you use the trapezoid rule for approximation? *Hint:* The volume of a tree trunk with changing radius is given by

$$V = \pi \int_0^h r^2(h)\,dh = \frac{1}{4\pi}\int_0^h C^2(h)\,dh$$

where V is the volume of the wood, $r(h)$ is the radius of the tree at height h, and $C(h)$ is the circumference of the tree at height h.

TABLE 15
Values for Problem 28

h (feet)	$C(h)$ (feet)
0	10.5
3	9.8
6	9.4
9	9.0
12	8.4
15	7.5
18	6.8
21	6.0
24	5.3
27	4.6
30	4.0
33	3.3

Simpson's Rule with Data Points

Simpson's Rule can also be used to evaluate integrals whose integrands are defined by data points. Suppose we are given the equally spaced data points in Table 16. If we interpret these data points as points on the graph of a function $y = f(x)$, then Simpson's Rule for approximating the integral

$$\int_{x_1}^{x_n} f(x)\,dx$$

is

$$\int_{x_1}^{x_n} f(x)\,dx \cong \frac{h}{3}[y_1 + 4y_2 + 2y_3 + 4y_4 + \cdots + 2y_{n-2} + 4y_{n-1} + y_n]$$

TABLE 16
Data Points for Simpson's Rule

x_i	y_i	
x_1	y_1	
x_2	y_2	
x_3	y_3	$(h = x_i - x_{i-1})$
⋮	⋮	
x_n	y_n	

29. Simpson's Rule with Data Points. Use Simpson's Rule to approximate the integral determined by the data points in Problem 27.

30. Simpson's Rule with Data Points. Use Simpson's Rule to approximate the integral determined by the data points in Problem 28.

Numerical Analysis to Find Producers' and Consumers' Surpluses

31. Producers' Surplus. The observations in Table 17 were taken by a marketing company to determine the supply and demand of a new product as a function of price p. These values are plotted in Figure 36. Using the trapezoid rule, use the necessary observations from Table 17 to approximate the producers' surplus. The equilibrium point is $(p_0, q_0) = (5, 8)$.

TABLE 17
Supply and Demand Data for Problems 31–36

Price, P	Supply, $q = S(p)$ (millions)	Demand, $q = D(p)$ (millions)
\$1	0	20
\$2	2	17
\$3	4	14
\$4	6	11
\$5	8	8
\$6	10	5
\$7	12	2

32. **Producers' Surplus.** Using Simpson's Rule, use the necessary observations from Table 17 to approximate the producers' surplus.
33. **Accuracy of the Trapezoid Rule.** The observations of the supply and demand in Table 17 are in reality the values of the functions

$$S(p) = 2p - 2$$
$$D(p) = 23 - 3p$$

Find the exact value of the producers' surplus and compare it to the approximation found in Problem 31.
34. **Consumers' Surplus.** Using the trapezoid rule, use the necessary observations in Table 17 to approximate the consumers' surplus with $p \leq 7$.

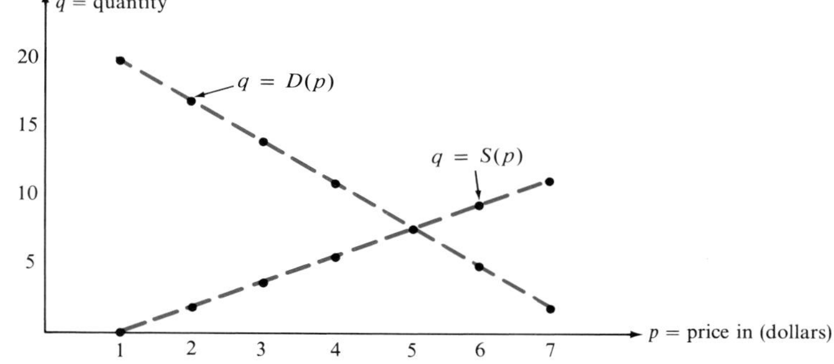

Figure 36
Supply and demand curves for Problem 31

35. **Consumers' Surplus.** Using Simpson's Rule, use the necessary observations in Table 17 to approximate the consumers' surplus with $p \leq 7$.
36. **Accuracy of Simpson's Rule.** The observations of the supply and demand in Table 17 are in reality the value of the functions

$$S(p) = 2p - 2$$
$$D(p) = 23 - 3p$$

Find the exact consumers' surplus with $p \leq 7$ and compare it to the approximations found in Problems 34 and 35.

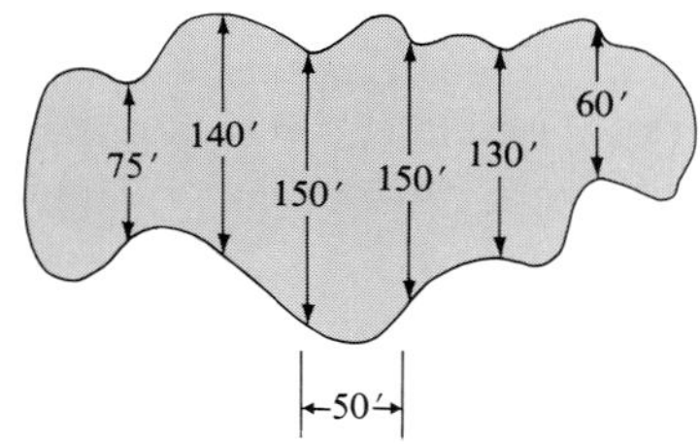

Figure 37
Distances across Harry's fish pond at equal intervals of 50 feet (see Problem 37).

Approximating Areas in the Real World

37. **Harry's Fish Pond.** Harry has just purchased a piece of land that contains a small fish pond. To determine the size of the pond, he and a friend measure the distance across the pond at equal intervals of 50 feet. (See Figure 37.) Use the trapezoid rule to estimate the area of Harry's fish pond.
38. **Sally's Cardiac Output.** Sally is having her cardiac output checked. Ten milligrams of dye are injected into a vein that leads directly to her heart. After the injection the concentration c of dye in her aortic artery (an artery leading from the heart) is measured every 2 seconds for 16 seconds. The results are shown in Table 18.

TABLE 18
Concentration (c) of Dye in the Aortic Artery

Seconds after injection	0	2	4	6	8	10	12	14	16
Concentration (mg/liter)	0	0	0.8	1.8	3.6	5.0	3.1	1.4	0.2

Sally's cardiac output R (liters of blood pumped per minute by the heart) can be approximated from the formula

$$R = \frac{600}{\int_0^{16} c(t)\,dt}$$

(a) Use the trapezoid rule to estimate the integral of $c(t)$.
(b) What is Sally's cardiac output?

5.5 Differential Equations (Growth and Decay)

PURPOSE

We introduce the basic concept of a differential equation and in particular the growth and decay equations. The important ideas introduced are

- The meaning of a differential equation
- The general solution of a differential equation
- The growth and decay equations

Basics of Differential Equations

A **differential equation** is an equation that contains at least one derivative of an unknown function. Differential equations are important because they are able to describe so many physical phenomena. Often the derivatives of a function represent physical phenomena (such as velocity, acceleration, force, or friction); hence equations that relate a function and its derivatives often describe natural laws of science. Differential equations were originally used by astronomers to describe planetary motion, but nowadays they are used to describe phenomena in such diversified areas as biology, economics, ecology, and genetics. Sending vehicles to the moon and the further exploration of space would be impossible without the solution of differential equations to guide the spaceships.

Until now, when you have been asked to find the solution of an equation such as

$$x^2 - x - 2 = 0$$

the unknown x has always been a real number. Now, however, we will solve a differential equation in which the unknown is not a number but a function. For example, to solve the differential equation

$$\frac{dy}{dt} + 3y = 0$$

which relates an unknown function $y(t)$ with its derivative dy/dt, we seek to find the function $y(t)$ whose derivative plus three times itself is identically zero. Such a function is called the **solution** of the differential equation, and t (which generally stands for time) is called the **independent variable**. For this differential equation, it is a simple matter to verify that

$$y(t) = e^{-3t}$$

is a solution, since

$$\underbrace{\frac{d}{dt}e^{-3t}}_{y'} + \underbrace{3e^{-3t}}_{3y} = -3e^{-3t} + 3e^{-3t} = 0$$

Furthermore, we can verify that

$$y_1(t) = 2e^{-3t}$$
$$y_2(t) = -3e^{-3t}$$
$$y_3(t) = \frac{1}{2}e^{-3t}$$

are also solutions. In fact, any function of the form

$$y(t) = Ce^{-3t}$$

where C is any real number is a solution of the differential equation. We call this collection of solutions, as we allow C to "run through" all the real numbers, the **general solution** of the differential equation. It constitutes all of the solutions of the differential equation. The name *general solution* is often misinterpreted by beginning students of differential equations and is thought to consist of only one solution; however, it is an entire family or set of solutions. Specific solutions, such as $2e^{-3t}$ and $-5e^{-3t}$, attained by assigning specific values of C in the general solution Ce^{-3t}, are called **particular solutions** of the differential equation.

This section does not attempt to study all types of differential equations but only an important class of differential equations called the growth and decay equations.

Growth and Decay Differential Equations

One of the simplest differential equations is the most important. It is called the **growth** and **decay equation**, and it is given by

$$\frac{dy}{dt} = ky \qquad \text{(growth/decay equation)}$$

More specifically, when $k > 0$ the equation is called the growth equation, and when $k < 0$ it is called the decay equation. In ordinary English it says that the rate of change in the variable y is always directly proportional to the value of y. In this equation, $y(t)$ is the dependent variable (which we denote simply by y) and t is the independent variable. Some phenomena that can be described by the growth and decay equations are described in Table 19. The graphs of a few of these phenomena are displayed in Figure 38.

TABLE 19
Common Phenomena Described by the Growth and Decay Equation

Growth Phenomena ($k > 0$)	**Decay Phenomena ($k < 0$)**
Bank account paying compound interest	Drug injected into bloodstream
Unchecked biological growth	Water temperature in a bathtub
Short-term human and animal populations	Radioactive decay
	Intensity of X-rays through the body
	Intensity of light passing through water

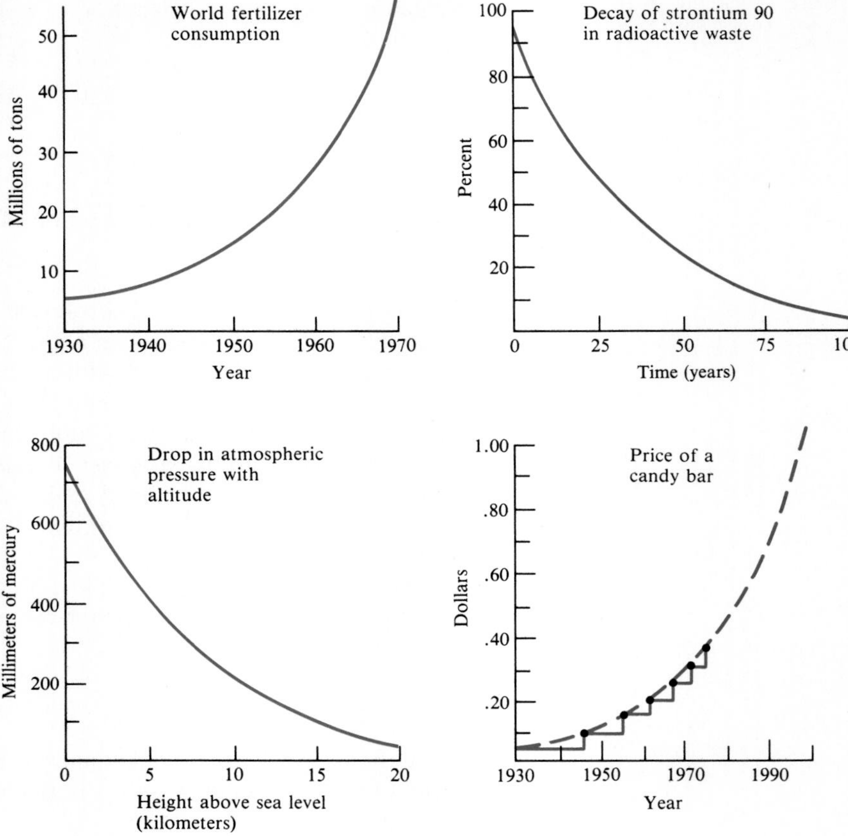

Figure 38
Typical growth and decay phenomena

Solution of the Growth and Decay Equation

To solve the growth and decay equation, we carry out the following steps:

Step 1: *Multiply by e^{-kt}.* We first write the equation as

$$\frac{dy}{dt} - ky = 0$$

We then multiply each side of the equation by e^{-kt}, getting

$$e^{-kt}\left(\frac{dy}{dt} - ky\right) = 0$$

However, the left-hand side of this equation is simply the derivative of the product $y(t)e^{kt}$ with respect to t. (Check it yourself.) Hence the equation can be rewritten as

$$\frac{d}{dt}\left[y(t)e^{-kt}\right] = 0$$

Step 2: *Find the antiderivative.* We now take the antiderivative of each side of this equation, getting

$$y(t)e^{-kt} = C$$

where C is an arbitrary constant.

Step 3: *Solve for y.* Solving for $y(t)$ gives the solution

$$y(t) = Ce^{kt}$$

We summarize this result below.

Solution of the Unlimited Growth and Decay Equation

For any constant k, the growth and decay equation

$$\frac{dy}{dt} = ky(t)$$

has an infinite number of solutions. They are

$$y(t) = Ae^{kt}$$

where A is any real number (the infinite number is a result of letting A be any real number). The constant k is positive for growth equations and negative for decay equations.

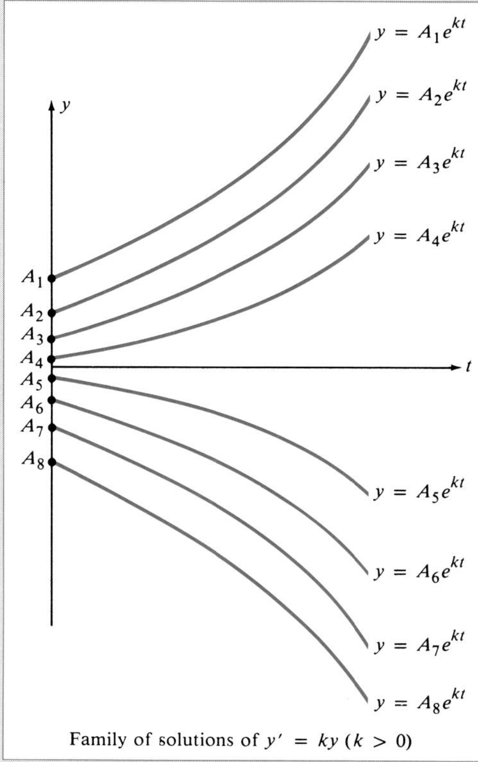

Family of solutions of $y' = ky$ $(k > 0)$

Check:

$$\frac{dy}{dt} = \frac{d}{dt}(Ae^{kt}) = Ake^{kt} = k(Ae^{kt}) = ky(t)$$

Unlimited Growth and Decay Curves

What do the growth of sunflowers, the growth of the total number of miles of railway tracks in the United States during the early 1900s, and the growth of money in a bank account in Lubbock, Texas, have in common? No, this is not a trick question; it is just that they can all be described by the exponential growth equation

$$y = Ae^{kt} \qquad (k > 0)$$

The graphs of these phenomena are displayed in Figure 39. Ready for another question? What does the decay of sunlight as one goes down into the ocean and the decay of the amount of alcohol in the blood after a person has stopped drinking have in common? Another trick question? No, it is just that these two phenomena can both be described by an exponential decay equation

$$y = Ae^{kt} \qquad (k < 0)$$

(See Figure 40.)

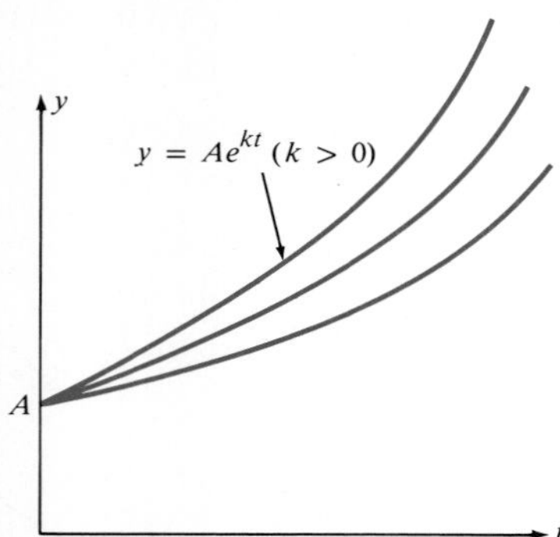

Figure 39
Typical growth curves

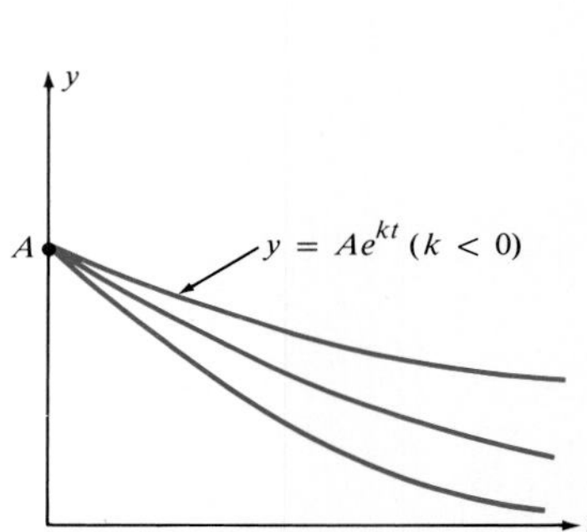

Figure 40
Typical decay curves

We illustrate some of the basic ideas of the growth and decay curves with the following examples.

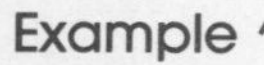

Example 1

Solution of a Growth Equation Verify that the growth curve $y = e^{0.05t}$ is a solution of the differential equation

$$\frac{dy}{dt} = 0.05y$$

Solution We first calculate dy/dt, getting

$$\frac{dy}{dt} = 0.05e^{0.05t}$$

Since $y = e^{0.05t}$, we have

$$\frac{dy}{dt} = 0.05e^{0.05t} = 0.05y$$

Hence, $y = e^{0.05t}$ is a solution of the differential equation. By the same argument, any function of the form $Ce^{0.05t}$, where C is a constant, will satisfy the above differential equation. Members of this family of solutions $Ce^{0.05t}$ are shown in Figure 41. □

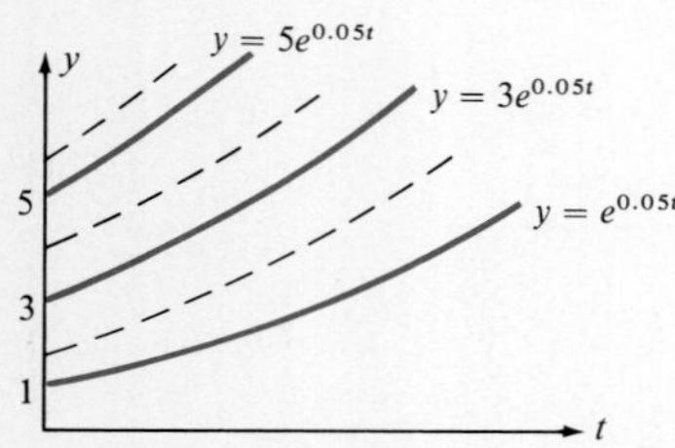

Figure 41
Family of curves $Ce^{0.05t}$ for $C > 0$

Example 2

Solution of a Decay Equation Find all the solutions of the decay equation

$$\frac{dy}{dt} = -3y$$

Solution The solutions consist of the functions

$$y = Ce^{-3t}$$

where C is any constant. Some of these decay curves are shown in Figure 42. □

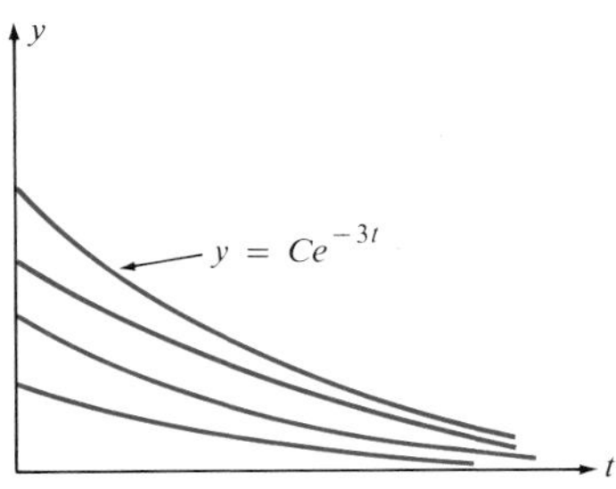

Figure 42
Typical particular solutions in the general solution

The Initial-Value Problem

Generally, when we solve the growth or the decay differential equation, our goal is not to find all the solutions, but that specific one that satisfies an additional initial condition $y(0) = y_0$. In order that the growth/decay curve $y = Ce^{kt}$ takes on a given value y_0 at $t = 0$, it is necessary that the constant C is y_0.

These ideas introduce the initial-value problem.

Initial-Value Problem and Solution

The **initial-value problem** for the unlimited growth and decay equation consists of finding the function $y(t)$ that satisfies the two equations:

$$\frac{dy}{dt} = ky \qquad \text{(growth/decay equation)}$$

$$y(0) = y_0 \qquad \text{(initial condition)}$$

where y_0 is a given constant.

The solution of this initial-value problem is the single function

$$y = y_0e^{kt}$$

It is called a growth curve when $k > 0$ and a decay curve when $k < 0$.

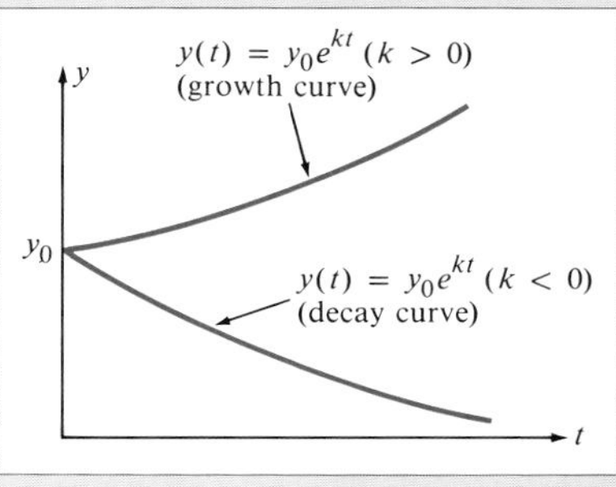

Example 3

Solution of Initial-Value Problem Find the solution of the initial-value problem

$$\frac{dy}{dt} = -0.15y$$

$$y(0) = 100$$

Solution We are given

$$k = -0.15$$
$$y_0 = 100$$

Hence, the solution is

$$\begin{aligned} y &= y_0 e^{kt} \\ &= 100e^{-0.15t} \end{aligned}$$

This decay curve is shown in Figure 43. □

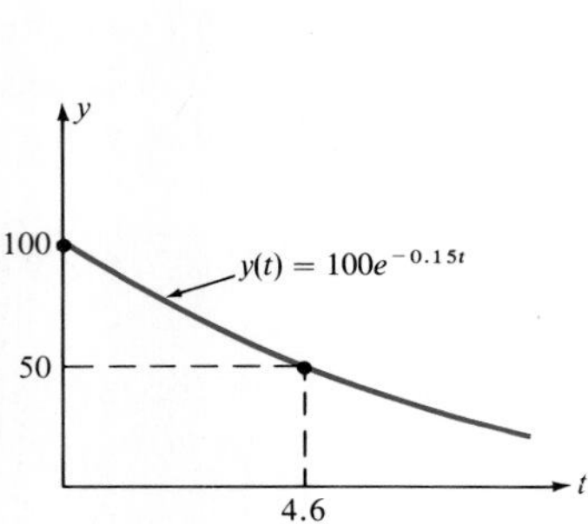

Figure 43
Solution of an initial-value problem

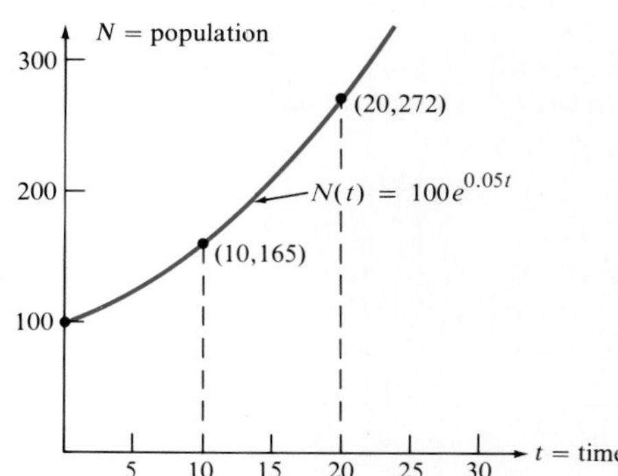

Figure 44
Growth curve with rate constant $k = 0.05$

Unrestricted Biological Growth

Consider the growth of a biological culture (such as a fungus, virus, bacteria, or cancer cells). We call the number of cells in the culture $N(t)$ and the number of cells when observations were begun N_0. If the culture is not contained in a crowded environment and has room to grow, then over the short run the rate of growth is often proportional to the number of cells present in the culture. This fact, along with the initial size N_0 of the culture, says that $N(t)$ must satisfy the initial-value problem

$$\frac{dN}{dt} = kN(t) \qquad (k > 0)$$

$$N(0) = N_0 \qquad \text{(initial population)}$$

The growth constant k varies from population to population. The larger the rate of growth, the larger the constant. Figure 44 shows the growth curve $N(t)$ for the rate constant $k = 0.05$ with an initial population of $N_0 = 100$.

Example 4

Unrestricted Biological Growth Assume the population of a certain culture of *Escherichia coli* grows at a rate proportional to its size N. A researcher has determined that every hour the size of the culture is 7% larger than it was the previous hour. Find the differential equation

$$\frac{dN}{dt} = kN(t)$$

that describes the size of this population.

Solution The fact that the size is increasing by 7% every hour means that the population size after t hours will be

$$N(t) = N_0(1.07)^t$$

where N_0 is the initial population size. To determine the growth constant k, we use a property of exponentials to rewrite the above equation as

$$\begin{aligned} N(t) &= N_0(1.07)^t \\ &= N_0 e^{\ln(1.07)t} \\ &\cong N_0 e^{0.068t} \end{aligned}$$

Hence, the growth equation is

$$\frac{dN}{dt} = 0.068N$$

The growth curve in Figure 45 gives the number of *Escherichia coli* at any time t when $N_0 = 1000$. □

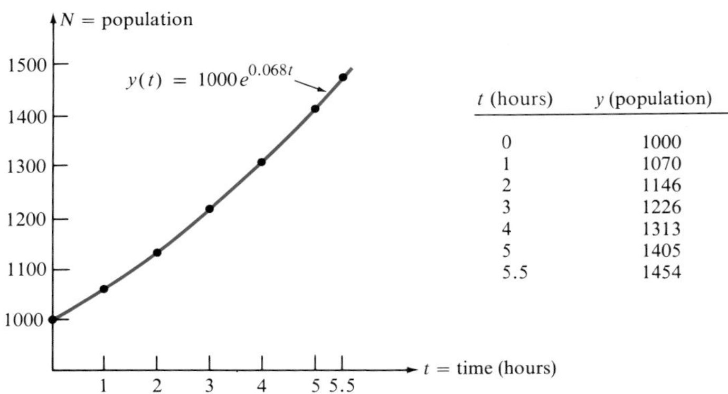

t (hours)	y (population)
0	1000
1	1070
2	1146
3	1226
4	1313
5	1405
5.5	1454

Figure 45
Growth of Escherichia coli

Example 5 Decay Problem in Biology Suppose N_0 milligrams of a drug are injected into the bloodstream of a patient. The drug is carried by the oxygen in the blood to organs that consume and eliminate it from the body. Researchers have determined that the rate of decay of the drug in the bloodstream is proportional to the amount of the drug present. Suppose they have also determined that the amount of drug present decreases at a rate of 5% every hour. What is the initial-value problem that describes the amount of drug in the bloodstream?

Solution Starting with N_0 milligrams of the drug in the bloodstream, the future amount is described by the decay curve

$$\begin{aligned} N(t) &= N_0(0.95)^t \\ &= N_0 e^{\ln(0.95)t} \\ &\cong N_0 e^{-0.051t} \end{aligned}$$

where t is measured in hours from the time the drug was injected.

Hence, the initial-value problem for $N(t)$ is given by

$$\frac{dN}{dt} = -0.051N \qquad \text{(decay equation)}$$

$$N(0) = N_0 \qquad \text{(initial condition)}$$

Interpretation Note that in order to find the decay constant k, we had to convert the hourly decay rate of 5% to the continuous decay rate of 5.1%. Figure 46 shows the amount of drug that will be in the bloodstream at any time if 9 milligrams are initially injected. □

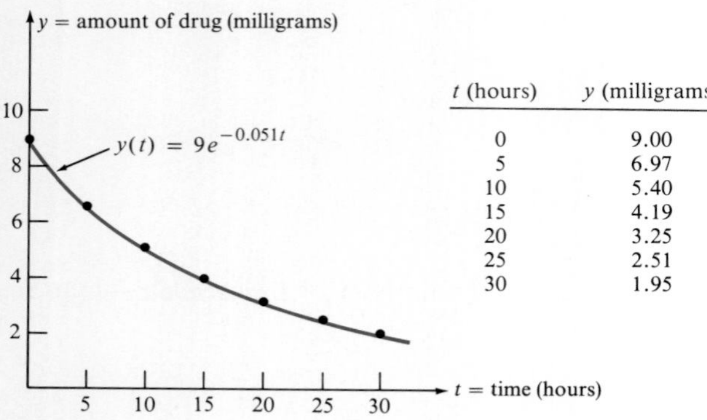

t (hours)	y (milligrams)
0	9.00
5	6.97
10	5.40
15	4.19
20	3.25
25	2.51
30	1.95

Figure 46
Decay of a drug in the bloodstream

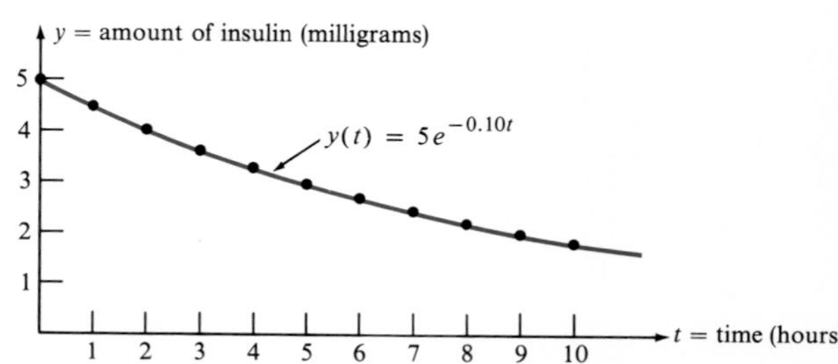

Figure 47
Continuous decay of insulin in the bloodstream

Example 6

Typical Decay Phenomenon A diabetic patient is injected with 5 milligrams of insulin directly into the bloodstream. From past experience, it is known that the insulin in the bloodstream decays exponentially and that the decay constant is $k = -0.10$.

- What initial-value problem describes the amount of insulin in the bloodstream?
- What is the solution of the initial-value problem?

Solution Calling $N(t)$ the number of milligrams of insulin in the blood after t hours, the initial-value problem is given by

$$\frac{dN}{dt} = -0.10N \qquad \text{(decay equation)}$$

$$N(0) = 5 \qquad \text{(initial condition)}$$

The solution of this problem is given by

$$N(t) = 5e^{-0.10t}$$

Figure 47 displays this decay curve; Table 20 displays the level of insulin in the bloodstream at various times. □

TABLE 20
Decay of Insulin Bloodstream

t (hours)	$N(t)$ = Amount of Drug (mg)
0	5.00
1	4.52
2	4.09
3	3.70
4	3.35
5	3.03
6	2.74
7	2.48
8	2.24
9	2.03
10	1.84
20	0.667
30	0.249
40	0.092
50	0.034
100	0.000227
250 (10.4 days)	0.00000000694

Money Growth by Continuous Compounding

When an initial amount of money P_0 is deposited in a bank that pays an annual interest of r percent compounded continuously, then the future value $P(t)$ of this account is known to grow exponentially according to the law

$$P(t) = P_0 e^{rt}$$

Another way of stating this exponential law is to say that the rate of growth dP/dt of the account is proportional to the amount present $P(t)$. Furthermore, the proportionality constant is the annual interest rate r. In other words,

$$\frac{dP}{dt} = rP$$

Hence, the future value $P(t)$ can be described by the initial-value problem

$$\frac{dP}{dt} = rP \qquad \text{(growth equation)}$$

$$P(0) = P_0 \qquad \text{(initial amount)}$$

Example 7

Compound Interest An initial amount of \$1000 is deposited in a bank that pays an annual interest of 12% compounded continuously.

- What initial-value problem describes the future value of this account?
- What is the future value of this account at time t?

Solution

- The initial-value problem is

$$\frac{dP}{dt} = 0.12P$$

$$P(0) = 1000$$

- The future value of the account is the solution of this initial-value problem, which is

$$P(t) = 1000e^{0.12t}$$

Table 21 shows the value of the above account for the first five years. □

TABLE 21
Future Value of a Bank Account that Pays an Annual Interest of 12% Compounded Continuously

t (years)	$P(t)$	
0	\$1000	← *initial deposit*
1	\$1127.50	
2	\$1271.25	
3	\$1433.33	
4	\$1616.07	
5	\$1822.12	

Problems

For Problems 1–10, find all the solutions of the following differential equations. Sketch the graphs of the solutions.

1. $\dfrac{dy}{dt} = 1$
2. $\dfrac{dy}{dt} = -1$
3. $\dfrac{dy}{dt} = 3y(t)$
4. $\dfrac{dy}{dt} = -3y(t)$
5. $\dfrac{dy}{dt} = y(t)$
6. $\dfrac{dN}{dt} = -0.01N(t)$
7. $\dfrac{dy}{dt} = 0.05y(t)$
8. $\dfrac{dy}{dt} = -y(t)$
9. $\dfrac{dy}{dt} = 10y(t)$
10. $\dfrac{dN}{dt} = 0.05N(t)$

For Problems 11–20, determine the exponential growth or decay curves that satisfy the following initial-value problems. Sketch the graph of the solution.

	Growth/Decay Equation	Initial Condition
11.	$\dfrac{dy}{dt} = y$	$y(0) = 100$
12.	$\dfrac{dN}{dt} = 2N$	$N(0) = 10$
13.	$\dfrac{dN}{dt} = -2N$	$N(0) = 50$
14.	$\dfrac{dy}{dt} = 0.08y$	$y(0) = 100$
15.	$\dfrac{dN}{dt} = -0.08N$	$N(0) = 50$
16.	$\dfrac{dN}{dt} = -0.05N$	$N(0) = 100$
17.	$\dfrac{dP}{dt} = 0.05P$	$P(0) = 1$

18. $\dfrac{dP}{dt} = 0.15P$ $\qquad P(0) = 50$

19. $\dfrac{dP}{dt} = 0.12P$ $\qquad P(0) = 1000$

20. $\dfrac{dP}{dt} = 0.50$ $\qquad P(0) = 50{,}000$

For Problems 21–25, the following derivatives dy/dt represent the velocity of a car along a road (miles per hour), where t is time measured in hours. The initial conditions $y(0) = y_0$ represent the initial position of the car when $t = 0$. Find the position $y(t)$ of the car at any time t by solving the initial-value problems.

	Differential Equation	Initial Condition
21.	$\dfrac{dy}{dt} = t^2$	$y(0) = 1$
22.	$\dfrac{dy}{dt} = t - 1$	$y(0) = 1$
23.	$\dfrac{dy}{dt} = t^2 + 2t + 1$	$y(0) = 3$
24.	$\dfrac{dy}{dt} = t^2 - t$	$y(0) = 0$
25.	$\dfrac{dy}{dt} = 1$	$y(0) = 0$

Relative Rate of Growth

Another way of stating the growth equation

$$\frac{dy}{dt} = ky$$

is to rewrite it as

$$\frac{1}{y}\frac{dy}{dt} = k$$

The left-hand side of this equation is called the relative rate of growth. This form of the growth equation says that the relative rate of growth is a constant. The relative rate is very useful because it does not depend on the amount present at a given time.

For Problems 26–31, find the populations $y(t)$ with the given relative rate of growth (RRG) and specified initial populations.

26. $RRG = 0.08;\quad y(0) = 100$
27. $RRG = 0.05;\quad y(0) = 1$
28. $RRG = 0.12;\quad y(0) = 50$
29. $RRG = 0.00;\quad y(0) = 100$
30. $RRG = 0.50;\quad y(0) = 1$
31. $RRG = 0.50;\quad y(0) = 1$

Finding the Rate Constant k

32. Yeast Growth. The size $P(t)$ of a yeast culture grows by 10% every week. What is the continuous growth constant k in the equation

$$P(t) = P_0e^{kt}$$

if t is time measured in weeks and P_0 is the initial size of the yeast population?

33. Decline of the Whales. It has been shown that a certain whale population $N(t)$ is decreasing at a rate of 5% per year. What is the continuous decay constant k in the curve

$$N(t) = N_0e^{kt}$$

if t is time measured in years and N_0 is the initial whale population?

34. Bacterial Growth. A bacteria culture grows in such a way that its growth rate at time t is equal to one-tenth its population. What is the initial-value problem that describes this phenomenon?

35. Yeast Growth. Yeast is growing in a medium at a rate equal to one-twentieth the amount present. If the initial amount present is 10 grams, determine the amount present at any time t.

36. Population Problem. Suppose the earth's human population is growing at the relative growth rate

$$\frac{1}{y}\frac{dy}{dt} = 0.02 \qquad \text{(2 percent)}$$

per year.

(a) What initial-value problem describes this population? Assume the population of the earth was 4.9 billion in in 1988 (set the time scale so $t = 0$ in 1988).

(b) What will the population of the earth be at any time t provided this relative growth rate holds?

37. Thorium Decay. Thorium is used to date coral and other marine life. After the death of a coral, the amount of radioactive thorium present in the coral decays according to the differential equation

$$\frac{dy}{dt} = (-9.2 \times 10^{-8})y$$

where t is time measured in years. What is the half-life of radioactive thorium? (*Hint:* Remember that the half-life of a substance is the time it takes for the substance to decrease to one-half of the current amount.)

38. Flu Epidemic. Flu often spreads at a rate proportional to the number y of infected individuals. Suppose the relative rate of increase in the number of infected individuals is 5% per week.

(a) What differential equation describes the number of infected individuals?

(b) If there are presently 100 infected individuals, how many will be infected after one week?

39. Decay Rate. The half-life of radioactive carbon 14 is approximately 5600 years.
(a) What is the differential equation that describes the amount present at any time $t > 0$?
(b) If the initial amount present is $y(0) = 10$ grams, how much will be present at any time $t > 0$?

40. Compound Interest. The growth of a bank account is always equal to one-twentieth of the amount present.
(a) What differential equation describes the future value of this account at any time $t > 0$?
(b) If the initial deposit is \$1, how much will be in the account after 10 years?

Epilogue: Population Curves in Biology

One area of mathematics that has been particularly useful in biology is the analysis of growth of cells, organisms, and other populations. We describe here some useful growth models.

Exponential Growth Curve

The **exponential growth curve** describes unrestricted growth and is often used to describe short-term populations of a whole host of phenomena such as multicellular organisms. (See Figure 48.) The main weakness of this model for long-term predictions of populations lies in the fact that the curve goes to infinity.

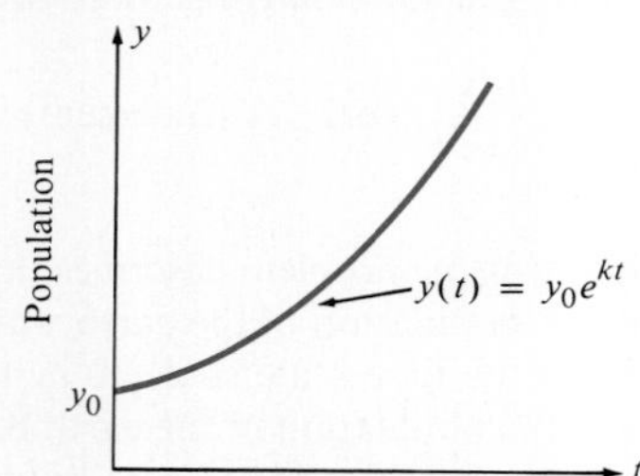

Figure 48
Unrestricted growth

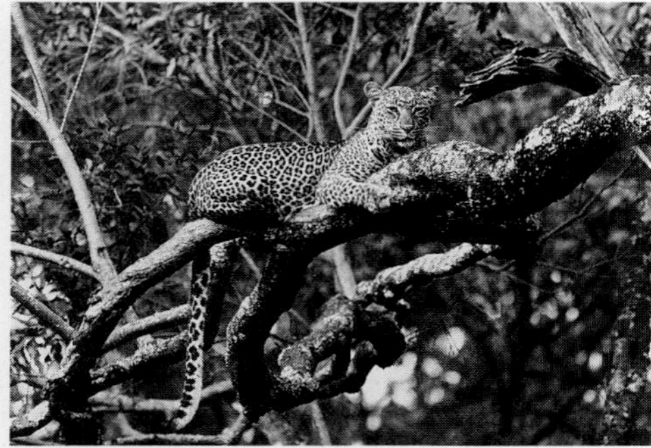

The Logistics Growth Curve

The **logistics growth curve** overcomes the major criticism of the exponential growth curve; the logistics growth curve does not go to infinity. It describes populations that grow slowly at first, then grow rapidly, and then grow slowly. (See Figure 49.) The rate of growth in this model is proportional to both the current population and the difference between the current population and some asymptotic value of the population. It is a very popular model in biology.

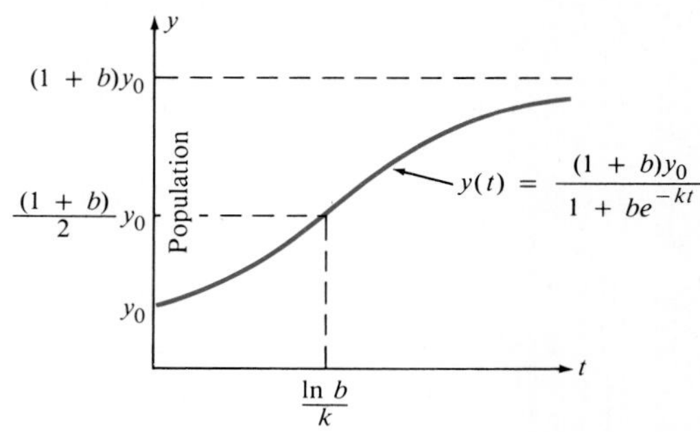

Figure 49
The logistic curve

The Gompertz Growth Curve

The **Gompertz growth curve** applies to those phenomena in which the relative growth rate is not a constant but a linear function of time. (See Figure 50.) It was

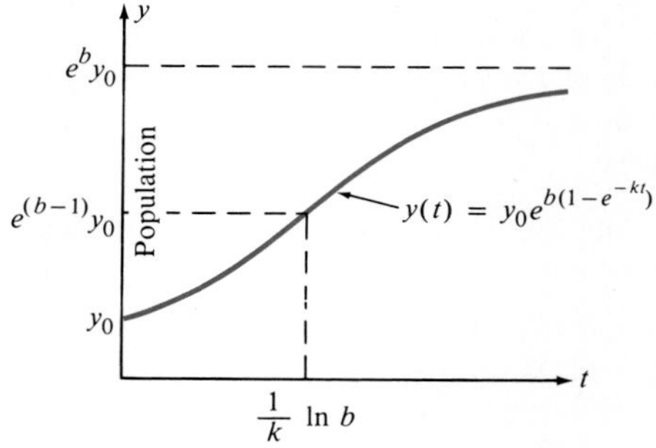

Figure 50
The Gompertz growth curve

formulated in 1825 by the German mathematician of the same name for work in actuarial (life insurance) studies. In 1940, P. B. Medawar published a paper in which he theorized that the growth of an embryo chicken heart should follow this type of function. Since then, other biological organisms have been accurately described by the Gompertz curve.

The von Bertalanffy Growth Curve

The **von Bertalanffy growth curve** is often used to describe the growth of a cell. The curve starts fast and reaches an upper limit. (See Figure 51.)

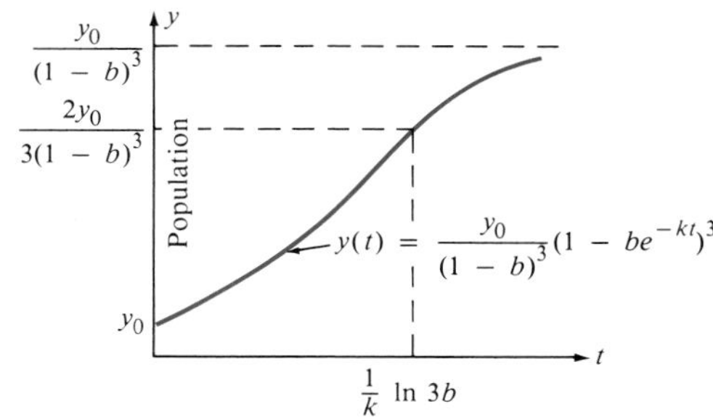

Figure 51
The von Bertalanffy growth curve

Key Ideas for Review

areas between curves, 376
consumers' surplus, 378
decay equation, 405
differential equations, 404
growth equation, 405
improper integrals, 357
initial-value problem, 409
integration by parts, 367
paint can paradox, 384
producers' surplus, 378
Simpson's Rule, 399
solid of revolution, 381
trapezoid rule, 391
trapezoid rule with data points, 396

Review Exercises

For Problems 1–9, find the antiderivative of the given functions.

1. $\int xe^{3x}\,dx$ **2.** $\int x\ln x\,dx$

3. $\int \ln(x^2)\,dx$ **4.** $\int xe^{-x}\,dx$

5. $\int x\sqrt{x+4}\,dx$ **6.** $\int (5x-9)e^{-3x}\,dx$

7. $\int \frac{x^3}{\sqrt{x^2+1}}\,dx$ **8.** $\int \frac{x}{\sqrt{2x+1}}\,dx$

9. $\int x^3\ln x\,dx$

For Problems 10–14, find the area of the regions bounded by the curve $y = f(x)$ and the x-axis for x defined on the indicated interval. Draw the indicated regions.

10. $y = x^2$ on $[-1, 1]$ **11.** $y = \sqrt{x}$ on $[0, 1]$
12. $y = xe^{-x}$ on $[0, 2]$ **13.** $y = e^x + e^{-x}$ on $[0, 1]$
14. $y = \ln(x^2)$ on $[1, 2]$

For Problems 15–19, find the area of the regions bounded by the curves $y = f(x)$ and $y = g(x)$. Draw the indicated regions.

15. $y = x^2$, $y = \sqrt{x}$. **16.** $y = x^3$, $y = x^2$
17. $y = x^2$, $y = 2x + 1$ **18.** $y = x^2$, $y = 2 - x$
19. $y = x^2$, $y = 1 - x^2$

For Problems 20–24, find the volumes of the solids of revolution formed by rotating the functions around the x-axis. Draw a rough picture of the function along with the solid of revolution.

20. $y = x^2$ on $[0, 1]$ **21.** $y = x$ on $[0, 1]$
22. $y = \sqrt{4 - x^2}$ on $[0, 2]$ **23.** $y = x^{1/3}$ on $[0, 1]$
24. $y = 1 - x$ on $[-1, 1]$

For Problems 25–28, use the given number of subintervals n to approximate the given integral by both the trapezoid method and Simpson's Rule.

25. $\int_0^1 x^2\,dx$, $n = 4$ **26.** $\int_0^1 e^{-x}\,dx$, $n = 4$

27. $\int_0^2 \frac{dx}{x+1}$, $n = 2$ **28.** $\int_0^4 \frac{dx}{\sqrt{x+1}}$, $n = 4$

For Problems 29–38, evaluate the indicated improper integral.

29. $\int_0^\infty e^{-ax}\,dx$ **30.** $\int_1^\infty \frac{1}{x}\,dx$

31. $\int_1^\infty \frac{1}{x^{3/2}}\,dx$

32. $\int_0^\infty e^{-2t}\,dt$

33. $\int_0^\infty xe^{-x^2}\,dx$

34. $\int_0^\infty \frac{dx}{x+1}$

35. $\int_{-\infty}^0 e^x\,dx$

36. $\int_1^\infty \frac{dx}{(1+x)^{1/2}}$

37. $\int_1^\infty \frac{x}{(1+x^2)^2}\,dx$

38. $\int_1^\infty \frac{1}{x^p}\,dx \quad (p > 1)$

For Problems 39–44, find the volume of the solid of revolution formed by revolving the indicated functions about the x-axis.

39. $y = e^{-x}$ $\quad 0 \le x \le 5$

40. $y = x^3$ $\quad 0 \le x \le 2$

41. $y = x^{3/2}$ $\quad 0 \le x \le 1$

42. $y = (1 - x^{2/3})^{3/2}$ $\quad 0 \le x \le 1$ (hypocycloid)

43. $y = \sqrt{4 - x^2}$ $\quad -2 \le x \le 2$ (ellipsoid)

44. $y = \frac{b^2}{a^2}\sqrt{b^2 - x^2}$ $\quad -b \le x \le b$ (general ellipsoid)

For Problems 45–50, determine the exponential growth and decay curves that satisfy the given initial-value problem.

	Growth/Decay Equation	Initial Condition
45.	$\frac{dy}{dt} = -0.01y$	$y(0) = 10$
46.	$\frac{dy}{dt} = 0.08y$	$y(0) = 1$
47.	$\frac{dP}{dt} = -0.08P$	$P(0) = 100$
48.	$\frac{dN}{dt} = 0.15N$	$N(0) = 50$
49.	$\frac{dP}{dt} = 0.25P$	$P(0) = 100$
50.	$\frac{dP}{dt} = 0.10P$	$P(0) = 15$

The Integral in Business

51. **Real Value of a Lottery.** Ed has won the New York Lottery, which will pay him \$100,000 per year for the next 20 years. If banks pay 8% interest, compounded continuously, what is the present value of Ed's winnings?

52. **Present Value of an Ore Deposit.** A coal mine is expected to earn an income of

$$p(t) = 100e^{-0.05t}$$

during the next ten years where p is measured in thousands of dollars and t is time measured in years. If money is discounted at 10% a year, what is the present value of the mine?

53. **Producers' Surplus.** If the supply and demand for a given commodity are given by

$$S(p) = p^2 - 4$$
$$D(p) = 10 - p$$

what is the producers' surplus?

54. **Consumers' Surplus.** For Problem 53, what is the consumers' surplus?

55. **Finding the Continuous Rate Constant.** Suppose the size of a bacteria culture is growing according to the exponential function

$$P(t) = P_0(1.15)^t$$

Rewrite this growth equation as

$$P(t) = P_0e^{kt}$$

Differential Equations in Science

56. **Urinary Infection.** The *Escherichia coli* bacteria often grows in the human bladder and causes discomfort when the number of bacteria reaches about 10^8 cells. Suppose the current number of *E. coli* bacteria present is 100 and that the number of bacteria grows exponentially, doubling every 30 minutes. How long will it be until discomfort is felt? (Realize, of course, that we have not considered the complication that the bladder is periodically emptied and refilled, thus complicating the problem.)

57. **Stocking Fish in San Francisco Bay.** In 1880 a total of 500 striped bass from the Atlantic Ocean were placed in San Francisco Bay. Twenty years later, in 1900, the commercial catch indicated that 12 million bass were present in the bay. Assuming the growth over this period was exponential, what are the differential equation and initial condition that described the growth of this fish population?

58. **Stocking Caribou in Maine.** In 1987 a total of 25 Canadian caribou were relocated in Maine in an attempt to bring back caribou to Maine. Suppose the growth of the caribou herd is exponential and increases by 3% per year.
   (a) What is the equation that describes the size of the caribou herd after n years?
   (b) What is the initial-value problem that describes the size of the herd?
   (c) What is the expected size of the herd in the year 2000?

Chapter Test

1. Evaluate

$$\int_0^1 xe^{6x}\,dx$$

2. Approximate the following integral using Simpson's Rule with four subintervals

$$\int_0^4 x^2\,dx$$

3. Find the area bounded by the curves $y = x^2 + x - 1$ and $y = x$.

4. Suppose the supply and demand curves for a commodity are

$$S(p) = p - 5$$

$$D(p) = \frac{5}{p} - 1$$

What are the consumers' and producers' surpluses? Sketch the supply and demand curves.

5. Evaluate the improper integral

$$\int_0^\infty e^{-3x}\,dx$$

6. **Trazezoid Rule.** Approximate the integral

$$\int_0^1 x^2\,dx$$

using the trapezoid rule with $n = 4$ subintervals. What is the error in this approximation?

7. **A Difficult Area.** Find the area bounded by the two curves

$$y = 2x^2$$

$$y = x^3 - 3x$$

8. **Solid of Revolution.** Find the volume of the solid of revolution obtained by revolving the curve

$$y = e^x \qquad 0 \le x \le 1$$

about the x-axis.

9. **Volume of a Cone.** It is possible to find a formula for the volume of a **right circular cone** (the form of an ice cream cone) by revolving a straight line about the x-axis. Use Figure 52 as a guide to find a formula for the volume of a right circular cone with height h and radius r.

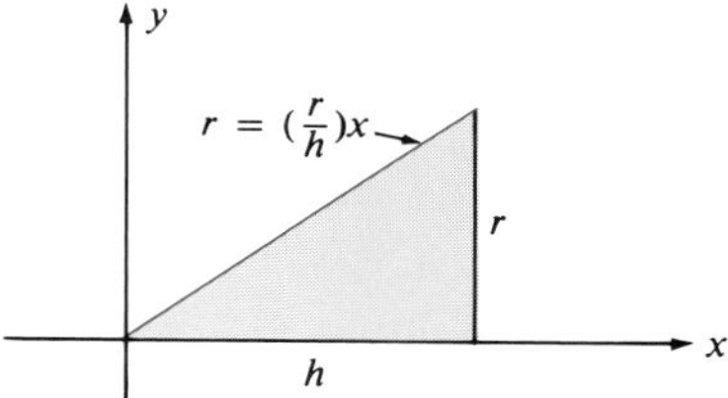

(a) How can you use this graph...

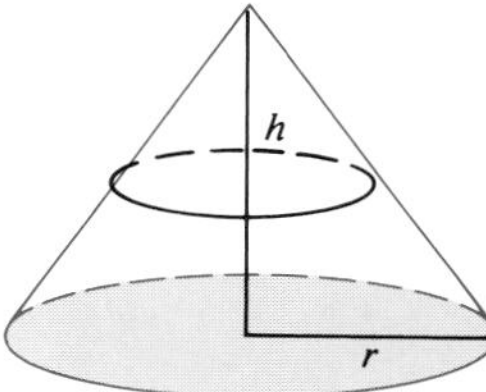

(b) ... to find the volume of this cone?

Figure 52
Finding the volume of a cone using the volume of revolution

10. **Return of the Sea Lion.** Sea lions have been returning to islands off the coast of California for several years at an increase of 12% per year.
    (a) What is the initial-value problem that describes the sea lion population?
    (b) What is the continuous growth curve for the number of sea lions

$$N(t) = N_0 e^{kt}$$

where t is time in years and N_0 is the current size of the sea lion population?

There are many interesting differences between functions of one variable and functions of several variables, but several concepts from single-variable calculus carry over to the study of multivariable calculus.

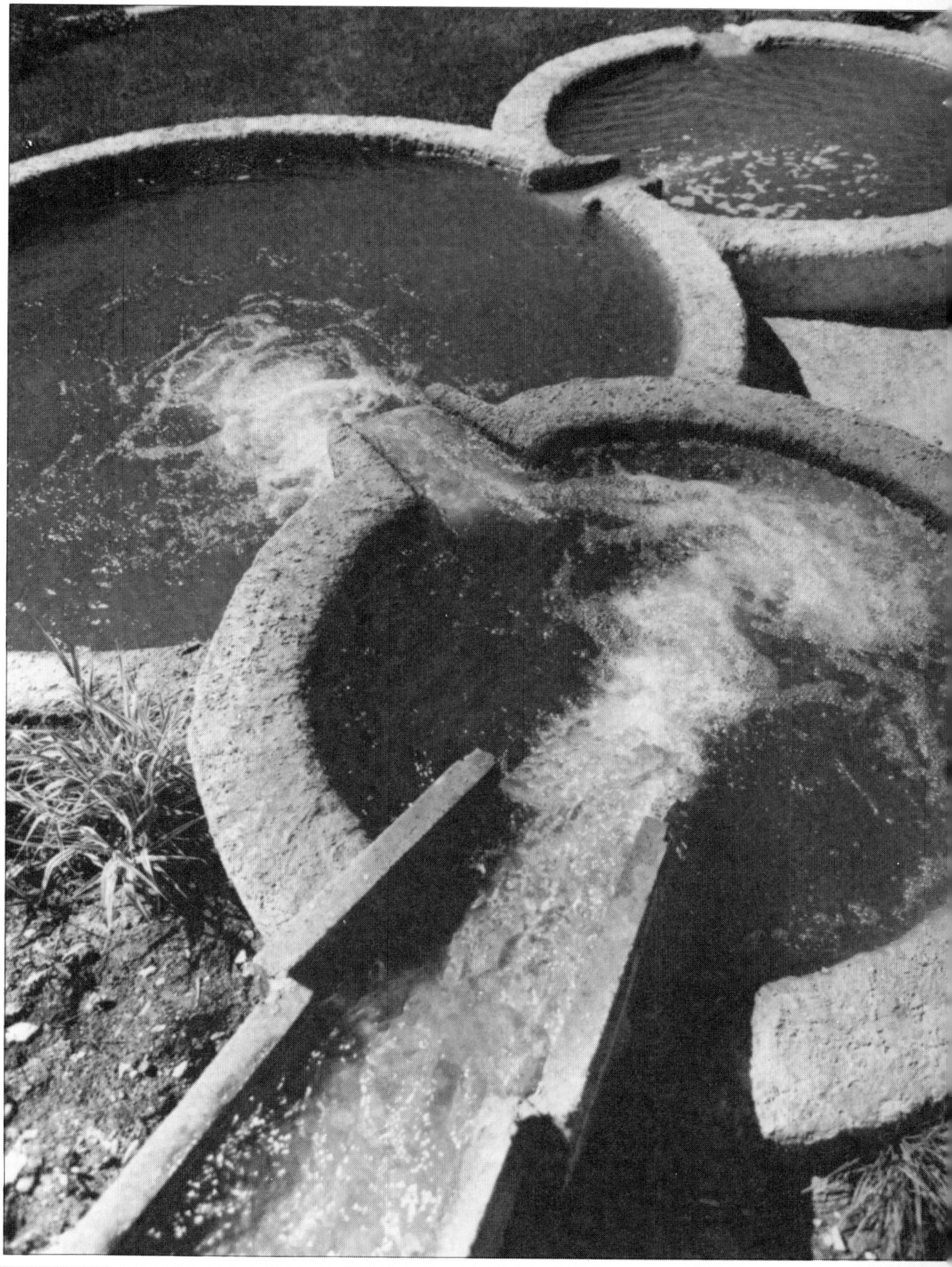

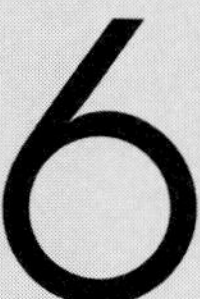

Multivariable Calculus

In this chapter we introduce the concept of a function of more than one variable and present some of the important problems related to such functions. In Section 6.1 we show how a function of two variables, $z = f(x, y)$, is graphed as a surface in three dimensions. In Section 6.2 we define the partial derivatives of a function of several variables that are the natural extensions of the ordinary derivative of a function of a single variable. In Sections 6.3 and 6.4 we find the maximum and minimum of functions of two variables and show how such optimization problems are useful in business management problems. In Section 6.5 we introduce the method of least squares. Finally, in Section 6.6 we show how functions of two variables can be integrated as double integrals in much the same way that functions of one variable are integrated.

6.1 Functions of Several Variables

PURPOSE

We introduce functions of two or more variables and show how such functions arise in business and science. We also show how functions of two variables can be illustrated in three dimensions by means of surfaces.

Typical Functions of Two Variables

Until now we have considered only functions of one independent variable, say x, of the form $y = f(x)$. However, many situations arise in which a value depends on several variables. In biology, for example, the growth of an organism may depend on many variables, while in economics the price of a given commodity depends on many factors as well.

For instance, a company like the Owens Corning Fiberglass Corporation manufactures literally dozens of products that we use every day. Two of its products are roofing shingles and ceiling systems. Suppose the company earns a profit of \$75 for each unit of a given type of roofing shingle sold and \$350 for each unit of a given type of ceiling system. (We use hypothetical numbers for purposes of illustration. The precise values are not important for our discussion.) The total profit from the sale of x units of roofing shingles and y units of ceiling systems is a function of two variables $P(x, y)$. In this case it is the function

$$P(x, y) = 75x + 350y$$

Another company, the *Ralston Purina Company* of St. Louis, produces a wide variety of products ranging from pet foods to bakery goods. Two of its well-known products are *Chuck Wagon* dog food and *Cat Chow* cat food. Suppose the cost to produce a certain size bag of Chuck Wagon dog food is \$1.40 and the cost to produce a given size bag of Cat Chow is \$1.10. Suppose, too, that the plant that produces these two products has a fixed cost of \$10,000 per week. Then if the plant produces x bags of Chuck Wagon per week and y bags of Cat Chow, the total weekly cost $C(x, y)$ to produce these products is given by the function of two variables:

$$C(x, y) = 1.4x + 1.1y + 10{,}000$$

In reality, of course, both the *Owens Corning Fiberglass Corporation* and the *Ralston Purina Company* produce dozens of products, and hence their revenues, costs, and profits will be functions of dozens of variables.

In this section we will consider only functions that depend on two variables. We begin by describing the cartesian coordinate system in three dimensions.

Three-Dimensional Coordinate Systems

For a function $y = f(x)$ of one variable a simple graph in the xy-plane provides an excellent way to visualize its properties. For a function that we can graph accurately, we can easily see where the function is increasing or decreasing, where the curve is concave upward or downward, and where the maximum and minimum points are located. However, to visualize properties of two variables

$$z = f(x, y)$$

we must use three-dimensional space.

In three dimensions we construct three coordinate axes, the x-, y-, and z-axes, each of which is perpendicular to each of the others, and the three axes intersect at a point. We make it our convention in this book to have the positive x-axis pointing toward us, the positive y-axis pointing to our right, and the positive z-axis pointing upward. (See Figure 1a.)

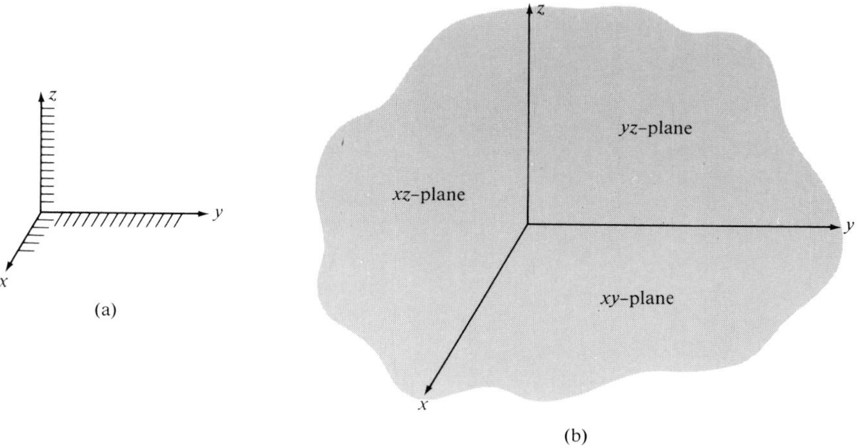

Figure 1
Basic ideas of the cartesian coordinate system. Each of the three axes is perpendicular to each of the others, and all three intersect at a point

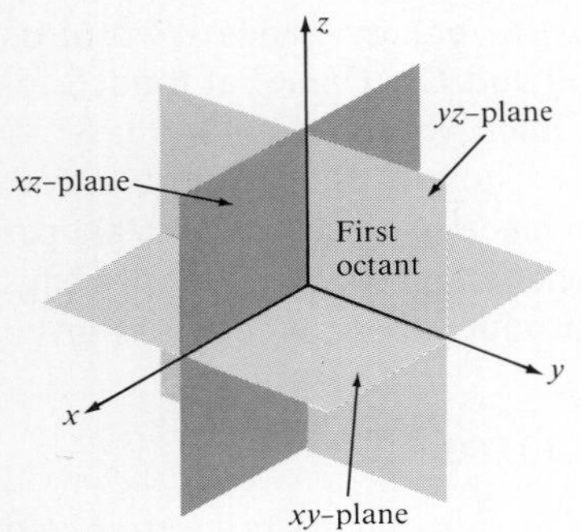

Figure 2
The eight octants of the three-dimensional coordinate system

These three coordinate axes form a three-dimensional rectangular or **cartesian coordinate system**. The point of intersection of the three axes is called the **origin** of the coordinate system. Each pair of axes determines a plane; these planes are called the ***xy*-plane**, the ***xz*-plane**, and the ***yz*-plane**, as shown in Figure 1b.

For each point in three dimensions we assign a **triple** of numbers (a, b, c), called the **coordinates** of the point. For instance, to locate the point with coordinates $(3, 3, -2)$, start at the origin and go three units along the positive x-axis (out of the page). Then go three units in the positive y-direction (to the right) and finally two units in the negative z-direction (downward).

Another difference between two and three dimensions is that while the x- and y-axes in two dimensions divide the plane into four quadrants, the three coordinate planes in three dimensions divide three-dimensional space into eight **octants**. The points in three-dimensional space having all three of their coordinates positive form the first octant. (See Figure 2.)

Some of the important planes and lines in a three-dimensional cartesian coordinate system are described in Table 1.

TABLE 1
Important Lines and Planes in Three Dimensions

Region	Mathematical Description
x-axis	Points of the form $(x, 0, 0)$
y-axis	Points of the form $(0, y, 0)$
z-axis	Points of the form $(0, 0, z)$
xy-plane	Points of the form $(x, y, 0)$
xz-plane	Points of the form $(x, 0, z)$
yz-plane	Points of the form $(0, y, z)$

Distance Between Points in Three Dimensions

In two dimensions the distance D between two points (x_1, y_1) and (x_2, y_2) is determined by the Pythagorean theorem

$$D = \sqrt{(x_1 - x_2)^2 + (y_1 - y_2)^2}$$

To understand how to find the distance between two points in three dimensions, consider the three-dimensional box drawn in Figure 3. By use of the Pythagorean theorem the diagonal of the base of this box has the length

$$\text{Diagonal length of base} = \sqrt{a^2 + b^2}$$

Now note that the diagonal of the three-dimensional box is the hypotenuse of a right triangle; the triangle having one leg as the diagonal of the base and the

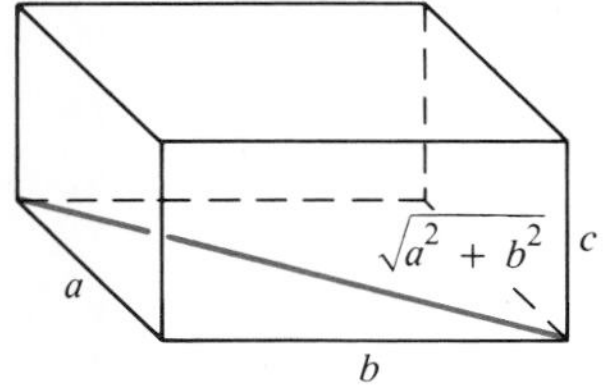

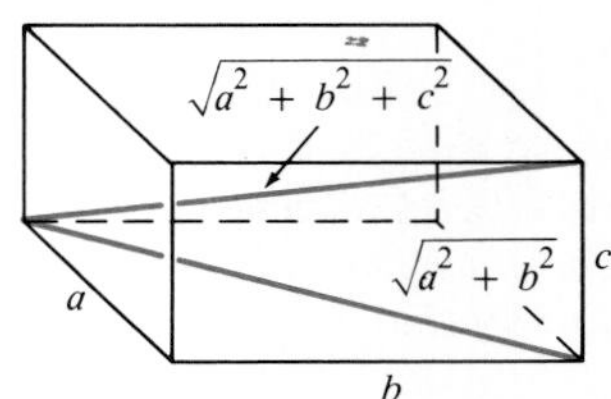

Figure 3
Finding distances in three dimensions

other leg as one of the vertical edges of the box. Hence we can apply the Pythagorean theorem again to find the length of the diagonal of the box. We have

$$(\text{Diagonal length of box})^2 = (\sqrt{a^2 + b^2})^2 + c^2$$

Hence we have

$$\text{Diagonal length of box} = \sqrt{a^2 + b^2 + c^2}$$

This discussion leads to the general formula for the distance between two points in three-dimensional space.

Distance in Three Dimensions

The distance D between any two points (x_1, y_1, z_1) and (x_2, y_2, z_2) in three-dimensional space is given by the generalized Pythagorean theorem

$$D = \sqrt{(x_1 - x_2)^2 + (y_1 - y_2)^2 + (z_1 - z_2)^2}$$

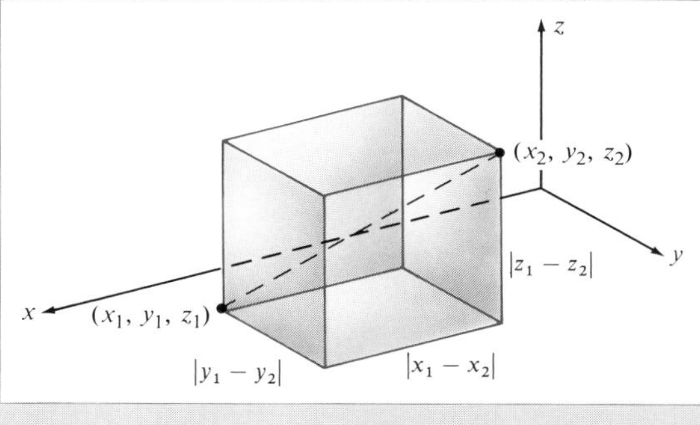

Example 1

Distance Between Points Find the distance between the two points (1, 2, 3) and (1, 3, −4).

Solution

$$\begin{aligned} D &= \sqrt{(1 - 1)^2 + (2 - 3)^2 + (3 + 4)^2} \\ &= \sqrt{50} \end{aligned}$$

□

Function of Two Variables

From our understanding of the meaning of a function we would say that the expression

$$z = f(x, y)$$

defines a function f of two variables x and y if a unique value of z is obtained for each pair of values of x and y in a set, called the **domain** of the function. The domain of f is often taken as all points (x, y) where $f(x, y)$ makes mathematical sense. The **range** of a function is the set of values

$$\{f(x, y) \mid (x, y) \text{ is in the domain of } f\}$$

The variable z is called the dependent variable, and x and y are called the independent variables.

We have already seen a few functions of two variables. We list a few additional ones in Table 2.

TABLE 2
Functions of Two Variables

Subject	Function	Variables
Area of a rectangle	$A(x, y) = xy$	x = Width y = Length
Volume of a cylinder	$V(r, h) = \pi r^2 h$	r = Radius h = Height
Future value of simple interest of \$1	$F(r, t) = 1 + rt$	r = Annual interest t = Time period
Future value of continuous compounding of \$1	$F(r, t) = e^{rt}$	r = Annual interest t = Time period
Revenue	$R(p, q) = pq$	p = Price per item q = Number of items sold
Profit	$P(R, C) = R - C$	R = Revenue C = Cost

Graphing Surfaces in Three Dimensions

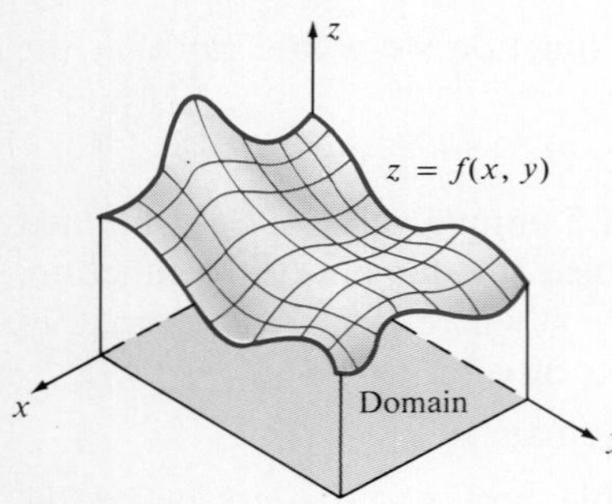

Figure 4
A function of two variables represented by a surface

The graph of a function of one variable $y = f(x)$ consists of the points $(x, f(x))$ in the xy-plane such that x belongs to the domain of f. To find the graph of a function, the usual strategy is to plot a few well-selected points, find the first and second derivatives at these points, and use all this information to draw the graph.

Analogously, the graph of a function of two variables $z = f(x, y)$ in three dimensions consists of the points $(x, y, f(x, y))$ such that (x, y) is a point in the domain of f. Geometrically, the graphs of functions of two variables represent surfaces in three-dimensional space. It should be noted that for every point (x, y) in the domain of the function the vertical line passing through the point (x, y) should intersect the surface exactly once. Figure 4 shows a typical surface drawn in three dimensions.

It is often difficult to draw the graph of a function $z = f(x, y)$. With the introduction of computer graphics packages the task has become much easier. Figure 5 shows computer drawings of several surfaces.

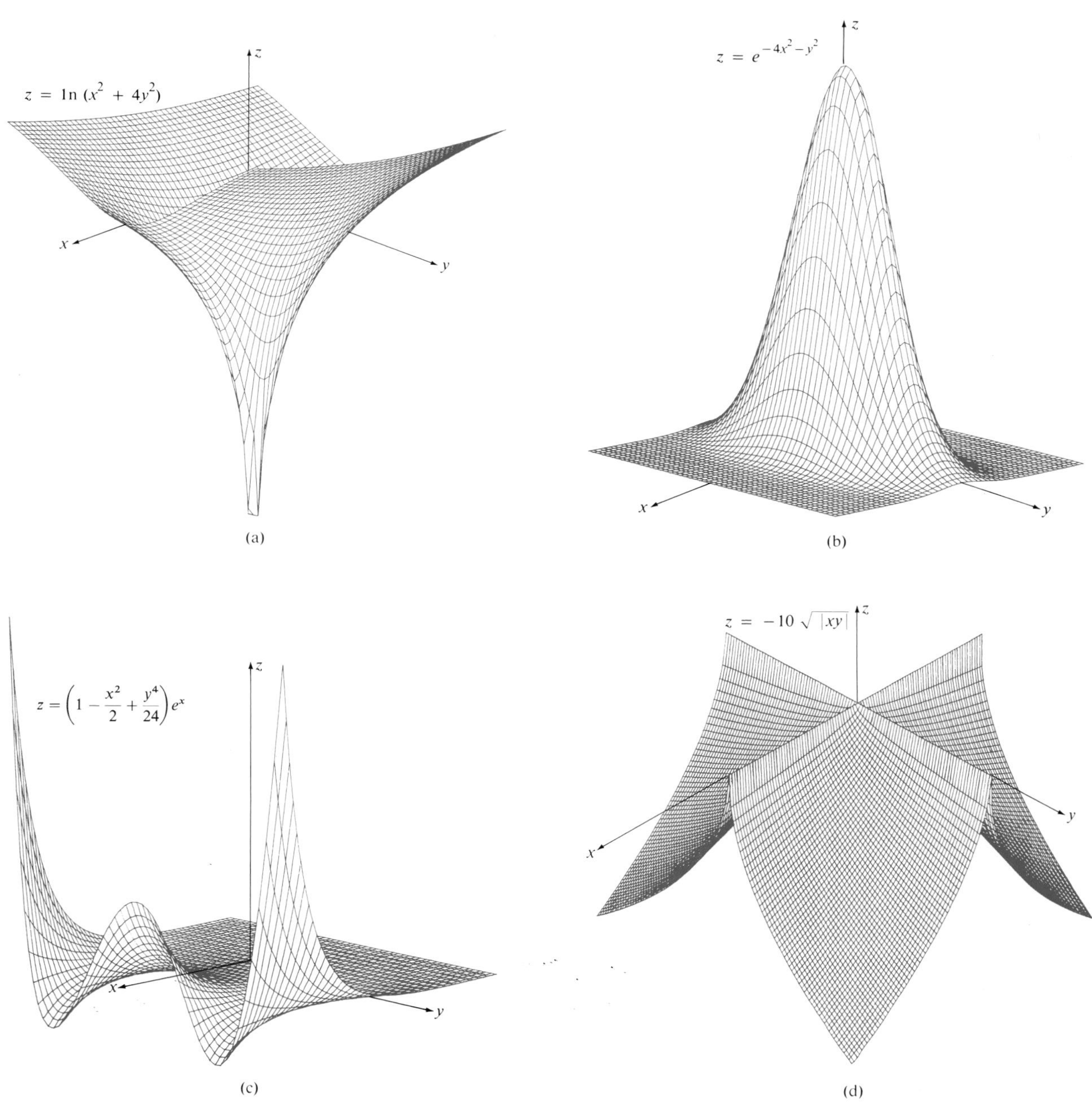

Figure 5
Computer-generated graphs of six surfaces

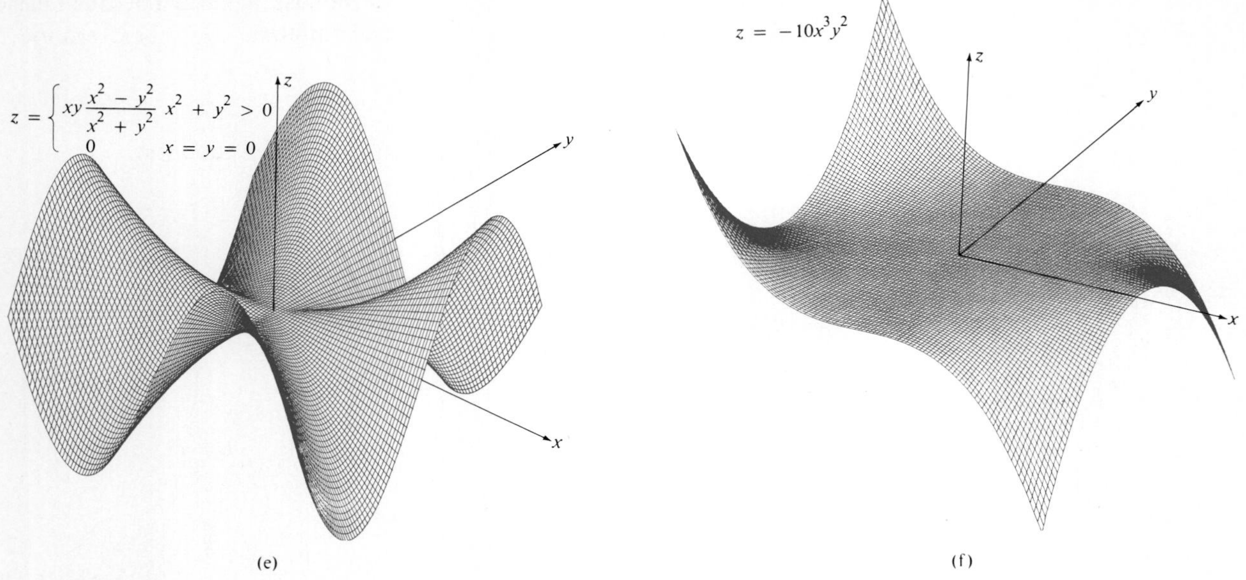

Figure 5
(continued)

Spheres in Three Dimensions

A **sphere** in three-dimensional space with **center** (a, b, c) and **radius** r consists of all points (x, y, z) at a distance of r units from the center (a, b, c). This fact can be stated by writing

$$\sqrt{(x-a)^2 + (y-b)^2 + (z-c)^2} = r$$

Squaring each side of this equation leads to the equation for a sphere.

Equation of a Sphere

The equation of a sphere of radius r with center (a, b, c) is given by

$$(x-a)^2 + (y-b)^2 + (z-c)^2 = r^2$$

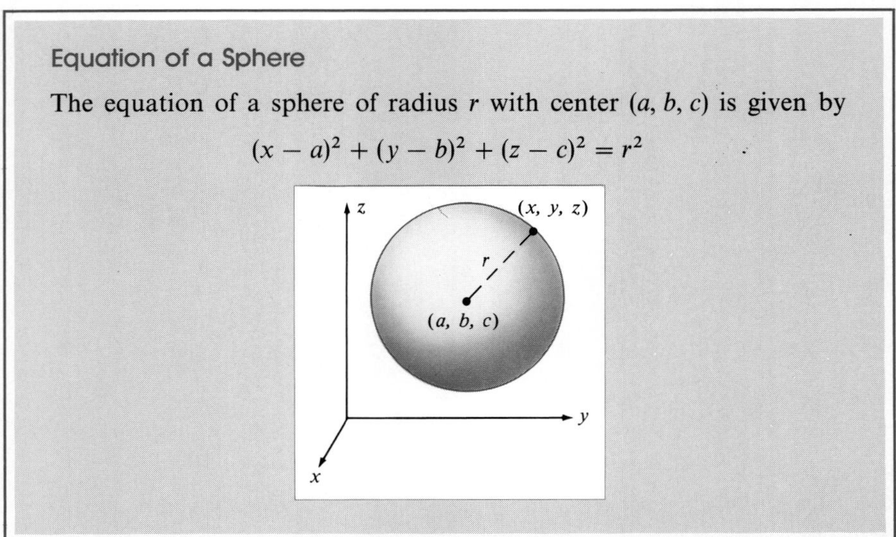

Note, however, that a sphere does not define a function, since vertical lines (parallel to the z-axis) that intersect the sphere intersect the sphere at two points (with the exception of those vertical lines that intersect the sphere around the outer rim).

Example 2

Typical Sphere Sketch the surface described by the equation

$$(x-1)^2 + (y-5)^2 + (z+2)^2 = 1$$

Solution First observe that the equation represents a sphere. The sphere is centered at $(1, 5, -2)$ and has radius 1. (See Figure 6.) □

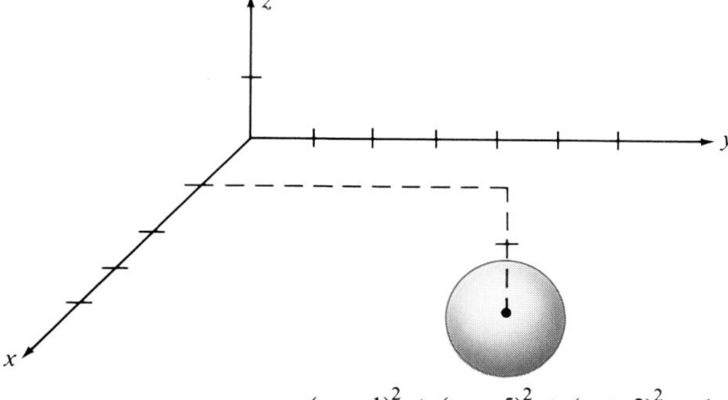

Figure 6
The equation of a sphere

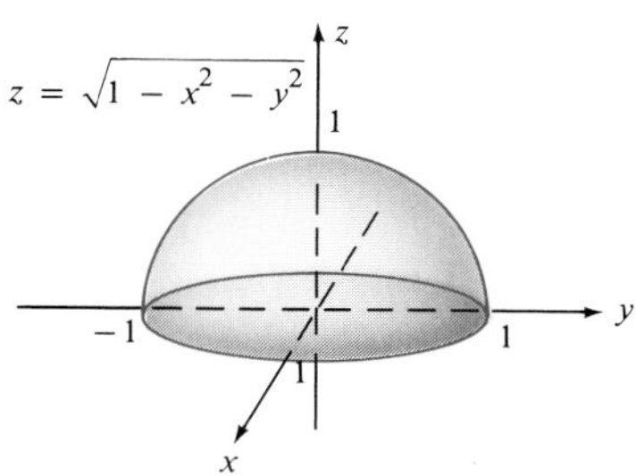

Figure 7
The upper part of a sphere

Example 3

Graphing a Function of Two Variables Sketch the surface described by the function

$$z = \sqrt{1 - x^2 - y^2} \qquad (x^2 + y^2 \le 1)$$

Solution We first note that in the domain of the function $x^2 + y^2 \le 1$ we have $z \ge 0$. If we now square each side of the equation, we obtain the equation of a sphere with center at the origin

$$x^2 + y^2 + z^2 = 1$$

Hence the graph of the function is the upper half of the sphere shown in Figure 7. □

Planes in Three Dimensions

We learned in the Calculus Preliminaries that the general formula for a straight line in two dimensions is given by

$$ax + by = c$$

This equation generalizes to the equation of a plane in three dimensions.

Plane in Three Dimensions

Let a, b, c, and d be constants where not all a, b, and c are zero. The points (x, y, z) in three dimensions that satisfy the equation

$$ax + by + cz = d$$

define a plane.

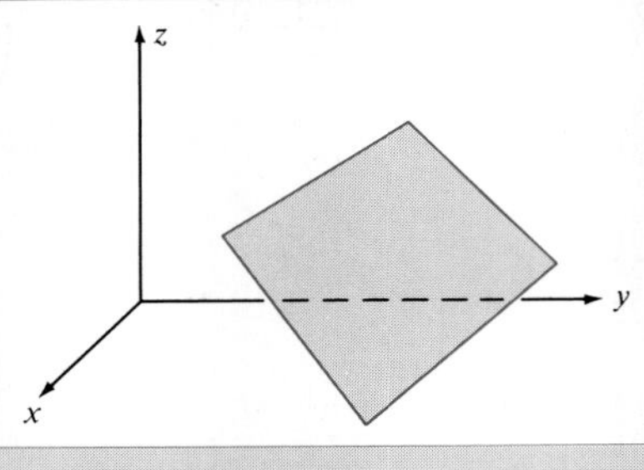

Example 4

Sample Plane Graph

$$x + 2y + z = 2$$

Solution A convenient way to graph planes in three dimensions is to find the points at which the plane crosses each of the x-, y-, and z-axes. By letting the values $x = y = 0$ we see that $z = 2$. Likewise, if we let $x = z = 0$, then we have $y = 1$. Finally, if we let $y = z = 0$, we get $x = 2$. Hence the plane passes through the three points (0, 0, 2), (0, 1, 0), and (2, 0, 0). We can draw a portion of the plane by connecting these points in the manner shown in Figure 8. □

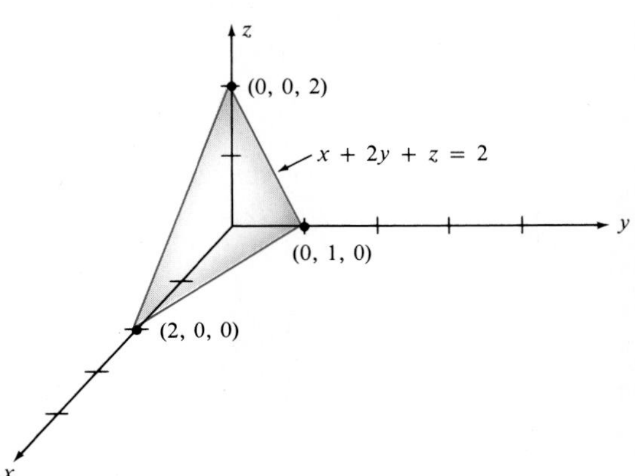

Figure 8
Graphing a plane in the first octant

Another graphing hint is the following.

> **Hint for Graphing Functions in Three Dimensions**
>
> It is often useful when graphing a surface $z = f(x, y)$ to let $x = 0$ and graph the intersection of $z = f(x, y)$ on the yz-plane. Then let $y = 0$ and graph the intersection of $z = f(x, y)$ on the xz-plane.

Example 5

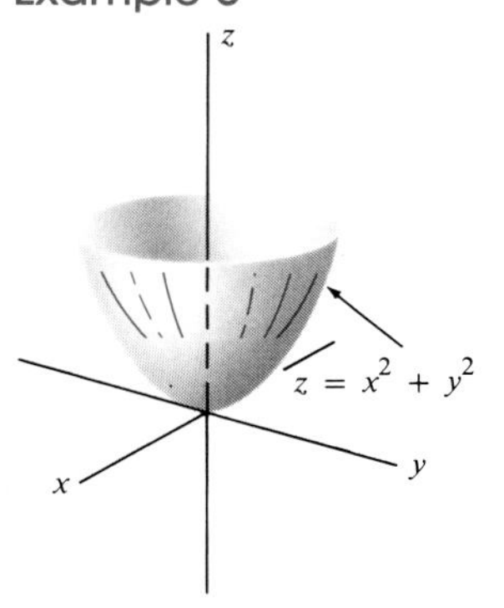

Figure 9
The graph of a paraboloid

Paraboloid Graph the function

$$z = x^2 + y^2$$

Solution Using the above hint, we begin by letting $x = 0$ and graph

$$z = 0^2 + y^2 = y^2$$

on the yz-plane. This is the equation that represents a parabola. We then let $y = 0$ and graph the parabola

$$z = x^2 + 0^2 = x^2$$

in the xz-plane. Both of these individual graphs drawn on the yz- and xz-planes are parabolas (see the Calculus Preliminaries). It can be shown that the surface $z = x^2 + y^2$ is the one that is formed when one rotates either of these two parabolas around the z-axis. This resulting cup-shaped surface is called a **paraboloid**. (See Figure 9.) □

Contour Maps

A useful way to visualize a surface $z = f(x, y)$ is to draw a contour map of the surface. We begin by slicing the surface with planes $z = c$ of various heights. (See Figure 10.) Each plane $z = c$ intersects the surface $z = f(x, y)$ along a curve.

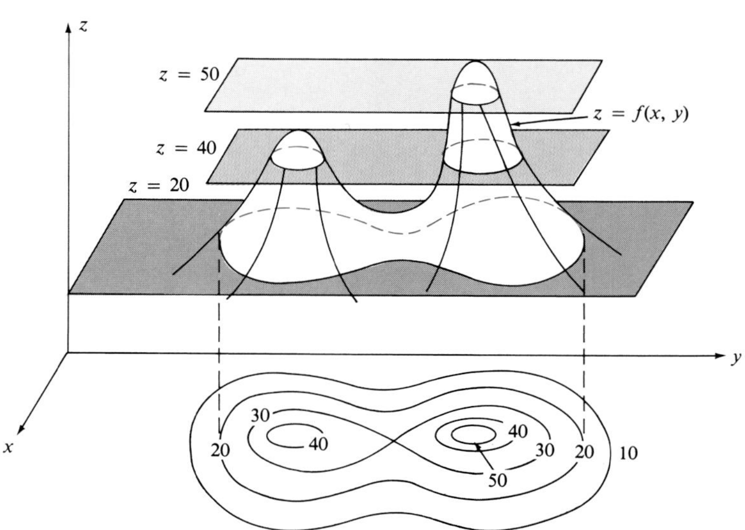

Figure 10
A contour map of a function of two variables

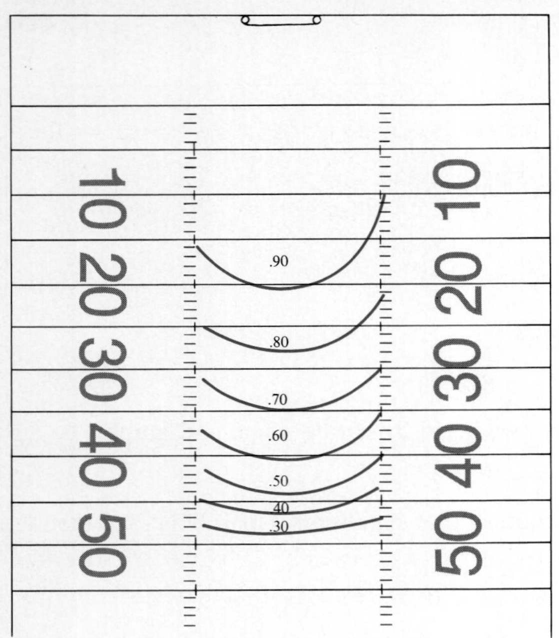

(a) Contour curves showing equal probability curves of success for an NFL field goal kicker.

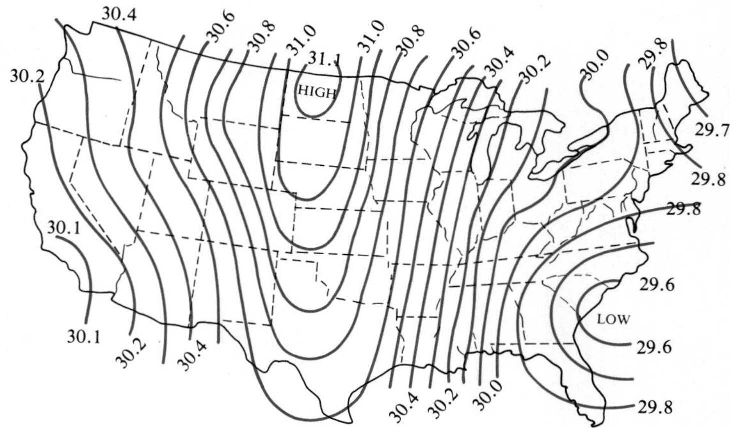

(b) Distribution of air pressure (in inches) during a strong norther in Gulf of Mexico

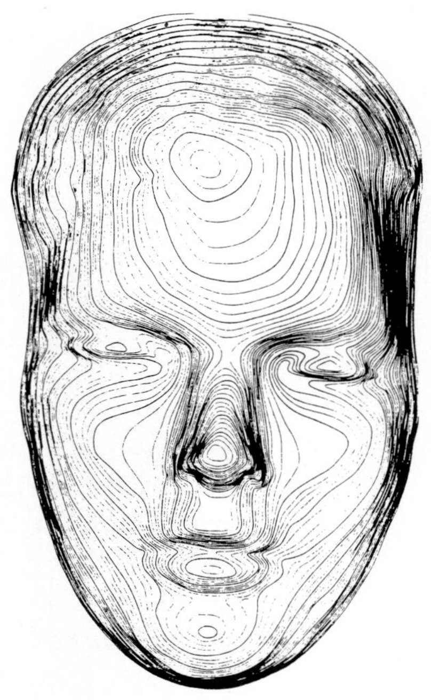

(c) Contour curves of the human face. Today an image of the human face can be stored in a computer as a complicated function of two variables.

Figure 11
A few sample contour curves

The projection of this curve onto the xy-plane is called the **contour curve** at level c. It is this set of points (x, y) in the xy-plane that satisfies $f(x, y) = c$ that indicates where the surface has a "height" of c. Finally, a collection of contour curves forms what is called a **contour map**, in which the contour curves are close together when the surface is steep, and where they are far apart, the surface is relatively flat. Figure 11 shows some typical contour maps.

Example 6

Making a Contour Map Make a contour map for the surface defined by

$$z = 100 - (x^2 + y^2) \qquad (x^2 + y^2 \leq 100)$$

Solution Since the surface clearly lies on or above the xy-plane, we slice the surface by planes $z = c$ for positive c. Hence the contour curves are simply circles

$$x^2 + y^2 = 100 - c$$

A few of these curves are shown in Figure 12. □

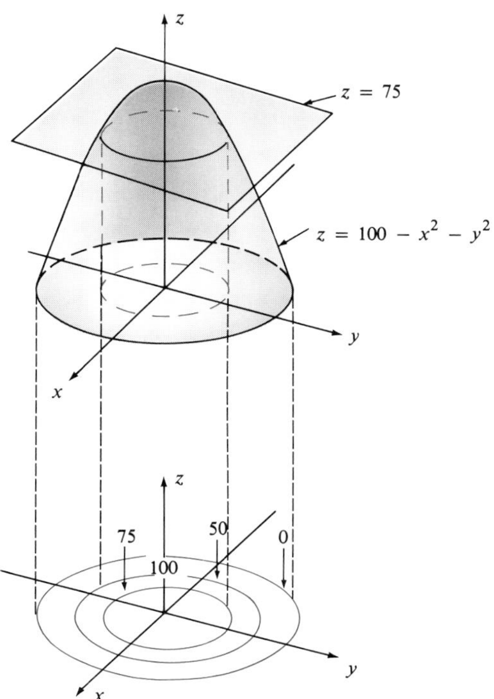

Figure 12
A contour map of $z = 100 - x^2 - y^2$

Problems

Problems 1–5 are concerned with the three common functions that occur in the theory of the firm (revenue, cost, and profit) where we assume that the firm produces two products. For each problem, evaluate the function at the indicated point.

1. $R(x, y) = 50x + 25y$ $\quad R(10, 15)$
2. $C(x, y) = 10{,}000 + 5x + 7y$ $\quad C(10, 20)$
3. $P(x, y) = 7x + 5y$ $\quad P(100, 50)$
4. $C(x, y) = x^2 + xy + y^2$ $\quad C(10, 5)$
5. $C(x, y) = 2x^2 + y^2$ $\quad C(5, 10)$

For Problems 6–14, evaluate the given functions of two variables at the indicated points.

6. $f(x, y) = \sqrt{x^2 + y^2}$ $\quad f(1, 2), f(3, 4)$
7. $f(x, y) = \dfrac{e^x + e^y}{e^x}$ $\quad f(0, \ln 3), f(\ln 4, \ln 5)$
8. $f(x, y) = \ln(x - 2y + 4)$ $\quad f(7, 1), f(11, 4)$
9. $f(x, y) = \dfrac{x + y}{x - y}$ $\quad f(2, 4), f(3, 7)$
10. $f(x, y) = x^2 + y^2 - 2x + 4y + 1$ $\quad f(-2, 3), f(4, -2)$
11. $f(x, y) = \dfrac{x}{x + y}$ $\quad f(-3, 1), f(2, 5)$
12. $f(x, y) = \dfrac{2xy}{x^2 + y^2}$ $\quad f(-3, 2), f(4, -3)$
13. $f(x, y) = xy + x^2 - 1$ $\quad f(1, 3), f(5, 7)$
14. $f(x, y) = \log\left(\dfrac{x}{\sqrt{x^2 + y^2}}\right)$ $\quad f(2, 3), f(5, 4)$

For Problems 15–19, calculate the distance between the given pairs of points.

15. $(3, 1, 5), (8, 2, -3)$
16. $(2, 2, 5), (-3, 2, 1)$
17. $(4, -3, 1), (2, 3, -2)$
18. $(3, 1, 5), (-1, -4, 2)$
19. $(0, 1, 3), (2, 7, -1)$

Identify the Sphere

For Problems 20–23, determine the center (a, b, c) and the radius r of the spheres. You may have to review the technique of completing the square.

20. $x^2 + (y - 1)^2 + (z + 1)^2 = 16$
21. $x^2 + y^2 - 2y + z^2 + 2z = 14$
22. $x^2 + 2x + y^2 + 4y + z^2 + 8z = 25$
23. $x^2 + y^2 - 2y + z^2 + 2z - 7 = 0$

Graphing Equations in Three Dimensions

For Problems 24–30, draw the surfaces in three dimensions described by the following equations. Systematically let $x = 0$ and $y = 0$ to determine what the surfaces look like in the yz- and xz-planes, respectively.

24. **Plane.** $x + 2y + z = 2$
25. **Plane.** $y = 3x$
26. **Mystery Figure.** $x = 5$
27. **Plane.** $x + y + 2z = 5$
28. **Paraboloid.** $z = x^2 + y^2$
29. **Paraboloid.** $z = x^2 + 4y^2$
30. **Upper Hemisphere.** $z = \sqrt{1 - x^2 - y^2}$

Functions of Two Variables in the Publishing Industry

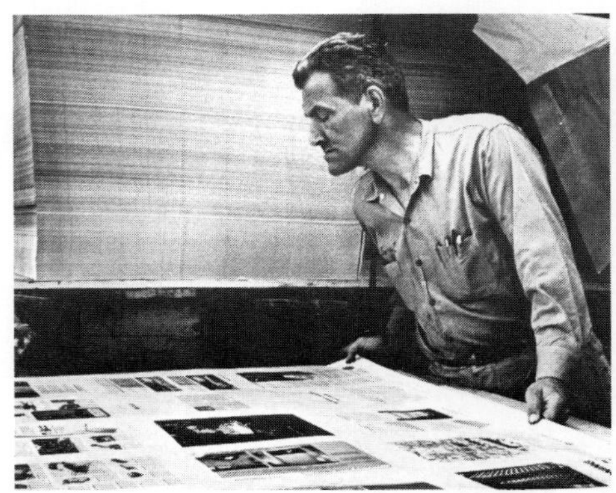

31. **Cost to Produce Textbooks.** Suppose a certain publishing company produces a calculus textbook and a finite math textbook. Suppose the cost to produce a single calculus book is \$20, and the cost to produce a single finite math book is \$25. If we neglect fixed costs (electricity, taxes, general expenses, and so on), then the total cost in dollars of producing x calculus books and y finite math books is the function of two variables

$$C(x, y) = 20x + 25y$$

Find $C(500, 750)$.

32. **Revenue for Calculus and Finite Math Texts.** A certain publishing company sells its calculus and finite math books to college bookstores for \$27 for each calculus book and \$30 for each finite math book. Hence the total revenue in dollars taken in by the company will be the function of two variables

$$R(x, y) = 27x + 30y$$

Suppose the company sells 750 calculus textbooks and 1000 finite math textbooks to the University of Louisville. What is the revenue obtained from this sale?

33. **Profit on Calculus and Finite Math Textbooks.** Based on the cost and revenue functions in Problems 31 and 32, the publishing company's profit in dollars for selling x

calculus books and y finite math books will be

$$\begin{aligned} P(x, y) &= R(x, y) - C(x, y) \\ &= (27x + 30y) - (20x + 25y) \\ &= 7x + 5y \end{aligned}$$

If the company sells 500 calculus books and 750 finite math books to Florida State University, what will be the company's profit from this sale?

34. Author's Royalties. Suppose the author of a certain calculus and finite math sequence earns \$2.25 for each calculus textbook sold and \$2.75 for each finite math textbook sold. If the publisher sells x calculus textbooks and y finite math textbooks, then the author's collective royalties will be

$$P(x, y) = 2.25x + 2.75y$$

Suppose the publisher sells the following numbers of textbooks to the following universities. How much are these sales worth to the author?

University of Colorado:
1000 calculus, 750 finite math textbooks

Colorado State University:
750 calculus, 900 finite math textbooks

35. Isoprofit Lines. Suppose Figure 13 illustrates the number of calculus and finite math textbooks bought by some colleges and universities. We have seen that the profit from the sale of x calculus books and y finite math books is

$$P(x, y) = 7x + 5y$$

Draw the isoprofit lines in the xy-plane defined by

$$7x + 5y = c \qquad (x \geq 0, y \geq 0)$$

for $c =$ \$10,000, \$15,000, and \$20,000. Each of these lines will define different combinations of sales x and y that yield profits of \$10,000, \$15,000, and \$20,000, respectively. Of course x and y are really integers, but the numbers x and y are large, and so the error in this approximation is small.

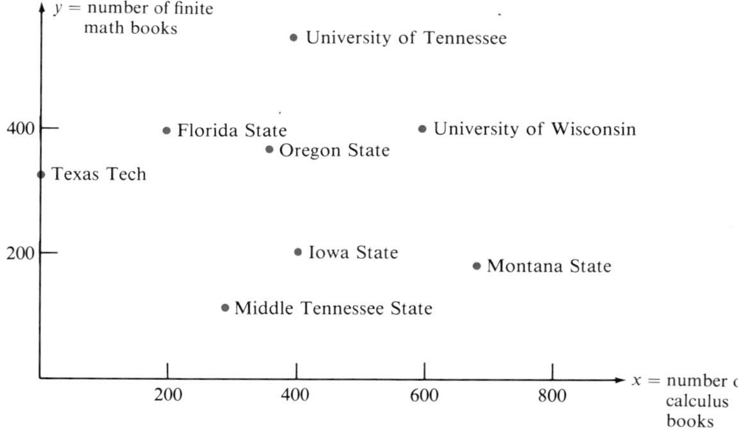

Figure 13
Textbook sales for Problem 35

Functions of Two Variables Are Everywhere

36. Cost of Producing Jogging and Racing Shoes. Suppose a sporting goods manufacturer produces two types of running shoes, jogging shoes and racing shoes. If it costs \$15 to produce each pair of jogging shoes and \$20 to produce each pair of racing shoes, what is the general function $C(x, y)$ that describes the cost of producing x pairs of jogging shoes and y pairs of racing shoes? Neglect any fixed costs.

37. Cobb-Douglas Production Function. The **Cobb-Douglas production function**

$$p(x, y) = Ax^k y^{1-k}$$

where $A > 0$ and $0 < k < 1$ can be used to predict the number p of units of a product produced as a function of x hours of labor and y dollars of capital expenses. By capital expenses we mean the cost of machinery, buildings, supplies, and so on. Suppose that it has been determined that the monthly production of automobiles in a given plant is described by the Cobb-Douglas function

$$p(x, y) = 1.2x^{2/3}y^{1/3}$$

where

$p =$ Number of cars produced (in thousands)

$x =$ Number of hours of labor (in thousands of hours)

$y =$ Capital expenses (in millions of dollars)

Find $p(10, 30)$. What does the value of this function mean?

38. How Big Are You? A biologist has constructed a mathematical model that predicts the surface area (measured in square feet) of a person's body. The model is given by

$$S(w, h) = 0.67w^{0.4}h^{0.7}$$

where w is the person's weight in pounds and h is the person's height in feet. What is the surface area of your body? How would you estimate the accuracy of this model?

39. Measuring Your Weight with a Ruler. On the basis of years of collecting observations a physician has constructed a mathematical model that can predict a person's weight from the person's height and waist size. The formula is

$$W(h, w) = 6.4h + 4.2w - 450$$

where

h = Person's measured height (in inches)

w = Person's measured waist size (in inches)

W = Person's predicted weight (in pounds)

On the basis of your own height and waist size, compute your predicted weight from this model. What is the error in this prediction?

40. Predicting Verbal Test Scores. The U.S. Office of Education has conducted a study to determine the factors that contribute to verbal test scores of high school students. A mathematical model was constructed that depended on two variables. The model is

$$V(s, t) = 0.50s + 0.75t + 15$$

where

s = Measure of the student's socioeconomic environment (ranges from -20 to $+20$)

t = Measure of the teacher's verbal scores

V = Predicted student's verbal scores

Evaluate $V(5, 20)$. What is the interpretation of this value?

41. What Is Your Cephalic Index? A useful measurement for anthropologists is the ratio of width W in inches of the human skull to its length L in inches expressed as a percentage (Figure 14). This measurement is called the **cephalic index** and is given by

$$C(W, L) = 100\frac{W}{L}$$

A cephalic index of over 80 is called *brachycephalic*, and a measurement below 75 is called *dolicocephalic*. What is your cephalic index? What is the cephalic index of a person whose head has a width of 9 inches and a length of 12 inches?

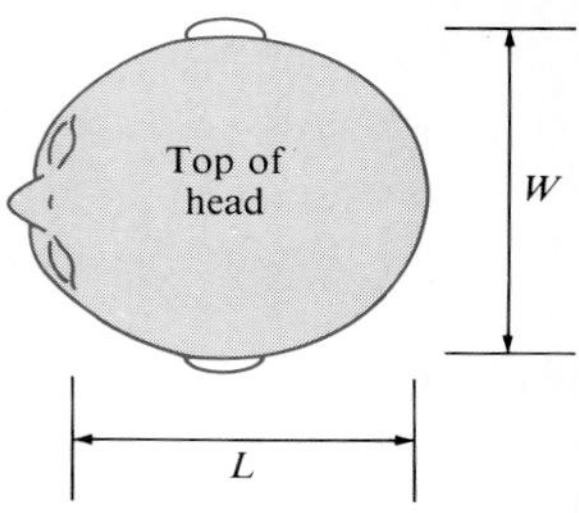

Figure 14
Head measurements for the cephalic index

42. Brrrrr. Anne must decide whether to get out of bed and go to her 8 A.M. business math class or go back to sleep. The temperature outside is -15°F, and the wind is blowing at 30 miles per hour. What's more, according to the local meteorologist, the **wind chill temperature** is -71°F. Anne is curious about this wind chill temperature, so she calls the local TV station and asks for the exact equation used to find it. The meteorologist tells her that the wind chill temperature WC is a quantity proposed by meteorologists Siple and Passel to describe the relative discomfort resulting from a combination of wind and temperature. The value of WC can be found by evaluating the function of two variables

$$WC(V, T) = 91 + (0.44 + 0.325\sqrt{V} - 0.023V)(T - 91)$$

where $5 \le V \le 45$ and

WC = Wind chill temperature (°F)

T = Temperature without wind (°F)

V = Wind speed (mph)

(a) What will be the wind chill temperature if the temperature remains at -15°F and the wind speed falls to 10 mph?
(b) What will be the wind chill temperature if the temperature rises to 0°F but the wind blows at 40 mph?
(c) Suppose the temperature has risen to 5°F and the wind is now blowing at only 5 mph. Anne decides to go to her business math class if the wind chill temperature is above -20°F. Will Anne go to class?

43. Making Your Own Wind Chill Table. Write a computer program using the wind chill function $WC(V, T)$ given in Problem 42 to make your own table of wind chill temperatures. Since the wind chill function makes sense only for wind speeds $5 \le V \le 45$, evaluate $WC(V, T)$ at

$$T = -40, -35, -30, \ldots, 25, 30$$
$$V = 5, 10, 15, \ldots, 40, 45$$

As a check, your computed table should look like Table 3.

TABLE 3
Wind Chill Temperature (°F)

Wind Velocity (mph)	Still Air Temperature (°F)																	Wind Velocity (mph)
	−45	−40	−35	−30	−25	−20	−15	−10	−5	0	5	10	15	20	25	30	35	
5	−52	−47	−42	−38	−31	−26	−21	−15	−10	−5	0	6	11	16	22	27	32	5
10	−77	−71	−64	−58	−52	−46	−40	−34	−27	−22	−15	−9	−3	3	10	16	22	10
15	−92	−85	−78	−72	−65	−58	−51	−45	−38	−31	−25	−18	−11	−5	2	9	16	15
20	−103	−95	−88	−81	−74	−67	−60	−53	−46	−39	−31	−24	−17	−10	−3	4	12	20
25	−112	−104	−100	−89	−82	−74	−67	−59	−52	−45	−37	−30	−22	−15	−7	0	8	25
30	−117	−109	−102	−94	−86	−79	−71	−64	−56	−48	−41	−33	−25	−18	−10	−2	5	30
35	−121	−113	−105	−97	−90	−82	−74	−66	−59	−51	−43	−35	−27	−20	−12	−4	4	35
40	−123	−115	−108	−100	−92	−84	−76	−68	−60	−52	−44	−37	−29	−21	−13	−5	3	40
45	−125	−117	−109	−101	−93	−85	−77	−69	−61	−53	−45	−37	−29	−22	−14	−6	2	45

What are the different values of V and T that give a wind chill temperature of $-60°$F? These values given an approximation to the points (V, T) on the contour curve

$$WC(V, T) = -60°\text{F}$$

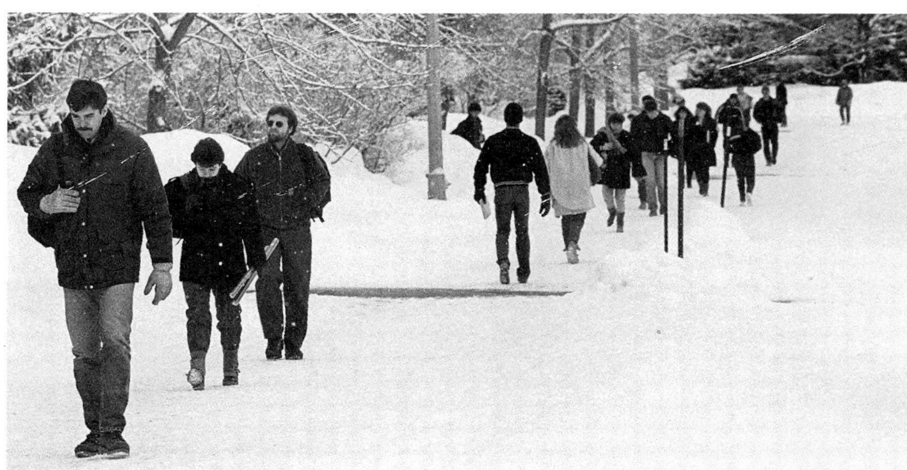

Although most students are probably unaware of the exact formula that determines the wind chill factor, most students are aware of its effects.

6.2 Partial Derivatives

PURPOSE

We introduce the partial derivatives of a function of two variables. The major topics are

- the definition of a partial derivative and
- a geometric interpretation of partial derivatives.

We close this section by showing how partial derivatives can be used to study ideas in a multicommodity economy.

Introduction

We have seen that the derivative of a function of a single variable $y = f(x)$ gives the rate of change of the dependent variable y with respect to the independent variable x. When we study functions of two variables $z = f(x, y)$, we are interested in knowing how the function changes with respect to x (keeping y fixed) and how the function changes with respect to y (keeping x fixed). This brings us to the concept of the partial derivative.

Meaning of Partial Derivatives

Let f be a function of two variables x and y. If y is held constant, say $y = y_0$, then $f(x, y_0)$ can be viewed as a function of x alone. If this function is differentiable at $x = x_0$, then this derivative is called the **partial derivative of f with respect to x** at the point (x_0, y_0) and is denoted

$$f_x(x_0, y_0)$$

On the other hand, if x is held constant, say $x = x_0$, then $f(x_0, y)$ can be viewed as a function of y alone. If this function is differentiable at $y = y_0$, then this derivative is called the **partial derivative of f with respect to y** at the point (x_0, y_0) and is denoted by

$$f_y(x_0, y_0)$$

The partial derivatives $f_x(x_0, y_0)$ and $f_y(x_0, y_0)$ are generally found by first finding expressions for $f_x(x, y)$ and $f_y(x, y)$ at an arbitrary point (x, y) and then letting $x = x_0$ and $y = y_0$. To find $f_x(x, y)$ simply differentiate $f(x, y)$ with respect to x, treating y as a constant. To find $f_y(x, y)$, simply differentiate $f(x, y)$ with respect to y, treating x as a constant.

Example 1 Partial Derivatives Find $f_x(1, 3)$ and $f_y(0, 0)$ for

$$f(x, y) = x^2y + y^2 + 3xy + 4$$

Solution Treating y as a constant and differentiating with respect to x, we obtain

$$f_x(x, y) = 2xy + 3y$$

Evaluating this partial derivative at the point (1, 3), we have

$$\begin{aligned} f_x(1, 3) &= 2(1)(3) + 3(3) \\ &= 15 \end{aligned}$$

To find the partial derivative with respect to y, we treat x as a constant and differentiate with respect to y, getting

$$f_y(x, y) = x^2 + 2y + 3x$$

Hence the partial derivative $f_y(x, y)$ at the origin (0, 0) is

$$\begin{aligned} f_y(0, 0) &= (0)^2 + 2(0) + 3(0) \\ &= 0 \end{aligned}$$

□

Notation for Partial Derivatives

Table 4 lists some of the common ways for denoting the partial derivative of $z = f(x, y)$ with respect to x and y. Table 5 lists the common ways for denoting the partial derivatives of $z = f(x, y)$ evaluated at a point (x_0, y_0).

TABLE 4
Notation for Partial Derivatives

Partial Derivative of f (or z) with Respect to x	Partial Derivative of f (or z) with Respect to y
$f_x(x, y)$	$f_y(x, y)$
$\dfrac{\partial f(x, y)}{\partial x}$	$\dfrac{\partial f(x, y)}{\partial y}$
z_x	z_y
$\dfrac{\partial z}{\partial x}$	$\dfrac{\partial z}{\partial y}$

TABLE 5
Notation for Partial Derivatives (x_0, y_0)

Partial Derivative of f (or z) with Respect to x Evaluated at (x_0, y_0)	Partial Derivative of f (or z) with Respect to y Evaluated at (x_0, y_0)
$f_x(x_0, y_0)$	$f_y(x_0, y_0)$
$\left.\dfrac{\partial f}{\partial x}\right\|_{\substack{x=x_0\\y=y_0}}$	$\left.\dfrac{\partial f}{\partial y}\right\|_{\substack{x=x_0\\y=y_0}}$
$z_x(x_0, y_0)$	$z_y(x_0, y_0)$
$\left.\dfrac{\partial z}{\partial x}\right\|_{\substack{x=x_0\\y=y_0}}$	$\left.\dfrac{\partial z}{\partial y}\right\|_{\substack{x=x_0\\y=y_0}}$

Example 2

Partial Derivatives Find z_x and z_y for

$$z = x^2 + y^2 + 5xy + 1$$

Solution To find z_x, we treat y as a constant and differentiate z with respect to x, getting

$$z_x = 2x + 5y$$

To find z_y, we treat x as a constant and differentiate z with respect to y, getting

$$z_y = 2y + 5x$$

□

Example 3 Partial Derivatives Find f_x and f_y for

$$f(x, y) = x \ln y + ye^x$$

Solution Just remember that when finding f_x, we treat y as a constant and differentiate with respect to x. This gives

$$f_x(x, y) = \ln y + ye^x$$

Likewise, we have

$$f_y(x, y) = \frac{x}{y} + e^x$$

□

Example 4 Partial Derivatives Find f_x and f_y for

$$f(x, y) = \frac{x + 2y}{4x - 3y}$$

Solution We use the quotient rule in each case, getting

$$f_x(x, y) = \frac{(4x - 3y)(1) - (x + 2y)(4)}{(4x - 3y)^2}$$

$$= \frac{-11y}{(4x - 3y)^2}$$

$$f_y(x, y) = \frac{(4x - 3y)(2) - (x + 2y)(-3)}{(4x - 3y)^2}$$

$$= \frac{11x}{(4x - 3y)^2}$$

□

HISTORICAL NOTE

The first calculus book, *Analyse des infiniment petis,* was written in 1696 by the French mathemaician, Marquis de L'Hôpital (1661–1704). The book was so popular that it influenced mathematics during the eighteenth century. During the latter part of the eighteenth century, L'Hôpital's text gradually gave way to a new calculus text, *Traité èlèmentaire du calcul diffèrentiel et du calcul intégral,* written by another French mathematician, S. F. Lacroix (1765–1843). This book was to the nineteenth century what L'Hôpital's text had been to the eighteenth century. The concepts of functions and limits now took over calculus, which the infinitesimal "ghosts of departed quantities" had so long dominated. During the twentieth century, no calculus textbook has been dominant for more than a few years.

Geometric Interpretation of Partial Derivatives

When we studied the derivative of a function of one variable, we learned that it represented the slope of the tangent line. We now see that partial derivatives also represent slopes of tangent lines.

Let P be a point on the surface

$$z = f(x, y)$$

If y is held constant, $y = y_0$, and x is allowed to vary, then the point P will move along the curve C_1, which is the intersection of the surface $z = f(x, y)$ and the vertical plane $y = y_0$. (See Figure 15a.) Hence the partial derivative $f_x(x_0, y_0)$ can be interpreted as the slope of the tangent line (the change in z per unit change in x) to the curve C_1 at the point (x_0, y_0, z_0). In other words, it tells the rate of change of z with respect to x.

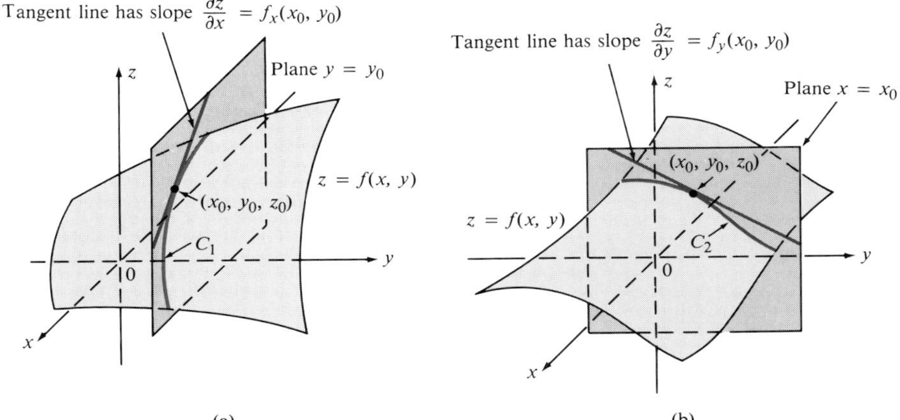

Figure 15
Geometric interpretation of the partial derivatives

On the other hand, if x is held constant, $x = x_0$, and y varies, then the point P moves along the curve C_2, which is the intersection of the surface $z = f(x, y)$ and the vertical plane $x = x_0$. (See Figure 15b.) Hence the partial derivative $f_y(x_0, y_0)$ can be interpreted as the slope of the tangent line (the change in z per unit change in y) to the curve C_2 at the point (x_0, y_0, z_0). In other words, it tells the rate of change in z with respect to y.

Higher-Order Partial Derivatives

Since the partial derivatives $\partial f/\partial x$ and $\partial f/\partial y$ are themselves functions of x and y, we can differentiate these functions and find higher-order partial derivatives. However, unlike the case of functions of one variable for which we had one second derivative, we now have four second-order partial derivatives.

Second-Order Derivatives

For $z = f(x, y)$ the four **second-order partial derivatives** are

$$z_{xx} = f_{xx} = \frac{\partial^2 f}{\partial x^2} = \frac{\partial}{\partial x}\left(\frac{\partial f}{\partial x}\right) \quad \text{(second partial with respect to } x\text{)}$$

$$z_{yx} = f_{yx} = \frac{\partial^2 f}{\partial x\,\partial y} = \frac{\partial}{\partial x}\left(\frac{\partial f}{\partial y}\right) \quad \text{(cross partial, first with respect to } y\text{, then with respect to } x\text{)}$$

$$z_{xy} = f_{xy} = \frac{\partial^2 f}{\partial y\,\partial x} = \frac{\partial}{\partial y}\left(\frac{\partial f}{\partial x}\right) \quad \text{(cross partial, first with respect to } x\text{, then with respect to } y\text{)}$$

$$z_{yy} = f_{yy} = \frac{\partial^2 f}{\partial y^2} = \frac{\partial}{\partial y}\left(\frac{\partial f}{\partial y}\right) \quad \text{(second partial with respect to } y\text{)}$$

Note that f_{xy} means that the partial derivative of f is taken with respect to x first, and then the resulting partial derivative f_x is differentiated with respect to y. This is in contrast to f_{yx}, where the partial derivative of f is taken with respect to y first, and the resulting partial derivative f_y is then differentiated with respect to x. You can remember which partial derivative to compute first by reading the x and y in the symbol f_{xy} as you would read a book (from left to right). Although it is not always true that f_{xy} is equal to f_{yx}, for all functions seen in this course the two partial derivatives will be the same.

Example 5 Higher-Order Partial Derivatives Find the partial derivatives f_x, f_y, f_{xx}, f_{xy}, f_{yx}, and f_{yy} of

$$f(x, y) = x^2 + y \ln x + e^{xy}$$

Solution We have

$$f_x = 2x + \frac{y}{x} + ye^{xy} \quad \text{(treating } y \text{ as a constant)}$$

$$f_y = \ln x + xe^{xy} \quad \text{(treating } x \text{ as a constant)}$$

$$f_{xx} = \frac{\partial}{\partial x}(f_x) = \frac{\partial}{\partial x}\left(2x + \frac{y}{x} + ye^{xy}\right)$$

$$= 2 - \frac{y}{x^2} + y^2e^{xy}$$

$$f_{yx} = \frac{\partial}{\partial x}(f_y) = \frac{\partial}{\partial x}(\ln x + xe^{xy})$$

$$= \frac{1}{x} + e^{xy} + xye^{xy}$$

$$f_{xy} = \frac{\partial}{\partial y}(f_x) = \frac{\partial}{\partial y}\left(2x + \frac{y}{x} + ye^{xy}\right)$$
$$= \frac{1}{x} + e^{xy} + xye^{xy}$$

$$f_{yy} = \frac{\partial}{\partial y}(f_y) = \frac{\partial}{\partial y}(\ln x + xe^{xy})$$
$$= x^2e^{xy}$$

□

Multicommodity Theory in Business

Until now we have studied the theory of the firm for companies that only produce one product. However, most companies produce several products, and for that reason a serious study of revenue, cost, and profit should consider multicommodity firms.

A typical multicommodity firm is the *A. H. Robbins Company* of Richmond, Virginia, which produces literally dozens of different products from pharmaceutical goods (Robitussin, Dimetapp, Chap Stick) to medical instruments and pet products. Although a serious study of revenue, cost, and profit conducted by a company such as this would involve many products, for mathematical simplicity we will focus our attention on only two products.

Multicommodity Costs

Suppose the A. H. Robbins Company has determined the cost $C(x, y)$ to produce x units of a given Item 1 and y units of a given Item 2. The two partial derivatives C_x and C_y are called the marginal costs of the two commodities. The interpretation of these partial derivatives is

$$C_x(x, y) = \text{Cost to make one additional unit of Item 1}$$
$$C_y(x, y) = \text{Cost to make one additional unit of Item 2}$$

when the production level is x units of Item 1 and y units of Item 2. For example, if

$$C_x(100, 50) = \$500$$
$$C_y(100, 50) = \$200$$

then at the production level of 100 units of Item 1 and 50 units of Item 2, it would cost the company \$500 to produce the next unit of Item 1 and \$200 to produce the next unit of Item 2.

Multicommodity Revenues

If the prices that the company charges for the two products are p_1 and p_2, respectively (and assuming that the company sells all that it produces), then the firm's total revenue is given by

$$R(x, y) = p_1x + p_2y$$

The two partial derivatives R_x and R_y are called the marginal revenues of the two products. These partial derivatives have the following interpretations:

$$R_x(x, y) = \text{Increase in revenue as a result of selling one more unit of Item 1}$$
$$R_y(x, y) = \text{Increase in revenue as a result of selling one more unit of Item 2}$$

when sales levels are at x units of Item 1 and y units of Item 2. Note that if the company charges \$100 and \$50 for each unit of Items 1 and 2, respectively, then the revenue function will be

$$R(x, y) = 100x + 50y$$

Hence the marginal revenues will be

$$R_x(x, y) = \$100$$
$$R_y(x, y) = \$50$$

Ordinarily the marginal revenue functions represent the prices the company charges for the two products.

Multicommodity Profits

Finally, the profit the company makes when producing x and y units of Items 1 and 2, respectively, is the revenue minus the cost. That is,

$$\begin{aligned} P(x, y) &= R(x, y) - C(x, y) \\ &= p_1x + p_2y - C(x, y) \end{aligned}$$

Just as there are marginal costs and revenues, there are marginal profits. The two partial derivatives P_x and P_y of the profit functions are called the marginal profits. They have the economic interpretation

$$P_x(x, y) \cong \text{Increase in profit from selling one more unit of Item 1}$$
$$P_y(x, y) \cong \text{Increase in profit from selling one more unit of Item 2}$$

when the sales level is x units of Item 1 and y units of Item 2.

Example 6

Multicommodity Firm *Cincinnati Milicron* of Cleveland, Ohio, manufactures different types of robots for industrial use. Suppose the monthly cost $C(r, s)$ of producing two models of robots at a certain plant is

$$C(r, s) = 20r^2 + 10rs + 10s^2 + 300{,}000$$

where C is measured in dollars and

$$r = \text{Number of Model R robots made per month}$$
$$s = \text{Number of Model S robots made per month}$$

Suppose the company charges

$$p_1 = \$5000 \text{ for each Model R robot}$$
$$p_2 = \$8000 \text{ for each Model S robot}$$

Find

(a) the monthly cost and marginal costs,

(b) the monthly revenue and marginal revenues, and

(c) the monthly profit and marginal profits,

when the monthly production of robots is

50 Model R robots
70 Model S robots

Solution

(a) **Cost and marginal costs:** The monthly cost to produce 50 Model R and 70 Model S robots is

$$\begin{aligned} C(50, 70) &= 20 \cdot 50^2 + 10(50)(70) + 10 \cdot 70^2 + 300{,}000 \\ &= \$434{,}000 \end{aligned}$$

The marginal costs are

$$\begin{aligned} C_r(r, s) &= 40r + 10s \\ C_s(r, s) &= 10r + 20s \end{aligned}$$

An economist would say that these partial derivatives give the "marginal costs" to produce more robots. For instance, if the company is currently producing 50 Model R robots and 70 Model S robots per month, the marginal costs are

$$\begin{aligned} C_r(50, 70) &= 40(50) + 10(70) = \$2700 \\ C_s(50, 70) &= 10(50) + 20(70) = \$1900 \end{aligned}$$

In other words, it will cost the company approximately \$2700 to make the next Model R robot and \$1900 to make the next Model S robot. Note from the marginal revenue formulas that as the monthly production levels r and s rise, it costs more to make each of the two types of robots. This may be partly due to the fact that overtime wages must be paid and special ordering of materials is necessary.

(b) **Revenue and marginal revenues:** The firm's monthly revenue R is given by

$$R(r, s) = \$5000r + \$8000s$$

At the production level of 50 Model R robots and 70 Model S robots per month the firm will have a monthly revenue of

$$\begin{aligned} R(50, 70) &= \$5000(50) + \$8000(70) \\ &= \$810{,}000 \end{aligned}$$

The marginal revenues are the partial derivatives of the revenue function R. Hence

$$\begin{aligned} R_r(r, s) &= \$5000 \\ R_s(r, s) &= \$8000 \end{aligned}$$

These values simply represent the prices charged for the two products.

(c) **Profit and marginal profits:** The firm's monthly profit is found by computing the money taken in minus the money expended in costs. That is,

$$\begin{aligned} P(r, s) &= R(r, s) - C(r, s) \\ &= 5000r + 8000s - (20r^2 + 10rs + 10s^2 + 300{,}000) \end{aligned}$$

At the production level of 50 Model R robots and 70 Model S robots the company will earn a monthly profit of

$$\begin{aligned} P(50, 70) &= \$810{,}000 - \$434{,}000 \\ &= \$376{,}000 \end{aligned}$$

The marginal profits are given by

$$\begin{aligned} P_r(r, s) &= 5000 - 40r - 10s \\ P_s(r, s) &= 8000 - 10r - 20s \end{aligned}$$

This means that when the production level is 50 Model R robots and 70 Model S robots per month, the company will make a profit on each additional Model R robot sold of

$$\begin{aligned} P_r(50, 70) &= 5000 - 40(50) - 10(70) \\ &= \$2300 \end{aligned}$$

while the profit on each additional Model S robot will be

$$\begin{aligned} P_s(50, 70) &= 8000 - 10(50) - 20(70) \\ &= \$6100 \end{aligned}$$

□

Deeper Interpretation

As the production levels r and s increase, the revenue increases only linearly (first-order polynomial), whereas the cost increases quadratically (second-order polynomial). This means that costs will eventually grow faster than revenues (more money going out than coming in). When this happens, it makes sense that the company should not increase its level of production. This means that there will be an optimum production level that will maximize the company's profit. Of course, if the company can actually sell more than this optimum amount produced, it should consider a number of alternatives, such as raising prices or building a new factory to change the present cost structure.

PROBLEMS

For Problems 1–20, find $f_x(x, y)$ and $f_y(x, y)$ for the given functions.

1. $f(x, y) = 2x - xy + y + 3x^2$

2. $f(x, y) = (x - 3y)^2$

3. $f(x, y) = x/y$

4. $f(x, y) = xy^3 - yx^3$

5. $f(x, y) = \dfrac{x + y}{x - y}$

6. $f(x, y) = \sqrt{x^2 - 3y^2}$

7. $f(x, y) = \dfrac{x + y}{x^2 + y^2}$

8. $f(x, y) = \dfrac{3xy + y^2}{x^3 - y^3}$

9. $f(x, y) = e^{xy}$

10. $f(x, y) = xe^y + ye^x$

11. $f(x, y) = \dfrac{e^x + e^y}{e^x - e^y}$

12. $f(x, y) = e^y \ln x$

13. $f(x, y) = e^x \ln y + e^y \ln x$

14. $f(x, y) = xe^{-y/2} + xy + \dfrac{x}{y}$

15. $f(x, y) = e^{(x^2+y^2)}$

16. $f(x, y) = \dfrac{(3x - 2y)^3}{y^2 - x^2}$

17. $f(x, y) = (x^2e^y - 2xye^x + y^2e^y)^{2/3}$

18. $f(x, y) = x^y + y^x$

19. $f(x, y) = \ln \sqrt{x^2 + 2xy + y^2}$ (Sometimes a little preliminary algebra will go a long, long way.)

20. $f(x, y) = \ln\left(\dfrac{x + y}{x - y}\right)$ (The same hint is true here, too.)

For Problems 21–25, evaluate the indicated partial derivatives.

21. $f(x, y) = 9 - y^2 - 5x^2$	$f_x(3, 1)$	$f_y(2, 3)$
22. $f(x, y) = y^2 + y^3x$	$f_x(2, 3)$	$f_y(3, 2)$
23. $f(x, y) = e^{(2x+3y)}$	$f_x(0, 1)$	$f_y(-3, 2)$
24. $f(x, y) = \dfrac{3xy}{x^2 + y^2}$	$f_x(-1, -1)$	$f_y(-1, 0)$
25. $f(x, y) = (x + 3y)(\ln x + e^y)$	$f_x(3, 4)$	$f_y(2, 5)$

For Problems 26–35, find $f_x(x, y)$, $f_y(x, y)$, $f_{xx}(x, y)$, $f_{xy}(x, y)$, and $f_{yy}(x, y)$ for the given functions.

26. $f(x, y) = 4xy - 5y + 4$

27. $f(x, y) = x^2 + 2xy - 3y^2 - 2y + 10x - 3$

28. $f(x, y) = e^{(x+y)}$

29. $f(x, y) = (x^2 + 2xy - y^2)^2$

30. $f(x, y) = \dfrac{xy}{x + y}$

31. $f(x, y) = (x + y) \ln (x + y)$

32. $f(x, y) = x^3 - x^3y + yx^2 - y^3$

33. $f(x, y) = (x + 2y)(3x - y)$

34. $f(x, y) = \sqrt{x + y}$

35. $f(x, y) = \dfrac{(x + y)^2}{(x - y)^3}$

Geometric Interpretation of Partial Derivatives

For Problems 36–39, give rough approximations of the partial derivatives f_x and f_y of the functions $f(x, y)$ at the indicated points A, B, and C. Your answers do not have to be accurate to the nearest tenth, but you should at least be able to determine whether the partial derivatives are positive or negative at the points.

36.

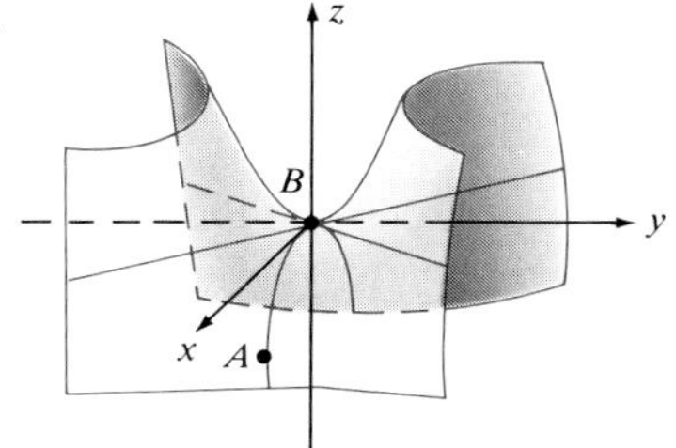

37.

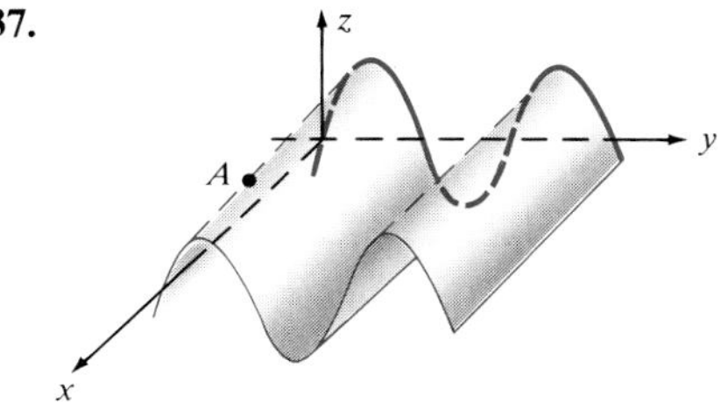

38.

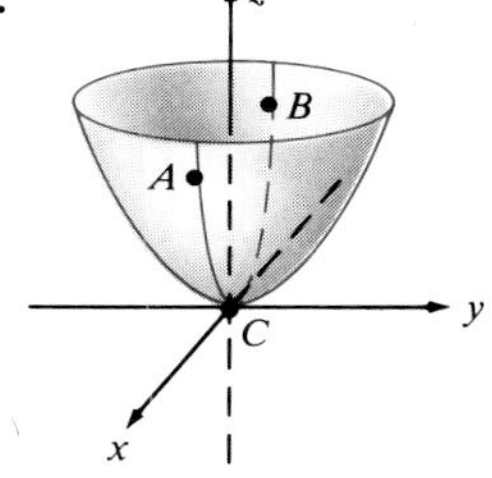

39.

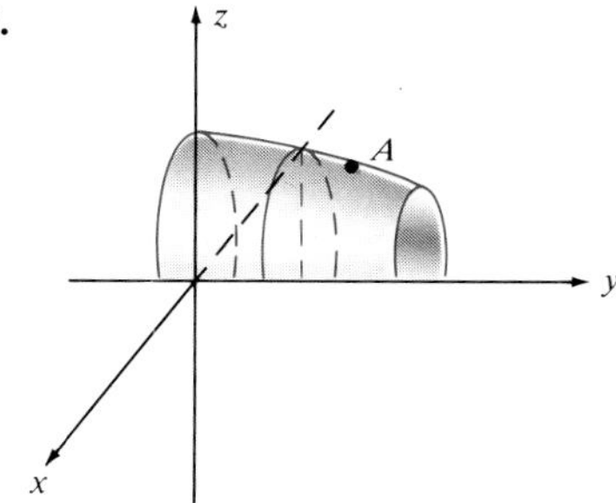

Marginal Functions in a Multicommodity Firm

The functions in Problems 40–48 represent common revenue, cost, and profit functions found in the theory of the multicommodity firm. For each function, find the two marginal functions. Evaluate all the marginal functions when $x = 10$, $y = 5$, and interpret the results.

40. $R(x, y) = 30x + 50y$

41. $R(x, y) = 5x + 10y - 0.05x^2$

42. $R(x, y) = 10x + 20y - 0.2x^2 - 0.3y^2$

43. $C(x, y) = x^2 + xy + y^2 + 10$

44. $C(x, y) = 10x + 20y + x^2 + xy + y^2 + 5000$

45. $C(x, y) = 100x + 50y + 5x^2 + xy + 10{,}000$
46. $P(x, y) = 100x + 200y - x^2 - xy - y^2 - 5000$
47. $P(x, y) = 50x + 200y - x^2 - 5000$
48. $P(x, y) = 2x + 2y - xy - 100$

Partial Derivatives in Mathematical Economics

49. **Marginal Cost.** Suppose the cost to a firm to produce x units of Product A and y units of Product B is given by

$$C(x, y) = 50x + 100y + x^2 + xy + y^2 + 10{,}000$$

Find $C_x(10, 20)$ and $C_y(10, 20)$. What is the interpretation of your answer?

50. **Marginal Revenue.** The revenue from the production of x units of Product A and y units of Product B is given by

$$R(x, y) = 50x + 100y - 0.01x^2 - 0.01y^2$$

Find $R_x(10, 20)$ and $R_y(10, 20)$. What is the interpretation of your answer?

51. **Marginal Profit.** A firm's profit $P(x, y)$ for producing x units of Product A and y units of Product B is given by

$$P(x, y) = 10x + 20y - x^2 + xy - 0.5y^2 - 10{,}000$$

Find $P_x(10, 20)$ and $P_y(10, 20)$. What is the interpretation of your answer?

52. **Change in Present Value.** The present value of an annuity for which R dollars are to be paid every year for t years is given by

$$\text{Present value} = \frac{R}{i}\left[1 - \left(\frac{1}{1+i}\right)^t\right]$$

where i is the annual rate of interest. If the length t of the annuity is fixed, how does the present value change as the annual rate of interest i changes? Evaluate this change when $R = \$750$ and $i = 0.10$. What is the interpretation of your answer?

53. **Cobb-Douglas Production Function.** The Cobb-Douglas production function describes the production output p of a firm in terms of the cost x of capital and the cost y of labor. It is given by

$$p(x, y) = Ax^k y^{1-k}$$

where $A > 0$ and $0 < k < 1$. Show that a Cobb-Douglas production function $p(x, y)$ satisfies the relations

$$\frac{p_x(x, y)}{p(x, y)} = \frac{k}{x}$$

$$\frac{p_y(x, y)}{p(x, y)} = \frac{1-k}{y}$$

Cobb and Douglas were able to see the economic significance of these two equations. Can you interpret these two equations?

54. **Marginal Productivity.** The partial derivative $p_x(x, y)$ of the Cobb-Douglas production function is called the **marginal productivity of capital** and $p_y(x, y)$ is the **marginal productivity of labor.** Find the points (x, y) for which the marginal productivity of capital is equal to the marginal productivity of labor if the Cobb-Douglas function is given by

$$p(x, y) = 40x^{2/3}y^{1/3}$$

Problems 55–57 concern themselves with three important **partial differential equations** (equations that contain partial derivatives) that describe natural phenomena.

Some Interesting Partial Derivatives

55. **Partial Differential Equation.** If

$$u(x, y) = \frac{2x + y}{x - y}$$

show that $u(x, y)$ satisfies the partial differential equation

$$xu_x + yu_y = 0$$

56. **Laplace's Equation.** If

$$u(x, y) = \ln(x^2 + y^2)$$

show that $u(x, y)$ satisfies Laplace's equation

$$u_{xx} + u_{yy} = 0$$

57. **Cauchy-Riemann Equations.** If

$$u(x, y) = x^2 - y^2$$
$$v(x, y) = 2xy$$

show that $u(x, y)$ and $v(x, y)$ satisfy the Cauchy-Riemann equations

$$u_x(x, y) = v_y(x, y)$$
$$u_y(x, y) = -v_x(x, y)$$

Partial Derivatives in Biology

58. **Just How Big Are You Getting?** A biologist has determined that the surface area in square inches of the human body can be reasonably approximated by

$$S(h, w) = 16h^{0.4}w^{0.7}$$

where h is a person's height in inches and w is a person's weight in pounds.

(a) Compute $S_w(64, 100)$. For a person who is 64 inches tall (5′4″) and weighs 100 pounds this partial derivative with respect to w will tell roughly how many square inches that person's surface area changes if height remains constant but weight increases by one pound. It will have units of square inches of surface area per pound of increase.

(b) Evaluate the partial derivative S_w at your own height and weight to estimate your own increase in surface area as a function of weight increase (assuming that you are not growing in height). If you gain x pounds (assuming that x is small), you can approximate your actual increase in surface area by using the differential approximation by multiplying the computed partial derivative by the weight increase x.

59. Cooling of an Elephant. The amount of heat an animal loses because of surface convection can be estimated in terms of the diameter of the animal and the wind velocity. The exact function is given by

$$h(v, d) = k\frac{v^{1/3}}{d^{2/3}}$$

where k depends on the species of animal. Find the partial derivatives h_v and h_d. Why would a biologist be interested in knowing these values?

6.3 Unconstrained Optimization

PURPOSE

We show how the first- and second-partial derivatives can be used to find relative maximum and minimum points of a function of two variables. We do this by using the following two-step process:

- **Step 1.** Use the first-partial derivatives to find the critical points.
- **Step 2.** Use the second-partial derivatives to determine if the critical points are relative maximum or relative minimum points (or neither).

Introduction

One of the major applications of differential calculus is in finding maximum and minimum points of a function. Earlier, we used the first and second derivatives to find the maximum and minimum points of a function of a single variable. Now we will see how partial derivatives can be used to find maximum and minimum points of a function $z = f(x, y)$ of two variables.

We assume that the surface $z = f(x, y)$ is "continuous and smooth" as shown in Figure 16a, which means it does not have any jumps, sharp corners, or edges of the type shown in Figure 16b.

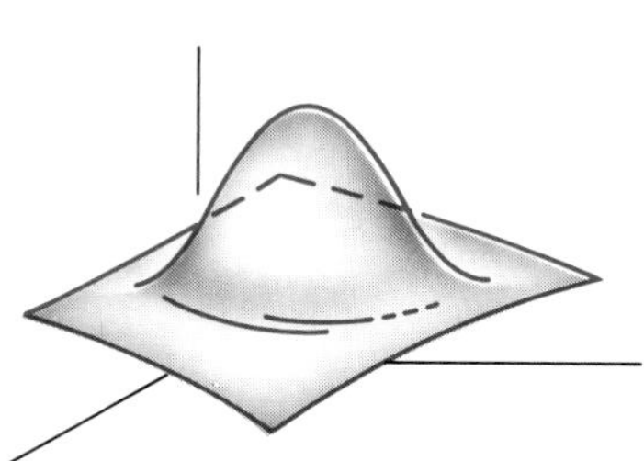

The surface should be smooth

(a)

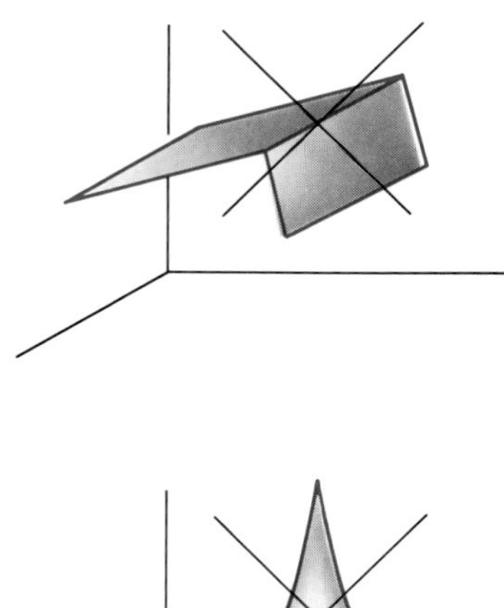

The surface should not have jumps or corners

(b)

Figure 16
Surfaces that we will and will not study

Relative Maximum and Minimum Points

What does it mean for a point (a, b) to be a relative maximum or minimum point of a function f of two variables? Roughly, it means that the surface $z = f(x, y)$ has a "high point" or a "low point" at (a, b) as shown in Figure 17.

If we were to state more precisely what our intuition tells us, we would say the following.

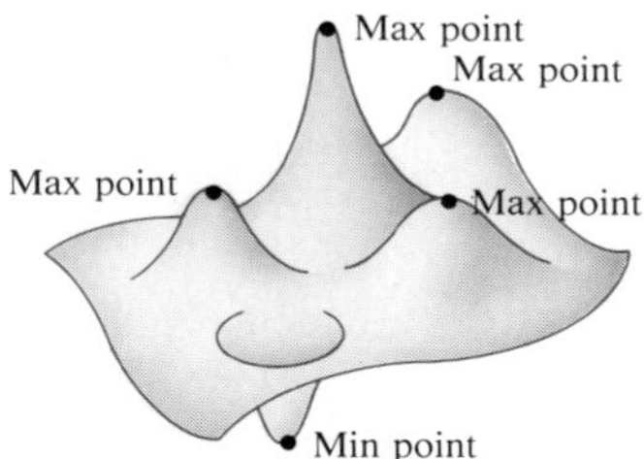

Figure 17
Relative maximum and minimum points

Definition of Relative Maximum and Minimum Points

A function f of two variables is said to have a **relative maximum** at a point (a, b) if there is a circle centered at (a, b) such that

$$f(a, b) \geq f(x, y)$$

for all points (x, y) inside the circle. Similarly, a function f of two variables has a **relative minimum** at a point (a, b) if there is a circle centered at (a, b) such that

$$f(a, b) \leq f(x, y)$$

for all points (x, y) inside the circle.

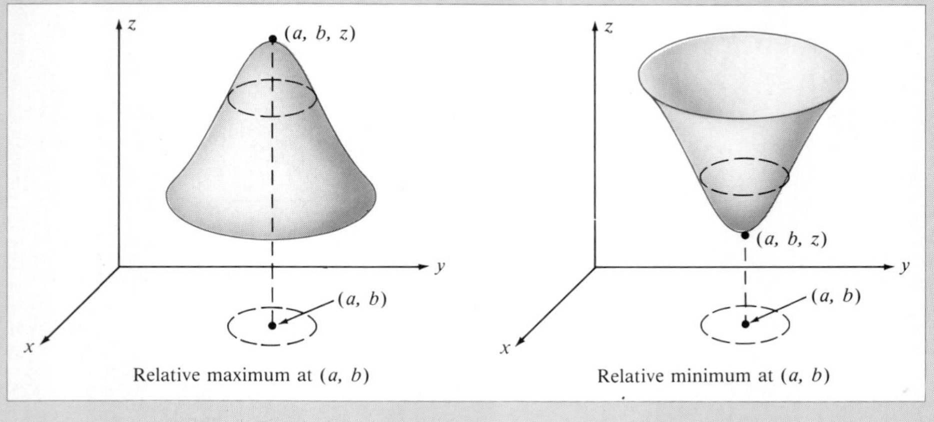

Relative maximum at (a, b) Relative minimum at (a, b)

What is true about the partial derivatives $f_x(a, b)$ and $f_y(a, b)$ at a point (a, b) where $f(a, b)$ is a relative maximum or minimum point? The above diagram indicates that both partial derivatives $f_x(a, b)$ and $f_y(a, b)$ are zero, since the slopes of the tangent lines in the x- and y-directions are both zero. The following theorem indicates that our intuition is correct.

Test Conditions for Relative Maximum and Minimum Points

If $f(a, b)$ is a relative maximum or minimum value of a function f and if the first partial derivatives f_x and f_y exist at (a, b), then it must hold that the two partial derivatives are zero at that point. That is,

$$f_x(a, b) = 0$$
$$f_y(a, b) = 0$$

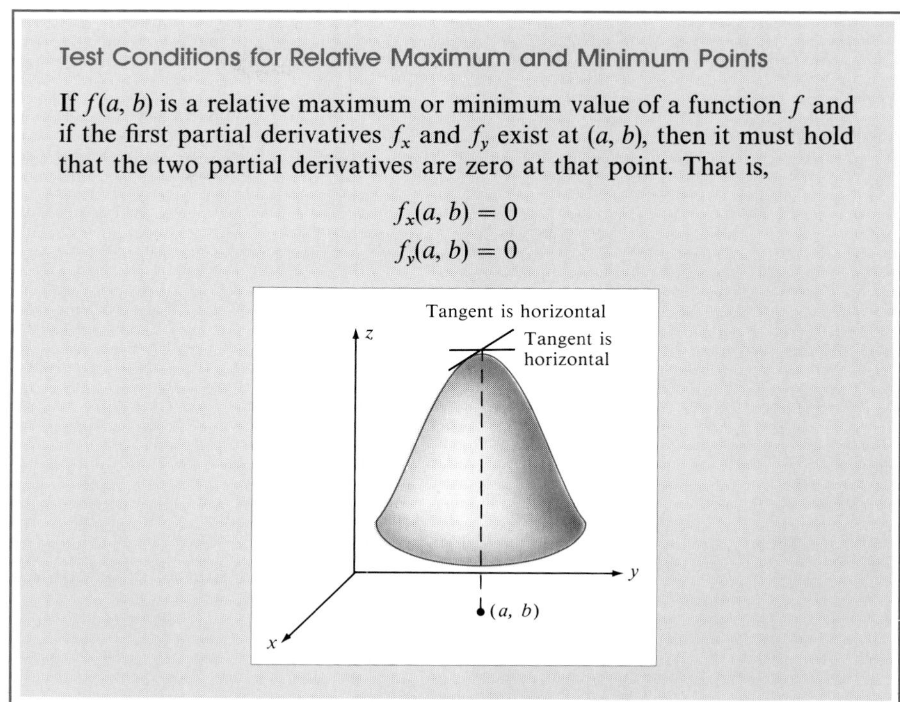

The points (a, b) where both partial derivatives f_x and f_y are zero are called **critical points**. It is important to understand that if (a, b) is a relative maximum or minimum point, then

$$f_x(a, b) = 0$$
$$f_y(a, b) = 0$$

but not vice versa. That is, just because $f_x(a, b)$ and $f_y(a, b)$ are both zero at (a, b), it is not necessarily true that $f(a, b)$ is a relative maximum or minimum value. Figure 18 shows an example of a function $f(x, y)$ that has the property

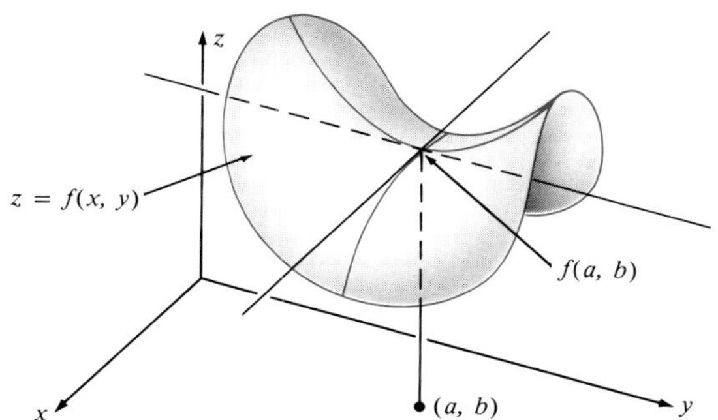

Figure 18
$f_x(a, b)$ and $f_y(a, b)$ are both zero, but (a, b) is not a relative maximum or minimum point

that both partial derivatives $f_x(a, b)$ and $f_y(a, b)$ are zero but $f(x, y)$ does not have a relative maximum or minimum value at (a, b). We call the point (a, b) a **saddle point**. The reason for the name is that the surface $z = f(x, y)$ at the point (a, b) is shaped somewhat like a saddle.

Example 1

Finding Critical Points Find the critical points of the function

$$f(x, y) = x^2 - xy + y^2 + 3x + 10$$

and determine which critical points are relative maximum or minimum points.

Solution To find the critical points, we look for solutions (a, b) of the system of equations

$$f_x(x, y) = 0$$
$$f_y(x, y) = 0$$

Setting the partial derivatives to zero, we get

$$f_x(x, y) = \frac{\partial}{\partial x}(x^2 - xy + y^2 + 3x + 10) = 2x - y + 3 = 0$$

$$f_y(x, y) = \frac{\partial}{\partial y}(x^2 - xy + y^2 + 3x + 10) = -x + 2y = 0$$

This gives us the two simultaneous equations

$$\begin{aligned} 2x - y &= -3 \\ -x + 2y &= 0 \end{aligned}$$

which have the unique solution

$$x = -2$$
$$y = -1$$

The above solution gives the single critical point $(-2, -1)$. Of course, we cannot be absolutely sure that this point is a relative maximum or minimum point. What we can say, however, is that every other point can be eliminated as a candidate for a relative maximum or minimum point (where f_x and f_y are defined). If we now evaluate the function $f(x, y)$ at the critical point $(-2, -1)$ and at several nearby points, we get a pretty good indication that $(-2, -1)$ is a relative maximum or minimum point. Figure 19 illustrates the value of $f(x, y)$ at the critical point $(-2, -1)$ and at four nearby points.

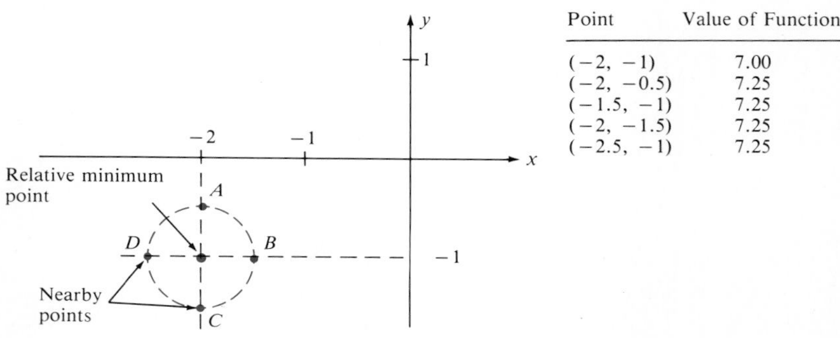

Point	Value of Function
$(-2, -1)$	7.00
$(-2, -0.5)$	7.25
$(-1.5, -1)$	7.25
$(-2, -1.5)$	7.25
$(-2.5, -1)$	7.25

Figure 19
Testing to determine a relative minimum point

A computer-driven plotter was also used by Professor Norton Starr of Amherst University to draw the surface that is shown in Figure 20. This surface also indicates that $(-2, -1)$ is a relative minimum point. Later, when we study the second-partials test, we will confirm this conclusion. □

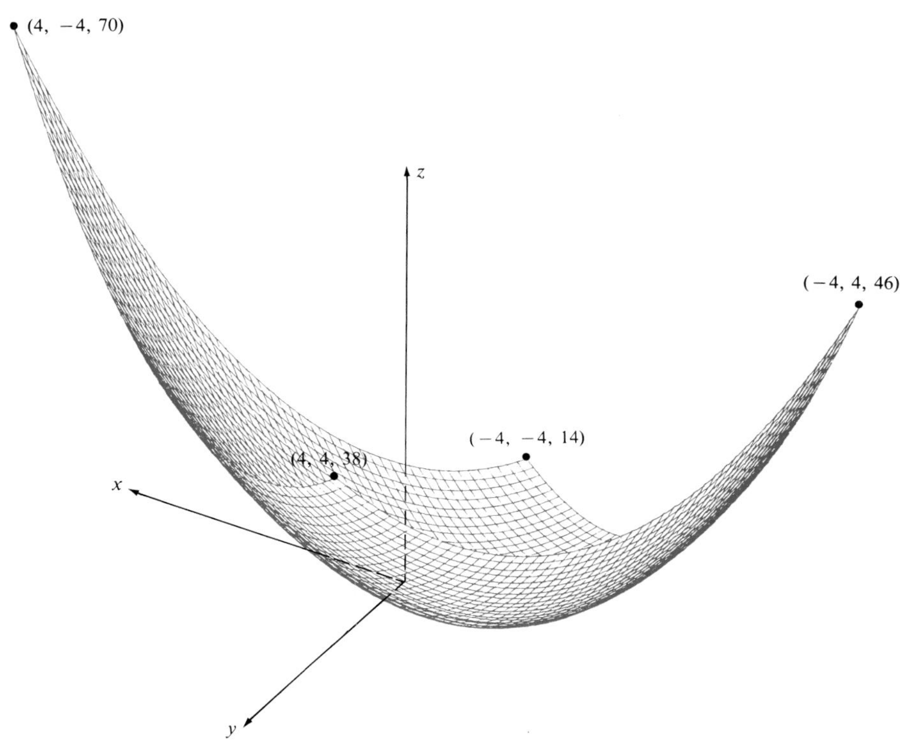

Figure 20
Graph of
$z = x^2 - xy + y^2 + 3x + 10$

Example 2

Finding Critical Points Find the critical point(s) of

$$f(x, y) = 2x^2 + y^2 + 2$$

and determine whether they are relative maximum or minimum points.

Solution Setting the partial derivatives f_x and f_y to zero, we have

$$f_x(x, y) = \frac{\partial}{\partial x}(2x^2 + y^2 + 2) = 4x = 0$$

$$f_y(x, y) = \frac{\partial}{\partial y}(2x^2 + y^2 + 2) = 2y = 0$$

Since $x = 0$ and $y = 0$ is the only solution of the system of equations, we conclude that the origin $(0, 0)$ is the only critical point. Hence this point is the only candidate for a relative maximum or minimum point. In this case it is clear that the value of the function

$$f(x, y) = 2x^2 + y^2 + 2$$

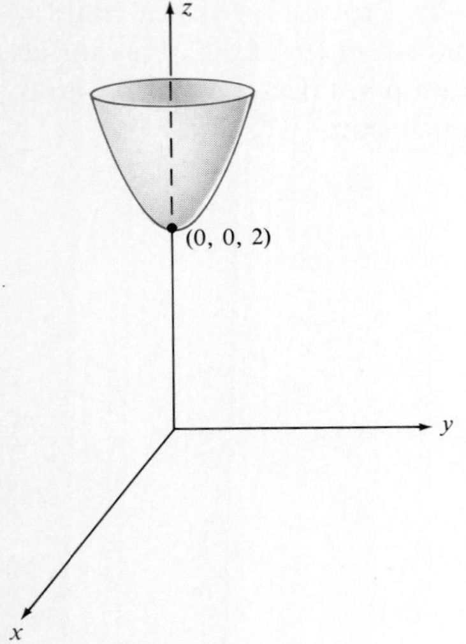

Figure 21
Relative and absolute minimum at (0, 0, 2)

is always greater than the value of the function at the origin. Hence we can conclude that $f(0, 0) = 2$ is a relative minimum value of the function. In fact, since $f(0, 0) = 2$ is smaller than any other value of $f(x, y)$, this means that $f(0, 0)$ is the absolute minimum value of the function. This surface is shown in Figure 21. □

The Second-Partials Test

Knowing the critical points of a function of two variables narrows the search for the relative maximum and minimum points. However, the critical point may be a saddle point and not a relative maximum or minimum point. To determine whether a critical point is in fact a relative maximum or minimum point, there is a convenient test involving the second-partial derivatives f_{xx}, f_{xy}, and f_{yy}. The only price we pay for using this test is the computation of the second derivatives. We state the test here without proof.

Second-Partials Test for Relative Maximum and Minimum Points

Let $z = f(x, y)$ be a function of two variables with a critical point (a, b). That is, $f(x, y)$ satisfies

$$f_x(a, b) = 0$$
$$f_y(a, b) = 0$$

Define the **discriminant** D as

$$D = f_{xx}(a, b) \cdot f_{yy}(a, b) - f_{xy}^2(a, b)$$

The nature of the critical point (a, b) depends on the following values of D:

$$\mathbf{D = f_{xx}(a, b) \cdot f_{yy}(a, b) - f_{xy}^2(a, b)}$$

$D < 0$	$D = 0$	$D > 0$	
Saddle point	Nothing can be said (test fails)	$f_{xx}(a, b) < 0$ Relative maximum point	$f_{xx}(a, b) > 0$ Relative minimum point

It might be pointed out here that when $D > 0$, it is impossible that the second partial derivative $f_{xx}(a, b)$ is zero. (This is why this possibility is not included in the table.)

Figure 22 shows the steps that should be taken in finding relative maximum and minimum points of a function.

Example 3 Second-Partials Test Use the second-partials test to find the relative maximum and minimum points of the function

$$f(x, y) = x^2 - xy + y^2 + 3x + 10$$

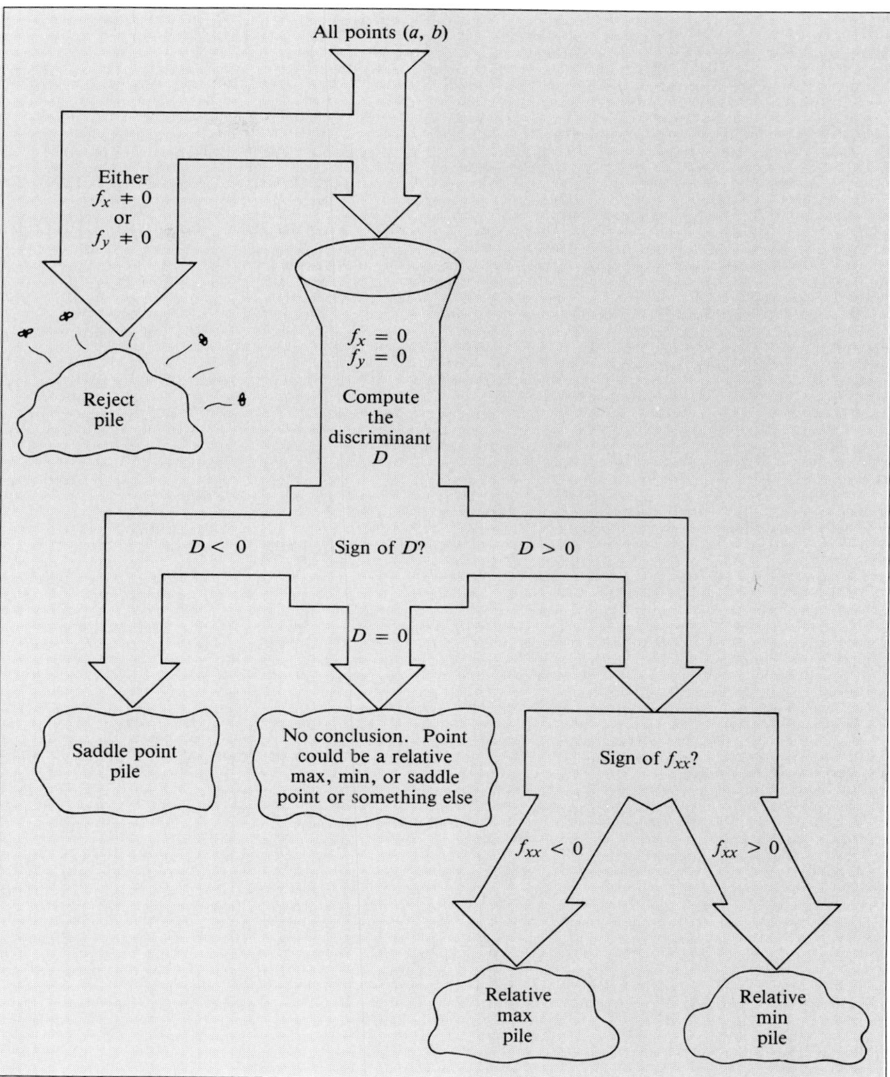

Figure 22
The "classification machine"

Solution

- **Step 1** (find first-partial derivatives). Computing the first-partial derivatives, we get

$$f_x(x, y) = \frac{\partial}{\partial x}(x^2 - xy + y^2 + 3x + 10) = 2x - y + 3$$

$$f_y(x, y) = \frac{\partial}{\partial y}(x^2 - xy + y^2 + 3x + 10) = -x + 2y$$

- **Step 2** (find the critical points). Setting the first-partial derivatives to zero gives the simultaneous equations

$$f_x(x, y) = 2x - y + 3 = 0$$
$$f_y(x, y) = -x + 2y = 0$$

Solving for x and y, we have

$$x = -2$$
$$y = -1$$

Hence the only critical point is $(-2, -1)$. This provides one candidate for a relative maximum or minimum point.

- **Step 3** (compute the discriminant). Computing $f_{xx}(x, y)$, $f_{yy}(x, y)$, and $f_{xy}(x, y)$, we get

$$f_{xx}(x, y) = \frac{\partial}{\partial x} f_x = \frac{\partial}{\partial x}(2x - y + 3) = 2$$

$$f_{xy}(x, y) = \frac{\partial}{\partial y} f_x = \frac{\partial}{\partial y}(2x - y + 3) = -1$$

$$f_{yy}(x, y) = \frac{\partial}{\partial y} f_y = \frac{\partial}{\partial y}(-x + 2y) = 2$$

Thus the discriminant is

$$\begin{aligned} D &= f_{xx}(-2, -1) \cdot f_{yy}(-2, -1) - f_{xy}^2(-2, -1) \\ &= (2)(2) - (-1)^2 \\ &= 3 \end{aligned}$$

- **Step 4** (apply the second-partials test). Since the discriminant D is positive and $f_{xx}(-2, -1) = 2$ is positive, we conclude from the second-partials

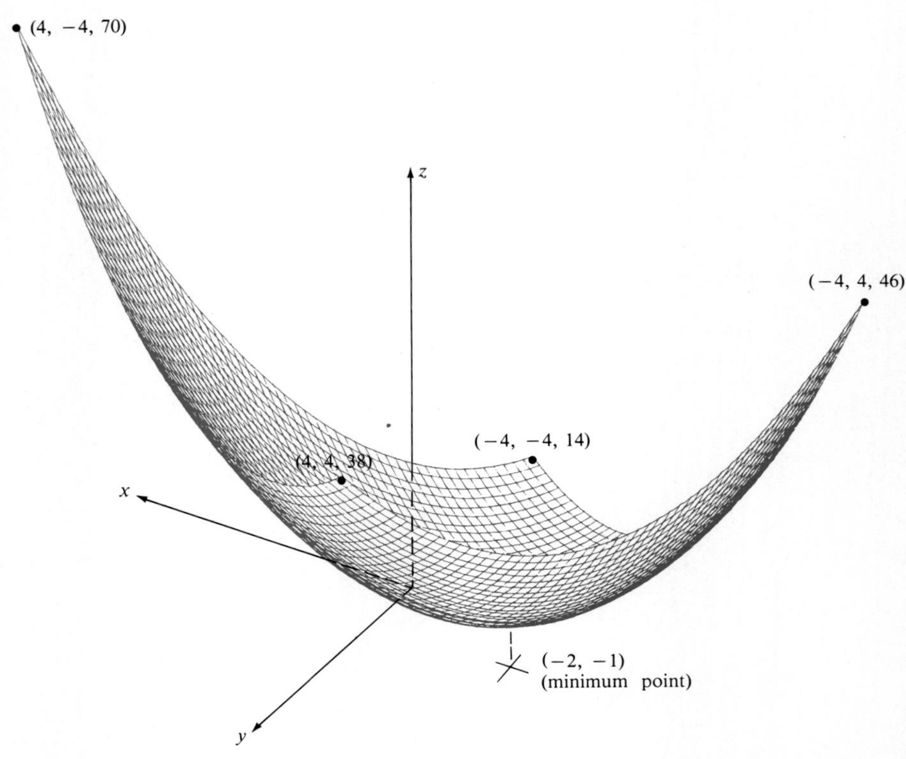

Figure 23
Minimum point of $z = x^2 - xy + y^2 + 3x + 10$

test that the critical point $(-2, -1)$ is a relative minimum point. We would also say that the value $f(-2, -1) = -3$ is a relative minimum value.

The graph of

$$f(x, y) = x^2 - xy + y^2 + 3x + 10$$

is shown in Figure 23. □

Example 4

Second-Partials Test Use the second-partials test to find the relative maximum and minimum points of the function

$$f(x, y) = x^3 + y^3 - 3xy + 10$$

Solution

- **Step 1** (find the first-partial derivatives). Computing f_x and f_y, we have

$$f_x(x, y) = \frac{\partial}{\partial x}(x^3 + y^3 - 3xy + 10) = 3x^2 - 3y$$

$$f_y(x, y) = \frac{\partial}{\partial y}(x^3 + y^3 - 3xy + 10) = 3y^2 - 3x$$

- **Step 2** (find the critical points). Setting f_x and f_y to zero gives

$$3x^2 - 3y = 0$$
$$3y^2 - 3x = 0$$

or

$$x^2 = y$$
$$y^2 = x$$

Substituting $y = x^2$ into the second equation gives

$$x^4 = x$$
$$x^4 - x = 0$$
$$x \cdot (x^3 - 1) = 0$$

The solutions of this equation are $x = 0$ and 1. Substituting these values into the equation for y in terms of x gives $x = 0$, $y = 0$, and $x = 1$, $y = 1$ as solutions. Therefore the critical points are $(0, 0)$ and $(1, 1)$.

- **Step 3** (compute the discriminant). First we find $f_{xx}(x, y)$, $f_{xy}(x, y)$, and $f_{yy}(x, y)$:

$$f_{xx}(x, y) = \frac{\partial}{\partial x} f_x = \frac{\partial}{\partial x}(3x^2 - 3y) = 6x$$

$$f_{xy}(x, y) = \frac{\partial}{\partial y} f_x = \frac{\partial}{\partial y}(3x^2 - 3y) = -3$$

$$f_{yy}(x, y) = \frac{\partial}{\partial y} f_y = \frac{\partial}{\partial y}(3y^2 - 3x) = 6y$$

We then evaluate the above second-partial derivatives and the discriminant at each of the two critical points (0, 0) and (1, 1). We display these values in Table 6.

TABLE 6
Second-Partial Derivatives and Discriminant at the Critical Points

Critical Point	$f_{xx}(x, y)$	$f_{xy}(x, y)$	$f_{yy}(x, y)$	$D = f_{xx}f_{yy} - f_{xy}^2$
(0, 0)	0	−3	0	−9
(1, 1)	6	−3	6	27

- **Step 4** (apply the second-partials test). Since the discriminant is negative at the critical point (0, 0), the point (0, 0) is a saddle point. On the other hand, since the discriminant is positive at the critical point (1, 1) and $f_{xx}(1, 1)$ is positive, we conclude that (1, 1) is a relative minimum point.

The graph of

$$z = x^3 + y^3 - 3xy + 10$$

is shown in Figure 24. □

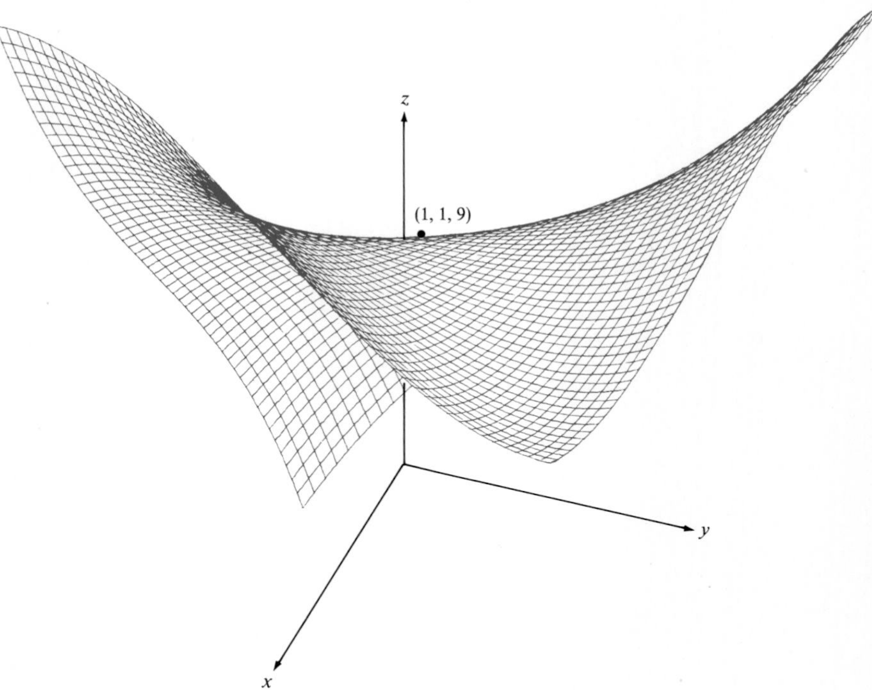

Figure 4
Graph of $z = x^3 + y^3 - 3xy + 10$

Profit Maximization in the Multicommodity Theory of the Firm

We saw in the previous section that the theory of the firm can be extended to multicommodity companies. We present an example that shows how production levels can be determined to maximize a company's profits.

Example 5

Profit Maximization Suppose a company that produces x units of Product A per day and y units of Product B per day makes a daily profit (in dollars) of

$$P(x, y) = 200x + 300y - x^2 - 2xy - 2y^2 - 2000$$

Find the production levels x and y of the two products that will maximize the profit. What is the maximum profit that the company can earn?

Solution To find the relative maximum value of the function

$$P(x, y) = 200x + 300y - x^2 - 2xy - 2y^2 - 2000$$

we carry out the following steps:

- **Step 1** (find the first-partial derivatives). Computing P_x and P_y, we have

$$P_x(x, y) = 200 - 2x - 2y$$
$$P_y(x, y) = 300 - 2x - 4y$$

- **Step 2** (find the critical points). Setting P_x and P_y to zero, we find

$$2x + 2y = 200$$
$$2x + 4y = 300$$

Solving for x and y, we get

$$x = 50$$
$$y = 50$$

This gives the critical point (50, 50) as the sole candidate for a relative maximum point of $P(x, y)$.

- **Step 3** (find the discriminant). Computing the second-order partial derivatives $P_{xx}(x, y)$, $P_{xy}(x, y)$, and $P_{yy}(x, y)$, we find

$$P_{xx}(x, y) = -2$$
$$P_{xy}(x, y) = -2$$
$$P_{yy}(x, y) = -4$$

Evaluating these partial derivatives at the critical point (50, 50) gives the values

$$P_{xx}(50, 50) = -2$$
$$P_{xy}(50, 50) = -2$$
$$P_{yy}(50, 50) = -4$$

Hence the discriminant is given by

$$\begin{aligned} D &= P_{xx}(50, 50) \cdot P_{yy}(50, 50) - P_{xy}^2(50, 50) \\ &= (-2)(-4) - (-2)^2 \\ &= 4 \end{aligned}$$

- **Step 4** (apply the second-partials test). Since the discriminant is positive and $P_{xx}(50, 50)$ is negative, the second-partials test says that (50, 50) is a relative maximum point. The value of the profit function $P(x, y)$ at this point is

$$P(50, 50) = \$10{,}500$$

In Figure 25 we see a drawing of the profit surface $z = P(x, y)$ as a function of the production levels x and y. It is clear from this graph that \$10,500 is in fact the absolute maximum profit.

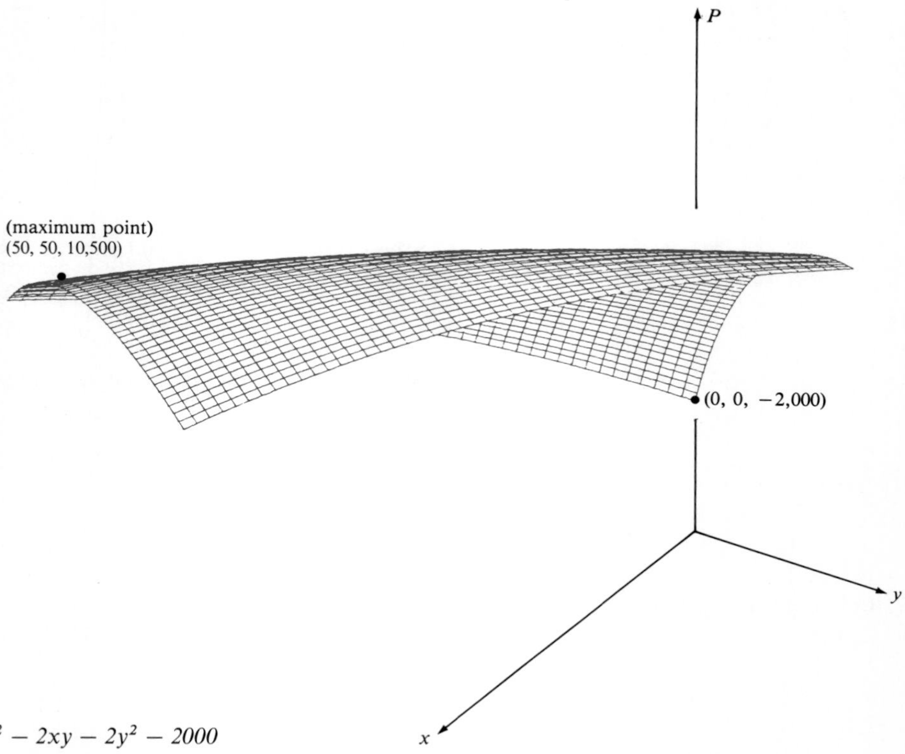

Figure 25
Graph of $P(x, y) = 200x + 300y - x^2 - 2xy - 2y^2 - 2000$

Interpretation: The optimal production level for this company is 50 units of Product A and 50 units of Product B per day. This production level results in a maximum daily profit of \$10,500. □

Problems

For Problems 1–20, find all the critical points of the given functions.

1. $f(x, y) = x^2 - 2xy + 2y^2 - 3y - x$
2. $f(x, y) = 3 + 2x - 3x^2 - y^2$
3. $f(x, y) = x + 2y + x^2 - 3y^2$
4. $f(x, y) = -2x + xy^3 + 2x^3$
5. $f(x, y) = -2x + 4y + 3xy$
6. $f(x, y) = 3x - 7xy + x^2 + y^2$
7. $f(x, y) = 5x^2 + 2y^3 - 12y - 3y^2$
8. $f(x, y) = 6 + 3x - 4y + x^2 - 2y^2$
9. $f(x, y) = 7 + 6x - 3y + x^3 - y^2$
10. $f(x, y) = 6xy - 2x^2 - 3y^2$
11. $f(x, y) = 4 + 5x - 6y + 3xy + 2x^2 - 3y^2$
12. $f(x, y) = -7 - 3x + 2y + 4xy + 3x^2 + 4y^2$
13. $f(x, y) = -3 + 5x + 4y + 3xy + y^2$
14. $f(x, y) = 5xy + x^2 - 3y^2$
15. $f(x, y) = -8 - 5x + 12y + x^3 - 4y^3$
16. $f(x, y) = 4xy - xy^2 + 3x^2y$
17. $f(x, y) = 5 - 12xy + 3x^3 + 2y^3$
18. $f(x, y) = 8xy + 2xy^2 - 3x^2y$
19. $f(x, y) = ye^x$
20. $f(x, y) = xe^y$

For Problems 21–40, use the second-partials test to classify the critical points as relative maximum or minimum points, saddle points, or unclassified.

21. $f(x, y) = x^2 - 2xy + 4y^2 + 6x$
22. $f(x, y) = 5 + 2xy - 6x + 4y - x^2 - 2y^2$

23. $f(x, y) = 7 + 24x - 3x^2 + 8y - 2y^2$
24. $f(x, y) = x^4 + y^4 - 4xy$
25. $f(x, y) = (x - 2)(y - 2)(x + y - 2)$
26. $f(x, y) = 120x + 120y - xy - x^2 - y^2$
27. $f(x, y) = y^2 - 3x^2y + 2x^4$
28. $f(x, y) = 3x^2 + 4xy + y^2 - 6y$
29. $f(x, y) = x^2 - 3xy + 2y^2 + 5x$
30. $f(x, y) = y^3 - 3xy + x^2 + x - 4$
31. $f(x, y) = 8x^3 + y^3 - 6x^2 - 6y^2 + 4$
32. $f(x, y) = 7 + 4x - 3y - x^2 + y^3$
33. $f(x, y) = -x^3 - y^3 + 9xy + 7$
34. $f(x, y) = xy - y^2 - x^2 - 3y + 4x$
35. $f(x, y) = xy + \frac{8}{y} + \frac{2}{x}$
36. $f(x, y) = 2xy + \frac{10}{y}$
37. $f(x, y) = x^3 - y^3 - 9x$
38. $f(x, y) = 2 + x^4 + y^4 - 32y$
39. $f(x, y) = e^x + e^{-y}$
40. $f(x, y) = xe^y$

Finding Minimum Distances

41. **Closest Point to the Origin.** Find the point on the plane

$$x + 2y + 2z = 4$$

that is the closest to the origin (0, 0, 0). What is this distance? *Hint:* The square of the distance D is

$$D^2 = x^2 + y^2 + z^2$$

Solve for z in the above equation of the plane, substitute this value into the formula for D^2, and find the minimum of D^2. This strategy is valid, since D is minimized when D^2 is minimized.

42. **Closest Point to the Origin.** Using the strategy discussed in Problem 41, find the point on the plane

$$x + y + z = 1$$

that is the closest to the origin. What is this distance?

43. **Closest Point to the Origin.** Using the strategy discussed in Problem 41, find the point on the plane

$$x = 2$$

that is the closest to the origin. What is this distance? Is it the same distance that you suspected?

Maximizing Problems in a Multicommodity Economy

44. **Pricing Candy Bars.** A company produces two kinds of candy bars, Gold Blocks and Wildbars. It costs the company \$0.20 to make each Gold Block and \$0.25 for each Wildbar. The demand for Gold Blocks and Wildbars has been determined to be

$$D_G(g, w) = \frac{10{,}000}{g^2 w} \quad \text{(demand for Gold Blocks)}$$

$$D_W(g, w) = \frac{50{,}000}{gw^2} \quad \text{(demand for Wildbars)}$$

where g is the price for a Gold Block and w is the price of a Wildbar.

(a) Find the company's revenue

$$R(g, w) = gD_G(g, w) + wD_W(g, w)$$

in terms of the prices g and w.

(b) Find the cost

$$C(g, w) = 0.20D_G(g, w) + 0.25D_W(g, w)$$

in terms of the prices g and w.

(c) Find the profit $P(g, w)$ in terms of g and w.

(d) Find the price of each candy bar g and w that will maximize the profit.

(e) What is the maximum profit?

45. **Profit Maximization.** A company's revenue and cost function are given by

$$R(x, y) = 25x + 35y$$

$$C(x, y) = \frac{3}{2}x^2 - 3xy + \frac{5}{2}y^2$$

Find the company's profit-maximizing output level and its maximum profit.

46. **General Formulation of Production Levels.** A firm markets two products and charges p_1 for the first product and p_2 for the second product. Hence the revenue from the sale of x and y units of these two products will be

$$R(x, y) = p_1x + p_2y$$

Suppose the cost function to produce these products is given by

$$C(x, y) = 2x^2 + xy + 2y^2$$

Determine as a function of p_1 and p_2 the number of items the company should produce to maximize profits. How many items should the company produce when the prices are $p_1 = \$5$ and $p_2 = \$2$?

47. **Finding Maximum Profits from Demand Functions.** A company markets two products. The demands for these two products x and y depend on the prices p_1 and p_2 that the company charges for the products. The two demand functions are

$$x = 40 - 2p_1 + p_2$$
$$y = 25 + p_1 - p_2$$

Suppose the cost to the company to produce x and y units of each product is

$$C(x, y) = x^2 + xy + y^2$$

(a) Solve the demand functions for p_1 and p_2 in terms of x and y.

(b) Find the revenue function $R(x, y) = xp_1 + yp_2$ in terms of x and y.
(c) Find the profit function $P(x, y)$ in terms of x and y.
(d) Find the production levels x and y that maximize the profit.

48. Optimal Pricing of Candy Bars. The Mr. NiceBar Company produces two kinds of candy bars, Mr. NiceBar Jr. and Mr. NiceBar Sr. The cost to produce each of these candy bars is \$0.15 for Mr. NiceBar Jr. and \$0.25 for Mr. NiceBar Sr. The weekly demands x and y (in thousands) for Mr. NiceBar Jr. and Mr. NiceBar Sr. are

$$x = 10(p_2 - p_1) \qquad \text{(Mr. NiceBar Jr.)}$$
$$y = 5 + 3p_1 - 5p_2 \qquad \text{(Mr. NiceBar Sr.)}$$

respectively, where p_1 and p_2 are the prices in cents for Mr. NiceBar Jr. and Mr. NiceBar Sr., respectively.

(a) Find the revenue function $R(p_1, p_2) = p_1x + p_2y$ as a function of the prices p_1 and p_2.
(b) Find the cost function $C(p_1, p_2) = 0.15x + 0.25y$ as a function of the prices p_1 and p_2.
(c) Find the profit $P(p_1, p_2)$ function as a function of the prices p_1 and p_2.
(d) Find the prices that maximize the profit.

49. Spreading Fertilizer. An experiment measures the results of applying two fertilizers A and B to an artichoke field. The yield of artichokes in bushels per acre is given by

$$V(x, y) = 10x + 5y + 2x^2 + y^2 - 8xy + 10$$

where x is the number of pounds of fertilizer A used and y is the number of pounds of fertilizer B used. What is the maximum yield of artichokes that can be produced? How many pounds of each fertilizer should be used?

6.4 Constrained Optimization (Lagrange Multipliers)

PURPOSE

We show how to find the maximum and the minimum of a function $y = f(x, y)$ where x and y are restricted to satisfy an additional "side condition" or constraint equation $g(x, y) = 0$. The major topics studied are

- a comparison between constrained and unconstrained optimization problems and
- the Lagrange multiplier rule for transforming constrained optimization problems into unconstrained optimization problems.

We close the section by showing how constrained optimization problems can be applied to the economic topic of consumer or utility theory.

Geometry of Constrained Problems

Consider the two optimization problems illustrated in Table 7. Note that the **unconstrained maximization** problem, which here consists of finding the maximum value of the function

$$f(x, y) = \sqrt{4 - x^2 - y^2}$$

has a larger maximum value (maximum value of 2) than does the **constrained maximization** problem, which consists of finding the maximum value of

$$f(x, y) = \sqrt{4 - x^2 - y^2}$$

where now x and y are **constrained** to lie on the plane

$$x + 2y = 1$$

As one might imagine, optimization problems with constraints are generally much more difficult to solve than problems without constraints. One approach for attacking optimization problems with constraints goes back 200 years to a method devised by the brilliant mathematician Joseph Louis Lagrange. Today, the method is called the **method of Lagrange multipliers**.

Table 7
Unconstrained and Constrained Optimization Problems

Unconstrained Optimization Problem	Constrained Optimization Problem
Find the maximum point on the surface $$f(x, y) = \sqrt{4 - x^2 - y^2}$$	Find the maximum point on the surface $$f(x, y) = \sqrt{4 - x^2 - y^2}$$ where x and y are constrained to lie on the plane $$x + 2y = 1$$

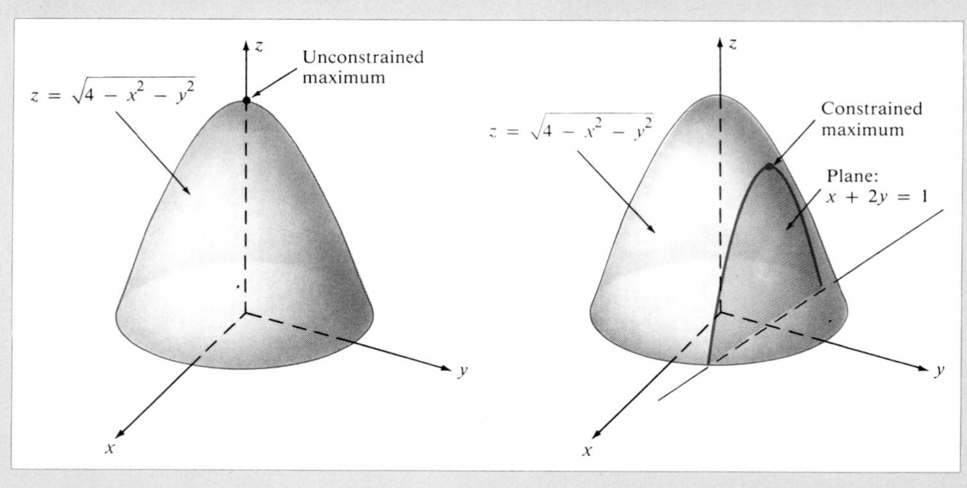

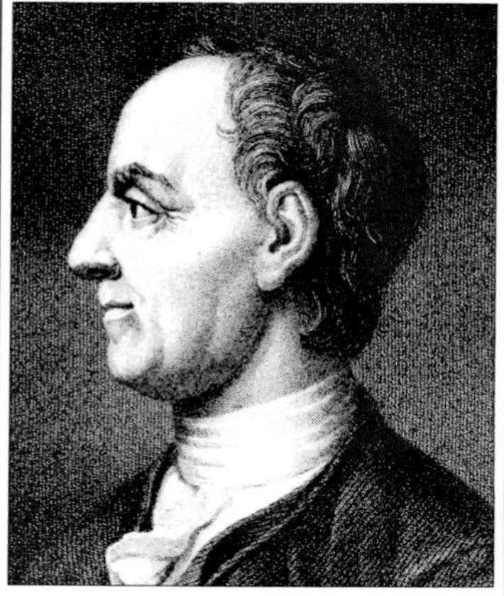

HISTORICAL NOTE

Joseph Louis Lagrange (1736–1813) was born in Turin, Italy, and is considered to be one of the two "great mathematicians" of the eighteenth century (the Swiss mathematician Leonhard Euler being the other). Lagrange was one of the first mathematicians to bring a rigorous level of precision to mathematics and was responsible for introducing our moden notation $f(x)$ to denote a function.

Constraints and the Lagrange Multiplier

A typical constrained optimization problem would be to find the minimum value of a function, called the **objective function**,

$$z = x^2 + y^2$$

subject to the **constraint**

$$x + y = 2$$

From a geometric point of view we seek to find the lowest point (smallest value of z) on the intersection of the plane $x + y = 2$ and the paraboloid $z = x^2 + y^2$ as shown in Figure 26.

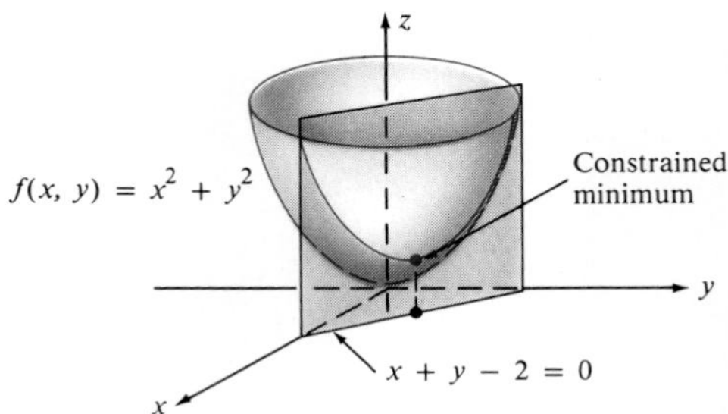

Figure 26
Constrained minimum problem

Finding a maximum or a minimum point of a constrained optimization problem is generally quite difficult, since the constraint equation makes it hard to describe the domain of the problem. However we now introduce a method known as the Lagrange multiplier method, which transforms a constrained optimization problem into an unconstrained optimization problem. In this way the maximum and minimum points of the original constrained problem can be found by finding the maximum and minimum points of the unconstrained problem. For example, consider minimizing the objective function.

$$z = x^2 + y^2$$

subject to the constraint

$$x + y = 2$$

The method of Lagrange multipliers uses the above functions to define a new function

$$L(x, y, \lambda) = x^2 + y^2 + \lambda(x + y - 2)$$

known as the **Lagrange function**. It is important that you understand a few things about this function.

Observe how the constraint equation $x + y = 2$ enters into the Lagrange function.

The Lagrange function $L(x, y, \lambda)$ is a function of three variables x, y, and λ. The variables x and y are the same variables as in the original constrained problem, but the variable λ is a new variable. We could just as well call them x, y, and z, but convention dictates that we call them x, y, and λ. The new variable λ is called the **Lagrange multiplier**.

The reason the Lagrange function $L(x, y, \lambda)$ is important is the interesting fact that when the point (x_0, y_0, λ_0) is a relative minimum point of the Lagrange function of three variables $L(x, y, \lambda)$, then (x_0, y_0) is a relative minimum point of the original constrained problem. Since minimizing a function without constraints is easier than minimizing a function with constraints, Lagrange in effect discovered a powerful rule for solving constrained optimization problems. His rule is stated here without proof.

Lagrange's Method for Solving Constrained Optimization Problems

If we define the Lagrange function as

$$L(x, y, \lambda) = f(x, y) + \lambda g(x, y)$$

then all the relative maximum and minimum points of $f(x, y)$ with x and y constrained to satisfy the equation $g(x, y) = 0$ will be among those points (x_0, y_0) for which (x_0, y_0, λ_0) is a maximum or minimum point of $L(x, y, \lambda)$. These points (x_0, y_0, λ_0) will be solutions of the system of simultaneous equations

$$L_x(x, y, \lambda) = 0$$
$$L_y(x, y, \lambda) = 0$$
$$L_\lambda(x, y, \lambda) = 0 \qquad [\text{this is just } g(x, y) = 0]$$

We assume that all indicated partial derivatives exist.

Example 1

Constrained Optimization Find the maximum and the minimum values of

$$z = x + 3y$$

where x and y satisfy the side condition

$$x^2 + y^2 = 1$$

Solution Geometrically, we seek to find the highest and lowest points on the plane

$$z = x + 3y$$

that also lies on the cylinder

$$x^2 + y^2 = 1$$

Think of slicing the inner cardboard core of a roll of paper towels at an angle. When the core is held vertically, the highest and lowest points on the core's cut will be analogous to the maximum and the minimum points. (See Figure 27.)

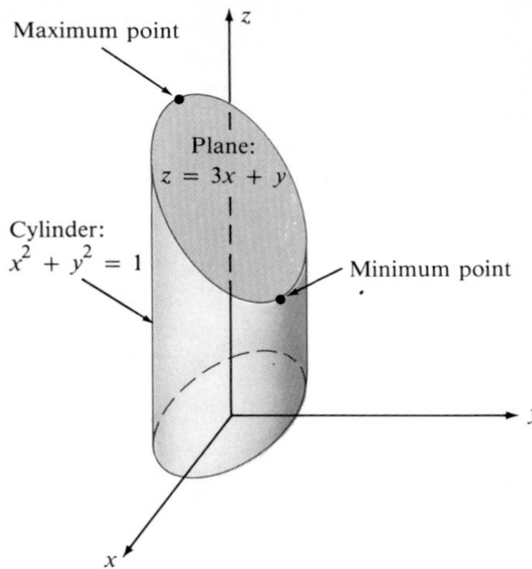

Figure 27
Constrained maximum and minimum problem

- **Step 1** (define the Lagrange function). We begin by writing the Lagrange function

$$\begin{aligned} L(x, y, \lambda) &= f(x, y) + \lambda g(x, y) \\ &= x + 3y + \lambda(x^2 + y^2 - 1) \end{aligned}$$

  Note that the constraint $x^2 + y^2 = 1$ is written in the Lagrange function as $x^2 + y^2 - 1$ (and not $x^2 + y^2$).

- **Step 2** (solve the equations $L_x = 0$, $L_y = 0$, $L_\lambda = 0$). Computing the partial derivatives L_x, L_y, and L_λ, we have

$$L_x(x, y, \lambda) = \frac{\partial}{\partial x}[(x + 3y) + \lambda(x^2 + y^2 - 1)] = 1 + 2x\lambda$$

$$L_y(x, y, \lambda) = \frac{\partial}{\partial y}[(x + 3y) + \lambda(x^2 + y^2 - 1)] = 3 + 2y\lambda$$

$$L_\lambda(x, y, \lambda) = x^2 + y^2 - 1$$

  Setting these partial derivatives to zero, we have

$$\begin{aligned} L_x(x, y, \lambda) &= 1 + 2x\lambda = 0 \\ L_y(x, y, \lambda) &= 3 + 2y\lambda = 0 \\ L_\lambda(x, y, \lambda) &= x^2 + y^2 - 1 = 0 \qquad \text{(constraint equation)} \end{aligned}$$

These equations are nonlinear algebraic equations and cannot be solved by using the usual methods for solving systems of linear equations. In this problem (and in many problems of this kind) the strategy is to solve for x and y in terms of the Lagrange multiplier λ in the two equations $L_x = 0$ and $L_y = 0$. Doing this, we find

$$x = -\frac{1}{2\lambda}$$

$$y = -\frac{3}{2\lambda}$$

Substituting these values into the constraint equation

$$x^2 + y^2 = 1$$

we obtain

$$\frac{1}{4\lambda^2} + \frac{9}{4\lambda^2} = 1$$

Solving for λ, we get

$$\lambda = \pm\frac{1}{2}\sqrt{10}$$

Now, by direct substitution of these values into the above equations for x and y, we get the two critical points of $L(x, y, \lambda)$:

$$\text{Critical point 1} = (x_0, y_0, \lambda_0) = \left(-\frac{1}{\sqrt{10}}, -\frac{3}{\sqrt{10}}, \frac{\sqrt{10}}{2}\right)$$

$$\text{Critical point 2} = (x_0, y_0, \lambda_0) = \left(\frac{1}{\sqrt{10}}, \frac{3}{\sqrt{10}}, -\frac{\sqrt{10}}{2}\right)$$

- **Step 3** (interpret the results). The values of the Lagrange multiplier λ_0 were needed so that the values of x_0 and y_0 could be found. However, once the values of x_0 and y_0 are known, the values of λ_0 can be ignored. We conclude that the two points

$$\left(-\frac{1}{\sqrt{10}}, -\frac{3}{\sqrt{10}}\right) \quad \text{and} \quad \left(\frac{1}{\sqrt{10}}, \frac{3}{\sqrt{10}}\right)$$

are the only candidates for relative maximum and minimum points of the constrained optimization problem. If we remember the physical analogy of slicing the inner core of a roll of paper towels (Figure 27), then it is clear that the maximum value of $z = x + 3y$ will occur at one of these points and the minimum value at the other point. By simply evaluating $z = x + 3y$ at these two points we find that the larger value occurs at the point

$$\left(\frac{1}{\sqrt{10}}, \frac{3}{\sqrt{10}}\right)$$

Hence we conclude that

$$\text{Maximum point} = \left(\frac{1}{\sqrt{10}}, \frac{3}{\sqrt{10}}\right) \qquad \text{Maximum value} = \frac{10}{\sqrt{10}}$$

$$\text{Minimum point} = \left(-\frac{1}{\sqrt{10}}, -\frac{3}{\sqrt{10}}\right) \qquad \text{Minimum value} = -\frac{10}{\sqrt{10}}$$

□

We summarize the steps that should be carried out when using the Lagrange multiplier method.

Steps in the Lagrange Method

To find candidates for the relative maximum and minimum points of $f(x, y)$ subject to the constraint

$$g(x, y) = 0$$

perform the following steps.

Step 1. Write the Lagrange function

$$L(x, y, \lambda) = f(x, y) + \lambda g(x, y)$$

Step 2. Solve the system of equations

$$L_x(x, y, \lambda) = 0$$
$$L_y(x, y, \lambda) = 0$$
$$L_\lambda(x, y, \lambda) = 0 \qquad [\text{same as } g(x, y) = 0]$$

Step 3. Interpret the results. The relative maximum and minimum points (x_0, y_0) for $z = f(x, y)$ subject to $g(x, y) = 0$ will be among the solutions (x_0, y_0, λ_0) of the three equations listed in Step 2 (among the critical points of the Lagrange function).

Comments on Lagrange's Method

Note that the Lagrange function $L(x, y, \lambda)$ is a function of *three* variables, and hence we cannot find its maximum and minimum points by using the discriminant function as we did in the previous section. (In that section we found maximum and minimum points of functions of *two* variables.) The power of Lagrange's method lies in its ability to find candidates for maximum and minimum points of constrained problems. It does not say, "This is a maximum point or this is a minimum point," as did the discriminant function of the previous section.

Sometimes, if the functions $f(x, y)$ and $g(x, y)$ are fairly simple, a rough graph might be drawn to determine whether a critical point is a relative maximum or minimum point. Also, by evaluating the function $f(x, y)$ at the points that are candidates for relative maximum and minimum points and at nearby points (nearby points that satisfy $g(x, y) = 0$) it is often possible to determine which points are relative maximum points and which points are relative minimum points.

Example 2

Lagrange Multiplier Method Find the absolute maximum value of

$$f(x, y) = xy$$

subject to the constraint

$$x + y = 4$$

Solution

- **Step 1** (find the Lagrange function). The Lagrange function is

$$L(x, y, \lambda) = f(x, y) + \lambda g(x, y)$$
$$= xy + \lambda(x + y - 4)$$

- **Step 2** (solve the equations $L_x = 0$, $L_y = 0$, $L_\lambda = 0$). Computing the partial derivatives L_x, L_y, and L_λ and setting them to zero, we have

$$L_x(x, y, \lambda) = y + \lambda = 0$$
$$L_y(x, y, \lambda) = x + \lambda = 0$$
$$L_\lambda(x, y, \lambda) = x + y - 4 = 0$$

Solving these equations for x, y, and λ, we have

$$x = 2$$
$$y = 2$$
$$\lambda = -2$$

- **Step 3** (interpret the results). The only critical point or candidate for a relative maximum or minimum point is (2, 2). To determine whether (2, 2) is a relative maximum or minimum point, we evaluate the objective function

$$z = xy$$

at this point and at several nearby points (points that satisfy $x + y = 4$). Table 8 shows the results of these computations. The values lead us to believe that (2, 2) is the absolute maximum point and that $z = 4$ is the absolute maximum value. □

TABLE 8
Value of an Objective Function in a Neighborhood of a Critical Point

Point on $x + y = 4$	Value of $z = xy$	
(0, 4)	0	
(0.5, 3.5)	1.75	
(1, 3)	3.00	
(1.5, 2.5)	3.75	
(2, 2)	**4.00**	← *Maximum value*
(2.5, 1.5)	3.75	
(3, 1)	3.00	
(3.5, 0.5)	1.75	
(4, 0)	0	

Consumer or Utility Theory in Economics

Suppose that you are in a bakery that has just replenished its shelves with fresh doughnuts, cookies, cakes, and pies. The major problem for you is to decide what to buy. The secondary problem is that you have only $1.00 to spend. You, the consumer, are trying to maximize your pleasure (or, as economists say, utility) under given budgetary constraints. You are not the first person to face such a problem. In fact, millions of people try to solve some variation of this problem every day. No doubt you have tried to solve a similar problem already today.

In consumer theory, economists try to determine how consumers should spend a given amount of their money to maximize what economists call "**utility**." For instance, would you be happier (get more utility) spending your dollar on three doughnuts, or on two doughnuts and a cookie, or on one doughnut and two cookies, or some other possibility?

To make these ideas more precise, assume that a consumer has the option to buy two products, which we call Product A and Product B. We denote

$$x = \text{Number of units of Product A purchased}$$
$$y = \text{Number of units of Product B purchased}$$

Suppose that the cost of each product is given by

$$c_1 = \text{Cost per unit of Product A}$$
$$c_2 = \text{Cost per unit of Product B}$$

Under these circumstances, economists define a **utility function** $U(x, y)$ that gives a "measure" of the desirability of purchasing x and y units of the two products. Although a utility function is not as precise a measurement as other quantitative concepts, such as profit, revenue, and cost, general qualitative results can be obtained from an analysis of this function. Some typical utility functions of two variables that economists have found useful are the following:

$$U(x, y) = \ln x + \ln y \qquad \text{(logarithmic utility)}$$
$$U(x, y) = x + y \qquad \text{(linear utility)}$$
$$U(x, y) = x + y - 0.05x^2 - 0.05y^2 \qquad \text{(quadratic utility)}$$

Note that each of these utility functions will increase as the consumer buys more and more of the two products (although the quadratic utility will eventually start to decrease).

Quite often a consumer's utility will start to increase at a fast rate as the consumer starts buying but will grow at a slower rate for larger values of x and y. What this means is that although the consumer will always receive more "enjoyment" for larger purchases, the enjoyment is not proportional to the amount of goods bought. For instance, a consumer might get a great deal of enjoyment from eating the first doughnut, but not twice as much from eating two doughnuts, and certainly not ten times as much enjoyment from eating ten doughnuts (at least for most people). With this general concept of the utility function a typical problem in consumer or utility theory is to maximize a utility function subject to the budgetary constraint that the total amount of money spent by the consumer is some fixed amount. Mathematically, we can state the consumer problem as finding x and y in order to

$$\text{maximize} \quad U(x, y)$$

where x and y are subject to the budgetary constraint

$$c_1x + c_2y = M$$

with c_1 and c_2 defined as above and

$$M = \text{Total amount of money the consumer has to spend}$$

We illustrate this idea with the following example.

Example 3

Utility Theory Hannah has \$50 to spend. She has decided to spend it on record albums and computer diskettes. She has determined that her utility from the purchase of x record albums and y boxes of computer diskettes is

$$U(x, y) = 3 \ln x + \ln y$$

where

$$\text{Cost per record album} = \$6$$
$$\text{Cost per box of computer diskettes} = \$4$$

How many record albums and boxes of computer diskettes should Hannah buy to maximize her utility while at the same time spending a total amount of \$50?

Solution We must find the purchase levels x and y that maximize

$$U(x, y) = 3 \ln x + \ln y$$

subject to the spending constraint

$$6x + 4y = 50$$

- **Step 1** (find the Lagrange function). The Lagrange function is

$$\begin{aligned} L(x, y, \lambda) &= U(x, y) + \lambda g(x, y) \\ &= 3 \ln x + \ln y + \lambda(6x + 4y - 50) \end{aligned}$$

- **Step 2** (solve the equations $L_x = 0$, $L_y = 0$, and $L_\lambda = 0$). Computing the partial derivatives L_x, L_y, and L_λ and setting them to zero, we have

$$L_x(x, y, \lambda) = \frac{3}{x} + 6\lambda = 0$$

$$L_y(x, y, \lambda) = \frac{1}{y} + 4\lambda = 0$$

$$L_\lambda(x, y, \lambda) = 6x + 4y - 50 = 0$$

Solving for x and y in the first two equations in terms of λ, we find

$$x = -\frac{1}{2\lambda}$$

$$y = -\frac{1}{4\lambda}$$

Substituting these values into the third (constraint) equation

$$6x + 4y - 50 = 0$$

gives

$$-\frac{6}{2\lambda} - \frac{4}{4\lambda} = 50$$

or

$$\lambda_0 = -\frac{2}{25}$$

Finally, substituting this value of λ_0 back into the previous equations for x and y in terms of λ gives the values of x_0 and y_0:

$$x_0 = \frac{25}{4} = 6.250$$

and

$$y_0 = \frac{25}{8} = 3.125$$

Hence the candidate for a constrained maximum point is (6.250, 3.125).

- **Step 3** (interpret the results). By evaluating the utility function $U(x, y)$ at nearby points on the line

$$6x + 4y = 50$$

we convince ourselves that the utility function attains its relative maximum value at the point (6.250, 3.125).

Interpretation: Hannah should purchase 6.25 record albums and 3.125 boxes of computer diskettes to maximize her utility while at the same time spending exactly \$50. (You can check to see that Hannah has spent exactly \$50.) Of course, it is impossible to purchase either a fractional number of record albums or a fractional number of boxes of computer diskettes. Hannah would have to resolve this dilemma by rounding off to some integer values (as long as she does not overspend her \$50). Generally, in utility theory the numbers are only meant to give a rough guide to the spending strategy and not meant to be read to the last decimal. Hannah might conclude that six record albums and three boxes of computer diskettes would be appropriate.

Also note that the value of the utility function at the relative maximum point is

$$\begin{aligned} U(6.25, 3.125) &= 3 \ln (6.25) + \ln (3.125) \\ &= 6.64 \end{aligned}$$

This relative maximum value of $U(x, y)$ is not significant in our analysis. The more important aspect of this problem to economists is the point (6.25, 3.125).

□

Problems

For Problems 1–10, find the critical point(s) for the functions such that the given constraint is satisfied.

	Function	Constraint
1.	$f(x, y) = x + 2xy$	$x - y = 3$
2.	$f(x, y) = -3x - 2y$	$x + xy = 1$
3.	$f(x, y) = 2x - y$	$x^2 - 2y^2 = 3$
4.	$f(x, y) = 5x + 3y + 4$	$x^2 + y^2 = 1$
5.	$f(x, y) = x^2 - y^2$	$x^2 - 2y^2 = 3$
6.	$f(x, y) = 2x^2 - 3y^2 + 2xy$	$x + 3y = 5$
7.	$f(x, y) = x^2 + y^2 + xy$	$x + 2y = 4$
8.	$f(x, y) = x^2 + y^2 - 3x - 4y$	$x^2 + y^2 = 1$
9.	$f(x, y) = 2x^2 - 3y^2 + 5x - 3y$	$3x - 5y = 2$
10.	$f(x, y) = x^2 - y^2 - 3xy$	$5x - 3y = 2$

General Optimization Problems with Constraints

Problems 11–13 concern themselves with finding the optimal shapes of various solids under certain constraints.

11. **Minimum Surface Area.** A box with a square base and a top with volume 125 cubic feet is to be constructed to minimize the surface area. What should be the dimensions of the box?
12. **Maximum Volume.** A box with a square base and no top with surface area of 125 square feet is to be constructed to maximize the volume. What should be the dimensions of the box?
13. **Minimum Surface Area.** A cylindrical tank with an open top has a volume of 256 cubic inches. What should its dimensions be to minimize the surface area? *Note:* Compare this problem to the cat food problem (Section 2.4).

Constrained Optimization Problems in Business

14. **Cobb-Douglas Production Function.** Maximize the Cobb-Douglas production function

$$u(x, y) = x^{1/2}y^{1/2}$$

in the case when the resources that are available satisfy the constraint

$$7x + 3y = 84$$

15. **Minimum Cost.** The cost of producing x units of Product A and y units of Product B is given by

$$C(x, y) = 100 + 3x^2 + 5y^2$$

The production capacity for both products together is 75 units. How many units of each product should be produced to minimize costs?

16. **Doughnuts Versus Cookies.** George is trying to decide how many doughnuts and cookies to buy. Each doughnut costs \$0.35, and each cookie costs \$0.25. He decides that his "index of enjoyment" or utility function is

$$U(x, y) = \ln x + \ln y$$

where

$$x = \text{Number of doughnuts he buys}$$

$$y = \text{Number of cookies he buys}$$

If George can spend \$1.50, how many doughnuts and cookies should he buy to maximize his pleasure?

17. **Maximizing a Logarithmic Utility Function.** A consumer's utility function is given by

$$U(x, y) = 2 \ln x + \ln y$$

with budget constraints

$$2x + 4y = 50$$

Find the values of x and y that maximize the utility function, subject to the budgetary constraints.

18. **Marginal Utility of Money.** In the consumer problem the value of the Lagrange multiplier λ is called by economists the **marginal utility of money**. Find the marginal utility of money for Problem 17. It can be shown that the marginal utility of money is the change in the optimal value of the utility with respect to the total amount of money spent. In other words, if the total amount spent of \$50 in Problem 17 were to be increased to \$51, then the change in the maximum utility would be approximately equal to the marginal utility of money (or the value of the Lagrange multiplier λ).
19. **Consumer Problem.** A consumer's utility function is given by

$$U(x, y) = xy$$

with budgetary constraints

$$5x + 10y = 100$$

Find the values of x and y that maximize this utility function subject to the budgetary constraint. What is the marginal utility of money? (See Problem 18 for the definition of marginal utility.)

20. **General Consumer Problem.** A consumer's utility function is given by

$$U(x, y) = xy$$

with budgetary constraints

$$c_1x + c_2y = M$$

Find the values of x and y that maximize this utility function subject to the general constraints. The answers, of course, will depend on c_1, c_2, and M.

Max/Min Problems Solved by the Lagrange Multiplier Technique

Back in Section 2.4, Optimization Problems (Max–Min Problems), we maximized (and minimized) functions of two variables, where the variables were related by a constraint equation. We solved those problems by solving the constraint equation for one variable and then substituting that value into the function to be maximized (or minimized). In that way we reduced the maximizing (or minimizing) function to a function of only one variable. It is possible to solve those same problems by the method of Lagrange multipliers.

For Problems 21–32, solve the indicated problems in Section 2.4 using Lagrange multipliers.

21. Solve Problem 1 (Maximum Product).
22. Solve Problem 2 (Minimum Sum of Squares).
23. Solve Problem 3 (Constrained Maximum).
24. Solve Problem 11 (Optimal Pricing).
25. Solve Problem 14 (Minimum-Cost Box).
26. Solve Problem 16 (Minimum Surface Area).
27. Solve Problem 18 (Maximum Volume).
28. Solve Problem 20 (Minimum-Cost Box).
29. Solve Problem 21 (Wire Problem).
30. Solve Problem 26 (Maximum Surface Area).
31. Solve Problem 27 (Telephone Lines).
32. Solve Problem 31 (Maximum Area of Field).

Some Interesting Container Problems

33. Harry's Chocolate Box. Harry is trying to win a trip to Disneyland by entering a contest sponsored by the Cholesterol Chocolate Company. The goal is to design a 48-cubic-inch rectangular box with no top and a partition down the middle that contains the least amount of material (surface area on the bottom, outsides, and partition). In other words, how should Harry pick the length (l), width (w), and height (h) of the box shown in Figure 28 such that the total surface area of the bottom, sides, and partition is minimized but the volume of the box (we assume that the partition doesn't take up any space in the box) is fixed at 48 cubic inches?

(a) What is your guess for the dimensions of the minimum surface area box? We will see whether your guess is close to optimal.

(b) Use calculus to find the dimensions of the box that require the least amount of material. How many square inches of material are actually required to make this box of minimum surface area?

34. Harry's New Box. Harry won the trip to Disneyland described in Problem 33 and is now trying to win a trip to Disney World. To win this new contest, he must design a topless rectangular box with a volume of 576 cubic inches similar in design to the one shown in Figure 29 with the least amount of material. In other words, he is seeking the length (l), width (w), and height (h) of the box that minimize the total surface area of the bottom, outsides, and partitions.

(a) What is your guess for the dimension of the minimum surface area box? We will see whether your guess is optimal.

(b) Use calculus to find the dimensions of the box that require the least amount of material. How many square inches of material are actually required to make this box of minimum surface area?

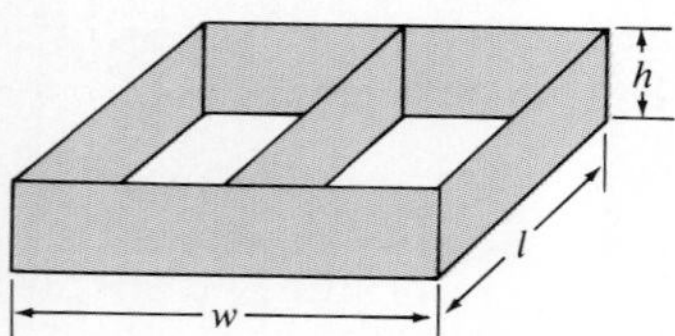

Figure 28
What is your guess for the dimensions of a box of this design with a volume of 48 cubic inches using minimum material?

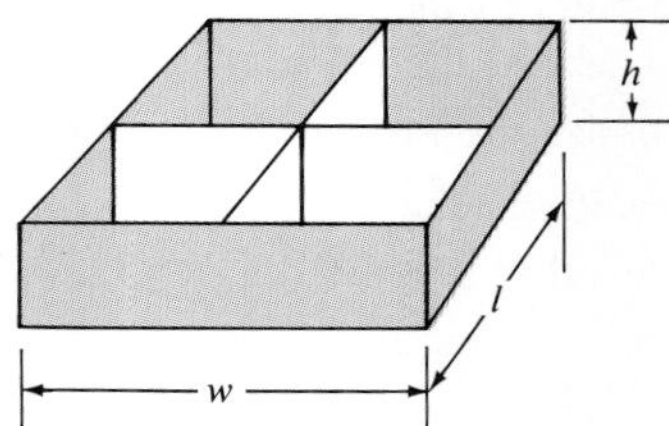

Figure 29
What is your guess for the dimensions of a box of this design with a volume of 576 cubic inches using minimum material?

6.5 Curve Fitting (Least Squares)

PURPOSE

We will show how to "fit" a first-order polynomial (straight line) to a set of data points by the method of least squares. To find this line, we will need to solve an unconstrained optimization problem.

Introduction

The reader might wonder how economists and management scientists determine the formulas for revenue, cost, and profit that are used in the theory of the firm. For example, how does a management scientist know that the cost $C(q)$ to produce q items of a given product is a given quadratic polynomial, say,

$$C(q) = 5q - 0.01q^2$$

Or how is it determined that the profit from the manufacture of q items of a product is

$$P(q) = 10q - 0.2q^2$$

One way to find a **mathematical model** (equation) that describes real-world situations is to approximate observed data points by some type of "approximating" curve. We often say that we "fit a curve" to the observed data points.

For example, Table 9 gives the daily cost to produce q typewriters at a given factory. By plotting the values in Table 9 on graph paper (Figure 30) it is possible to see a general trend. It appears that these data points lie more or less on some quadratic polynomial. By carrying out a least squares analysis, the best (least squares) quadratic approximation is

$$C(q) = 10{,}000 + 0.10q^2$$

TABLE 9
Daily Cost to Produce a Given Number of Typewriters

Number of Typewriters Produced	Total Daily Cost
0	\$10,000
100	\$11,250
200	\$14,150
300	\$18,800
400	\$26,100
500	\$34,900

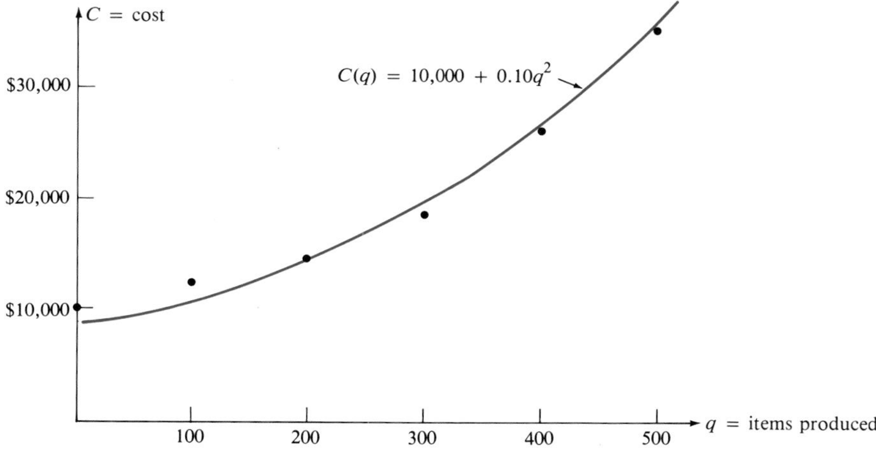

Figure 30
A least squares quadratic approximation of some data points

We will show how to approximate data points by linear polynomials. The same ideas are used to approximate polynomials of higher degree.

First-Order Least Squares Approximation

Suppose the year is 1993 and you have just accepted a challenging position in the operations research department of a major corporation. The net income for this company for the three years 1991–1993 is shown in Figure 31. Your job is to forecast the net income for 1994.

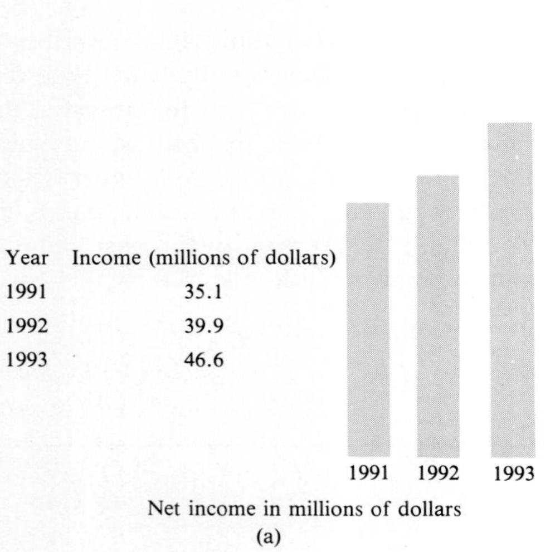

Year	Income (millions of dollars)
1991	35.1
1992	39.9
1993	46.6

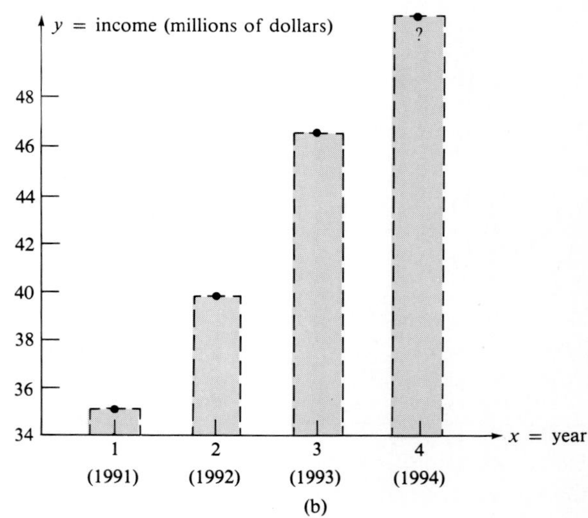

Figure 31
Typical business data

We call the observations in Figure 31 (x_1, y_1), (x_2, y_2), and (x_3, y_3) where it is convenient to denote the years 1991–1993 by the numbers 1, 2, and 3, respectively (Figure 31b).

Year	**Income (millions)**
$x_1 = 1(1991)$	$y_1 = 35.1$
$x_2 = 2(1992)$	$y_2 = 39.9$
$x_3 = 3(1993)$	$y_3 = 46.6$

The goal is to approximate these observations with a first-order polynomial of the form

$$y = ax + b$$

See Figure 32.

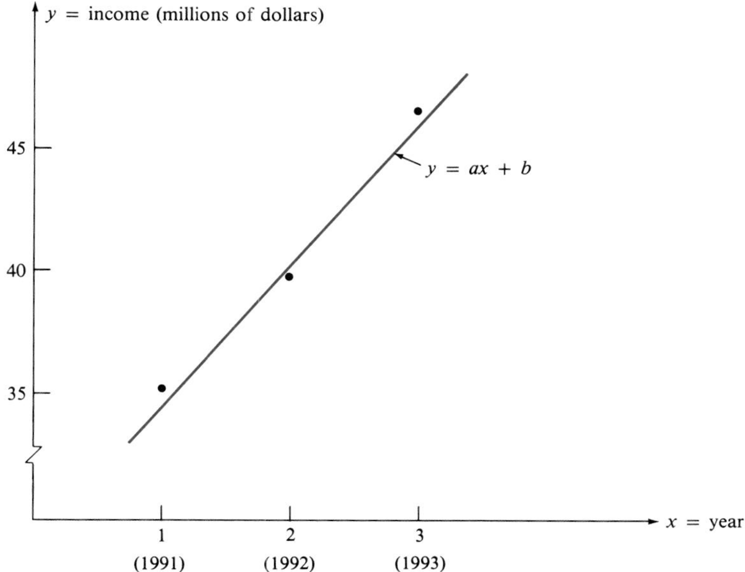

Figure 32
First-order least squares approximation

To find a line that approximates these observations, it is always possible to simply use a ruler and draw by hand a straight line that "passes down the middle" of the points. A more exacting procedure, however, is the **method of least squares**. The least squares strategy picks the specific line that minimizes the sum of squares of the vertical distances from the data points to the points on the line. For instance, to find the least squares line

$$y = ax + b$$

that approximates the three given data points

$$\begin{aligned}(x_1, y_1) &= (1, 35.1)\\(x_2, y_2) &= (2, 39.9)\\(x_3, y_3) &= (3, 46.6)\end{aligned}$$

we define the three **residuals** r_1, r_2, and r_3. The residuals are the vertical distances between the data points y_1, y_2, and y_3 and the points on the straight line. That is,

$$\begin{aligned}r_1 &= y_1 - (ax_1 + b) = 35.1 - (a + b)\\r_2 &= y_2 - (ax_2 + b) = 39.9 - (2a + b)\\r_3 &= y_3 - (ax_3 + b) = 46.6 - (3a + b)\end{aligned}$$

The residuals represent discrepancies or "errors" between the data points and the points on the line as shown in Figure 33.

The goal of the method of least squares is to find the constants a and b in the function $y = ax + b$ that minimize the sum of squares of the residuals

$$S = r_1{}^2 + r_2{}^2 + r_3{}^2$$

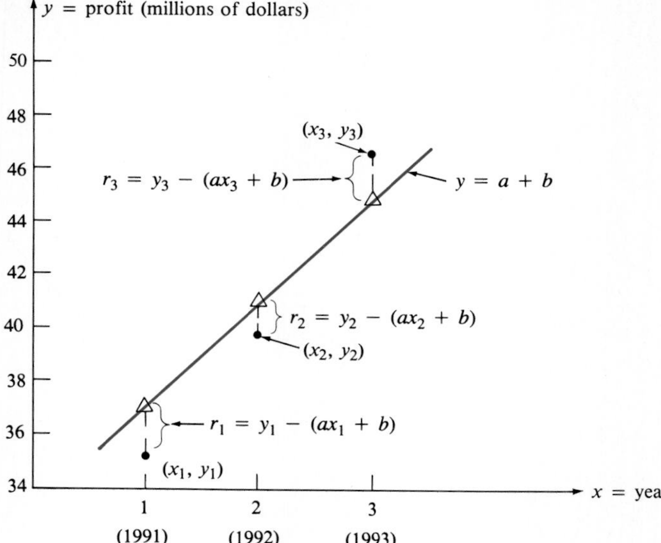

Figure 33
A linear least squares curve showing the residuals, which measure the difference between the data points and the least squares curve

It is important to realize that S is a function of the two variables a and b. This can be seen more clearly by substituting the values for $r_1{}^2$, $r_2{}^2$, and $r_3{}^2$ into S. Doing this, we get

$$\begin{aligned} S(a, b) &= r_1{}^2 + r_2{}^2 + r_3{}^2 \\ &= [y_1 - (ax_1 + b)]^2 + [y_2 - (ax_2 + b)]^2 + [y_3 - (ax_3 + b)]^2 \\ &= [35.1 - (a + b)]^2 + [39.9 - (2a + b)]^2 + [46.6 - (3a + b)]^2 \end{aligned}$$

The reader should realize that $S(a, b)$ is a quadratic polynomial in the variables a and b. The reader could square each of the three terms in $S(a, b)$ and simplify the resulting expression to see this.

The problem now is to find the values of a and b that minimize $S(a, b)$. This problem is an unconstrained optimization problem of the kind we have seen before. To find the minimum point (a, b), we find the critical points by taking the partial derivatives of $S(a, b)$ with respect to a and b. Using the chain rule, we get

$$\begin{aligned} \frac{\partial S}{\partial a} &= 2[35.1 - (a + b)](-1) + 2[39.9 - (2a + b)](-2) + 2[46.6 - (3a + b)](-3) \\ &= 28a + 12b - 509.4 \end{aligned}$$

$$\begin{aligned} \frac{\partial S}{\partial b} &= 2[35.1 - (a + b)](-1) + 2[39.9 - (2a + b)](-1) + 2[46.6 - (3a + b)](-1) \\ &= 12a + 6b - 243.2 \end{aligned}$$

Setting these derivatives to zero, we get

$$\begin{aligned} 28a + 12b &= 509.4 \\ 12a + 6b &= 243.2 \end{aligned}$$

Finally, solving for a and b, we find the only critical point

$$a = 5.75$$
$$b = 29.03$$

Although we will not carry out the second-partials test here, it can be used to confirm that this critical point is in fact a relative minimum point. It can also be shown that this point

$$(a, b) = (5.75, 29.03)$$

is the absolute minimum point of $S(a, b)$. Hence the least squares line is given by

$$\begin{aligned} y &= ax + b \\ &= 5.75x + 29.03 \end{aligned}$$

This line in drawn in Figure 34.

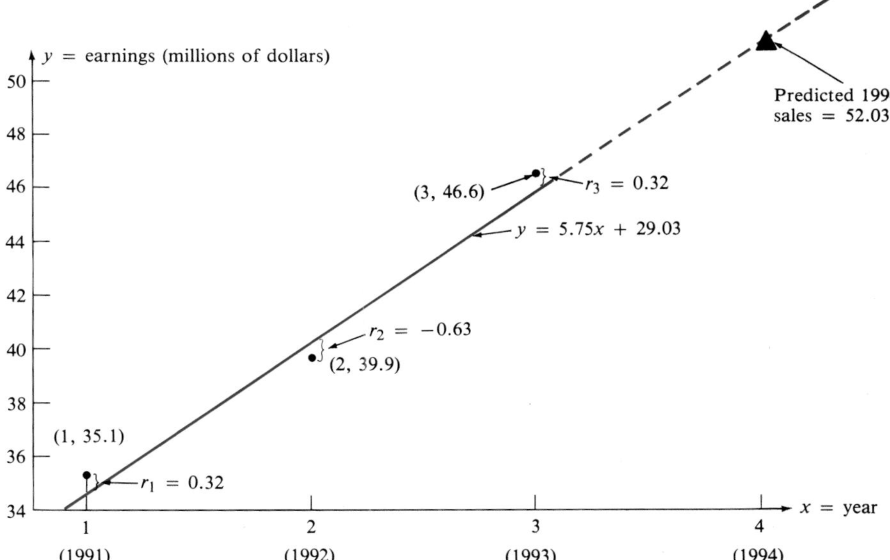

Figure 34
Least squares line passing under two data points and above the other points

Interpretation

The least squares line shown in Figure 34 will have a smaller sum of squares of residuals than any other straight line. The actual value of this minimum sum of squares can be found by direct substitution into the equation for S and is

$$S(5.75, 29.03) = 0.60$$

This number provides a measure of how well the line "fits" the data points. If the data points were all lying on a straight line, then the least squares line would pass exactly through all of these points, and the minimum value of $S(a, b)$ would be zero.

The forecasted income for the company in 1994 ($x = 4$) is

$$\begin{aligned} y &= ax + b \\ &= 5.75(4) + 29.03 \\ &= 52.03 \quad \text{million dollars} \end{aligned}$$

The above analysis can be carried out for any number of data points (x_1, y_1), $(x_2, y_2), \ldots, (x_n, y_n)$ with the following results.

Least Squares Line

The first-order least squares approximation to the n points (x_1, y_1), $(x_2, y_2), \ldots, (x_n, y_n)$ is given by

$$y = ax + b$$

where

$$a = \frac{(\sum x_i)(\sum y_i) - n \sum x_i y_i}{(\sum x_i)^2 - n(\sum x_i^2)}$$

$$b = \frac{\sum y_i - a(\sum x_i)}{n}$$

and

$$\begin{aligned} \textstyle\sum x_i &= \text{Sum of the } x \text{ values} \\ \textstyle\sum y_i &= \text{Sum of the } y \text{ values} \\ \textstyle\sum x_i y_i &= \text{Sum of the } x \text{ values times the } y \text{ values} \\ \textstyle\sum x_i^2 &= \text{Sum of squares of the } x \text{ values} \end{aligned}$$

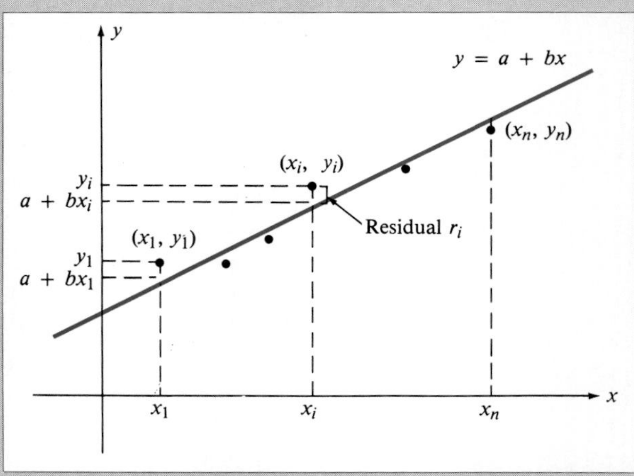

Example 1

Least Squares Fit Find the least squares line $y = ax + b$ that best fits the eight data points in Table 10.

TABLE 10
Observed Data Points

x	y
1.23	0.70
1.93	0.77
2.40	0.93
3.10	1.14
3.70	1.26
4.50	1.51
5.70	1.76
6.30	1.89

Solution To use the formula for finding the least squares line, it is convenient to construct Table 11.

TABLE 11

i	x_i	y_i	x_i^2	x_iy_i
1	1.23	0.70	1.51	0.86
2	1.93	0.77	3.72	1.49
3	2.40	0.93	5.76	2.23
4	3.10	1.14	9.61	3.53
5	3.70	1.26	13.69	4.66
6	4.50	1.51	20.25	6.79
7	5.70	1.76	32.49	10.03
8	6.30	1.89	39.69	11.91
Totals:	$\sum x_i = 28.86$	$\sum y_i = 9.96$	$\sum x_i^2 = 126.72$	$\sum x_iy_i = 41.50$

Using the least squares formulas for a and b, we have

$$
\begin{aligned}
a &= \frac{(\sum x_i)(\sum y_i) - n(\sum x_iy_i)}{(\sum x_i)^2 - n(\sum x_i^2)} \\
&= \frac{(28.86)(9.96) - 8(41.50)}{(28.86)^2 - 8(126.72)} \\
&= 0.25 \\
b &= \frac{(\sum y_i) - a(\sum x_i)}{n} \\
&= \frac{9.96 - 0.25(28.86)}{8} \\
&= 0.34
\end{aligned}
$$

Hence the least squares line is

$$y = 0.25x + 0.34$$

This line is drawn in Figure 35. Using a calculator, we can easily compute the residuals in Figure 35 at each of the data points, as shown in Table 12.

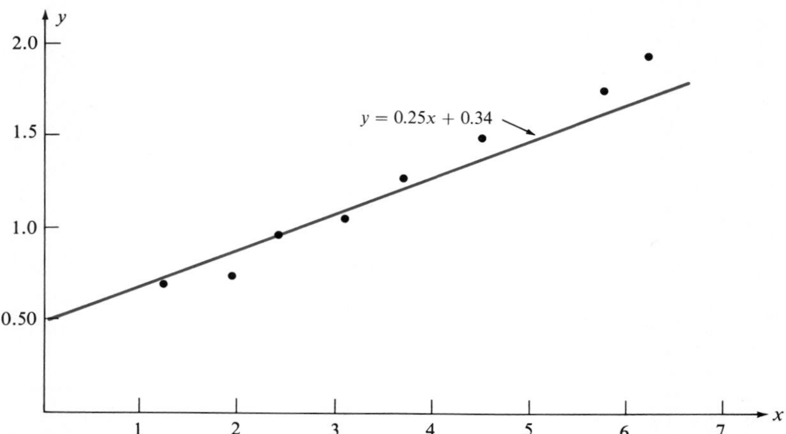

Figure 35
A least squares line

TABLE 12
Predicted Values and Errors

Observed x_i	**Observed** y_i	**Predicted** $Y_i = 0.25x_i + 0.34$	**Residuals** $r_i = y_i - Y_i$	**Squared Residual**
1.23	0.70	0.65	0.05	0.0025
1.93	0.77	0.82	−0.05	0.0025
2.40	0.93	0.94	−0.01	0.0001
3.10	1.14	1.11	0.03	0.0009
3.70	1.26	1.26	0	0
4.50	1.51	1.46	0.05	0.0025
5.70	1.76	1.76	0	0
6.30	1.89	1.92	−0.03	0.0009
		Sum of Squares of Residuals =		0.0094

Example 2

Olympic 100-Meter Freestyle Times Table 13 shows the 100-meter freestyle winning times for men and women in the Olympic Games from 1956 to 1984. On the basis of these data, predict the 1988, 1992, and 1996 winning times for both men and women by modeling these winning times with a first-order least squares approximation.

TABLE 13
Olympic Games 100-Meter Freestyle Winning Times

Year	Men: Winner		Men: Time (sec)	Women: Winner		Women: Time (sec)
1956	Hendricks	(Aus.)	55.4	Fraser	(Aus.)	62.0
1960	Devitt	(Aus.)	55.2	Fraser	(Aus.)	61.2
1964	Schollander	(U.S.)	53.4	Fraser	(Aus.)	59.5
1968	Wenden	(Aus.)	52.2	Henne	(U.S.)	60.0
1972	Spitz	(U.S.)	51.22	Neilsen	(U.S.)	58.59
1976	Montgomery	(U.S.)	49.99	Ender	(G.D.R.)	55.65
1980	Wothe	(G.D.R.)	50.40	Krauss	(G.D.R.)	54.79
1984	Gaines	(U.S.)	49.80	Steinseifer	(U.S.)	55.92

Solution It is convenient to relabel the years as $x = 1$ (1956), $x = 2$ (1960), . . . , $x = 11$ (1996). We begin by constructing Table 14. From these values we first find the men's least squares line:

TABLE 14
Computations for Finding the Least Squares Line

Men				Women			
x_i	y_i	x_i^2	x_iy_i	x_i	y_i	x_i^2	x_iy_i
1	55.4	1	55.4	1	62.0	1	62.0
2	55.2	4	110.4	2	61.2	4	122.4
3	53.4	9	160.2	3	59.5	9	178.5
4	52.2	16	208.8	4	60.0	16	240.0
5	51.22	25	256.10	5	58.59	25	292.95
6	49.99	36	299.94	6	55.65	36	333.90
7	50.40	49	352.80	7	54.79	49	383.53
8	49.80	64	398.40	8	55.92	64	447.36
36	417.61	204	1842.04	36	467.65	204	2060.64

$$
\begin{aligned}
a &= \frac{(\sum x_i)(\sum y_i) - n(\sum x_iy_i)}{(\sum x_i)^2 - n(\sum x_i^2)} \\
&= \frac{(36)(417.61) - (8)(1842.04)}{(36)^2 - (8)(204)} \\
&= -0.89 \\
b &= \frac{(\sum y_i) - a(\sum x_i)}{n} \\
&= \frac{(417.61) - (-0.89)(36)}{8} \\
&= 56.21
\end{aligned}
$$

Hence the least squares line for the men's times is

$$y = -0.89x + 56.21$$

We can carry out the least squares analysis for the women's times in exactly the same way and arrive at the least-squares line

$$y = -1.04x + 63.14$$

The two least squares lines are plotted in Figure 36.

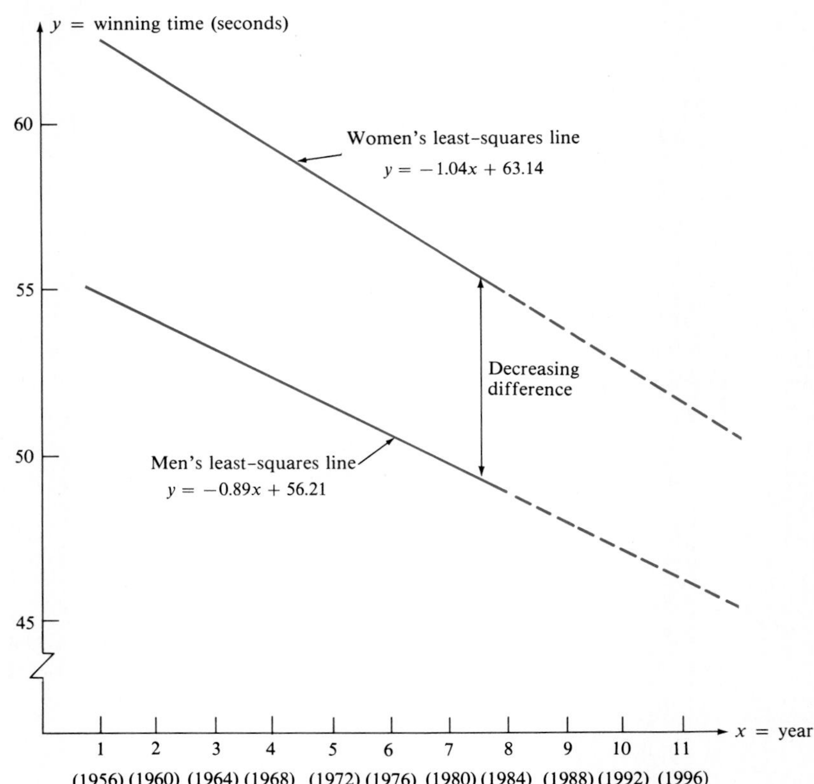

Figure 36
Comparison of mens' and women's Olympic 100-meter freestyle times from 1956 to 1984

If we evaluate the two linear least squares functions for the 1988, 1992, and 1996 Olympic Games, we get the results in Table 15.

TABLE 15
Predicted Olympic 100-Meter Freestyle Times Using a Least Squares Line

Year	Men's Predicted Times (seconds)	Women's Predicted Times (seconds)
1988 ($x = 9$)	48.20	53.78
1992 ($x = 10$)	47.31	52.74
1996 ($x = 11$)	46.42	51.70

Interpretation

One might be tempted to say that if the present trend continues, the women's times in the 100-Meter Freestyle will surpass the men's times (have a lower Olympic record) when $x = 96.2$. This corresponds to 96.2 Olympic Games after the Olympic Games of 1952, or during the Olympic Games of 2142. Whether you believe that this will ever happen depends on whether you believe that the linear model will accurately describe the men's and women's times in the future.

It should be pointed out here that many scientific and business calculators have least squares keys that allow one to enter the data points and then press "a" and "b" keys to find the values in the least squares line $y = ax + b$.

Problems

For Problems 1–4, fill in the tables and use this information to determine the least squares line.

1.

x_i	y_i	x_i^2	x_iy_i
1	3		
2	4		
3	7		
4	9		

2.

x_i	y_i	x_i^2	x_iy_i
−1	3		
1	4		
3	6		
5	4		

3.

x_i	y_i	x_i^2	x_iy_i
−2	−3		
0	4		
1	7		
2	9		

4.

x_i	y_i	x_i^2	x_iy_i
1	3		
2	5		
3	6		
4	8		
5	11		

5. **Finding Residuals.** For the data points and line in Figure 37, find the residuals r_1, r_2, r_3, r_4, and r_5.

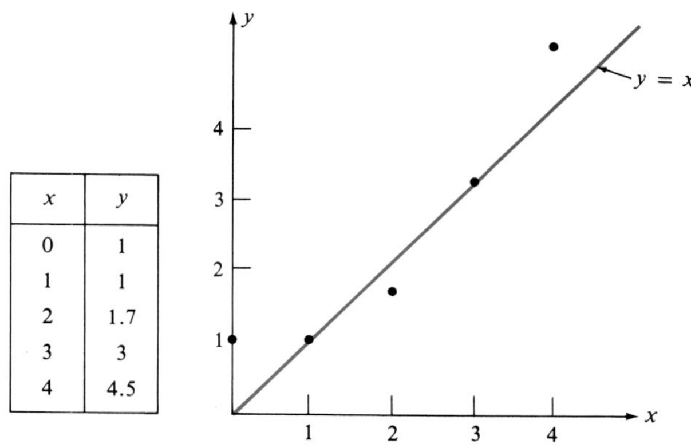

Figure 37
Can you find the residuals?

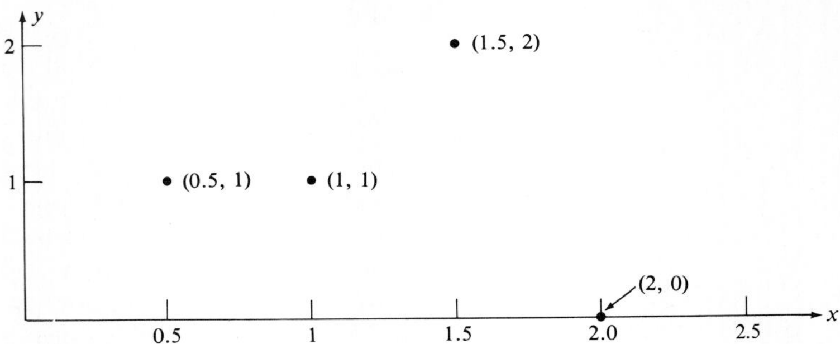

Figure 38
Typical data points

Problems 6–8 refer to the following data points in Figure 38.

6. Find the sum of squares of the residuals for the line $y = x$.
7. Find the sum of squares of the residuals for the line $y = 1$.
8. Find the sum of squares of the residuals for the line $y = 2 - x$.

9. For the data points in Figure 39, which of the lines $y = 1$, $y = 0.5$, or $y = 0$ has the smallest sum of squares of residuals?

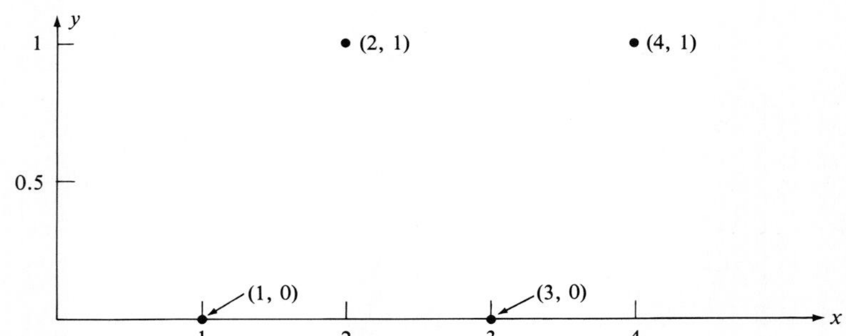

Figure 39
Typical data points

10. **Adequacy of Linear Least Squares Line.** The heights and weights of five men were recorded, and the following results were obtained:

Height (inches)	Weight (pounds)
68	160
70	145
71	190
74	180
75	190

Plot the data points. Do you believe it is possible to fit these data points accurately with a straight line? Why?

11. **Picking the Form of Least Squares Line.** What is the degree of the least squares polynomial that would best describe the phenomena illustrated in Figure 40?

For the observations in Problems 12–18, find the linear least squares line. Plot the data and the least squares line and compute the residuals.

12. (1, 1), (2, 3)
13. (0, 0), (1, 1), (2, 1)
14. (1, 1), (2, 2), (3, 1)
15. (0, 0), (1, 2), (2, 3), (3, 6)
16. (1, 1), (2, 1), (3, 2), (4, 4)
17. (1, 0), (2, 1), (3, 4), (4, 6)
18. (1, 1), (2, 2), (3, 3), (4, 3)
19. **Find the Least Squares Horizontal Line.** Find the least squares line of the form $y = c$ for the three data points (1, 1), (2, 2), and (3, 1). *Hint:* Write the expression for the sum of squares of the residuals and observe that it depends on only one variable c.

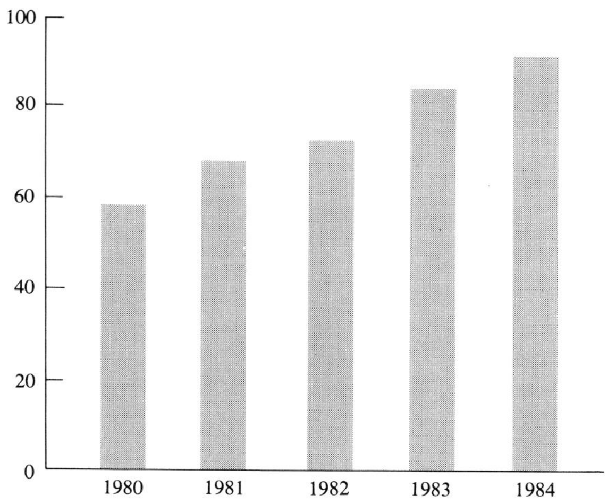

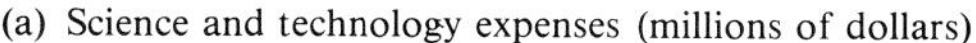
(a) Science and technology expenses (millions of dollars)

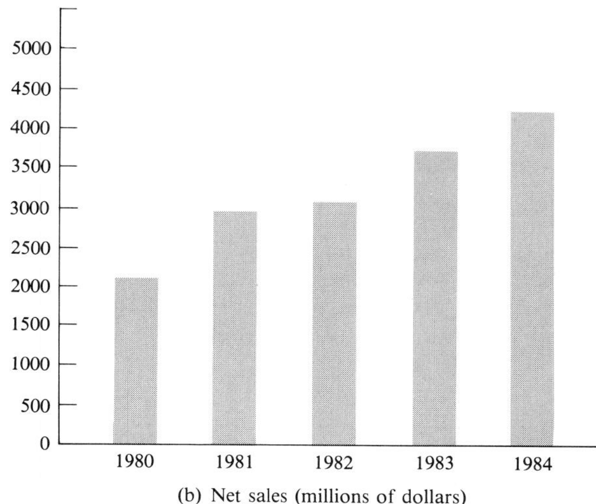

(b) Net sales (millions of dollars)

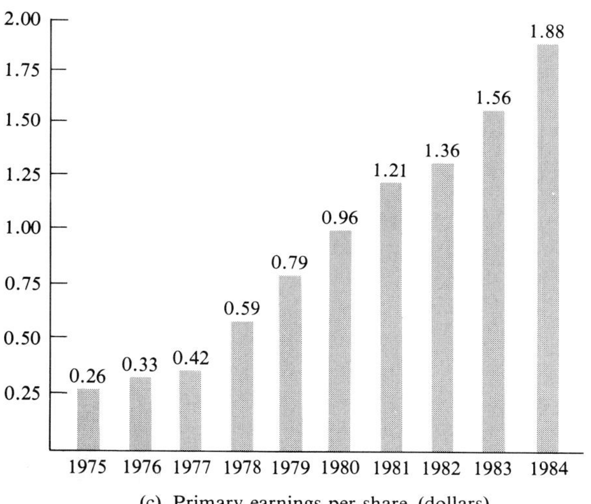

(c) Primary earnings per share (dollars)

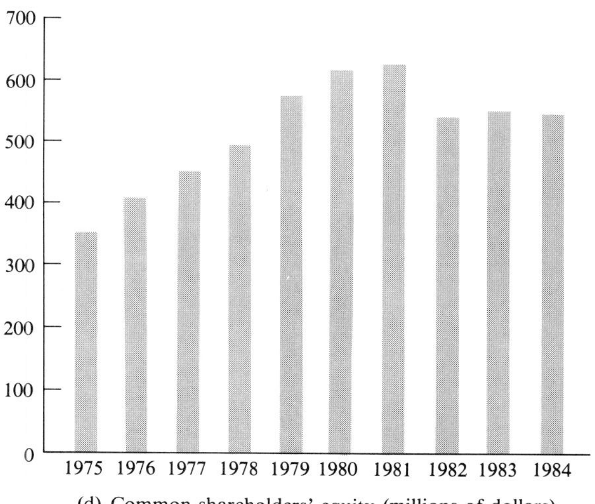

(d) Common shareholders' equity (millions of dollars)

Figure 40
Typical business data

20. Nonlinear Least Squares. Find the least squares curve of the form

$$y = Ae^{kx}$$

for the following data points:

x	y
1	1.15
2	0.41
3	0.15
4	0.05

Hint: If we take the natural logarithm of each side of the above equation, we get

$$\ln y = \ln A + kx$$

Hence the strategy is to construct a new column of numbers $Y = \ln y$, getting

x	$Y = \ln y$
1	0.1398
2	−0.8916
3	−1.8971
4	−2.9957

Now find the least squares line

$$Y = B + kx$$

that best fits these new data points (find B and k). Finally, since $B = \ln A$, the value of A in the original function can be found from the equation $A = e^B$.

Least Squares in the Business World

21. Finding the Revenue Curve. A company has determined that the revenue obtained when it sells q items of a given product can be described by the following table. From these observations, find the least squares line of the form

$$R(q) = aq + b$$

Amount Produced (q)	10	20	30
Revenue (R)	\$30	\$55	\$90

22. Finding the Cost Curve. A company has collected information relating the cost $C(q)$ to produce q items of a given product. Use the following table to find the least squares model of the form

$$C(q) = aq + b$$

Amount Produced (q)	5	10	15
Cost (C)	17	24	30

23. Finding the Demand Curve. The following observations were collected relating the demand D of a given product to the price p per unit of this product. Use these observations to determine the least squares curve of the form

$$D(p) = ap + b$$

Price (p)	\$10	\$20	\$30
Demand (D)	10	6	1

24. Weighing Yourself with a Ruler. A rough rule of thumb for weighing yourself with a ruler is the following:*

Females: Multiply your height in inches by 3.5 and subtract 108.

Males: Multiply your height in inches by 4 and subtract 128. For individuals with

Small-bone structure: Adjust the above value by subtracting 10% of the value.

Large-bone structure: Adjust the above value by adding 10% of the value.

Average-bone structure: No adjustment is necessary.

(a) Does the above rule of thumb predict your weight accurately?

(b) Gather some data on the height and weight of friends of different ages and sizes. Restrict yourself to one sex and to individuals having the same bone structure. Find the least squares line that fits your data. Does your least squares line agree with the rule of thumb?

* This problem is based on a problem taken from the text, Frank Giordano and Maurice Weir, *A First Course in Mathematical Modeling*, Brooks/Cole, A division of Wadsworth, Inc., Belmont, Calif. 1985, p. 107.

6.6 Double Integrals

PURPOSE

We introduce the concept of the double integral and show how to integrate functions $f(x, y)$ of two variables. The major topics discussed are

- the antiderivatives of functions of two variables,
- the iterated integral,
- the double integral, and
- the computation of volumes using double integrals.

Introduction

Earlier in this chapter, we extended the concept of the derivative from functions of one variable to functions of two variables (three in the case of the Lagrange multiplier). We now see how the integral can be extended with the introduction of the double integral. We start by showing how to find antiderivatives of functions of two variables.

Antiderivatives of Functions of Two Variables

When we found a partial derivative of a function of two variables, we differentiated with respect to one of the two variables while treating the other variable as a constant. We can also find the antiderivative of a function of two variables in much the same way. That is, we take the antiderivative with respect to one of the two variables while treating the other variable as a constant. When we take the antiderivative or indefinite integral of a function $f(x, y)$ with respect to x (treating y as a constant), we denote this by

$$\int f(x, y)\, dx$$

Similarly, the antiderivative or indefinite integral of a function $f(x, y)$ with respect to y (treating x as a constant) is denoted by

$$\int f(x, y)\, dy$$

Example 1

Antiderivative with Respect to x Find the antiderivative of

$$f(x, y) = 2xy + 3y^2 + 3x^2$$

with respect to x.

Solution Taking the antiderivative with respect to x while treating y as a constant, we have

$$\int (2xy + 3y^2 + 3x^2)\, dx = x^2y + 3xy^2 + x^3 + C(y)$$

The constant of integration $C(y)$ is not really a constant but can, in fact, be any function of y.

Check:

$$\frac{\partial}{\partial x}[x^2y + 3xy^2 + x^3 + C(y)] = 2xy + 3y^2 + 3x^2$$

Note that any function $C(y)$ of y alone has a derivative of zero when differentiated with respect to x. □

Example 2

Antiderivative with Respect to y Find the antiderivative

$$\int (x^2 + y^2)\, dy$$

Solution Integrating with respect to y while treating x as a constant, we get

$$\int (x^2 + y^2)\, dy = x^2y + \frac{1}{3}y^3 + C(x)$$

Check:

$$\frac{\partial}{\partial y}\left[x^2y + \frac{1}{3}y^3 + C(x)\right] = x^2 + y^2$$

Note that any function $C(x)$ of x alone has a derivative of zero when differentiated with respect to y. □

Definite Integral of Functions of Two Variables

Just as the concept of the antiderivative or the indefinite integral can be extended to functions of two variables, so can the definite integral. Consider the two definite integrals of the form

$$\int_a^b f(x, y)\,dx \qquad \text{and} \qquad \int_a^b f(x, y)\,dy$$

The limits of integration refer to limits of integration for the variable for which integration is being performed. For example, in the integral involving dx the limits of integration refer to limits for x, while in the integral involving dy the limits of integration refer to limits for y.

Example 3 Definite Integrals Evaluate the definite integral

$$\int_0^1 (x^2 + y^2)\,dy$$

Solution In Example 2 we saw that

$$\int (x^2 + y^2)\,dy = x^2y + \frac{1}{3}y^3 + C(x)$$

Hence we have

$$\begin{aligned}\int_0^1 (x^2 + y^2)\,dy &= \left[x^2y + \frac{1}{3}y^3 + C(x)\right]\Bigg|_{y=0}^{y=1}\\ &= \left[x^2 + \frac{1}{3} + C(x)\right] - [0 + 0 + C(x)]\\ &= x^2 + \frac{1}{3}\end{aligned}$$

Note that the function $C(x)$ "canceled," as it always will. In the future we will choose it to be zero. □

Iterated Integrals

In Example 3 the definite integral with respect to y resulted in a function of x. On the other hand, if we integrated a function $f(x, y)$ with respect to x, we would get a function of y. In either case the resulting function is simply a continuous function of one variable and can be integrated a second time. This process of first integrating a function $f(x, y)$ with respect to one of the two variables and then integrating the resulting function with respect to the remaining variable is called **iterated integration**. The two successive integrals are called an **iterated integral**.

Example 4

Iterated Integration Evaluate the iterated integral

$$\int_1^2 \left[\int_0^1 (x^2 + y^2)\, dy \right] dx$$

Solution We first evaluate the inside or **inner integral**. We evaluated this integral in Example 3 and found

$$\begin{aligned}\int_0^1 (x^2 + y^2)\, dy &= \left(x^2 y + \frac{1}{3} y^3 \right) \Bigg|_{y=0}^{y=1} \\ &= x^2 + \frac{1}{3}\end{aligned}$$

Hence this function now acts as the integrand in the second or **outer integral**. Hence we write

$$\begin{aligned}\int_1^2 \left[\int_0^1 (x^2 + y^2)\, dy \right] dx &= \int_1^2 \left(x^2 + \frac{1}{3} \right) dx \\ &= \left(\frac{1}{3} x^3 + \frac{x}{3} \right) \Bigg|_{x=1}^{x=2} \\ &= \left(\frac{8}{3} + \frac{2}{3} \right) - \left(\frac{1}{3} + \frac{1}{3} \right) \\ &= \frac{8}{3}\end{aligned}$$

In the above iterated integral, integration was performed first with respect to y (inner integral) and then with respect to x (outer integral). We wonder what would happen if we integrated the same function $f(x, y)$ in the opposite order. The following example gives the answer. □

Example 5

Interchanging the Order of Integration Evaluate the iterated integral in Example 4 in the opposite order. That is, instead of integrating with respect to y first and x second, integrate with respect to x first and y second as in the iterated integral

$$\int_0^1 \left[\int_1^2 (x^2 + y^2)\, dx \right] dy$$

Solution Evaluating the inner integral, we get

$$\begin{aligned}\int_1^2 (x^2 + y^2)\, dx &= \left(\frac{1}{3} x^3 + xy^2 \right) \Bigg|_{x=1}^{x=2} \\ &= y^2 + \frac{7}{3}\end{aligned}$$

Substituting this value into the outer integral gives

$$\int_0^1 \left[\int_1^2 (x^2 + y^2)\,dx\right] dy = \int_0^1 \left(y^2 + \frac{7}{3}\right) dy$$

$$= \left(\frac{1}{3}y^3 + \frac{7y}{3}\right)\Bigg|_{y=0}^{y=1}$$

$$= \left(\frac{1}{3} + \frac{7}{3}\right) - \left(\frac{0}{3} + \frac{0}{3}\right)$$

$$= \frac{8}{3}$$

Note that although the order of integration is changed in Examples 4 and 5, the values of the iterated integrals are still the same. □

Sometimes the inner integral in an iterated integral has variable limits of integration. The following example illustrates how this type of integration is carried out.

Example 6

Variable Limits of Integration Evaluate the iterated integral

$$\int_0^1 \left[\int_{x^2}^{x} xy\,dy\right] dx$$

Solution We evaluate this integral using basically the same steps we used when we evaluated iterated integrals with constant limits of integration. The variable x that occurs in the inner limits of integration is treated as a constant, while the inner integration is carried out with respect to y. We carry out this process here.

$$\int_0^1 \left[\int_{x^2}^{x} xy\,dy\right] dx = \int_0^1 \left[\frac{1}{2}xy^2\Bigg|_{y=x^2}^{y=x}\right] dx$$ (find the antiderivative with respect to y)

$$= \int_0^1 \left[\frac{x^3}{2} - \frac{x^5}{2}\right] dx$$ (substitute the limits of integration)

$$= \frac{1}{2}\int_0^1 (x^3 - x^5)\,dx$$ (x is now the variable in the outer integral)

$$= \frac{1}{2}\left[\frac{x^4}{4} - \frac{x^6}{6}\Bigg|_{x=0}^{x=1}\right]$$ (find the antiderivative with respect to x)

$$= \left(\frac{1}{8} - \frac{1}{12}\right) - 0$$

$$= \frac{1}{24}$$ □

The Double Integral

The notion of the definite integral for functions of a single variable can be extended to functions of two variables, called the **double integral**. Whereas the

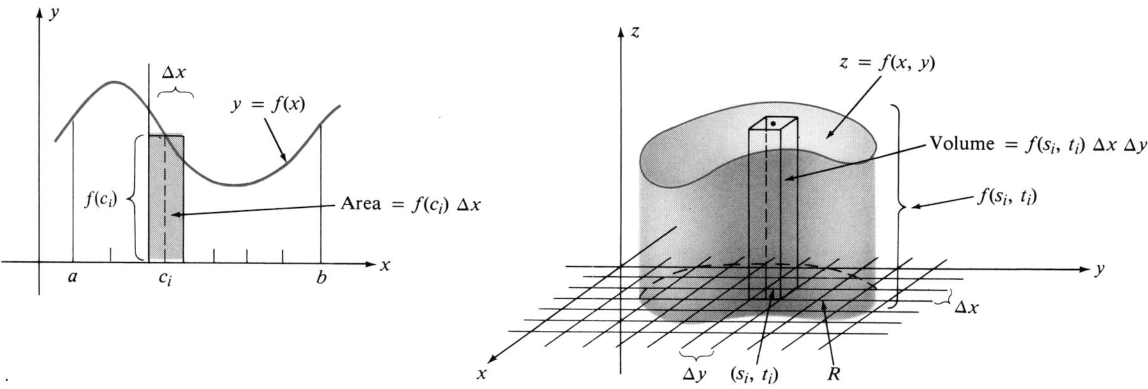

(a) The definite integral can be interpreted as the limiting value of the sum of areas of rectangles.

(b) The double integral can be interpreted as the limiting value of the sum of volumes of rectangular cylinders.

Figure 41
Comparison of the definite and double integrals for nonnegative functions

definite integral of a function of one variable can be used to find the area of a region in the plane, the double integral of a function of two variables can be used to find the volume of a solid in three dimensions. To understand the double integral of a function $f(x, y)$ of two variables, it is useful to compare it with the definite integral of a function $f(x)$ of a single variable. For instance, for a function of a single variable we integrate the function over an interval $[a, b]$. If the function $f(x)$ is nonnegative throughout the interval, the value of the definite integral represents the area under the graph of $y = f(x)$ for $a \le x \le b$. (See Figure 41a.) To generalize this idea to nonnegative functions $f(x, y)$ of two variables, consider finding the volume of a solid under the surface $z = f(x, y)$ above a region R in the xy-plane. (See Figure 41b.) To find this volume, we do the following:

1. Subdivide the region R into small rectangles, each having area $\Delta A = \Delta x\, \Delta y$.
2. Within each rectangle that lies completely in R, select an arbitrary point (s_i, t_i) and evaluate the product

$$f(s_i, t_i)\, \Delta x\, \Delta y$$

   Each product will give the volume of a rectangular solid that lies above one of the rectangles. (See Figure 41b.)
3. Compute the sum of the volumes found in Step 2:

$$\sum_{i=1}^{n} f(s_i, t_i)\, \Delta x\, \Delta y$$

   This sum will be an approximation to the desired volume.
4. Find the limit of the approximating sum found in Step 3 as the number of terms n becomes infinite while at the same time the dimensions Δx and Δy of each of the rectangles approach zero.

Without going into the technical details of how the above limiting process is performed, we appeal to your intuition to visualize that the approximating sum found in Step 3 will approach the exact volume of the solid as more and more, thinner and thinner rectangular solids are added. This limiting sum is called the **double integral** of the function $f(x, y)$ over the region R. This discussion gives rise to the formal definition of the double integral.

Definition of the Double Integral

If a function $z = f(x, y)$ of two variables is defined on a region R in the xy-plane, then the **double integral** of $f(x, y)$ over R, denoted

$$\iint_R f(x, y)\,dA$$

is defined by

$$\iint_R f(x, y)\,dA = \lim_{n\to\infty} \sum_{i=1}^{n} f(s_i, t_i)\,\Delta x\,\Delta y$$

provided that the limit exists.

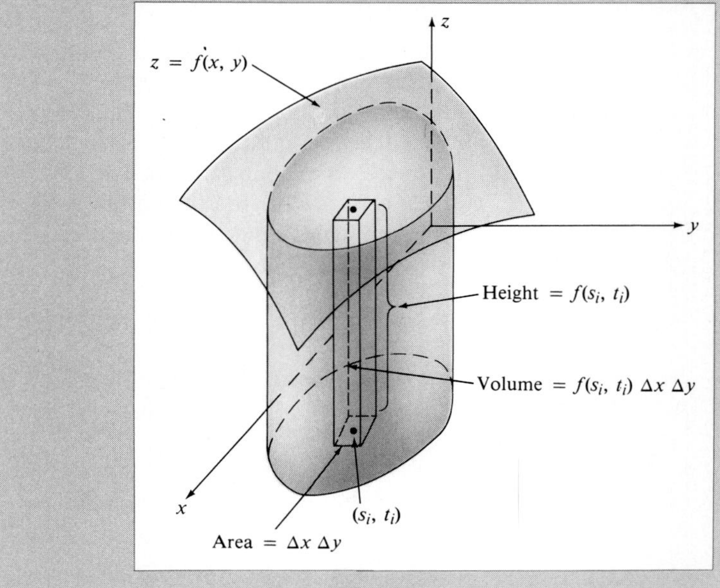

How to Evaluate the Double Integral

If you remember, it was difficult (impossible for all practical purposes) to find the definite integral of a function $f(x)$ of a single variable using the limit definition. Fortunately, we were able to use the fundamental theorem of calculus and find the definite integral by first finding the antiderivative $F(x)$ of the integrand and then evaluating the difference $F(b) - F(a)$. Now when we come to the double integral, we again face an almost impossible limit. Fortunately, we are saved again from the process of evaluating a complicated limit. In this case we can evaluate the double integral by evaluating two definite integrals in succession, that is, an iterated integral.

The Double Integral as an Iterated Integral

To set the groundwork for the evaluation of the double integral in terms of an iterated integral, we first introduce two special regions, called **type I** and **type II** regions.

Type I Region (Bounded by Vertical Lines)

A type I region is a region in the xy-plane bounded on the left and right by vertical lines $x = a$ and $x = b$ and bounded below and above by smooth curves $y = g_1(x)$ and $y = g_2(x)$, where $g_1(x) \le g_2(x)$ for $a \le x \le b$. (See Figure 42a.)

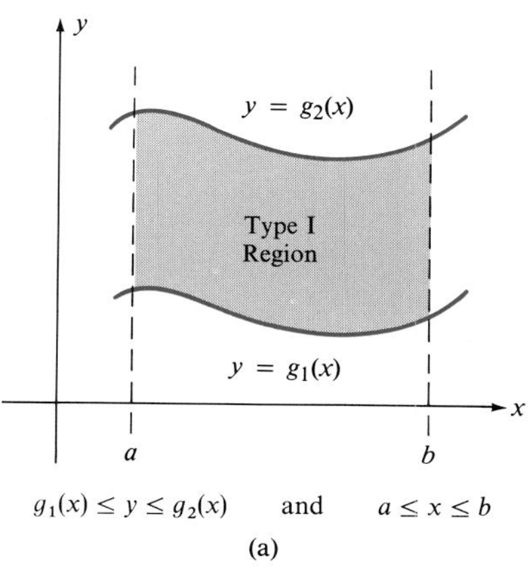

$g_1(x) \le y \le g_2(x)$ and $a \le x \le b$

(a)

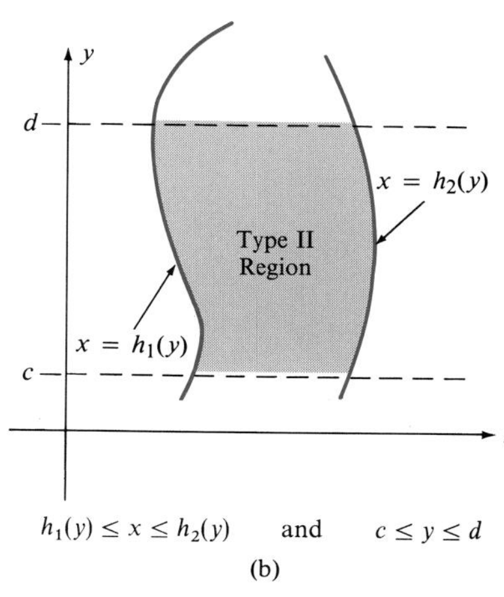

$h_1(y) \le x \le h_2(y)$ and $c \le y \le d$

(b)

Figure 42
Typical regions over which we can find a double integral

Type II Region (Bounded by Horizontal Lines)

A type II region is a region in the xy-plane bounded below and above by horizontal lines $y = c$ and $y = d$ and bounded on the left and right by smooth curves $x = h_1(y)$ and $x = h_2(y)$, where $h_1(y) \le h_2(y)$ for $c \le y \le d$. (See Figure 42b.)

We now state the important theorem that shows how a double integral over type I and type II regions can be written as an iterated integral.

The Double Integral as an Iterated Integral

Let $z = f(x, y)$ be a function of two variables.

If R is a *type I region* defined by

$$g_1(x) \leq y \leq g_2(x) \qquad \text{and} \qquad a \leq x \leq b$$

then the double integral of f over R can be found by evaluating the iterated integral

$$\iint_R f(x, y)\, dA = \int_a^b \left[\int_{g_1(x)}^{g_2(x)} f(x, y)\, dy \right] dx$$

If R is a *type II region* defined by

$$h_1(y) \leq x \leq h_2(y) \qquad \text{and} \qquad c \leq x \leq d$$

then the double integral of f over R can be found by evaluating the iterated integral

$$\iint_R f(x, y)\, dA = \int_c^d \left[\int_{h_1(y)}^{h_2(y)} f(x, y)\, dx \right] dy$$

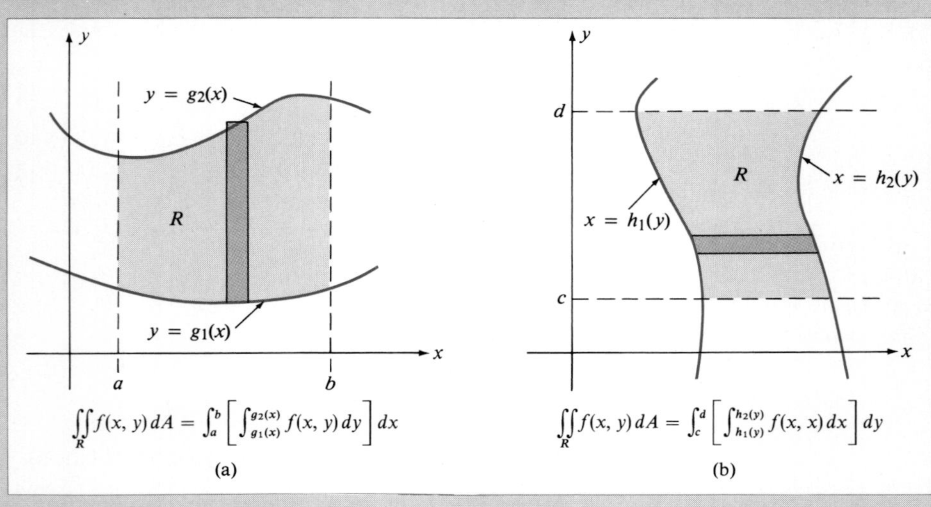

(a) (b)

The rectangles drawn inside the regions in the definition of the double integral are meant to illustrate the order in which the integration is performed.

Many regions can be thought of as either type I or type II regions. The following example illustrates this idea.

Example 7

A Region of Both Types Show why the region R bounded by the curves

$$y = x$$
$$y = x^2$$

can be interpreted as either a type I or a type II region.

Solution The region R is illustrated in Figure 43. Clearly, the points (x, y) in R can be described by either of the following sets of inequalities:

Type I description: $x^2 \le y \le x$, $0 \le x \le 1$

Type II description: $y \le x \le \sqrt{y}$, $0 \le y \le 1$

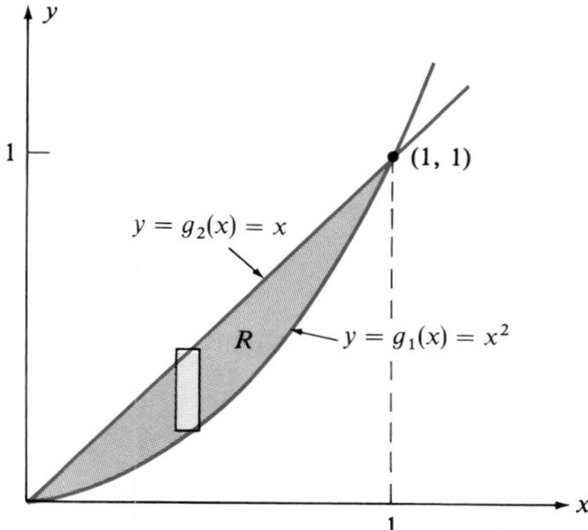

Figure 43
Region bounded by $y = x$ and $y = x^2$

In other words, if we wished to evaluate a double integral over this region, we could either integrate with respect to x first and y second or vice versa. The following example illustrates this idea. □

Example 8

Evaluating a Double Integral Evaluate the double integral

$$\iint_R xy\,dA$$

where R is the region bounded by the curves

$$y = x$$
$$y = x^3$$

Solution It is possible to interpret R as a type I region bounded below and above by

$$g_1(x) = x^3$$
$$g_2(x) = x$$

and on the left and right by

$$x = 0$$
$$x = 1$$

In this case we would evaluate the double integral as the iterated integral

$$\iint_R xy\,dA = \int_0^1 \left[\int_{x^3}^{x} xy\,dy\right] dx$$

$$= \int_0^1 \left[\frac{xy^2}{2}\Bigg|_{y=x^3}^{y=x}\right] dx \qquad \text{(find the antiderivative of the inner integral with respect to } y\text{)}$$

$$= \int_0^1 \left[\frac{1}{2}x^3 - \frac{1}{2}x^7\right] dx \qquad \text{(substitute the limits of integration of the inner integral for } y\text{)}$$

$$= \left[\left(\frac{1}{8}x^4 - \frac{1}{16}x^8\right)\Bigg|_{x=0}^{x=1}\right] \qquad \text{(find the antiderivative of the remaining integral with respect to } x\text{)}$$

$$= \left[\frac{1}{8}(1)^4 - \frac{1}{16}(1)^8\right] - \left[\frac{1}{8}(0)^4 - \frac{1}{16}(0)^8\right]$$

$$= \left[\frac{1}{8} - \frac{1}{16}\right] - 0$$

$$= \frac{1}{16}$$

□

Which Order of Integration Is Best?

For a region that can be interpreted as either a type I or type II region, it is theoretically possible to evaluate a double integral over the region by evaluating either of the two iterated integrals. However, it is often the case that one of the iterated integrals is far easier to evaluate than the other. The following example illustrates this idea.

Example 9

Changing the Order of Integration Evaluate the integral

$$\iint_R e^{-x^2}\,dA$$

where R is the region in the xy-plane bounded by the lines $y = x$, $y = 0$, and $x = 1$. (See Figure 44.)

Solution We see from Figure 44 that the region R can be interpreted as either a type I or a type II region. Hence the double integral can be evaluated by integrating either with respect to x first and y second or vice versa. However,

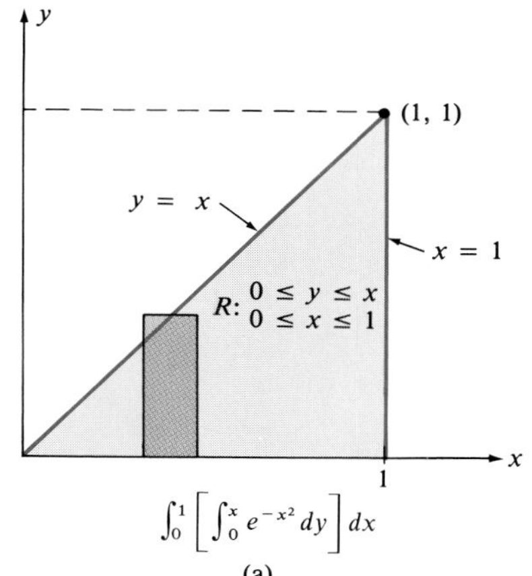

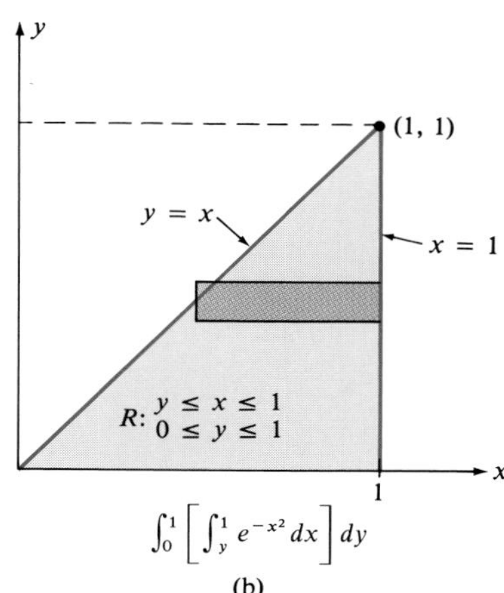

Figure 44
We can find the double integral over the region R by evaluating either of these interated integrals

difficulties arise if we integrate with respect to x first, since we must find

$$\iint_R e^{-x^2}\,dA = \int_0^1 \left[\int_x^1 e^{-x^2}\,dx\right] dy$$

Unfortunately, the function $f(x, y) = e^{-x^2}$ has no elementary antiderivative with respect to x. On the other hand, however, if we integrate with respect to y first, we get the iterated integral

$$\begin{aligned}\iint_R e^{-x^2}\,dA &= \int_0^1 \left[\int_0^x e^{-x^2}\,dy\right] dx \\ &= \int_0^1 \left[ye^{-x^2}\Big|_{y=0}^{y=x}\right] dx \\ &= \int_0^1 xe^{-x^2}\,dx \\ &= -\frac{1}{2}e^{-x^2}\Big|_0^1 \\ &= -\frac{1}{2}e^{-1} + \frac{1}{2} \\ &= \frac{e-1}{2e}\end{aligned}$$

□

Finding Volumes with Double Integrals

One of the major applications of the double integral lies in finding volumes of solid regions in three-dimensional space. Consider the solid region in Figure 45a. Here the solid is bounded below by a region R in the xy-plane and above by a portion of the surface $z = f(x, y)$.

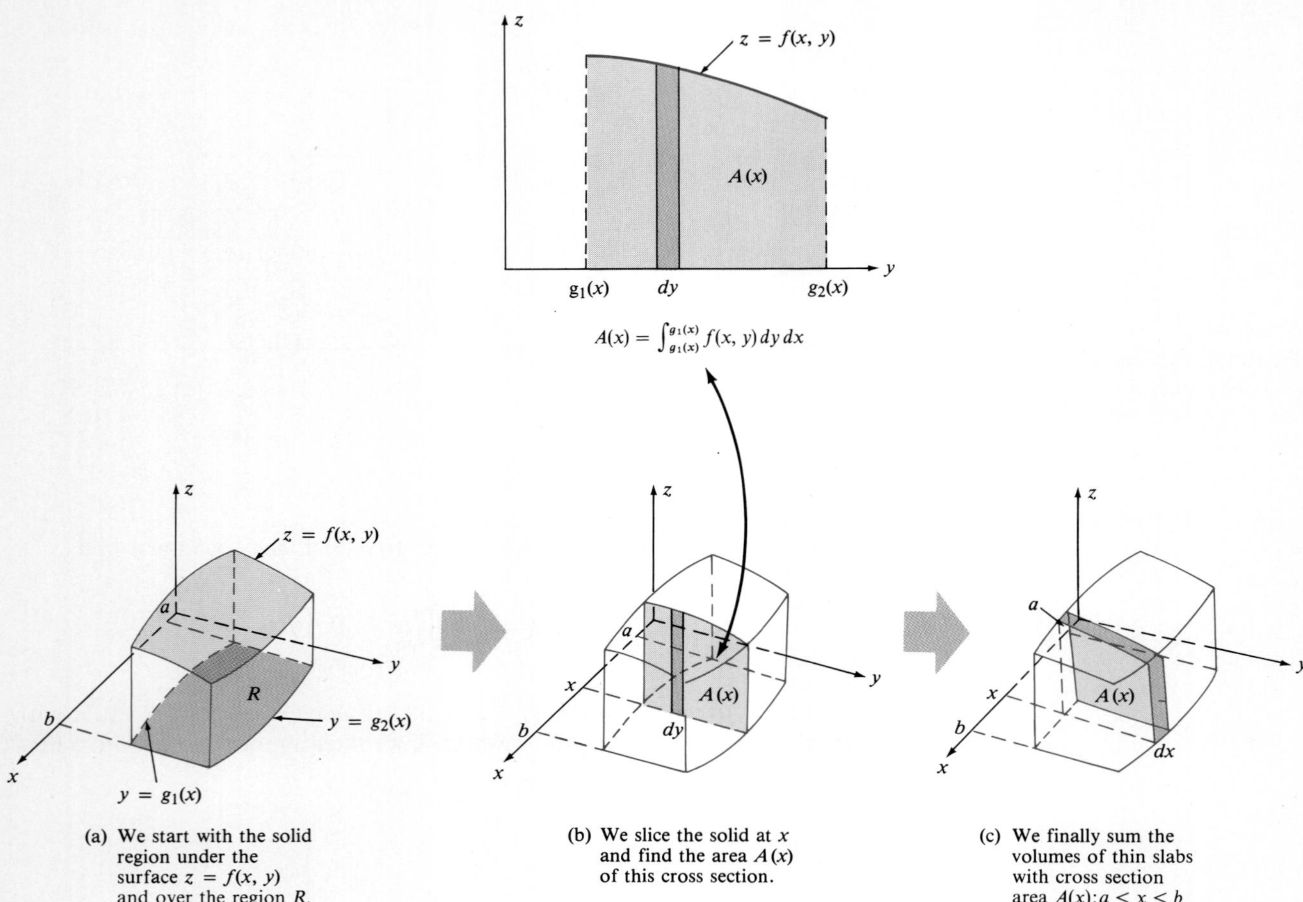

(a) We start with the solid region under the surface $z = f(x, y)$ and over the region R.

(b) We slice the solid at x and find the area $A(x)$ of this cross section.

(c) We finally sum the volumes of thin slabs with cross section area $A(x): a \le x \le b$ and thickness dx.

Figure 45
Finding the volume of a solid using a double integral

To visualize how we might find the volume of this solid using an iterated integral, observe the following steps:

Step 1: First compute the area $A(x)$ of a cross-sectional slice of the solid at some x in the interval $a \le x \le b$. (See Figure 45b.) To find $A(x)$, realize that for each fixed x the function $f(x, y)$ is now a function of y alone and that $A(x)$ can be viewed as the area under the surface $z = f(x, y)$ along the interval $a \le x \le b$. Hence

$$A(x) = \int_{g_1(x)}^{g_2(x)} f(x, y)\, dy$$

Step 2: The volume of the solid can now be found by integrating (the process of summing) these cross-sectional areas for $a \le x \le b$, getting

$$V = \int_a^b A(x)\, dx$$
$$= \int_a^b \left[\int_{g_1(x)}^{g_2(x)} f(x, y)\, dy \right] dx$$

This discussion motivates the following formulas for finding the volume of a solid region.

Finding a Volume from a Double Integral

Let $z = f(x, y) \geq 0$ over a region R in the xy-plane. The volume V of the solid region that lies above R and below the surface $z = f(x, y)$ is given by one of the following formulas:

Type I region:

$$V = \iint_R f(x, y)\, dA = \int_a^b \left[\int_{g_1(x)}^{g_2(x)} f(x, y)\, dy \right] dx$$

Type II region:

$$V = \iint_R f(x, y)\, dA = \int_c^d \left[\int_{h_1(y)}^{h_2(y)} f(x, y)\, dx \right] dy$$

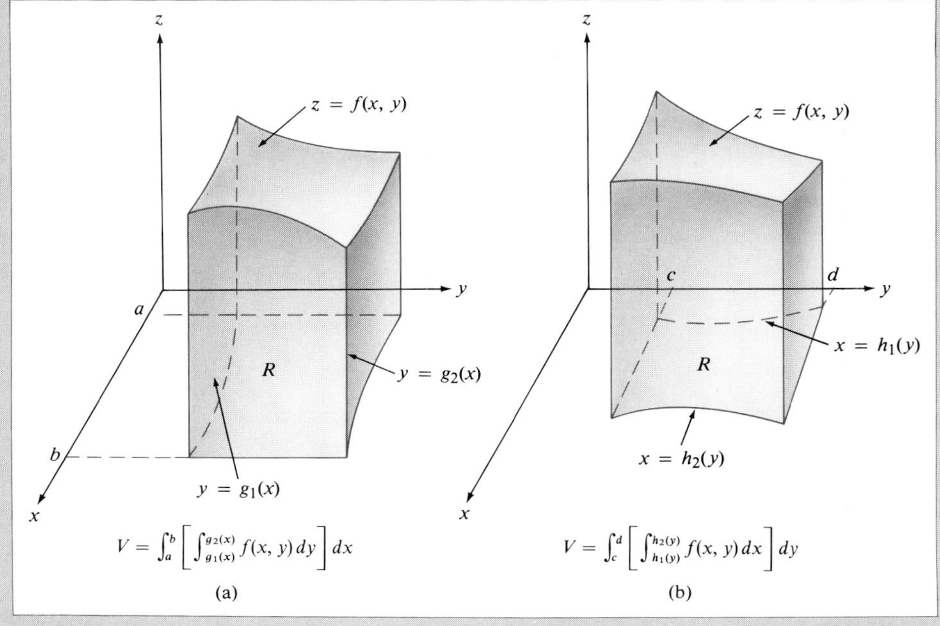

Example 10 Volumes from Double Integrals Find the volume of the solid that lies below the surface

$$z = x^2 + y^2$$

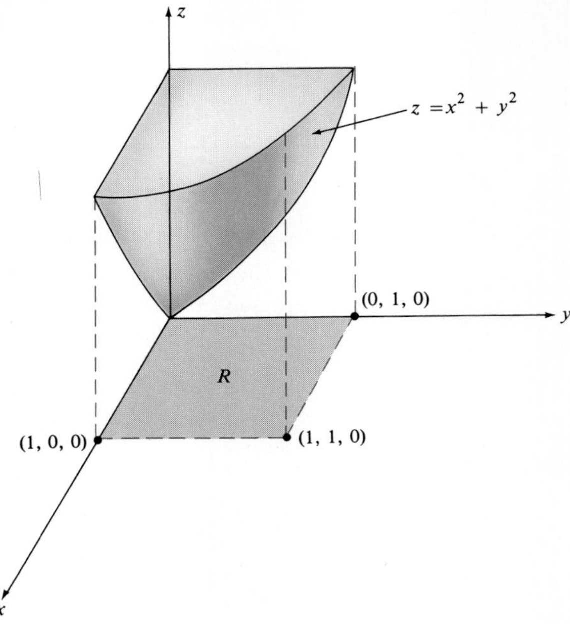

Figure 46
The solid under the surface $z = x^2 + y^2$ over the region R

and above the square R defined by

$$0 \leq x \leq 1 \qquad \text{and} \qquad 0 \leq y \leq 1$$

(See Figure 46.)

Solution The square R can be interpreted as either a type I or a type II region. Hence we can find the volume by integrating either with respect to x first and y second or vice versa. For no special reason we integrate with respect to x first, getting

$$\begin{aligned} V &= \iint_R (x^2 + y^2)\,dA \\ &= \int_0^1 \left[\int_0^1 (x^2 + y^2)\,dx \right] dy \\ &= \int_0^1 \left[\left(\frac{1}{3}x^3 + xy^2 \right) \Bigg|_0^1 \right] dy \\ &= \int_0^1 \left(\frac{1}{3} + y^2 \right) dy \\ &= \left(\frac{y}{3} + \frac{y^3}{3} \right) \Bigg|_0^1 \\ &= \left(\frac{1}{3} + \frac{1}{3} \right) - 0 \\ &= \frac{2}{3} \end{aligned}$$

□

Example 11

Volumes from Double Integrals Find the volume of the solid that lies under the surface

$$z = e^{-x}e^{-y}$$

and over the triangular region R with vertices (0, 0), (1, 0), (0, 1).

Solution We first draw the solid region as shown in Figure 47. It is possible to find the volume by evaluating either of the iterated integrals:

$$V = \int_0^1 \left[\int_0^{1-x} e^{-x}e^{-y}\,dy\right]dx \qquad (y \text{ first, } x \text{ second})$$

$$V = \int_0^1 \left[\int_0^{1-y} e^{-x}e^{-y}\,dx\right]dy \qquad (x \text{ first, } y \text{ second})$$

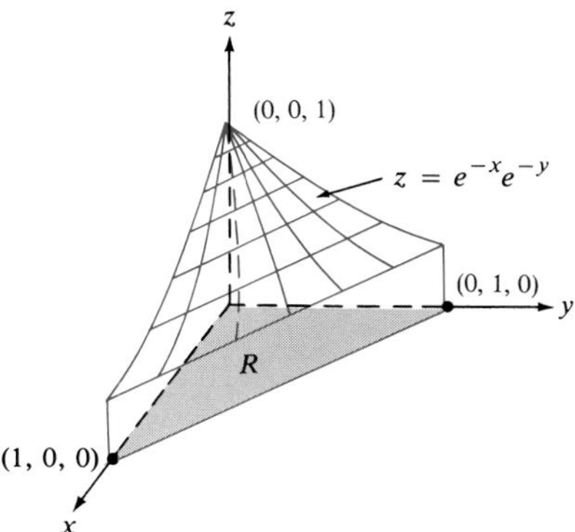

Figure 47
The solid under the surface $z = e^{-x}e^{-y}$ *over the region* R

Since both of these integrals can be easily evaluated, we arbitrarily select the first integral for evaluation, getting

$$\begin{aligned} V &= \int_0^1 \left[\int_0^{1-x} e^{-x}e^{-y}\,dy\right]dx \\ &= \int_0^1 \left[-e^{-x}e^{-y}\Big|_{y=0}^{y=1-x}\right]dx \\ &= \int_0^1 (-e^{-x}e^{x-1} + e^{-x})\,dx \\ &= \int_0^1 (-e^{-1} + e^{-x})\,dx \\ &= \left(-xe^{-1} - e^{-x}\right)\Big|_0^1 \\ &= 1 - 2e^{-1} \end{aligned}$$

□

Problems

In Problems 1–10, calculate the indicated antiderivative with respect to each of the two variables. Check the answers by differentiating.

1. $\int (x^2 + xy - 2y + y^2)\,dx$ $\qquad \int (x^2 + xy - 2y + y^2)\,dy$
2. $\int (x^3 - y^3 + 3xy)\,dx$ $\qquad \int (x^3 - y^3 + 3xy)\,dy$
3. $\int xy\sqrt{x^2 + y^2}\,dx$ $\qquad \int xy\sqrt{x^2 + y^2}\,dy$
4. $\int (x + xy - 2x^2y)\,dx$ $\qquad \int (x + xy - 2x^2y)\,dy$
5. $\int (2x^2y + 1)\,dx$ $\qquad \int (2x^2y + 1)\,dy$
6. $\int r(r + s)\,dr$ $\qquad \int r(r + s)\,ds$
7. $\int x^2y^2\,dx$ $\qquad \int x^2y^2\,dy$
8. $\int \frac{2t}{(s + t)^2}\,ds$ $\qquad \int \frac{2t}{(s + t)^2}\,dt$
9. $\int e^x \ln y\,dx$ $\qquad \int e^x \ln y\,dy$
10. $\int xe^{xy}\,dx$ $\qquad \int xe^{xy}\,dy$

In Problems 11–25, calculate the value of the iterated integrals.

11. $\int_0^1 \left[\int_0^1 4\,dx\right] dy$
12. $\int_0^1 \left[\int_0^1 dy\right] dx$
13. $\int_{-2}^1 \left[\int_{-1}^2 (x + y)^2\,dy\right] dx$
14. $\int_1^3 \left[\int_0^3 xy\,dx\right] dy$
15. $\int_0^3 \left[\int_1^3 xy\,dy\right] dx$ (see Problem 14)
16. $\int_0^{\ln 2} \left[\int_0^1 xe^y\,dx\right] dy$
17. $\int_0^1 \left[\int_0^{\ln 2} xe^y\,dy\right] dx$ (see Problem 16)
18. $\int_0^1 \left[\int_0^1 \frac{x^2y}{x^3 + 3}\,dx\right] dy$
19. $\int_{-2}^1 \left[\int_{-1}^2 (x + y)^3\,dx\right] dy$
20. $\int_{-1}^1 \left[\int_0^1 (x^2 + y^2)xy\,dx\right] dy$
21. $\int_0^1 \left[\int_{-1}^1 (x^2 + y^2)xy\,dy\right] dx$ (see Problem 20)
22. $\int_0^1 \left[\int_0^1 \frac{x}{(xy + 1)^2}\,dy\right] dx$
23. $\int_0^{\ln 2} \left[\int_0^1 xye^{y^2x}\,dy\right] dx$
24. $\int_0^{\ln 2} \left[\int_0^{\ln 3} e^{(x+y)}\,dx\right] dy$
25. $\int_{-1}^1 \left[\int_0^1 (x^4y + y^2)\,dy\right] dx$

Which Type of Region?

For Problems 26–35, find the inequalities that describe the region bounded by the given curves and tell whether the region is a type I or type II region. For regions that can be interpreted as either type I or type II regions, find both sets of inequalities that describe the region.

26. $y = x$ $\quad y = 1 - x$ $\quad x = 0$
27. $y = x$ $\quad y = 1$ $\quad x = 0$
28. $y = 2x$ $\quad y = -1$ $\quad x = 1$
29. $y = x + 1$ $\quad y = 1 - x$ $\quad y = 3$
30. $y = x^2$ $\quad y = x + 1$
31. $y = x^2$ $\quad y = 1 - x^2$
32. $y = \frac{x}{2}$ $\quad y = \sqrt{x}$
33. $y = \frac{x^2}{2}$ $\quad y = 2x$
34. $y = \ln x$ $\quad y = x - 1$
35. $y^2 = 9 - x$ $\quad y^2 = 9 - 9x$

Finding Volumes

For Problems 36–45, find the volume under the given surface over the indicated region R in the xy-plane.

	Surface	Region		
36.	$f(x, y) = 1$	$0 \le x \le 1$	and	$0 \le y \le 1 - x^2$
37.	$f(x, y) = 1$	$0 \le x \le 1$	and	$x \le y \le 2x$
38.	$f(x, y) = 1$	$0 \le x \le 1$	and	$x^3 \le y \le x^2$
39.	$f(x, y) = e^y$	$1 \le x \le 2$	and	$1 \le y \le x + 3$
40.	$f(x, y) = x + y^2$	$-1 \le x \le 1$	and	$-x \le y \le 1$
41.	$f(x, y) = e^xe^y$	$1 \le x \le 2$	and	$0 \le y \le \ln x$
42.	$f(x, y) = x^2$	$0 \le y \le 1$	and	$0 \le x \le y$
43.	$f(x, y) = x + 2y$	$0 \le y \le 2$	and	$-y \le x \le y$
44.	$f(x, y) = 1$	$-1 \le y \le 1$	and	$-1 \le x \le y^2$
45.	$f(x, y) = 1$	$0 \le y \le 2$	and	$y \le x \le e^y$

Can You Find the Volumes of These Solids?

For Problems 46–55, find the volume of the indicated solid region.

46.

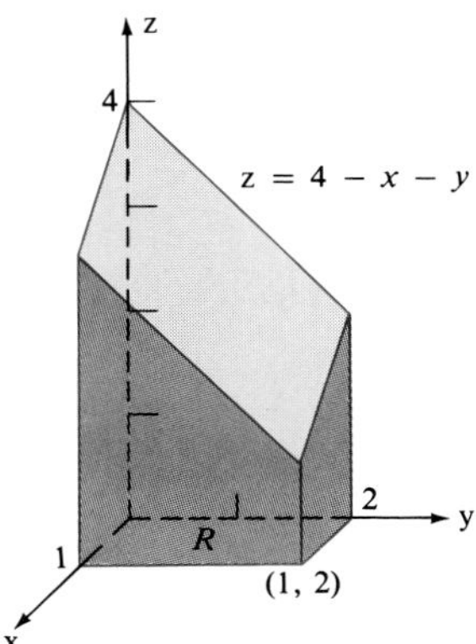

R: $0 \le x \le 1$, $0 \le y \le 2$

47.

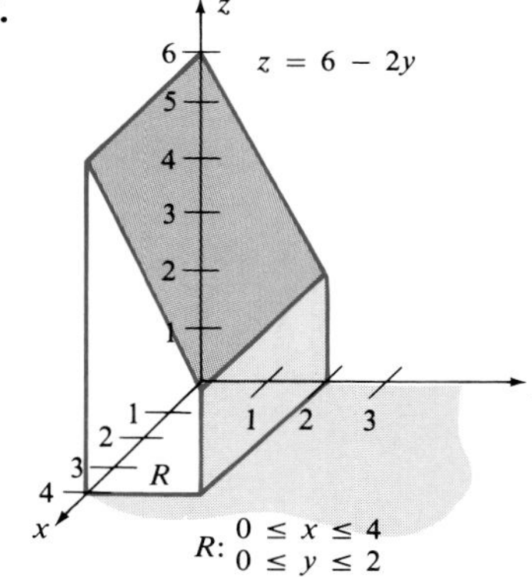

R: $0 \le x \le 4$, $0 \le y \le 2$

48.

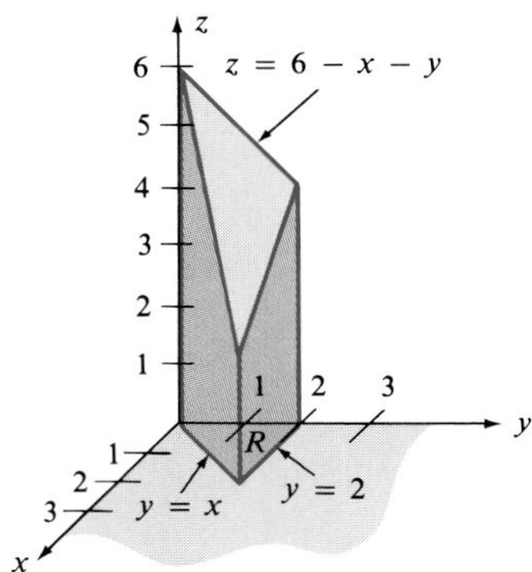

49.

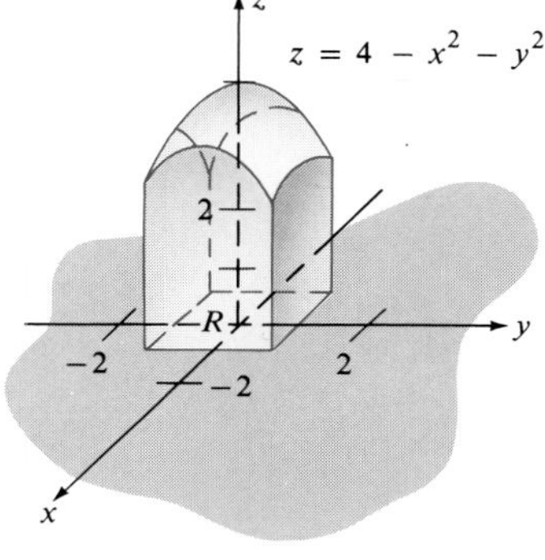

R: $-1 \le x \le 1$, $-1 \le y \le 1$

50.

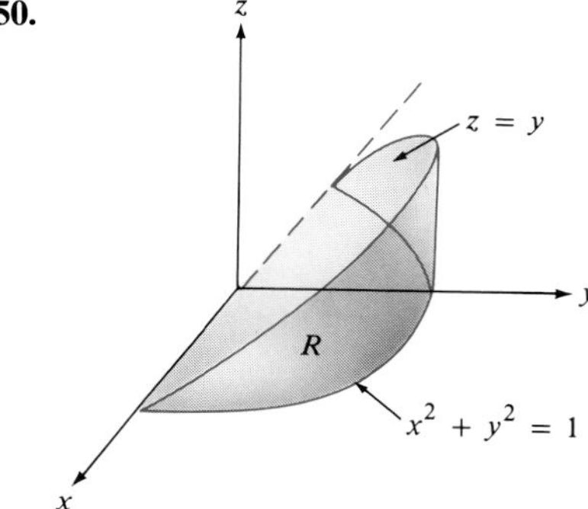

51.

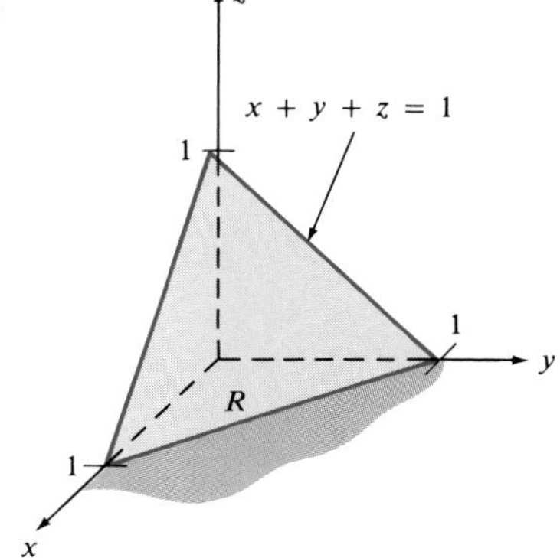

52.

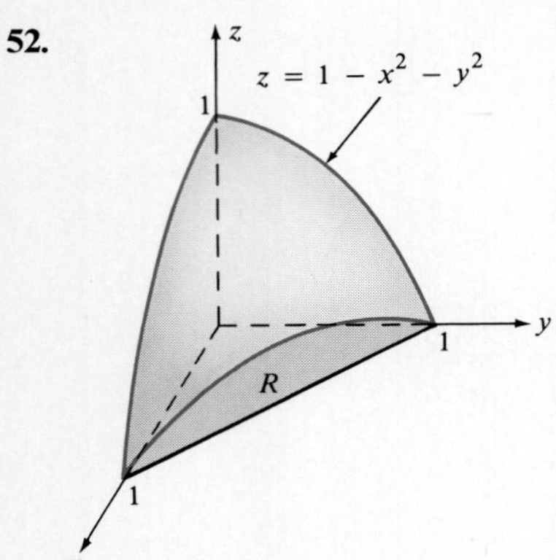

53.

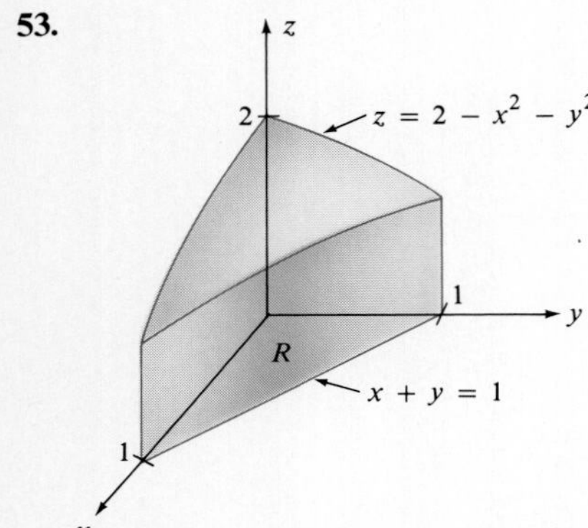

54.

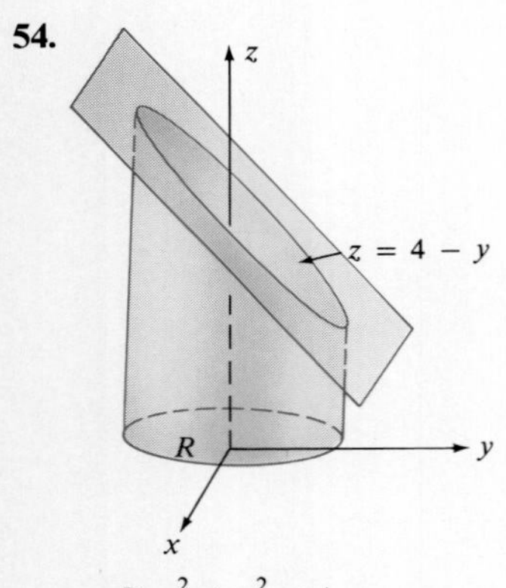

55.

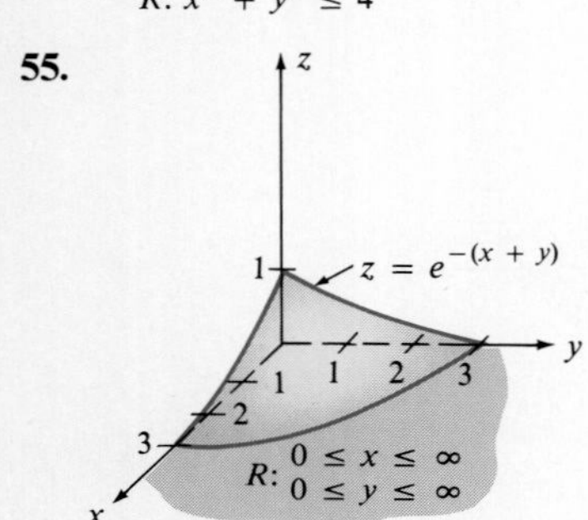

Finding Areas from the Double Integral

It is possible to find the area of a region R in the xy-plane by evaluating the appropriate double integral. If we simply let $f(x, y) = 1$ in the double integral formula for the volume of a solid under the surface $z = f(x, y)$ and over the region R, we will obtain a formula for the area of R. (See Figure 48.)

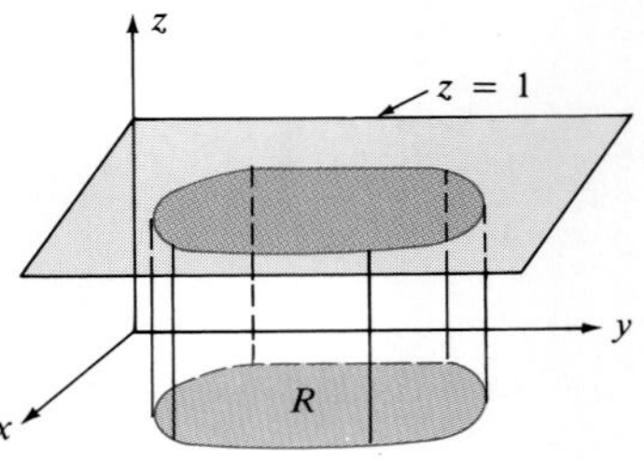

Figure 48
The volume of the solid region under the surface z = 1 with a base R is numerically the same as the area of R

For Problems 56–67, find the area of the indicated region R by evaluating the appropriate double integral. Draw the region R in the xy-plane.

56. $0 \leq x \leq 1 \qquad x^2 \leq y \leq x$
57. $0 \leq x \leq 1 \qquad x \leq y \leq 2x$
58. $0 \leq x \leq 2 \qquad x^2 \leq y \leq \sqrt{x}$
59. $3 \leq x \leq 5 \qquad -x \leq y \leq x^2$
60. $1 \leq x \leq 3 \qquad 0 \leq y \leq x + 1$
61. $0 \leq x \leq 2 \qquad 0 \leq y \leq x + 1$
62. $0 \leq y \leq 3 \qquad 0 \leq x \leq 3y$
63. $1 \leq y \leq 3 \qquad -y \leq x \leq 2y$
64. The region bounded by $y = \ln x$, $y = x$, $y = 0$, and $y = 1$
65. The region bounded by $y = x^2$, $y = 2 - x$, $x = 0$
66. The region bounded by $y = x^2$, $y = 1 - x^2$, $y = 0$
67. The region bounded by $y = -x + 1$, $y = x + 1$, $y = 3$

Double Integrals in Business

A company's production (say per day) in goods or services often can be estimated from the number of employees x and the company's invested capital y according to the Cobb-Douglas production function

$$P(x, y) = Cx^k y^{1-k} \qquad (0 < k < 1)$$

where C and k depend on the company. If over a given period of time the amount of labor x varies more or less uniformly between a and b while capital y varies between c and d, then the average daily production is given by the double integral

$$\text{Average production} = \frac{1}{A} \iint_R P(x, y)\, dA$$

where R is the rectangular region

$$R = \{(x, y): a \leq x \leq b, c \leq y \leq d\}$$

and A is the area of R. Use the above formula to find the average production in units per day for the Cobb-Douglas functions in Problems 68–70.

68. $P(x, y) = 100x^{0.2}y^{0.8}$,
$R = \{(x, y): 0 \leq x \leq 10, 0 \leq y \leq 10\}$

69. $P(x, y) = 50x^{0.5}y^{0.5}$,
$R = \{(x, y): 0 \leq x \leq 25, 5 \leq y \leq 20\}$

70. $P(x, y) = 10x^{0.9}y^{0.1}$,
$R = \{(x, y): 0 \leq x \leq 20, 20 \leq y \leq 30\}$

Physical Applications of the Double Integral

Suppose a sheet of material with varying density covers a given region R of the plane where at each point (x, y) in the region the density (in pounds per square inch) of the material is given by a function $f(x, y)$. (See Figure 49.) It can be shown that the total mass of the sheet in pounds is given by the double integral

$$M = \iint_R f(x, y)\, dA$$

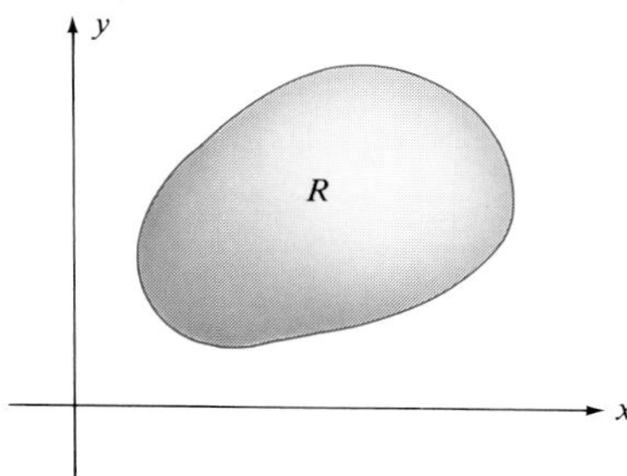

Figure 49
The double integral can be used to determine the mass of a nonhomogeneous region in the plane

For Problems 71–76, find the mass of the drawn figures with given density function.

71. $f(x, y) = 3$

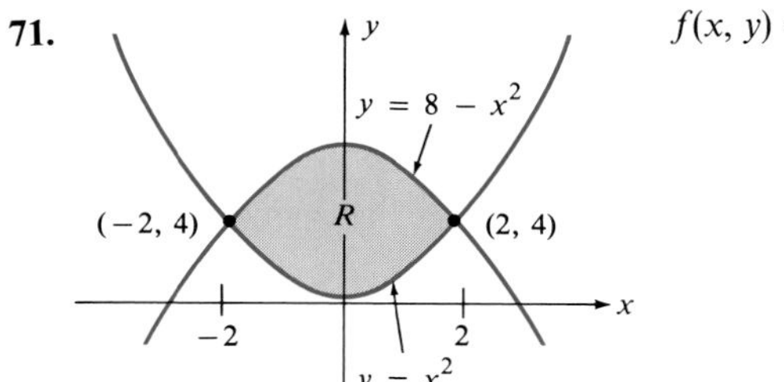

72. $f(x, y) = y$

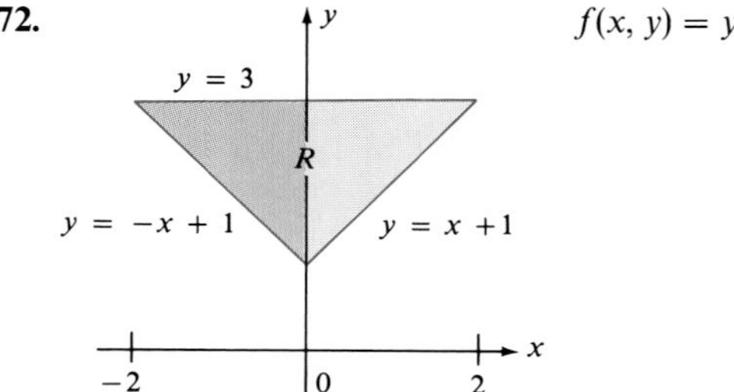

73. $f(x, y) = y^2$

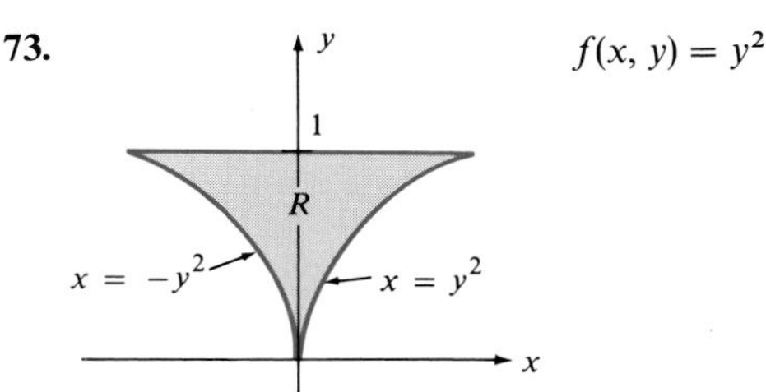

74. $f(x, y) = x^2$

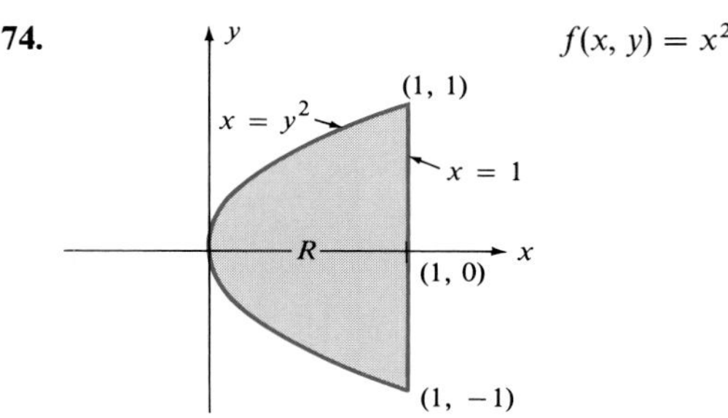

75. $f(x, y) = x + 1$

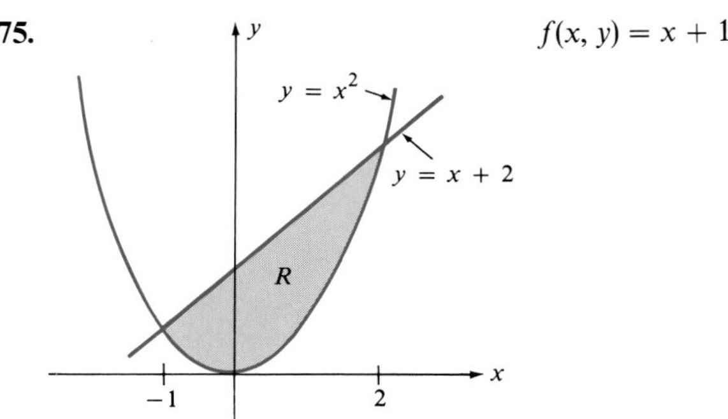

76. $f(x, y) = x^2 + 1$

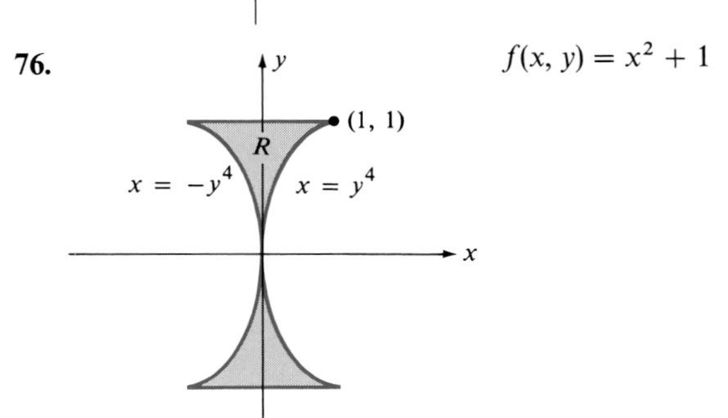

Epilogue: Calculus Crossword Puzzle*

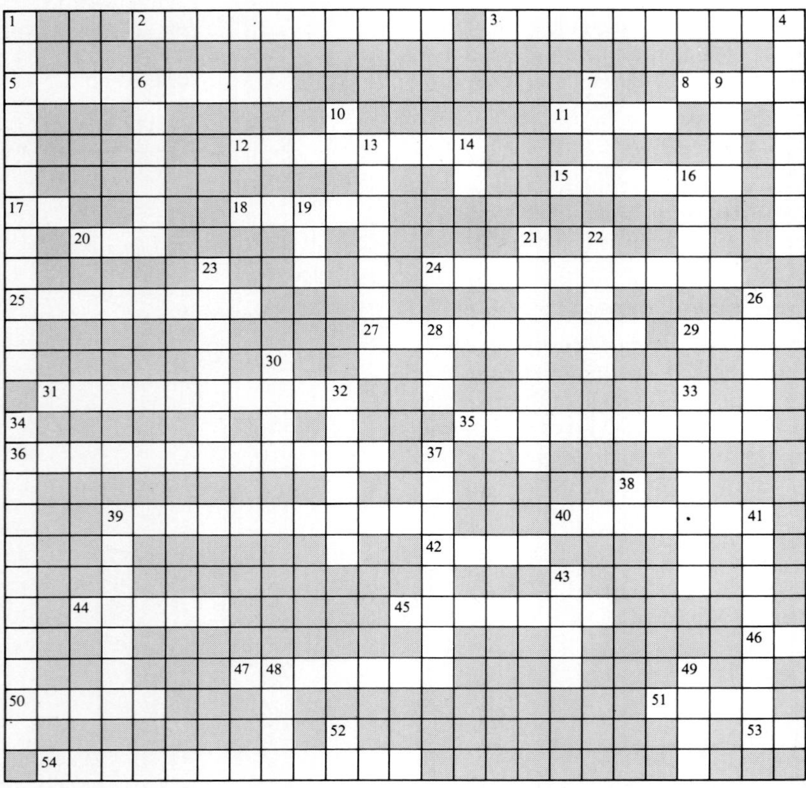

Across

2. Something that gives the rate of change of a function.

3. The point at which a function changes its concavity, spelled backward.

5. The rule for differentiating compositions.

8. The number 2 is a ________ of the equation $x^2 - 3x + 2 = 0$.

11. The number 1 is a ________ of the equation $x^2 - 3x + 2 = 0$.

12. To find the derivative dy/dx given the expression $x^3 + y^3 = 0$, we use ________ differentiation.

15. The logarithm to base 10 is called the ________ logarithm.

17. Initials of the founder of analytical geometry.

18. Probably the single most important concept in the calculus is the ________.

20. If $f'(a) = 0$ and $f''(a) > 0$, then the point a is a relative ________ point.

24. If $f'(a) > 0$ then f is ________ at a.

25. To find areas of unbounded regions, we use the ________ integral.

28. The line $y = 0$ is a horizontal ________ of the curve $y = e^{-x}$.

29. The lines $x = 0$ and $y = 0$ are called ________ for the cartesian plane.

31. Functions whose graphs can be drawn without lifting the pencil from the paper are ________ functions.

35. If $f'(a) = 0$, then a is called a ________ point.

36. The kinds of problems that involve finding the maximum or minimum of functions are called ________ problems.

* Answers are given in the Chapter Review.

39. Many growth phenomena are described mathematically by __________ functions.
40. If $f'(a) = 0$ and $f''(a) > 0$, then a is a relative __________ point.
42. The integral gives the __________ of a nonnegative function.
44. The method of __________ allows us to find the volume of solids of revolution.
45. The name of the mathematician whose name is associated with the numerical method for approximating integrals.
46. The initials of one of the founders of the calculus.
47. If $f''(a) > 0$, then the function f is __________ up at a.
50. The Swiss mathematician who introduced the symbol e.
51. The integral often represents the __________ under the graph of a function.
53. Initials of a famous Swiss mathematician.
54. When we wish to approximate the real change in the functional value, we can use the __________.

Down

1. The derivative of the velocity is the __________.
4. The inverse of the derivative is the __________.
6. One of the two founders of the calculus.
7. When the tangent line is horizontal, the derivative is __________.
9. An interval without its endpoints is called an __________ interval.
10. The initials of one of the founders of the calculus.
13. A famous limiting sum in calculus.
14. The initials of the supposed discoverer of a numerical method for evaluating integrals.
16. An interval without its endpoints is called an __________ interval.
19. A point a is an absolute __________ point if the function is greater at this point than at any other point in the domain of the function.
22. When we integrate functions such as $f(x) = xe^x$, it is convenient to use integration by __________.
23. The German mathematician who cofounded the calculus.
26. The curve $y(t) = Ae^{-kt}$ decribes __________ phenomena.
28. A type of tree.
30. The equation $x^2 + 1 = 0$ does not have a real __________.
32. If a function is differentiable, the graph will appear __________.
33. If $f'(a) = 0$ and $f''(a) < 0$, then a is a relative __________ point.
34. Lagrange multipliers help one to solve __________ optimization problems.
37. If a function is greater at a certain point than at neighboring points, then the point is called a __________ maximum point.
38. The initials of the inventor of the logarithm.
39. An oblong circle is called an __________.
41. The derivative of the revenue is the __________ revenue.
43. The number 2 is the only __________ of the equation $3x - 4 = 2$.
48. An interval without its endpoints is called an __________ interval.
49. The integral is often used to find an __________.
52. The ratio of the circumference of a circle to the diameter is the number __________.

Key Ideas for Review

constrained optimization, 462
contour maps, 431
critical points, 451
discriminant, 454
double integral, 492
iterated integral, 490
Lagrange multiplier method, 464
Least squares, 474
partial derivatives
definition, 438
economic applications, 443
geometric interpretation, 441
relative maximum points, 450
relative minimum points, 450
saddle point, 452
second-partials test, 454
three dimensions, graphing, 426
unconstrained optimization, 449
utility theory, 469
volumes with double integrals, 499

Review Exercises

For Problems 1–12, find the indicated partial derivatives.

1. $f(x, y) = x^2y + y$ — $f_x(x, y)$
2. $f(x, y) = \ln x + x$ — $f_{xx}(x, y)$
3. $f(x, y) = \log_{10} x + \ln x$ — $f_x(x, y)$
4. $f(x, y) = x^2 + 1$ — $f_{xy}(x, y)$
5. $f(x, y) = \sqrt{x^2 + y}$ — $f_{xx}(x, y)$
6. $f(x, y) = e^{xy}$ — $f_{yy}(x, y)$
7. $f(x, y) = x^2y + y$ — $f_{xy}(x, y)$
8. $f(x, y) = x^2y$ — $f_{xy}(x, y)$
9. $f(x, y) = (x^2 + y^2)^2$ — $f_x(x, y)$
10. $f(x, y) = \ln (x + y)$ — $f_y(x, y)$
11. $f(x, y) = x^y$ — $f_x(x, y)$
12. $f(x, y) = x^y$ — $f_y(x, y)$

13. **Price-Earnings Ratio.** The price-earnings ratio of a stock is given by

$$R(P, E) = \frac{P}{E}$$

where P is the price per share of the stock and E is the annual earnings per share of the stock. Draw the level curves for this function in the PE-plane. That is, draw curves of the form

$$R(P, E) = k$$

for different positive values of k. The following is a list of recent earnings and stock prices for five companies. Plot these companies in the PE-plane and compute their price-earnings ratio.

Company	Recent Price	Earnings per Share
A	\$20	\$4
B	\$45	\$6
C	\$81	\$8
D	\$34	\$2
E	\$146	\$49

For Problems 14–22, find the critical points and determine if they are relative maximum or minimum points.

14. $f(x, y) = 2xy - x^3 - y^2$
15. $f(x, y) = x^2 - y^2$
16. $f(x, y) = x^2 + y^2 - 2$
17. $f(x, y) = y^2 - 4x^2$
18. $f(x, y) = x^3 + y^3 - 3xy$
19. $f(x, y) = x + 2y + 1$
20. $f(x, y) = 5$
21. $f(x, y) = xy$
22. $f(x, y) = x$

Production Functions in Business

Problems 23–24 refer to a management tool called the **production function**. A company can often estimate the number N of items of a given product it can produce in terms of the amount of labor used to produce the product and the capital expended by the company to make the product. To illustrate this concept, suppose a company that manufactures teddy bears has determined that the number N of teddy bears (measured in hundreds) the company can produce per week is estimated by

$$N(L, C) = \sqrt{CL}$$

where L is the number of hours of labor required to produce the bears and C is the capital expenditure (measured in thousands of dollars per week) required.

23. **Marginal Production Functions.** The partial derivative of N with respect to L is called the **marginal production function** with respect to labor. The partial derivative of N with respect to C is called the marginal production function of N with respect to capital. Find these two marginal production functions and interpret the meaning of each.
24. **Marginal Production Functions.** Evaluate the production function N and the two marginal production functions with respect to L and C when
    (a) $L = 400$ hours, $C = 9$ (\$9,000)
    (b) $L = 900$ hours, $C = 4$ (\$4,000)
    (c) $L = 100$ hours, $C = 36$ (\$36,000)

Multicommodity Theory of the Firm

Problems 25–27 refer to the following two-commodity firm. A company makes

$$q_1 = \text{Number of units of Product 1}$$
$$q_2 = \text{Number of units of Product 2}$$

where

$$c_1 = \text{Price/unit of Product 1} = \$100$$
$$c_2 = \text{Price/unit of Product 2} = \$250$$

The cost to produce q_1 and q_2 units of these two products is given by

$$C(q_1, q_2) = 2q_1{}^2 + q_1q_2 + 4q_2{}^2$$

25. **Marginal Costs.** The partial derivatives of C with respect to q_1 and q_2 are called the **marginal costs** with respect to Product 1 and Product 2, respectively.
    (a) Find the marginal costs.
    (b) Evaluate the marginal costs when $q_1 = 100$, $q_2 = 100$.

26. **Total Cost.** Find the total profit when $q_1 = 100$ units of Product 1 and $q_2 = 200$ units of Product 2 are produced.
27. **Maximizing the Profit.** Find q_1 and q_2 so that the profit is maximized.
28. **Price Discrimination.** Consider a company that sells a product on both the foreign and domestic markets. For example, suppose the number q_f and q_d of computers of a given model that a company can sell on the foreign and domestic markets is given by

$$q_f = 10{,}000 - 2p_f \qquad \text{(foreign demand)}$$
$$q_d = 7000 - 3p_d \qquad \text{(domestic demand)}$$

respectively, where

p_f = Price charged per computer on the foreign market

p_d = Price charged per computer on the domestic market

Suppose the cost to produce the computers (in dollars) has been found to be

$$C = 100{,}000 - q_f - q_d$$

(a) What selling prices should the company adopt to maximize its profits?
(b) Can you think of a company that faces a problem such as this?

Multivariable Calculus in Medicine

Problems 29–32 refer to an important problem relating to what is called the cardiac shunt.* It is possible for a cardiologist to measure the percentage P of the total blood flow that passes through the right lung (and hence the left lung) by means of the equation

$$P = \frac{100ad}{ad + bc}$$

where

a = CO_2 output of the right lung

b = Arteriovenous CO_2 differences in the right lung

c = CO_2 output of the left lung

d = Arteriovenous CO_2 differences in the left lung

Without going into the details of what these variables mean and how this experiment is carried out, we simply say that the values of a, b, c, and d can be measured by a cardiologist.

29. **Sensitivity of *P*.** Find P_a (the partial derivative of P with respect to the CO_2 output of the right lung) and interpret its meaning.

* These problems are based on material from the fascinating book, J. G. Defares and I. N. Sneddon, *The Mathematics of Medicine and Biology*, Year Book Publishers, Chicago, 1960.

30. **Sensitivity of *P*.** Find the partial derivative P_b and interpret its meaning.
31. **Sensitivity of *P*.** Find the partial derivative P_c and interpret its meaning.
32. **Sensitivity of *P*.** Find the partial derivative P_d and interpret its meaning.
33. **Maximum Profits.** A company makes two kinds of baseball gloves. Model A gloves sell for \$15 each, and model B gloves sell for \$25 each. The total revenue in thousands of dollars from the sale of x thousand model A gloves and y thousand model B gloves will be given by

$$R(x, y) = 15x + 25y$$

The company determines that the total cost, in thousands of dollars, to produce x thousand model A gloves and y thousand model B gloves is given by

$$C(x, y) = x^2 + y^2 + 3x + 9y + 50$$

Find the amount of each type of glove that must be produced and sold to maximize their profit.

For Problems 34–47, find the critical points of the following functions and use the second-partials test to classify each of the critical points. Use any information you know about the surface to justify your answers.

34. $f(x, y) = x + y + 1$
35. $f(x, y) = -2x + y + xy$
36. $f(x, y) = xy$
37. $f(x, y) = x^2 + y^2$
38. $f(x, y) = 1 - x^2 - y^2$
39. $f(x, y) = x - x^2$
40. $f(x, y) = 10$
41. $f(x, y) = 120x + 60y - xy - x^2 - y^2$
42. $f(x, y) = \dfrac{1}{x^2} + \dfrac{1}{y^2}$
43. $f(x, y) = \dfrac{1}{x^2 + y^2}$
44. $f(x, y) = \ln(x^2 + y^2)$
45. $f(x, y) = e^{xy}$
46. $f(x, y) = e^{-(x^2+y^2)}$
47. $f(x, y) = \ln x + y$

For Problems 48–57, find the point(s), if any, at which the functions attain their relative maximum and minimum values subject to the given constraints. Try working the problems using what you know about the graphs of the functions before resorting to the method of Lagrange multipliers.

	Function	Constraint
48.	$f(x, y) = x + y$	$x - y = 1$
49.	$f(x, y) = x + y$	$x = 0$
50.	$f(x, y) = x^2 + y^2$	$x = 0$
51.	$f(x, y) = x^2 + y^2$	$x + y = 1$
52.	$f(x, y) = x^2 + y^2$	$x^2 + y^2 = 1$
53.	$f(x, y) = x^2 + y^2 + x$	$x + y = 1$
54.	$f(x, y) = x^2 + y^2 - 3x$	$x + y = 1$
55.	$f(x, y) = x^2 + y^2 + x + y$	$x^2 + y^2 = 1$
56.	$f(x, y) = 5$	$x \ln x + e^y = 1$
57.	$f(x, y) = x^2 + y^2$	$x - 3y = 0$

A				D	E	R	I	V	A	T	I	V	E		N	O	I	T	C	E	L	F	N	I
C																								N
C	H	A	I	N	R	U	L	E										Z			R	O	O	T
E				E						W							Z	E	R	O		P		E
L				W			I	M	P	L	I	C	I	T				R				E		G
E				T							N			S			C	O	M	M	O	N		R
R	D			O			L	I	M	I	T										P			A
A		M	I	N					A		E					C		P			E			L
T						L			X		G		I	N	C	R	E	A	S	I	N	G		
I	M	P	R	O	P	E	R				R					I		R					D	
O						I					A	S	Y	M	P	T	O	T	E		A	X	E	S
N						B		R			L		E			I		S					C	
	C	O	N	T	I	N	U	O	U	S			W			C					M		A	
C						I		O		M				S	T	A	T	I	O	N	A	R	Y	
O	P	T	I	M	I	Z	A	T	I	O	N		R			L					X			
N										O			E						J		I			
S			E	X	P	O	N	E	N	T	I	A	L				M	I	N	I	M	U	M	
T			L							H			A	R	E	A					U		A	
R			L										T				R				M		R	
A		D	I	S	K	S						S	I	M	P	S	O	N					G	
I			P										V				O						I	N
N			S				C	O	N	C	A	V	E				T				A		N	
E	U	L	E	R				P												A	R	E	A	
D								E		P											E		L	E
	D	I	F	F	E	R	E	N	T	I	A	L									A			

For Problems 58–64, find the volumes under the given surfaces above the region R in the xy-plane.

	Function	Region
58.	$f(x, y) = 1$	$R = \{(x, y): 0 \le x \le 1, 0 \le y \le 5\}$
59.	$f(x, y) = xy$	$R = \{(x, y): 0 \le x \le 2, 0 \le y \le 2\}$
60.	$f(x, y) = e^x + e^y$	$R = \{(x, y): 0 \le x \le 1, 0 \le y \le 1\}$
61.	$f(x, y) = e^y$	$R = \{(x, y): 0 \le x \le 1, 0 \le y \le 1\}$
62.	$f(x, y) = xe^y$	$R = \{(x, y): 0 \le x \le 1, -1 \le y \le 1\}$
63.	$f(x, y) = 1$	$R = \{(x, y): 5 \le x \le 7, -5 \le y \le 5\}$
64.	$f(x, y) = (x + 2y)^2$	$R = \{(x, y): 1 \le x \le 2, 1 \le y \le 2\}$

Chapter Test

1. For the function

$$f(x, y) = \ln (x + y)$$

find
(a) $f_x(x, y)$
(b) $f_y(x, y)$
(c) $f_{xx}(x, y)$
(d) $f_{xy}(x, y)$
(e) $f_{yy}(x, y)$

2. Find the critical points of

$$f(x, y) = x^3 + y^3 + 3xy$$

and use the second-partials test to classify them.

3. Of all numbers whose sum is 142, find the two that have a maximum product. Use the method of Lagrange multipliers to solve this problem.

4. Find the minimum value of

$$f(x, y) = x^2 + y^2$$

where x and y satisfy

$$x + y = 1$$

5. Evaluate the double integral

$$\iint_R (xy^2 + yx^2)\, dA$$

where

$$R = \{(x, y): 0 \le x \le 2, 0 \le y \le 1\}$$

6. **Iterated Integral.** Evaluate the iterated integral

$$\int_0^1 \left[\int_0^x e^{x-y}\, dy \right] dx$$

7. **Hmmmmm.** Show that the least squares lines that approximates the two data points (x_1, y_1), (x_2, y_2) is the straight line that passes through the two data points.
8. **Minimum Surface Area of a Box.** Mary is giving her boyfriend an assortment of candies for Valentine's Day and is sending them through the mail in a box with a square base. U.S. postal rules require that the girth (total length around the sides) plus length of the box be no more than 84 inches. (See Figure 50.) What is the maximum amount of candy (in cubic inches) that Mary can send? What are the dimensions of the box that maximize the volume?

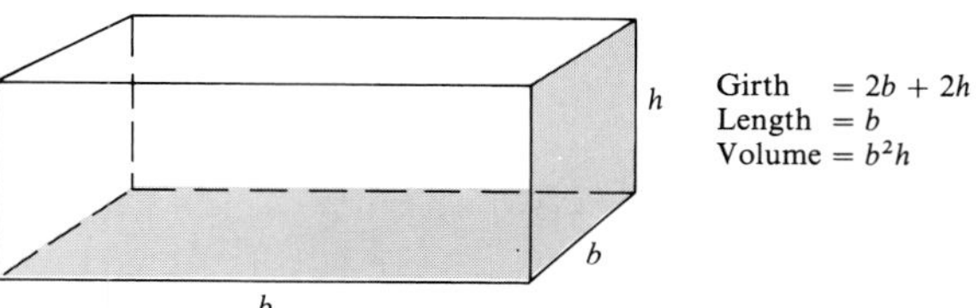

Figure 50
The length plus girth must not exceed 84 inches

9. **Sign of the Partial Derivative.** Suppose the demand for certain model car is given by a function of two variables $f(p,g)$ where p is the price of the car and g is the cost of gasoline. What can you say about the signs of the partial derivatives $\partial f/\partial p$ and $\partial f/\partial g$?

Projects and Problems: Chapters 4–6

Cumulative Exercises

For Problems 1–10, evaluate each of the definite integrals.

1. $\int_1^3 (x^2 + 3x + 4)\,dx$

2. $\int_{-2}^2 |x|\,dx$

3. $\int_0^1 \sqrt{5x + 4}\,dx$

4. $\int_1^2 \frac{x^2 + 1}{x}\,dx$

5. $\int_0^1 3^{2x}\,dx$

6. $\int_0^1 5^x\,dx$

7. $\int_0^{\ln 2} e^{-2x}\,dx$

8. $\int_{-1}^1 \frac{e^x - e^{-x}}{e^x + e^{-x}}\,dx$

9. $\int_0^4 (3e^x - 10)\,dx$

10. $\int_4^{12} (2x + 1)^{1/2}\,dx$

For Problems 11–15, compute all first-order partial derivatives.

11. $z = f(x, y) = xe^{xy}$

12. $z = f(x, y) = x^2 + 2xy + y^2$

13. $z = f(x, y) = x^3y^2 + 3xy$

14. $z = f(x, y) = \ln (xy)$

15. $z = f(x, y) = x \ln y$

Calculus and Computers

Much of calculus today is being influenced by the computer. In Problems 16–21 we ask the reader to write a computer program to carry out important calculations. Write these programs in the language of your choice (BASIC, Pascal, C, FORTRAN, etc.).

16. Trapezoid Rule and the Computer. Write a computer program to approximate the definite integral

$$\int_0^1 e^x\,dx$$

using the trapezoid rule with ten subintervals. Since it is possible to find the exact integral, what is the error in using the trapezoid rule?

17. Trapezoid Rule for Difficult Integrals. Write a computer program to approximate the definite integral

$$\int_0^1 e^{-x^2}\,dx$$

(Figure 1) using the trapezoid rule with ten trapezoids. Approximate the integral using the trapezoids with 20 subintervals.

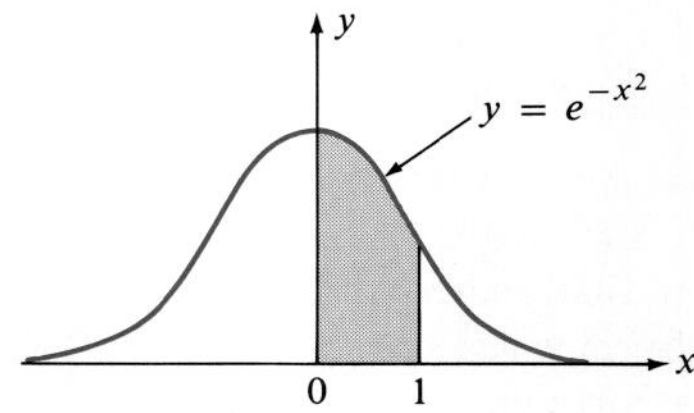

Figure 1
Approximating areas using the trapezoid rule

18. Simpson's Rule and the Computer. Write a computer program to approximate the definite integral

$$\int_0^1 e^{-x^2}\,dx$$

using Simpson's Rule with ten subintervals. Then approximate the integral using Simpson's Rule with 20 subintervals.

19. Average of a Function. The average of a function f on an interval $[a, b]$ is defined by

$$\bar{f} = \frac{1}{b - a}\int_a^b f(x)\,dx$$

Approximate the average of the function $f(x) = e^{-x^2}$ on the $[0, 1]$ using Simpson's Rule with 20 subintervals (Figure 2).

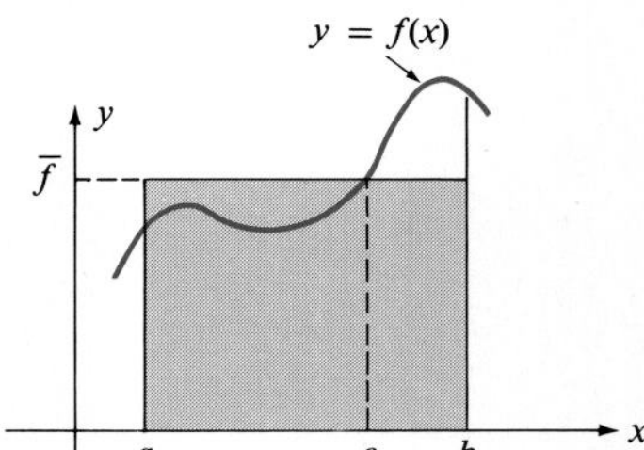

Figure 2
Illustration of the average of a function

20. Checking Table 11. Write a computer program to check the values in Table 11 in Chapter 5.

21. Checking Table 20. Write a computer program to check the values in Table 20 in Chapter 5.

Interesting Problems and Applications

22. An Integral Paradox. Let's prove that $1 = -1$. Clearly, we can write

$$\int \frac{dx}{x} = \int \frac{-dx}{-x}$$

Integrating each side of the equation, we get

$$\ln x = \ln(-x)$$

or

$$x = -x$$

Hence

$$1 = -1$$

What is wrong with this argument?

23. Another Type of Improper Integral. The function $f(x) = 1/\sqrt{x}$ can be integrated on the interval (0, 1) even though the region under the curve is unbounded. (See Figure 3.) We define this integral over the interval (0, 1) as

$$\int_0^1 \frac{1}{\sqrt{x}}\,dx = \lim_{a\to 0} \int_a^1 \frac{1}{\sqrt{x}}\,dx$$

(a) Evaluate

$$\int_a^1 \frac{1}{\sqrt{x}}\,dx$$

(b) Find the limit of the expression in part (a) as $a \to 0$. This gives the area under the curve in Figure 3.

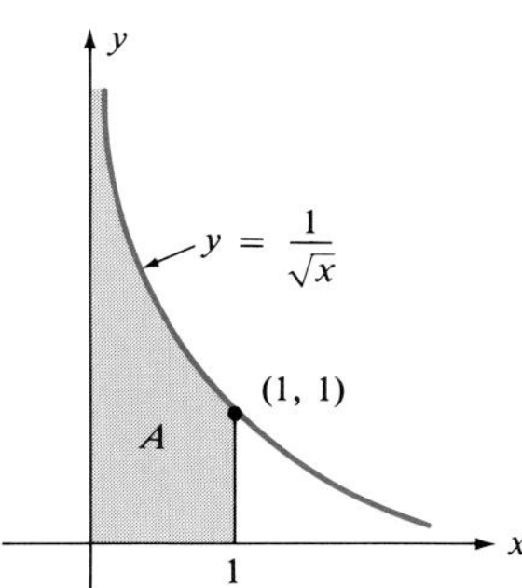

Figure 3
A different kind of improper integral

24. Integrals and Work. Anne is working out, trying to get in shape. She is exercising by repeatedly stretching a spring apparatus a distance of 1 foot. She knows that the force F (in pounds) required to stretch this spring x feet (or any fraction thereof) is $F = 50x$ (Figure 4). Anne is a physics major and knows that the work W (in foot-pounds) required to stretch this spring 1 foot is given by

$$W = \int_0^1 50x\,dx$$

How many foot-pounds of work does Anne perform every time she stretches the spring?

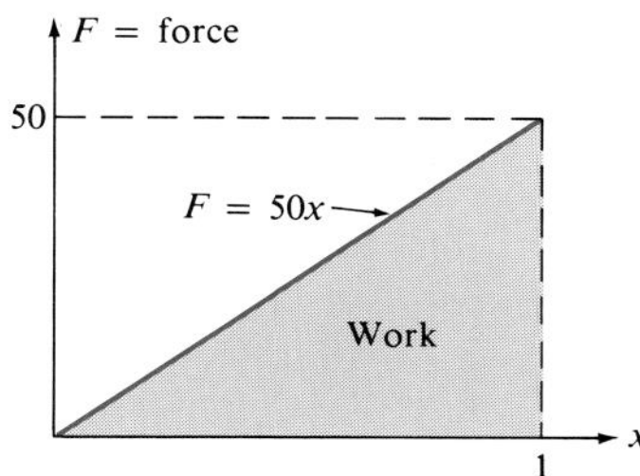

Figure 4
The area under a force curve is work

25. Mean of the Normal Distribution. The bell-shaped normal distribution curve in probability and statistics (Figure 5) is given by

$$f(x) = \frac{1}{\sqrt{2\pi}} e^{-x^2/2} \qquad (-\infty < x < \infty)$$

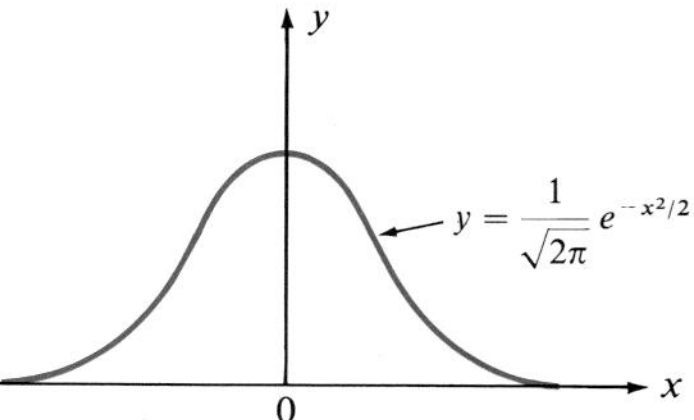

Figure 5
Normal distribution curve

The mean of the distribution is given by the integral

$$\text{Mean} = \int_{-\infty}^{\infty} xf(x)\,dx$$

Show that the mean is zero. *Hint:* This problem is easier than it looks.

26. **Total Costs.** Economists like to work with marginal costs, since they are often easy to find. Suppose an economist has determined the marginal cost for a particular product to be

$$\frac{dC}{dt} = \frac{1}{\sqrt{x+1}}$$

(a) Find the total cost if $C = 100$ when $x = 10$.
(b) Graph the total cost $C(x)$ for $0 \leq x < \infty$.

27. **Mary's Bowl.** Mary is taking a beginning pottery class and is making a soup bowl whose profile is described by the equation

$$f(x) = 1 - x^2 \qquad (0 \leq x \leq 1)$$

(Figure 6). How much soup will her bowl hold? We will assume negligible thickness for the sides of the bowl and the x-axis as the axis of revolution.

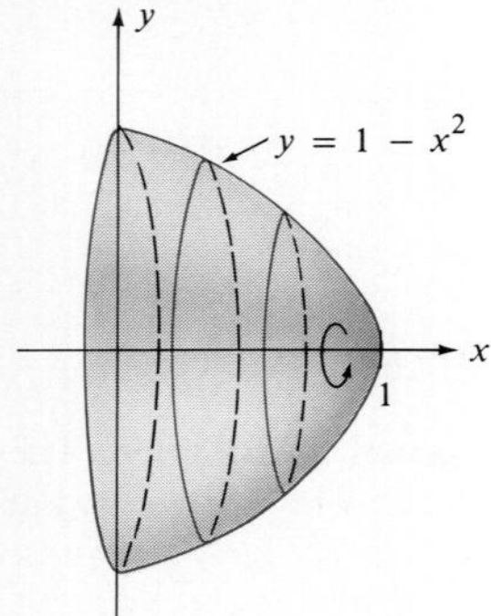

Figure 6
Mary's bowl on its side

28. **Volume of a Football.** The profile of a football is described roughly by the equation

$$f(x) = 1.5(x - x^2) \qquad (0 \leq x \leq 1)$$

where x is measured in feet (Figure 7). What is the volume of a football?

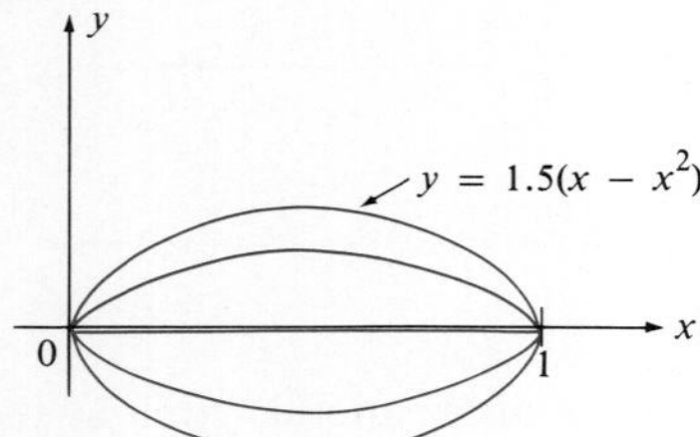

Figure 7
The equation of a football is roughly $y = 1.5(x - x^2)$

29. **Which Is Bigger?** Which of the two shaded areas, A_1 or A_2, in Figure 8 is the larger?

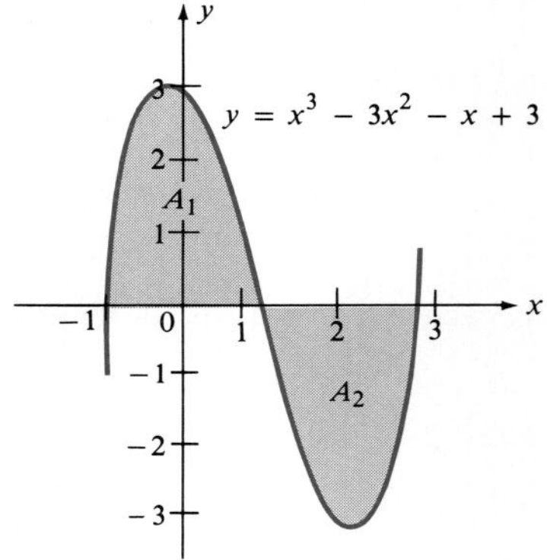

Figure 8
Which area is larger?

30. **Sally's Cardiac Output.** Sally would like to remeasure her cardiac output as discussed in Section 4.3. Write a computer program to approximate the integral of the concentration curve using the trapezoid rule and the observations in Table 1. Assuming that Sally was injected with 5 mg of dye, what is Sally's cardiac output?

TABLE 1
Results for Sally's Dye Dilution Test for Measuring Cardiac Output

Seconds After Injection	Concentration (mg/liter)	Seconds After Injection	Concentration (mg/liter)
1	0	11	4.1
2	0	12	4.0
3	0.2	13	3.6
4	0.5	14	3.4
5	0.8	15	2.7
6	1.3	16	2.0
7	1.9	17	1.5
8	2.6	18	1.0
9	3.5	19	0.4
10	4.0	20	0.0

31. **How Deep Is the Well?** Henry is exploring a cave and comes upon a seemingly bottomless pit (Figure 9). In an attempt to determine the depth of the pit he drops a stone into the pit and listens for the stone to strike the bottom. Henry knows that the velocity of the stone in-

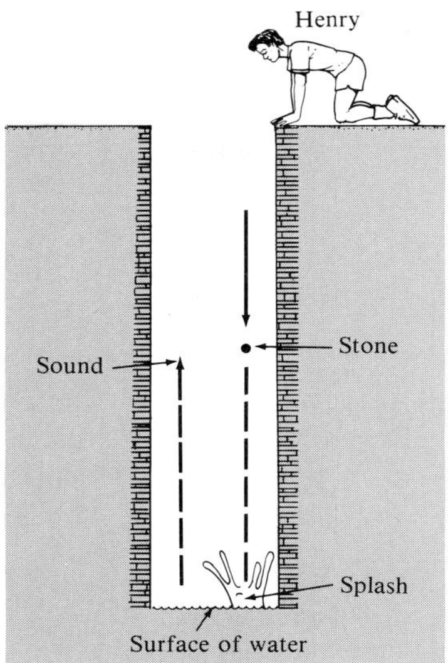

Figure 9
How deep is the pit?

creases by 32 feet per second every second. In other words, if $y(t)$ represents the number of feet the stone falls in t seconds, then the change in velocity (or acceleration) will always have the same value of

$$\frac{d^2y}{dt^2} = 32 \text{ ft/sec}^2$$

Ten seconds after Henry drops the stone, he hears a faint splash. Assuming that the time for the sound of the splash to travel from the bottom of the pit to Henry is negligible, how deep is the pit?

32. How Much Did You Win* You have just won the lottery and will collect R dollars each year for the next T years. If the interest rate paid by banks for deposits is r percent compounded continuously, then the value of your winnings in today's dollars (or the present value PV) is

$$PV = \int_0^T Re^{-rt}\,dr$$

(a) Show that this present value can be written as

$$PV = \frac{R}{r}(1 - e^{-rT})$$

(b) Why is it true that if you collect R dollars per year indefinitely, the present value of your winnings is R/r?
(c) If you are to collect \$50,000 per year for the next 10 years, and if banks pay interest on deposits of 10% compounded continuously, then what is the present value of your winnings?
(d) If you are to collect \$50,000 per year indefinitely, what is the present value of your winnings? Assume that interest rates remain constant at 10% compounded continuously.

33. Blood Flow Through an Artery. Experiments have determined that the speed (in centimeters per second) of blood through an artery r centimeters from the central axis is given by

$$S(r) = k(R^2 - r^2) \qquad (0 \le r \le R)$$

where R is the radius of the artery and $k > 0$ is a constant that depends on the individual. (See Figure 10.) The rate of flow F of blood (in cubic centimeters per second) through an artery can be found by computing the integral

$$F = 2\pi \int_0^R rS(r)\,dr$$

Find the general expression for the rate of flow F of an artery of radius R.

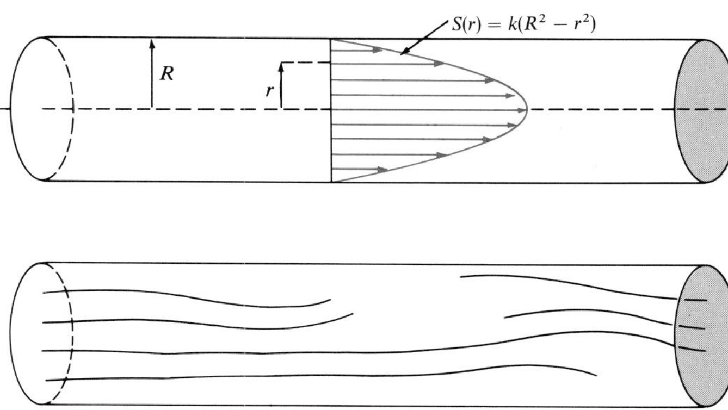

Figure 10
Profile showing the velocity of blood through a vein

34. Sledding Problem. Suppose you are sitting on a sled on a snowpacked surface described by a function $z = f(x, y)$ at the point $(a, b, f(a, b))$. Suppose that

$$f_x(a, b) = 0$$
$$f_y(a, b) = 0$$
$$f_{xx}(a, b) f_{yy}(a, b) - f_{xy^2}(a, b) = 1$$
$$f_{xx}(a, b) = 1$$

(a) What will the sled do?
(b) What will the sled do if $f_{xx}(a, b)$ is changed to -1?

35. Hmmmmm. Suppose we describe the surface of the earth (the northern hemisphere at least) by a function of two variables $z = f(x, y)$. Suppose you are standing at a point $(a, b, f(a, b))$ on the surface where

$$f_x(a, b) = 0$$
$$f_y(a, b) = 0$$
$$f_{xx}(a, b) f_{yy}(a, b) - f_{xy^2}(a, b) = 1$$
$$f_{xx}(a, b) = -1$$

All of a sudden you see a bear. What color is the bear?

36. A Strange Surface? Can you find a function $z = f(x, y)$ other than a constant function that satisfies the equation

$$f_x(x, y) = f_y(x, y)$$

for all x and y? What can you say about a surface described by such an equation?

37. A Strange Surface? Can you find a function $z = f(x, y)$ that satisfies the equation

$$f_x(x, y) = 1$$

for all x and y? What can you say about a surface that satisfies such an equation?

Learning Through Writing

38. Writing Lucid Mathematics. The authors must have written the definition of the integral on page 321 many, many times in order that it was defined precisely and easy to understand. We would like you to try to write a better definition.

39. You Can Be the Author. Compose an interesting word problem that illustrates some topic studied in Chapters 4–6. What important aspect does your problem illustrate?

40. You Make Up the Test. Most professors are criticized for giving exams that cover material that is not covered in the book. Write a sample exam covering the material in Chapters 4–6 and give it to a classmate for evaluation.

One of the more impressive applications of the calculus (mostly integral) lies in the modern development of probability.

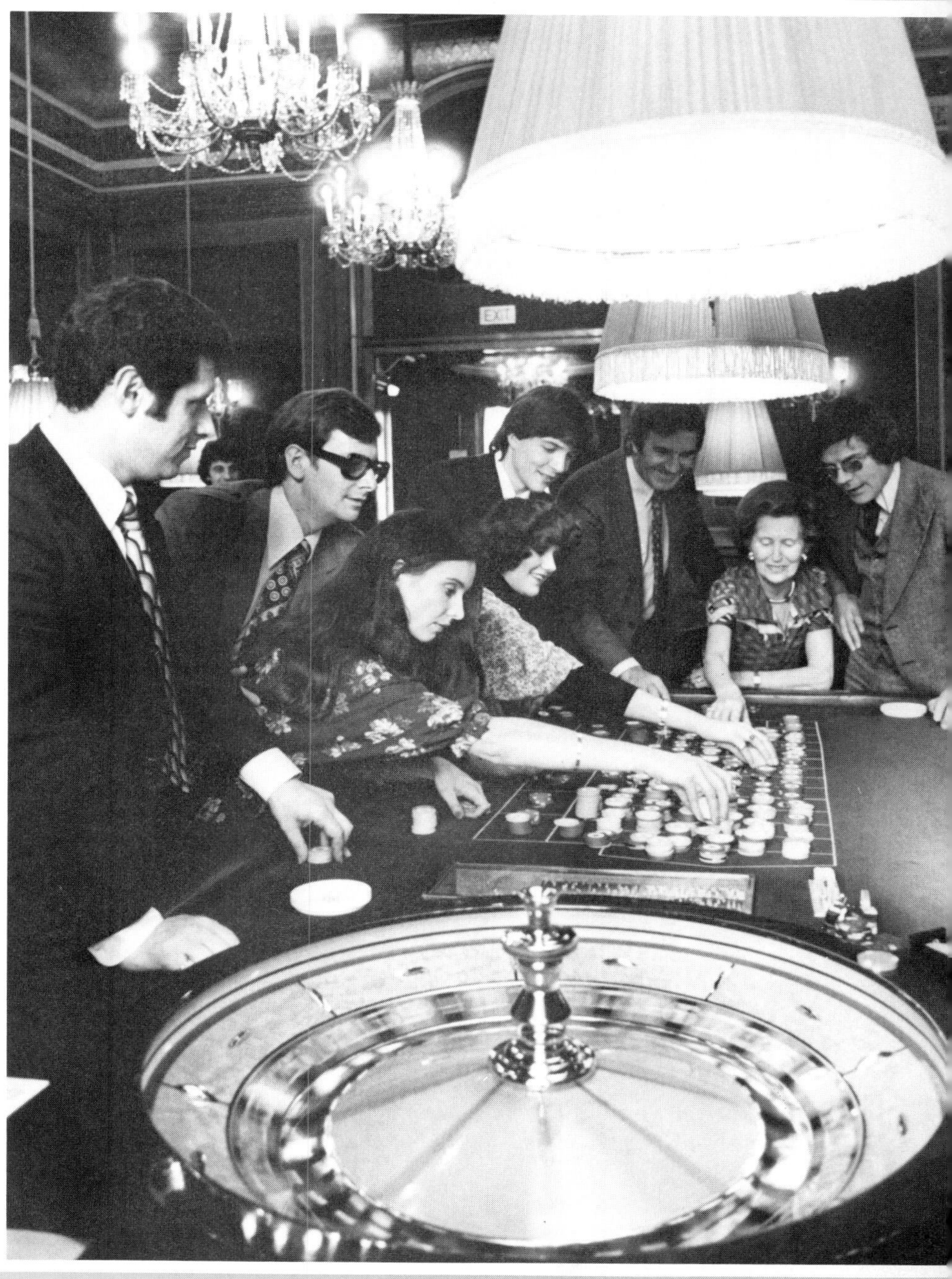

7 Calculus and Probability

This chapter introduces a few of the basic ideas of probability and shows how the integral calculus is used in the development of these ideas. In Section 7.1 we introduce the concepts of probability experiments, finite random variables, and probability functions of finite random variables. Although Section 7.1 does not require a knowledge of calculus, it is important for you to understand the ideas introduced here so that the material studied in the following sections can be better appreciated. In Section 7.2 we introduce the continuous random variable and the probability density function of a continuous random variable. Knowledge of integral calculus is necessary for a serious study of these topics. Finally, in Section 7.3 we study the two most important continuous random variables in probability, the exponential random variable and the normal random variable.

7.1 Basic Concepts: Finite Random Variables

PURPOSE

In this introductory section we present a few of the basic ideas of probability. Although this section does not rely on the calculus, it provides a useful introduction to the material that follows. In particular, we introduce

- the probability experiment,
- the sample space of a probability experiment,
- an event of a sample space,
- the probability that an event occurs, and
- the finite random variable and its expectation.

Introduction

The word “chance” is used so often that we generally do not give it a second thought. We talk about the chance that the Dow Jones average will reach 3000 by the end of the year or the chance that the Cleveland Indians will win the American League Pennant. The word “chance” is a synonym for “probability,” and the subject of probability attempts to give a precise meaning to this word. It is hard to believe that a subject such as probability, which had its origins in French gambling parlors, would become one of the most important intellectual developments of modern times.

Today, the subject of probability has outgrown its disreputable origins. It is extremely important in the fields of the natural and social sciences, business management, physics and engineering, and many more. For example, it has been said that the single most important result in population genetics is the Hardy-Weinberg Law, which is basically a theorem in probability.

The Probability Experiment

Central to the subject of probability is the probability experiment. Any experiment (such as a scientific experiment) that has two or more possible outcomes is called a **probability experiment**. Examples are tossing a coin, rolling a die, testing products on an assembly line, measuring some physical characteristic of a spruce budworm, and even asking a family its annual income. The set of all possible outcomes of a probability experiment is called the **sample space** of the experiment. Any collection of outcomes or subset of the sample space is called an **event** in the sample space. For instance, when we toss a coin and observe whether the coin is a head (H) or a tail (T), the sample space is $S = \{H, T\}$. The subset $\{H\}$ is an event in S and would be called "the event of tossing a head."

We summarize these basic definitions.

Probability Experiment, Sample Space, and Event

1. *Probability Experiment.* A probability experiment is an experiment that has two or more outcomes.
2. *Sample Space.* The set of all outcomes of a probability experiment is called the sample space of the experiment. It is denoted by S.
3. *Event.* A subset of a sample space is called an event.

Example 1

Rolling a Die Consider the experiment of rolling a die (singular of dice) and observing the number of dots that appear on the top face. What is the sample space of this experiment?

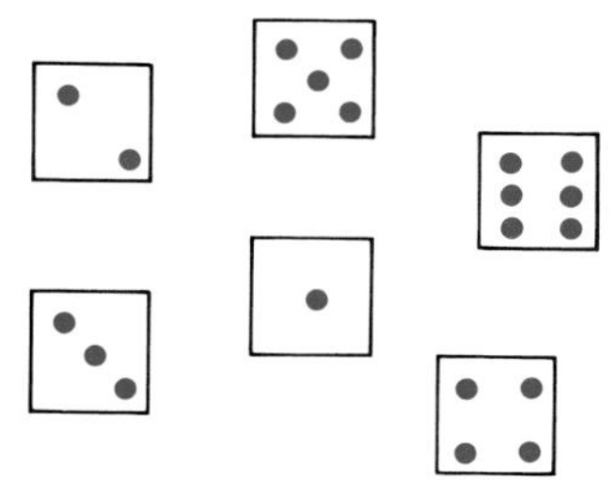

Figure 1
Sample space for tossing one die and observing the top face

Solution This experiment is a probability experiment because it has more than one possible outcome. The set of all possible outcomes or the sample space of the experiment would be denoted by $S = \{1, 2, 3, 4, 5, 6\}$. See Figure 1. Typical events in S would be

$A = \{1\}$ (event of rolling a 1)
$B = \{4, 5, 6\}$ (event of rolling a 4, 5, or 6)
$C = S$ (certain event: rolling a 1, 2, 3, 4, 5, or 6) □

Example 2

Pair of Dice Roll a pair of dice (one red die and one green die), and observe the sum of the dots that appear on the faces that turn up. What is the sample space of the event?

Solution This experiment has 36 possible outcomes. Each individual outcome is represented by an ordered pair (r, g), where

$$r = \text{Number of dots showing on the red die} \qquad r \in \{1, 2, 3, 4, 5, 6\}$$
$$g = \text{Number of dots showing on the green die} \qquad g \in \{1, 2, 3, 4, 5, 6\}$$

The 36 outcomes of this sample space are shown in Figure 2.

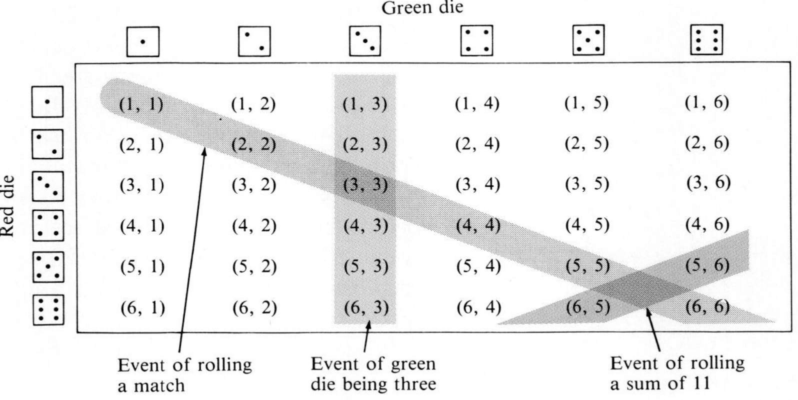

Figure 2
Sample space and three typical events when rolling a pair of dice

Figure 2 also shows the events:

Event of rolling a match:

$$MD = \{(r, g) \mid r = g\} = \{(1, 1), (2, 2), (3, 3), (4, 4), (5, 5), (6, 6)\}$$

Event that the total number of dots on the top faces is 11:

$$S11 = \{(r, g) \mid r + g = 11\} = \{(5, 6), (6, 5)\}$$

Event of rolling a pair of dice where the green die is a 3:

$$G3 = \{(r, g) \mid g = 3\} = \{(1, 3), (2, 3), (3, 3), (4, 3), (5, 3), (6, 3)\}$$ □

HISTORICAL NOTE

Probability had its origins during the fifteenth and sixteenth centuries when Italian mathematicians attempted to evaluate the odds in various games of chance. The great Italian mathematician Geronimo Cardano (1501–1576) wrote a gambler's guidebook in which he discussed how to cheat and how to detect cheaters. He later used probability theory to predict the exact date of his death. When the date of his prediction arrived and he seemed to be in good health, Cardano committed suicide to uphold his theory. Although Cardano's work was important, it is generally agreed that the rigorous origins of probability sprang from the minds of the two great French mathematicians, Pierre de Fermat (1601–1665) and Blaise Pascal (1623–1662) around 1654. By studying games of chance, they developed much of the elementary theory of probability.

Example 3

Typical Events The sample space of the experiment of flipping three different coins is illustrated by means of a tree diagram in Figure 3. Here each outcome of the experiment is illustrated by one of the paths of the tree as you move from left to right through the tree.

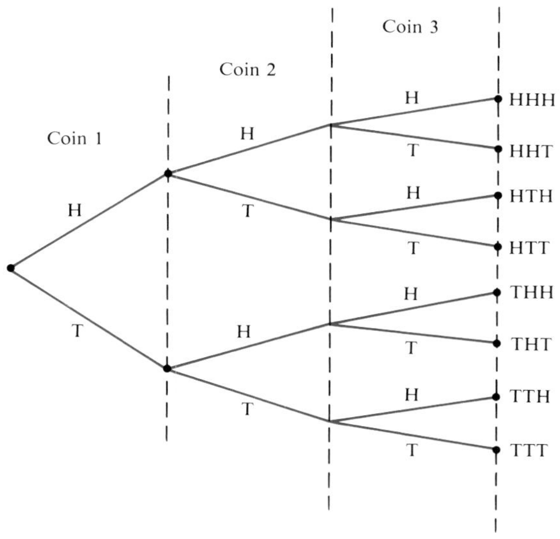

Figure 3
The sample space for tossing three coins

The sample space can be written mathematically as

$$S = \{\text{TTT, TTH, THT, THH, HTT, HTH, HHT, HHH}\}$$

Find the three different events:

(a) Event of getting one head,

(b) Event of getting two heads,

(c) Event of getting three heads.

Solution

(a) Event of getting one head = {TTH, THT, HTT}

(b) Event of getting two heads = {THH, HTH, HHT}

(c) Event of getting three heads = {HHH} □

Meaning of Probability

Probability has to do with our confidence about knowing whether something will happen. One often hears something like "There is a 40% chance of rain tomorrow" or "The chance that the Yankees will win the pennant is 1 in 100." The subject of **mathematical probability** provides a framework for making these ideas precise.

Consider a probability experiment that can have several possible outcomes. Suppose that none of the outcomes can be predicted with 100% accuracy but that a given "degree of confidence" P can be assigned to each outcome. The value of P measures the **likelihood** that a given outcome will occur. For instance, if we assign the value $P = .50$ to an outcome, this means that the likelihood that the outcome occurs on any trial of the experiment is 50% or one-half the time. The number P is called the **probability** that the outcome occurs. The concept of probability is made precise in the following definition.

> **Definition of Probability**
>
> Let S be the **finite sample space**
>
> $$S = \{s_1, s_2, s_3, \ldots, s_n\}$$
>
> Assign to each outcome s_i of S, any number $P(s_i)$ such that the value of $P(s_i)$ satisfies the two **fundamental laws of probability**:
>
> **1.** $0 \le P(s_i) \le 1 \qquad (i = 1, 2, \ldots, n)$
>
> **2.** $P(s_1) + P(s_2) + \cdots + P(s_n) = 1$
>
> The number $P(s_i)$ is called the **probability** that s_i occurs.

Example 4

Coin Toss Toss a coin and observe whether it turns up heads or tails. Assign probabilities to the sample space of this experiment in such a way that the likelihood of tossing a head is the same as tossing a tail. Such a coin is called a "fair" coin.

Solution The sample space of this probability experiment is

$$S = \{\mathrm{H}, \mathrm{T}\}$$

Since tossing a head has the same chance of occurring as tossing a tail, we assign the probabilities

$$P(\mathrm{H}) = 1/2$$
$$P(\mathrm{T}) = 1/2$$

Note that this assignment of probabilities satisfies the two fundamental laws of probability. □

When every outcome of a probability experiment has the same chance of occurring (as in the above example), the outcomes are called **equally likely**.

Example 5

Coin Toss Three Times Suppose a fair coin is tossed three times. How would you assign probabilities to each outcome of this experiment?

Solution The sample space of this experiment is

$$S = \{\mathrm{TTT, TTH, THT, THH, HTT, HTH, HHT, HHH}\}$$

Since each of these outcomes has the same chance of occurring, we would assign the equal probabilities

$$P(\mathrm{TTT}) = 1/8 = .125$$
$$P(\mathrm{TTH}) = 1/8 = .125$$
$$P(\mathrm{THT}) = 1/8 = .125$$
$$P(\mathrm{THH}) = 1/8 = .125$$

$$P(\text{HTT}) = 1/8 = .125$$
$$P(\text{HTH}) = 1/8 = .125$$
$$P(\text{HHT}) = 1/8 = .125$$
$$P(\text{HHH}) = 1/8 = .125$$
□

Probability of an Event

We have defined the probability P that an outcome of a probability experiment occurs. We can also define the probability that an event occurs. We have said before that an event occurs when the outcome of the experiment is one of the outcomes in the event. We can then define the **probability of an event** to mean the probability that the outcome of the experiment is one of the outcomes in the event. The following rules show how to find the probability of an event, both in an equally likely sample space and in a non–equally likely sample space.

Computation of Probabilities of Events

Let S be a sample space with n equally likely outcomes, and let A be an event in S that contains k of these outcomes. Then the probability that the event A occurs is

$$P(A) = \frac{k}{n}$$

In a non–equally likely sample space the probability of an event A can be found by adding the probabilities of each of the outcomes in A.

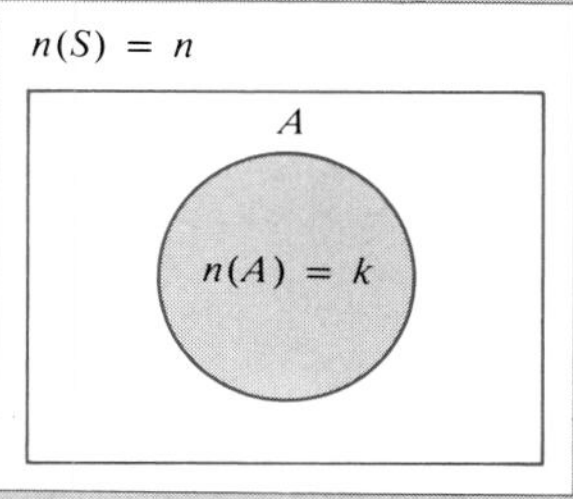

Example 6

Probabilities in Poker Figure 4 lists the ten different types of poker hands and the probability that a player will be dealt each type of hand. Using this table, find the probability of being dealt the following hands:

(a) Three of a kind or better

(b) Two pairs or better

(c) Full house or better

Solution In each of the above cases we are asked to find the probability of the union of various events. Since the ten events (hands) are *disjoint* (you have never been dealt two of the above hands at the same time, have you?), the probability of getting one hand *or* another hand is the sum of getting each hand. Hence we have

Poker hand	Hand	Number of favorable events	Probability
Royal flush	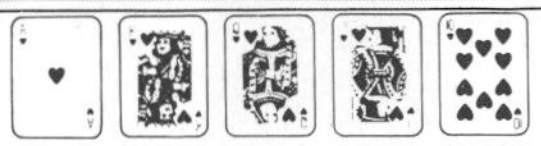	4	.00000153908
Other straight flush	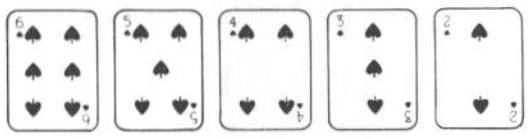	36	.00001385169
Four of a kind	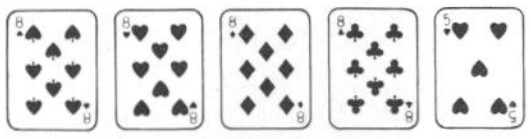	624	.00024009604
Full house	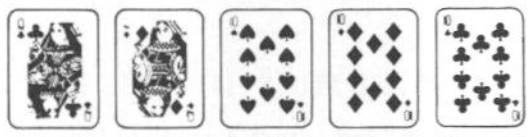	3,744	.00144057623
Flush	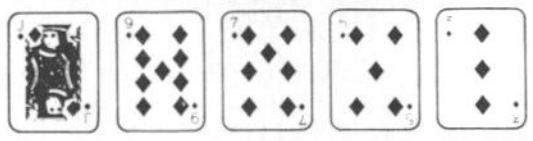	5,108	.00196540155
Straight	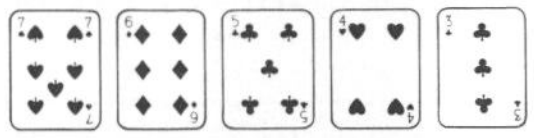	10,200	.00392464682
Three of a kind	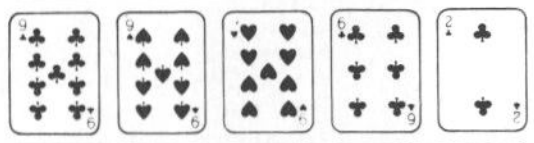	54,912	.02112845138
Two pairs	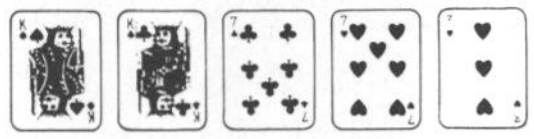	123,552	.04753901561
One pair	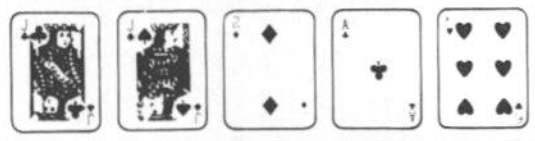	1,098,240	.42256902761
Other hands	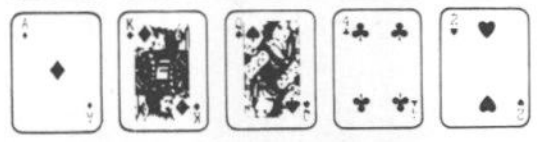	1,302,540	.50117739403
Totals		2,598,960	1.00000000000

Figure 4
Poker hands

(a) $P(\text{three of a kind or better}) = .0211285 + \cdots + .0000015 = .0287145$

(b) $P(\text{two pairs or better}) = .0475390 + \cdots + .0000015 = .0762535$

(c) $P(\text{full house or better}) = .0014406 + \cdots + .0000015 = .0016961$ □

Example 7

Equally Likely Outcomes Suppose you roll a pair of dice. What is the probability that the sum of the two numbers rolled is a 7 or 11?

Solution The desired event of rolling a 7 or 11 is

$$\text{Rolling a 7 or 11} = \{(6, 1), (5, 2), (4, 3), (3, 4), (2, 5), (1, 6), (5, 6), (6, 5)\}$$

which has $k = 8$ outcomes. Since the sample space has $n = 36$ equally likely outcomes (see Figure 5), we have

$$P(\text{Rolling 7 or 11}) = \frac{k}{n} = \frac{8}{36} = .22$$

Die II

Die I	⚀	⚁	⚂	⚃	⚄	⚅
⚀	(1, 1)	(1, 2)	(1, 3)	(1, 4)	(1, 5)	(1, 6)
⚁	(2, 1)	(2, 2)	(2, 3)	(2, 4)	(2, 5)	(2, 6)
⚂	(3, 1)	(3, 2)	(3, 3)	(3, 4)	(3, 5)	(3, 6)
⚃	(4, 1)	(4, 2)	(4, 3)	(4, 4)	(4, 5)	(4, 6)
⚄	(5, 1)	(5, 2)	(5, 3)	(5, 4)	(5, 5)	(5, 6)
⚅	(6, 1)	(6, 2)	(6, 3)	(6, 4)	(6, 5)	(6, 6)

Event of rolling a 7

Event of rolling an 11

Figure 5
Event of rolling a 7 or 11

In other words, there is a 22% chance of rolling a 7 or an 11. □

The Random Variable

When one performs probability experiments, such as tossing a coin, rolling a pair of dice, measuring vital signs of a patient, or measuring daily inventory, one generally records numbers. More often than not, when a probability experiment is performed, some real number is computed for each outcome of the experiment. This brings us to one of the most important ideas in probability, the **random variable**.

Definition of a Random Variable

A **random variable** is a function whose domain is the set of outcomes of a probability experiment and whose value for an outcome is a real number.

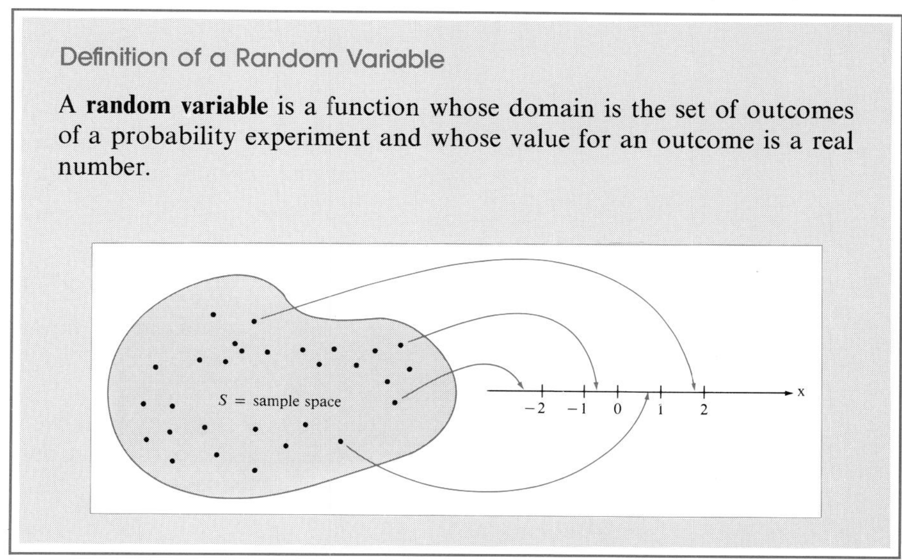

Random variables are generally denoted by the capital letters X, Y, and Z.

Example 8

Typical Random Variable Roll a pair of dice. What are some typical random variables that could be associated with this experiment?

Solution There are many ways to assign numbers to the 36 outcomes of this experiment. We list a few here.

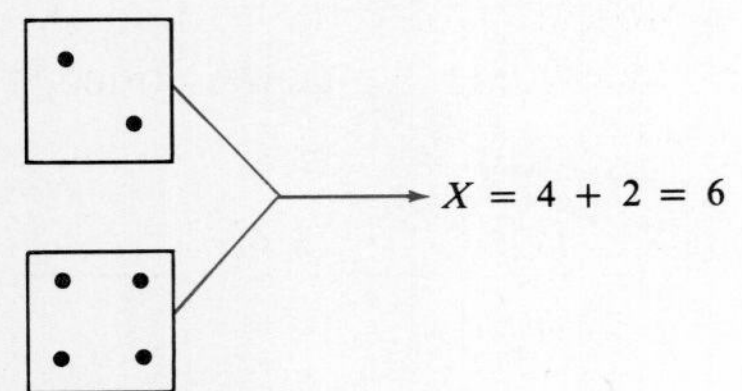

Figure 6
Sum of the numbers of the top faces

(a) One random variable is

$$X = \text{Total number of dots that appear on the top faces}$$

Figure 6 illustrates how the random variable X assigns a number to each outcome of the sample space of the experiment.

(b) Another random variable is

$$Y = \text{Difference between the larger and smaller numbers rolled}$$

Here the random variable Y would be 2 when the roll of the dice turned up 5 and 3, as in Figure 7.

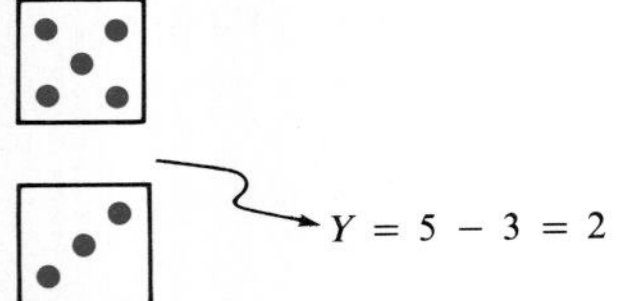

Figure 7
The difference between the larger and smaller numbers rolled is 2

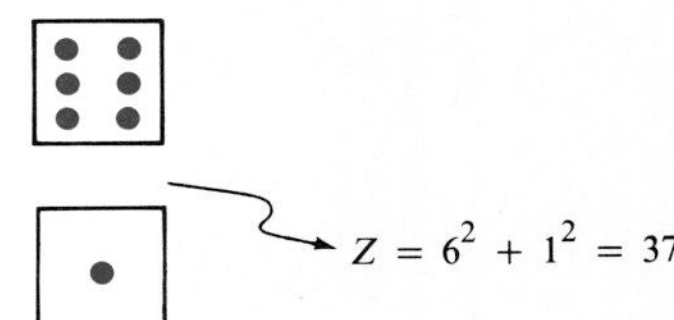

Figure 8
Dice showing a sum of squares equal to 37

(c) A third random variable is

$$Z = \text{Sum of squares of the numbers on the top faces}$$

The value of Z would be 37 when the roll of the dice turn up a 6 and 1, as in Figure 8. □

A random variable is called a **finite random variable** if it can take on only a finite number of different values. The following example illustrates this idea.

Example 9

Finite Random Variable Roll a pair of dice and define the random variable

$$X = \text{Sum of the two numbers on the top faces}$$

What are the possible values of X?

Solution The **range of values** of X, or the values that X can take on, are clearly the integers 2, 3, . . . , 12. Since these are the only 11 possible values for X, we call X a finite random variable. □

Probability Distribution of a Random Variable

Intuitively, we often think of a random variable as a variable "jumping" from number to number while the probability experiment is being performed over and over. For example, for repeated rolls of a pair of dice the sum of the numbers on the top faces "jumps" randomly among the values 2 through 12. The question we would like to answer is whether there is a pattern to the way in which this sum jumps from number to number. In other words, is it possible to find the probability that the sum takes on a given value? This brings us to the concept of the **probability distribution** of a random variable.

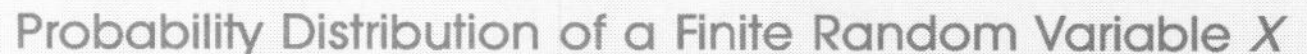

Probability Distribution of a Finite Random Variable X

Let X be a finite random variable that can take on values $x_1, x_2, \ldots, x_n$. The **probability distribution** of X is the function p defined for $1 \leq i \leq n$ by

$$p(x_i) = P(X = x_i)$$

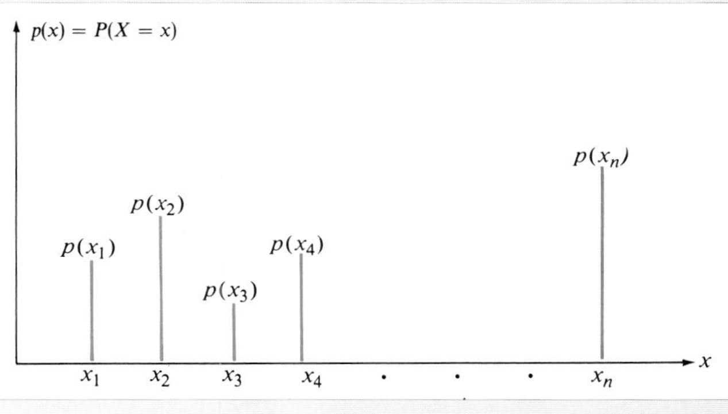

In other words, the probability distribution $p(x)$ at x of the random variable X is the probability that X takes on the value x. From this definition of the probability distribution the following two properties hold.

Two Properties of Probability Distributions

A probability distribution p of a random variable satisfies the properties

1. $0 \leq p(x) \leq 1$

2. $p(x_1) + p(x_2) + \cdots + p(x_n) = 1$

where $x_1, x_2, \ldots, x_n$ are all the possible values taken on by the random variable.

Example 10 Probability Distribution Roll a pair of dice, and define the random variable

$$X = \text{Total number of dots showing on the top faces}$$

The probability distribution for this random variable is graphed in Figure 9.

x	$p(x)$
2	1/36
3	2/36
4	3/36
5	4/36
6	5/36
7	6/36
8	5/36
9	4/36
10	3/36
11	2/36
12	1/36

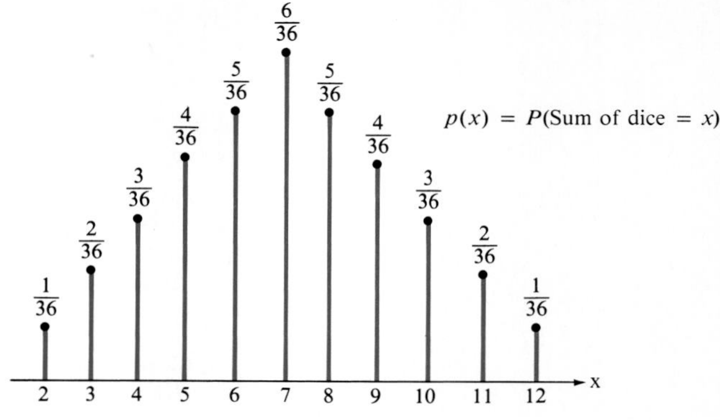

Figure 9
Probability distribution of the sum of rolled numbers of two dice

Expectation of a Random Variable

Suppose we perform a probability experiment several times, each time recording the value of a random variable X. When finished, we compute the arithmetic average of the values of X that have occurred. (Just add them up and divide by the number of terms.) This average value will approximate what is called the **expectation** or **expected value** of X. Sometimes people say intuitively that the expected value of X is the average value of an infinite number of X's. Of course we cannot find the average value of an infinite number of terms, but we can compute the average value of a large number of X's. A more precise definition of the expectation of X is now given.

Expectation of a Random Variable X

Let the **probability distribution** p of a finite random variable X be defined by the table:

Possible Values of X, x	**Probability of X Taking on This Value, $p(x)$**
x_1	$p(x_1)$
x_2	$p(x_2)$
$\vdots$	$\vdots$
x_n	$p(x_n)$

The **expectation** of X (or **expected value** of X), denoted by $E[X]$, is given by

$$E[X] = x_1p(x_1) + x_2p(x_2) + \cdots + x_np(x_n)$$

$$= \sum_{i=1}^{n} x_ip(x_i) \qquad \text{(summation notation)}$$

Steps for Finding $E[X]$

To find the expectation of a random variable X, perform the following steps:

- **Step 1.** Find the possible values $x_1, x_2, \ldots, x_n$ that X can take on.
- **Step 2.** Find the probabilities

$$p(x_1) = P(X = x_1)$$
$$p(x_2) = P(X = x_2)$$
$$\vdots$$
$$p(x_n) = P(X = x_n)$$

- **Step 3.** Compute

$$E[X] = x_1p(x_1) + x_2p(x_2) + \cdots + x_np(x_n)$$

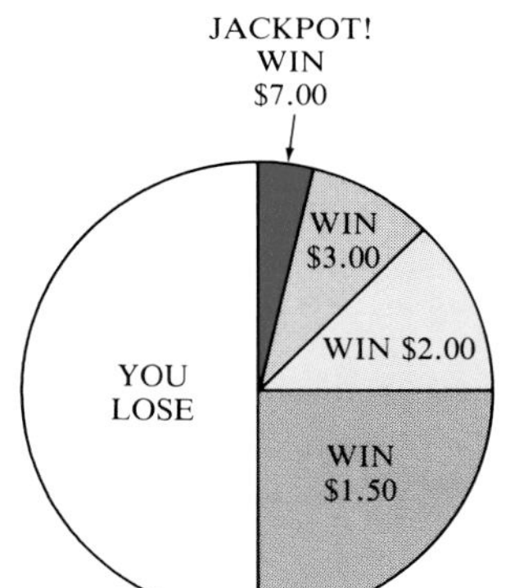

Figure 10
What are the average winnings?

The term *expectation* or *expected value* is often used in discussing games of chance. The following game illustrates this idea.

Example 11

Spin the Wheel Let's play Spin the Wheel. The player spins the wheel and waits for it to stop. The wheel is subdivided into five sectors, and the winnings for each sector are shown in Figure 10. Would you be willing to pay $1 for a spin of this wheel?

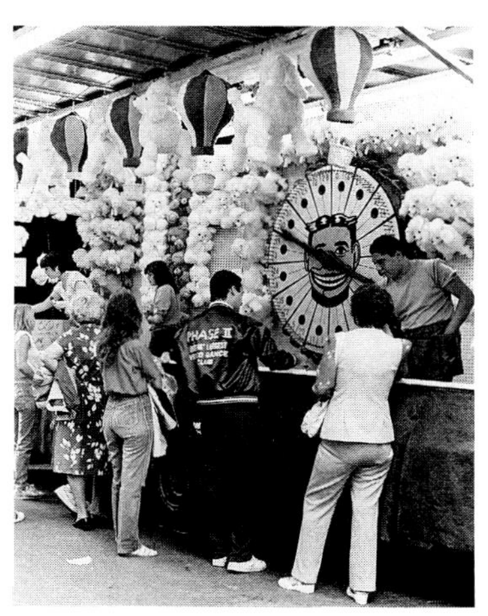

Solution Define the random variable

$$W = \text{Winnings from one spin of the wheel}$$

To find $E[W]$, we carry out the following steps:

- **Step 1** (find the values that W takes on). The possible winnings are 0, $1.50, $2, $3, and $7. These are listed in the first column of Table 1.
- **Step 2** (find the probability that W takes on its values). The probability that the winnings will take on any of these values is determined from Figure 10. These are listed in the second column of Table 1.
- **Step 3** (compute the expected value). Compute the product of the values in the first and second columns found in Steps 2 and 3 and put these products in the third column. Summing the values in the third column, we have the expected value.

TABLE 1
Steps in Finding an Expected Value

Winnings, x (Step 1)	**Probability of Winning, $p(x)$ (Step 2)**	**Expected Value, $x \cdot p(x)$ (Step 3)**
$0	.500	(0)(.500) = 0
$1.50	.250	(1.5)(.250) = $0.375
$2	.125	(2)(.125) = $0.250
$3	.092	(3)(.092) = $0.276
$7	0.33	(7)(.033) = $0.231
Total	1.000	$1.13

In other words, you will collect (on the average) \$1.13 per spin while playing this game. Of course, if it costs \$1 to play the game, then your expected net winnings per game will be reduced to \$0.13. This does not mean that you will win 13 cents on every game (in fact you never win 13 cents on a single game), but after, say, an entire weekend of playing this game, your average winnings per game will approximate this value. If you play 1000 games over the course of a weekend, your expected take will be \$130. The graph of the probability distribution of the winnings W is shown in Figure 11. □

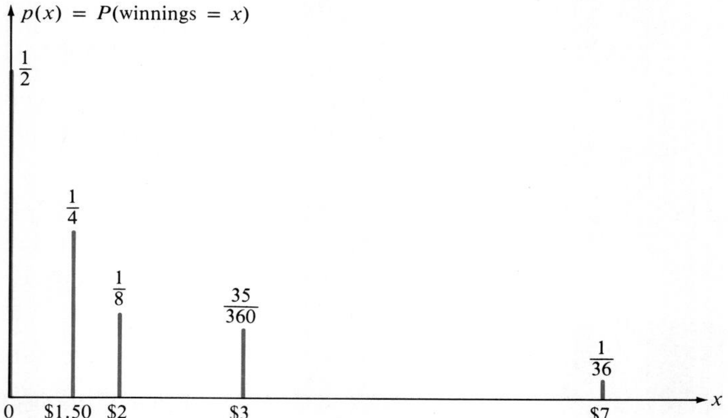

Figure 11
Distribution of winnings in Spin the Wheel

Example 12

Win Big Money We've got just the game for you. All you do is roll a pair of dice. The rules of the game are the following:

- You win \$10 if a 7 or 11 turns up.
- You win \$3 if a 8, 9, or 10 turns up.
- You lose \$8 otherwise.

What are your expected winnings per roll of the dice?

Solution To find your expected winnings, you simply ask yourself what the different amounts are that you can win (or lose) and the probabilities of winning these amounts; then just sum the products of these amounts. To carry out these steps, it is useful to draw a figure illustrating the possible winnings and the probability of achieving these winnings. Then to find the expected winnings, compute the values in Table 2 using Figure 12 as an aid.

Interpretation

In the long run, you will lose an average of \$0.33 on each roll of the dice. Stated another way, if you roll the dice 1000 times, you should expect to lose roughly (−\$0.33)(1000) = −\$333. □

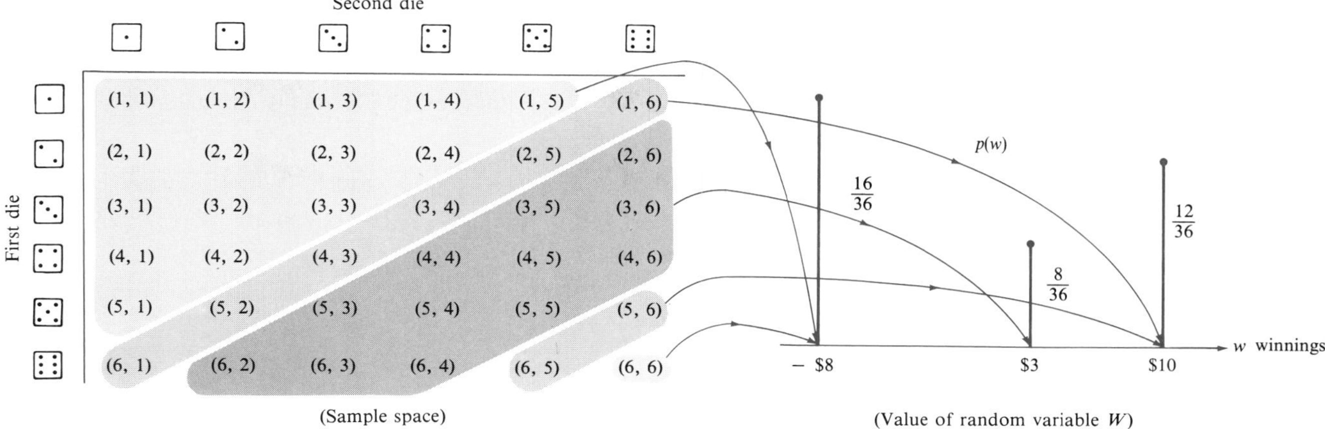

Figure 12
Sample space that results from rolling a pair of dice and the winnings associated with each outcome

TABLE 2
Steps in Finding Your Expected Winnings

Winnings, w (Step 1)	**Probability of Winning, $p(w)$ (Step 2)**	**Expected Value, $w \cdot p(w)$ (Step 3)**
\$3	$\frac{12}{36}$	$(3)\left(\frac{12}{36}\right) = 1$
\$10	$\frac{8}{36}$	$(10)\left(\frac{8}{36}\right) = \frac{80}{36}$
−\$8	$\frac{16}{36}$	$(-8)\left(\frac{16}{36}\right) = -\frac{128}{36}$
Totals	1	$E[W] = -\frac{12}{36} = -\$0.33$

Problems

For Problems 1–6, find the sample space when three coins are tossed if the following quantities are observed:

1. If we observe whether each coin is a head or a tail.
2. If we observe the number of heads tossed.
3. If we observe the sum when Head = 2 and Tail = 5.
4. If we observe the difference

$$\text{Number of tails} - \text{Number of heads}$$

5. If we observe the difference

$$(\text{Number of heads})^2 - (\text{Number of tails})^2$$

6. If we observe the number of "switches" from head to tail or tail to head (the first toss does not count as a switch).

For Problems 7–11, illustrate by means of a diagram the sample space of rolling a red and a green die. Shade the following events:

7. Shade the event that the sum of the two dice is greater than or equal to 10.
8. Shade the event that the number shown on the red die is two or more larger than the number shown on the green die.
9. Shade the event that the sum of squares of the numbers on the two dice is less than 9.
10. Shade the event that the sum of the two dice is 7 or 11 (winning roll in craps).
11. Shade the event that the difference (red die − green die) is two.
12. **Finding the Sample Space.** A physician measures a person's weight and systolic blood pressure (which is generally between 90 and 210 mg of mercury). What would seem to be a reasonable sample space for this experiment?

For Problems 13–14 a couple has three children.

13. Describe the sample space if one is interested in knowing the sex of each child (oldest, middle, youngest).
14. Describe the sample space if one is interested only in knowing the number of girls.

For Problems 15–19 a coin and a die are tossed simultaneously.

15. Enumerate the elements of the sample space of this experiment?
16. Enumerate the elements of the event that the coin turns up heads.
17. Enumerate the elements of the event that the die turns up a 3.
18. Enumerate the elements of the event that the die turns up a 3 or a 6?
19. Enumerate the elements of the event that the coin turns up a head and the die turns up a 2.

For Problems 20–23 a red die and a green die are rolled.

20. Enumerate the elements of the event that the sum is a 6 or a 9.
21. Enumerate the elements of the event that the sum is even.
22. Enumerate the elements of the event that the red die is a 2 or a 3.
23. Enumerate the elements of the event that the sum is a 7 or the red die is a 5.

Expected Values

24. **Quality Control.** Suppose you are the plant manager at a large shoe factory. A study has been conducted to determine the number of machines that fail each day. It has been determined that the random variable

$$X = \text{Number of machines that fail each day}$$

has the following probability distribution:

Failures, x	Probability of Failure, $p(x)$
0	.40
1	.35
2	.20
3	.05

What is the expected number of machines that will fail each day?

Problems 25–26 concern themselves with the game described by the diagram shown in Figure 13. The possible outcomes of this game are

$$S = \{\text{T, HT, HHT, HHH}\}$$

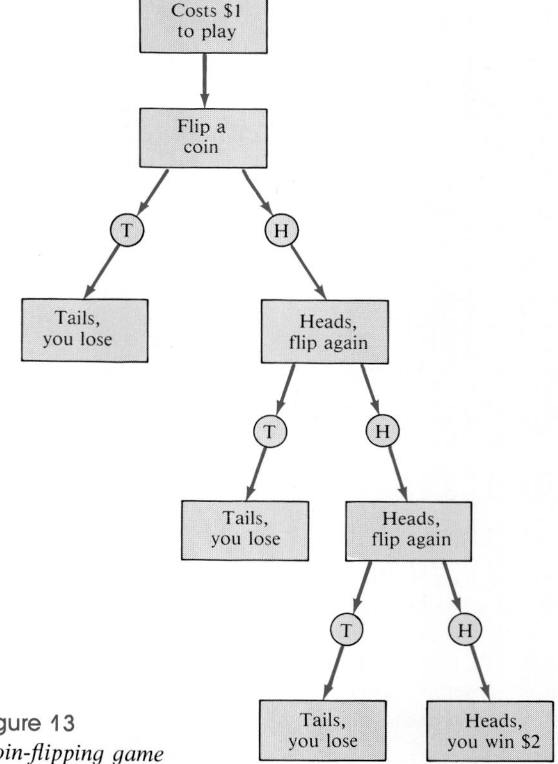

Figure 13
Coin-flipping game

Define the random variable

$$W = \text{Winnings per play}$$

25. What is the probability distribution of W?
26. What is the expected value of W?

Coin Toss

For Problems 27–28, toss two coins and define the random variable

$$H = \text{Total number of heads}$$

27. What is the probability distribution of H?
28. What is the expected value of H?

Rolling Dice

Roll a pair of dice and define the random variables:

$$D = \text{Difference between the high and low die}$$
$$P = \text{Product of the numbers on the dice}$$

29. What is the probability distribution of D?
30. What is the probability distribution of P?
31. What is the expected value of D?
32. What is the expected value of P?

Expected Values of Distributions

For Problems 33–38, what are the expectations of the indicated probability distributions?

33. $p(x)$ = probability of profits

1

.6

.4

x = Profit

0 $50,000

Investment cost = $15,000

34.

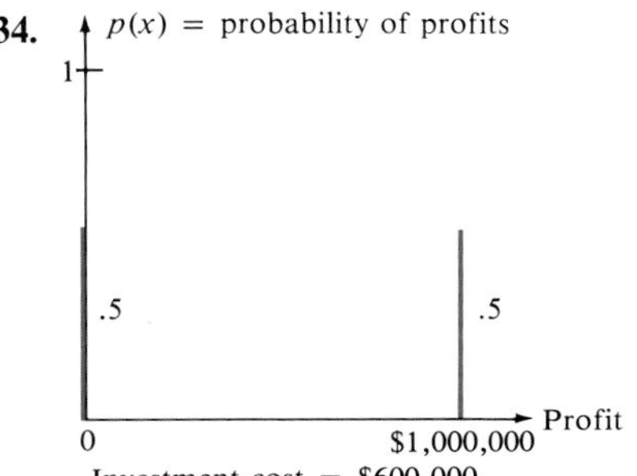

35.

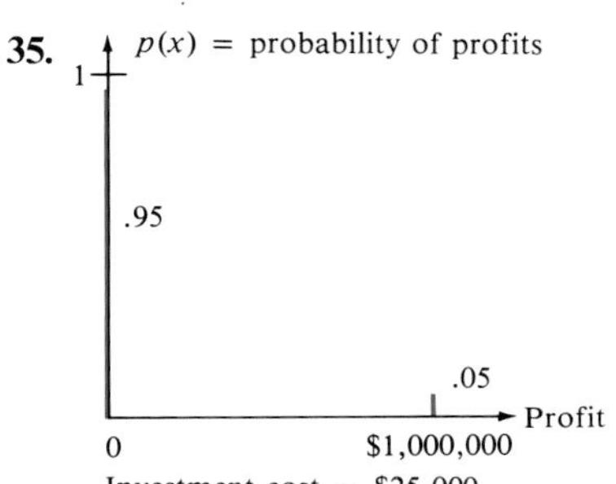

36.

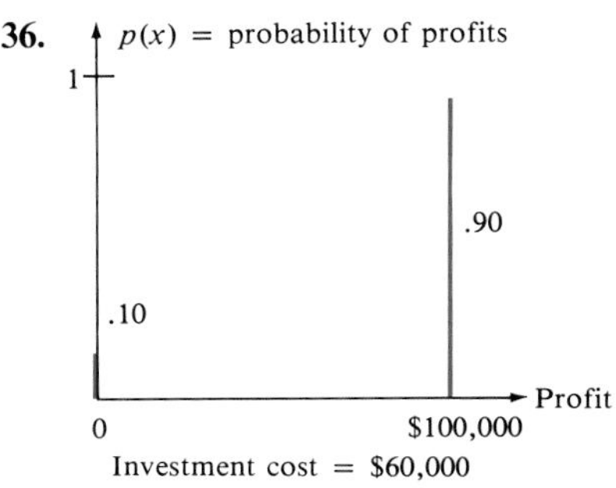

37.

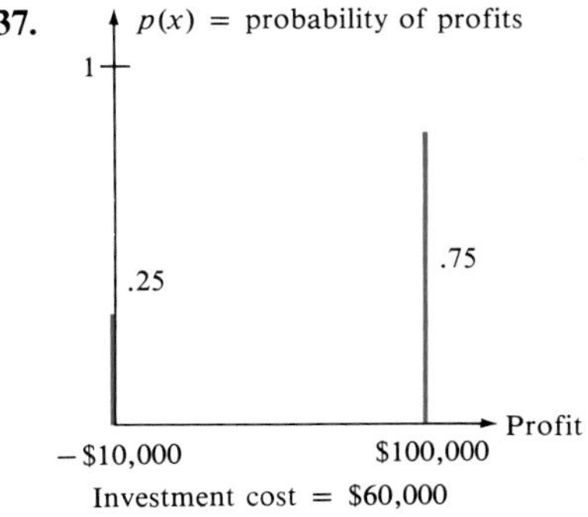

38.

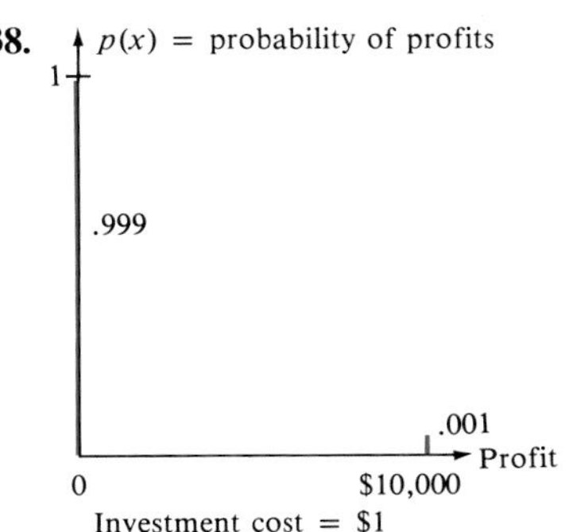

Odds and Ends

39. Baby Needs New Shoes. Take ten cards out a deck of 52 playing cards and mark them as follows:

$1 on four of them

$2 on three of them

$3 on two of them

$5 on one of them

Shuffle the ten cards and pick one at random. You win the value shown on the card. How much should you expect to win?

Probability in the Insurance Industry

Problems 40–43 are concerned with the insurance industry. Suppose an insurance company sells an accident insurance policy for $5000 per year. The policy pays policyholders $250,000 in the event of an accident. The probability that a policyholder will have a liable accident is $p = .01$.

40. Determine the probability distribution of the random variable

$$P = \text{Company's profit per policy each year}$$

41. Determine the probability distribution of the random variable

$$M = \text{Money paid to a policyholder}$$

42. What is the company's expected profit per policy each year?

43. What must the company charge for a policy in order for its expected profit to be $2000 on a policy?

Some Interesting Expected Values

44. Expected Value. Roll a pair of dice and define the random variable

$$SS = \text{Sum of squares of the rolled numbers}$$

What is the expected value of SS?

45. Expected Value. Suppose you have five nickels, four dimes, two quarters, two 50-cent pieces, and a Susan B. Anthony silver dollar in your pocket. Suppose you draw one coin at random from your pocket and tip a waitress. What is the expected tip?

46. Numbers Game. People still play "the numbers" in many parts of the country. "The numbers" consists of guessing a three-digit number, such as 391, that will occur in tomorrow's newspaper. Suppose the local bookie pays $250 on a $1 bet. What is a player's expected winnings?

47. Punch-Out Cards. Back in the 1940's a game that was popular was punch-out cards. A person could go into a drug store and pay the druggist a dollar for the privilege of punching out one hole in a gigantic board. Each hole contained a rolled-up wad of paper, which told the player whether he or she had won a prize. Unfortunately, most wads were blank. Suppose a board contains 1000 holes with one $100 prize, five $50 prizes, ten $25 prizes, and twenty-five $10 prizes. What is a player's expected winnings for this game?

48. Carnival Game. A carnival game offers $100 to anyone who can knock off three milk bottles on a stand. A player thinks she has a 25% chance of success. What is her expected payoff?

49. Coin Game. A game consists of tossing two coins. If both coins turn up heads, a player wins $10. If both coins turn up tails, the player wins $5. Finally, if one coin turns up a head and the other a tail, the player wins $2. What is the expected value of this game?

Maine Lottery

Problems 50–52 are concerned with the Maine Lottery. The following lottery ticket is sold in the state of Maine for $0.50. To win a Straight-type bet, which pays $2500, the player must select the correct four-digit number.

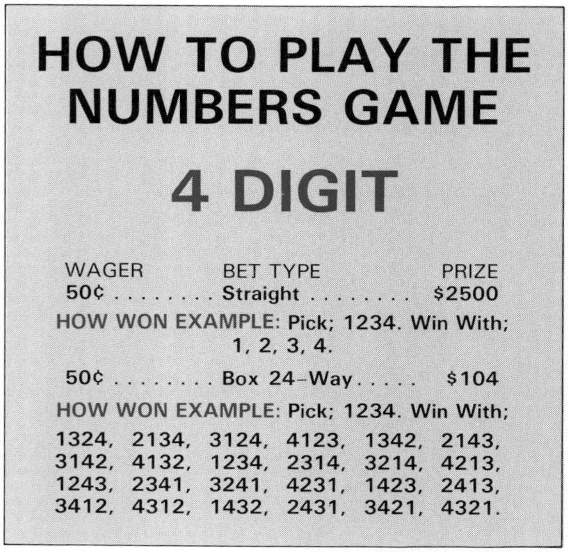

HOW TO PLAY THE NUMBERS GAME

4 DIGIT

WAGER	BET TYPE	PRIZE
50¢	Straight	$2500

HOW WON EXAMPLE: Pick; 1234. Win With; 1, 2, 3, 4.

WAGER	BET TYPE	PRIZE
50¢	Box 24–Way	$104

HOW WON EXAMPLE: Pick; 1234. Win With;

1324, 2134, 3124, 4123, 1342, 2143,
3142, 4132, 1234, 2314, 3214, 4213,
1243, 2341, 3241, 4231, 1423, 2413,
3412, 4312, 1432, 2431, 3421, 4321.

Figure 14
Maine lottery ticket

50. How much will a player expect to win on a Straight-type bet?

51. How much will the state of Maine expect to earn when a player makes a Straight-type bet?

52. How much will the state of Maine expect to earn if 50,000 people make the Straight-type bet?

7.2 Continuous Random Variables

PURPOSE

We introduce

- the continuous random variable,
- the probability density function, and
- the expected value of a continuous random variable.

Introduction

Since antiquity, many people, including the Greek philosopher Plato, have believed that a rectangle that has a height-to-width ratio of $1:\sqrt{3}$ is the most preferred esthetically. It seems that other rectangles appear either "too tall" or "too short," but rectangles with a height-to-width ratio of $1:\sqrt{3}$ appear "just right." Figure 15 shows various rectangles with different height-to-width ratios. You can pick your preference. In a recent study conducted by behavorial psychologists, 244 college students were asked to draw what they believed to be the most esthetically pleasing rectangle. The only constraint was that the height of the rectangle should not be any larger than the width of the rectangle.

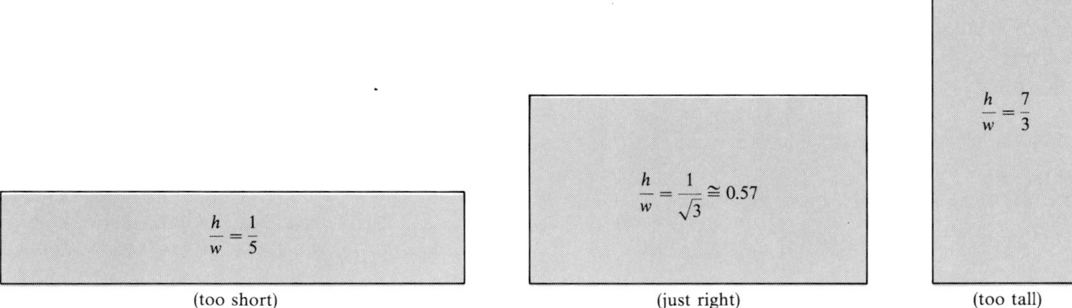

Figure 15
Which rectangle is most appealing?

There are various ways to measure the results from such an experiment. After the height (h) and width (w) are measured and the height-to-width ratio h/w of each rectangle computed, the ratios can then be placed in a number of different categories. As a first approximation, we could place the ratios in three categories, say,

- Category 1: $(0 < h/w \leq \frac{1}{3})$
- Category 2: $(\frac{1}{3} < h/w \leq \frac{2}{3})$
- Category 3: $(\frac{2}{3} < h/w \leq 1)$

as shown in the histogram drawn in Figure 16a.

The area of each of the three bars of the histogram represents the observed fraction of preferred height-to-width ratios in the category. Also, the sum of the areas of the three bars is 1. By classifying the preferred values of h/w in these three categories the researcher is interpreting the ratio h/w as a finite

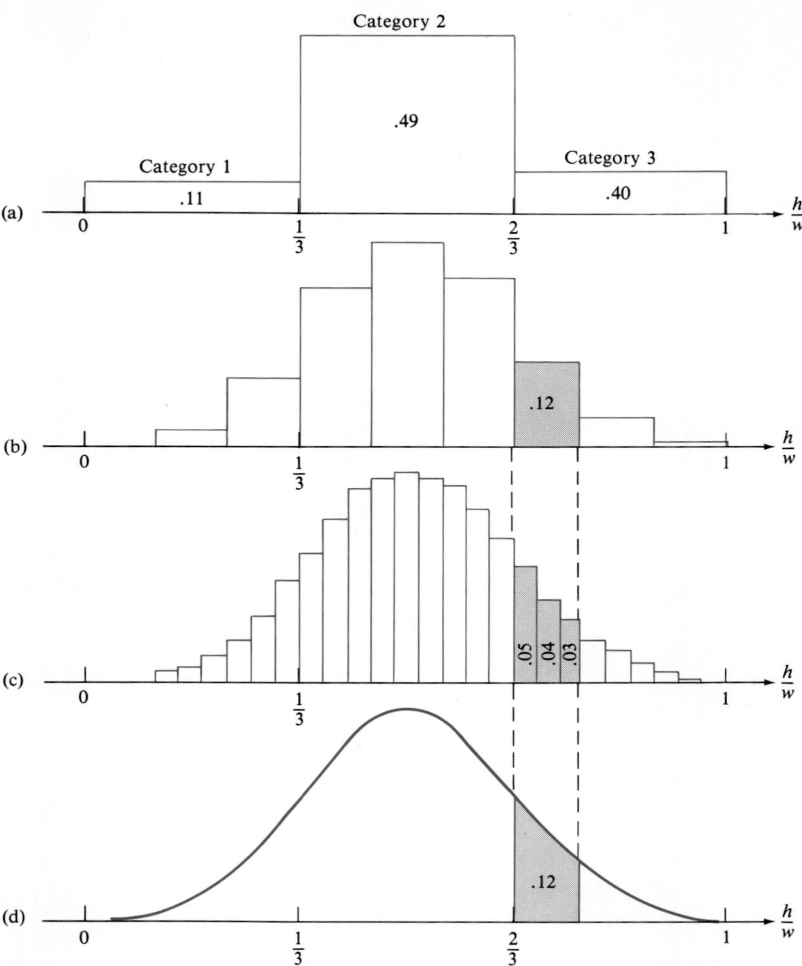

Figure 16
Histograms approaching the probability density function for h/w

random variable that can attain one of three values: Category 1, Category 2, or Category 3. For more precise information the psychologist may use a larger number of categories such as the eight categories shown in Figure 16b.

One of the major problems facing experimental scientists in any area of research is the determination of the number of categories in which to classify the observations. If the scientist had confidence in the accuracy of the observations, it might be possible to classify the observations into more categories as shown in Figure 16c. However, from a theoretical point of view the scientist might find it more instructive to interpret the measured quantity as something that changes continuously. For example, the psychologist might find it more insightful to interpret the height-to-width ratio h/w as a continuous random variable, say X, that can assume *any* real number in the interval $[0, 1]$. The psychologist would then replace the histograms as drawn in Figure 16a–16c by a smooth curve whose y-values indicate the "density of probability" at each point. This smooth curve $y = f(x)$ as shown in Figure 16d defines what is called the **probability density function** or the **probability distribution** curve of the continuous random variable X.

There are two important reasons why we are concerned with continuous random variables. First of all, many phenomena found in the social sciences, biology, business, and economics are more reasonably represented with continuous random variables than with discrete random variables. Quantities such as weight, length, and time are often interpreted as continuous variables. The second reason for the interest in continuous random variables lies in the fact that we can use the power of the integral calculus in the analyses of many technical problems.

We now show how the integral calculus plays an important role in the analysis of continuous random variables.

A Simple Probability Density Function

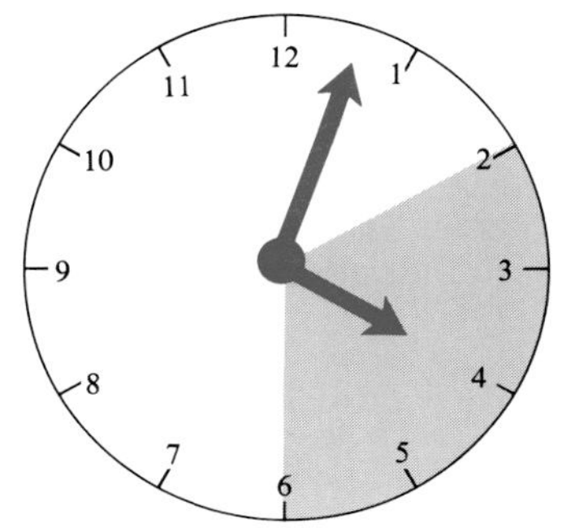

Figure 17
What is the probability that the hour hand stops between 2 and 6?

Each continuous random variable has its own probability density function. To introduce the idea of a probability density function, suppose your watch stops sometime during the day. What is the probability that the hour hand will come to rest somewhere between the numerals 2 and 6?

To answer this question, we interpret the stopping of the watch to be a probability experiment in which the time T when the hour hand stops is a continuous random variable whose value can assume any real number between the numerals 0 and 12. Our goal is to find the probability that T will take on some value between the values of 2 and 6. However, since there are an infinite number of real numbers in this interval, we are unable to proceed as we did in Section 7.1, when we simply counted the number of outcomes in the desirable event. However, there is a way out of this difficulty. Since the hour hand will stop equally likely at any time between 0 and 12, our strategy is to assign to each subinterval in the interval [0, 12] a probability proportional to the length of the subinterval. Hence we would conclude that the probability the hour hand will stop somewhere between 2 and 6 is

$$P(2 < T < 6) = \frac{\text{length of } [2, 6]}{\text{length of } [0, 12]} = \frac{4}{12} = \frac{1}{3}$$

However, there is a more instructive way to find the above probability, and that way is to interpret the probability as an area of a region under the probability density curve. This means that we must first find the probability density function of T. To find the probability density function of T, we realize that the watch is equally likely to stop at any time between 0 and 12. Hence the probability density function (the density of probability) of T will be a constant function on the interval [0, 12]. Since the area under the graph of a probability density function is analogous to the sum of the probability function taken over the entire sample space, we require the area to be 1. Hence

$$f(x) = \frac{1}{12} \qquad (0 \le x \le 12)$$

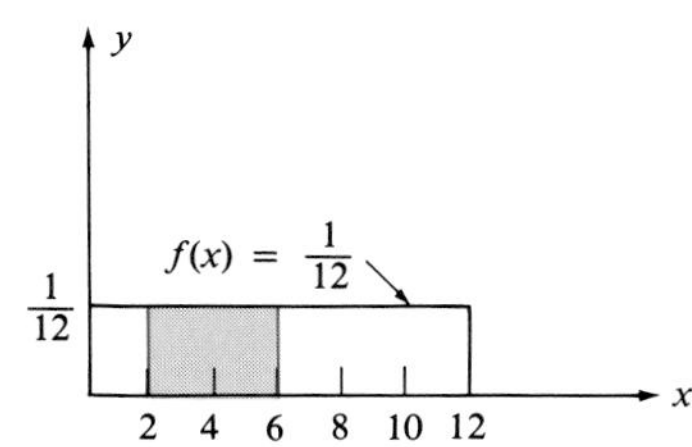

Figure 18
The shaded area represents the probability that the hour hand will stop between 2 and 6.

We now interpret the probability $P(2 \le T \le 6)$ as the area under the graph of $f(x)$ for x between 2 and 6. In terms of the definite integral we have

$$P(2 < T < 6) = \int_2^6 f(x)\,dx = \int_2^6 \frac{1}{12}\,dx = \frac{1}{3}$$

The above probability is represented in Figure 18.

The General Probability Density Function

To understand the probability density function more generally, realize that the probability density function $f(x)$ of a random variable X determines the probability that X lies in a given interval. Specifically, the probability that a random variable X with probability density function f lies in the interval $[a, b]$ is given by the definite integral

$$P(a \leq X \leq b) = \int_a^b f(x)\,dx$$

The probability that the outcome X of a random experiment lies between two numbers a and b gives a measure of the likelihood that the outcome lies in this interval. If the experiment were repeated many times, the proportion of times that X would lie in the interval $[a, b]$ would be close to this value. For many random phenomena it is possible to find a function $f(x)$ that satisfies

$$P(a \leq X \leq b) = \int_a^b f(x)\,dx$$

for every a and b in the range of values of X. In general we say that a function is a **probability density function** for some continuous random variable if it satisfies the following properties.

Definition of a Probability Density Function

A function $y = f(x)$ is a **probability density function** on an interval $[a, b]$ if it satisfies the conditions:

1. $f(x) \geq 0 \qquad a \leq x \leq b \qquad$ (nonnegative condition)
2. $\int_a^b f(x)\,dx = 1 \qquad$ (area under the graph is 1)

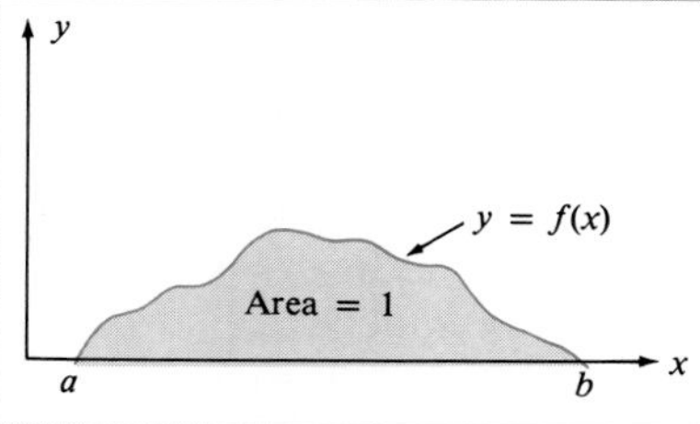

It is possible that the interval on which a probability density function is defined is the entire real line $(-\infty, \infty)$ or one of the half lines $[a, \infty)$ or $(-\infty, b]$.

Comments on Probability Density Functions

1. *Probability at a point is zero.* Note that for a continuous random variable the probability that the random variable attains any single real number a is zero. This can be seen by evaluating the integral

$$P(a \leq X \leq a) = \int_a^a f(x)\,dx = 0$$

2. *Endpoints do not affect probabilities.* The probability that a continuous random variable X lies in a given interval $[a, b]$ is not affected by whether or not the endpoints of the interval are included or excluded. Hence the following probabilities are all the same:

$$P(a \le X \le b) = P(a < X \le b) = P(a \le X < b) = P(a < X < b)$$

3. *Shorthand notation.* A convention that is often used in defining probability density functions is to define the function only when it is positive. The function is assumed to have the value zero at all other values of x. For example, when we write the uniform probability density function on $[0, 1]$ as

$$f(x) = 1 \qquad (0 \le x \le 1)$$

we really mean that

$$f(x) = \begin{cases} 1 & 0 \le x \le 1 \\ 0 & \text{all other values of } x \end{cases}$$

4. *Infinite domains.* Often an experiment in the real world will involve a random variable for which it is difficult to specify an upper bound on its value. For example, it is difficult to put an upper limit on the length of time T of a random telephone call passing through a switchboard. In this case we might find it convenient to say that T can take on values from 0 to ∞. On the other hand, some experiments involve variables that assume large negative numbers. Here we might say that these variables can assume values between $-\infty$ and some upper limit.

Example 1

Uniform Probability Density A continuous random variable X has a probability density function given by

$$f(x) = 1 \qquad (0 \le x \le 1)$$

The graph of this density function is shown in Figure 19. Find the following probabilities:

(a) $P(0 \le X \le .25)$

(b) $P(.25 \le X \le .75)$

(c) $P(.50 \le X \le .60)$

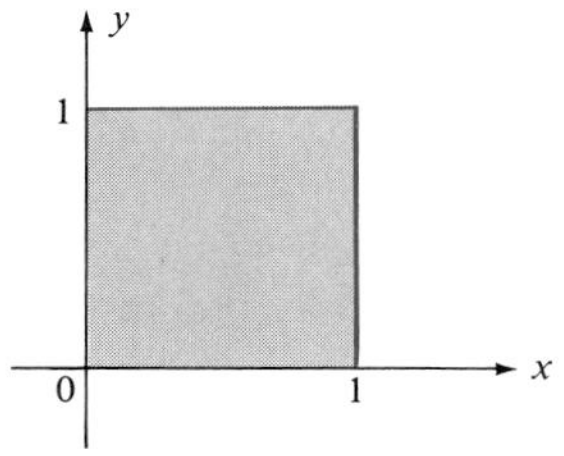

Figure 19
Uniform probability density function on the interval [0, 1]

Solution The probability density function drawn in Figure 19 is called the **uniform probability density** over $[0, 1]$. We refer to a random variable X having this density function as a **uniformly distributed random variable** over $[0, 1]$. To find the probability that a uniformly distributed random variable lies in the given intervals, we evaluate the following definite integrals:

(a) $P(0 \le X \le .25) = \int_0^{.25} f(x)\,dx = \int_0^{.25} 1\,dx = .25$

(b) $P(.25 \le X \le .75) = \int_{.25}^{.75} f(x)\,dx = \int_{.25}^{.75} 1\,dx = .50$

(c) $P(.50 \le X \le .60) = \int_{.50}^{.60} f(x)\,dx = \int_{.50}^{.60} 1\,dx = .10$ □

Example 2

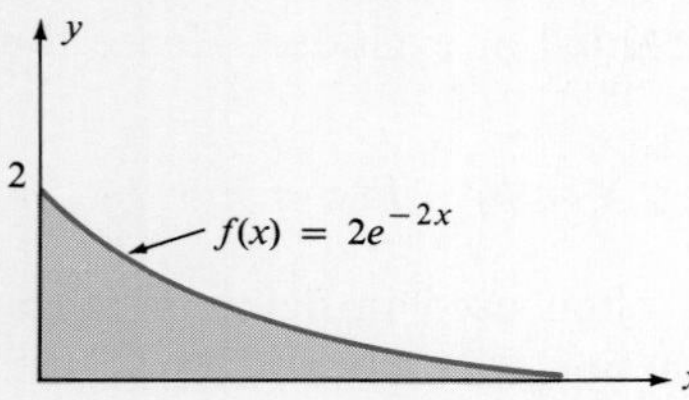

Figure 20
Exponential probability density function

Probability Density Function Consider the function

$$f(x) = 2e^{-2x} \qquad (0 \le x < \infty)$$

(a) Verify that $f(x)$ is a probability density function.

(b) Find $P(0 \le X \le 1)$, where X is a random variable whose probability density function is $f(x)$.

Solution

(a) To verify that $f(x)$ is a probability density function, we must show two things: first that $f(x) \ge 0$ for all x and second that the area under the graph of $f(x)$ is 1. First, since the exponential function is always nonnegative, we have $f(x) \ge 0$. Second, we find the area under the graph of $f(x)$. We get

$$\begin{aligned}\int_0^\infty 2e^{-2x}\,dx &= \lim_{b\to\infty} \int_0^b 2e^{-2x}\,dx \\ &= \lim_{b\to\infty} \left(-e^{-2x}\Big|_0^b\right) \\ &= \lim_{b\to\infty} (-e^{-2b} + 1) \\ &= 1\end{aligned}$$

(b) By definition we have

$$\begin{aligned}P(0 \le X \le 1) &= \int_0^1 2e^{-2x}\,dx \\ &= -e^{-2x}\Big|_0^1 \\ &= -e^{-2} + 1 \\ &\cong .865\end{aligned}$$

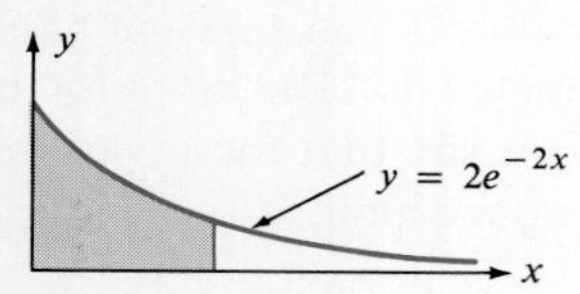

Figure 21
Shaded area is $P(0 \le X \le 1)$

This probability is illustrated by the shaded area in Figure 21. □

Expected Value of a Continuous Random Variable

In Section 7.1 we learned that when a probability experiment is performed repeatedly and the value of a random variable X recorded on each trial, the arithmetic average of the recorded values of X will approach some real number. This number is the expected value (or expectation) of the random variable X and is denoted by $E[X]$. We now introduce the expected value of a continuous random variable, or what is sometimes called the **mean** of a probability density function. The expected value of a continuous random variable is analogous to that of a finite random variable. Here if we perform a probability experiment repeatedly and the value of a continuous random variable X is recorded on each trial, then the arithmetic average of these recorded values of X will approach the expected value $E[X]$ of the continuous random variable.

We saw in Section 7.1 that the expected value of a finite random variable X with probability distribution $p(x)$ is given by

$$E[X] = x_1p(x_1) + x_2p(x_2) + \cdots + x_np(x_n)$$

where $x_1, x_2, \ldots, x_n$ are the values assumed by X. The expected value of a continuous random variable X with probability density function $f(x)$ has an analogous form.

> **Expected Value Formula of a Continuous Random Variable**
>
> Let X be a continuous random variable whose values lie in the interval $[a, b]$, and let $f(x)$ be the probability density function of X. The **expected value** of X is the real number given by
>
> $$E[X] = \int_a^b x\, f(x)\, dx$$
>
> The expected value is also called the **mean**, denoted μ, of the probability density function $f(x)$

We should point out that the lower limit a in the above expected value formula could be $-\infty$ or the upper limit b could be $+\infty$.

Example 3

Mean of a Probability Density Find the mean of the probability density function

$$f(x) = 2x \qquad (0 \le x \le 1)$$

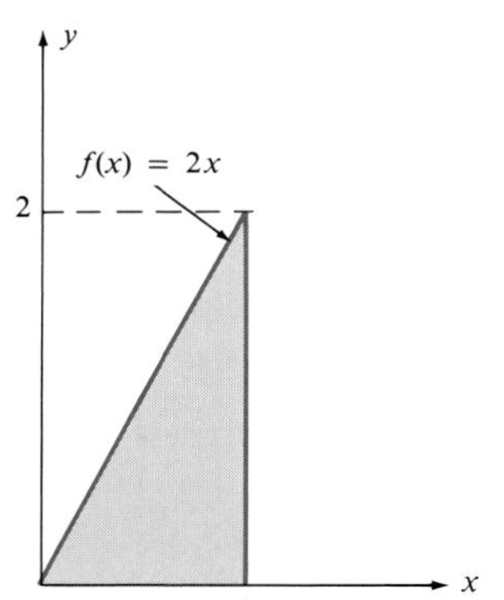

Figure 22
Probability density function $f(x) = 2x$, $0 \le x \le 1$

Solution The graph of the probability density function is shown in Figure 22. The mean μ of a probability density function $f(x)$ is the same as the expected value of a random variable X whose probability density function is $f(x)$. Hence we have

$$\begin{aligned}\mu = E[X] &= \int_0^1 xf(x)\, dx \\ &= \int_0^1 x(2x)\, dx \\ &= \int_0^1 2x^2\, dx \\ &= \frac{2}{3} x^3 \Big|_0^1 \\ &= \frac{2}{3}\end{aligned}$$

Interpretation

If a probability experiment were carried out for a large number of trials, and if a random variable X whose probability density function is $f(x) = 2x$, $0 \le x \le 1$, was observed on each trial, then the arithmetic average of the values of X would approach the mean of $\frac{2}{3}$.) □

Example 4

Expected Age of Plant Biologists have determined that the age T of a bacteria cell chosen at random from a given population is a random variable with probability density function

$$f(x) = 0.02e^{-0.02x} \qquad (x \ge 0)$$

where x is time measured in days. (See Figure 23.) Find the average age of a bacteria cell from this population.

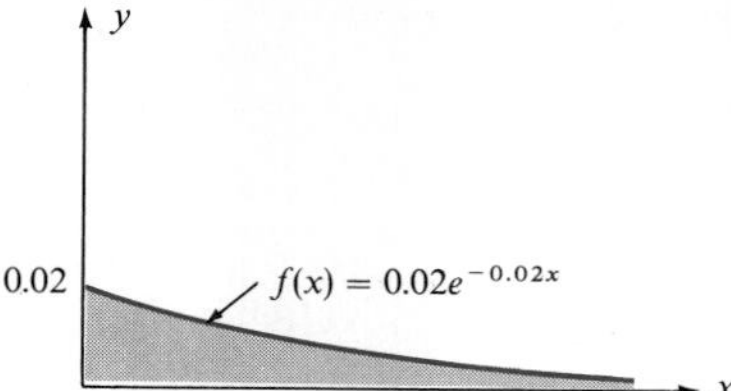

Figure 23
Exponential probability density function

Solution The average age of a bacteria cell is given by the expected value

$$E[T] = \int_0^\infty 0.02xe^{-0.02x}\,dx$$

To find this value, we first evaluate the following integral on $[0, b]$:

$$\int_0^b xe^{-0.02x}\,dx$$

Using the integration by parts technique, we let

$$u = x \qquad dv = e^{-0.02x}\,dx$$
$$du = dx \qquad v = -50e^{-0.02x}$$

This gives

$$\begin{aligned}\int_0^b xe^{-0.02x}\,dx &= -50xe^{-0.02x}\Big|_0^b + 50\int_0^b e^{-0.02x}\,dx \\ &= (-50be^{-0.02b} + 0) - 2500e^{-0.02x}\Big|_0^b \\ &= -50be^{-0.02b} - 2500(e^{-0.02b} - 1)\end{aligned}$$

Hence we have

$$\begin{aligned}E[T] &= \int_0^\infty 0.02xe^{-0.02x}\,dx \\ &= 0.02\int_0^\infty xe^{-0.02x}\,dx \\ &= 0.02 \lim_{b\to\infty} [-50be^{-0.02b} - 2500(e^{-0.02b} - 1)] \\ &= 0.02(2500) \\ &= 50 \quad \text{(days)}\end{aligned}$$

In other words, the average age of a bacteria cell from this population is 50 days. □

Problems

For Problems 1–5, determine which of the following variables are finite and which are continuous.

1. The number of delinquent accounts a utility company contends with every month.
2. The amount of sulfur (in milligrams per cubic foot of air) emitted from a smokestack.
3. The number of shoes a worker can stitch in a day.
4. The results (favorable, no opinion, or unfavorable) of a personal preference poll for a new product.

5. The length of time observed in a quality control study until a battery dies.

For Problems 6–20, determine if the given function is a probability density function.

6. $f(x) = 0.5$ $\quad -1 \le x \le 1$
7. $f(x) = 0.05$ $\quad 0 \le x \le 20$
8. $f(x) = 2x$ $\quad 0 \le x \le 1$
9. $f(x) = 2(x - 1)$ $\quad 1 \le x \le 2$
10. $f(x) = 3x^2$ $\quad 0 \le x \le 1$
11. $f(x) = 4x^3$ $\quad 0 \le x \le 1$
12. $f(x) = 6(x - x^2)$ $\quad 0 \le x \le 1$
13. $f(x) = 2(1 - x)$ $\quad 0 \le x \le 1$
14. $f(x) = \frac{3}{14}x^{1/2}$ $\quad 1 \le x \le 4$
15. $f(x) = \begin{cases} x & 0 \le x < 1 \\ 2 - x & 1 \le x \le 2 \end{cases}$
16. $f(x) = 2e^{-2x}$ $\quad 0 \le x < \infty$
17. $f(x) = 0.02e^{-0.02x}$ $\quad 0 \le x < \infty$
18. $f(x) = 0.05e^{-0.05x}$ $\quad 0 \le x < \infty$
19. $f(x) = \frac{1}{50}e^{-x/50}$ $\quad 0 \le x < \infty$
20. $f(x) = \frac{1}{100}e^{-0.01x}$ $\quad 0 \le x < \infty$

For Problems 21–35 a continuous random variable X has the given probability density function. Find the indicated probabilities.

21. $f(x) = \frac{1}{2}$ $\quad -1 \le x \le 1$ $\quad P(0 \le X \le 1)$
22. $f(x) = 0.05$ $\quad 0 \le x \le 20$ $\quad P(1 \le X \le 7)$
23. $f(x) = 2x$ $\quad 0 \le x \le 1$ $\quad P(0.5 \le X \le 1)$
24. $f(x) = 2(x - 1)$ $\quad 1 \le x \le 2$ $\quad P(1 \le X \le 1.5)$
25. $f(x) = 3x^2$ $\quad 0 \le x \le 1$ $\quad P(0.25 \le X \le 0.75)$
26. $f(x) = 4x^3$ $\quad 0 \le x \le 1$ $\quad P(0 \le X \le 0.75)$
27. $f(x) = 6(x - x^2)$ $\quad 0 \le x \le 1$ $\quad P(0 \le X \le 1)$
28. $f(x) = 6(x - x^2)$ $\quad 0 \le x \le 1$ $\quad P(0 \le X \le 0.5)$
29. $f(x) = \frac{3}{14}x^{1/2}$ $\quad 1 \le x \le 4$ $\quad P(1 \le X \le 3)$
30. $f(x) = \begin{cases} x & 0 \le x < 1 \quad P(0.5 \le X \le 1.5) \\ 2 - x & 1 \le x \le 2 \quad P(0.5 \le X \le 1.5) \end{cases}$
31. $f(x) = 2e^{-2x}$ $\quad 0 \le x < \infty$ $\quad P(0 \le X \le 0.5)$
32. $f(x) = 0.02e^{-0.02x}$ $\quad 0 \le x < \infty$ $\quad P(25 \le X \le 50)$
33. $f(x) = 0.05e^{-0.05x}$ $\quad 0 \le x < \infty$ $\quad P(0 \le X \le 30)$
34. $f(x) = \frac{1}{50}e^{-x/50}$ $\quad 0 \le x < \infty$ $\quad P(X \ge 50)$
35. $f(x) = \frac{1}{100}e^{-0.01x}$ $\quad 0 \le x < \infty$ $\quad P(X \ge 75)$

For Problems 36–46, find the mean of the indicated probability density function.

36. $f(x) = 1$ $\quad 0 \le x \le 1$
37. $f(x) = 0.5$ $\quad 1 \le x \le 3$
38. $f(x) = 2(x - 1)$ $\quad 1 \le x \le 2$
39. $f(x) = 3x^2$ $\quad 0 \le x \le 1$
40. $f(x) = 6(x - x^2)$ $\quad 0 \le x \le 1$
41. $f(x) = 12(x^2 - x^3)$ $\quad 0 \le x \le 1$
42. $f(x) = \begin{cases} x & 0 \le x \le 1 \\ 2 - x & 1 < x \le 2 \end{cases}$
43. $f(x) = e^{-x}$ $\quad 0 \le x < \infty$
44. $f(x) = 2e^{-2x}$ $\quad 0 \le x < \infty$
45. $f(x) = 0.05e^{-0.05x}$ $\quad 0 \le x < \infty$
46. $f(x) = 10e^{-10x}$ $\quad 0 \le x < \infty$

7.3 Exponential and Normal Random Variables

PURPOSE

We introduce the exponential and the normal random variables and study their probability density functions.

Exponential Density Function

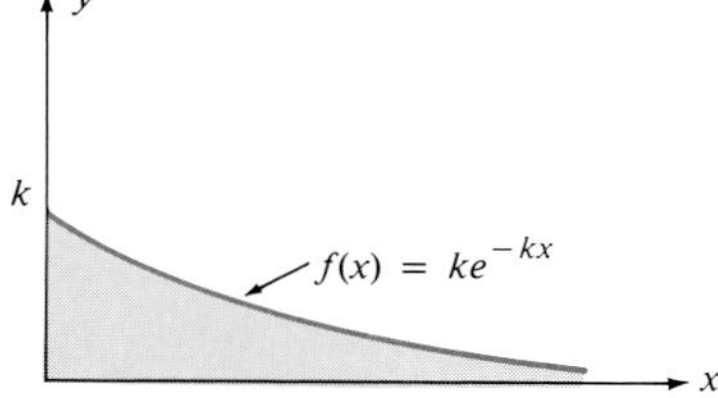

Figure 24
General shape of an exponential probability density function

Let k be a positive constant. Any function of the form

$$f(x) = ke^{-kx} \qquad (x \ge 0)$$

is called an **exponential probability density function** with parameter k. For each different value of the parameter k there is a different exponential density function. A typical exponential probability density function is shown in Figure 24. It is not hard to show that each exponential function satisfies the conditions of a probability density function. First, by the definition of the exponential function, each function satisfies the nonnegative condition $f(x) \geq 0$. Second, the area under each of these density curves is 1, since

$$\begin{aligned}\int_0^\infty ke^{-kx}\,dx &= \lim_{b\to\infty}\int_0^b ke^{-kx}\,dx \\ &= \lim_{b\to\infty}\left(-e^{-kx}\right)\Big|_0^b \\ &= \lim_{b\to\infty}\left(1 - e^{-kb}\right) \\ &= 1\end{aligned}$$

A random variable X whose probability density function is an exponential density function is called an **exponential random variable**.

Why Exponential Random Variables Are Important

Exponential random variables occur in random phenomena all around us. For example, the age T at which many species of plants die is an exponential random variable. Then too, the length of time T between two successive arrivals of customers at a business establishment, such as a McDonald's fast-food restaurant, is often an exponentially distributed random variable. Even the length of time between scores at a basketball game can be an exponential random variable.

Example 1

Exponential Lifetime Biologists have determined that the age T at which a given species of plant dies is an exponentially distributed random variable with probability density function

$$f(x) = \frac{1}{75}e^{-x/75} \qquad (x \geq 0)$$

where x is time measured in days. Find the probability that a plant of this species will

(a) Live less than 60 days
(b) Die at some time between 25 and 50 days
(c) Live longer than 75 days

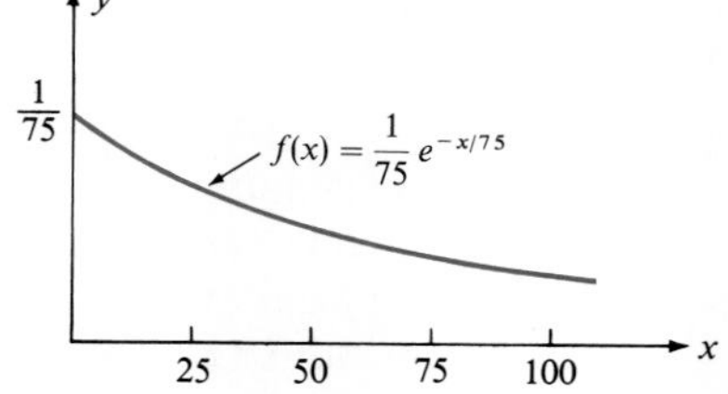

Figure 25
Distribution of the lifetime of a given species of plant

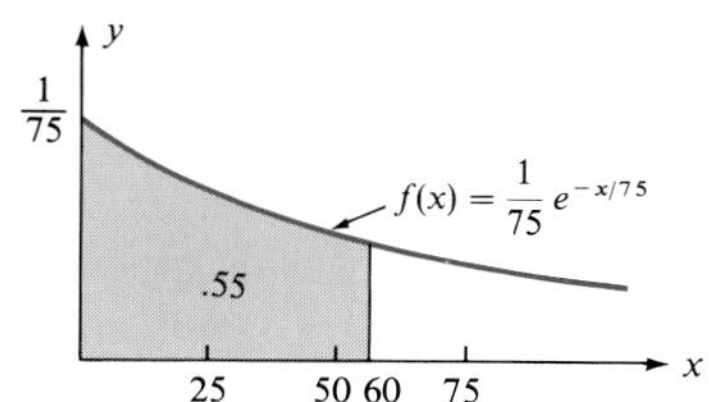

Figure 26
The shaded area represents $P(0 \le T < 60)$

Solution

(a)

$$P(0 \le T < 60) = \int_0^{60} \frac{1}{75} e^{-x/75}\, dx$$
$$= -e^{-x/75}\Big|_0^{60}$$
$$= -e^{-60/75} + 1$$
$$= 1 - e^{-0.8}$$
$$\cong 2.55$$

This probability is represented by the shaded area in Figure 26.

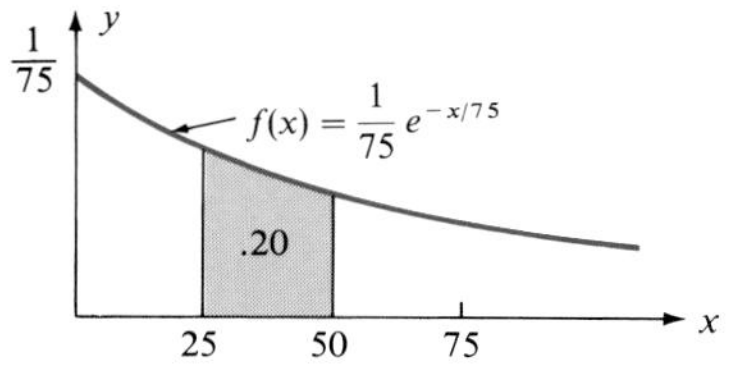

Figure 27
The shaded area represents $P(25 < T < 50)$

(b)

$$P(25 < T < 50) = \int_{25}^{50} \frac{1}{75} e^{-x/75}\, dx$$
$$= -e^{-x/75}\Big|_{25}^{50}$$
$$= -e^{-50/75} + e^{-25/75}$$
$$\cong .20$$

This probability is represented by the shaded area in Figure 27.

(c)

$$P(T > 75) = \int_{75}^{\infty} \frac{1}{75} e^{-x/75}\, dx$$
$$= \lim_{b\to\infty} \int_{75}^{b} \frac{1}{75} e^{-x/75}\, dx$$
$$= \lim_{b\to\infty} \left(-e^{-x/75}\Big|_{75}^{b}\right)$$
$$= \lim_{b\to\infty} (-e^{-b/75} + e^{-1})$$
$$= \frac{1}{e}$$
$$\cong .37$$

This probability is represent by the shaded area in Figure 28. □

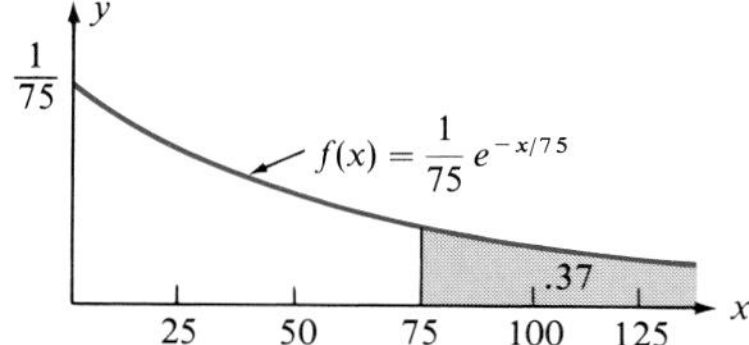

Figure 28
The shaded area represents

$P(T > 75)$

Comment on Example 1

We can also interpret the results of Example 1 by stating that

- 55% of the plants in this population will live less than 40 days.
- 20% of the plants in this population will live between 25 and 50 days.
- 37% of the plants in this population will live longer than 75 days.

Expected Value of the Exponential Density Function

The expected value of an exponentially distributed random variable can be found by integration by parts. Assuming that X is a random variable with probability density function $f(x) = ke^{-kx}$, the expected value of X is given by

$$E[X] = \int_0^\infty xf(x)\,dx = \int_0^\infty xke^{-kx}\,dx$$

To evaluate this integral, we first evaluate the integral

$$\int_0^b xke^{-kx}\,dx$$

We use the integration by parts technique letting

$$u = x \qquad dv = ke^{-kx}\,dx$$
$$du = dx \qquad v = -e^{-kx}$$

Hence we have

$$\begin{aligned}\int_0^b xke^{-kx}\,dx &= -xe^{-kx}\Big|_0^b + \int_0^b e^{-kx}\,dx \\ &= (-be^{-kb} + 0) - \frac{1}{k}e^{-kx}\Big|_0^b \\ &= -be^{-kb} - \frac{1}{k}e^{-kb} + \frac{1}{k}\end{aligned}$$

To find the limit of this expression as $b \to \infty$, we first examine the term $-be^{-kb}$. We will not prove it here, but this expression will approach zero as $b \to \infty$ for any constant k. You will find it interesting to use your calculator and evaluate some values of $-be^{-b}$ ($k = 1$) for larger and larger values of b. A few values are shown in Table 3.

TABLE 3
Illustration of $\lim_{b\to\infty} -(be^{-b}) = 0$

b	$-be^{-b}$
1	$-e^{-1} \cong -0.3678794$
5	$-5e^{-5} \cong -0.0336897$
10	$-10e^{-10} \cong -0.0004539$
15	$-15e^{-15} \cong -0.0000046$
20	$-20e^{-20} \cong -0.000000041$
25	$-25e^{-25} \cong -0.00000000035$

Hence we have

$$\begin{aligned}E[X] &= \int_0^\infty xke^{-kx}\,dx \\ &= \lim_{b\to\infty} \int_0^b xke^{-kx}\,dx \\ &= \lim_{b\to\infty} \left(-\frac{b}{e^{kb}} - \frac{1}{ke^{kb}} + \frac{1}{k}\right) \\ &= \frac{1}{k}\end{aligned}$$

Expected Value of the Exponential Random Variable

If X is a random variable with the exponential probability density function

$$f(x) = ke^{-kx} \qquad (x \geq 0)$$

then the expected value of X is

$$E[X] = \frac{1}{k}$$

The expected value of X is also called the **mean** of the probability density function, denoted by μ.

The expected value of an exponentially distributed random variable X is simply the reciprocal of the parameter k in the probability density function of X.

Example 2

Average Life of a Plant Species In Example 1 we said that the lifetime T of a given species of plant is an exponentially distributed random variable with probability density function

$$f(x) = \frac{1}{75}e^{-x/75} \qquad (x \geq 0)$$

What is the average lifetime expectancy of a plant of this species?

Solution The parameter k in the given distribution is

$$k = \frac{1}{75}$$

Hence the expected value of X is

$$E[X] = \frac{1}{k} = \frac{1}{\frac{1}{75}} = 75 \text{ days}$$

□

The Normal Random Variable

There are many phenomena in the world about us that give rise to random variables that produce the familiar "bell-shaped" curve shown in Figure 29a. For example, if you could measure the lengths of the leaves of a tree on your campus and subdivide these lengths into categories, you would discover a "distribution of lengths" of the general shape drawn in Figure 29b.

Quantities in almost every area of science in which you weigh, measure in length, or measure in time are generally interpreted as continuous random variables, which often give rise to bell-shaped probability curves. Some typical phenomena are shown in Figures 30a–30d.

Although such diverse phenomena as those shown in Figure 30 might not appear to have much in common, mathematically speaking, each phenomena

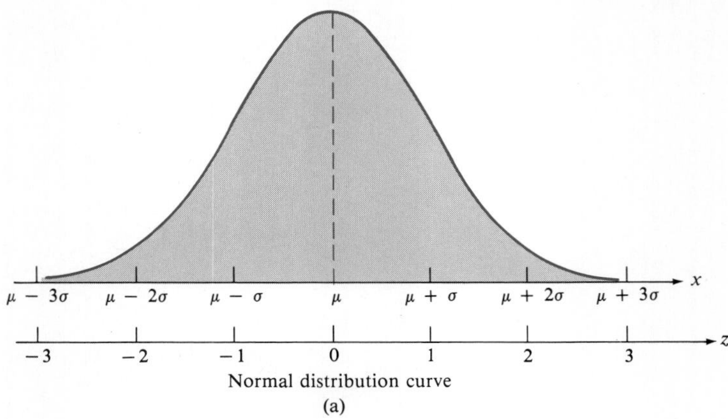

Normal distribution curve
(a)

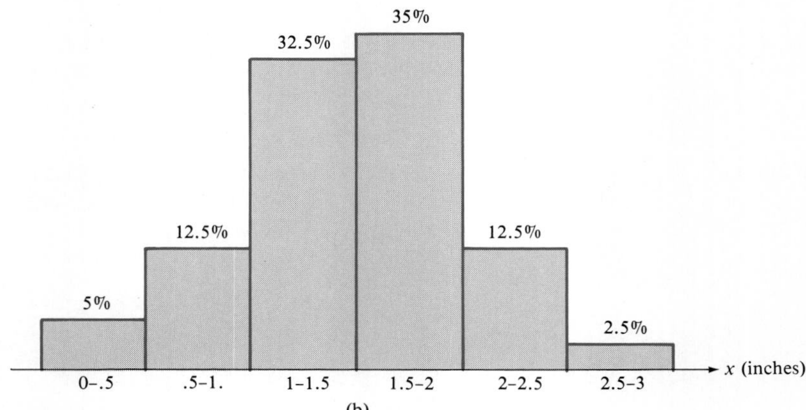

(b)

Figure 29
Lengths of leaves approximated by a normal distribution

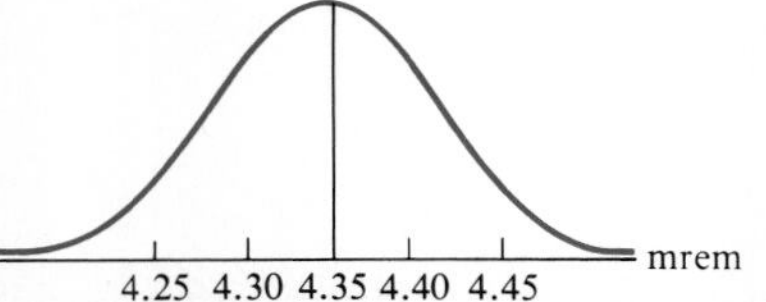

(a) The number of roentgens of radiation that a person receives when flying by jet across the United States is a normal random variable.

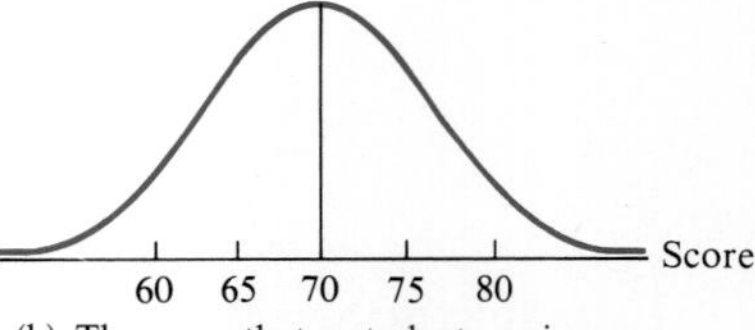

(b) The score that a student receives on a final exam is often approximated by a normal random variable.

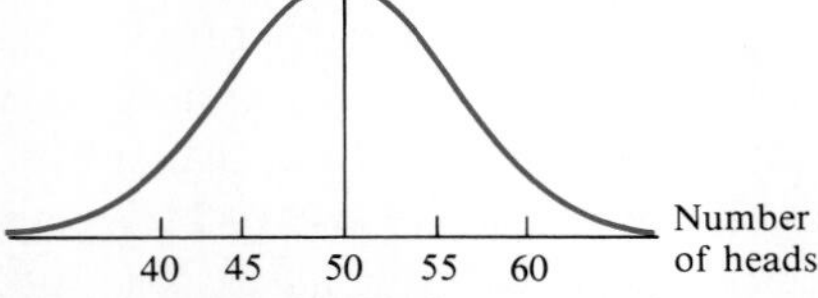

(c) The number of heads that turn up when you toss a coin 100 times is approximately a normal random variable.

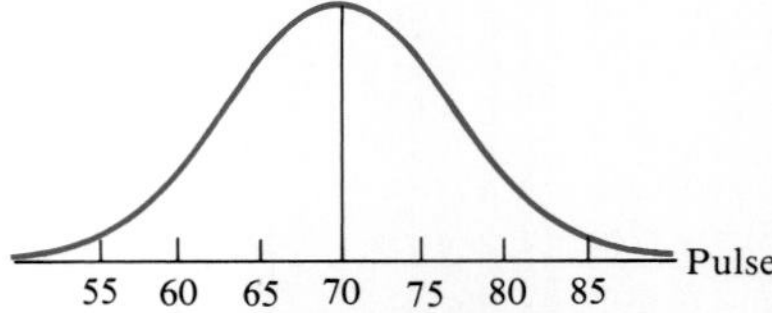

(d) The pulse rate of American females is a normal random variable.

Figure 30
Typical normal distributions in the real world

is characterized by a random variable X that has a normal probability density function (or normal distribution)

$$f(x) = \frac{1}{\sqrt{2\pi}\sigma} e^{-(x-\mu)^2/2\sigma^2} \qquad (-\infty < x < \infty)$$

where

μ = Mean of the normal distribution

σ = Standard deviation of the normal distribution

Observations on the Normal Distribution

We say that the random variable X is a normally distributed random variable. The values of μ and σ are called the **mean** and **standard deviation**, respectively, of the normal distribution. The mean μ can be any real number, whereas the standard deviation must always be a positive real number. We also call the square of the standard deviation, σ^2, the **variance** of the normal distribution. Although we refer to "the" normal distribution curve, we in fact obtain a different normal curve each time one of the values of the two parameters μ or σ is changed. Each one of these individual normal curves has a bell-shaped appearance and is symmetric about the vertical line $x = \mu$. (See Figure 31.) Also, if we move one standard deviation (1σ) to the left or right of the mean μ (to the points $x = \mu \pm 1\sigma$), we will find (using differential calculus) that these points are **inflection points** where the curve changes from being concave downward (inside the region) to concave upward (outside the region). Every normal curve extends from minus infinity to plus infinity, always lies above the x-axis, and always has an area of 1 under the curve. Hence the normal probability density function satisfies the conditions of being a probability function.

Whereas the mean μ of the normal distribution curve locates the "middle" of the normal curve, the standard deviation σ determines the "shape" of the curve. For instance, if we hold the mean μ fixed at some value, then a small value of the standard deviation σ will produce a "tall, skinny" normal curve, whereas a large standard deviation σ will produce a "short, flat" normal curve. (See Figure 31.)

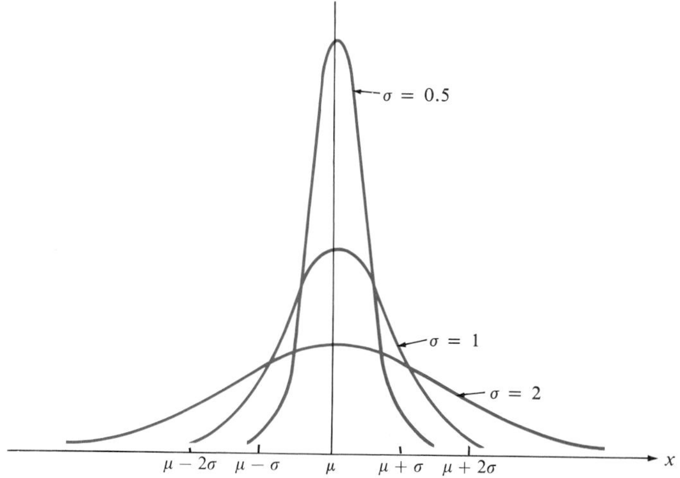

Figure 31
These three normal distributions have the same mean or middle, but different standard deviations, which gives them different shapes

The Standardized Normal Curve

A major problem in probability is determining the probability that a normal random variable lies between two numbers. Using integral calculus, we can find the probability that a normal random variable X with mean μ and standard deviation σ lies between two numbers a and b by evaluating the definite integral

$$P(a \le X \le b) = \int_a^b \frac{1}{\sqrt{2\pi}\sigma} e^{-(x-\mu)^2/2\sigma^2}\,dx$$

However, such an integral cannot be evaluated directly, since the normal probability density function has no elementary antiderivative. It is true, however, that integrals of the above type can be approximated by numerical methods and tables of probabilities have been compiled. To show how such probabilities can be found by means of tables, we introduce what is called the standardized normal random variable.

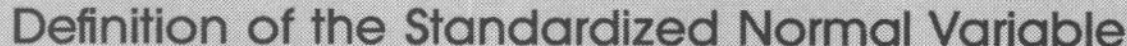

Definition of the Standardized Normal Variable

The **standardized normal random variable**, called Z, is a normal random variable that has a normal density function $f(x)$ with mean $\mu = 0$ and standard deviation $\sigma = 1$. That is,

$$f(x) = \frac{1}{\sqrt{2\pi}} e^{-x^2/2} \qquad (-\infty < x < \infty)$$

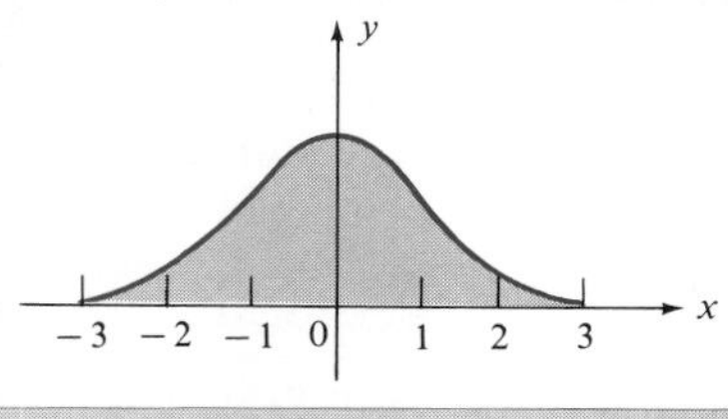

Using numerical methods, we can approximate the integral of the standardized probability density function over various intervals and compile a table of probabilities. A simplified list of probabilities is shown in Table 4.

Example 3

Probability of a Standardized Normal Variable What is the probability that a standardized normal random variable Z lies between 0.5 and 1.0?

Solution It is always useful when finding probabilities involving normal random variables to draw pictures illustrating various probabilities. In this problem we must find the area of the shaded region in Figure 32a, which represents the probability $P(0.5 < Z < 1.0)$. To find this probability, note that the area of the shaded region drawn in Figure 32*a* is simply the area of the shaded region shown in Figure 32*b* minus the area of the shaded region shown in Figure 32c.

TABLE 4
A(x) Is the Area Under the Standard Normal Curve from 0 to *x*

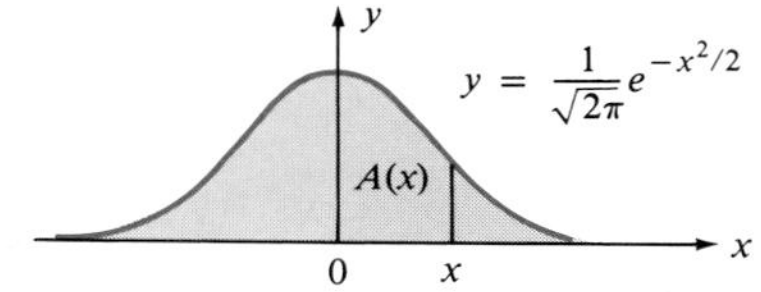

x	Area, $A(x)$	x	Area, $A(x)$
0.0	0.0000	2.1	0.4821
0.1	0.0398	2.2	0.4861
0.2	0.0793	2.3	0.4893
0.3	0.1179	2.4	0.4918
0.4	0.1554	2.5	0.4938
0.5	0.1915	2.6	0.4953
0.6	0.2257	2.7	0.4965
0.7	0.2580	2.8	0.4974
0.8	0.2881	2.9	0.4981
0.9	0.3159	3.0	0.4987
1.0	0.3413	3.1	0.4990
1.1	0.3643	3.2	0.4993
1.2	0.3849	3.3	0.4995
1.3	0.4032	3.4	0.4997
1.4	0.4192	3.5	0.4998
1.5	0.4332	3.6	0.4998
1.6	0.4452	3.7	0.4999
1.7	0.4554	3.8	0.4999
1.8	0.4641	3.9	0.5000
1.9	0.4713	4.0	0.5000
2.0	0.4772		

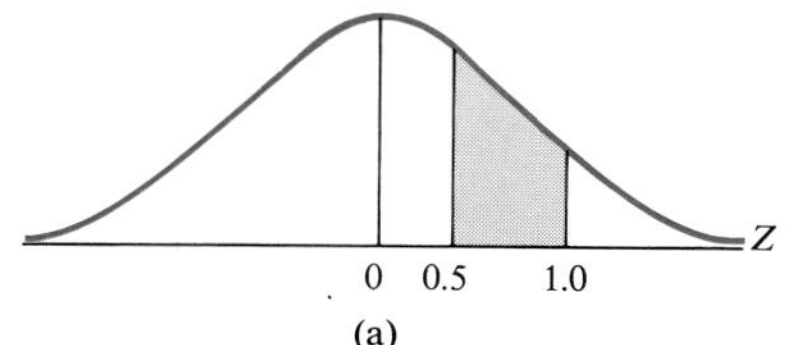

=

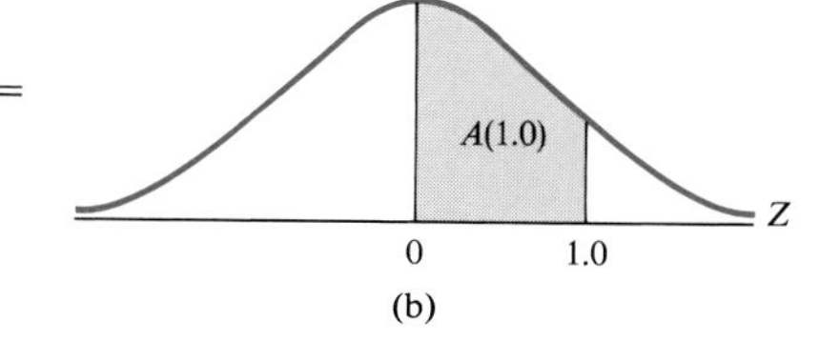

−

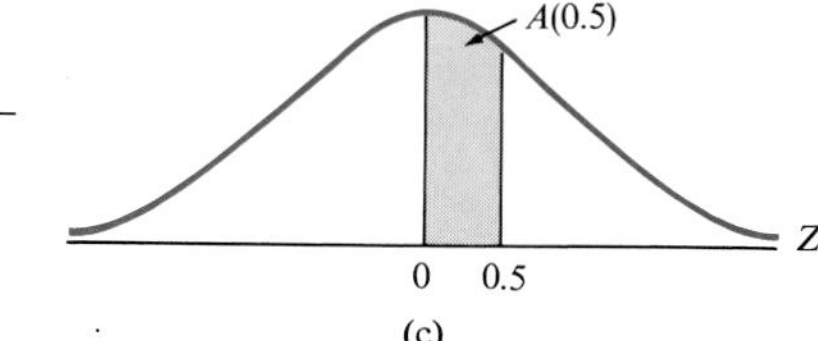

Figure 32
Geometric interpretation of normal probabilities

In other words, Figure 32 provides a geometric proof that

$$P(0.5 < Z < 1.0) = P(0 < Z < 1.0) - P(0 < Z < 0.5)$$

Stated in terms of the areas $A(x)$ given in Table 4, we can restate this fact as

$$\begin{aligned} P(0.5 < Z < 1.0) &= A(1.0) - A(0.5) \\ &= 0.3413 - 0.1915 \\ &= 0.1498 \end{aligned}$$

□

Example 4 Probability of a Standardized Normal Variable Find

$$P(-0.4 < Z < 0.3)$$

Solution By symmetry of the normal curve the area under the standardized normal curve between $Z = -0.4$ and $Z = 0$ is the same as the area under the standardized normal curve between 0 and 0.4. To this area we must add the area under the standardized normal curve between 0 and 0.3 (see Figure 33). These observations lead us to the conclusion that

$$\begin{aligned} P(-0.4 < Z < 0.3) &= A(0.4) + A(0.3) \\ &= 0.1554 + 0.1179 \\ &= 0.2733 \end{aligned}$$

□

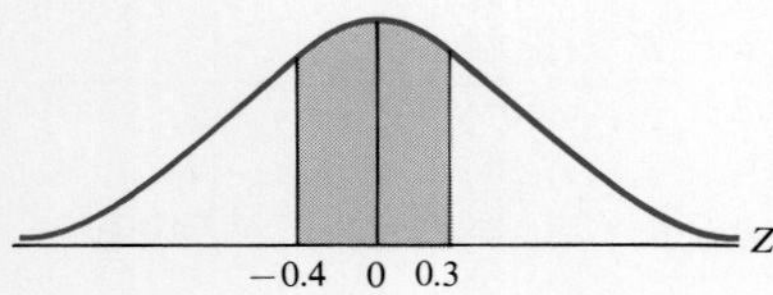

=

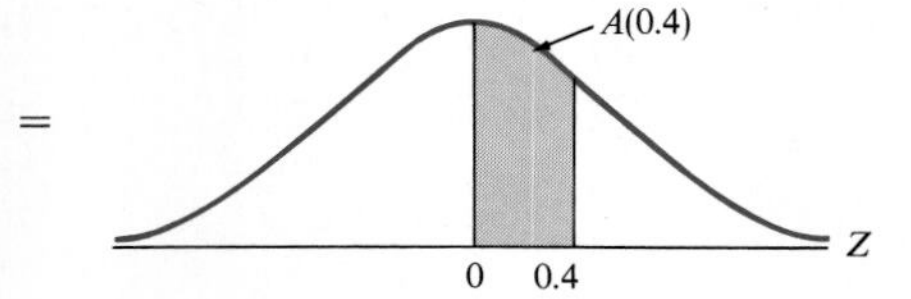

+

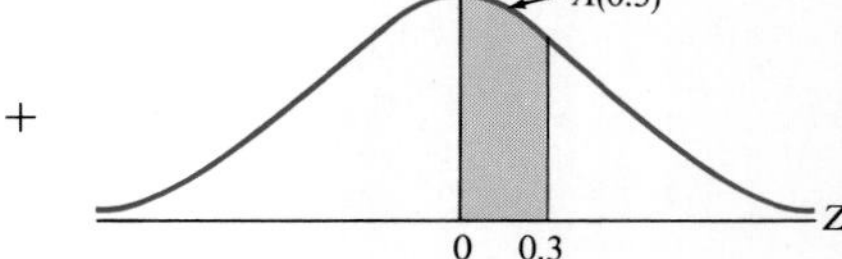

Figure 33
Geometric interpretation of $P(-0.4 < X < 0.3)$

Example 5 Probability of a Standardized Normal Variable Find

$$P(Z > 1)$$

Solution Using the fact that the total area under the standardized normal curve for $x > 0$ is 0.5, we can write

$$\begin{aligned} P(Z > 1) &= 0.5 - P(0 < Z < 1) \\ &= 0.5 - A(1) \\ &= 0.5 - 0.3413 \\ &= 0.1587 \end{aligned}$$

See Figure 34. □

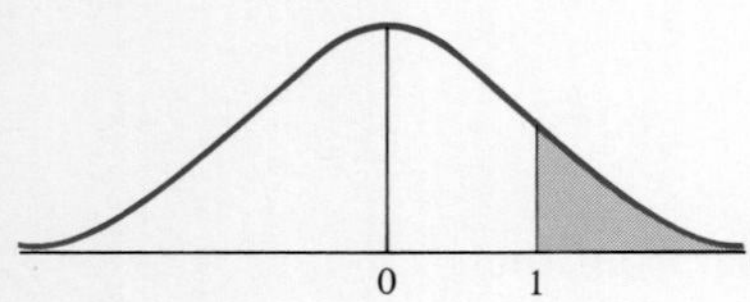

=

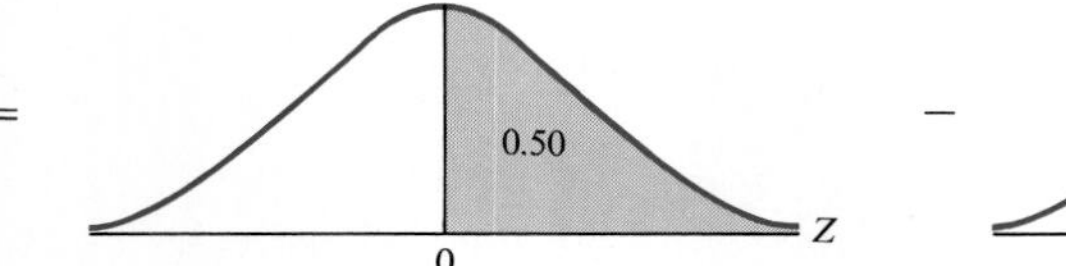

−

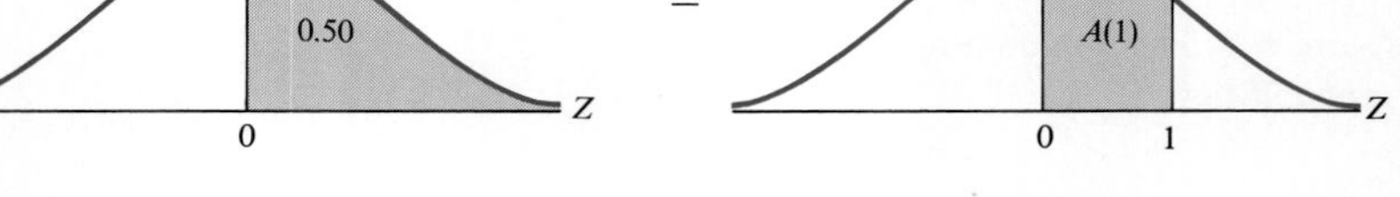

Figure 34
Geometric illustration of $P(Z > 1)$

Finding Probabilities of Other Normal Random Variables

We have found the probability that a standardized normal random variable lies in a given interval. We now show how to find the probability that other normal random variables with different means and standard deviations lie in given intervals. To do this, we use the following fact from the theory of probability.

Converting Normal Variables to Standardized Normal Variables

If X is a normal random variable with a normal probability density function with mean μ and standard deviation σ, then the variable Z found by

$$Z = \frac{X - \mu}{\sigma}$$

is a standardized normal random variable having the standardized normal probability density function.

We can use the above result to find the probability that any normal random variable will lie in any given interval.

Example 6

Finding Normal Probabilities Let X be a normal random variable with mean $\mu = 100$ and standard deviation $\sigma = 10$. Find

$$P(100 \le X \le 110)$$

Solution The strategy here is to first subtract the mean $\mu = 100$ from each of the three sides of the inequalities in $P(100 \le X \le 110)$ and then divide each of these three sides by the standard deviation $\sigma = 10$. In this way the normal random variable X in the expression $P(100 \le X \le 110)$ will be changed to the standardized normal variable $Z = (X - \mu)/\sigma$. Carrying out these elementary operations with inequalities, we get

$$\begin{aligned} P(100 \le X \le 110) &= P\left(\frac{100 - 100}{10} \le \frac{X - 100}{10} \le \frac{110 - 100}{10}\right) \\ &= P(0 \le Z \le 1) \\ &= 0.3413 \end{aligned}$$

The above steps are illustrated in Figure 35. □

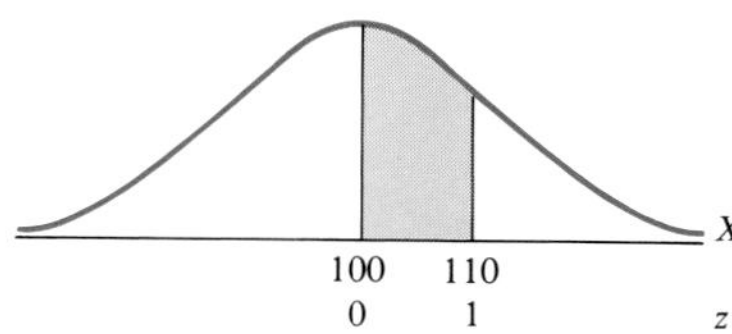

Figure 35
Area illustrating the probability of $P(100 \le X \le 110) = P(0 \le Z \le 1)$

Example 7

Normal Probabilities If X is a normal random variable with mean $\mu = 45$ and standard deviation $\sigma = 5$, find

$$P(35 \le X \le 55)$$

Solution Carrying out the steps described in Example 6, we find

$$P(35 \le X \le 55) = P\left(\frac{35-45}{5} \le \frac{X-45}{5} \le \frac{55-45}{5}\right)$$
$$= P(-2 \le Z \le 2)$$
$$= 2P(0 \le Z \le 2)$$
$$= 2(0.4772)$$
$$= 0.9544$$

The above steps are illustrated in Figure 36. □

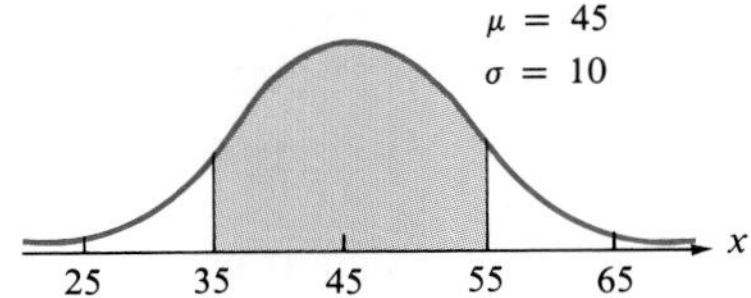

Figure 36
The shaded area represents $P(35 \le X \le 55)$

Example 8

Subway Problem Margaret has observed that the time T when the subway arrives at Kenmore Square every morning is a normal random variable with a mean of 8 A.M. and a standard deviation of 10 minutes. If Margaret is correct, what is the probability that the subway will arrive sometime between 7:55 A.M. and 8:05 A.M.?

Solution It is convenient to set the time of arrival T of the subway equal to zero when the actual time is 8 A.M. In this way the times of 7:55 A.M. and 8:05 A.M. correspond to $T = -5$ and $T = +5$, respectively. Hence the probability that the subway arrives between 7:55 A.M. and 8:05 A.M. is given by

$$P(-5 < T < 5) = P\left(\frac{-5-0}{10} < \frac{T-0}{10} < \frac{5-0}{10}\right)$$
$$= P(-0.5 < Z < 0.5)$$
$$= 2P(0 < Z < 0.5)$$
$$= 2(0.1915)$$
$$= 0.3830$$
□

Problems

For Problems 1–5, verify that the following functions are probability density functions. What is the mean of each probability function?

1. $f(x) = e^{-x}$ $\quad 0 \le x < \infty$
2. $f(x) = 0.001e^{-0.001x}$ $\quad 0 \le x < \infty$
3. $f(x) = 0.5e^{-0.5x}$ $\quad 0 \le x < \infty$
4. $f(x) = \frac{1}{2}e^{-x/2}$ $\quad 0 \le x < \infty$
5. $f(x) = 0.99e^{-0.99x}$ $\quad 0 \le x < \infty$

For Problems 6–13 a random variable X has an exponential distribution as indicated. Find the probability that X lies in the given interval.

	Exponential Density Function	Interval
6.	$f(x) = e^{-x}$	(0, 1)
7.	$f(x) = 0.01e^{-0.01x}$	(0, 50)
8.	$f(x) = 0.5e^{-0.5x}$	(0, 3)
9.	$f(x) = \frac{1}{3}e^{-x/3}$	(1, 3)
10.	$f(x) = \frac{1}{50}e^{-x/50}$	(10, 50)
11.	$f(x) = \frac{1}{100}e^{-0.1x}$	(100, 150)
12.	$f(x) = \frac{1}{25}e^{-x/25}$	$(25, \infty)$
13.	$f(x) = \frac{1}{4}e^{-0.25x}$	$(4, \infty)$

For Problems 14–20, draw a rough graph of the normal distribution curve with given mean and standard deviation. Be sure to draw the inflection point of the probability curve at the correct point.

	Mean	Standard Deviation
14.	$\mu = 0$	$\sigma = 1$
15.	$\mu = 0$	$\sigma = 2$
16.	$\mu = 1$	$\sigma = 3$
17.	$\mu = 5$	$\sigma = 1.5$
18.	$\mu = 2.5$	$\sigma = 0.5$
19.	$\mu = -1.0$	$\sigma = 1$
20.	$\mu = -2$	$\sigma = 2$

For Problems 21–35, find the probability that a standardized normal random variable Z lies in the given interval. Use Table 4 in the text to find the answers.

21. $P(0 \le Z \le 1.5)$
22. $P(0 \le Z \le 2.5)$
23. $P(1 \le Z \le 3.0)$
24. $P(-1 \le Z \le 1.5)$
25. $P(-1.5 \le Z \le 0.5)$
26. $P(-0.5 \le Z \le 1.0)$
27. $P(-1.5 \le Z \le -1.0)$
28. $P(-2.2 \le Z \le -2.0)$
29. $P(Z \le -1)$
30. $P(Z \le -0.5)$
31. $P(Z \le -1.2)$
32. $P(Z \ge 1.2)$
33. $P(Z \ge 0.8)$
34. $P(Z \ge -0.1)$
35. $P(Z \ge -2.1)$

For Problems 36–45, find the probability that a normal random variable X with given mean and standard deviation lies in the given interval.

	Probability	Mean	Standard Deviation
36.	$P(-1 \le X \le 1)$	0.0	0.5
37.	$P(0 \le X \le 3)$	0.0	2.0
38.	$P(0.3 \le X \le 1)$	0.5	1.0
39.	$P(0.8 \le X \le 1.5)$	1	1.0
40.	$P(20 \le X \le 30)$	25	5.0
41.	$P(140 \le X \le 160)$	150	15.0
42.	$P(700 \le X \le 770)$	750	50.0
43.	$P(-50 \le X \le -40)$	−50	5.0
44.	$P(-110 \le X \le -90)$	−100	5.0
45.	$P(-420 \le X \le 510)$	−500	100.0

Exponential Distributions in the Real World

46. Virus Problem. Researchers at the National Institutes of Health have made an extensive study of a certain type of virus and have discovered that the expected age of a virus chosen at random satisfies the exponential distribution

$$f(x) = 0.02e^{-0.02x} \qquad (0 \le x < \infty)$$

where x is time measured in weeks.

(a) What is the expected lifespan of a virus from this population?

(b) What fraction of virus from this population would one expect to have a lifespan over 8 weeks?

47. Threading a Needle. Thread a needle. After the needle is threaded, take the thread out of the needle and rethread it again, then again and again, and so on. It is often true that the time it takes to thread a needle is an exponential random variable. Suppose you thread a needle and the times satisfy the probability density function

$$f(x) = 0.25e^{-0.25x} \qquad (0 \le x < \infty)$$

where x is time measured in minutes. What is the probability that the time it takes to thread a needle is greater than 4 minutes?

48. Phone Calls. Suppose the time between successive phone calls arriving at a telephone exchange is an exponential random variable X with an expected value of 0.25 second.

(a) What is the probability density function of X?

(b) What is the probability that the elapsed time between two successive calls is between 0.25 second and 0.5 second?

49. Survival Analysis. A group of cancer patients has been treated with a new drug. It is known that the number of years X a person survives after receiving the treatment with this drug is a random variable with a probability density function of the form

$$f(x) = ke^{-kx} \qquad (0 \le x < \infty)$$

(a) If it has been determined experimentally that the expected survival time for a patient receiving the new drug is 4 years, what would you use for the probability density function for X?

(b) Find the probability that a new patient receiving the drug will survive for less than 3 years.

(c) The cumulative function $F(x)$ gives the probability that a patient survives for less than x years. Find $F(x)$.

(d) Find the probability that a patient will survive for more than 3 years.

(e) The reliability function $r(x)$ gives the probability that a patient will survive for more than x years. Find $r(x)$.

50. Tollbooth Problem. Suppose the length of time between two successive cars' arrivals at a certain tollbooth on the

New Jersey Turnpike is an exponential random variable with an expected value of 30 seconds.

(a) What is the exponential distribution of the length of time between successive cars?

(b) What is the probability that the length of time between two successive cars is greater than 45 seconds?

51. **Big Mac Problem.** Suppose the time required to prepare a Big Mac at a McDonalds fast-food restaurant has an exponential random variable with an expected value of 45 seconds.

(a) What is the exponential distribution of the time required to prepare a Big Mac?

(b) What is the probability that the time required to prepare a Big Mac is between 15 seconds and 1 minute?

Normal Distributions in the Real World

The following problems can be solved by using the table of standardized normal variables (Table 4) in the text.

52. **Normally Distributed Grades.** It was found that the distribution of grades in a calculus class could be approximated by a continuous normal distribution with a mean of 80 and a standard deviation of 5. What fraction of the class received a grade between 80 and 90?

53. **Height Problem.** The height of a male in the United States is approximately a normal random variable with a mean of 5′9″ (69 inches) and a standard deviation of 3″. What fraction of males in the United States have a height between 5′6″ (66 inches) and 6′0″ (72 inches)?

54. **Delinquent Accounts.** Delinquent charge accounts for a chain of department stores are approximately normally distributed with a mean of \$125 and a standard deviation of \$25. What is the probability that a delinquent account will be less than \$90?

55. **Fish Problem.** The lengths of an adult fish of a certain species are normally distributed with a mean of 9″ and a standard deviation of 2″. What fraction of fish from this species have lengths between 5″ and 11″?

56. **Tall Fish Story.** Anne claims that she caught a 25-pound salmon while fishing in Maine. State biologists know that the weights of adult salmon are normally distributed with a mean of 10 pounds and a standard deviation of 5 pounds. What is the probability that a person catching a salmon will catch one that weighs 25 pounds or more?

57. **Acidity of Blood.** The acidity of human blood measured on the pH scale is a normal random variable with a mean of 7.2 and a standard deviation of 0.15. What fraction of people have blood whose acidity is measured below 7.05?

58. **Baseball Averages.** The seasonal batting averages of major league players are roughly normally distributed with a mean of 0.262 and a standard deviation of 0.04. If this model is correct, what fraction of players will have a seasonal average between 0.222 and 0.302?

Epilogue: Why the Normal Distribution?

Many quantities in the natural sciences appear to be normally distributed. The question many people have asked is: Why the normal distribution? To answer this question, consider your own height. Many factors have gone into its determination. Biologists believe that genetic factors play a major role. Many genes are located at various loci upon chromosomes, and all contribute to your height. Also, many environmental factors such as nutrition, exercise, and environment contribute to your height. In other words, your total height is the net result of many independent factors.

The English scientist Sir Francis Galton (1822–1911) demonstrated by means of what we now call the **Galton board** that the net result of several independent factors often gives rise to a normal distribution. In a Galton board, when small balls roll onto a board that is inclined to the horizontal, the balls strike nails that are pounded into the board. Upon striking a nail, each ball deviates either to the left or to the right. At the bottom of the board are many slots in which the balls ultimately come to rest. After several balls pass through the Galton board, most of the balls come to rest in the slots at the middle of the board, the frequency of balls tapering off at the outer edges. The frequency of balls in the slots will approximate a normal distribution. The reason, as Galton reasoned, was due to the effect of a large number of independent random deviations, some acting in a positive manner (say, moving a ball to the right) and some acting in a negative manner (say, moving a ball to the left). Galton realized that many phenomena in the natural sciences, such as an individual's height, have similar characteristics.

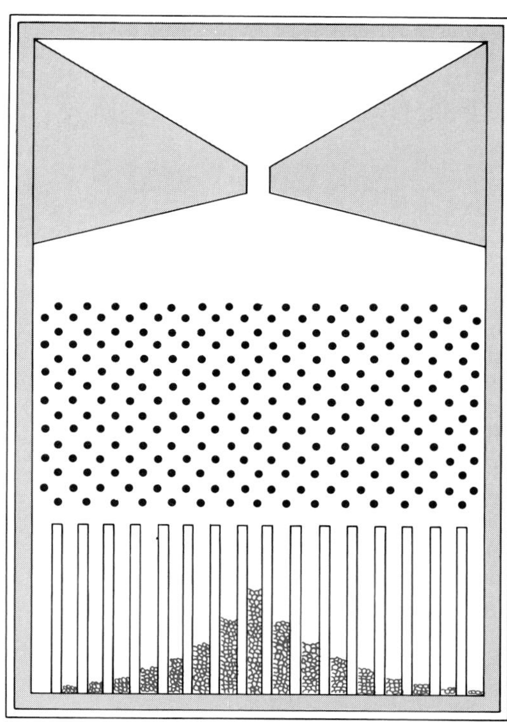

Figure 37
The Galton board

Key Ideas for Review

Review Exercises

For Problems 1–5, describe the sample space of the indicated probability experiments.

1. A couple have three children.
2. Two coins are tossed, and then a die is rolled.
3. Two letters are randomly chosen from the word *cats*.
4. From four books on a table, *A*, *B*, *C* and *D*, two books are randomly selected, one after the other, the first book being replaced on the table after it is selected.
5. Three letters are chosen from the word *little* (assume that the two t's and two l's are distinguishable).

For Problems 6–10, two dice are rolled.

6. What is the probability of not rolling a double?
7. What is the probability that the number on one die is three times the number on the other die?
8. What is the probability that the number on one die is twice the number on the other die?

9. What is the probability that one die is a 3 and the other die is a number greater than 3?
10. What is the probability that the top face of one die is an even number and the top face of the other die is an odd number?

Expected Values

11. **The Raffle.** The freshman class at Bentworth College decides to raise money by raffling off a portrait of an old university professor worth \$500. A total of 2500 tickets are sold for \$1 apiece. How much can you expect to win if you buy a ticket in this raffle?
12. **The Raffle Revisited.** Suppose the portrait in Exercise 11 has been found to be worth \$750. How much will you now expect to win if you buy a ticket in the raffle?
13. **Dice Problem.** If two dice are rolled, what is the expected sum of the two dice?
14. **Life Insurance.** The probability that a man aged 50 will live another year is 0.988. How large a premium should an insurance company charge a man this age for a \$5000 one-year policy in order to make a profit?
15. **World Series.** Suppose that the probability that the Mets will beat the Red Sox on a given game in a world series is 2/3 and assume that each game is independent from the others. Under these conditions it can be proved that the probability that the series will go 4, 5, 6, or 7 games is .21, .30, 27, and .22, respectively. Find the expected number of games in the series under these conditions.

Probability Density Functions

For Problems 16–20, verify that each of the given functions is a probability density function.

16. $f(x) = 0.25 \quad 3 \le x \le 7$
17. $f(x) = \dfrac{x}{18} \quad 0 \le x \le 6$
18. $f(x) = 5x^4 \quad 0 \le x \le 1$
19. $f(x) = \frac{3}{2}x - \frac{3}{4}x^2 \quad 0 \le x \le 2$
20. $f(x) = 0.5e^{-0.5x} \quad 0 \le x < \infty$

Finding Probabilities

For Problems 21–25 a continuous random variable X has the given probability density function. Find the indicated probability.

21. $f(x) = 0.25 \quad 3 \le x \le 7 \quad P(3 \le X \le 4)$
22. $f(x) = \dfrac{x}{18} \quad 0 \le x \le 6 \quad P(0 \le X \le 3)$
23. $f(x) = 5x^4 \quad 0 \le x \le 1 \quad P(0.25 \le X \le 1)$
24. $f(x) = \frac{3}{2}x - \frac{3}{4}x^2 \quad 0 \le x \le 2 \quad P(0 \le X \le 1)$
25. $f(x) = 0.5e^{-0.5x} \quad 0 \le x < \infty \quad P(0 \le X \le 1)$

Probabilities of Normal Random Variables

For Problems 26–35, find the indicated probabilities. The variable X is a normal random variable with indicated mean μ and standard deviation σ.

	Probability	Mean	Standard Deviation
26.	$P(1 \le X \le 2)$	$\mu = 0$	$\sigma = 1$
27.	$P(-2 \le X \le 1)$	$\mu = 0$	$\sigma = 1$
28.	$P(X \le -1)$	$\mu = 0$	$\sigma = 1$
29.	$P(X \ge 10)$	$\mu = 11$	$\sigma = 2$
30.	$P(500 \le X \le 700)$	$\mu = 550$	$\sigma = 100$
31.	$P(-10 \le X \le 0)$	$\mu = -5$	$\sigma = 2.5$
32.	$P(X \ge 0.5)$	$\mu = 0.8$	$\sigma = 0.1$
33.	$P(5000 \le X \le 7500)$	$\mu = 6000$	$\sigma = 1000$
34.	$P(-100 \le X \le 100)$	$\mu = 0$	$\sigma = 50$
35.	$P(-500 \le X \le 250)$	$\mu = -500$	$\sigma = 500$

Exponential Distributions in the Real World

36. **Light Bulbs.** The next time a lightbulb in your house burns out, just say, "There's another exponential random variable." It is well known that the lifespan of many electrical and electronic parts is an exponential random variable. Suppose the lifespan X of a given brand of lightbulbs is an exponential random variable with an expected value of 150 days.
    (a) What is the probability density function of X?
    (b) What is the probability that a randomly chosen lightbulb from this brand will last between 100 and 200 days?
    (c) What is the probability that a lightbulb of this brand will last for more than 100 days?
37. **Hockey Scores.** The elapsed time between successive points scored by a given hockey team during a season is often an exponential random variable. Suppose that the expected time X between successive scores for the University of North Dakota's hockey team is 10 minutes.
    (a) What is the probability distribution of X?
    (b) What is the probability that after one point is scored, another point will be scored within 5 minutes?
38. **Firehouse Calls.** The time X between successive calls to a firehouse is often an exponential random variable. Suppose that the expected length of time between successive calls to Station 41 is 3.5 hours.
    (a) What is the probability density function of X?
    (b) What is the probability that Station 41 will experience two calls within 1 hour of each other?

Normal Distributions in the Real World

39. **Wheat Munchies.** A cereal company sells a 12-ounce box of its major product, Wheat Munchies. The actual number of ounces of cereal that a machine puts in each box is a

normal random variable with a mean of 12 ounces and a standard deviation of 0.1 ounce. What fraction of boxes will contain between 11.8 and 12.2 ounces of Wheat Munchies?

40. Getting to Class on Time. A student with an 8:00 A.M. class at the University of Houston commutes to school. She has discovered that the arrival time for her bus is a normal random variable with a mean of 7:00 A.M. and a standard deviation of 30 minutes. What is the probability that the bus will be at least 30 minutes late?

41. SAT Scores. The SAT scores of a freshman class at a midwestern university is a normally distributed random variable with a mean of 580 and a standard deviation of 100. What percent of the scores from this class were greater than 500?

42. Minimum Temperature. The average daily minimum temperature in Duluth, Minnesota, in January is a normal random variable with a mean of -1.6 degrees and a standard deviation of 8 degrees. What is the probability that the minimum daily temperature in Duluth in January will be greater than 6.4 degrees?

Some Interesting Miscellaneous Problems

43. Chebyshev's Law. The Chebyshev inequality states that for any random variable X with expected value μ and any standard deviation σ, we have

$$P(\mu - n\sigma < X < \mu + n\sigma) \geq 1 - \frac{1}{n^2}$$

Let $n = 2$ and apply Chebyshev's inequality to the exponential distribution

$$f(x) = e^{-x} \qquad (x \geq 0)$$

44. One σ from μ. Show that roughly 68% of the area under a normal curve lies within one standard deviation from the mean.

45. Two σ's from μ. Show that roughly 95% of the area under the normal curve lies within two standard deviations from the mean.

46. Three σ's from μ. Show that roughly 99% of the area under the normal curve lies within three standard deviations from the mean.

Chapter Test

1. You write the numbers 1, 2, 3, and 4 separately on four slips of paper. You then put the slips of paper in a box. Without looking, you reach into the box and draw two slips of paper, one first and the other second. What is the sample space for this probability experiment?
2. To study the distribution of boys and girls in families having three children, a survey of such families is taken. What is the sample space of such a survey?
3. A pair of dice is rolled. What is the probability the dice do not turn up the same number?
4. A church bazaar sells 2000 tickets at \$1 a ticket to earn money for a new organ. There is one \$300 first prize, two \$200 second prizes, and four \$100 third prizes. Suppose Margaret buys a ticket. What are her expected winnings?
5. Let Z be a standardized normal variable. Find
   (a) $P(-2 \leq Z \leq -1)$
   (b) $P(Z \geq 2)$
6. A continuous random variable X has a probability density function

$$f(x) = \begin{cases} x & 0 \leq x \leq 1 \\ 2 - x & 1 < x \leq 2 \end{cases}$$

   Find

$$P(0.5 \leq X \leq 1.5)$$

7. The lifetime of a television set is an exponential random variable with an expected value of 10 years. The television set sells for \$500, and the company will give a customer a \$200 rebate if the television set burns out within 5 years. In this situation the revenue the company receives is a random variable R that can assume the two values \$500 and \$300. Find the expected value of R.
8. The time that Harry arrives at his 8:00 A.M. class is approximately normally distributed with a mean of 8:00 A.M. and a standard deviation of 5 minutes. What is the probability that Harry will be more than 5 minutes late for class on a given day?
9. Let X be a normal random variable with mean μ and standard devation σ. Find
   (a) $P(\mu - \sigma \leq X \leq \mu + \sigma)$
   (b) $P(\mu - 2\sigma \leq X \leq \mu + 2\sigma)$
   (c) $P(\mu - 3\sigma \leq X \leq \mu + 3\sigma)$
10. Roll a pair of dice (one red and one green). Let

$$RL3 = \text{Event the red die turns up larger than 3}$$

$$GL1 = \text{Event the green die turns up larger than 1}$$

   Verify the rule

$$P(RL3 \cup GL1) = P(RL3) + P(GL1) - P(RL3 \cap GL1)$$

11. Three coins are tossed. Define the random variable

$$X = \text{Total number of heads that turn up}$$

What is the probability distribution of X?

12. A student studying European history is asked to match three historical events with three dates (Columbus's discovery of America, the Great Plague of London, and the Treaty of Nantes with the three dates 1665, 1492, and 1685).

(a) If the student has no knowledge and guesses at the answers, what is the probability distribution of the random variable

$$X = \text{Number of answers the student gets correct}$$

(b) Suppose the student's professor gives the student 0, 50, 75, or 100 points if the student gets 0, 1, 2, or 3 matches. What will be this student's expected grade?

Appendix: Tables

- Table 1 Common Logarithms
- Table 2 The Natural Logarithm Function: $\ln x = \log_e x$
- Table 3 The Exponential Function: e^x
- Table 4 Trigonometric Functions

TABLE 1
Common Logarithms

N	0	1	2	3	4	5	6	7	8	9
1.0	0.0000	0.004321	0.008600	0.01284	0.01703	0.02119	0.02531	0.02938	0.03342	0.03743
1.1	0.04139	0.04532	0.04922	0.05308	0.05690	0.06070	0.06446	0.06819	0.07188	0.07555
1.2	0.07918	0.08279	0.08636	0.08991	0.09342	0.09691	0.1004	0.1038	0.1072	0.1106
1.3	0.1139	0.1173	0.1206	0.1239	0.1271	0.1303	0.1335	0.1367	0.1399	0.1430
1.4	0.1461	0.1492	0.1523	0.1553	0.1584	0.1614	0.1644	0.1673	0.1703	0.1732
1.5	0.1761	0.1790	0.1818	0.1847	0.1875	0.1903	0.1931	0.1959	0.1987	0.2014
1.6	0.2041	0.2068	0.2095	0.2122	0.2148	0.2175	0.2201	0.2227	0.2253	0.2279
1.7	0.2304	0.2330	0.2355	0.2380	0.2405	0.2430	0.2455	0.2480	0.2504	0.2529
1.8	0.2553	0.2577	0.2601	0.2625	0.2648	0.2673	0.2695	0.2718	0.2742	0.2765
1.9	0.2788	0.2810	0.2833	0.2856	0.2878	0.2900	0.2923	0.2945	0.2967	0.2989
2.0	0.3010	0.3032	0.3054	0.3075	0.3096	0.3118	0.3139	0.3160	0.3181	0.3201
2.1	0.3222	0.3243	0.3263	0.3284	0.3304	0.3324	0.3345	0.3365	0.3385	0.3404
2.2	0.3424	0.3444	0.3464	0.3483	0.3502	0.3522	0.3541	0.3560	0.3579	0.3598
2.3	0.3617	0.3636	0.3655	0.3674	0.3692	0.3711	0.3729	0.3747	0.3766	0.3784
2.4	0.3802	0.3820	0.3838	0.3856	0.3874	0.3892	0.3909	0.3927	0.3945	0.3962
2.5	0.3979	0.3997	0.4014	0.4031	0.4048	0.4065	0.4082	0.4099	0.4116	0.4133
2.6	0.4150	0.4166	0.4183	0.4200	0.4216	0.4232	0.4249	0.4265	0.4281	0.4298
2.7	0.4314	0.4330	0.4346	0.4362	0.4378	0.4393	0.4409	0.4425	0.4440	0.4456
2.8	0.4472	0.4487	0.4502	0.4518	0.4533	0.4548	0.4564	0.4579	0.4594	0.4609
2.9	0.4624	0.4639	0.4654	0.4669	0.4683	0.4698	0.4713	0.4728	0.4742	0.4757
3.0	0.4771	0.4786	0.4800	0.4814	0.4829	0.4843	0.4857	0.4871	0.4886	0.4900
3.1	0.4914	0.4928	0.4942	0.4955	0.4969	0.4983	0.4997	0.5011	0.5024	0.5038
3.2	0.5051	0.5065	0.5079	0.5092	0.5105	0.5119	0.5132	0.5145	0.5159	0.5172
3.3	0.5185	0.5198	0.5211	0.5224	0.5237	0.5250	0.5263	0.5276	0.5289	0.5302
3.4	0.5315	0.5328	0.5340	0.5353	0.5366	0.5378	0.5391	0.5403	0.5416	0.5428
3.5	0.5441	0.5453	0.5465	0.5478	0.5490	0.5502	0.5514	0.5527	0.5539	0.5551
3.6	0.5563	0.5575	0.5587	0.5599	0.5611	0.5623	0.5635	0.5647	0.5658	0.5670
3.7	0.5682	0.5694	0.5705	0.5717	0.5729	0.5740	0.5752	0.5763	0.5775	0.5786
3.8	0.5798	0.5809	0.5821	0.5832	0.5843	0.5855	0.5866	0.5877	0.5888	0.5899
3.9	0.5911	0.5922	0.5933	0.5944	0.5955	0.5966	0.5977	0.5988	0.5999	0.6010
4.0	0.6021	0.6031	0.6042	0.6053	0.6064	0.6075	0.6085	0.6096	0.6107	0.6117
4.1	0.6128	0.6138	0.6149	0.6160	0.6170	0.6180	0.6191	0.6201	0.6212	0.6222
4.2	0.6232	0.6243	0.6253	0.6263	0.6274	0.6284	0.6294	0.6304	0.6314	0.6325
4.3	0.6335	0.6345	0.6355	0.6365	0.6375	0.6385	0.6395	0.6405	0.6415	0.6425
4.4	0.6435	0.6444	0.6454	0.6464	0.6474	0.6484	0.6493	0.6503	0.6513	0.6522
4.5	0.6532	0.6542	0.6551	0.6561	0.6571	0.6580	0.6590	0.6599	0.6609	0.6618
4.6	0.6628	0.6637	0.6646	0.6656	0.6665	0.6675	0.6684	0.6693	0.6702	0.6712
4.7	0.6721	0.6730	0.6739	0.6749	0.6758	0.6767	0.6776	0.6785	0.6794	0.6803
4.8	0.6812	0.6821	0.6830	0.6839	0.6848	0.6857	0.6866	0.6875	0.6884	0.6893
4.9	0.6902	0.6911	0.6920	0.6928	0.6937	0.6946	0.6955	0.6964	0.6972	0.6981
5.0	0.6990	0.6998	0.7007	0.7016	0.7024	0.7033	0.7042	0.7050	0.7059	0.7067
5.1	0.7076	0.7084	0.7093	0.7101	0.7110	0.7118	0.7126	0.7135	0.7143	0.7152
5.2	0.7160	0.7168	0.7177	0.7185	0.7193	0.7202	0.7210	0.7218	0.7226	0.7235
5.3	0.7243	0.7251	0.7259	0.7267	0.7275	0.7284	0.7292	0.7300	0.7308	0.7316
5.4	0.7324	0.7332	0.7340	0.7348	0.7356	0.7364	0.7372	0.7380	0.7388	0.7396

TABLE 1
Common Logarithms (*continued*)

N	0	1	2	3	4	5	6	7	8	9
5.5	0.7404	0.7412	0.7419	0.7427	0.7435	0.7443	0.7451	0.7459	0.7466	0.7474
5.6	0.7482	0.7490	0.7497	0.7505	0.7513	0.7520	0.7528	0.7536	0.7543	0.7551
5.7	0.7559	0.7566	0.7574	0.7582	0.7589	0.7597	0.7604	0.7612	0.7619	0.7627
5.8	0.7634	0.7642	0.7649	0.7657	0.7664	0.7672	0.7679	0.7686	0.7694	0.7701
5.9	0.7709	0.7716	0.7723	0.7731	0.7738	0.7745	0.7752	0.7760	0.7767	0.7774
6.0	0.7782	0.7789	0.7796	0.7803	0.7810	0.7818	0.7825	0.7832	0.7839	0.7846
6.1	0.7853	0.7860	0.7868	0.7875	0.7882	0.7889	0.7896	0.7903	0.7910	0.7917
6.2	0.7924	0.7931	0.7938	0.7945	0.7952	0.7959	0.7966	0.7973	0.7980	0.7987
6.3	0.7993	0.8000	0.8007	0.8014	0.8021	0.8028	0.8035	0.8041	0.8048	0.8055
6.4	0.8062	0.8069	0.8075	0.8082	0.8089	0.8096	0.8102	0.8109	0.8116	0.8122
6.5	0.8129	0.8136	0.8142	0.8149	0.8156	0.8162	0.8169	0.8176	0.8182	0.8189
6.6	0.8195	0.8202	0.8209	0.8215	0.8222	0.8228	0.8235	0.8241	0.8248	0.8254
6.7	0.8261	0.8267	0.8274	0.8280	0.8287	0.8293	0.8299	0.8306	0.8312	0.8319
6.8	0.8325	0.8331	0.8338	0.8344	0.8351	0.8357	0.8363	0.8370	0.8376	0.8382
6.9	0.8388	0.8395	0.8401	0.8407	0.8414	0.8420	0.8426	0.8432	0.8439	0.8445
7.0	0.8451	0.8457	0.8463	0.8470	0.8476	0.8482	0.8488	0.8494	0.8500	0.8506
7.1	0.8513	0.8519	0.8525	0.8531	0.8537	0.8543	0.8549	0.8555	0.8561	0.8567
7.2	0.8573	0.8579	0.8585	0.8591	0.8597	0.8603	0.8609	0.8615	0.8621	0.8627
7.3	0.8633	0.8639	0.8645	0.8651	0.8657	0.8663	0.8669	0.8675	0.8681	0.8686
7.4	0.8692	0.8698	0.8704	0.8710	0.8716	0.8722	0.8727	0.8733	0.8739	0.8745
7.5	0.8751	0.8756	0.8762	0.8768	0.8774	0.8779	0.8785	0.8791	0.8797	0.8802
7.6	0.8808	0.8814	0.8820	0.8825	0.8831	0.8837	0.8842	0.8848	0.8854	0.8859
7.7	0.8865	0.8871	0.8876	0.8882	0.8887	0.8893	0.8899	0.8904	0.8910	0.8915
7.8	0.8921	0.8927	0.8932	0.8938	0.8943	0.8949	0.8954	0.8960	0.8965	0.8971
7.9	0.8976	0.8982	0.8987	0.8993	0.8998	0.9004	0.9009	0.9015	0.9020	0.9025
8.0	0.9031	0.9036	0.9042	0.9047	0.9053	0.9058	0.9063	0.9069	0.9074	0.9079
8.1	0.9085	0.9090	0.9096	0.9101	0.9106	0.9112	0.9117	0.9122	0.9128	0.9133
8.2	0.9138	0.9143	0.9149	0.9154	0.9159	0.9165	0.9170	0.9175	0.9180	0.9186
8.3	0.9191	0.9196	0.9201	0.9206	0.9212	0.9217	0.9222	0.9227	0.9232	0.9238
8.4	0.9243	0.9248	0.9253	0.9258	0.9263	0.9269	0.9274	0.9279	0.9284	0.9289
8.5	0.9294	0.9299	0.9304	0.9309	0.9315	0.9320	0.9325	0.9330	0.9335	0.9340
8.6	0.9345	0.9350	0.9355	0.9360	0.9365	0.9370	0.9375	0.9380	0.9385	0.9390
8.7	0.9395	0.9400	0.9405	0.9410	0.9415	0.9420	0.9425	0.9430	0.9435	0.9440
8.8	0.9445	0.9450	0.9455	0.9460	0.9465	0.9469	0.9474	0.9479	0.9484	0.9489
8.9	0.9494	0.9499	0.9504	0.9509	0.9513	0.9518	0.9523	0.9528	0.9533	0.9538
9.0	0.9542	0.9547	0.9552	0.9557	0.9562	0.9566	0.9571	0.9576	0.9581	0.9586
9.1	0.9590	0.9595	0.9600	0.9605	0.9609	0.9614	0.9619	0.9624	0.9628	0.9633
9.2	0.9638	0.9643	0.9647	0.9652	0.9657	0.9661	0.9666	0.9671	0.9675	0.9680
9.3	0.9685	0.9689	0.9694	0.9699	0.9703	0.9708	0.9713	0.9717	0.9722	0.9727
9.4	0.9731	0.9736	0.9741	0.9745	0.9750	0.9754	0.9759	0.9763	0.9768	0.9773
9.5	0.9777	0.9782	0.9786	0.9791	0.9795	0.9800	0.9805	0.9809	0.9814	0.9818
9.6	0.9823	0.9827	0.9832	0.9836	0.9841	0.9845	0.9850	0.9854	0.9859	0.9863
9.7	0.9868	0.9872	0.9877	0.9881	0.9886	0.9890	0.9894	0.9899	0.9903	0.9908
9.8	0.9912	0.9917	0.9921	0.9926	0.9930	0.9934	0.9939	0.9943	0.9948	0.9952
9.9	0.9956	0.9961	0.9965	0.9969	0.9974	0.9978	0.9983	0.9987	0.9991	0.9996

TABLE 2
The Natural Logarithm Function: $\ln x = \log_e x$

x	$\ln x$	x	$\ln x$	x	$\ln x$
0.0	—	4.5	1.5041	9.0	2.1972
0.1	−2.3026	4.6	1.5261	9.1	2.2083
0.2	−1.6094	4.7	1.5476	9.2	2.2192
0.3	−1.2040	4.8	1.5686	9.3	2.2300
0.4	−0.9163	4.9	1.5892	9.4	2.2407
0.5	−0.6931	5.0	1.6094	9.5	2.2513
0.6	−0.5108	5.1	1.6292	9.6	2.2618
0.7	−0.3567	5.2	1.6487	9.7	2.2721
0.8	−0.2231	5.3	1.6677	9.8	2.2824
0.9	−0.1054	5.4	1.6864	9.9	2.2925
1.0	0.0000	5.5	1.7047	10	2.3026
1.1	0.0953	5.6	1.7228	11	2.3979
1.2	0.1823	5.7	1.7405	12	2.4849
1.3	0.2624	5.8	1.7579	13	2.5649
1.4	0.3365	5.9	1.7750	14	2.6391
1.5	0.4055	6.0	1.7918	15	2.7081
1.6	0.4700	6.1	1.8083	16	2.7726
1.7	0.5306	6.2	1.8245	17	2.8332
1.8	0.5878	6.3	1.8405	18	2.8904
1.9	0.6419	6.4	1.8563	19	2.9444
2.0	0.6931	6.5	1.8718	20	2.9957
2.1	0.7419	6.6	1.8871	25	3.2189
2.2	0.7885	6.7	1.9021	30	3.4012
2.3	0.8329	6.8	1.9169	35	3.5553
2.4	0.8755	6.9	1.9315	40	3.6889
2.5	0.9163	7.0	1.9459	45	3.8067
2.6	0.9555	7.1	1.9601	50	3.9120
2.7	0.9933	7.2	1.9741	55	4.0073
2.8	1.0296	7.3	1.9879	60	4.0943
2.9	1.0647	7.4	2.0015	65	4.1744
3.0	1.0986	7.5	2.0149	70	4.2485
3.1	1.1314	7.6	2.0281	75	4.3175
3.2	1.1632	7.7	2.0412	80	4.3820
3.3	1.1939	7.8	2.0541	85	4.4427
3.4	1.2238	7.9	2.0669	90	4.4998
3.5	1.2528	8.0	2.0794	95	4.5539
3.6	1.2809	8.1	2.0919	100	4.6052
3.7	1.3083	8.2	2.1041	200	5.2983
3.8	1.3350	8.3	2.1163	300	5.7038
3.9	1.3610	8.4	2.1282	400	5.9915
4.0	1.3863	8.5	2.1401	500	6.2146
4.1	1.4110	8.6	2.1518	600	6.3069
4.2	1.4351	8.7	2.1633	700	6.5511
4.3	1.4586	8.8	2.1748	800	6.6846
4.4	1.4816	8.9	2.1861	900	6.8024

TABLE 3
The Exponential Function: e^x

x	e^x	e^{-x}	x	e^x	e^{-x}
0.00	1.0000	1.0000	3.0	20.086	0.0498
0.05	1.0513	0.9512	3.1	22.198	0.0450
0.10	1.1052	0.9048	3.2	24.533	0.0408
0.15	1.1618	0.8607	3.3	27.113	0.0369
0.20	1.2214	0.8187	3.4	29.964	0.0334
0.25	1.2840	0.7788	3.5	33.115	0.0302
0.30	1.3499	0.7408	3.6	36.598	0.0273
0.35	1.4191	0.7047	3.7	40.447	0.0247
0.40	1.4918	0.6703	3.8	44.701	0.0224
0.45	1.5683	0.6376	3.9	49.402	0.0202
0.50	1.6487	0.6065	4.0	54.598	0.0183
0.55	1.7333	0.5769	4.1	60.340	0.0166
0.60	1.8221	0.5488	4.2	66.686	0.0150
0.65	1.9155	0.5220	4.3	73.700	0.0136
0.70	2.0138	0.4966	4.4	81.451	0.0123
0.75	2.1170	0.4724	4.5	90.017	0.0111
0.80	2.2255	0.4493	4.6	99.484	0.0101
0.85	2.3396	0.4274	4.7	109.95	0.0091
0.90	2.4596	0.4066	4.8	121.51	0.0082
0.95	2.5857	0.3867	4.9	134.29	0.0074
1.0	2.7183	0.3679	5.0	148.41	0.0067
1.1	3.0042	0.3329	5.1	164.02	0.0061
1.2	3.3201	0.3012	5.2	181.27	0.0055
1.3	3.6693	0.2725	5.3	200.34	0.0050
1.4	4.0552	0.2466	5.4	221.41	0.0045
1.5	4.4817	0.2231	5.5	244.69	0.0041
1.6	4.9530	0.2019	5.6	270.43	0.0037
1.7	5.4739	0.1827	5.7	298.87	0.0033
1.8	6.0496	0.1653	5.8	330.30	0.0030
1.9	6.6859	0.1496	5.9	365.04	0.0027
2.0	7.3891	0.1353	6.0	403.43	0.0025
2.1	8.1662	0.1225	6.5	665.14	0.0015
2.2	9.0250	0.1108	7.0	1096.6	0.0009
2.3	9.9742	0.1003	7.5	1808.0	0.0006
2.4	11.023	0.0907	8.0	2981.0	0.0003
2.5	12.182	0.0821	8.5	4914.8	0.0002
2.6	13.464	0.0743	9.0	8103.1	0.0001
2.7	14.880	0.0672	9.5	13,360	0.00007
2.8	16.445	0.0608	10.0	22,026	0.00004
2.9	18.174	0.0550			

Answers to Selected Problems

CALCULUS PRELIMINARIES

SECTION P1: THE REAL NUMBERS

Properties of the Real Numbers

1. Rational **3.** Rational **5.** Rational **7.** Irrational **9.** Irrational
11. Since $2 \cdot 0 = 1 \cdot 0$ if we were allowed to divide by zero, we could show that $2 = 1$.
13. No largest real number less than 1 **15.** No smallest real number **17.** No largest rational number
19. They have the "same" number of members. **21.** Substitute n for age and c for cents in $100n + c$.

Exponents and Roots

1. 125 **3.** -1 **5.** $\frac{5}{2}$ **7.** Undefined **9.** $-\frac{1}{16}$ **11.** $-\frac{1}{16}$ **13.** -1 **15.** 1024 **17.** 0.0816327

19. 1.6446318 **21.** $\frac{1}{25}$ **23.** 10^8 **25.** ab^4 **27.** $\frac{1}{8m}$ **29.** $\frac{y}{x}$ **31.** 2 **33.** $2^{22} = 4{,}194{,}307$, yes, 222

35. 9^{9^9} **37.** 2 **39.** 2 **41.** 4 **43.** 1.1486984 **45.** 2 **47.** $5x\sqrt{x}$ **49.** $3\sqrt{x}$ **51.** $\frac{\sqrt{xy}}{xy}$ **53.** $z^3\sqrt{z}$

55. uv^2 **57.** If a and b are both negative, then $\sqrt{ab} = \sqrt{a}\sqrt{b}$ does not hold. **59.** $10\sqrt{2}\sqrt{5}$ **61.** $100x^2y^3$
63. $a^2b^2(\sqrt{ab} + b\sqrt{b})$ **65.** $5\sqrt{3}$ **67.** $2xy(2y)^{1/4}$ **69.** $2x\sqrt[5]{2}$ **71.** $5\sqrt{2} + 2\sqrt{3}\sqrt{5}$

Inequalities and Intervals

1. $x > -4$ **3.** $x \leq -\frac{1}{2}$ **5.** $x \leq -\frac{5}{8}$ **7.** $x \geq 0$ **9.** $x > 1$ **11.** (Hmmmmm.) Remember that $b - a$ is negative.

Algebraic Fractions and Rationalization

1. $\frac{2 + x^2}{2x}$ **3.** $\frac{-x^2 + 2x + 2}{(x - 1)(x + 2)}$ **5.** $\frac{x - 1}{x - 2}$ **7.** $\frac{x^{3/2} + x - x^{1/2} + 1}{x(1 - \sqrt{x})}$ **9.** $\frac{\sqrt{x} - \sqrt{y}}{x - y}$ **11.** $\frac{\sqrt{x + a} + \sqrt{x}}{a}$

13. $\frac{\sqrt{x + 2} - \sqrt{x - 2}}{4}$ **15.** $\frac{1}{\sqrt{2 + h} + \sqrt{2}}$ **17.** $\frac{4}{x(\sqrt{x + 2} + \sqrt{x - 2})}$ **19.** $\frac{x^2 - y}{x(x + \sqrt{y})}$

SECTION P2: FUNCTIONS AND THEIR GRAPHS

Functional Notation

1. -1 **3.** -2 **5.** $x^2 - 2$ **7.** $x^2 - 1$ **9.** $4x - 2$ **11.** 1 **13.** Undefined **15.** $\frac{1}{x^2}$ **17.** $\frac{1 + x^2}{x^2}$

19. $\frac{1 + 4x^2}{2x}$ **21.** 1 **23.** 0 **25.** x^4 **27.** $x^4 + 1$ **29.** $4x^2 + 2x$ **31.** All real numbers, $\{1\}$

33. All real numbers, all nonnegative real numbers **35.** All nonnegative real numbers, all nonnegative real numbers
37. All real numbers, all real numbers ≥ 1 **39.** All real numbers, $(0, 1]$

Cartesian Coordinate System

1.

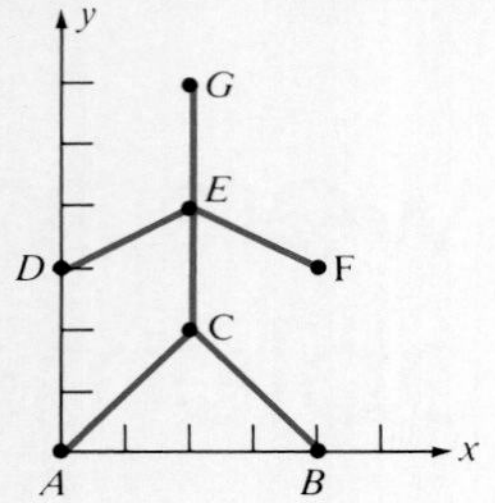

3.

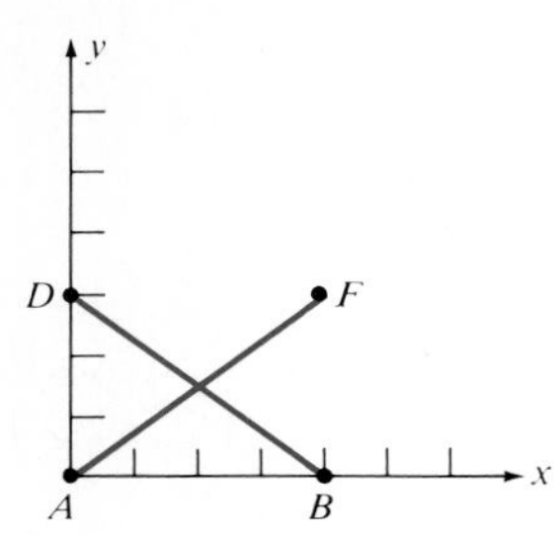

5.

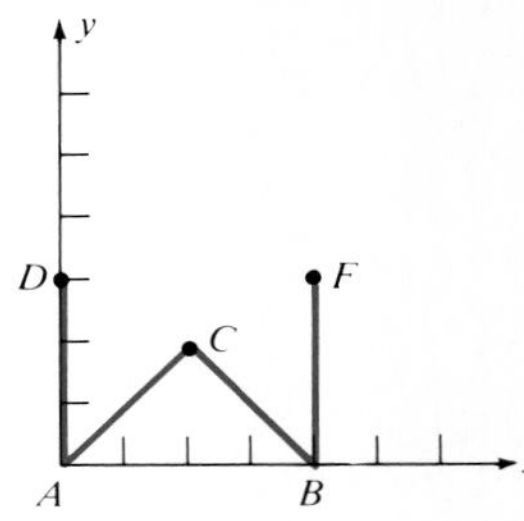

7.

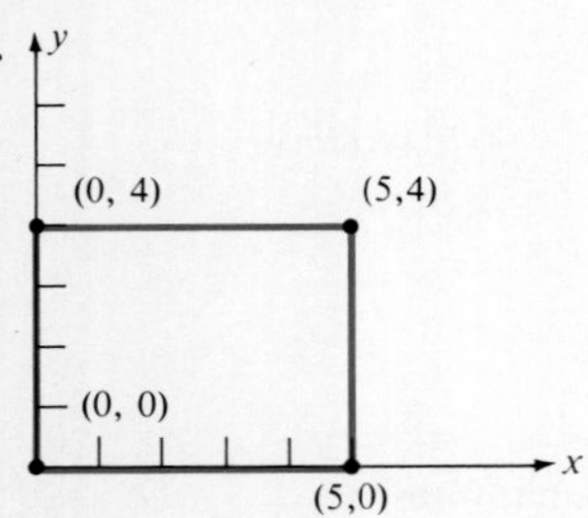

9.

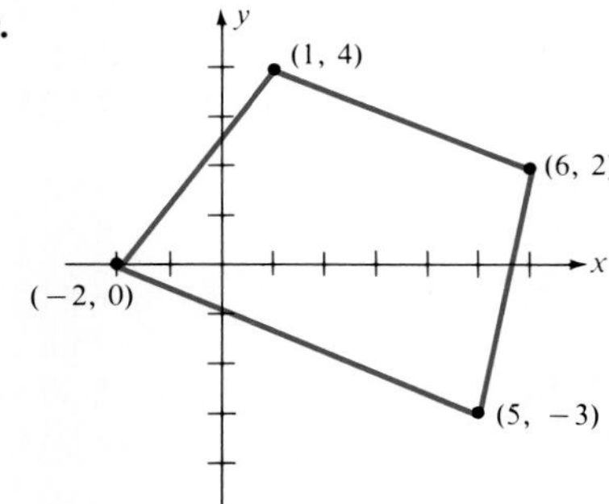

11.

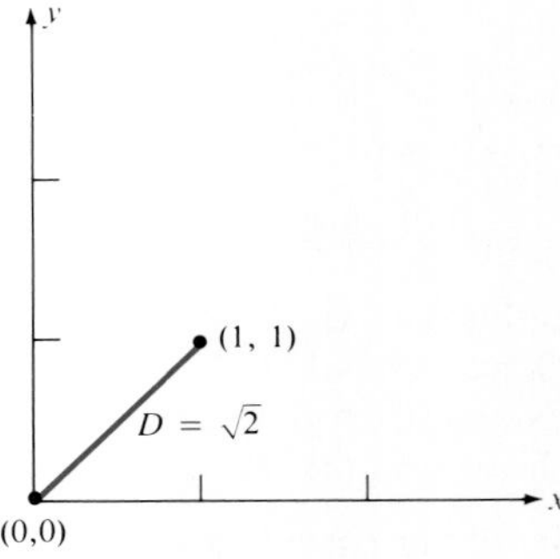

13.

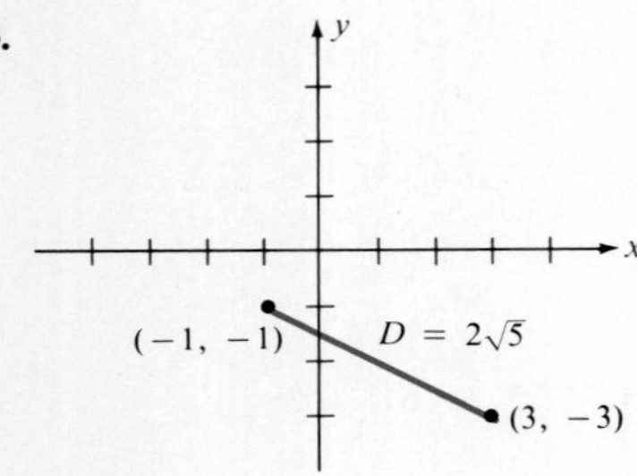

15. $D[(1, 1), (2, 3)] = \sqrt{1^2 + 2^2} = \sqrt{5}$
$D[(2, 3), (4, -1)] = \sqrt{2^2 + (-4)^2} = 2\sqrt{5}$
$D[(4, -1), (1, 1)] = \sqrt{(-3)^2 + 2^2} = \sqrt{13}$
Total distance $= 3\sqrt{5} + \sqrt{13}$

Graphs of Functions

1.

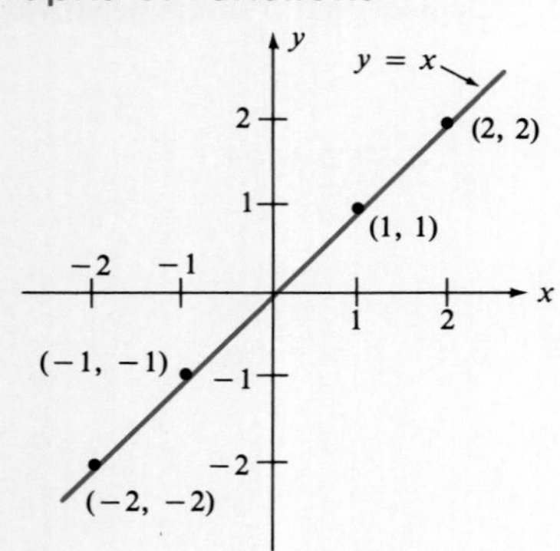

3.

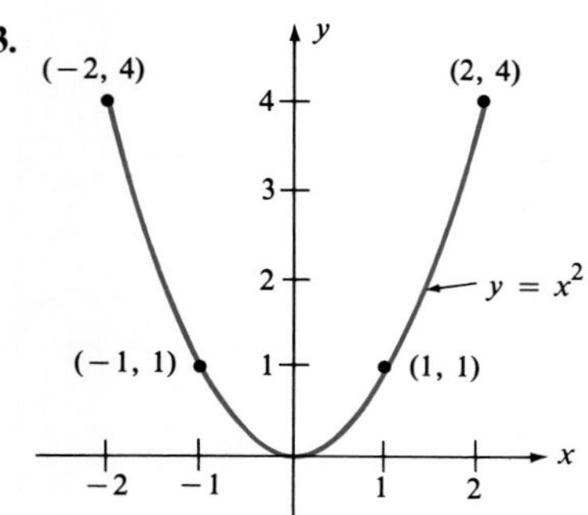

5.

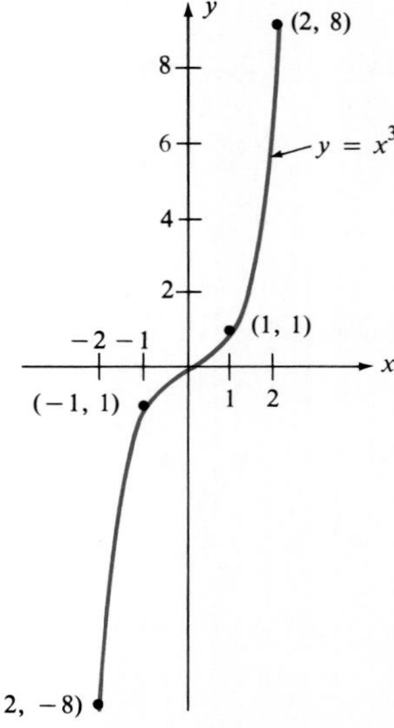

7.

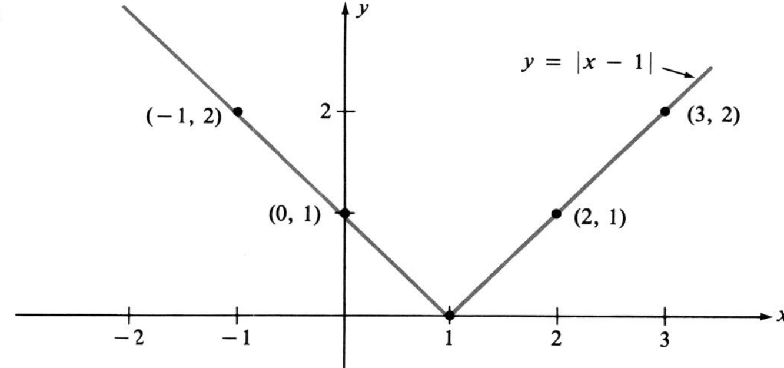

9.

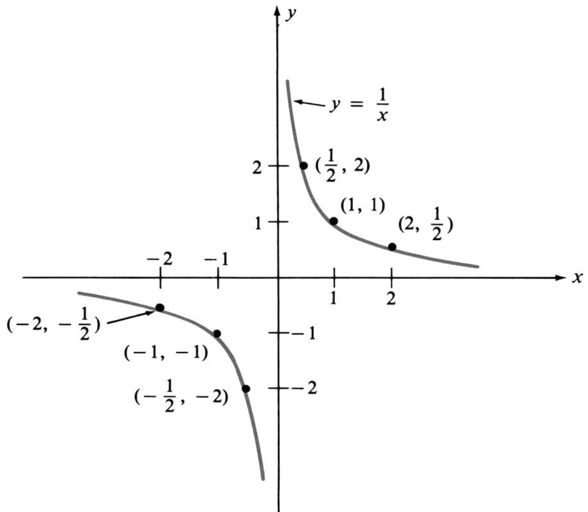

11. (Wind Chill Factor) $WC(30) = -78.8$ degrees

First-Order Polynomials: Straight Lines

1.

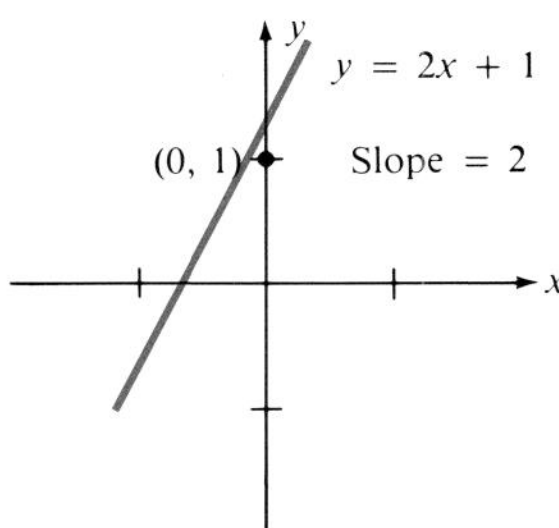

3.

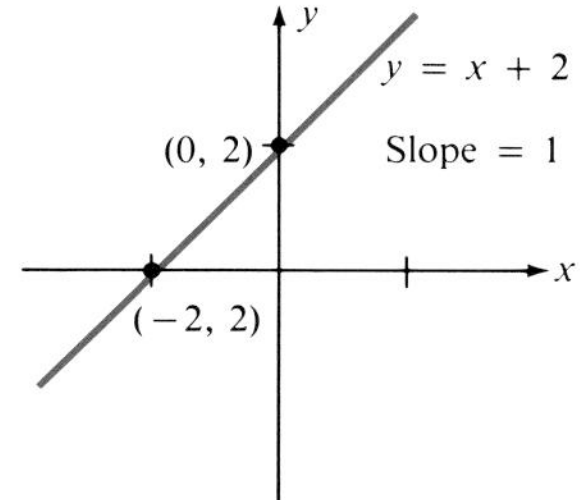

5.

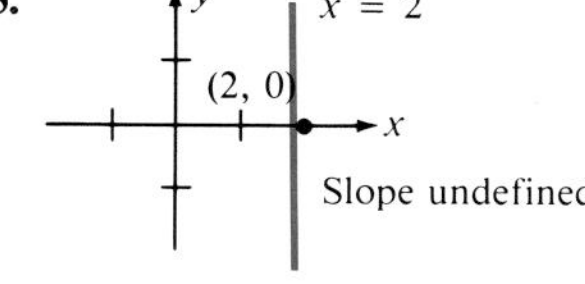

7. Slope = 2, y-intercept = 0

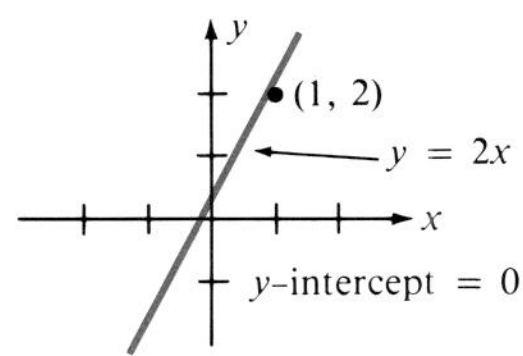

9. Slope = 3, y-intercept = 5

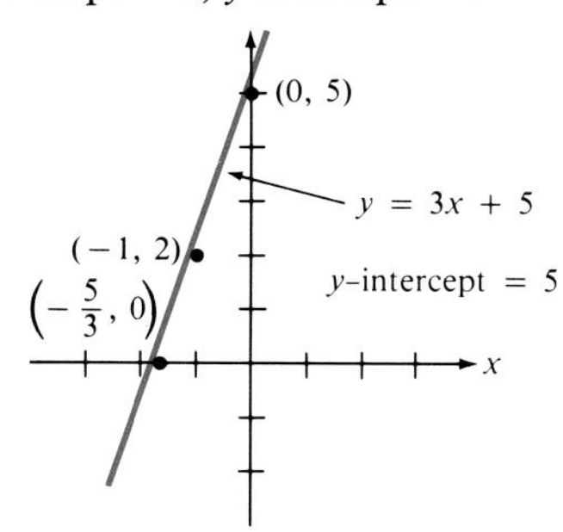

11. Slope = 1, y-intercept = 0

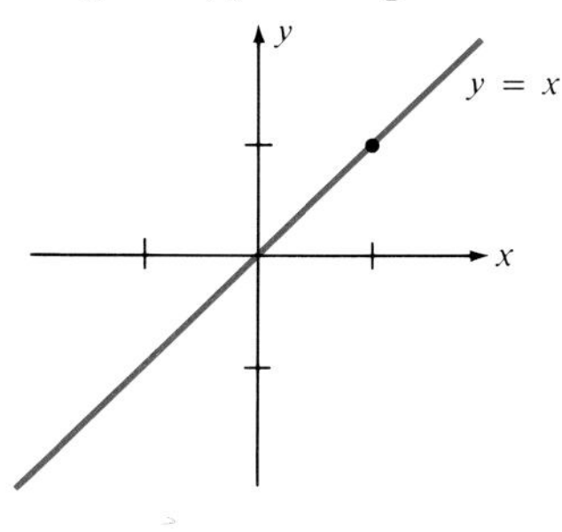

13. Slope $= -1$, y-intercept $= 0$

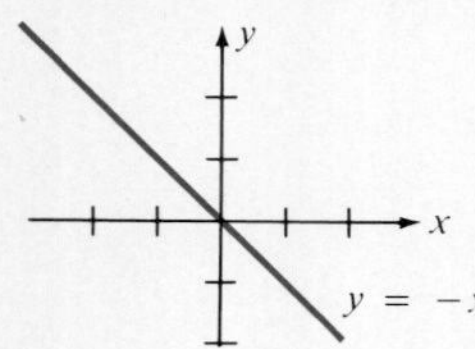

15. Slope $= -1$, y-intercept $= 4$

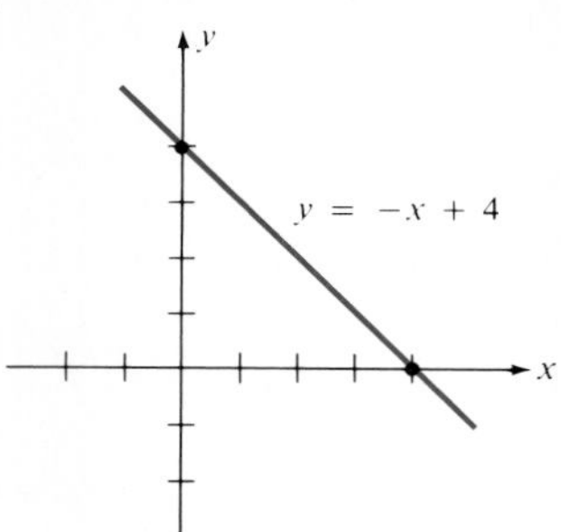

17.

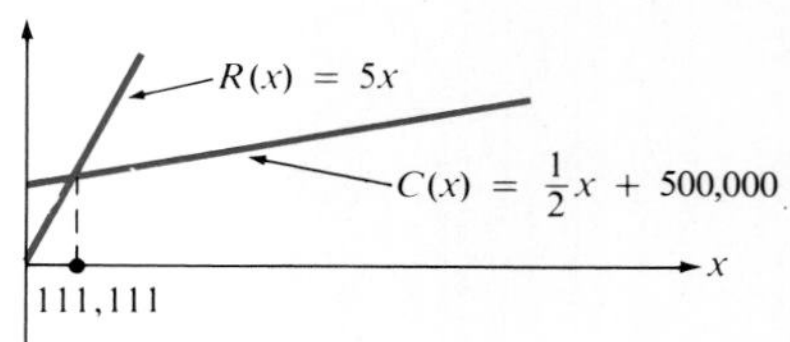

19.

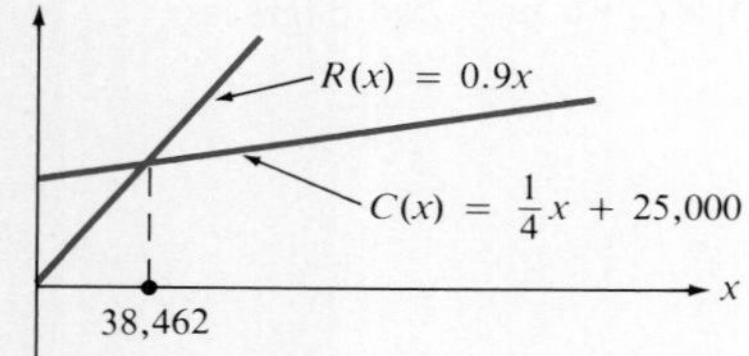

21.

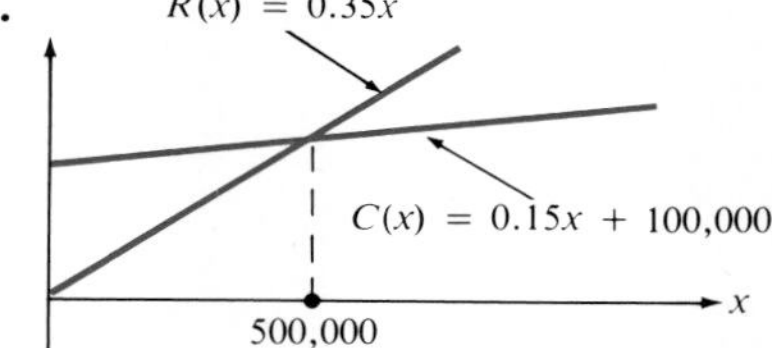

23. (a) 50 **(b)** Fixed costs are generally larger than \$200

25. (a)

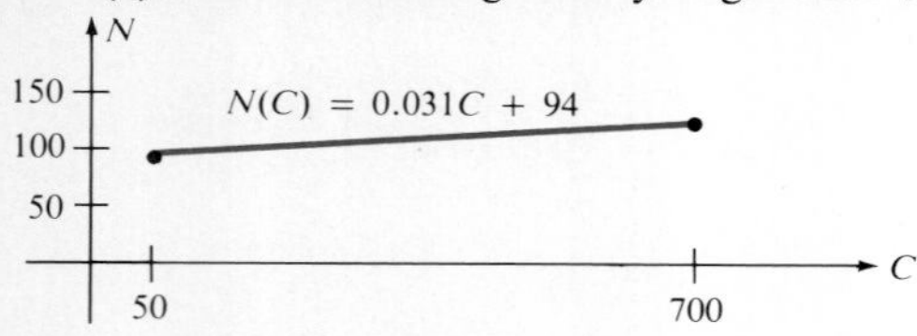

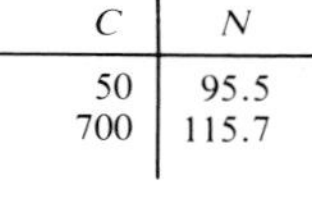

C	N
50	95.5
700	115.7

(b) 97.1

27. $T(1995) = 3.731$ minutes (3 min, 43.86 sec)

29. The rope will be 1.59 feet above the ground, and hence the mouse can crawl under the rope.

Higher-Order Polynomials

1. First-order polynomial **3.** Fourth-order polynomial **5.** Not a polynomial **7.** First-order polynomial

9. Not a polynomial

11.

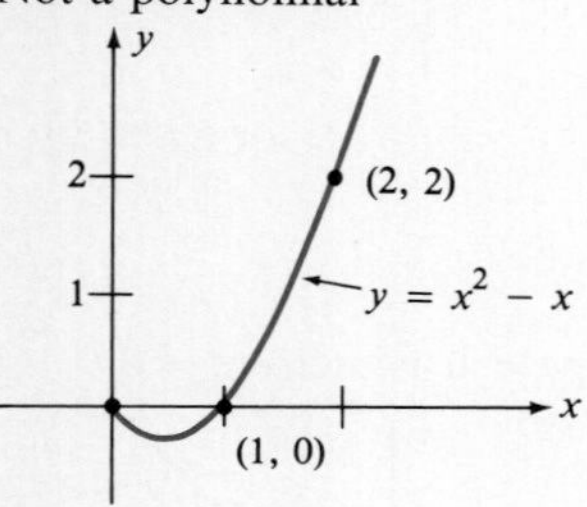

13.

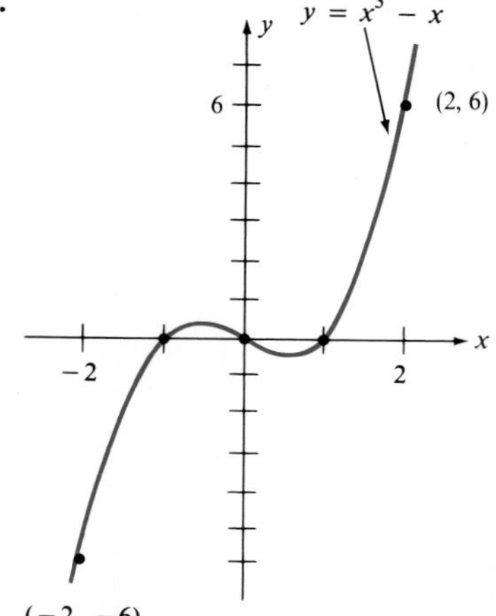

15.

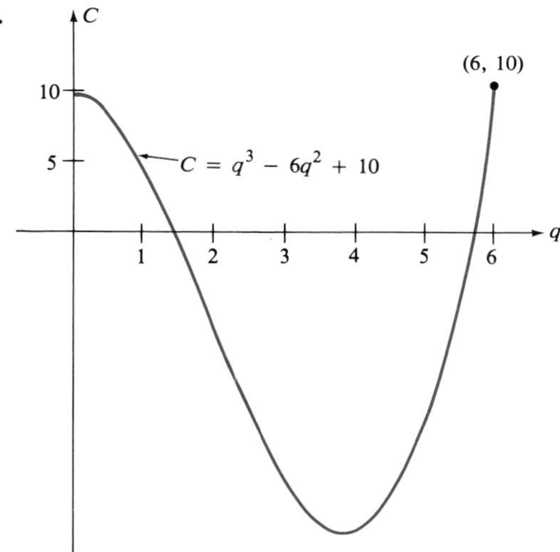

17.

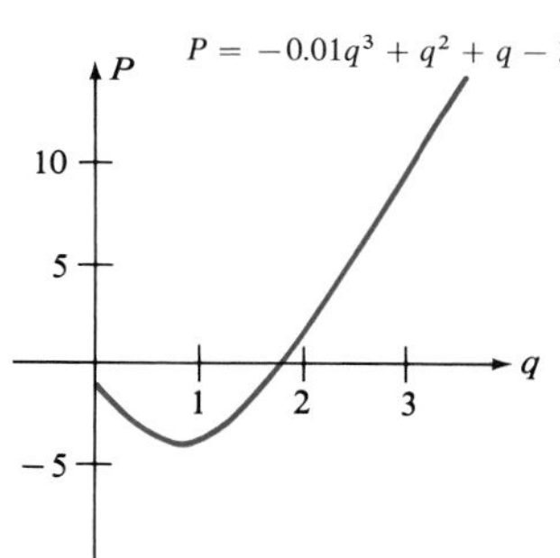

19.

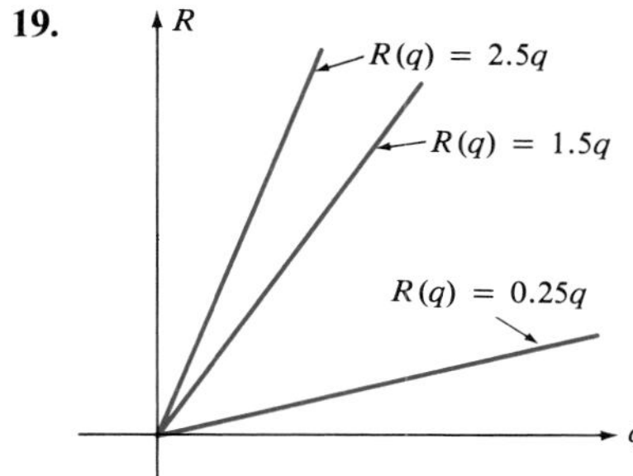

21. $C(q) = 0.5q^3 - 0.5q^2 + 100q + 500$

C

100

q

Absolute Value Function

1. Verify that the equation holds for $x < 0$, $= 0$, > 0.
3. Verify that the equation holds for x and y each less than, equal to, or greater than 0.
5. Verify that the equation holds for $x < 0$, $= 0$, > 0. **7.** $x \geq 3$ or $x \leq -3$ **9.** $0 < x < 2$ **11.** $-8 < x < 2$
13. No number satisfies the inequality. **15.** All real numbers satisfy the inequality.
17. $|x + y|$ is always larger. **19.** $|x + y| \leq |x| + |y|$ holds for all real numbers. **21.** The two values are always the same.

SECTION P3: ZEROS OF LINEAR AND QUADRATIC FUNCTIONS

Zeros of Linear Functions

1. $\frac{13}{3}$ **3.** $\frac{11}{13}$ **5.** $\frac{2}{5}$ **7.** -4 **9.** -1 **11.** $\frac{3}{4}$ **13.** -3

Zeros of Quadratic Functions

1. $2, -7$ **3.** $3, -3$ **5.** $\frac{3}{4}, -\frac{3}{4}$ **7.** $\frac{3}{5}, -1$ **9.** $2, 4$ **11.** $1, -1, 2$ **13.** $\frac{-1 \pm \sqrt{31}}{3}$ **15.** $\frac{4}{3}, \frac{2}{3}$

17. $-4 \pm \sqrt{14}$ **19.** $2m \pm \sqrt{4m^2 - m}$ **21.** $\frac{1 \pm \sqrt{13}}{6}$

SECTION P4: FUNCTION OPERATIONS

Manipulation of Graphs of Functions

1.

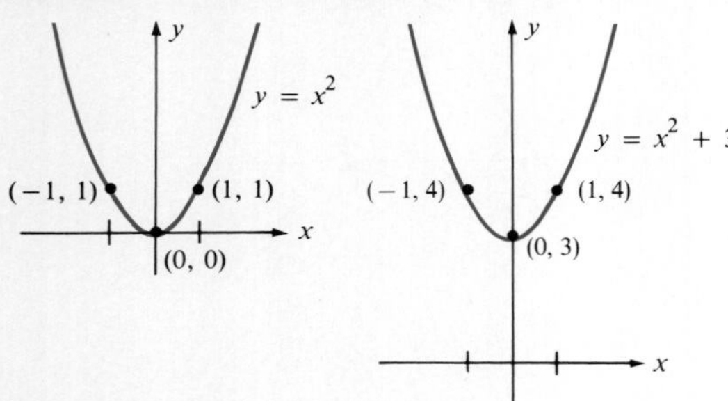

3.

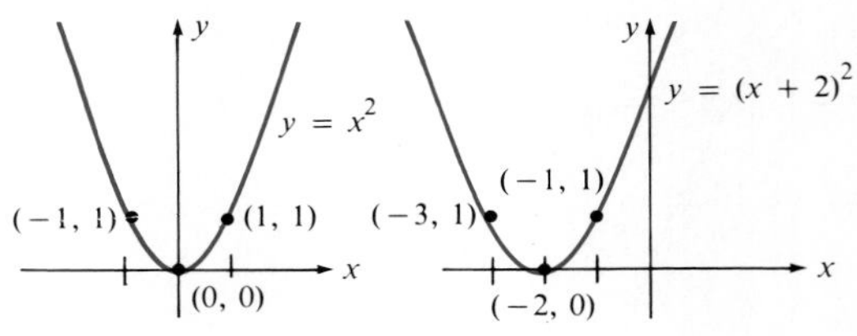

5.

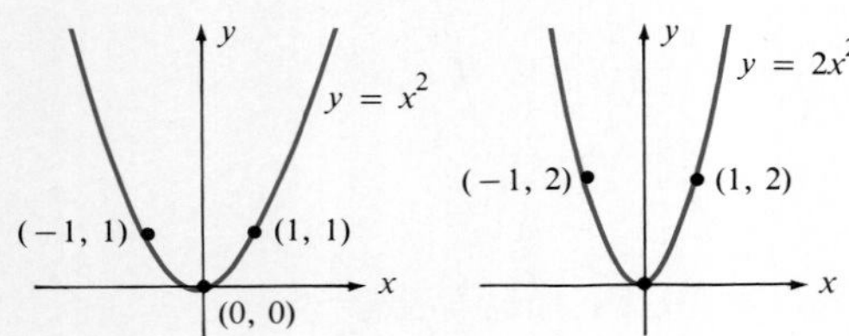

7.

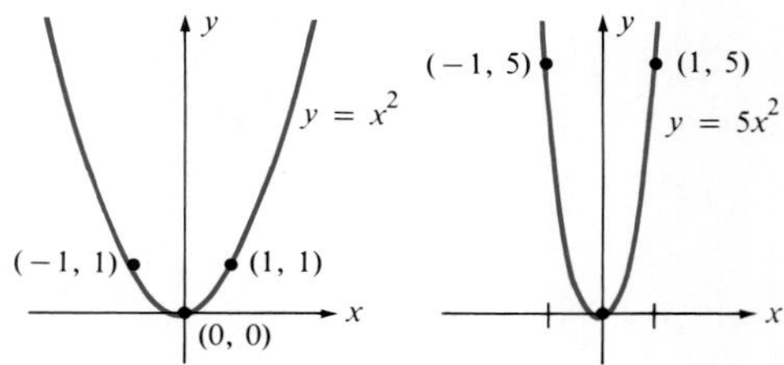

9.

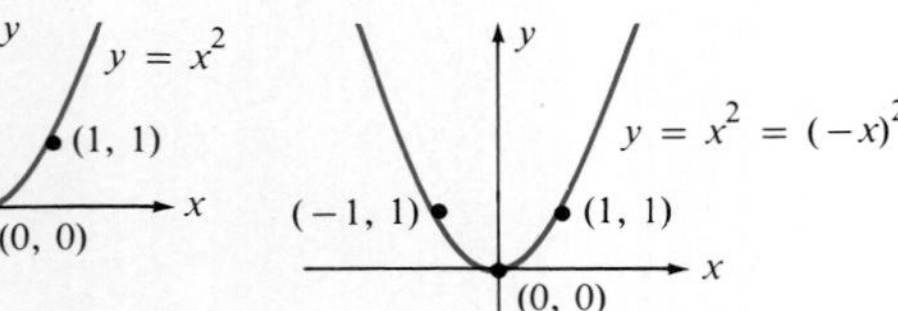

11.

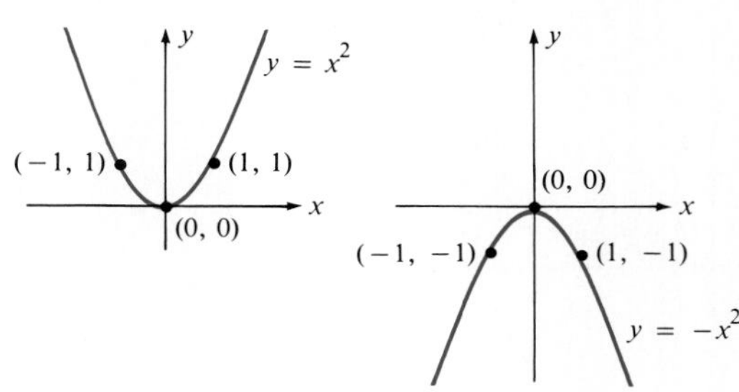

Zeros of Quadratic Functions

1. $(f + g)(x) = 2x + 1$ (the real numbers)
$(f - g)(x) = 2x - 1$ (the real numbers)
$(f \cdot g)(x) = 2x$ (the real numbers)
$\left(\dfrac{f}{g}\right)(x) = 2x$ (the real numbers)

3. $(f + g)(x) = |x| + |x| - 1$ (the real numbers)
$(f - g)(x) = |x| - x + 1$ (the real numbers)
$(f \cdot g)(x) = |x|(x - 1)$ (the real numbers)
$\left(\dfrac{f}{g}\right)(x) = \dfrac{|x|}{x - 1}$ (all real numbers except $x = 1$)

5. $(f + g)(x) = \sqrt{1 - x^2} + \sqrt{x}$ $(0 \le x \le 1)$
$(f - g)(x) = \sqrt{1 - x^2} - \sqrt{x}$ $(0 \le x \le 1)$
$(f \cdot g)(x) = \sqrt{x}\sqrt{1 - x^2}$ $(0 < x \le 1)$
$\left(\dfrac{f}{g}\right)(x) = \dfrac{\sqrt{1 - x^2}}{\sqrt{x}}$ $(0 \le x \le 1)$

7. $(f + g)(x) = \dfrac{x - 1}{x^2 + 1} + x^2 + 1$ (the real numbers)
$(f - g)(x) = \dfrac{x - 1}{x^2 + 1} - x^2 - 1$ (the real numbers)
$(f \cdot g)(x) = x - 1$ (the real numbers)
$\left(\dfrac{f}{g}\right)(x) = \dfrac{x - 1}{(x^2 + 1)^2}$ (the real numbers)

Composition of Functions

1. $f[g(x)] = 3(x^2 + 2x + 1)$ **3.** $g[f(x)] = 9x^2 + 6x + 1$ **5.** $h[f(x)] = 1 + \dfrac{1}{3x}$
7. $f[g(x)] = \sqrt{x^2 + 1}$ (all real numbers) **9.** $g[f(x)] = x + 1,\ x \ge 0$ **11.** $h[f(x)] = \sqrt{x} - 1,\ x \ge 0$
13. $f[f(x)] = x^{1/4},\ x \ge 0$ **15.** $h[h(x)] = x - 2$ (all real numbers)

Practice Test

1. **(a)** 2 **(b)** $\frac{1}{2}\frac{1}{\sqrt[5]{2}}$ **(c)** 4 **(d)** Does not exist, since the fourth powers are positive. **(e)** 9

2. **(a)** $4x$ **(b)** $ab + c$ **(c)** $2xy^2$ **3.** **(a)** $(x - 3)(x + 3)$ **(b)** $(x - 4)(x + 3)$ **4.** $\frac{-5 \pm \sqrt{33}}{2}$ **5.** $\frac{x - 3}{(x + 1)(x + 3)}$

6. $\frac{\sqrt{x} + \sqrt{y}}{x - y}$ **7.** **(a)** $-\infty < x \leq \frac{4}{3}$ **(b)** $-\infty < x \leq -\frac{1}{2}$ or $0 < x < \infty$ **8.**

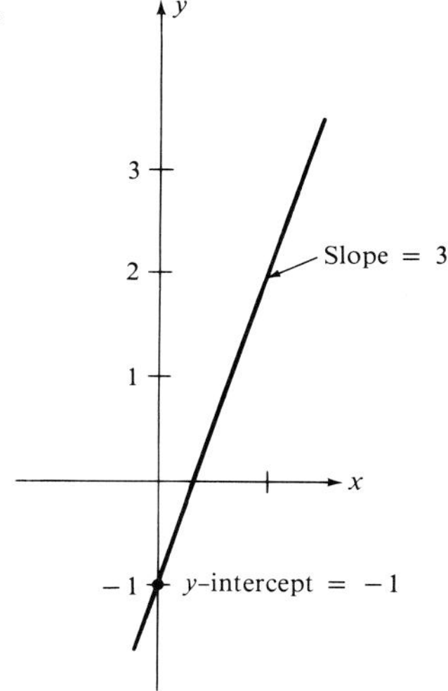

9. $y = 2x + 1$ **10.** $y = -x + 2$ **11.** $f[g(x)] = (2x + 1)^2$
$g[f(x)] = 2x^2 + 1$

CHAPTER 1

Section 1.2

1. 6

3. $\frac{1}{3}$

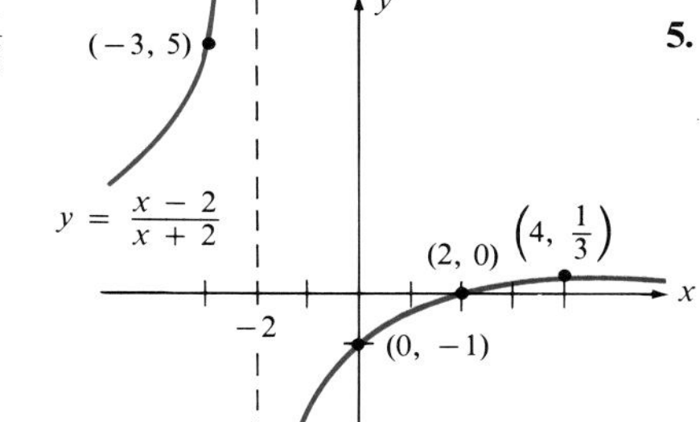

5. $\sqrt{5}$

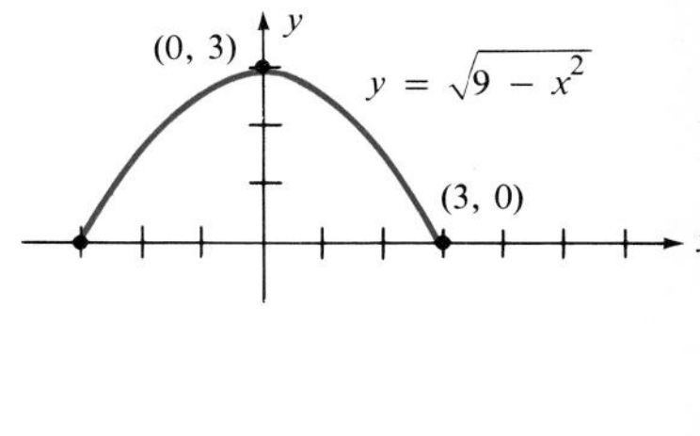

7. $\frac{1}{4}$

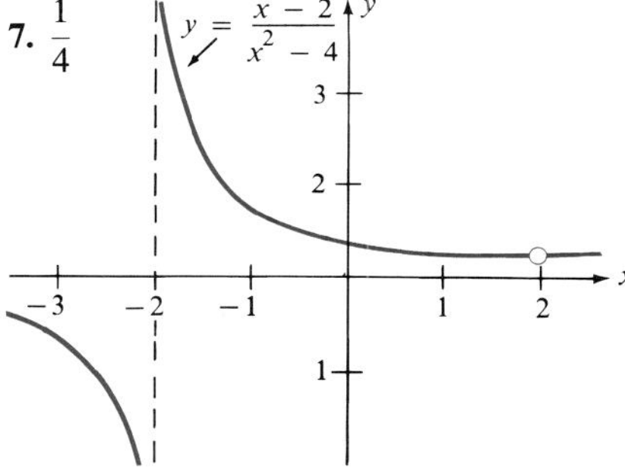

9. $\frac{1}{2}$

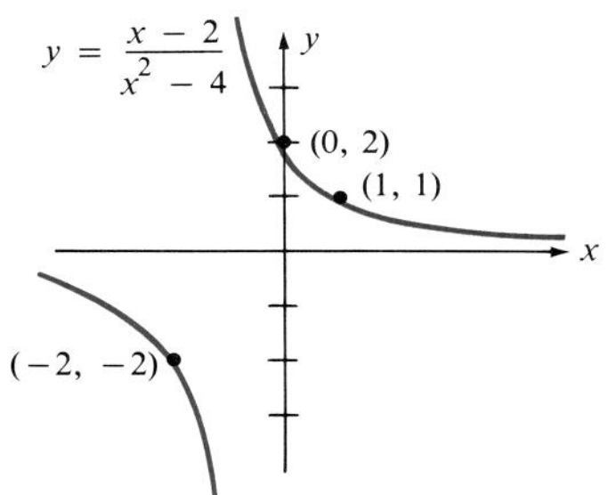

11. 2

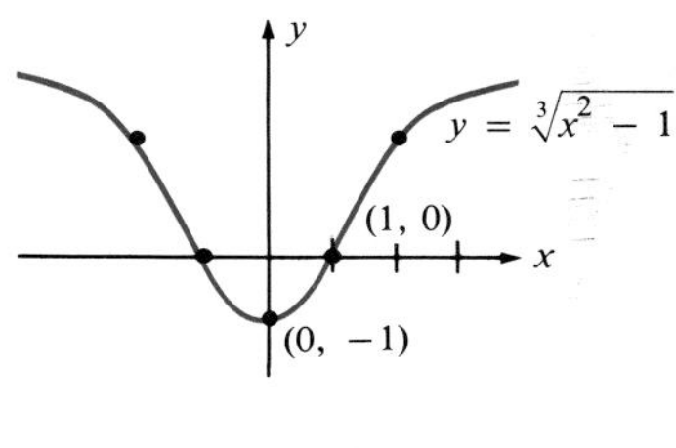

13. 0 **15.** No limit **17.** No limit **19.** Not limit **21.** −1 **23.** 0 **25.** 6 **27.** 10 **29.** 12
31. Discontinuous **33.** Continuous **35.** Discontinuous **37.** Discontinuous **39.** $(-\infty, \infty)$ **41.** $(-\infty, \infty)$

43. Discontinuous at $x = -1$ **45.** $(-\infty, \infty)$ **47.** Discontinuous at $-1, 3$ **49.** $-3, -1, 2$ **51.** -1

53. $f(x) = \begin{cases} 25 & 0 < x < 1 \\ 25 + 20n & n < x \leq n + 1 \ (n = 1, 2, 3, \ldots, 11) \end{cases}$

Discontinuous at each integer value of x for $0 < x < 12$

Section 1.3

1. 8 **3.** 3 **5.** 3 **7.** 3 **9.** 1 **11.** 8 **13.** -4 **15.** 2 **17.** 0 **19.** 2 **21.** -2 **23.** 144 ft

25. 96 ft/sec **27.** 2.5 sec **29.** 1 **31.** $2t$ **33.** **(a)** $s'(0) = v$, $s''(0) = -32$ **(b)** $v/32$ sec **(c)** $\frac{v^2}{64}$ feet

35. 2π **37.** $-\frac{128}{5}$ **39.** $-\frac{81}{10}$ **41.** -5.1 **43.** -2.9 **45.** -2.2 **47.** $-\frac{1}{2}$ **49.** $\frac{-9}{10}$

51. $-0.00234(-0.234\%)$ **53.** $-0.189 \frac{\text{sec}}{\text{year}}$ **55.** 10.5¢/year **57.** 330 million

Section 1.4

1. $y = 3x - 1$ **3.** $2 + h$

5. $f'(x) = 1$, $f'(0) = 1$, $f'(1) = 1$

7. $f'(x) = 2$, $f'(0) = 2$, $f'(1) = 2$

9. $f'(x) = 2x$, $f'(0) = 0$, $f'(1) = 2$

11. $f'(x) = 2x + 1$, $f'(0) = 1$, $f'(1) = 3$

13. $f'(x) = 14x + 5$, $f'(0) = 5$, $f'(1) = 19$

15. $f'(x) = -1/x^2$, $f'(0)$ undefined, $f'(1) = -1$

17. $f'(x) = -2/x^3$, $f'(0)$ undefined, $f'(1) = -2$

19. $f'(x) = \frac{1}{2\sqrt{x}} + 1$, $f'(0)$ undefined, $f'(1) = \frac{3}{2}$

21. $f'(x) = 2x$, $f'(2) = 4$, $y = 4x - 4$

23. $f'(1) = -\frac{2}{x^3}$, $y = -2x + 3$

25. $f'(0) = 0$ **27.** $f'(-1) = -2$ **29.** $\left.\frac{dy}{dx}\right|_{x=4} = 8$ **31.** $\left.\frac{dy}{dx}\right|_{x=16} = \frac{1}{8}$ **33.** $y = 3x + 5$ **35.** $y = 6x - 4$

37. **(a)** **39.** **(a)** **41.** **(a)**

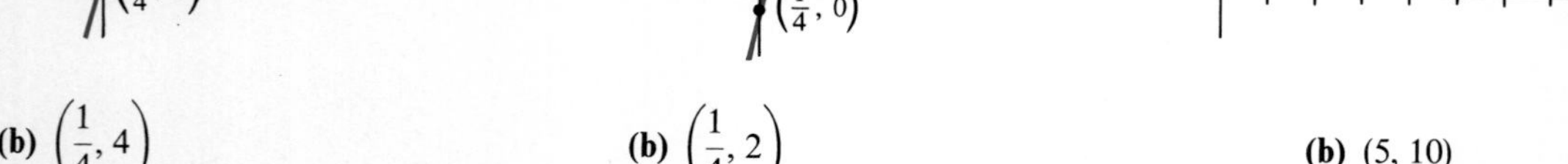

37. **(b)** $\left(\frac{1}{4}, 4\right)$
(c) (1, 3)
(d) $S'(p) = 4$, $D'(p) = -1$
$S'(0.5) = 4$, $D'(0.5) = -1$

39. **(b)** $\left(\frac{1}{4}, 2\right)$
(c) (1, 3)
(d) $S'(p) = 4$, $D'(p) = -2p$
$S'(1) = 4$, $D'(1) = -2$

41. **(b)** (5, 10)
(c) (8.10, 34.4)
(d) $S'(p) = 2p - 2$, $D'(p) = -2p$
$S'(7.5) = 13$, $D'(7.5) = -15$
For each dollar increase in price there will be an increase of 13 units supplied and a decrease of 15 units in demand.

43. **(a)** $D'(p) = -2p$
$E(p) = \frac{2p^2}{16 - p^2}$
(b) $E(2) = \frac{2}{3}$

45. $x = 0$ **47.** $x = 2$

Section 1.5

1. $f'(x) = 0$ **3.** $f'(x) = 2.5x^{1.5}$ **5.** $f'(x) = -2x^{-3}$ **7.** $f'(x) = \frac{3}{2}x^{1/2}$ **9.** $f'(x) = -3x^{-4}$ **11.** $f'(x) = 0$

13. $f'(x) = 0$ **15.** $f'(x) = 2$ **17.** $f'(x) = 2(x + 2)$ **19.** $f'(x) = 2ax + b$ **21.** $f'(x) = \frac{3}{2}x^{1/2}$ **23.** $f'(x) = 2x - \frac{1}{x^2}$

25. $f'(x) = -40x^{-5} + 6x + 2$

27. $s'(t) = 32t$
$s''(t) = 32$
$s''(1) = 32$
$s''(2) = 32$

29. $h'(t) = 12 - 32t$
$h'(1) = -20$
$h'(t) = 0$ if $t = \frac{3}{8}$

31. $M'(t) = 6t + \frac{1}{2}$
$M'(1) = \frac{13}{2}$
$M'(2) = \frac{25}{2}$

33. $p_1(t) = 100t - 20$
$p_1(4) = 380$
$p_1(6) = 580$

35. $p_1'(t) + p_2'(t) = 160t - 100$ **37.** $y = 3x + 3$

39. $s'(t) = 4t + 4$
$s'(10) = 44$
$s'(20) = 84$

41. **(a)** $P(q) = -0.01q^2 + 5q - 5000$ **(b)** $R'(q) = 10 - 0.02q$, $C'(q) = 5$, $P'(q) = -0.02q + 5$ **(c)** $P'(q) = 0$ if $q = 250$

43. $R(q) = \frac{q^2 + 10q}{4}$

45. $C'(q) = 6q - 3$
$C'(100) = 597$
The cost to produce the 101st unit is approximately \$597.

Section 1.6

1. $f'(x) = 4x^3 + 3x^2 + 6x$ **3.** $f'(x) = 4x^3$ **5.** $f'(t) = 4t^3$ **7.** $f'(u) = 4u^3 + 3u^2 + 1$ **9.** $f'(x) = -2x^{-3}$

11. $f'(x) = \frac{-15x^2}{(x^3 + 5)^2}$ **13.** $h'(x) = \frac{x^2 + 4x + 1}{(x + 2)^2}$ **15.** $f'(x) = \frac{2x(x + 1)^2 - 2}{(x + 1)^2}$ **17.** $y' = \frac{-2x^4 + 4x - 6}{(2x + 1)^2(x^2 + 3)^2}$

19. $y = -\frac{1}{2}x^{-3/2}$ **21.** $\frac{d}{dx}[f(x)g(x)h(x)] = f(x)g(x)h'(x) + f(x)g'(x)h(x) + f'(x)g(x)h(x)$

23. $R'(x) = P(x) + xP'(x)$
by the product rule

25. $C'(t) = -\frac{100{,}000}{(t + 2)^2}$
$C'(1) = -11{,}111$
$C'(2) = -6250$
$C'(3) = -4000$

27. $s'(t) = -\frac{100}{(t + 1)^2}$
$s'(1) = -25$
$s'(2) = -11\frac{1}{9}$
$s'(3) = -6\frac{1}{4}$

29. $R'(x) = 60 - 6x$

31. $C'(x) = \frac{50}{\sqrt{x}}$
$C'(100) = 5$

33. $AC(x) = \frac{100\sqrt{x} + 100{,}000}{x}$ **35.** $AC(10{,}000) = 11$ **37.** $\frac{d}{dx}\left[\frac{C(x)}{x}\right]\Bigg|_{x=100} = \frac{-50\sqrt{x} - 100{,}000}{x^2}\Bigg|_{x=100} = -10.05$

39. $\frac{d}{dr}R(r)\Big|_{r=0.2} = \frac{-kL}{0.00008}$ **41.** $y' = \frac{(x^2 + 3)^2(x^2 + 1) + 2x^2(x^2 + 3)^2 - 4x^2(x^2 + 1)(x^2 + 3)}{(x^2 + 3)^4}$

43. $W(t) = (0.5t^2 + t + 1000)(0.3t^2 + 2t + 1)$
$W'(t) = (t + 1)(0.3t^2 + 2t + 1) + (0.5t^2 + t + 1000)(0.6t + 2)$
$W'(1) = 2610.5$
$W'(2) = 3231.4$

45. Student project

Section 1.7

1. $f'(x) = 4(x^2 + 3x + 1)^3(2x + 3)$ **3.** $f'(x) = \frac{2x + 3}{2\sqrt{x^2 + 3x + 1}}$ **5.** $f'(x) = -\frac{3}{2}(2x + 1)(x^2 + x + 1)^{-5/2}$

7. $f'(x) = 3\left(x^2 + \frac{1}{x}\right)^2\left(2x - \frac{1}{x^2}\right)$ **9.** $f'(x) = 3[(x + 1)^2 + x]^2[2(x + 1) + 1]$ **11.** $f'(x) = -\frac{20x}{(x^2 + 1)^{11}}$

13. $f'(x) = \frac{(x+5)^4}{(x+4)^4}(2x+5)$ **15.** $g[f(x)] = 3(x^2+1)^3 - 4$ **17.** $\frac{d}{dx} g[f(x)] = 18x(x^2+1)^2$ **19.** $\frac{d}{dx} g[f(x)]\Big|_{x=1} = 72$

21. $y = 24x - 16$ **23.** $y = 81x - 54$ **25.** $y' = 10x(x^2+1)^4$ **27.** $y' = \frac{1}{\sqrt{2x+1}}$ **29.** $R'(q) = -4\left(2 - \frac{q}{500}\right)$

31. $N'(t) = \frac{25}{\sqrt{t+4}}$ **33.** $y' = \frac{1}{3}k(x-a)^{-2/3}$ **35.** $y' = \frac{7}{2}k(x-a)^{5/2}$

37. $\frac{dB}{dt} = 2\frac{dM}{dt}, \frac{dM}{dt} = 3\frac{dJ}{dt}$ then $\frac{dB}{dt} = 2\left(3\frac{dJ}{dt}\right) = 6\frac{dJ}{dt}$ **39.** $\frac{dy}{dx} = 24x(3x^2 - 7)$ **41.** $P'(q) = \frac{1200 - 3q^2}{2(1200q - q^3)^{1/2}}$

$P'(10) = \frac{450}{\sqrt{11{,}000}}$

$P'(20) = 0$

No profit in making more than 20 units

Chapter 1 Review

1. 4 **3.** $\sqrt{2} - 1$ **5.** $\frac{11}{24}$ **7.** 0 **9.** $\frac{1}{6}$ **11.** $2 - \frac{1}{x^2}$ **13.** $f'(x) = 18x(3x^2+4)^2$ **15.** $f'(t) = \frac{3}{2\sqrt{t}} - \frac{1}{2t^{3/2}}$

17. $f'(z) = \frac{1}{2}(z + \sqrt{z})^{-1/2}\left(1 + \frac{1}{2\sqrt{z}}\right)$ **19.** $f'(r) = 8r$ **21.** $y' = 0$ **23.** $g'(x) = t^{-1/2} - \frac{1}{2}t^{-3/2}$ **25.** $h'(t) = 0$

27. $h'(t) = 4t^3$ **29.** $f'(t) = -\frac{1}{4}t^{-5/4}$ **31.** $y' = \frac{1}{2} - \frac{2}{x^2}$ **33.** $h'(z) = \frac{-5(5z^2-1)}{(5z^2+1)^2}$ **35.** $f'(t) = \frac{3t-1}{2\sqrt{t-2}}$

37. $y' = 15x^2 + 26x - 9$ **39.** $y' = -\frac{1}{3}y^{-4/3}$ **41.** $f'(t) = 6t, f'(2) = 12$ **43.** 0 **45.** 1.5 **47.** 5 **49.** $-\frac{2}{9}$

51. $32t$ **53.** $12(2t+1)$ **55.** $\frac{1}{4}$ **57.** $2x[(x^2-1)(x^2+1) + (x^2+1)(x^2+2) + (x^2+1)(x^2-1)]$ **59.** $y = -\frac{3}{2}x + 4$

61. $x = 1, -1$ **63.** Use the product rule to differentiate.

$S(t) = \pi\left(3t + \frac{1}{t}\right)^2(2t^2 + 3t - 1)$

$S'(1) = 176\pi$

65. $R'(x) = 9$ **67.** $P(x) = -x^2 + 8x - 5$
$P'(x) = -2x + 8$
$P'(x) = 0$, if $x = 4$

69. $P'(x) = -0.72x + 7.20$

Chapter 1 Test

1. 0 **2.** $\frac{-1}{(x-3)^2}$ **3.** $\frac{1}{4\sqrt{x}\sqrt{x^{1/2}+1}}$ **4.** $15x^2 - 2x + 5$ **5.** $f'(x) = \frac{4}{3}x^{1/3} + \frac{3}{4}x^{-1/4}$ **6.** $s'(t) = -4 - 10t$
$s'(1) = -14$
$s'(2) = -24$

7. Does not exist **8. (a)** Yes **(b)** Yes **(c)** No

9. $B'(d) = 0.015(d-6)^2$; you can monitor the growth rate.
$B'(16) = 15$ board ft/inch

10. (a) 30 ft/sec
(b) -34 ft/sec
(c) $\frac{15}{8}$ sec
(d) -30 ft/sec

11. 10; the cost is growing as fast as the revenue.

CHAPTER 2

Section 2.1

1. (a, b), (c, d), (e, f), (g, h), (i, j) **3.** $b, c, d, e, f, g, h, i, j$ **5.** b, c, d, e, f, h

7.

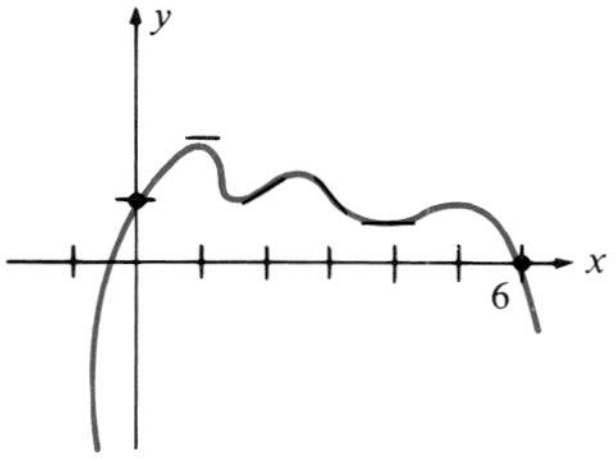

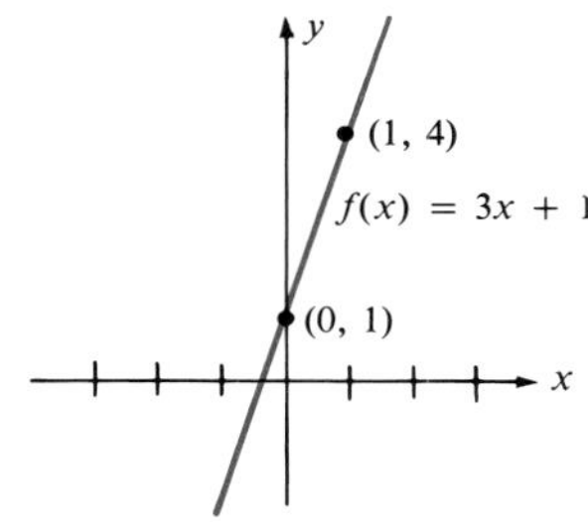

9.

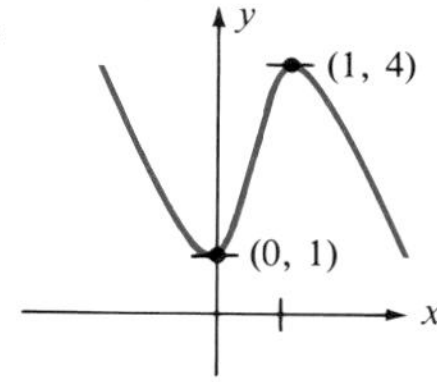

11. **(a)** + **(b)** − **(c)** + **(d)** 0

13. f has no critical or stationary points
f is increasing on $(-\infty, \infty)$

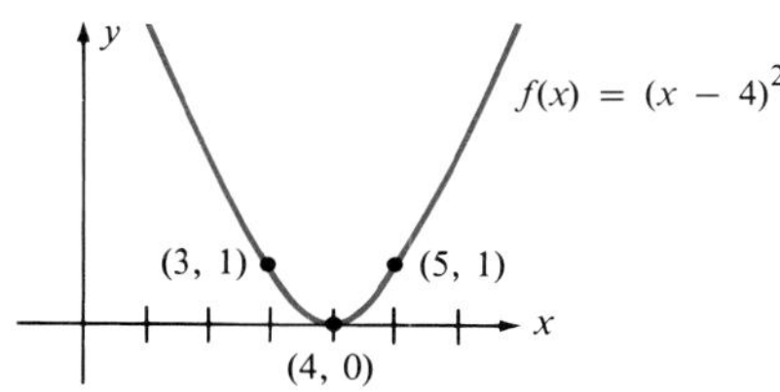

15. f has a critical and stationary point at 0
f is decreasing on $(-\infty, 0)$
f is increasing on $(0, \infty)$

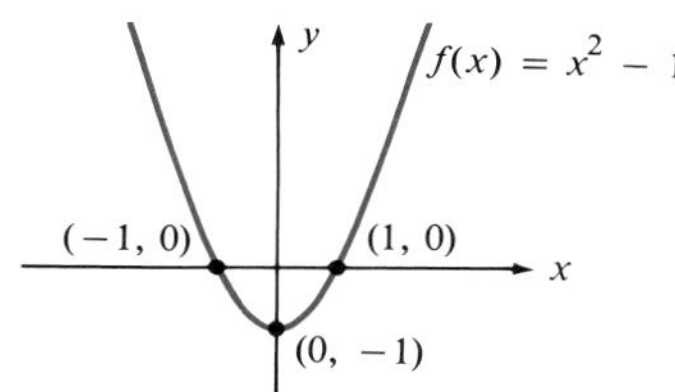

17. f has a critical and stationary point at 4
f is decreasing on $(-\infty, 4)$
f is increasing on $(4, \infty)$

19. f has a critical and stationary point at 0
f is increasing on $(-\infty, 0)$ and $(0, \infty)$

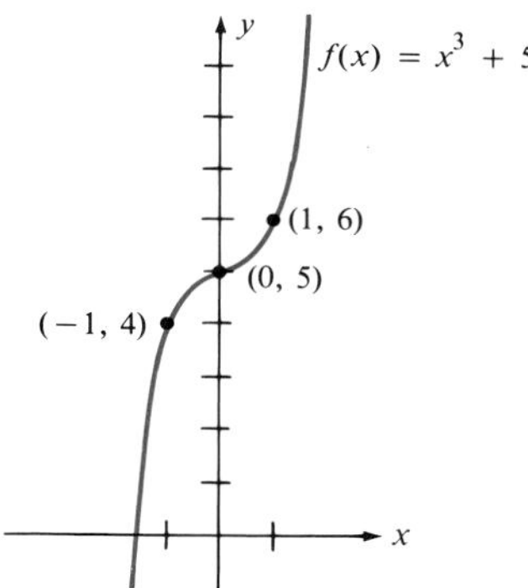

21. f has a critical and stationary point at 3
f is increasing on $(-\infty, 3)$ and $(3, \infty)$

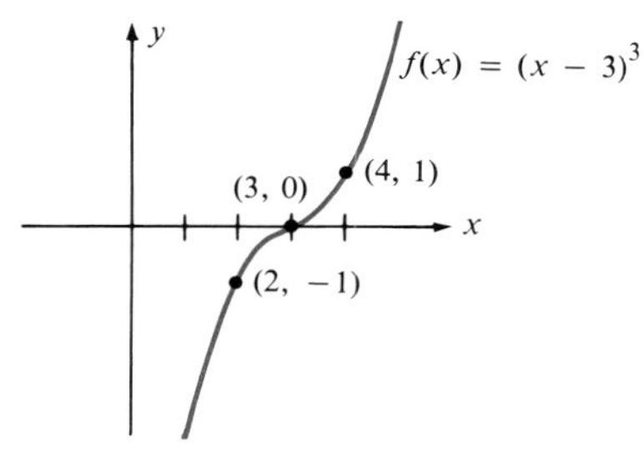

23. 0 is a critical point, $2^{1/3}$ is a critical and stationary point
f is increasing on $(-\infty, 0)$ and $(2^{1/3}, \infty)$
f is decreasing on $(0, 2^{1/3})$

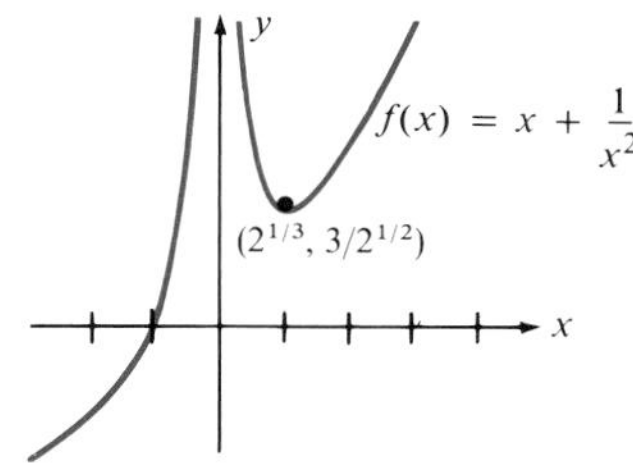

25. 0 is a critical and stationary point
f is decreasing on $(-\infty, 0)$
f is increasing on $(0, \infty)$

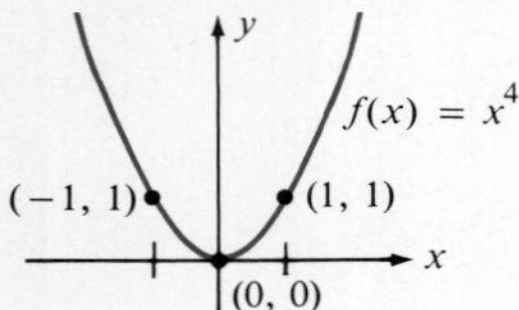

27. -2 is a critical and stationary point
f is decreasing on $(-\infty, -2)$
f is increasing on $(-2, \infty)$

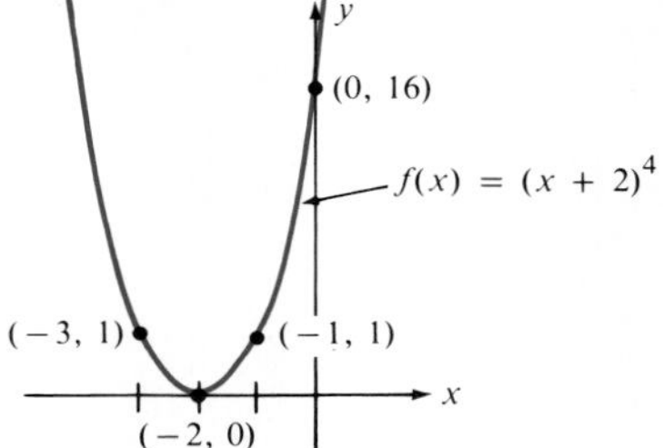

29. 0 is a critical point
f is increasing on $(0, \infty)$

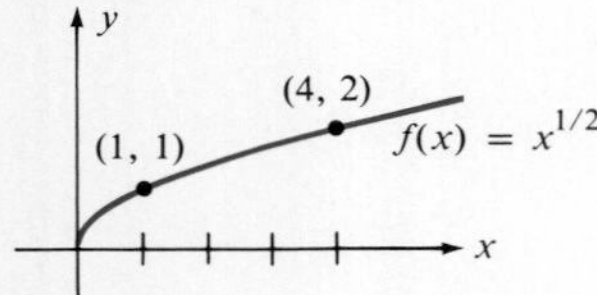

31. 0 is a critical point
f is increasing on $(-\infty, \infty)$

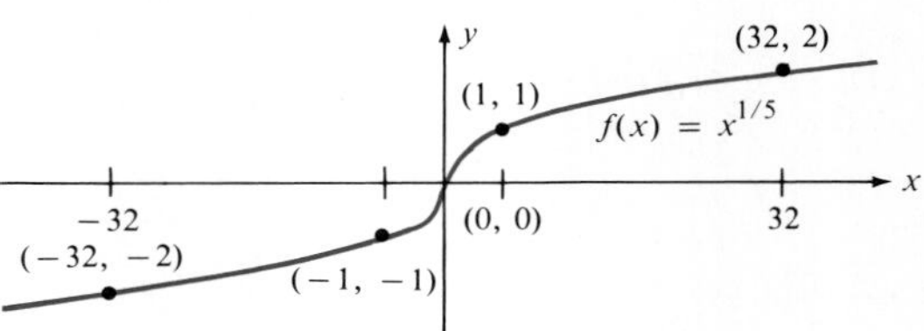

33. 4 is a critical point
f is decreasing on $(-\infty, 4)$
f is increasing on $(4, \infty)$

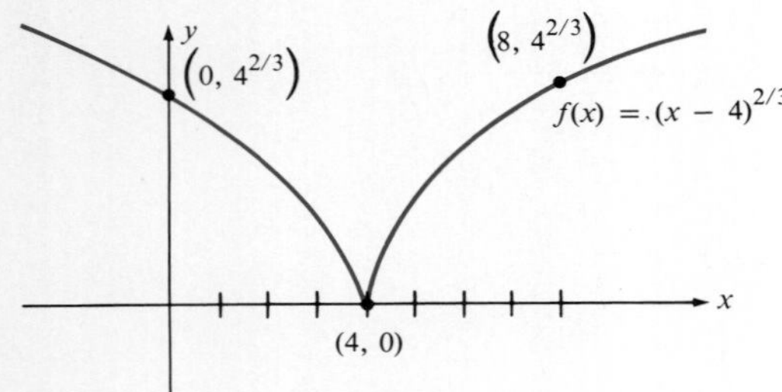

35. 0 is a critical point
f is increasing on $(-\infty, 0)$
f is decreasing on $(0, \infty)$

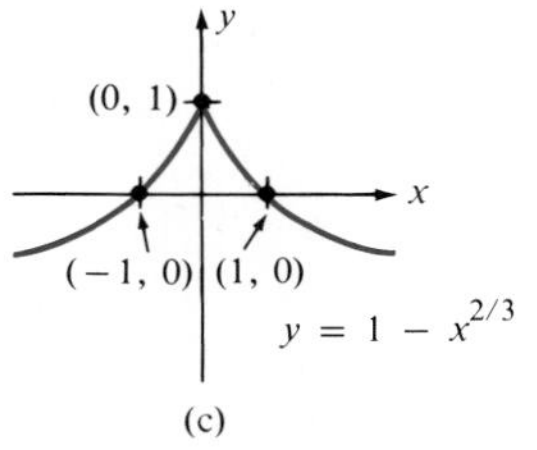

37. Increasing: $(0, \infty)$
Decreasing: $(-\infty, 0)$
Critical points: $x = 0$
Stationary points: $x = 0$

39. Increasing: $(-\infty, -1)$, $(-1, 0)$
Decreasing: $(0, 1)$, $(1, \infty)$
Critical points: $x = -1, 0, 1$
Stationary points: $x = 0$

41. Increasing: $(-\infty, -1)$, $(3, \infty)$
Decreasing: $(-1, 3)$
Critical points: $x = -1, 3$
Stationary points: $x = -1, 3$

43. The slope is positive from $x = -4$ to $x = 0$. At $x = 0$ the slope is 0. From $x = 0$ to $x = 4$ the slope is negative. The slope decreases from $x = -4$ to $x = 4$.

45. The slope is positive for all x different from zero. The slope increases from $x = -\infty$ to $x = 0$ and decreases from $x = 0$ to $x = \infty$.

47. $R(p) = p(9 - p^2)$ **49.** $P(q) = q\sqrt{36 - q} - 5 - 0.5q$

51. $R'(q) = \sqrt{64 - q} - \dfrac{q}{2\sqrt{64 - q}}$

$P'(q) = \sqrt{64 - q} - \dfrac{q}{2\sqrt{64 - q}} - 0.5 - 0.002q$

Section 2.2

1. $f''(x) = 6x + 2$
$f''(0) = 2$
$f''(1) = 8$
$f''(2) = 14$

3. $f''(x) = 2a$
$f''(0) = 2a$
$f''(1) = 2a$
$f''(2) = 2a$

5. $f''(x) = -\frac{1}{4}x^{-3/2}$
$f''(0)$ undefined
$f''(1) = -\frac{1}{4}$
$f''(2) = -\frac{1}{4}(2)^{-3/2}$

7. $f''(x) = \frac{4}{(x-1)^3}$
$f''(0) = -4$
$f''(1)$ undefined, since $f(1)$ is undefined
$f''(2) = 4$

9. $f''(x) = 2$
$f''(0) = 2$
$f''(1) = 2$
$f''(2) = 2$

11. $f''(x) = 6x + 4$
$f''(0) = 4$
$f''(1) = 10$
$f''(2) = 16$

13. $f''(x) = 18x + 8$
$f'''(x) = 18$
$f^{(4)} = 0$

15. $f''(x) = n(n-1)x^{n-2}$
$f'''(x) = n(n-1)(n-2)x^{n-3}$
$f^{(4)}(x) = n(n-1)(n-2)(n-3)x^{n-4}$

17. $f''(x) = 12x^{-5} - \frac{1}{4}x^{-3/2}$
$f'''(x) = -60x^{-6} + \frac{3}{8}x^{-5/2}$
$f^{(4)}(x) = 360x^{-7} - \frac{15}{16}x^{-7/2}$

19. $f'(x) = 2x$
$f''(x) = 2$
(a) Critical points: 0
(b) Stationary points: 0
(c) Increasing: $(0, \infty)$
(d) Decreasing: $(-\infty, 0)$
(e) Inflection points: none
(f) Concave up: $(-\infty, \infty)$
(g) Concave down: never

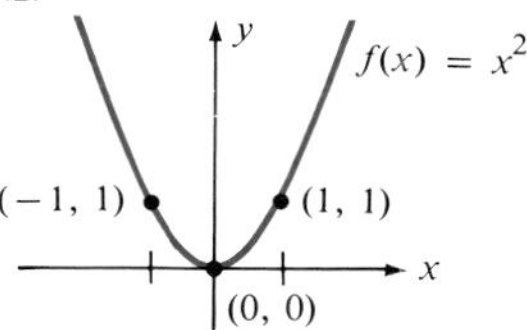

21. $f'(x) = 2x - 4$
$f''(x) = 2$
(a) Critical points: 2
(b) Stationary points: 2
(c) Increasing: $(2, \infty)$
(d) Decreasing: $(-\infty, 2)$
(e) Inflection points: none
(f) Concave up: $(-\infty, \infty)$
(g) Concave down: never

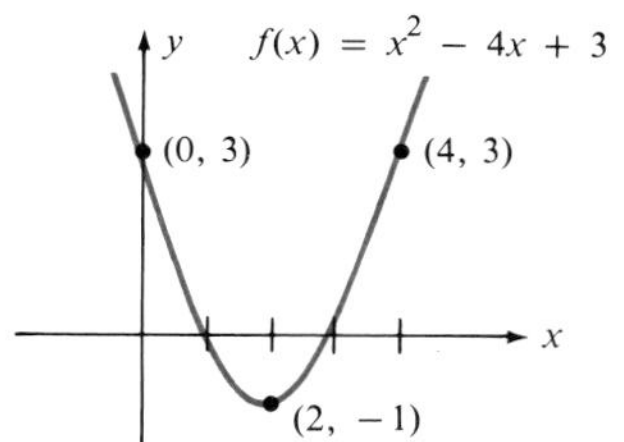

23. $f'(x) = 3x^2$
$f''(x) = 6x$
(a) Critical points: 0
(b) Stationary points: 0
(c) Increasing: $(-\infty, 0)$, $(0, \infty)$
(d) Decreasing: never
(e) Inflection points: 0
(f) Concave up: $(0, \infty)$
(g) Concave down: $(-\infty, 0)$

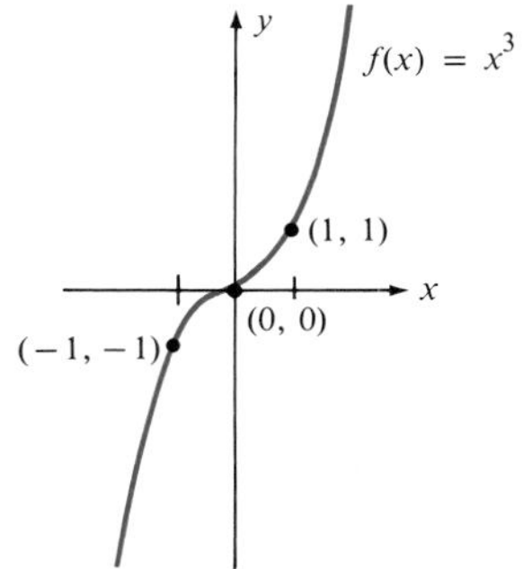

25. $f'(x) = 3x^2 - 1$
$f''(x) = 6x$
(a) Critical points: $\pm\sqrt{1/3}$
(b) Stationary points: $\pm\sqrt{1/3}$
(c) Increasing: $(-\infty, -\sqrt{1/3})$, $(\sqrt{1/3}, \infty)$
(d) Decreasing: $(-\sqrt{1/3}, \sqrt{1/3})$
(e) Inflection points: 0
(f) Concave up: $(0, \infty)$
(g) Concave down: $(-\infty, 0)$

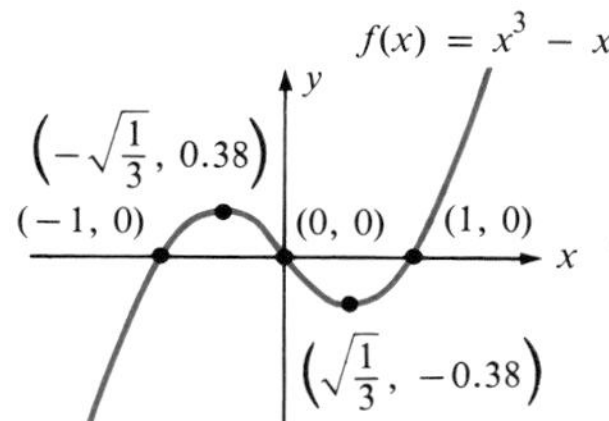

27. $f'(x) = 1 - \dfrac{2}{x^3}$

$f''(x) = \dfrac{6}{x^4}$

(a) Critical points: 0, $2^{1/3}$
(b) Stationary points: $2^{1/3}$
(c) Increasing: $(-\infty, 0)$, $(2^{1/3}, \infty)$
(d) Decreasing: $(0, 2^{1/3})$
(e) Inflection points: none
(f) Concave up: $(-\infty, 0)$, $(0, \infty)$
(g) Concave down: never

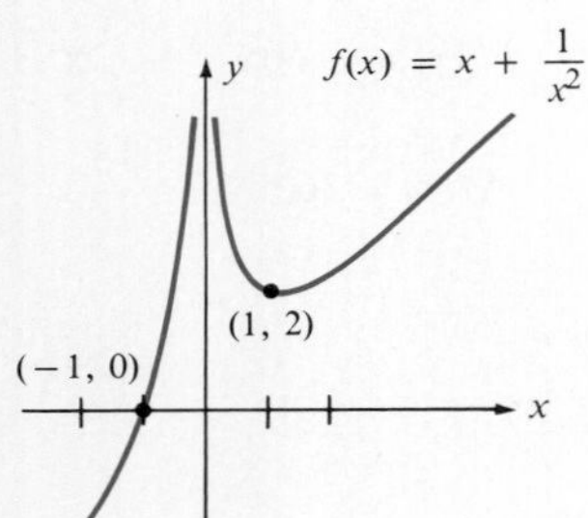

29. $f'(x) = 3(x - 2)^2$
$f''(x) = 6(x - 2)$
(a) Critical points: 2
(b) Stationary points: 2
(c) Increasing: $(-\infty, \infty)$
(d) Decreasing: never
(e) Inflection points: 2
(f) Concave up: $(2, \infty)$
(g) Concave down: $(-\infty, 2)$

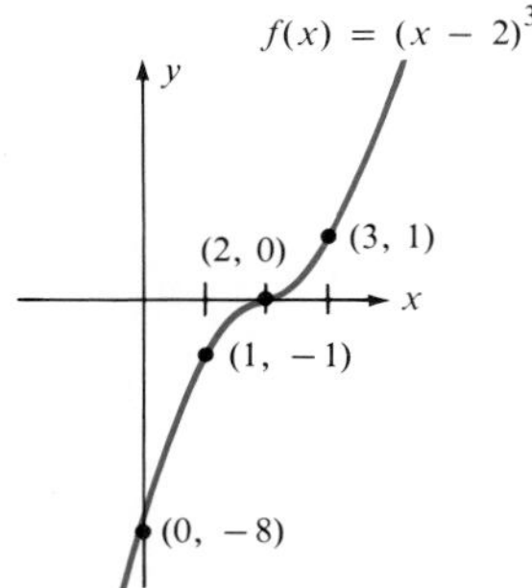

31. $f'(x) = 4(x + 2)^3$
$f''(x) = 12(x + 2)^2$
(a) Critical points: -2
(b) Stationary points: -2
(c) Increasing: $(-2, \infty)$
(d) Decreasing: $(-\infty, -2)$
(e) Inflection points: none
(f) Concave up: $(-\infty, \infty)$
(g) Concave down: never

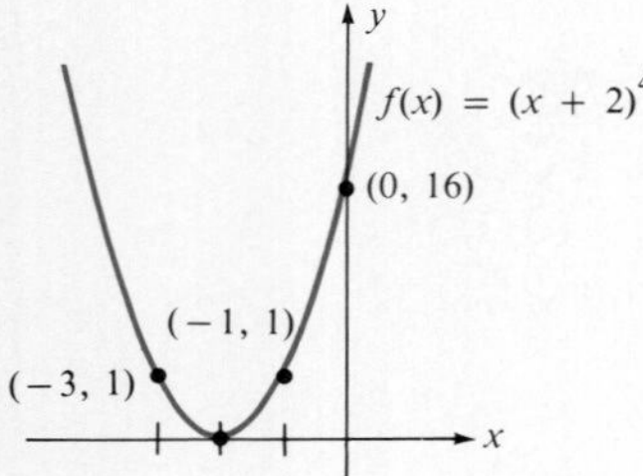

33. $f'(x) = \dfrac{1}{5} x^{-4/5}$

$f''(x) = -\dfrac{4}{25} x^{-9/5}$

(a) Critical points: 0
(b) Stationary points: none
(c) Increasing: $(-\infty, 0)$, $(0, \infty)$
(d) Decreasing: never
(e) Inflection points: 0
(f) Concave up: $(-\infty, 0)$
(g) Concave down: $(0, \infty)$

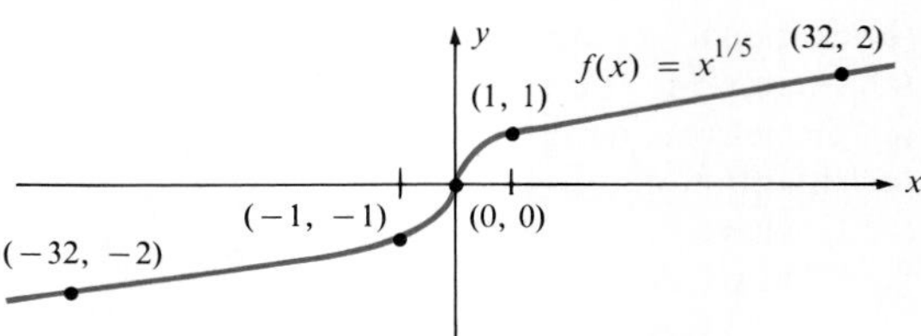

35. Concave down: $(-\infty, 1)$
Inflection point: none

37. Concave up: $(0, \infty)$
Concave down: $(-\infty, 0)$
Inflection point: 0

39. Concave up: $(1, \infty)$
Concave down: $(-\infty, 1)$
Inflection point: 1

41. Plus infinity: 3
Minus infinity: 3
Horizontal asymptote: $y = 3$

43. Plus infinity: 3
Minus infinity: 3
Horizontal asymptote: $y = 3$

45. Plus infinity: 0
Minus infinity: 0
Horizontal asymptote: $y = 0$

47. Plus infinity: 9
Minus infinity: 9
Horizontal asymptote: $y = 9$

49. Plus infinity: ∞
Minus infinity: $-\infty$
No horizontal asymptote

51. Vertical asymptote: $x = -1$
Horizontal asymptote: $y = 0$

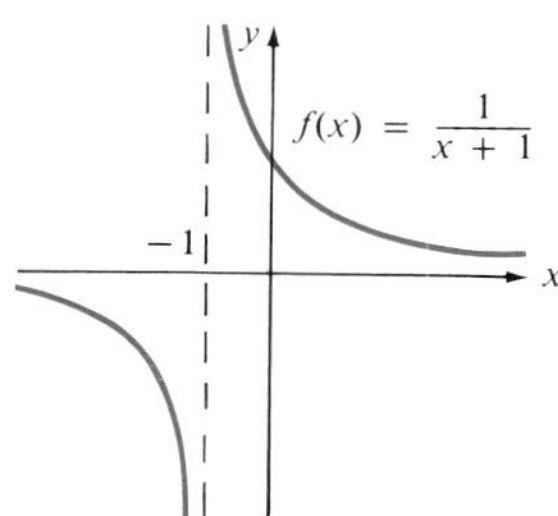

53. Vertical asymptote: $x = -1$
Horizontal asymptote: $y = 1$

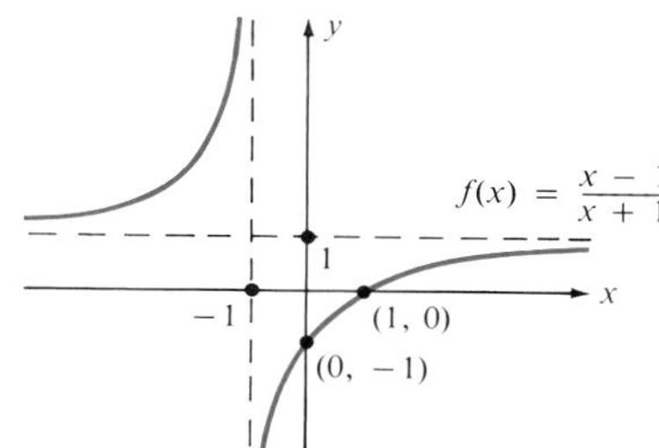

55. Vertical asymptote: $x = 1, -1$
Horizontal asymptote: $y = 0$

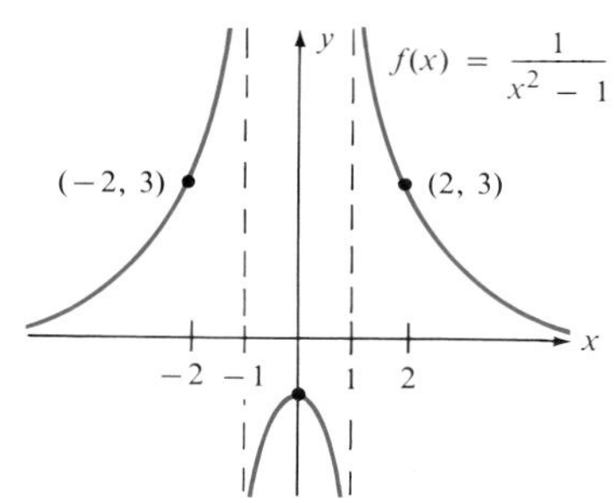

57. Vertical asymptote: $x = 2$
Horizontal asymptote: $y = 1$

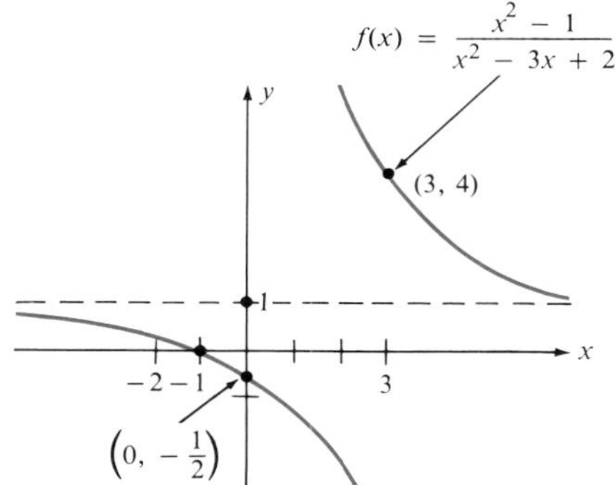

59. Vertical asymptote: $x = 1, 2, 3$
Horizontal asymptote: $y = 0$

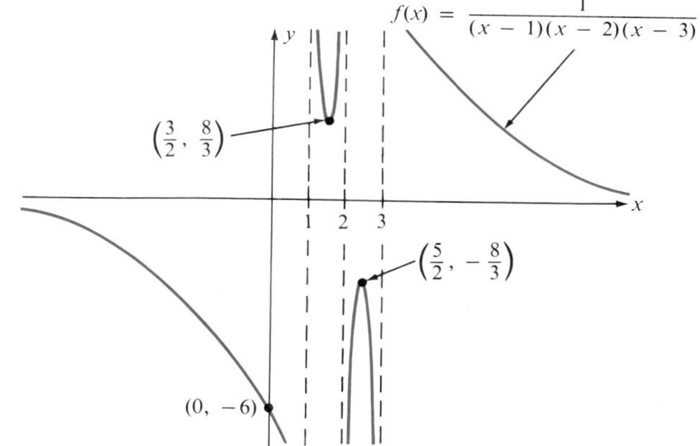

Section 2.3

1. $(a, b), (c, d), (e, f), (g, h)$ **3.** g, i **5.** c, e, g **7.** e **9.** i **11.**

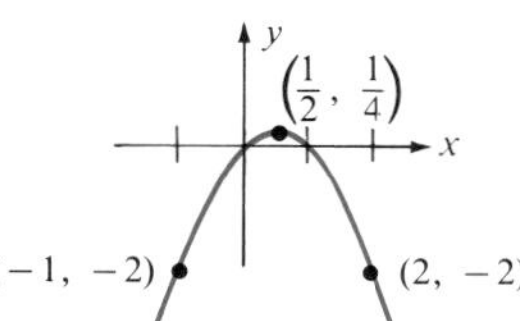

13.

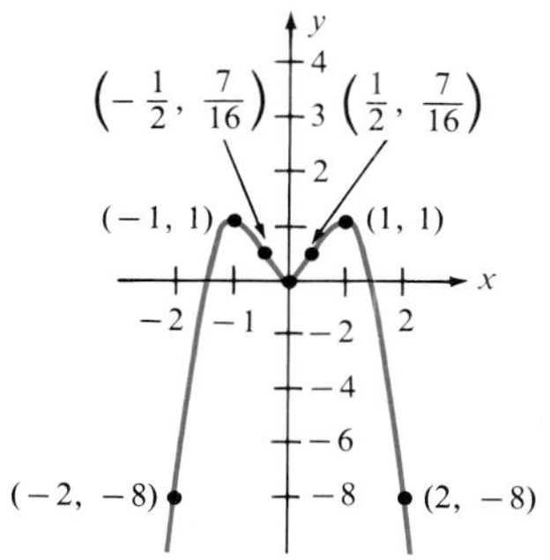

15. No relative max or min points

17. Relative minimum: $x = \frac{1}{2}$

19. Relative maximum: $-\sqrt{\frac{1}{3}}$

Relative minimum: $\sqrt{\frac{1}{3}}$

21. Relative minimum: $x = 12$

23. Relative maximum: $x = -2$

Relative minimum: $x = \frac{1}{2}$

25. First derivative test does not apply at $x = 0$; however, $x = 0$ is a relative minimum

27. No relative maximum or minimum

29. Relative minimum at $x = 0$

31. Second derivative test does not apply, since $f'(x)$ is never zero.

33. Critical point $x = 0$ is a relative minimum

35. Critical point $x = 1$ is a relative minimum

37. Critical point $x = 1$ (relative minimum)
Critical point $x = -2$ (relative minimum)
Critical point $x = -1$ (relative maximum)

39. Critical point $x = \sqrt{2}$ (relative maximum)
Critical point $x = -\sqrt{2}$ (relative minimum)

41. Critical point $x = 0$ (second derivative does not apply)
Critical point $x = 1$ (relative maximum)

43. Critical point $x = 3$ (relative minimum)

45. Absolute maximum: $x = 2$
Absolute minimum: $x = -1$

47. Absolute maximum: $x = 2$
Absolute minimum: $x = 5$

49. Absolute maximum: $x = 0$
Absolute minimum: $x = 3$

51. Absolute maximum: $x = 1$
Absolute minimum: $x = -\frac{1}{2}$

53. Absolute maximum: $x = 4$
Absolute minimum: $x = 2$

55. Absolute maximum: $x = 2$
Absolute minimum: $x = 3$

57. Absolute maximum: $x = -1, 1$
Absolute minimum: $x = 0$

59. **(a)** 79 (approximately) **(b)** Evaluate the cost at the nearest integer values.

61. 6

63. Maximum at $q = \frac{98}{3}$
Maximum profit = \$17,179.98

65. Maximum profit $= \frac{25}{8}$, $q = \frac{5}{4}$

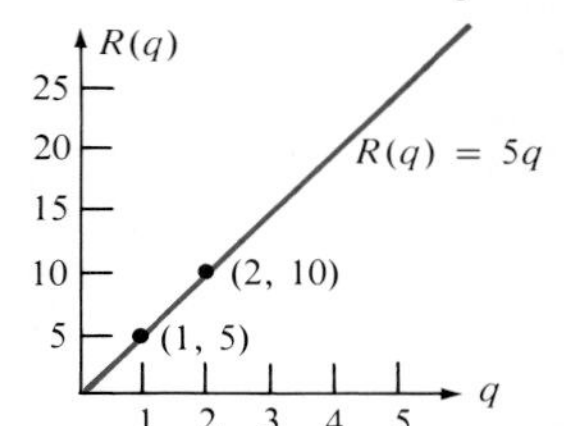

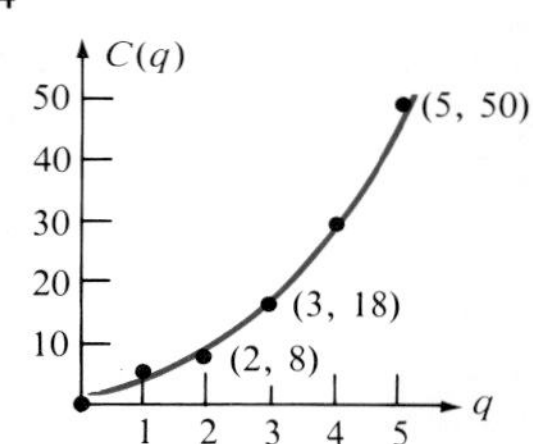

67. The function has no maximum on the open interval (0, 1).

69. Student project

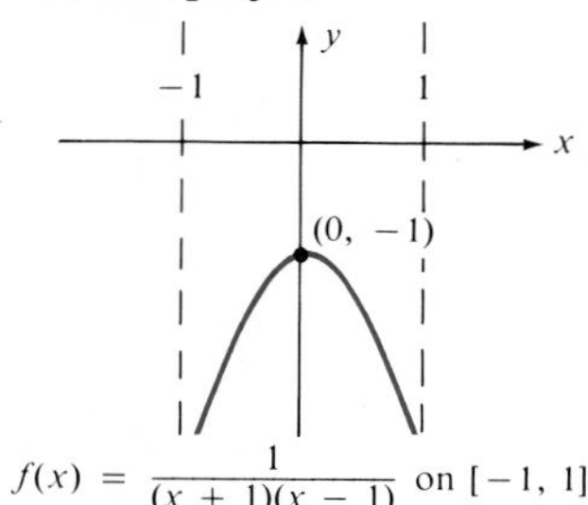

$f(x) = \frac{1}{(x+1)(x-1)}$ on $[-1, 1]$

71. **(a)** $t = \frac{3}{2}$ sec
(b) 76 ft
(c) -32 ft/sec²
(d) 3.68 sec
(e) -165.7 ft/sec

73. **(a)** 16.25 mph
(b) 9.3 cars/sec

Section 2.4

1. $x = y = 7.5$ **3.** $x = 25$, $y = 50$ **5.** 70.7 **7.** \$50 **9.** \$1250 **11.** \$1750 **13.** 25 trees

15. 10 by 10 by 10 feet **17.** 10 by 10 by 20 feet **19.** 1.79 by 3.79 by 0.607
$V(0.607) = 4.104$

21. $x = \dfrac{25}{4+\pi} \cong 3.5$ inches, $4x \cong 14$ inches
$r = \dfrac{25}{8+2\pi} \cong 1.75$ inches, $2\pi r \cong 11$ inches

23. $x = \sqrt{120}$ inches (10.9 inches)
$y = 7.3$ inches
(page is 11.3×16.95 inches)

25. 18 square inches

27. $x = \dfrac{14}{\sqrt{5}}$ (x as given in figure) **29.** \$7.50 **31.** 500 by 1000 feet **33.** $t = 5\sqrt{2}$ weeks
Maximum size $= 250\sqrt{2} \cong 353.6$

Section 2.5

1. $\dfrac{dy}{dx} = 2x$ **3.** $\dfrac{dy}{dx} = -\dfrac{2y}{x}$ **5.** $\dfrac{dy}{dx} = -\dfrac{1+y}{x}$ **7.** $\dfrac{dy}{dx} = \dfrac{1-y-3x^2}{x}$ **9.** $\dfrac{dy}{dx} = \dfrac{1-y}{x+2y}$ **11.** $\dfrac{dy}{dx} = -\dfrac{9x}{16y}$

13. $\dfrac{dy}{dx} = \dfrac{x-y}{x+y}$ **15.** $\dfrac{dy}{dx} = \dfrac{-x}{y(x^2-1)^2}$ **17.** $\dfrac{dy}{dx} = \dfrac{3x^2+4x-2xy-y^2}{2xy+x^2}$ **19.** $\dfrac{dy}{dx} = \dfrac{-2xy}{x^2+1}, 0$ **21.** $\dfrac{dy}{dx} = \dfrac{-2y}{x}, -2$

23. $\dfrac{dy}{dx} = \dfrac{2x-3y}{3x}, \dfrac{7}{6}$ **25.** $\dfrac{dy}{dx} = -\dfrac{\sqrt{y}(\sqrt{y}+1)}{\sqrt{x}(\sqrt{x}+1)}, -3$ **27.** $y = -2x+3$ **29.** $y = x-2$ **31.** $y = 3$

33. $y = -3x+5$ **35.** $y = \dfrac{2x}{\sqrt{3}} - \dfrac{1}{\sqrt{3}}$ **37.** $\dfrac{dy}{dt} = 4$ **39.** $\dfrac{1}{\pi} \cong 0.32 \dfrac{\text{inch}}{\text{sec}}$ **41.** $\dfrac{50\pi}{3} \cong 52.4 \dfrac{\text{cubic feet}}{\text{min}}$ **43.** 4.2 ft/sec

Section 2.6

1. $dy = 0$ **3.** $dy = 0.02$ **5.** $dy = -0.1$ **7.** $dy = -0.09$ **9.** $dy = 0.0375$ **11.** 0.3 million **13.** 1.96%
15. 0.04 **17.** 0.03 **19.** 0.06 **21.** 1.29 **23.** 0 **25.** 2500.7 **27.** 0.55 **29.** 0.91

31. Profit = \$2000
Relative error = 0.01

33. Revenue = \$100,000
Relative error = 0.075

35. Actual change: $I(r_0 + dr) - I(r_0)$
Approximate change: $dI = 2cr_0\,dr$

37. $\dfrac{-2x}{k_2 - x}\%$

Chapter 2 Review

1. $x = -\dfrac{2}{3}$ (relative max)
$x = 2$ (relative min)

3. $x = \sqrt{2}$ (relative max)
$x = -\sqrt{2}$ (relative min)

5. $x = \dfrac{1}{2}$ (relative min)

7. $x = 1$ (relative max)
$x = 3$ (relative min)

9. $x = -2$ (relative min)
$x = 2$ (relative max)

11. $x = 3$ (relative min)
$x = -1$ (relative max)

13. $x = 1$ (stationary point);
second derivative test inconclusive.

15. $x = 0$ (stationary point);
second derivative test inconclusive.

17. No critical points **19.** $x = 0$ (relative max)

21. Absolute max: $f(0) = 12$
Absolute min: $f(3) = -69$

23. Absolute max: $f(4) = 16$
Absolute min; $f(2) = 0$

25. Absolute max: $f(1) = 23$
Absolute min: $f(0) = 0$

27. Absolute max: $f(4) = \sqrt{3}$
Absolute min: $f(1) = 0$

29. Absolute max: $f(1) = 1$
Absolute min: $f(0) = 0$

31. $\dfrac{dy}{dx} = -\dfrac{x}{y}$ **33.** $\dfrac{dy}{dx} = -2\dfrac{y}{x}$ **35.** $\dfrac{dy}{dx} = 1$

37. 0.95 **39.** 10.00333 **41.** 1.009 **43.** 0.01001 **45.** $\dfrac{dA}{dt} = 2\pi r \dfrac{dr}{dt}$ **47.** Shadow is shortening by $\dfrac{28}{3} \dfrac{\text{ft}}{\text{sec}}$

49. Produce 450 items; maximum profit = \$20,210 **51.** $4 \dfrac{\text{ft}}{\text{sec}}$ **53.** $\dfrac{dV}{d\tau} = \dfrac{r}{2} \dfrac{dS}{d\tau}$

55. 35 trees/acre, yielding $12{,}250 \dfrac{\text{bushels}}{\text{acre}}$ **57.** $x = \dfrac{-b}{3a}$ **59.** 0.3 **61.** $x = y = 5$

Chapter 2 Test

1. Increasing: $\left(\dfrac{1}{2}, \infty\right)$,
Decreasing: $\left(-\infty, \dfrac{1}{2}\right)$

2. $x = \dfrac{1}{2}$ **3.** $x = \dfrac{1}{2}$ **4.** Relative min: $x = \dfrac{1}{2}$ **5.** No inflection points

6. Concave up: $(-\infty, \infty)$ **7.** Absolute max: $x = 5$ **8.** $\dfrac{dy}{dx} = \dfrac{-2y^{3/2}}{2xy^{1/2} + 1}$ **9.** $\dfrac{dy}{dx} = 3x^2 \dfrac{dx}{dt}$ **10.** 50 and 50

11. 0.10 **12.** Length = 28 in., radius = $\dfrac{28}{\pi}$ in., volume = $\dfrac{21{,}952}{\pi}$ in.^{3}

13. Decreasing by 33 cases per day

CHAPTER 3

Section 3.1

1. 1, 3, 9, 27, 81, 243 **3.** $\frac{1}{2}$, 2, 8, 32, 128, 512 **5.** 2, 6, 18, 54, 162, 486 **7.** 1, 0.1, 0.01, 0.001, 0.0001, 0.00001

9. 3, −9, 27, −81, 243, −729 **11.** Almost, $\dfrac{226}{199} = 1.13$, $\dfrac{252}{226} = 1.11$ **13.** 1990: 283.61 million
2000: 319.17 million

15.

(−2, 4) (−1, 2) (0, 1) $\left(1, \frac{1}{2}\right)$ $\left(2, \frac{1}{4}\right)$ y x

17.

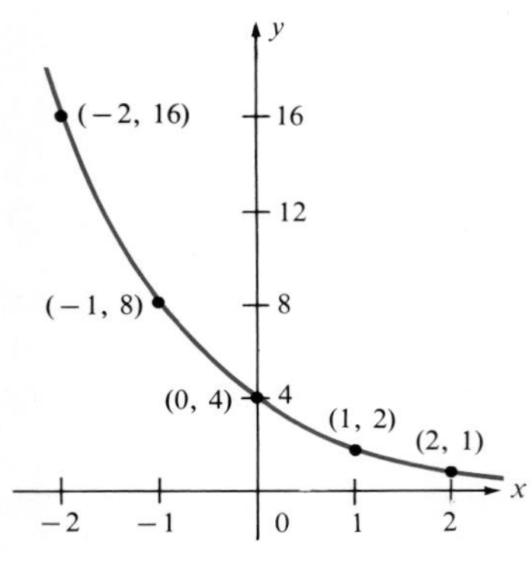

19.

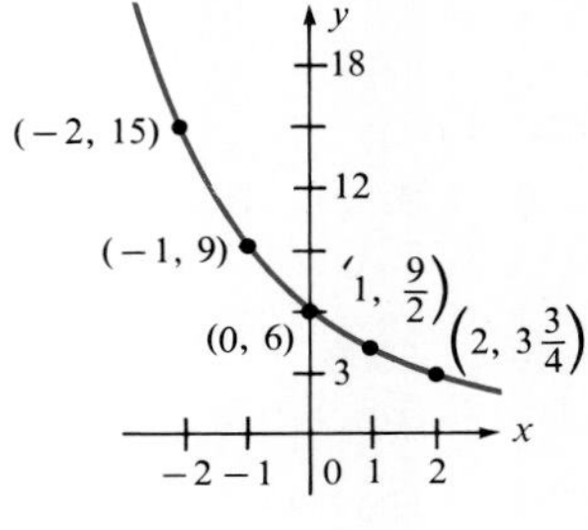

21. −1 **23.** 1 **25.** 0, $\frac{5}{3}$ **27.** −1, 2 **29.** $y_n = 3662(1.035)^n$ **31.** Japan: \$2337 billion
United States: \$5928 billion

33. Six months: \$105
One year: \$110.25
18 months: \$115.76
Two years: \$121.55

35. 4.95, 4.90, 4.85, 4.80, 4.75 billion **37.** $G(t) = 500(0.8)^t$ **39.** $V(t) = 20(0.9)^t = 20e^{-0.105t}$
$V(60) = 3.6 \times 10^{-2}$ mile/hr

41. $E(1) = 511.7$
$E(2) = 523.6$
$E(3) = 535.9$
$E(4) = 548.4$
$E(10) = 630.0$

43. $P(1) = 800$
$P(2) = 1600$
$P(4) = 6400$
$P(10) = 409{,}600$
$P(2) = 4.19 \times 10^8$

45. $P(t) = \$500e^{0.09t}$
$P(1) = \$547.09$
$P(1.5) = \$572.27$

47. $P(t) = \$10e^{0.05t}$
$P(75) = \$425.21$

49. Week 1: 9.5 units
Week 2: 18.1 units
Week 3: 25.9 units
Week 4: 33.0 units
Week 5: 39.3 units

51. Present: 1 g
1000 years: 0.84 g
2000 years: 0.71 g
4000 years: 0.50 g
800 years: 0.25 g

53. $y(-1) = 1.54$
$y(-0.5) = 1.13$
$y(0) = 1$
$y(0.5) = 1.13$
$y(1) = 1.54$

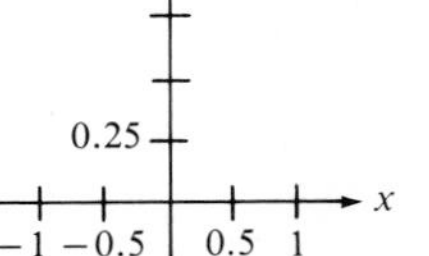

55. After 25 years: $500(250)^{24}$ (huge)

Section 3.2

1. 1.55 **3.** 0.19 **5.** −0.7 **7.** 7.05 **9.** 2.1 **11.** 4.075 **13.** 1.00 **15.** $\frac{3}{4}$ **17.** 9 **19.** $3 \log e - \log a$

21. $2^3 \cdot 3^2$ **23.** 2^{14} **25.** −1 **27.** 3 **29.** $\frac{3}{2}$ **31.** $\frac{4}{3}$ **33.** $\frac{\log 2}{2 - \log 2} \cong 0.17$ **35.** $\frac{-\log 6}{3 \log 5 - \log 6} \cong -0.59$

37. 6.94 years **39.** 6.60 years **41.** Double: 4.6 years
Triple: 7.3 years **43.** 9.78% **45.** Decrease an average of 0.26% per year

47. Increased an average of 7.73% per year **49.** Increased an average of 7.82% per year

51. Increased an average of 6.75% per year **53.** Student project

55. (a)

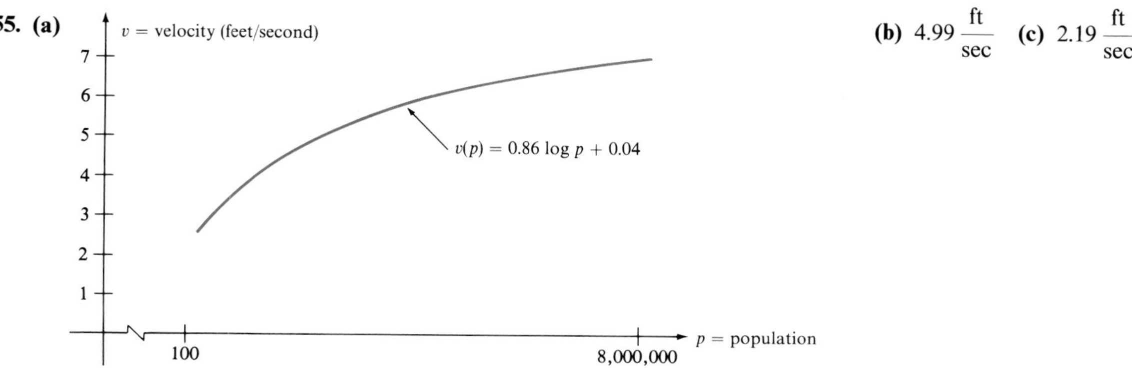

(b) $4.99 \frac{\text{ft}}{\text{sec}}$ **(c)** $2.19 \frac{\text{ft}}{\text{sec}}$

57. 1.58 hours **59.** 12.88 days **61.** 3960 units **63. (a)** 5.38 acid
(b) 5.10 acid
(c) 7.22 base
(d) 3.20 acid
65. $10^{4.5} \cong 31{,}623$ **67.** 30 decibels

Section 3.3

1. $e^{x \ln 2}$ **3.** $e^{x \ln 4}$ **5.** $e^{x \ln 1.5}$ **7.** $e^{x \ln 0.9}$ **9.** $e^{x \ln 100}$ **11.** $y' = 6e^{3x}$ **13.** $y' = 5e^{5x}$ **15.** $y' = 2xe^{x^2}$

17. $y' = \frac{e^{\sqrt{x}}}{2\sqrt{x}}$ **19.** $y' = \frac{xe^x - e^x}{x^2}$ **21.** $y' = (2x + 1)e^{x^2 + x}$ **23.** $y' = e^x - e^{-x}$ **25.** $y' = 2 - 4e^{4x} + 6xe^{x^2}$

27. $y' = (\ln 5)\, 5^x$ **29.** $y' = (\ln 2)\, 2^x$ **31.** $y' = (2x \ln 2)2^{x^2}$ **33.** $y' = (2 \ln 9)9^{(2x+5)}$ **35.** $y'' = e^x > 0$ for all x
(y concave up for all x)

37. $y' = (\ln 2)e^{x \ln 2} > 0$ for all x
$y'' = (\ln 2)^2 e^{x \ln 2}$ (y concave up for all x)
39. $y = x$ **41.** 9.8 years **43.** 14.8 years

45. Now (put money in bank) **47.** $\frac{dw}{dt} = \frac{(500)49ke^{-kt}}{(1 + 49ke^{-kt})^2}$ **49.** $\frac{dN}{dt} = 3bkN_0e^{-kt}(1 - be^{-kt})^2$ **51. (a)** $\frac{2A}{3B}$
(b) $\frac{A}{3B}$

53. (a) $\frac{dp}{dt} = -bke^{-kt}$
(b) $\frac{d^2p}{dt^2} = bk^2e^{-kt}$

Section 3.4

1. $\frac{dy}{dx} = \frac{3}{3x + 5}$ **3.** $\frac{dy}{dx} = \frac{-x}{4 - x^2}$ **5.** $\frac{dy}{dx} = \frac{1}{x + 1}$ **7.** $\frac{dy}{dx} = \frac{e^x - e^{-x}}{e^x + e^{-x}}$ **9.** $\frac{dy}{dx} = \frac{-2}{x}$ **11.** $\frac{dy}{dx} = \frac{2(1 - \ln x^2)}{x^3}$

13. $\frac{dy}{dx} = \ln x$ **15.** $\frac{dy}{dx} = e^x \ln(2x) + \frac{e^x}{x}$ **17.** $\frac{\ln x}{\ln 5}$ **19.** x **21.** $\frac{\ln(x^2+3x+5)}{\ln 10}$ **23.** $\frac{\ln(e^x+1)}{\ln 2}$

25. $\frac{\left(\frac{\ln x}{\ln 10}\right)+1}{\ln 2}$ **27.** $\frac{dy}{dx} = \frac{1}{\ln 10(x+1)}$ **29.** $\frac{dy}{dx} = \frac{2x}{\ln 10(x^2+1)}$ **31.** $\frac{dy}{dx} = \frac{-1}{x \ln 10}$

33. $\frac{dy}{dx} = \frac{2x+3}{\ln 10(x^2+3x+1)}$ **35.** $\frac{dy}{dx} = \frac{-1}{x \ln 2}$ **37.** Yes, $y' = y$ **39.** e^2 **41.** $y' = 1/x$ (x different from 0)

43. $E(p) = \frac{p}{200-p}$
Elastic: $\$100 < p < \$200$
Inelastic: $\$0 < p < \$100$

45. $E(p) = 3$
Always elastic

47. $E(p) = \frac{p}{1600-2p}$
Elastic: $\$533.33 < p < \$800$
Inelastic: $0 < p < \$533.33$

49. **(a)** $E(p) = 2$ **(b)** $R'(p) = -5000/p^2$ **(c)** Yes; as p decreases, revenue decreases.

51. **(a)** $E(p) = \frac{p}{10(1600-0.2p)}$ **(b)** Elastic **(c)** Elastic **(d)** Raised **(e)** Raised **53.** $\frac{y'}{y} = r$

55.

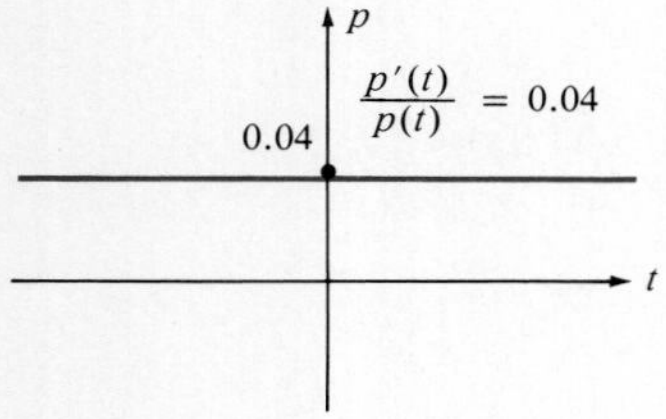

57. $y' = \left(\frac{3}{x} - \frac{2x}{x^2+1} - \frac{3}{3x-4}\right)\left[\frac{x^3}{(x^2+1)(3x-4)}\right]$

Chapter 3 Review

1. 2 **3.** -2 **5.** 2 **7.** 4 **9.** e^{-1} **11.** 0 **13.** $f'(x) = 2e^{(2x+1)}$ **15.** $f'(x) = \frac{e^x}{\ln 10}\left(\ln x + \frac{1}{x}\right)$

17. $f'(x) = \frac{1}{2x}$ **19.** $f'(x) = 1$ **21.** $f'(x) = \frac{e^x - e^{-x}}{2}$ **23.** $f'(x) = \frac{1}{x \ln 2}$ **25.** $f'(x) = \frac{-4x}{(x^2+1)(x^2-1)}$ **27.** $\frac{n}{x}$

29. $\frac{\sqrt{x^2+1}+x}{x\sqrt{x^2+1}+x^2+1}$ **31.** $\frac{e^{\sqrt{x}}}{2\sqrt{x}}$ **33.** $-\frac{\log e}{x}$ **35.** $\frac{2}{x}+1$ **37.** 0 **39.** $\frac{2-4\ln x}{x^3}$ **41.** $y' = (\ln 2)2^x$

43. $y' = 12x(x+1)^2$ **45.** $y' = (2x+1)^x\left[\ln(2x+1) + \frac{2x}{2x+1}\right]$ **47.** $y' = \frac{\sqrt{x+1}(x-3)}{x^2+1}\left[\frac{1}{2(x+1)} + \frac{1}{x-3} - \frac{2x}{x^2+1}\right]$

49. $R'(100) = 0$ **51.** After 1.56 years **53.** 3.16% **55.** $r = \ln(1+i)$ **57.** **(a)** $E(p) = \frac{2p}{-2p+110}$

(b) Elastic: $p > \$27.50$
Inelastic: $0 < p < \$27.50$
(c) $R(p) = -2p^2 + 110p$ **(d)** $R'(p) = -4p + 110$ **59.** $P(t) = 65e^{t \ln(0.85)}$

61. 13,055 **63.** 15.8 times stronger

Chapter 3 Test

1. $\frac{dy}{dx} = 2x \ln(x^2+1) + \frac{2x^3}{x^2+1}$ **2.** $\frac{dy}{dx} = \frac{1}{2 \ln 10}\left[\frac{x-1}{x(x+1)}\right]$ **3.** $P(t) = P_0 e^{0.049t}$ **4.** 27.73 months **5.** $x = e$

6. 11.61% **7.** $\frac{dy}{dx} = \frac{x^{\sqrt{x}}}{2\sqrt{x}}(\ln x + 2)$ **8.** $k = 0.0277$ **9.** After 18.8 years

10. **(a)** e^x is positive for any x; hence e^{-x^2} is positive for any x.

(b) Computing e^{-x^2} for x large and x small will convince you that the limit value is zero. $e^{-x^2} = \frac{1}{e^{x^2}}$ since $e^{x^2} > e^x \to \infty$, $\frac{1}{e^{x^2}} \to 0$ as $x \to \infty$ and by symmetry as $x \to -\infty$

(c) Since $y'(0) = 0$ and $y''(0) = -2$, we have that e^{-x^2} has a relative maximum at $x = 0$. Since $y'(x) > 0$ for $x < 0$ and $y'(x) < 0$ for $x > 0$, we have that $y(0) = 1$ is the absolute maximum.

(d) Since $y''(x)$ changes sign from negative to positive at $\frac{-1}{\sqrt{2}}$ and then from positive to negative at $\frac{1}{\sqrt{2}}$, we have that e^{-x^2} has inflection points at $\frac{-1}{\sqrt{2}}$ and $\frac{1}{\sqrt{2}}$.

PROJECTS AND PROBLEMS

Chapters 1–3

1. $y' = 2xe^{x^2} - 2xe^{-x^2}$ **3.** $y' = 20x^3 \ln x + 5x^3$ **5.** $y' = \frac{1}{x \ln x}$ **7.** $y' = 1$ **9.** $y' = \frac{1}{2}x^{-1/2} - \frac{1}{2}x^{-3/2}$

11. $y = 4 - 3x$ **13.** $y = \frac{1}{4}(x + 1)$ **15.** Increasing for $x > -\frac{3}{2}$, Decreasing for $x < -\frac{3}{2}$ **17.** Increasing for $x > e^{-1/2}$, Decreasing for $0 < x < e^{-1/2}$

19. Student project **21.** Student project **23.** 2 **25.** 4 **27.** Student project **29.** $\frac{dy}{dx} = x^x(1 + \ln x)$

31. $y = x$ on $(0, 1)$ **33.** $f(x) = x$ on $(0, 1)$ **35.** $f(x) = -(x - 1)^2$ **37.** Student project **39.** Student project

41. 3 hr 27 min **43. (a)** Height: 10.16″ Width: 7.61″ **(b)** No **45. (a)** 16.4 sec **(b)** 70.4 miles/hr **47.** 12.2 ft/sec **49.** $\frac{dI}{dt} = -kI$

51. Student project **53.** Student project

CHAPTER 4

Section 4.1

1. $y(x) = \frac{x^2}{2} + 3x + C$ **3.** $y(x) = \frac{1}{8}x^4 - \frac{2}{9}x^3 + \frac{x}{5} + C$ **5.** $y(x) = x^4 + 3x^{-1} + \frac{x^2}{2} - 3x + C$

7. $y(t) = \frac{1}{2}e^{2t} - e^{-3t} + C$ **9.** $y(x) = \frac{14}{3}x^{3/2} - e^{-2x} + C$ **11.** $y(t) = -\frac{1}{3}e^{-3t} + C$ **13.** $y(t) = -2e^{-0.5t} + C$

15. $F(x) = \frac{2}{3}(x^3 + 2x + 3)^{3/2} + C$ **17.** $F(x) = \frac{2}{3}x^3 + \frac{5}{4}x^4 + \frac{1}{5}x^5 + C$ **19.** $F(t) = \frac{4}{3}t^3 + 6t^2 + 9t + C$

21. $F(x) = -\frac{1}{2}(x^6 - 3)^{-2} + C$ **23.** $F(x) = \frac{1}{5}e^{5x} + C$ **25.** $F(t) = -25e^{-0.04t} + C$ **27.** $F(x) = \frac{2}{3}(3x + 2)^{3/2} + C$

29. $F(x) = \frac{1}{4}(x^2 + 1)^4 + C$ **31.** $f(x) = 1$ **33.** $f(s) = -s + 1$ **35.** $f(x) = \frac{3}{2}x^2 + 4x - 8$ **37.** $f(u) = \frac{1}{3}(u - 2)^3 - \frac{2}{3}$

39. $f(u) = u^2 - u^{-1} - 1$ **41.** $f(x) = \frac{3}{4}x^{4/3} + 48x^{1/3} - 96.6$ **43.** $f(t) = \frac{t^2}{2} + \frac{2}{3}t^{3/2} - \frac{34}{3}$

45. $f(t) = -100e^{-0.01t} + 101$ **47.** $f(x) = \frac{2}{3}(x^2 - 9)^{3/2} - \frac{113}{3}$ **49.** $f(x) = \frac{(x^2+1)^4}{4} - \frac{1}{4}$

51. $C(q) = 20q^2 - \frac{0.01}{3}q^3 + 100q + 100$ **53.** $C(q) = q^2 - \frac{0.02}{3}q^3 + 500$ **55.** $C(q) = 50e^{0.15q} + 30$

57. $P(q) = 10q - \frac{1}{4}q^2$ **59.** $R(q) = 10q - 0.04q^2 - \frac{0.10}{3}q^3$ **61.** $C(100) = \$9166.66$; $C(200) = \$48{,}333.33$; $C(300) = \$157{,}500$ **63.** $p(t) = -50e^{-0.02t} + 50$

65. $s(1) = 50$ miles **67.** $s(5) = 400$ feet **69.** $f(x) = e^x + 1$

Section 4.2

1. Left endpoint: $A = 16$
Right endpoint: $A = 80$
Midpoint: $A = 32$

3. Left endpoint: $A = 30$
Right endpoint: $A = 46$
Midpoint: $A = 37$

5. Left endpoint: $A = \frac{189}{8}$
Right endpoint: $A = \frac{81}{8}$
Midpoint: $A = \frac{297}{16}$

7. Left endpoint: $A = 0$
Right endpoint: $A = 8$
Midpoint: $A = 4$

9. Left endpoint: $A = 3$
Right endpoint: $A = 5$
Midpoint: $A = 4$

11. 2 subintervals: $A = 2$
4 subintervals: $A = 2$

13. 2 subintervals: $A = 16$
4 subintervals: $A = 16$

15. 2 subintervals: $A = 56.5$
4 subintervals: $A = 56.625$

17. 2 subintervals: $A = 0.6857$
4 subintervals: $A = 0.6912$

19. 15 **21.** $\frac{1}{3}$ **23.** \$3,100,000

Section 4.3

1. 10 **3.** 19.5 **5.** 1016.75 **7.** 12 **9.** 60 **11.** 29.6 **13.** 384 **15.** $\frac{e^2}{2} - \frac{1}{e} + \frac{1}{2}$ **17.** $\frac{65}{12}$ **19.** $\frac{33}{10}$

21. $4(\sqrt{33} - 2\sqrt{3})$ **23.** $\frac{1}{12}$ **25.** $\frac{(a+b+c)^2}{2} - \frac{c^2}{2}$ **27.** 24 **29.** 12 **31.** 6 **33.** $\frac{200}{3}$ **35.** $\frac{67 - 16\sqrt{2}}{12}$

37. $e - 1$ **39.** $-15e^{(-\ln 2)/5} + 15$ **41.** $3 - e^{-2}$ **43.** $\frac{1}{2}(e - 1)$ **45.** $3e^2 - 3e + 1$ **47.** Revenue increase: \$1662.50

49. Increase in profits: 880 units **51.** Total revenue: \$1,036,800 **53.** 256 feet

Section 4.4

1. $F(x) = \frac{1}{24}(3x^2 - 5)^4 + C$ **3.** $F(w) = \frac{(w^2+3)^3}{3} + C$ **5.** $F(x) = \frac{6}{5}(2x - 5)^{5/2} + C$ **7.** $F(t) = \ln|t + 3| + C$

9. $F(x) = 2\ln|x - 3| + C$ **11.** $F(x) = \frac{(\sqrt{x}+2)^6}{3} + C$ **13.** $F(x) = \frac{2}{3}(x^3 + 12x^2 + 3)^{3/2} + C$

15. $F(x) = \frac{2}{3}(e^x + 1)^{3/2} + C$ **17.** $F(u) = \frac{1}{2}\ln(e^{2u} + e^{-2u}) + C$ **19.** $\frac{[\ln(x^2+4)]^2}{2} + C$

21. $F(x) = -\frac{1}{2}e^{-x^2} + C$ **23.** $F(x) = x - 2\ln|x + 2| + C$ **25.** $F(u) = \frac{2}{5}(u - 1)^{5/2} - \frac{2}{3}(u - 1)^{3/2} + C$

27. $\frac{715}{4}$ **29.** $\frac{3}{2}\ln 2$ **31.** $\frac{1}{2}\ln 11 - \frac{1}{2}\ln 5$ **33.** $\frac{2}{3}$ **35.** 9 **37.** $\frac{2}{9}(56\sqrt{7} - 64)$

39. $\frac{1}{15}(1281^{3/2} - 6^{3/2})$ **41.** $\frac{2}{3}[8(17)^{3/4} - 24^{3/4}]$ **43.** $3(2 - \sqrt{3})$ **45.** $\frac{1}{2}$ **47.** $\frac{7}{24}$ **49.** Direct computation

51. Student project **53.** **(a)** Ratio of advantage $= 1.5x + 0.25$ **(b)** 0.55 **55.** 0.50

Chapter 4 Review

1. $F(x) = 7x + C$ **3.** $F(u) = \frac{2}{7}u^{7/2} + \frac{2}{3}u^{3/2} + C$ **5.** $F(x) = e^x - e^{-x} + C$ **7.** $F(x) = \frac{3}{2}x^{2/3} + C$

9. $F(x) = \frac{6}{5}x^{5/2} - \frac{4}{3}x^{3/2} + C$ **11.** $f(t) = t^2 + 5t$ **13.** $f(x) = e^x$ **15.** $f(u) = \frac{1}{3}(u^2 - 9)^{3/2} - \frac{64}{3}$

17. $C(q) = \frac{45}{2}q^2 - \frac{2}{3}q^3 + 10{,}000$ **19.** $C(q) = 10q + 4e^{-0.5q} + 996$ **21.** $\frac{4}{3}$ **23.** $\frac{3}{2} - e^{-1}$ **25.** e **27.** $\frac{a^4}{4}$

29. $\frac{8}{3}$

31. $\int_0^5 (x + 1)\,dx = \frac{35}{2}$

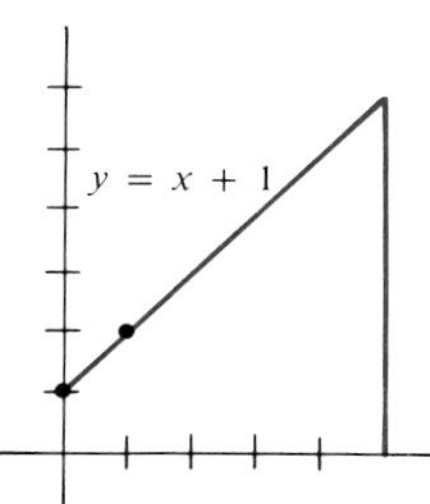

33. $\int_0^2 (4 - x^2)\,dx = \frac{16}{3}$

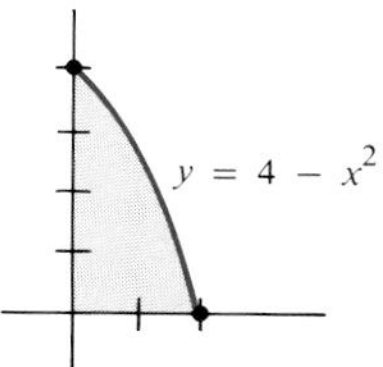

35. $\int_{-1}^1 (e^x + e^{-x})\,dx = 2\left(e - \frac{1}{e}\right)$

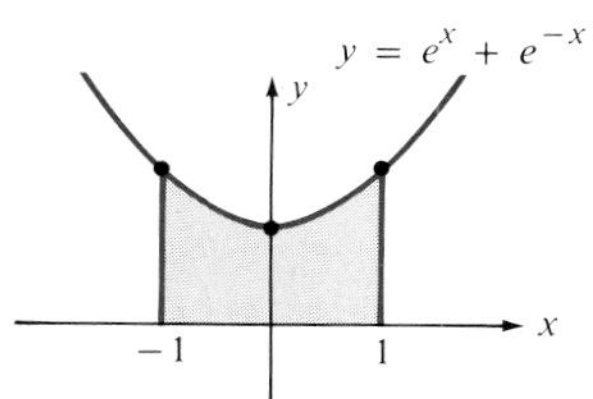

37. $\int_1^2 x^{-n}\,dx = \frac{2^{1-n} - 1}{1 - n}$

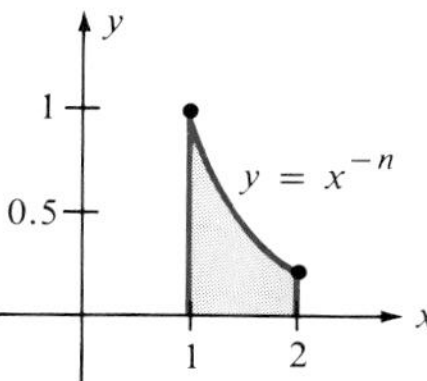

39. $F(x) = \frac{1}{8}(x^2 - 1)^4 + C$ **41.** $F(u) = \frac{(u + 1)^7}{7} - \frac{(u + 1)^6}{6} + C$ **43.** $F(x) = \frac{5(x + 1)^{11}}{11} + C$

45. $F(x) = 5\ln|x - 1| + C$ **47.** $F(t) = \ln|t + 1| + C$ **49.** $F(x) = \frac{x}{2} + \frac{5}{4}\ln|2x + 3| + C$ **51.** $\frac{1}{3}17^{3/2} - \frac{1}{3}$

53. $\frac{2}{3}[64 - (11)^{3/2}]$ **55.** $\frac{14}{3}$ **57.** 0 **59.** $R(q) = 100q - \frac{5}{2}q^2$ **61.** \$5000 **63.** **(a)** 1.9% **(b)** 27.5% **(c)** $L(x)$ is increasing. $L'(x) = 1.8x + 0.1 > 0$ for $x \in [0, 1]$ **(d)** $L(x)$ is concave up. $L''(x) = 1.8 > 0$ **(e)** $CI = 0.3$

65. **(a)** $s(t) = -5.5t^2 + 88t$ **(b)** 214.5 ft **(c)** 352 ft **67.** 0.81 meter **69.** 4793 whales

Chapter 4 Test

1. $F(t) = \frac{1}{2}t^2 + t + \ln|t| + C$ **2.** $\frac{3}{16}$ **3.** $F(u) = -\frac{2}{9}(1 - u^3)^{3/2} + C$ **4.** $10[10 + 2(e^{-1} - e^{-2})]$

5. $-\$29{,}500$ (loss) **6.** 1863 billion barrels **7.** 204 feet **8.** 14 words/min **9.** Amount = 289.5 million cubic feet

Chapter 5

Section 5.1

1. ∞ **3.** ∞ **5.** ∞ **7.** ∞ **9.** $-\frac{1}{2}$ **11.** ∞ **13.** $-\infty$ **15.** ∞ **17.** 0 **19.** ∞ **21.** $\frac{1}{k}$

23. $-\frac{1}{2}$ **25.** ∞ **27.** $\frac{15{,}000}{0.07}(1 - e^{-1.75}) = \$177{,}048.44$ **29.** $\frac{100{,}000}{0.06}(1 - e^{-3}) = \$1{,}583{,}688.20$

31. $\frac{10{,}000}{0.13} = \$76{,}923.08$ **33.** \$125 **35.** Scenario 1: \$1489.89
Scenario 2: \$1000
Scenario 1 is better.

Section 5.2

1. $F(x) = \frac{1}{3}xe^{3x} - \frac{1}{9}e^{3x} + C$ **3.** $F(x) = x(\ln x)^2 - 2(x \ln x - x) + C$

5. $F(x) = \frac{x^2}{3}(x^2 + 2)^{3/2} - \frac{1}{3}\left[\frac{2}{5}(x^2 + 2)^{5/2}\right] + C$ **7.** $F(x) = \frac{x^2}{2}(\ln x)^2 - \frac{x^2}{2}\ln x + \frac{x^2}{4} + C$

9. $F(x) = -x^2\sqrt{1 - x^2} - \frac{2}{3}(1 - x^2)^{3/2} + C$ **11.** $F(x) = -\frac{ax}{b}e^{-bx} - \frac{a}{b^2}e^{-bx} + C$ **13.** $F(x) = \frac{ax^2 \ln(bx)}{2} - \frac{ax^2}{4} + C$

15. $F(x) = -\frac{ax^2}{b}e^{-bx} + \frac{2}{b}\left(-\frac{ax}{b}e^{-bx} - \frac{a}{b^2}e^{-bx}\right) + C$ **17.** $\frac{1}{4}(e^2 + 1) \cong 2.0973$ **19.** $10.25e^{10} - 0.25e^2$ **21.** $e^e(e - 1)$

23. $12{,}500 + 2500e^{-10}$ **25.** $\frac{12{,}500}{e} = 4598$ hits in 50 hours
Batting average: $\frac{1}{e} = 0.368$ (not bad)

27. 500 million dollars (*Hint:* $ne^{-0.1n}$ approaches 0 as n gets large.)

Section 5.3

1. Area: 42

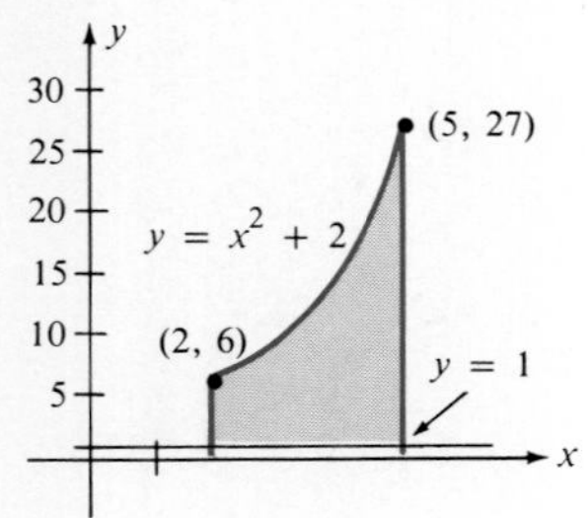

3. Area: $7\frac{7}{8}$

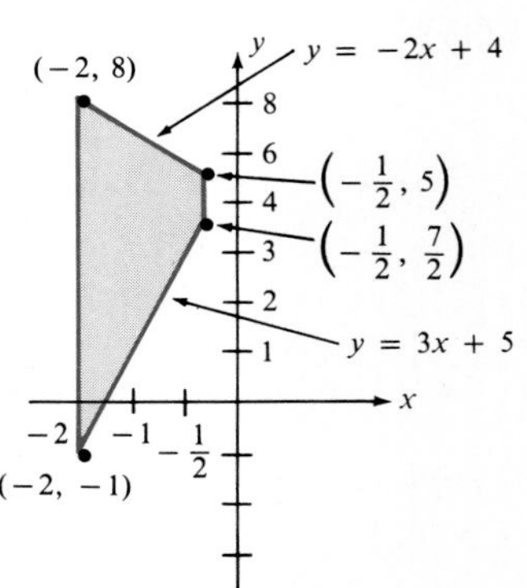

5. Area: $\frac{93}{2} - \frac{2}{3}(6^{3/2} - 3^{3/2})$

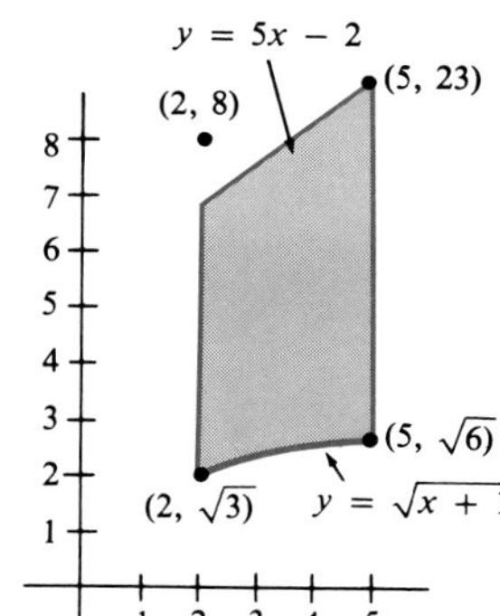

7. Area: $e^2 - 2\ln 2 + \frac{3}{4}$

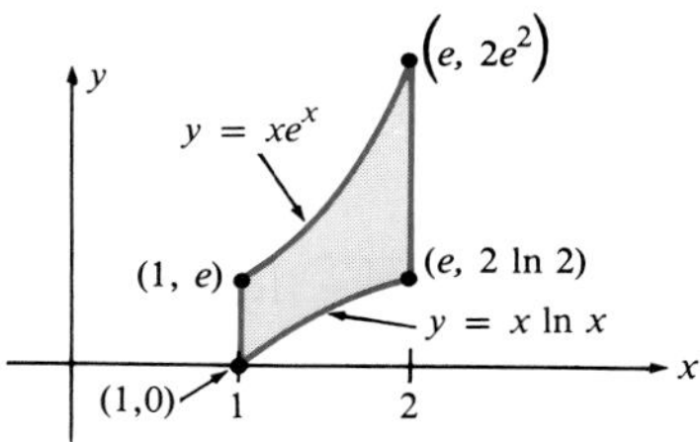

9. Area: 4

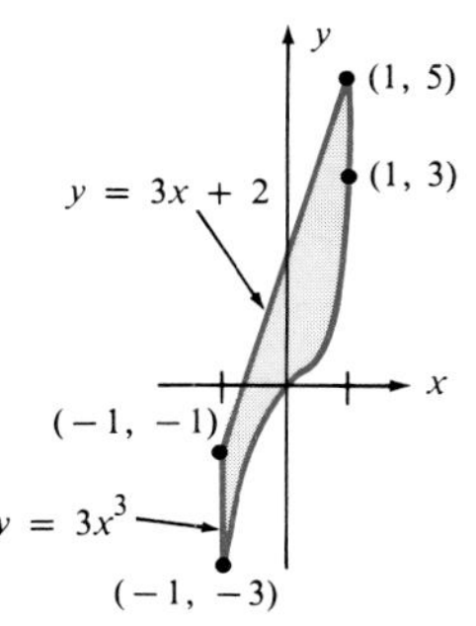

11. Area: 16.5

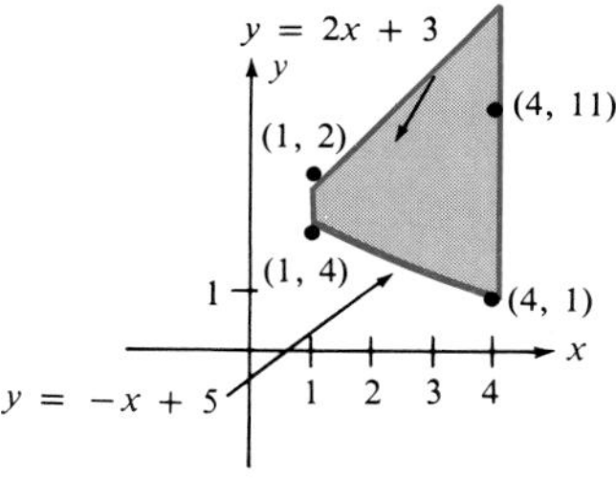

13. Area: $\frac{40}{3}$

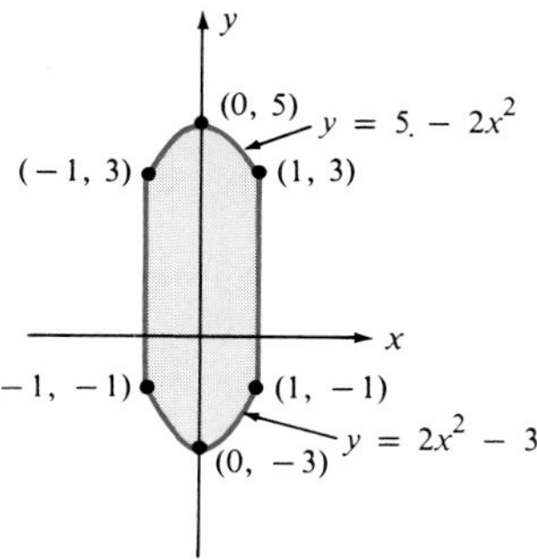

15. $\frac{128\sqrt{2}}{3}$

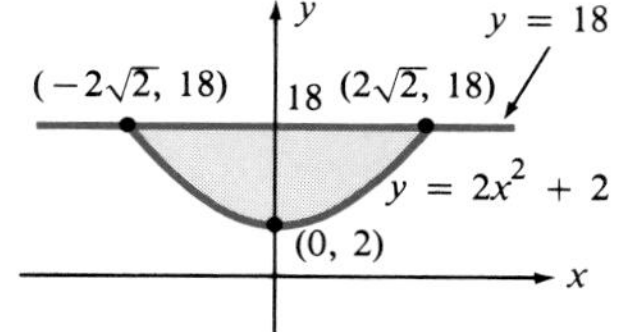

17. $\frac{1}{12}$

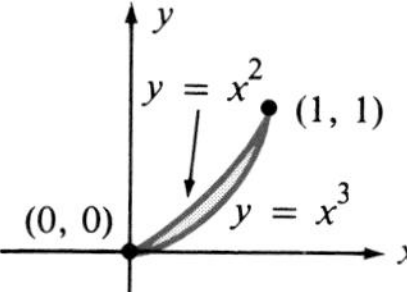

19. $\frac{125}{6}$

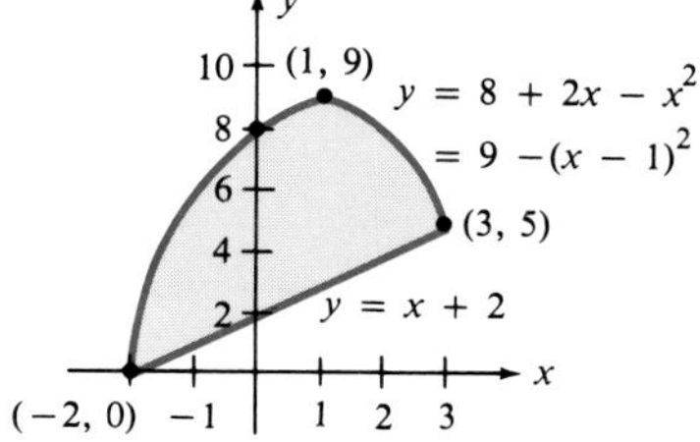

21. $18\sqrt{2}$

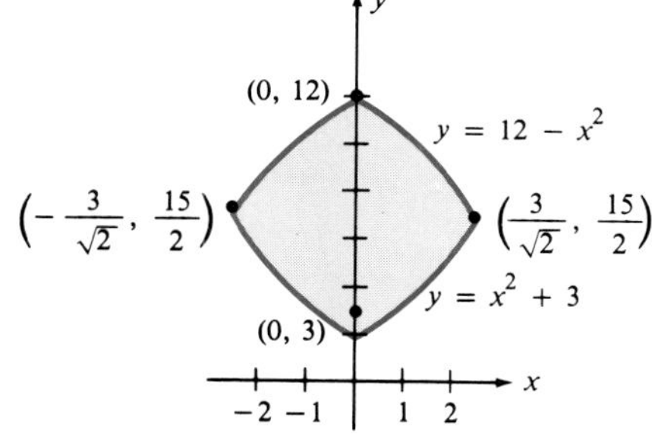

23. $\frac{1647}{5}\pi$

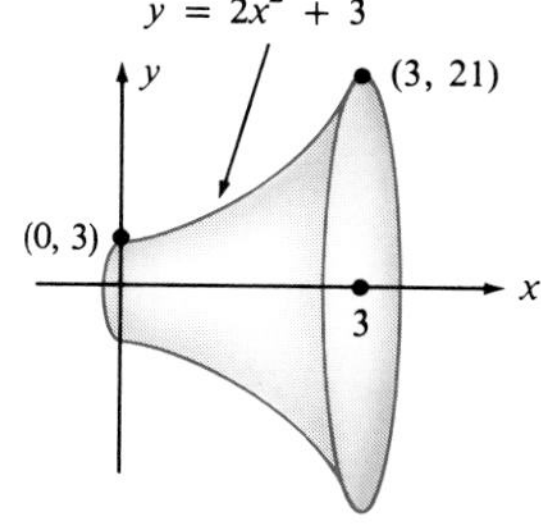

25. $\frac{2}{3}\pi$

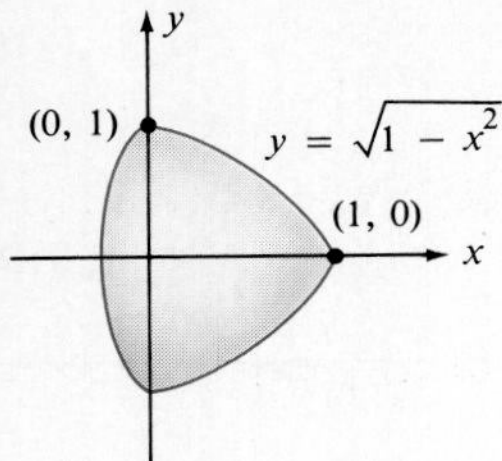

27. $\frac{1}{4}e^{-4}(1 - e^{-12})\pi$

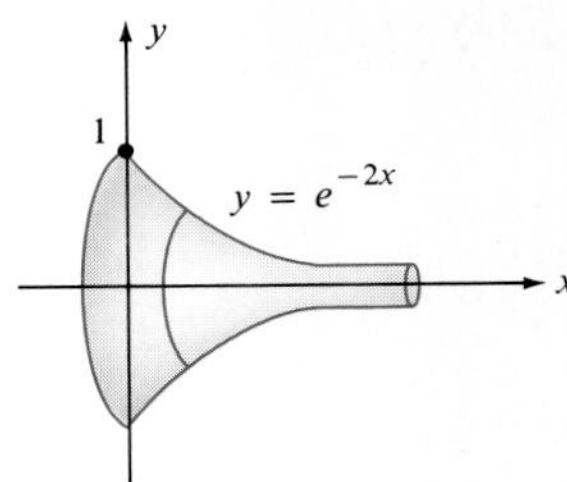

29. $P_S = \frac{224}{9} = 24.88$

$C_S = \frac{484}{9} = 53.78$

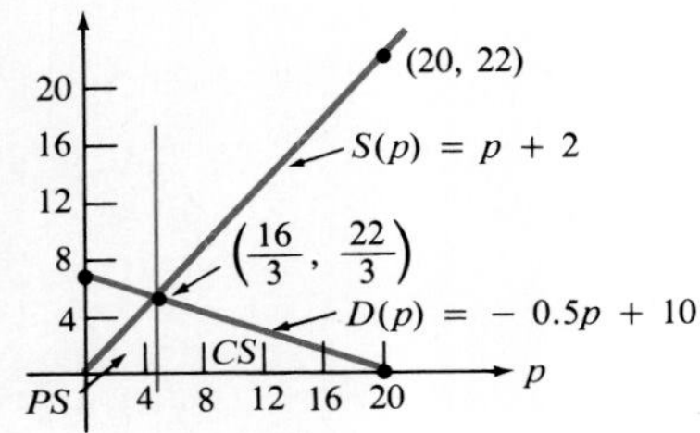

31. $P_S = \frac{200}{3}$

$= 66.67$

$C_S = 400$

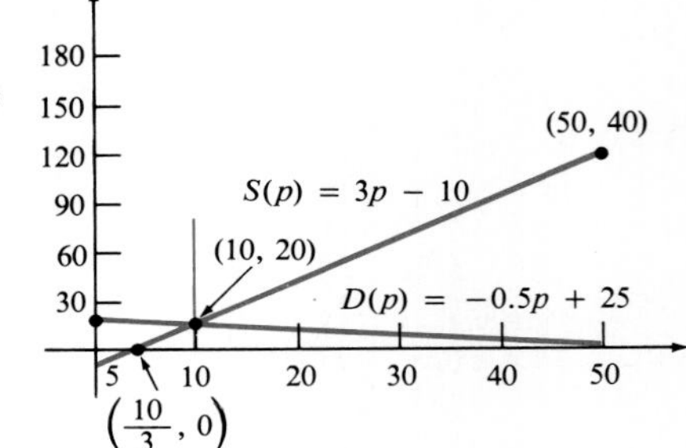

33. $P_S = 38.9$

$C_S = 35.1$

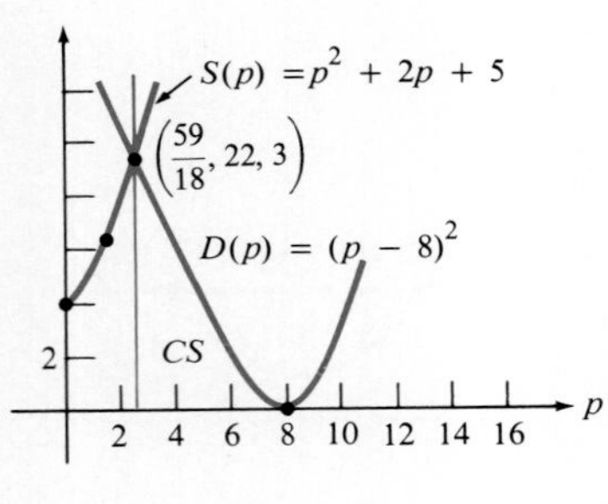

PS

35. $P_S = 9$

$C_s = 5.79$

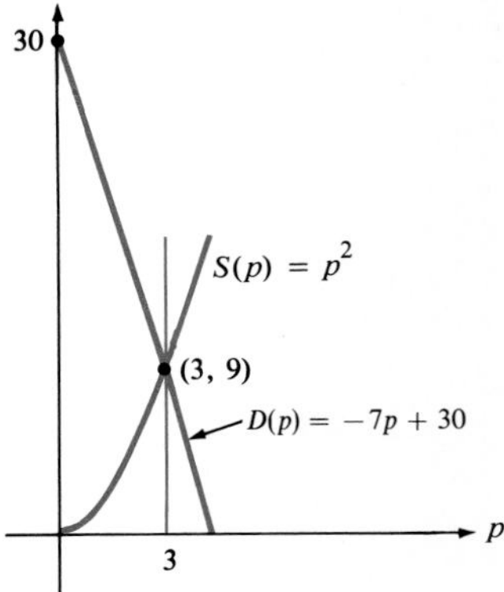

37. $P_S = 0$

$C_S = 0$

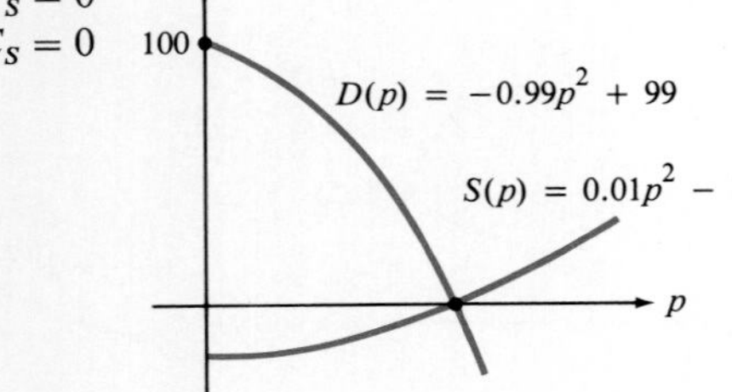

39. **(a)** (5, 7)
(b) 35 million dollars
(c) 25 surplus
(d) 13 demand

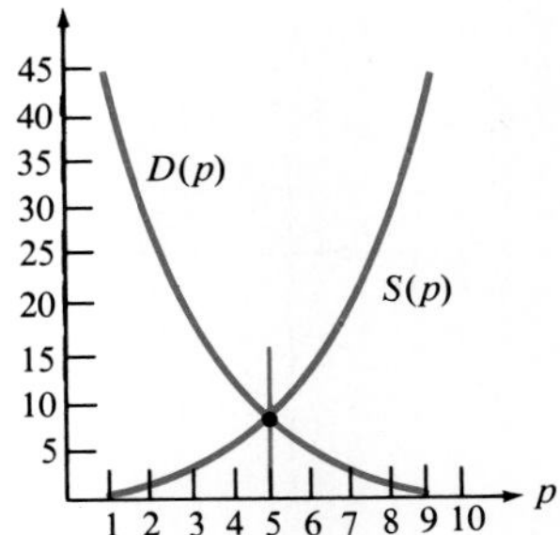

Section 5.4

1. Exact value: 8
Trapezoid rule: 8
Simpson's rule: 8

3. Exact value: 28
Trapezoid value: 28
Simpson's rule: 28

5. Exact value: $\frac{1}{3}$
Trapezoid rule: 0.34375
Simpson's rule: $\frac{1}{3}$

7. Exact value: 64
Trapezoid rule: 68
Simpson's rule:64

9. Exact value: 8
Trapezoid rule: 8
Simpson's rule: 8

11. Exact value: $\ln 2 \cong 0.6931472$
Trapezoid rule: 0.69702
Simpson's rule: 0.69325

13. Exact value: We cannot integrate
Trapezoid rule: 1.4907
Simpson's rule: 1.4637

15. Exact value: 1
Trapezoid rule: 1.023
Simpson's rule: 1.00017

17. Trapezoid rule: 2.205
Simpson's rule: 2.179

19. Trapezoid rule: 1.106
Simpson's rule: 1.107

21. Trapezoid rule: 1.260
Simpson's rule: 1.289

23. 1.106 **25.** 0.004152 **27.** 225.25 **29.** 232.5 **31.** P_S (trapezoid rule) = 16 **33.** P_S (exact) = 16
35. C_S (Simpson's rule) = 10 **37.** 35,250 ft²

Section 5.5

1. $y(t) = t + C$

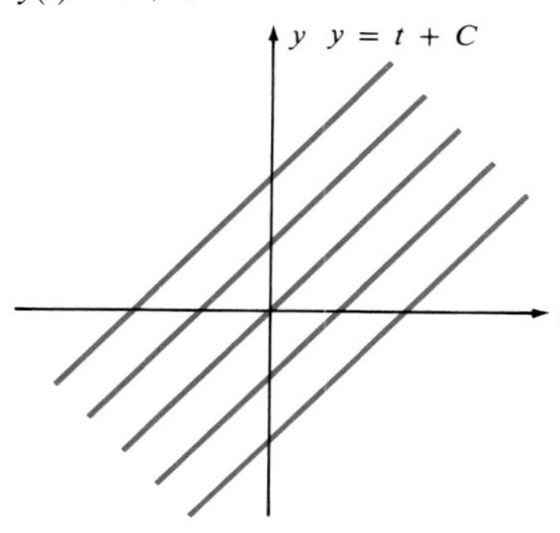

3. $y(t) = Ce^{3t}$

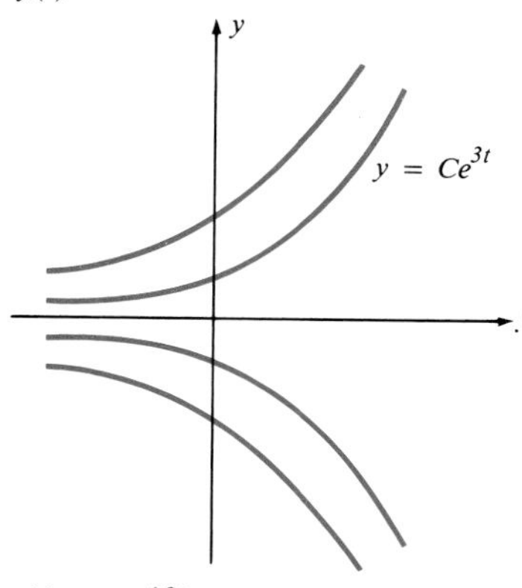

5. $y(t) = Ce^{t}$

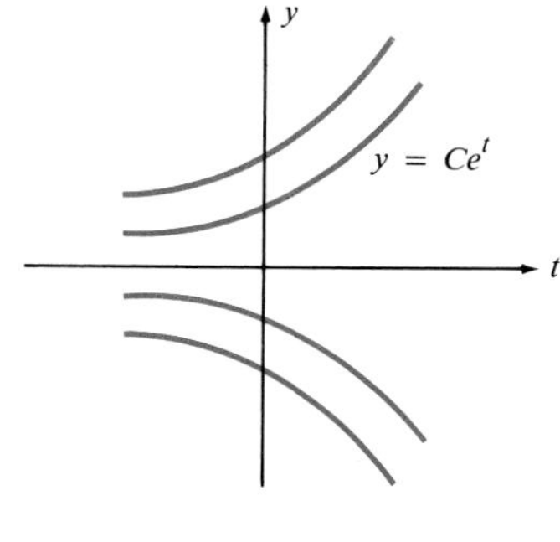

7. $y(t) = Ce^{0.05t}$

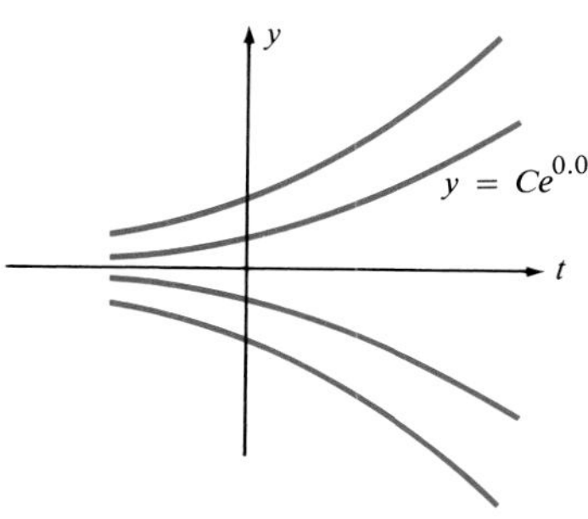

9. $y(t) = Ce^{10t}$

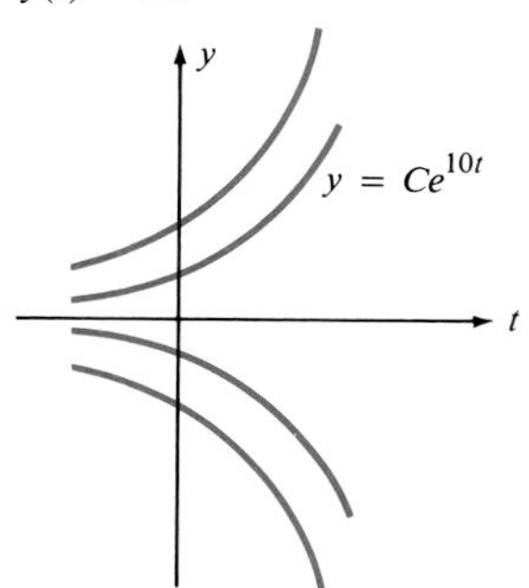

11. $y(t) = 100e^{t}$

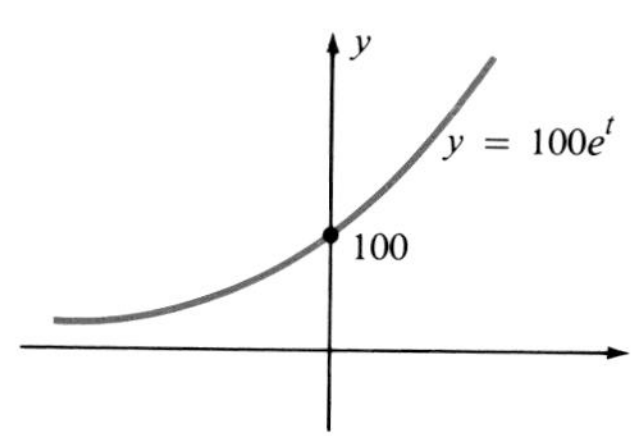

13. $N(t) = 50e^{-2t}$

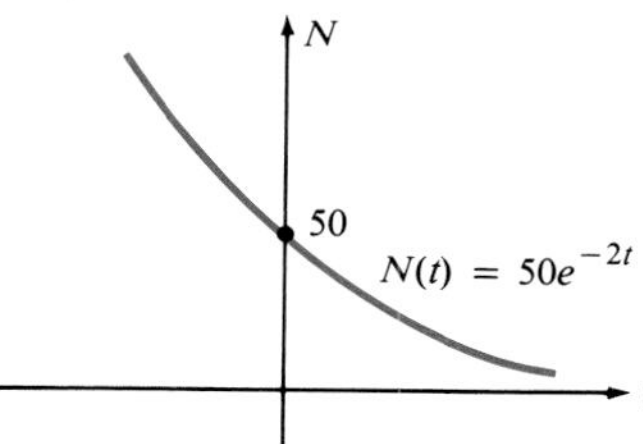

15. $N(t) = 50e^{-0.08t}$

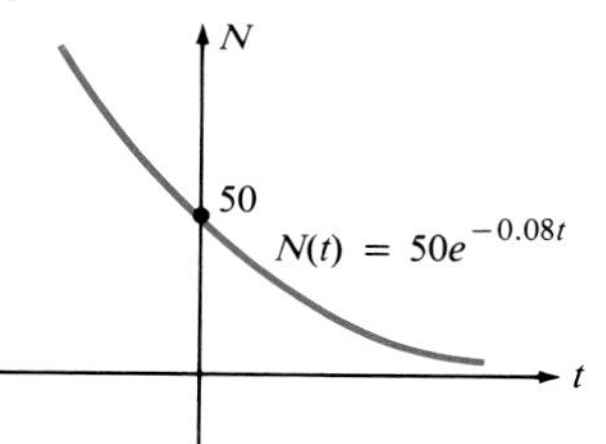

17. $P(t) = e^{0.05t}$

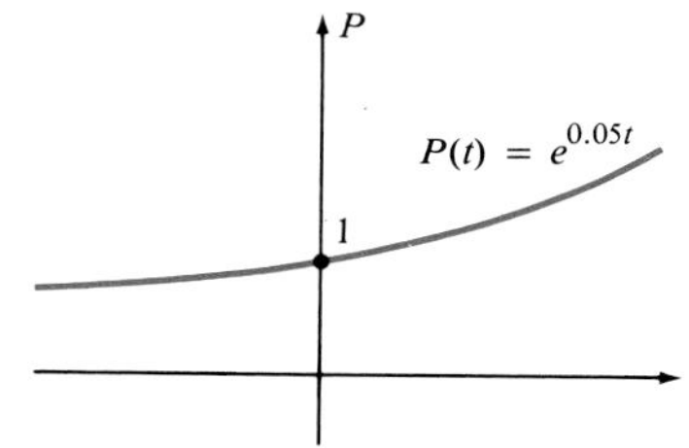

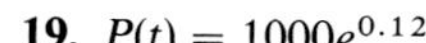

19. $P(t) = 1000e^{0.12t}$

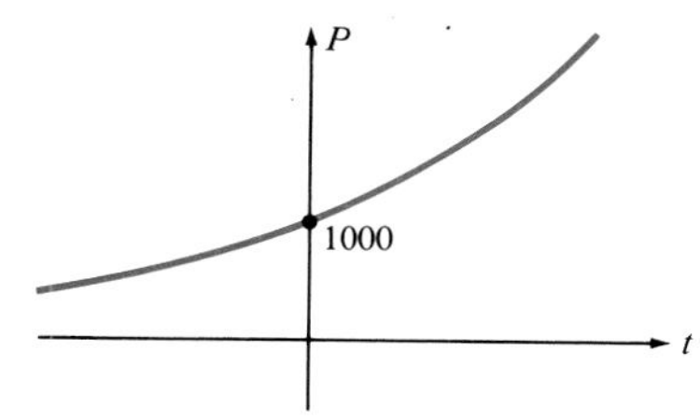

21. $y(t) = \frac{t^3}{3} + 1$ **23.** $y(t) = \frac{t^3}{3} + t^2 + t + 3$ **25.** $y(t) = t$ **27.** $y(t) = e^{0.05t}$ **29.** $y(t) = 100$

31. $y(t) = e^{0.5t}$ **33.** $k = \ln(.95) = -0.051$ **35.** $P(t) = 10e^{0.05t}$, $\frac{dP}{dt} = \frac{1}{20}P$ **37.** $t_h = \frac{\ln 2}{9.2} \times 10^8 = 7{,}500{,}000$ years

39. **(a)** $\frac{dP}{dt} = -0.0001238P$ **(b)** $P(t) = 10e^{-0.0001238t}$

Chapter 5 Review

1. $F(x) = \frac{x}{3}e^{3x} - \frac{1}{9}e^{3x} + C$ **3.** $F(x) = 2x \ln x - 2x + C$ **5.** $F(x) = \frac{2}{5}(x+4)^{5/2} - \frac{8}{3}(x+4)^{3/2} + C$

7. $-\sqrt{x^2+1} + \frac{1}{3}(x^2+1)^{3/2} + C$ **9.** $\frac{x^4(4\ln x - 1)}{16} + C$

11. $\frac{2}{3}$

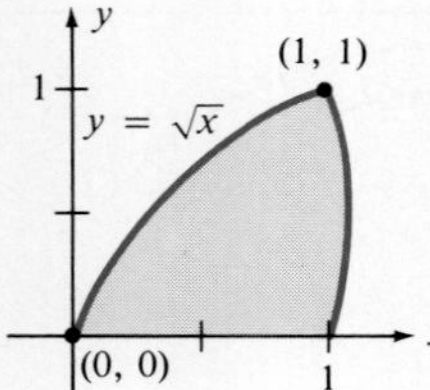

13. $e - \frac{1}{e}$

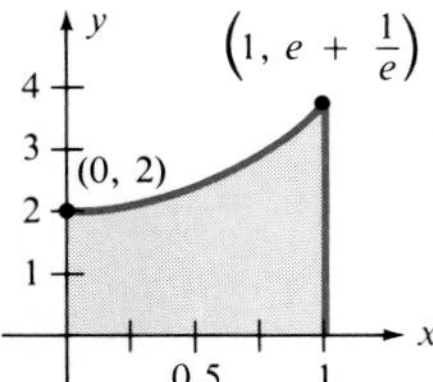

15. $\frac{1}{3}$

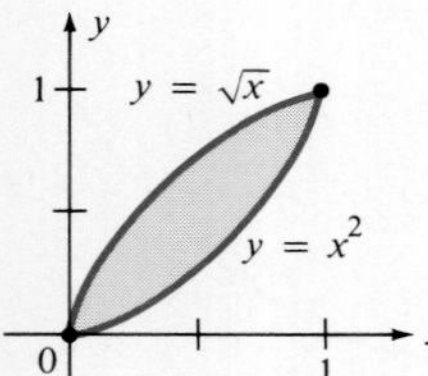

17. $\frac{8}{3}\sqrt{2}$

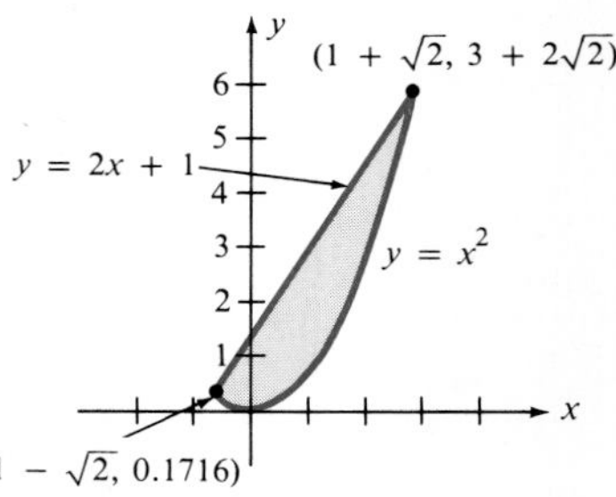

19. $\frac{4}{3\sqrt{2}}$

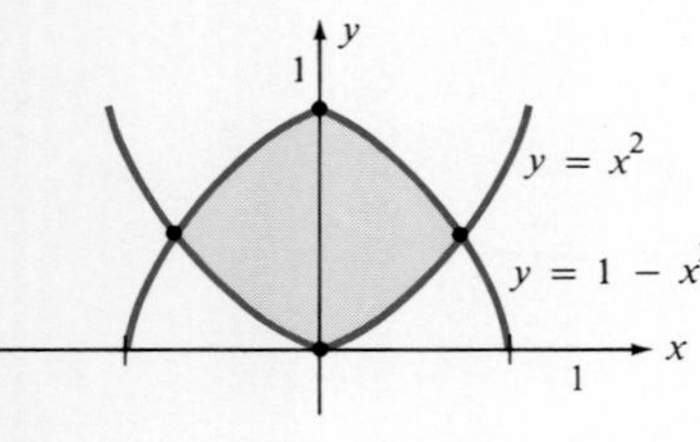

21. $\frac{\pi}{3}$

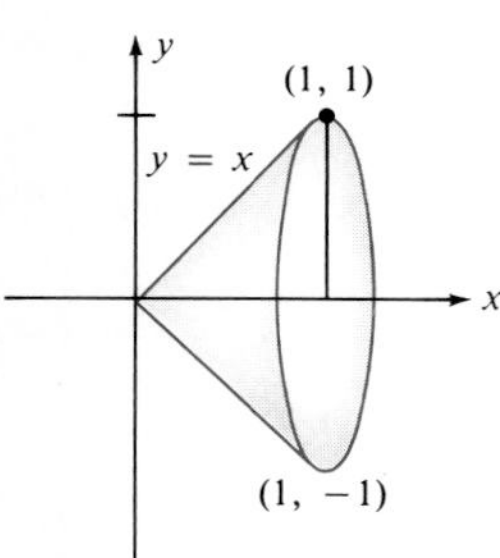

23. $\frac{3}{5}\pi$

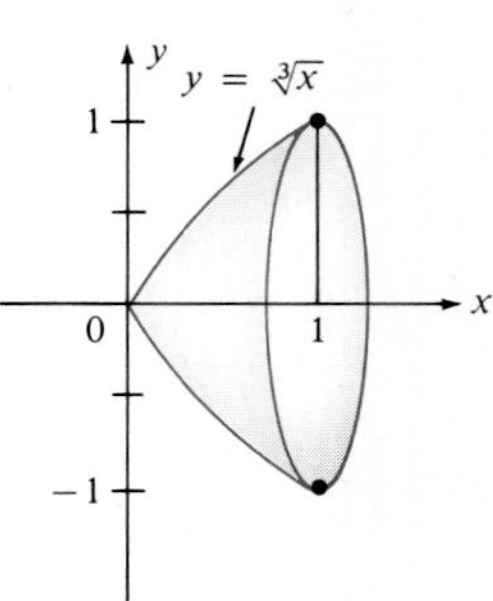

25. Trapezoid rule: 0.3437
Simpson's rule: 0.3333

27. Trapezoid rule: 1.1667
Simpson's rule: 1.1111

29. $\frac{1}{a}$ **31.** 2 **33.** $\frac{1}{2}$ **35.** 1 **37.** $\frac{1}{4}$

39. $\frac{1}{2}\pi(1 - e^{-10})$ **41.** $\frac{\pi}{4}$ **43.** $\frac{32\pi}{3}$ **45.** $y(t) = 10e^{-0.01t}$ **47.** $P(t) = 100e^{-0.08t}$ **49.** $P(t) = 100e^{0.25t}$

51. \$997,629.35 **53.** Producer's surplus = \$3.94 **55.** $P(t) = P_0e^{0.1398t}$ **57.** $\frac{dy}{dt} = 0.504y$
$y(0) = 500$

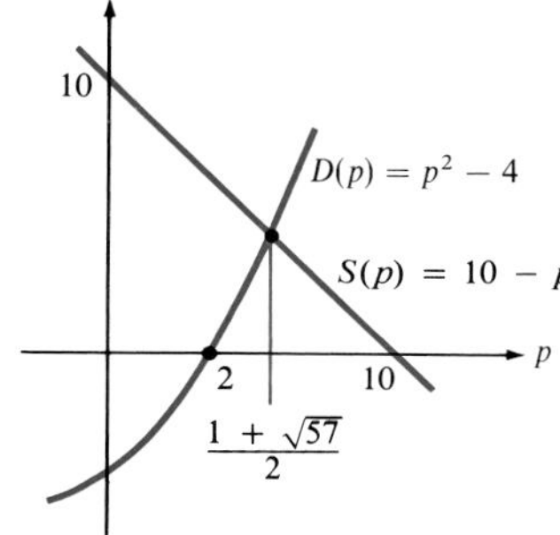

Chapter 5 Test

1. $\frac{1}{36}(1 + 5e^6)$ **2.** $\frac{64}{3}$ **3.** $\frac{4}{3}$ **4.** The consumers' and producers' surplus are both zero. **5.** $\frac{1}{3}$

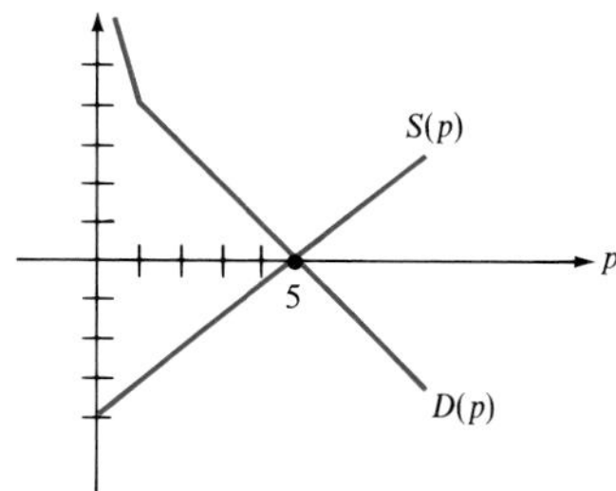

6. 0.34375 to five places (error is $\cong .0104$) **7.** $\frac{71}{6}$ (11.8333 to four places) **8.** $\frac{\pi}{2}(e^2 - 1)$ (10.0359 to four places)

9. $v = \frac{\pi}{3}rh^2$ **10. (a)** $\frac{dN}{dt} = 0.113N$ **(b)** $N(t) = N_0e^{0.113t}$
$N(0) = N_0$

CHAPTER 6

Section 6.1

1. \$875 **3.** \$950 **5.** \$150 **7.** $f(0, \ln 3) = 4$
$f(\ln 4, \ln 5) = \frac{9}{4}$
9. $f(2, 4) = -3$
$f(3, 7) = -\frac{5}{2}$
11. $f(-3, 1) = \frac{3}{2}$
$f(2, 5) = \frac{2}{7}$
13. $f(1, 3) = 3$
$f(5, 7) = 59$

15. $3\sqrt{10}$ **17.** 7 **19.** $2\sqrt{14}$ **21.** Center: $(0, 1, -1)$
Radius: 4
23. Center: $(0, 1, -1)$
Radius: 3

25.

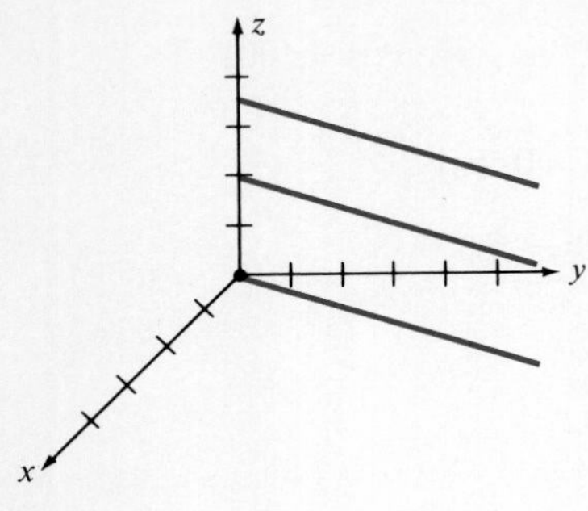

27.

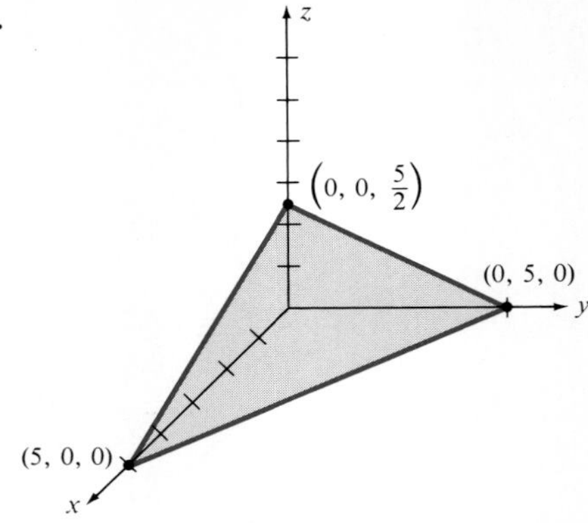

29.

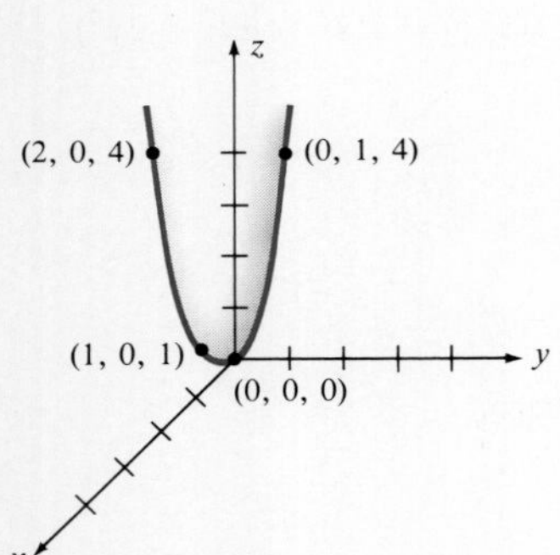

31. $C(500, 750) = \$28{,}750$ **33.** $P(500, 750) = \$7250$

35. Isoprofit lines: $7x + 5y = c$ **37.** $p(10, 30) = 17.31$ thousand cars **39.** Student project **41.** $C(9, 12) = 75$ **43.** Student project

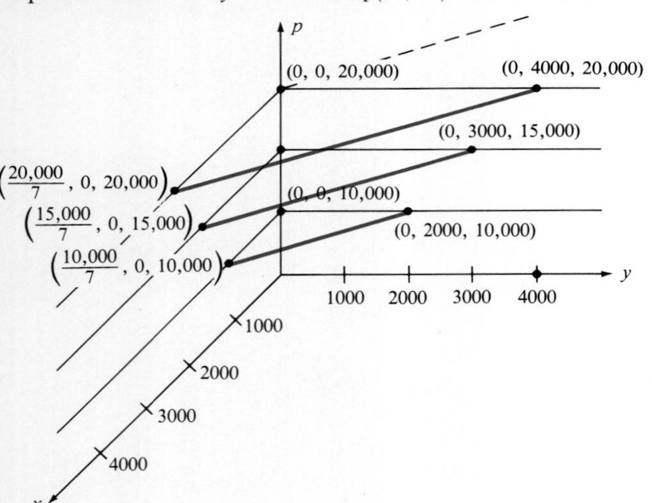

Section 6.2

1. $f_x(x, y) = 2 - y + 6x$
$f_y(x, y) = -x + 1$

3. $f_x(x, y) = \dfrac{1}{y}$
$f_y(x, y) = -\dfrac{x}{y^2}$

5. $f_x(x, y) = -\dfrac{2y}{(x - y)^2}$
$f_y(x, y) = \dfrac{2x}{(x - y)^2}$

7. $f_x(x, y) = \dfrac{y^2 - x^2 - 2xy}{(x^2 + y^2)^2}$
$f_y(x, y) = \dfrac{x^2 - y^2 - 2xy}{(x^2 + y^2)^2}$

9. $f_x(x, y) = ye^{xy}$
$f_y(x, y) = xe^{xy}$

11. $f_x(x, y) = -\dfrac{2e^{x+y}}{(e^x - e^y)^2}$
$f_y(x, y) = \dfrac{2e^{x+y}}{(e^x - e^y)^2}$

13. $f_x(x, y) = e^x \ln y + \dfrac{e^y}{x}$
$f_y(x, y) = \dfrac{e^x}{y} + e^y \ln x$

15. $f_x(x, y) = 2xe^{(x^2+y^2)}$
$f_y(x, y) = 2ye^{(x^2+y^2)}$

17. $f_x(x, y) = \dfrac{2}{3}(2xe^y - 2ye^x - 2xye^x)(x^2e^y - 2xye^x + y^2e^y)^{-1/3}$
$f_y(x, y) = \dfrac{2}{3}(x^2e^y - 2xe^x + 2ye^y + y^2e^y)(x^2e^y - 2xye^x + y^2e^y)^{-1/3}$

19. $f_x(x, y) = \dfrac{1}{x+y}$
$f_y(x, y) = \dfrac{1}{x+y}$

21. $f_x(3, 1) = -30$
$f_y(2, 3) = -6$

23. $f_x(0, 1) = 2e^3$
$f_y(-3, 2) = 3$

25. $f_x(3, 4) = \ln 3 + e^4 + 5$
$f_y(2, 5) = 3 \ln 2 + 20e^5$

27. $f_x(x, y) = 2x + 2y + 10$
$f_y(x, y) = 2x - 6y - 2$
$f_{xx}(x, y) = 2$
$f_{xy}(x, y) = 2$
$f_{yy}(x, y) = -6$

29. $f_x(x, y) = 4(x + y)(x^2 + 2xy - y^2)$
$f_y(x, y) = 4(x - y)(x^2 + 2xy - y^2)$
$f_{xx}(x, y) = 4(3x^2 + 6xy + y^2)$
$f_{xy}(x, y) = 4(3x^2 + 2xy - 3y^2)$
$f_{yy}(x, y) = 4(x^2 - 6xy + 3y^2)$

31. $f_x(x, y) = \ln(x + y) + 1$
$f_y(x, y) = \ln(x + y) + 1$
$f_{xx}(x, y) = \dfrac{1}{x+y}$
$f_{xy}(x, y) = \dfrac{1}{x+y}$
$f_{yy}(x, y) = \dfrac{1}{x+y}$

33. $f_x(x, y) = 6x + 5y$
$f_y(x, y) = 5x - 4y$
$f_{xx}(x, y) = 6$
$f_{xy}(x, y) = 5$
$f_{yy}(x, y) = -4$

35. $f_x(x, y) = -\dfrac{(x + y)(x + 5y)}{(x - y)^4}$
$f_y(x, y) = \dfrac{(x + y)(5x + y)}{(x - y)^4}$
$f_{xx}(x, y) = -\dfrac{2(x^2 + 10xy + 13y^2)}{(x - y)^5}$
$f_{xy}(x, y) = -\dfrac{2(5x^2 + 14xy + 5y^2)}{(x - y)^5}$
$f_{yy}(x, y) = \dfrac{2(13x^2 + 10xy + y^2)}{(x - y)^5}$

37. $f_x(A) = 0$
$f_y(A) = 0$

39. $f_x(A) = 0$
$f_y(A) < 0$

41. $R_x(10, 5) = 4$
$R_y(10, 5) = 10$

43. $C_x(10, 5) = 25$
$C_y(10, 5) = 20$

45. $C_x(10, 5) = 205$
$C_y(10, 5) = 60$

47. $P_x(10, 5) = 30$
$P_y(10, 5) = 200$

49. $C_x(10, 20) = 90$
$C_y(10, 20) = 150$

51. $P_x(10, 20) = 10$
$P_y(10, 20) = 10$

53. Direct computation

55. Direct computation

57. Direct computation

59. $h_v(v, d) = \dfrac{k}{3}\dfrac{1}{v^{2/3}d^{2/3}}$, $h_d(v, d) = -\dfrac{2k}{3}\dfrac{v^{1/3}}{d^{5/3}}$

Section 6.3

1. $\left(\dfrac{5}{2}, 2\right)$

3. $\left(-\dfrac{1}{2}, \dfrac{1}{3}\right)$

5. $\left(-\dfrac{4}{3}, \dfrac{2}{3}\right)$

7. $(0, 2)$, $(0, -1)$

9. No critical points

11. $\left(-\dfrac{4}{11}, -\dfrac{13}{11}\right)$

13. $\left(-\dfrac{2}{9}, -\dfrac{5}{3}\right)$

15. $\left(\sqrt{\dfrac{5}{3}}, 1\right), \left(\sqrt{\dfrac{5}{3}}, -1\right), \left(-\sqrt{\dfrac{5}{3}}, 1\right), \left(-\sqrt{\dfrac{5}{3}}, -1\right)$

17. $(0, 0)$, $\left(2\left(\dfrac{4}{9}\right)^{1/3}, 2\left(\dfrac{2}{3}\right)^{1/3}\right)$

19. No critical points

21. Relative minimum: $(-4, -1)$

23. Relative maximum: $(4, 2)$

25. Saddle points: $(2, 2)$, $(2, 0)$, $(0, 2)$, $(\frac{4}{3}, \frac{4}{3})$
Relative maximum: $\left(\dfrac{4}{3}, \dfrac{4}{3}\right)$

27. Test fails at $(0, 0)$

29. Saddle point: $(20, 15)$

31. Saddle points: $(0, 4)$, $\left(\dfrac{1}{2}, 0\right)$
Relative minimum: $\left(\dfrac{1}{2}, 4\right)$
Relative maximum: $(0, 0)$

33. Saddle point: $(0, 0)$
Relative maximum: $(3, 3)$

35. Relative minimum: $(2^{-1/3}, 2^{5/3})$

37. Test fails at $(\sqrt{3}, 0), (-\sqrt{3}, 0)$ **39.** No critical points **41.** $\left(\frac{4}{9}, \frac{8}{9}, \frac{8}{9}\right)$, distance $= \frac{4}{3}$ **43.** (2, 0, 0), distance = 2

45. Output level: $\left(\frac{115}{3}, 30\right)$

Maximum profit: $1004.17

47. **(a)** $p_1(x, y) = 65 - x - y$
$p_2(x, y) = 90 - x - 2y$
(b) $R(x, y) = 65x - x^2 - 2xy + 90y - 2y^2$ **(c)** $P(x, y) = 65x - 2x^2 - 3xy + 90y - 3y^2$

(d) Maximum production levels: (8, 11) **49.** Pounds A $= \frac{15}{7}$

Pounds B $= \frac{10}{7}$

Section 6.4

1. $\left(\frac{5}{4}, -\frac{7}{4}\right)$ **3.** $x = -\sqrt{\frac{24}{7}}, y = -\frac{1}{4}\sqrt{\frac{24}{7}}$
$x = \sqrt{\frac{24}{7}}, y = \frac{1}{4}\sqrt{\frac{24}{7}}$
5. $(\sqrt{3}, 0)$
$(-\sqrt{3}, 0)$
7. (0, 2) **9.** $\left(-\frac{58}{23}, -\frac{44}{23}\right)$

11. Sides and height both 5 feet **13.** Radius and height both $\left(\frac{256}{\pi}\right)^{1/3} \cong 4.33$ feet **15.** $x = \frac{375}{8}, y = \frac{225}{8}$

17. $x = \frac{50}{3}, y = \frac{25}{6}$ **19.** $x = 10, y = 5$
marginality $= -1$
21. Maximum product: minimize
$L(x, y, \lambda) = xy + \lambda(x + y - 15)$
23. Constrained minimum
$L(x, y, \lambda) = xy^2 + \lambda(x + y - 75)$

25. Minimum cost box
$L(x, y, \lambda) = 6x^2 + 4xy + \lambda(x^2y - 1600)$
27. Maximum volume
$L(x, y, \lambda) = x^2y + \lambda(y + 4x - 108)$

29. Wire problem
$L(x, r, \lambda) = x^2 + \pi r^2 + \lambda(4x + 2\pi r - 25)$
31. Telephone lines
$L(x, y, \lambda) = 2000y + 3000\sqrt{49 + x^2} + \lambda(x + y - 12)$

Section 6.5

1.

x_1	y_1	x_1^2	x_1y_1
1	3	1	3
2	4	4	8
3	7	9	21
4	9	16	36
10	23	30	68

$a = 2.1$
$b = 0.5$
$y = 2.1x + 0.5$

3.

x_1	y_1	x_1^2	x_1y_1
−2	−3	4	6
0	4	0	0
1	7	1	7
2	9	4	18
1	17	9	31

$a = 3.06$
$b = 3.485$
$y = 3.06x + 3.485$

5. $r_1 = 1$
$r_2 = 0$
$r_3 = -0.3$
$r_4 = 0$
$r_5 = 0.5$

7. 2 **9.** $y = 0.5$

11. **(a)** Basically linear
(b) Basically linear
(c) Quadratic
(d) Quadratic

13. $y = 0.5x + 0.17$

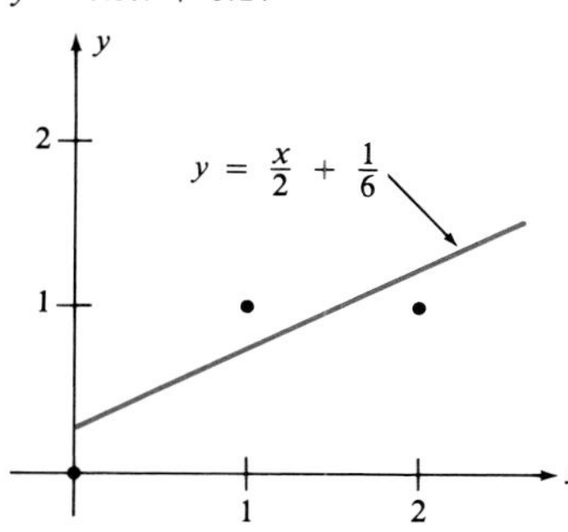

15. $y = 1.9x - 0.1$

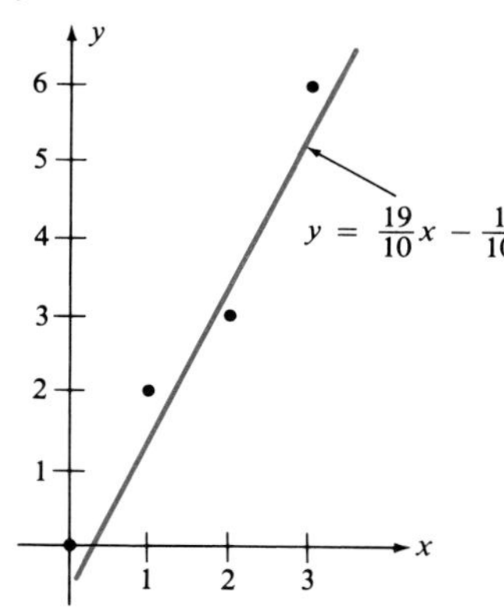

17. $y = 2.1x - 2.5$

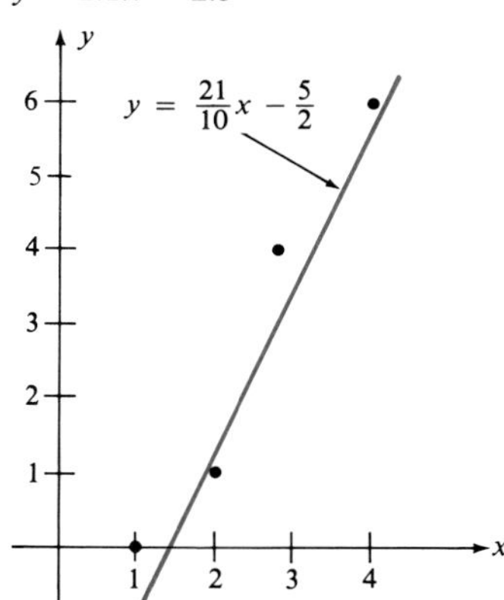

19. $y = \frac{4}{3}$ **21.** $R(q) = 3q - \frac{5}{3}$ **23.** $D(q) = -0.45q + 14.67$

Section 6.6

1. x-antiderivative: $\frac{x^3}{3} + \frac{x^2y}{2} - 2xy + xy^2 + C(y)$
y-antiderivative: $x^2y + \frac{xy^2}{2} - y^2 + \frac{y^3}{3} + C(x)$

3. x-antiderivative: $\frac{y}{3}(x^2 + y^2)^{3/2} + C(y)$
y-antiderivative: $\frac{x}{3}(x^2 + y^2)^{3/2} + C(x)$

5. x-antiderivative: $\frac{2}{3}x^3y + x + C(y)$
y-antiderivative: $x^2y^2 + y + C(x)$

7. x-antiderivative: $\frac{x^3}{3}y^2 + C(y)$
y-antiderivative: $x^2\frac{y^3}{3} + C(x)$

9. x-antiderivative: $e^x \ln y + C(y)$
y-antiderivative: $e^x(y \ln y - y) + C(x)$

11. 4 **13.** $\frac{27}{2}$ **15.** 18 **17.** $\frac{1}{2}$ **19.** 0 **21.** 0 **23.** $\ln 2 - \frac{1}{2} - \frac{(\ln 2)^2}{4}$ **35.** $\frac{13}{15}$

27. Type I: $x \le y \le 1$, $0 \le x \le 1$ or Type II: $0 \le x \le y$, $0 \le y \le 1$

29. Type II: $1 - y \le x \le y - 1$, $1 \le y \le 3$

31. Type I: $x^2 \le y \le 1 - x^2$, $\frac{-1}{\sqrt{2}} \le x \le \frac{1}{\sqrt{2}}$

33. Type I: $\frac{x^2}{2} \le y \le 2x$, $0 \le x \le 4$ or Type II: $\frac{y}{2} \le x \le \sqrt{2y}$, $0 \le y \le 8$

35. Type II: $1 - \frac{y^2}{9} \le x \le 9 - y^2$, $-3 \le y \le 3$

37. $\frac{1}{2}$ **39.** $e^5 - e^4 - e$

41. e **43.** $\frac{32}{3}$ **45.** $e^2 - 3$ **47.** 32 **49.** $\frac{40}{3}$ **51.** $\frac{1}{6}$ **53.** $\frac{5}{6}$ **55.** 1 **57.** $\frac{1}{2}$ **59.** $\frac{122}{3}$ **61.** 4

63. 12 **65.** $\frac{7}{6}$ **67.** 4 **69.** $\frac{200}{27}(20^{3/2} - 5^{3/2})$ (roughly 579.7) **71.** 64 **73.** $\frac{2}{5}$ **75.** $\frac{27}{4}$

Chapter 6 Review

1. $f_x(x, y) = 2xy$ **3.** $f_x(x, y) = \frac{1}{x}\left(\frac{\ln 10 + 1}{\ln 10}\right)$ **5.** $f_{xx}(x, y) = \frac{y}{(x^2 + y)^{3/2}}$ **7.** $f_{xy}(x, y) = 2x$ **9.** $f_x(x, y) = 4x(x^2 + y^2)$

11. $f_x(x, y) = yx^{y-1}$

13.

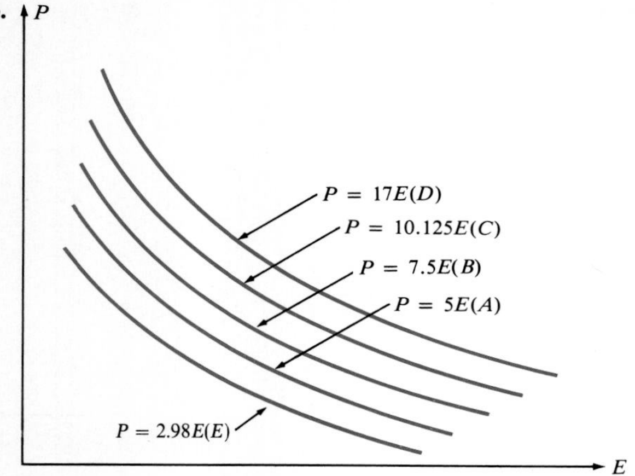

15. Saddle point: (0, 0)

17. Saddle point: (0, 0) **19.** No critical points **21.** Saddle point: (0, 0)

23. $N_C(L, C) = \frac{1}{2}\sqrt{\frac{L}{C}}$ [$N_C(L, C)$ gives the approximate increase in N brought about by increasing C one unit.]

$N_L(L, C) = \frac{1}{2}\sqrt{\frac{C}{L}}$ [$N_L(L, C)$ gives the approximate increase in N brought about by increasing L one unit.]

25. **(a)** $\frac{\partial C}{\partial q_1}(q_1, q_2) = 4q_1 + q_2$

$\frac{\partial C}{\partial q_2}(q_1, q_2) = q_1 + 8q_2$

(b) $\frac{\partial C}{\partial q_1}(100, 100) = 500$

$\frac{\partial C}{\partial q_2}(100, 100) = 900$

27. $q_1 = 17.74$
$q_2 = 29.03$

29. $P_a = \frac{100\ bcg}{(ag + bc)^2}$

31. $P_c = \frac{-100\ abg}{(ag + bc)^2}$

33. Maximum profit $x = 6$, $y = 8$ **35.** Saddle point: $(-1, 2)$ **37.** Relative minimum: (0, 0)

39. Test fails: $\left(\frac{1}{2}, y \text{ arbitrary}\right)$ **41.** Relative maximum: (60, 0) **43.** No critical points **45.** Saddle point: (0, 0)

47. No critical points **49.** No critical points **51.** Relative minimum: $\left(\frac{1}{2}, \frac{1}{2}\right)$ **53.** Relative minimum: $\left(\frac{1}{4}, \frac{3}{4}\right)$

55. $\left(\frac{\sqrt{2}}{2}, \frac{\sqrt{2}}{2}\right)$ is the maximum point

$\left(-\frac{\sqrt{2}}{2}, -\frac{\sqrt{2}}{2}\right)$ is the minimum point

57. (0, 0) is the minimum point **59.** 4 **61.** $e - 1$ **63.** 20

Chapter 6 Test

1. **(a)** $f_x(x, y) = (x + y)^{-1}$ **(b)** $f_y(x, y) = (x + y)^{-1}$ **(c)** $f_{xx}(x, y) = -(x + y)^{-2}$ **(d)** $f_{xy}(x, y) = -(x + y)^{-2}$
(e) $f_{yy}(x, y) = -(x + y)^{-2}$

2. Saddle point: (0, 0)
Relative maximum point $(-1, -1)$

3. $x = y = 71$ **4.** $\left(\frac{1}{2}, \frac{1}{2}\right)$ **5.** 2 **6.** $e - 2$

7. Direct computation of the least squares line from the formulas in the book. $a = \dfrac{-x_1y_1 - x_2y_2 + x_2y_1 + x_1y_2}{-(x_1^2 - 2x_1x_2 + x_2^2)} = \dfrac{y_2 - y_1}{x_2 - x_1}$

$$b = y_1 + y_2 - \frac{y_2 - y_1}{x_2 - x_1}(x_1 + x_2)$$
$$= \frac{x_2y_1 - x_1y_2}{x_2 - x_1}$$

8. Height = 14 in., base = $\dfrac{168}{9}$ in., volume = 4878.2 in.^{3} **9.** Both are negative.

Projects and Problems

Chapters 4–6

1. $\dfrac{172}{6}$ **3.** $\dfrac{28}{15}$ **5.** $\dfrac{4}{\ln 3}$ **7.** $\dfrac{3}{8}$ **9.** $3e^4 - 43$ **11.** $z_x = e^{xy} + xye^{xy}$, $z_y = x^2e^{xy}$ **13.** $f_x = 3x^2y^2 + 3y$, $f_y = 2x^3y + 3x$ **15.** $f_x = \ln y$, $f_y = \dfrac{x}{y}$

17. Student project **19.** Student project **21.** Student project **23.** **(a)** $2(1 - a^{1/2})$ **(b)** 2 **25.** 0 **27.** $\dfrac{8\pi}{15}$

29. Both areas are 4. **31.** 1600 feet **33.** $\dfrac{\pi k R^4}{2}$ **35.** White (you are at the north pole).

37. Any function of the form $f(x, y) = x + g(y)$, where $g(y)$ is any differentiable function of y. The slope of the surface is 1 in the x-direction.

39. Student project

CHAPTER 7

Section 7.1

1. {TTT, TTH, THT, THH, HTT, HTH, HHT, HHH} **3.** {6, 9, 12, 15} **5.** $\{-9, -3, 3, 9\}$

7. $\left\{\begin{array}{cccccc} (1,1) & (1,2) & (1,3) & (1,4) & (1,5) & (1,6) \\ (2,1) & (2,2) & (2,3) & (2,4) & (2,5) & (2,6) \\ (3,1) & (3,2) & (3,3) & (3,4) & (3,5) & (3,6) \\ (4,1) & (4,2) & (4,3) & (4,4) & (4,5) & \underline{(4,6)} \\ (5,1) & (5,2) & (5,3) & (5,4) & \underline{(5,5)} & \underline{(5,6)} \\ (6,1) & (6,2) & (6,3) & \underline{(6,4)} & \underline{(6,5)} & \underline{(6,6)} \end{array}\right\}$ (event underlined)

9. $\left\{\begin{array}{cccccc} \underline{(1,1)} & \underline{(1,2)} & (1,3) & (1,4) & (1,5) & (1,6) \\ \underline{(2,1)} & \underline{(2,2)} & (2,3) & (2,4) & (2,5) & (2,6) \\ (3,1) & (3,2) & (3,3) & (3,4) & (3,5) & (3,6) \\ (4,1) & (4,2) & (4,3) & (4,4) & (4,5) & (4,6) \\ (5,1) & (5,2) & (5,3) & (5,4) & (5,5) & (5,6) \\ (6,1) & (6,2) & (6,3) & (6,4) & (6,5) & (6,6) \end{array}\right\}$ (event underlined)

11. $\left\{\begin{array}{cccccc} (1,1) & (1,2) & (1,3) & (1,4) & (1,5) & (1,6) \\ (2,1) & (2,2) & (2,3) & (2,4) & (2,5) & (2,6) \\ \underline{(3,1)} & (3,2) & (3,3) & (3,4) & (3,5) & (3,6) \\ (4,1) & \underline{(4,2)} & (4,3) & (4,4) & (4,5) & (4,6) \\ (5,1) & (5,2) & \underline{(5,3)} & (5,4) & (5,5) & (5,6) \\ (6,1) & (6,2) & (6,3) & \underline{(6,4)} & (6,5) & (6,6) \end{array}\right\}$ (event underlined)

13. {FFF, FFM, FMF, FMM, MFF, MFM, MMF, MMM}

15. {(1, H), (2, H), (3, H), (4, H), (5, H), (6, H) (1, T), (2, T), (3, T), (4, T), (5, T), (6, T)} **17.** {(3, H), (3, T)} **19.** {(2, H)}

21. GREEN (columns), RED (rows)

$$\text{RED}\left\{\begin{array}{cccccc} (1,1) & & (1,3) & & (1,5) & \\ & (2,2) & & (2,4) & & (2,6) \\ (3,1) & & (3,3) & & (3,5) & \\ & (4,2) & & (4,4) & & (4,6) \\ (5,1) & & (5,3) & & (5,5) & \\ & (6,2) & & (6,4) & & (6,6) \end{array}\right\}$$

23. GREEN (columns), RED (rows)

$$\text{RED}\left\{\begin{array}{cccccc} & & & & & (1,6) \\ & & & & (2,5) & \\ & & & (3,4) & & \\ & & (4,3) & & & \\ (5,1) & (5,2) & (5,3) & (5,4) & (5,5) & (5,6) \\ (6,1) & & & & & \end{array}\right\}$$

25. $P(\text{T}) = \frac{1}{2}$

$P(\text{HT}) = \frac{1}{4}$

$P(\text{HHT}) = \frac{1}{8}$

$P(\text{HHH}) = \frac{1}{8}$

27. $P(\text{Number of heads} = 0) = \frac{1}{4}$

$P(\text{Number of heads} = 1) = \frac{1}{2}$

$P(\text{Number of heads} = 2) = \frac{1}{4}$

29. $P(\text{Difference} = 0) = \frac{6}{36}$

$P(\text{Difference} = 1) = \frac{10}{36}$

$P(\text{Difference} = 2) = \frac{8}{36}$

$P(\text{Difference} = 3) = \frac{6}{36}$

$P(\text{Difference} = 4) = \frac{4}{36}$

$P(\text{Difference} = 5) = \frac{2}{36}$

31. $E = \frac{35}{18}$

33. $E = \$20{,}000$ $5000 profit **35.** $E = \$50{,}000$ $25,000 profit **37.** $E = \$72{,}500$ $12,500 **39.** $E = \$2.10$

41. $P(M = -\$5{,}000) = \frac{99}{100}$

$P(M = +\$245{,}000) = \frac{1}{100}$

43. $4500 **45.** $E = \$0.22$ **47.** $-\$0.15$ **49.** $E = \$4.75$

51. Maine's expected earnings per ticket sold = 0.4 cents

Section 7.2

1. Finite **3.** Finite **5.** Continuous **7.** $0.05 \geq 0$, $\int_0^{20} 0.05\,dx = 1$ **9.** $2x - 2 \geq 0$ if $x \geq 1$, $\int_1^2 (2x - 2)\,dx = 1$ **11.** $4x^3 \geq 0$ if $x \geq 0$, $\int_0^1 4x^3\,dx = 1$

13. $1 - x \geq 0$ if $0 \leq x \leq 1$, $\int_0^1 (1 - x)\,dx = 1$ **15.** $x \geq 0$ on $[0, 1]$ $2 - x \geq 0$ on $[1, 2]$, $\int_0^1 x\,dx + \int_1^2 (2 - x)\,dx = 1$ **17.** $\int_0^\infty 0.02e^{-0.02x}\,dx = 1$ **19.** See Problem 7

21. 0.50 **23.** 0.75 **25.** 0.40625 **27.** 1 **29.** 0.5994503 **31.** 0.6321206 **33.** 0.7768698 **35.** 0.4723666
37. 2 **39.** 0.75 **41.** 0.6 **43.** 1 **45.** 20

Section 7.3

For Problems 1–5 the integrals are all 1.

1. Mean = 1 **3.** Mean = 2 **5.** Mean = $\frac{100}{99}$ **7.** $-\frac{1}{e^{0.5}} + 1$ (0.3935) **9.** $-e^{-1} + e^{-1/3}$ (0.3487)

11. $-e^{-1.5} + e^{-1}$ (0.1445) **13.** $1/e$ (0.3678)

15.

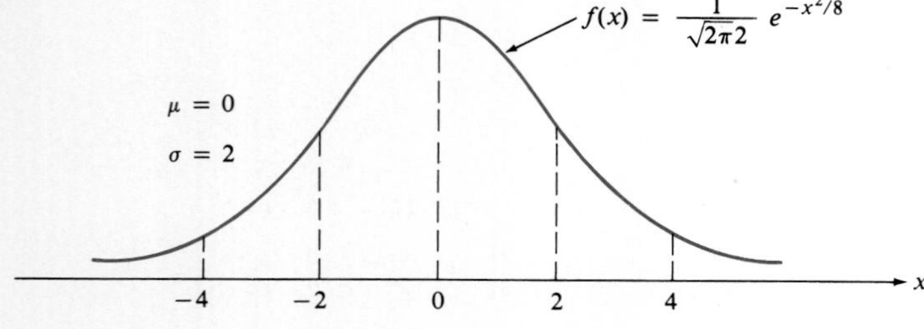

17.

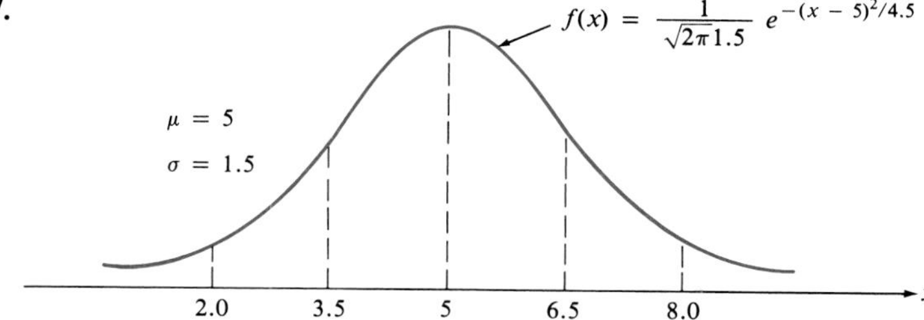

19.

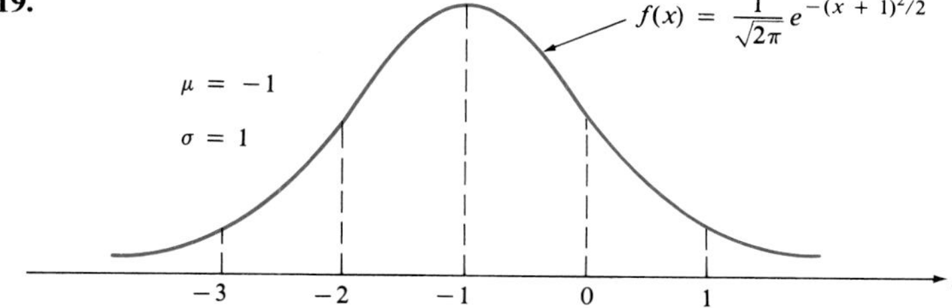

21. 0.4332 **23.** 0.1574 **25.** 0.6247 **27.** 0.0919 **29.** 0.1587 **31.** 0.1151 **33.** 0.2119 **35.** 0.9821
37. 0.4332 **39.** 0.2708 **41.** 0.4972 **43.** 0.4772 **45.** 0.2119 **47.** $1/e$ (roughly 0.3679)

49. **(a)** $f(x) = 0.25e^{-0.25x}$
(b) 0.53
(c) $F(x) = 1 - e^{0.25x}$
(d) 0.47
(e) $r(x) = 1 - F(x)$
$= e^{-0.25x}$

51. **(a)** $f(t) = \frac{1}{45} e^{-45t}$
(b) $-e^{-4/3} + e^{-1/3}$ (0.45)

53. 0.6826 **55.** 0.8185 **57.** 0.1587

Chapter 7 Review

1. If we are interested in the sex of the first-, second-, and third-born children, then the sample space is {(G, G, G), (G, G, B), (G, B, G), (G, B, B), (B, G, G), (B, G, B), (B, B, G), (B, B, B)} where B = boy and G = girl.
3. {ca, ct, cs, at, as, ts, cc, aa, tt, ss}
5. $\{l_1it_1, l_1it_2, l_1il_2, l_1ie, l_1t_1t_2, l_1t_1l_2, l_1t_1e, l_1t_2l_2, l_1t_2e, l_1l_2e, it_1t_2, it_1l_2, it_1e, it_2l_2, it_2e, il_2e, t_1t_2l_2, t_1t_2e, t_1l_2e, t_2l_2e\}$

7.
$$\begin{array}{c} \text{Green} \\ \left\{\begin{array}{cccccc} (1,1) & (1,2) & \underline{(1,3)} & (1,4) & (1,5) & (1,6) \\ (2,1) & (2,2) & (2,3) & (2,4) & (2,5) & \underline{(2,6)} \\ \underline{(3,1)} & (3,2) & (3,3) & (3,4) & (3,5) & (3,6) \\ (4,1) & (4,2) & (4,3) & (4,4) & (4,5) & (4,6) \\ (5,1) & (5,2) & (5,3) & (5,4) & (5,5) & (5,6) \\ (6,1) & \underline{(6,2)} & (6,3) & (6,4) & (6,5) & (6,6) \end{array}\right\} \end{array} \text{Prob} = \frac{4}{36} = \frac{1}{9}$$

9. Event = {(3, 4), (3, 5), (3, 6), (4, 3), (5, 3), (6, 3)}, Probability $= \frac{1}{6}$ **11.** −$0.80 **13.** $E = 7$ **15.** $E = 5.50$

For Problems 17 and 19, show that the function is nonnegative and the area under the graph of the function is 1.

21. $\frac{1}{4}$ **23.** $\frac{1023}{1024}$ **25.** $-e^{-0.5} + 1$ **27.** 0.8185 **29.** 0.6915 **31.** 0.9544 **33.** 0.7745 **35.** 0.4332

37. **(a)** $0.1e^{-0.1t}$
(b) $1 - e^{-0.5} \cong 0.3934693$

39. $P(11.8 \leq X \leq 12.2) = 0.9544$

41. $P(x \geq 500) = 0.7881$

43. The expected value is 1. Hence $P(1 - 2\sigma \leq x \leq 1 + 2\sigma) \geq \frac{3}{4}$

45. $P(-2 \leq Z \leq 2) = 0.9544 \cong 95\%$

Chapter 7 Test

1. {(1, 2), (1, 3), (1, 4), (2, 1), (2, 3), (2, 4), (3, 1), (3, 2), (3, 4), (4, 1), (4, 2), (4, 3)}

2. {(G, G, G), (G, G, B), (G, B, G), (G, B, B), (B, G, G), (B, G, B), (B, B, G), (B, B, B)} Here we are interested in whether the first, second, or third child is a boy (B) or girl (G).

3. $\frac{5}{6}$

4. $-\$0.45$

5. **(a)** 0.1395
(b) 0.0228

6. $\frac{3}{4}$

7. \$422

8. 0.1587

9. **(a)** 0.6826
(b) 0.9544
(c) 0.9974

10. $P(\text{RL3} \cup \text{GL1}) = \frac{33}{36}$

$P(\text{RL3}) = \frac{18}{36}$

$P(\text{GL1}) = \frac{30}{36}$

$P(\text{RL3} \cap \text{GL1}) = \frac{15}{36}$

Hence $P(\text{RL3} \cup \text{GL1}) = P(\text{RL3}) + P(\text{GL1}) - P(\text{RL3} \cap \text{GL1})$

11. $P(\text{Number of heads} = 0) = \frac{1}{8}$

$P(\text{Number of heads} = 1) = \frac{3}{8}$

$P(\text{Number of heads} = 2) = \frac{3}{8}$

$P(\text{Number of heads} = 3) = \frac{1}{8}$

12. **(a)** $P(X = 0) = \frac{2}{6}$

$P(X = 1) = \frac{3}{6}$

$P(X = 2) = 0$

$P(X = 3) = \frac{1}{6}$

(b) $E = \frac{250}{6} = 41.67$ (rounded off to 42%)

Credits

Calculus Preliminaries: page 1, The Bettmann Archive; pages 11 and 15, Sidney Harris; page 23, Culver Pictures; page 32, Sidney Harris; page 36, courtesy of Royal Carribean Cruise Lines; page 41, Sidney Harris; page 52, The Bettmann Archive.

Chapter 1: page 63, Dr. Harold Edgerton, MIT, Cambridge, MA; pages 66 and 67, North Wind Picture Archives; page 103, Boston Public Library; page 107, courtesy of New York Stock Exchange; page 130, courtesy of The Aetna Life Insurance Company and Aetna Casualty and Surety Company, Hartford, CT.

Chapter 2: page 146, George Gardner/Stock, Boston; page 153, Omikron/Photo Researchers; page 184, Peter Menzel/Stock, Boston; page 193, George Bellerose/Stock, Boston.

Chapter 3: page 233, Don W. Fawcett/Photo Researchers; page 241, Charles Gupton/Stock, Boston; page 252, The Bettmann Archive; page 259, UPI/Bettmann Newsphotos; page 271, Karen Preuss/Taurus Photos.

Chapter 4: page 301, Ellis Herwig/Stock, Boston; page 310, Suzanne Szasz/Photo Researchers; page 344, Owen Franken/Stock, Boston.

Chapter 5: page 355, Jean-Claude Lejeune/Stock, Boston; page 374, courtesy of Chevron Corporation; page 380, John Coletti/Stock, Boston; page 396, photo by Bruce Iverson for Random House; page 416, Leonard Lee Rue III/Photo Researchers.

Chapter 6: page 421, Mark Antman/The Image Works; page 434, Herb Levar/Photo Researchers; page 437, courtesy of the Public Information Center of the University of Maine, Orono, ME; page 459, Tom McHugh/Photo Researchers; page 463, North Wind Picture Archives; page 471, Arthur Glauberman/Photo Researchers.

Chapter 7: page 519, Robin Laurance/Photo Researchers; page 522, Culver Pictures; page 531, Barbara Reis/Photo Researchers.

Index of Applications

Biological Sciences and Medicine

Business

Ecology

Economics

General Interest

Physical Sciences

Social Sciences

Index

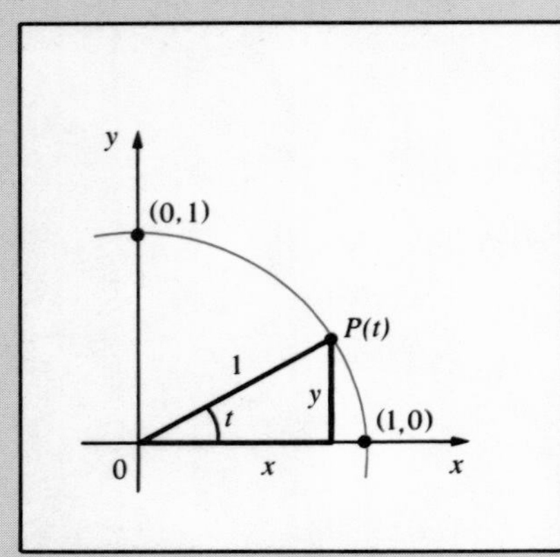

$\sin t = y$

$\cos t = x$

$\tan t = \dfrac{\sin t}{\cos t} = \dfrac{y}{x}$

$\cot t = \dfrac{\cos t}{\sin t} = \dfrac{x}{y}$

$\sec t = \dfrac{1}{\cos t} = \dfrac{1}{x}$

$\csc t = \dfrac{1}{\sin t} = \dfrac{1}{y}$

$\sin(-t) = -\sin t$
$\cos(-t) = \cos t$
$\tan(-t) = -\tan t$

$\cot(-t) = -\cot t$
$\sec(-t) = \sec t$
$\csc(-t) = -\csc t$

$$\sin^2 t + \cos^2 t = 1$$
$$1 + \tan^2 t = \sec^2 t$$
$$1 + \cot^2 t = \csc^2 t$$

$\sin(t_1 \pm t_2) = \sin t_1 \cos t_2 \pm \cos t_1 \sin t_2$

$\cos(t_1 \pm t_2) = \cos t_1 \cos t_2 \mp \sin t_1 \sin t_2$

$\tan(t_1 \pm t_2) = \dfrac{\tan t_1 \pm \tan t_2}{1 \mp \tan t_1 \tan t_2}$

$\sin 2t = 2 \sin t \cos t$

$\cos 2t = \cos^2 t - \sin^2 t = 1 - 2\sin^2 t = 2\cos^2 t - 1$

t	0	$\frac{\pi}{6}$	$\frac{\pi}{4}$	$\frac{\pi}{3}$	$\frac{\pi}{2}$	$\frac{2\pi}{3}$	$\frac{3\pi}{4}$	$\frac{5\pi}{6}$	π	$\frac{3\pi}{2}$	2π
$\sin t$	0	1/2	$\sqrt{2}/2$	$\sqrt{3}/2$	1	$\sqrt{3}/2$	$\sqrt{2}/2$	1/2	0	−1	0
$\cos t$	1	$\sqrt{3}/2$	$\sqrt{2}/2$	1/2	0	−1/2	$-\sqrt{2}/2$	$-\sqrt{3}/2$	−1	0	1
$\tan t$	0	$\sqrt{3}/3$	1	$\sqrt{3}$	—	$-\sqrt{3}$	−1	$-\sqrt{3}/3$	0	—	0
$\csc t$	—	2	$\sqrt{2}$	$2\sqrt{3}/3$	1	$2\sqrt{3}/3$	$\sqrt{2}$	2	—	−1	—
$\sec t$	1	$2\sqrt{3}/3$	$\sqrt{2}$	2	—	−2	$-\sqrt{2}$	$-2\sqrt{3}/3$	−1	—	1
$\cot t$	—	$\sqrt{3}$	1	$\sqrt{3}/3$	0	$-\sqrt{3}/3$	−1	$-\sqrt{3}$	—	0	—